Oxford Medical Publications

Textbook of musculoskeletal medicine

Textbook of musculoskeletal medicine

Edited by

Michael Hutson

Consultant Musculoskeletal Physician
Park Row Clinic
Nottingham

and

Richard Ellis

Consultant in Rheumatology and Rehabilitation
Southampton General Hospital
Southampton

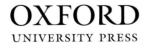
OXFORD
UNIVERSITY PRESS

OXFORD

UNIVERSITY PRESS

Great Clarendon Street, Oxford OX2 6DP

Oxford University Press is a department of the University of Oxford.
It furthers the University's objective of excellence in research, scholarship,
and education by publishing worldwide in

Oxford New York

Auckland Cape Town Dar es Salaam Hong Kong Karachi Kuala Lumpur
Madrid Melbourne Mexico City Nairobi New Delhi Taipei Toronto
Shanghai

With offices in
Argentina Austria Brazil Chile Czech Republic France Greece Guatemala
Hungary Italy Japan South Korea Poland Portugal Singapore Switzerland
Thailand Turkey Ukraine Vietnam

Oxford is a registered trade mark of Oxford University Press
in the UK and in certain other countries

Published in the United States
by Oxford University Press Inc., New York

A catalogue record for this title is available from the British Library

Library of Congress Cataloging in Publication Data
Textbook of musculoskeletal medicine / [edited by Michael Hutson and
Richard Ellis].
Includes bibliographical references and index.
1. Musculoskeletal system–Diseases. 2. Manipulation (Therapeutics)
3. Orthopedics. 4. Osteopathic medicine.
[DNLM: 1. Musculoskeletal Diseases–physiopathology. 2. Musculoskeletal
Diseases–therapy. 3. Pain. WE 140 T3548 2005] I. Hutson, M. A.
II. Ellis, Richard M.
RC925.T49 2005 616.7–dc22 2004019759

ISBN 0 19 263050 4 (Hbk) 978 0 19 263050 6

10 9 8 7 6 5 4 3 2 1

Typeset by EXPO Holdings Sdn Bhd., Malaysia.
Printed in Italy
on acid-free paper

Foreword

Musculoskeletal pain in the community

Vert Mooney, M. D.

This is a much needed textbook. It is an attempt to bring into the tent representatives of varied clinical perspectives in the evaluation and treatment of soft tissue pain. We all recognize there is often misunderstanding, and even distrust, of those clinical perspectives that are different from that in which we have been trained and are experienced. We are all wandering somewhat in the wilderness, which resides at the periphery of the fertile land of evidence based 'scientific medicine'. Why is that? We clinicians are treating the unmeasurable entity, pain. And we all certainly know that if we can't measure it, we have trouble comparing it. That is the essential reason why our varied clinical perspective has not been united into a uniform evaluation and therapeutic protocol. That is why so many specialties are represented here.

This book tries to integrate the body knowledge of numerous clinical specialties: orthopaedics, rheumatology, pain control, physical medicine and rehabilitation, osteopathic medicine, psychology, and physiotherapy. Elements from all these produce the discipline of musculoskeletal medicine. Although all these specialties have a base for their treatment in human anatomy and pathophysiology as emphasized in the introductory section of this book, we know each has ended up with a contrasting treatment approach. And in addition to the physical treatment based on physical deficit there is the interactive biosocial and psychological phenomenon. Measurement here becomes even more complex. Does the pain persist for non-anatomic reasons?

We are all treating disordered human anatomy and function of some type. Thus, the reasonable baseline of understanding anatomic deviation has to be the starting point of the discussion. Some of this is measurable by radiography and physical examination, but most of the functional disorders under consideration, alas, are not truly measurable, such as muscle spasms, tenderness, or induration. We all have a feel for these phenomena, but the significance and severity of the palpatory findings is varied. On the other hand, plain radiographs and MRIs may even be misleading in their attempt to supply objective evidence of skeletal and articular abnormality. More specific analysis of pain sources is available from anatomically specific injections, and this certainly will be covered in the text. Even that information can be misleading due to placebo factors, overlapping innervation, misplaced injections, and inconsistent analysis of results. What a problem!

Yet, only by continued communication and emphasis on the similarities of our approach can the effectiveness of dissimilar methods of analysis and treatment be understood. That is the value of this book. Naturally, as much evidence as is available will be presented, but we each have to be wary of excessive enthusiasm for a belief system without supporting data. Sometimes we have to admit that the treatments advocated are only a current conceptual framework. We all have to be wary of belief in the religion of our experience and training, rather than the reality of what works and does not.

Fortunately the editors have gathered a very balanced crew of authorities who are willing to discuss and listen. They all see this as a journey, with the final destination not yet achieved. This 'tent' of discussion is a temporary stopping point on the journey to full understanding of the sources of persistent pain secondary to soft tissue injury and deterioration. To have all of these experts 'under one roof' is a most important milestone of progress on this journey. I look forward to the education.

Preface

Multi-author textbooks take some years to come to fruition. Hopefully, the wait will have been worthwhile, both for those readers who have been aware of the impending completion of the text and for the authors themselves. When 'penning' this first paragraph of the draft preface, I wrote: 'Musculoskeletal medicine is a relatively new term, encompassing much if not all of orthopaedic medicine, manual medicine and osteopathic medicine'. Several years on, in 2005, the terms 'musculoskeletal medicine' and 'neuromusculoskeletal medicine' are in common usage. Service provision is well advanced in the UK for instance, where a new category of intermediate care provider has been established at the initiative of the Department of Health and the Royal College of General Practitioners — the general practitioner with a special interest (GPwSI) in musculoskeletal conditions. The International Federation for Manual/Musculoskeletal Medicine (FIMM) incorporated 'musculoskeletal medicine' into its title in 1995, and numerous national societies do the same: the British Institute of Musculoskeletal Medicine (BIMM) was established in 1991 when the British Association of Manipulative Medicine (BAMM) merged with the Institute of Orthopaedic Medicine (IOM). (Neuro)musculoskeletal medicine comprises the theoretical basis, diagnosis, and treatment of disorders of the musculoskeletal system, incorporating manual diagnostics, a variety of therapeutic techniques such as manipulation and injections, preventive and rehabilitative procedures.

The intrinsic components of disorders of the musculoskeletal system are twofold: structural (pathomorphological) and functional (pathophysiological). Within the text a comprehensive account is provided of both structural and functional disorders of the spine, and of the extremities.

Early pathomorphological changes reflect adaptive processes to biomechanical stresses. **Advanced structural pathology** such as intervertebral disc prolapse, meniscus derangements, and tendonopathies are the consequences of the failure of adaptation of the soft tissues to postural and dynamic stresses. They are described in some detail in the text. When appropriate the relevant stressors, particularly but not exclusively biomechanical, are identified and discussed.

Pathophysiological (neuromuscular) disturbances are classified using the accepted international term 'somatic (or 'segmental' when applied to the spine) dysfunction'. The recognition, diagnosis and management of these reversible dysfunctional states, manifesting clinically as reduced joint mobility, tight muscles, disturbances of the autonomic nervous system and abnormal neurodynamics, differentiate the discipline of musculoskeletal medicine from rheumatology. The non-surgical management of these disorders, both structural and functional, differentiates the discipline from orthopaedic surgery.

Clinical evaluation of musculoskeletal disorders demands specific expertise that is developed by 'hands-on' experience. Accordingly, it is recognized that there is no substitute for continued honing of these evaluative skills by repeated practice. For those clinicians who are new to the discipline, welcome – interesting insights await those with a receptive mental attitude (Mooney 1995).

Inexperienced physicians may experience initial difficulty accepting dysfunction as a 'dis-ease' model. It does not have 'hard' physical signs such as those associated with gross trauma seen in orthopaedic surgical practice as a predominant feature (Gargan 1995). However, the detection of relatively subtle soft tissue signs, such as loss of joint play, (troph)oedema, myofascial disturbance and abnormal neural tension, which requires patience and much practice, brings its own rewards.

The contributors to this book have international reputations in musculoskeletal medicine, particularly in those topics with which they are identified in the text. Inevitably there is some overlap between the individual contributions, but a common theme has been maintained throughout – the absolute requirement for the predication of a clinical diagnosis upon manual examining skills.

The concept of 'syndromes' is eschewed, although some would argue that many diagnoses, especially spinal dysfunction, are inherently syndromic. Whenever possible, the specific soft tissues associated with the dysfunctional process, their anatomical location, and aetiological factors are identified. The interaction between a decompensated musculoskeletal system and the human environment is explored with particular reference to behavioural responses to chronic pain.

A major development in recent years has been our increased knowledge of the mechanisms involved in the perception of pain, particularly pathological pain. The neurophysiological and neurodynamic abnormalities associated with (chronic) regional pain syndromes are correlated with their clinical expression in the text.

Management strategies are explored in considerable detail. The association between specific diagnoses and patients' responses to pain and dysfunction is developed. Inappropriate advice from inadequate training in musculoskeletal medicine (Hutson 1993) causes iatrogenic disease. Conversely, an active approach to management predicated upon expertise and experience, reaps its own rewards and reduces the likelihood of progression from acute musculoskeletal dysfunctions to chronic pain, distress and disability.

Although patient education is recognized as a priority, and given appropriate exposure in the text, a change in attitudes of doctors, particularly to back pain, is seen as essential (Ellis 1995). Emphasis is placed on keeping patients at work whenever possible. Specific therapeutic options, including spinal and peripheral joint manipulation, and injection techniques are described in detail, and their role identified in the wider strategem of resolution of dysfunction, pain relief, and rehabilitation.

Finally, the inclusion in the text of the best available documented research in this field provides the reader with an opportunity to integrate clinical expertise and scientific evidence, and thereby to pursue evidence-based musculoskeletal medicine as far as this is possible.

References

Ellis, R. M. (1995) Back pain. *BMJ*, **310**, 1220.

Gargan, M. F. (1995) What is the evidence for an organic lesion in whiplash injury? *J. Psychosomatic Medicine*, **39** (6), 777–81.

Hutson, M. A. (1993) *Back pain: recognition and management.* Butterworth Heinemann, Oxford, p. vii.

Mooney, V. (1995) Prolotherapy in the spine and pelvis: an introduction. *Spine: State of the art reviews*, **9**(2), 309–11.

Michael Hutson
2005

Contents

Contributors

Mark E. Batt
Centre for Sports Medicine
Queens Medical Centre
Nottingham, UK

Derek Bickerstaff
The Sheffield Centre of Sports Medicine
Sheffield, S.Yorks, UK

Stefan Blomberg
Stockholm Clinic — Stay Active
Lidingö, SWEDEN

Keith Bush
Consultant Orthopaedic Physician;
formerly of the Royal National
Orthopaedic Hospital Trust, London UK

David Butler
Neuro-Orthopaedic Institute Pty Ltd
Unley, Australia

Milton L. Cohen
Darlinghurst Arthritis and Pain Research Clinic
St Vincent's Medical Centre
Darlinghurst, NSW, Australia

Mark Comerford
Kinetic Control
Southampton, UK

Cyrus Cooper
University of Southampton
Southampton General Hospital
Southampton, UK

Thomas Dorman
Internal Medicine
Paracelsus Clinic
WA, USA

Richard M. Ellis
University of Southampton and Salisbury District
Hospital
Salisbury, UK

Bryan English
Northern General Hospital
Sheffield, UK

C. Chan Gunn
iSTOP - The Institute for the Study and
Treatment of Pain
Vancouver, BC, Canada

Roger Hackney
Leeds Nuffield Hospital
Leeds, UK

Richard Higgins
Hathersage, UK

Michael Hutson
Park Row Clinic
Nottingham, UK

Vladimír Janda*

Bruce L. Kidd
Bone & Joint Research Unit
Bart's & London School of Medicine
London, UK

Jennifer Klaber Moffett
Institute of Rehabilitation
University of Hull
Hull, UK

Martin T. N. Knight
The Spinal Foundation
Oldham, UK

Michael L. Kuchera
Philadelphia College of Osteopathic Medicine
USA

Stephen Levin
Potomac Back Center
McLean, VA, USA

Chris J. Main
Department of Behavioural Medicine
Hope Hospital
Salford, UK

Sarah Mottram
Kinetic Control
Southampton, UK

Jacob Patijn
University Hospital Maastricht
Dept Anaesthesiology
Pain Management and Research Centre
Maastricht, The Netherlands

Elva Pearson
Christiana Spine Center
Newark, DE, USA

Nicholas Peirce
Department of Orthopaedics
Nottingham City Hospital
Nottingham, UK

Charles Pither
Department of Anaesthetics
St Thomas' Hospital
London, UK

Malcolm Read
Pirbright, UK

Hugh Smythe
Department of Medicine
University of Toronto
Ontario, Canada

John Tanner
Oving Clinic
Oving, W Sussex, UK

Adam Ward
Royal London Homeopathic Hospital
London, UK

Paul J. Watson
University of Leicester
Division of Anaesthesia and Pain Management
Leicester, UK

*Deceased

Part 1

Introduction

1.1 Fundamentals

Michael Hutson

Concepts

Readers with limited knowledge of the history of the development of the diverse 'schools' of manual medicine, the core components of which are manual diagnosis and treatment of neuromusculoskeletal disorders, may be somewhat confused by the plethora of terminology used to describe the medical discipline embraced by these schools and the conceptual variants themselves. This diversity is the beauty and perhaps the frustration of musculoskeletal medicine. It epitomizes its eclecticism.

The distinctiveness of musculoskeletal medicine is undoubted and perhaps unparalleled in the medical sciences. At its heart is the recognition and management of dysfunctional states of the neuromusculoskeletal system, now formally defined as somatic dysfunction. The characteristics of somatic dysfunction are further described in Chapter 2.2.1. I confine myself here to the development of musculoskeletal medicine in the broadest sense.

I wish to address the characteristics of orthopaedic medicine, osteopathic medicine, manual medicine, and musculoskeletal medicine. By this means it will become apparent that there are a number of important conceptual models common to and underpinning these disciplines: structural (pathomorphological), pathophysiological ('functional'), biomechanical, and biopsychosocial.

Orthopaedic medicine

Orthopaedic medicine was founded upon the structural (anatomic or morphological) disturbances of the neuromusculoskeletal system as defined by James Cyriax. Orthopaedic medicine may be seen as the natural consequence of the application of the disease–illness model (which has provided the framework for most medical disciplines for several centuries) to orthopaedic derangements that come under the province of the physician. It is archetypically 'allopathic' (for those readers who wish to distinguish between allopathic and osteopathic medicine).

Cyriax (1969) envisaged derangements of the intervertebral disc as the primary spinal pathology to account for the vast majority of 'simple' back pain and nerve root pain. He described the capsular and non-capsular patterns of articular disturbances at peripheral joints, and devised selective tissue tension tests to differentiate between articular, ligamentous, contractile and neural lesions. Based on reductionist principles his views represented a seminal breakthrough in the evaluation of lesions of the soft tissues. Conceptually (in the 1940s) this was the first time since the work of Sir William Gowers at the end of the 19th century that allopathic medicine was able to throw off the mantle of soft tissue rheumatism and the somewhat nebulous conditions it embraced such as fibrositis.

Although distinct by definition (with respect to management of musculoskeletal problems) from orthopaedic surgery a further breakthrough made by orthopaedic medicine was in nosology. Orthopaedic medicine became recognized as the application of a unique systematized clinical evaluation (including inspection, active movements, passive movements, resisted muscle contraction, and palpation) to the soft tissues of the locomotor system. Predicated primarily on pathomorphology (such as degenerative, histopathologic, inflammatory, neoplastic, or infective lesions) with a relatively simple view of loss of function (pain, weakness, loss of movement), terminology accorded to the disease–illness model of scientific modernism. Specific diagnoses such as tendinitis, bursitis, ligament sprains and peripheral nerve entrapment replaced fibrositis and associated syndromes.

According to Cyriax, the principal challenges to osteopathy were the basic morphological concepts of annular disc tear, nuclear disc prolapse, and dural tension as the pathologies underlying the vast majority of spinal derangements. Although Cyriax soon discarded the theory of sacroiliac derangement (a mobilization technique for which was illustrated in his first textbook only) he allowed Barbor to describe the development of sclerotherapy (prolotherapy) for ligamentous disturbances of the spine, including sacroiliac ligamentous insufficiency, in the subsequent editions of his textbook. As will be seen later, the adoption by osteopathic physicians of the concept of fibroproliferative treatment techniques for ligamentous disturbances is an example of the increasingly 'broad church' attitudes adopted by both allopathic and osteopathic medicine and demonstrated with increasing maturity by musculoskeletal medicine over recent years.

Osteopathic medicine

Osteopathic medicine, founded on the work of Andrew Taylor Still who 'threw the banner (of osteopathy) to the breeze' in 1874, represented a seminal breakthrough in conceptual thinking. It provided a radical model for ill health and dis-ease. Although revised and redefined, Still's basic concepts continue to underpin osteopathic principles and practice. Interestingly there has been a resurgence of interest at Kirksville Osteopathic Medical School (founded by Still) in his original manual techniques.

Stated simplistically, the rationale was that health and ill health are related to spinal function and dysfunction. However, somatic dysfunction should never be considered in isolation. Viscerosomatic reflex patterns are the very essence of osteopathic medicine.

Originally described as the 'osteopathic lesion', somatic dysfunction is now the accepted international term for the dysfunctional lesion. It is more formally defined as 'impaired or altered function of related components of the somatic (body framework) system: skeletal, arthrodial, and myofascial structures, and related vascular, lymphatic, and neural elements'.

Somatic dysfunction is essentially a pathophysiological phenomenon. Anatomic derangements should always be considered as contributory factors, as should adverse posture and abnormal biomechanics. Of interest is that at the height of James Cyriax's influence in the UK in the middle and later decades of the twentieth century there could not be two more diametrically opposed schools than osteopathic manipulative (now renamed neuromusculoskeletal) training (the branch of osteopathic medicine that focuses particularly on neuromuscular problems) on the one hand and the structuralism of orthopaedic medicine on the other. However within the last two decades of the twentieth century there has been a gradual convergence of these schools, for instance the acceptance by allopathic medicine of dysfunctional neuromusculoskeletal states characterized by somatic dysfunction, and the incorporation of prolotherapy into advanced osteopathic training.

Manual medicine

In Europe, manual medicine was substantively influenced by osteopathic medicine. Chiropractic also played a role (Neumann 1989). An emphasis on articular dysfunction, using 'blockage' as old terminology, is a distinguishing characteristic. In this regard there is much in common with the theories and practice advanced by John Mennell (Zohn and Mennell, 1976) who, having trained in London, based his work (in the USA) on the concepts of his father (James Mennell) and the elder (Edgar) Cyriax. However, muscle hypertonus/contraction and the associated features of somatic dysfunction are consistent features in European manual medicine. The Czech school of manual medicine, led by Karel Lewit and Vladimir Janda places a particular emphasis on muscle dysfunction. A contrubution by Vladimir Janda is included in this book (2.2.2).

In general terms, 'manual medicine' has come to be regarded recently as the relatively pure core model of manual diagnostics and manual therapeutics. To practitioners of manual medicine in some European countries 'musculoskeletal medicine' is a somewhat wider subject, incorporating other management strategies such as injections.

Musculoskeletal medicine

Musculoskeletal medicine has emerged from a background of orthopaedic medicine (as previously described, developed by James Cyriax at St. Thomas' Hospital, London), manual medicine, and osteopathic manipulative medicine. Musculoskeletal medicine may easily be distinguished from allied specialties such as rheumatology and orthopaedic surgery. The distinctive and underlying concepts of musculoskeletal medicine are:

- The scientific basis of function of the neuromusculoskeletal system.

- The pathophysiological and structural basis of dysfunction of the neuromusculoskeletal system.

With respect to management strategies there is an overlap with other disciplines such as pain management and rehabilitation. There is a close working relationship with allied non-medical professions, particularly physiotherapy. Knowledge of functional anatomy, ergonomics, biomechanics, podiatry, exercise physiology, and general medicine is essential. Clinical application of this knowledge is reflected in distinctive manual diagnostic techniques. Management skills include spinal mobilization and manipulation (both allopathic and osteopathic), injections and a wide range of other manual techniques. Complementary, mind–body, and holistic approaches to health are particularly relevant to chronic musculoskeletal disorders (see Ward, Chapter 4.3.10).

In short, musculoskeletal medicine has accepted the concept of neuromusculoskeletal dysfunction, as developed by osteopathic medicine and manual medicine, but retains many of the allopathic characteristics of orthopaedic medicine. It has an established evidence base (upon which this textbook has been constructed) yet it retains the art and compassion of the healthcare professional that is well versed in the biopsychosocial as well as the biomechanical, pathophysiological and pathomorphological models of care. It incorporates holism and eclecticism and is an archetypal postmodern medical discipline.

Biosocial model of Engel (and other health care constructs)

George Engel, Professor of Psychiatry and Medicine at University of Rochester School of Medicine, Rochester, New York threw down a challenge by identifying the need for a new medical model. In a seminal article (Engel 1977) he stated that the adherence to a model of disease was no longer adequate for the scientific tasks and social responsibilities of either medicine or psychiatry. The existing biomedical model, with molecular biology as its basic scientific discipline, embraced reductionism and mind-body dualism. It developed as medicine became 'scientific', particularly as taxonomy and other analytical scientific methods were applied to disease and suffering.

Engel proposed a biosocial model that 'takes account of the patient', the social context in which he lives, and the complementary system devised by society to deal with the disruptive effects of illness – that is, the physician role and the healthcare system. Clearly it embraces psychosocial factors, including the status of the patient and the sick role, and addresses the apparent paradox that illness and wellness may not be related closely to 'positive' laboratory findings. It explains the variations of response by patients to health issues – from 'illness' or 'injury' to 'problems of living'.

Henrik Wulff developed a somewhat different view in 1999 when he described the two cultures of medicine: objective facts versus subjectivity and values. In clinical practice there are scientific components (reasoning from theoretical knowledge, and reasoning from past experience – evidence-based medicine for instance) and humanistic components based on wisdom and personal interpretation of findings from patient psychology and ethical reasoning.

McDonald (1996) went further when he suggested that physicians often make clinical decisions based on insufficient evidence-based medicine from randomized trials or epidemiological studies, and by the use of rules of thumb (or 'medical heuristics'), derived from personal theories, assumptions, experience, traditions, and lore.

My own views are similar to those of Suarez-Almazor and Russell (1998) who wrote that 'the art of medicine' is not about applying anecdotal experiences to the solution of clinical problems, it is about critically appraising the evidence in front of us and linking to our focus of interest, the individual patient.

The biopsychosocial model of Waddell is discussed later in the chapter.

Distinctiveness of musculoskeletal medicine

Numerous references are made in this textbook to the distinctiveness of musculoskeletal medicine. This is associated with improved and more widespread understanding of neural plasticity and neuromuscoloskeletal dysfunction, and the application of appropriate diagnostic manual techniques to problems that more often than not present as pain syndromes.

The clinician who acquires knowledge of neuromusculoskeletal dysfunction gains insight into conditions such as whiplash and upper limb pain that may be manifest in diverse ways, defy the established disease–illness model, and present to the 'uninitiated' a substantive diagnostic challenge.

By way of illustration some of those dysfunctional problems that commonly cause epistemological errors in conceptual thinking, diagnosis, and management in the absence of insight into neural plasticity are discussed in the following text.

Whiplash

Traumatic injuries to the musculoskeletal system caused by vehicular collisions are universal, apparently becoming more prevalent or at the very least more frequently complained of. However they are by no means a modern phenomenon. 'Railway spine' was just as much a suitable topic for the honing and application of polemical skills in the second half of the nineteenth century as whiplash and whiplash-associated disorders are today. In the nineteenth century opinion was divided between those physicians who were aligned to neurobiological explanations for traumatic backache and associated symptoms and those who identified psychosomatic fundamentalism as more congruent with their own beliefs (Cohen and Quintner 1996). In many respects the debate has not moved on to any substantive degree other than for the increasing recognition of the neurophysiological basis for many symptoms that were previously unexplained. Even so, 'spinal concussion' was not too far off the mark as an expression of a disturbed spinal cord when contrasted with the modern views regarding neuronal activity in the dorsal horns (see Kidd, Chapter 2.3.1).

A recognition of the concept and features of somatic dysfunction facilitates an understanding of the myriad complaints in whiplash-associated disorders ranging from dizziness, visual disturbances, and headaches, pain and dysaesthesiae in the upper limbs, discomfort in the lower back, sacroiliac regions, and buttocks – to name but a few. Temporomandibular joint dysfunction (jawlash) occurs in a significant subgroupof patients. The symptoms of vertigo, dizziness, visual disturbances, etc. are sometimes grouped together as the Barré–Lieou syndrome (Barré 1926). Proximal thoracic spinal dysfunctions are common, as are sacroiliac disturbances.

The Lithuanian experience of the low incidence of symptomatic whiplash 1 year after the index event (Schrader et al. 1996) is not surprising given the intrinsic modulating effect on pain pathways of the descending cerebrospinal tracts operating outside a medicolegal context. By contrast, it is hypothesized that the inhibitory function of these tracts is often compromised by perpetuating factors that are associated with the 'advanced' culture of the Western world.

The lack of 'hard physical signs' (Gargan 1995) inhibits most orthopaedic surgeons from making a meaningful evaluation within a biopsychosocial model of 'injury' in those who continue to complain 1 year after the index event. Without appropriate manual diagnostics, the absence of identifiable 'organic' pathology invites a suspicion (in the clinician's mind) of wilful exaggeration by the patient or frank malingering, thereby contributing (should the scepticism of the examiner be obvious to the patient) in some to distress, chronicity of symptoms, and disability.

Upper limb pain

The concept of neuropathic arm pain is explored in Chapter 3.5. Regional pain syndromes are relatively incomprehensible without an understanding of neural function and dysfunction. The application of neurodynamics to a functional assessment of the neck and upper limb is a fruitful exercise without which diagnoses are presumptive and based on exclusion. The medical profession is indebted to the work of Australian physiotherapists such as David Butler (see Chapters 2.2.4; 4.3.7) who have improved our understanding of the application of basic anatomy and physiology to neuronal circuitry between the neck and the hand. Musculoskeletal physicians should at the very least become acquainted with and hopefully skilled at evaluative diagnostic manual tests for neural dysfunction.

Although 'adverse neural tension' may soon become somewhat dated as medical shorthand and medical jargon (in deference to improving knowledge of neural plasticity) it should meanwhile become as familiar a concept for the expression of neural sensitivity or irritability as 'dural tension' in the lower limbs (as assessed by the straight leg raise and femoral stretch test).

Back pain

That appropriate diagnostic skills are prerequisites for meaningful and effective management strategies is a theme throughout this textbook. Nowhere is this more relevant than in the diagnosis and management of back pain, particularly lower back pain.

A time-consuming but potentially rewarding part of my own work over the last 5–10 years has been to disabuse many patients of misconceptions regarding the nature of their back pain and to reverse the effects of its past mismanagement, instilled by 'conventional wisdom' of the medical profession over the last 20 or so years. These misconceptions so often arise from the discussion of 'crumbling spine', 'worn out discs', and 'arthritis' arising from X-ray appearances, paying no heed to the findings of a competent musculoskeletal examination. Old habits die hard. The inculcation of healthy attitudes, appropriate rehabilitation programmes, and early return to premorbid levels of daily activities is predicated on evaluation strategies that differentiate nociceptive and neuropathic pain, and recognize the role of red flags (for serious disease), yellow flags (for psychosocial factors with particular relevance to chronicity), and illness behaviour.

Tender points

The concept of tender points and trigger points is explored throughout the textbook. Proponents of myofascial pain syndromes as an important diagnostic group propose a primary dysfunctional state within the muscle as the explanation for tenderness, muscle hypertonus, the jump sign, and referred pain phenomena. By contrast, Hugh Smythe (Chapter 2.2.3) relates tender/trigger points around the pectoral girdle and upper limbs to cervical spinal pathology.

A hypothesis with which I personally am comfortable is that tender/trigger points are, for the most part, a manifestation of secondary hyperalgesia. As such, they reflect the process of neurosensitization, whether locally, regionally, or generally.

Fibromyalgia may be considered to be an expression of a widespread pain syndrome. Regional pain syndromes abound, for instance neuropathic arm pain (type II work-related upper limb disorder). At a more local level, neurosensitization may well be an expression of local dysfunction, infection, or inflammation.

Allodynia indicates a reduced threshold to potentially nociceptive stimuli; hyperalgesia indicates reduced tolerance of nociceptive stimuli; and hyperpathia indicates a prolonged nociceptive response to provocative stimuli.

Practitioners of musculoskeletal medicine will be familiar with the ubiquitous tenderness and muscle hypertonus in the proximal scapular fixator muscles, and also in the glutei, which are common accompaniments (or responses) to gravitational or postural cervicodorsal spinal stresses and lower back stresses respectively.

Red flags and yellow flags

The terms 'red flags' and 'yellow flags' refer to the relevant factors that emerge at interview or examination of a patient that act as 'markers' for serious spinal pathology (red flags) or psychosocial factors and coping mechanisms associated with chronicity (yellow flags). Red flags include onset of back pain in the elderly, thoracic spinal pain, a history of malignancy, general ill health, weight loss, etc. Psychosocial yellow flags include social deprivation, poor job satisfaction, incorrect beliefs, a history of inappropriate or ineffective coping strategies, abnormal behaviour, and fear/pain-avoidance.

Illness behaviour

The behavioural responses to illness and injury are manifold. Accordingly, it is not unusual for emotional responses to be manifest by patients during contact with others, including examining clinicians. As a consequence, it is somewhat arbitrary as to when behavioural reactions identified by the examiner at interview or on clinical examination are 'abnormal'. The more common findings of established illness behaviour are hesitancy on movement (particular in response to instructions during examination), pain gesturing and vocalization, dizziness, and other somewhat inappropriate reactions.

Abnormal illness behaviour (first described by Pilowsky in 1969) is 'an inappropriate or maladaptive mode of experiencing, perceiving, evaluating or responding to one's own state of health'. It is sometimes, mistakenly, assumed to have a conscious aspect. However, a more ap-

Symptoms of inappropriate illness behaviour

- Non-dermatomal numbness and pain
- Non-myotomal ('global') weakness in the leg
- Constant symptoms
- Refractoriness to and often intolerance of treatments

Signs relating to low back pain complaints

- Lumbar pain on axial loading
- Lumbar pain on simulated rotation
- Improvement of straight leg raise on distraction
- Regional sensory changes
- Superficial widespread non-anatomical tenderness
- Regional jerky resisted muscle contraction
- Over-reaction generally

propriate interpretation is that abnormal illness behaviour with its accompanying concept 'the sick role' is the overt expression of distress, misattribution, and maladaptation, often reflecting poor or exhausted coping mechanisms.

Inappropriate signs

'Inappropriate' signs in assessment of low back pain were described by Waddell in 1980, but have been open to abuse. Waddell was instrumental in distinguishing 'non-organic' or 'inappropriate' symptoms and signs of abnormal illness behaviour from the symptoms and signs of 'organic pathology', or 'physical impairment' (see box). The signs in particular have been used extensively by orthopaedists.

Unfortunately the detection of inappropriate features, particularly inappropriate clinical signs, sometimes leads to inappropriate interpretation of the underlying clinical problem. 'Non-organic' does not necessarily equate to deliberate exaggeration or fabrication of symptoms. It should mean what it sets out to state: that there is probably no significant or relevant abnormality of tissue morphology – which, in the context of the underlying concept of neuromusculoskeletal dysfunction in this textbook, should come as no great surprise in many disorders. Additionally, in the light of our present understanding of neurosensitization, the sensory signs and possibly most of the other 'inappropriate' signs are capable of interpretation as abnormal neural processing.

Disability

Disability is the adverse effect on activities of daily living, particularly work, caused by illness or injury. It has a large subjective component, which makes it difficult if not impossible for the examining clinician to forecast or quantify in an individual. Reliance on demonstrable pathology (for instance by radiography or MRI) is epistemologically unsound because it ignores the behavioural responses to life's problems, illnesses, and injuries.

Disability should be contrasted with impairment of function. Loss of function may be relatively easy to quantify (for instance the loss of movements at a peripheral joint in a compliant patient), sometimes more difficult (such as the evaluation of loss of movement at the lumbar spine). Nevertheless, it represents an objective assessment made by the examiner. Naturally impairment of function is often a major contributor to disability but it may not be the most important factor. As previously stated psychosocial factors are often paramount in the development of and chronicity of disability.

In addition to societal factors, the role of the medical profession is often contributory. It is a truism to state that patients sometimes recover despite the 'best' attentions of the medical profession. In patients with neck and back pain, iatrogenesis is often a major aetiological, perpetuating, or aggravating factor (see next section). Disability is commonly the product of dysfunction, fear-avoidance, distress, and iatrogenesis.

Iatrogenesis

The following factors are often relevant to the role of the medical profession:

- failure to understand somatic dysfunction
- failure to distinguish between neuropathic and nociceptive pain
- failure to recognize illness behaviour and psychosocial factors
- failure to differentiate impairment from disability
- inappropriate labelling, misattribution and medical jargon
- catastrophizing (by the doctor)
- unjustified restriction of activity
- buck passing (for instance, delaying therapy by use of tests or secondary referral)
- a readiness or willingness to provide sickness certification.

The non-medical professions are not exempt: the domination of spinal manipulation at the expense of the inculcation of positive self-help and self-stabilization strategies in some osteopathic and chiropractic regimes leads to patient dependency. (An example of the biopsychosocial model cast aside in favour of the biomedical model.) The lack of mobilizing or manipulating techniques in some physiotherapists' armamentarium is a contrasting deficiency.

In some countries the ill-defined status of musculoskeletal medicine, and the uncertain role of the musculoskeletal physician within the medical community, are factors that affect the credibility of the examining doctor, hence the effectiveness of his management strategy.

Evidence-based medicine

Evidence-based medicine has been defined by Sackett as the conscientious, explicit, and judicious use of the current best evidence in making decisions about the care of individual patients (Sackett 1998). Universally accepted as concordant with best and most cost-effective practice at the turn of the millennium, it is equally applicable to musculoskeletal medicine. By definition, evidence-based medicine is reliant upon the best available evidence being brought to bear on a patient's problems. Physicians are expected to use diagnostic techniques that are both reliable and valid, and therapies that have proven efficacy. Sackett softened his approach to evidence-based medicine by stating that inherent in its practice is integration of the best available external clinical evidence from systematic research with individual clinical expertise.

The use of mathematics in musculoskeletal medicine has been refined by Bogduk (1999). Interobserver reliability for diagnostic examining techniques is crucial if sense is to be made of dysfunctional neuromusculoskeletal conditions. Unlike other branches of medicine, there are few gold standards for dysfunctional states. Serological, radiological, neurophysiological, and histopathological investigations may be normal in somatic dysfunction. As a consequence, validation of diagnostic techniques is dependent upon agreement on the basic characteristics of dysfunction. Despite the difficulties, critical appraisal of the evidence for its validity and usefulness is possible (see Patijn, Chapter 1.2).

The development and testing of hypotheses, allowing them to stand unless proven false (Popper 1959), combined with clinical observations has provided the empiric basis of advancement of knowledge in musculoskeletal medicine in the past (Dorman 1995). Hopefully evidence-based medicine will not stultify hypothesis and innovation.

Sometimes, in the frequent absence of 'gold standard' diagnoses in functional disorders, it is only when a putative syndromic diagnosis (that is 'recognized' by a specific test) responds to a specific therapeutic procedure that the test may be considered to be valid. This is essentially a pragmatic approach to diagnosis and management (see Blomberg, Chapter 4.4). For example, some clinicians (including myself) are satisfied that the three features – tenderness of the posterior superior iliac spine, reduced mobility of the sacroiliac joint, and gluteal hyperalgesia – constitute, in combination, an appropriate diagnostic test for sacroiliac joint dysfunction; but, in the absence of a gold standard diagnostic test for this condition, the subjective (patient's) approval of the results of appropriate therapy and the objective (observer's) assessment of improved sacroiliac mobility immediately after the procedure provide second-best validity for the diagnostic test.

Models of care in neuromusculoskeletal medicine

Four conceptual models are described: biomechanical, pathomorphological, pathophysiological, and biopsychosocial.

Biomechanical model

The biomechanical model of dynamic stability in which the components of the musculoskeletal system (bones, joints, ligaments, muscles, fascia, and other soft tissues) contribute to efficient load transference and, as a consequence, to movement of the body with least energy expenditure and injury risk, underpins the text of this book. However, the emphasis is on the clinical aspects of somatic disorders that arise when the body's adaptive processes to physical stresses (for instance gravitational, environmental, work- and sports-related) are overwhelmed – rather than biomechanics. For a greater understanding of basic biomechanics of the musculoskeletal system the reader is referred to other texts. The more advanced biomechanical concepts and their clinical application to the pelvis, developed in the last decade or so by Levin and Dorman (see Chapters 2.2.5 and 2.2.6) and by researchers in the Netherlands, prompts me to make reference to sacroiliac dysfunction, and to provide a short summary of recent 'trends' by way of illustration.

The concepts of **form closure** and **force closure** at the sacroiliac joint were introduced by Vleeming et al. (1990). Form closure is due to the close apposition of the joint surfaces, their 'irregular' but complementary pits, ridges, and grooves, and the wedge shape of the sacrum. Force closure is the biomechanical contribution to stability (maximal in nutation – forward movement of the base, or 'promontory', of the sacrum), made by the muscles, ligaments, and fascial systems. When shear forces at the sacroiliac joint are adequately controlled by the stabilizing effects of form closure and force closure, loads can be transmitted between the lower limbs and the trunk in a cost-effective manner. When pelvic functional stability is not achieved, and shear is uncontrolled, the 'cost' to the body is the state of functional and biomechanical decompensation, manifest as painful syndromes, particularly (but not exclusively) low back pain and somatic pelvic pain. The reader is also directed to Chapter 4.3.12 in which Mottram and Comerford address the motor control of the lower back and pelvis, the relationship between muscular balance and pain syndromes, and rehabilitation strategies for a return to dynamic stability.

The 'pathobiomechanics' of disorders in the upper and lower limbs is often of primary importance. This applies particularly to sport-related problems in the pelvis and lower limbs (dealt with comprehensively by Read, Chapter 3.6; Peirce, Chapter 3.7.2; English, Chapter 3.8.1; and Higgins, Chapter 3.8.2) and to both sports- and work-related problems in the shoulder and upper limbs (covered by Tanner, Chapter 3.4.3; Hackney, Chapter 3.4.4; and Hutson, Chapter 3.5). Ergonomics is an associated healthcare model worthy of study in patients with shoulder and arm pain due to repetitive or stereotyped movements. Knowledge of sports technique is essential for the diagnosis, rehabilitation, and prevention of further injury in overuse conditions of the lower limb.

Pathomorphological ('structural') model

One cannot consider the nature of musculoskeletal disorders without reference to structural abnormalities. After all, 'organic pathology' has always been, and indeed continues to be, the primary focus for orthopaedists (and surgeons in general, from which corporate body orthopaedic surgeons have emerged during the last 100 years). Disorders of bone, other than stress fractures, receive scant attention in this textbook; they are dealt with very adequately in numerous orthopaedic texts. However, physicians with expertise in neuromusculoskeletal disciplines should always consider bone pathology in the differential diagnosis of axial and peripheral pain, both traumatic (or 'acute') and overuse (or 'chronic'). Examples are to be found in the text: avulsion fractures, osteochondral injuries, epiphyseal fractures, and metastatic carcinoma for instance.

Traumatic injuries to the soft tissues, particularly in the limbs, may arise primarily as a consequence of external factors. A trip or stumble leading to a fall may cause a ligament sprain, joint dislocation, or muscle tear in the fittest; of course constitutional factors may increase vulnerability to injury and reduce the rate of recovery. When repetitive stresses cause failure of the adaptive processes inherent in collagenized tissues, the degree of decompensation may be assessed functionally by clinical examination, assisted when necessary by a variety of investigative tools. Experience is required in decision-making as to whether or when further investigations (with the inevitable financial cost) are desirable or necessary. Experience is essential with regard to the interpretation and relevance of pathomorphological findings (for instance disc degeneration, disc bulge, or even frank disc prolapse in back pain, or increased uptake in bone scans of the lower limbs in runners).

Terminology changes over time to keep abreast of improved understanding of pathomorphology. An example is the current use of the term tendinosis (replacing 'tendinitis') as the consequence of overuse. Disruption of collagen with histological features of degeneration, rather than an invasion of inflammatory cells, is seen in Achilles tendinopathy, patellar tendinopathy, and rotator cuff tendinopathy. Evidence is accumulating (Khan *et al.* 1999, 2002) that rehabilitation for tendinopathy affecting the weightbearing tendons (Achilles, patellar) should comprise eccentric contraction regimes. At the shoulder, assessment and rehabilitation of rotator cuff lesions demand an evaluation of the provocative factors (associated with shoulder girdle biomechanics, ergonomics, posture, sports dynamics) involved in subacromial impingement. Ligamentous laxity at the glenohumeral joint, often acquired by sportspeople as a consequence of repeated or forceful stretching at the shoulder, is often a confounding factor in sports that demand substantive upper limb activity (Hutson 2001).

Meniscus derangements, particularly at the knee, require careful evaluation. The 'classical' presentation of a twisting sprain, joint effusion, and locking of the knee is an indication for the attention of the traumatologist or orthopaedic surgeon. Recurrent, self-resolving bouts of knee pain in the young may be assessed most effectively by arthroscopy, but in middle life and beyond critical appraisal of the patient by the application of clinical examination techniques of the type devised by Cyriax, augmented by stress tests for cruciate insufficiency (see Bickerstaff, Chapter 3.7.1), will serve the musculoskeletal physician best. When degenerative tears of the menisci, as evident on MRI, become symptomatic, the clinician becomes increasingly reliant on a sound knowledge of functional rehabilitation. As degenerative changes in the soft tissues advance, tissue preservation and maximization of functional capacity become paramount.

Pathophysiological model

The pathophysiological model provides the framework for the construct of somatic dysfunction. As neurobiology and pathoneurobiological processes are further elucidated and defined, it becomes conceptually easier (even for allopathically trained physicians) to take a leaf out of the manual therapist's book in appreciating the limitations of chasing the (nociceptive source of the) pain, and to think in terms of evaluating the reasons behind the overt manifestations of dysfunction. Kuchera eloquently provides both an overview and an in-depth analysis of the factors associated with the pathophysiological model in Chapters 2.2.1 and 3.3.

The analgesic response to manual therapy is very probably associated with significant neurophysiological effects in addition to the effects on joint mechanics and the chemical environment of injured tissue. Although unproven as yet, it is postulated that for treatment of spinal dysfunction to be successful activation of descending pain inhibitory systems may be as important as local responses at (spinal) segmental and peripheral levels. Neurodynamics is also an important consideration in disorders of the upper and lower limbs. Neural dysfunction may be the primary or a contributory cause of shoulder and/or elbow pain or of buttock and/or posterior thigh pain. No musculoskeletal examination is complete, whether for axial or peripheral pain, without a neural assessment.

Butler (Chapters 2.2.4 and 4.3.7) refers to 'an emerging new construct in neurodynamics' (Butler 2000) by advising that the neurophysiological aspects of mechanosensitivity should be considered when undertaking neural tension tests. The changing concepts over recent years with respect to the upper limb neural tension tests provide the reader with an insight into how increasing recognition of neural plasticity affects our thinking. The Australian manual therapist Robert Elvey revived the concept of neural tension in the upper limb at an international manual therapy conference (Elvey 1979). 'Revival' perhaps does not do Elvey justice, but it is a fact that the London neurologist Vivian Poore wrote of arm pain in the 1870s and 1880s (100 years before Elvey's introduction of the term brachial plexus tension test). Poore (1887) included details of tension tests for the median, ulnar and radial nerves. The upper limb tension test was introduced by Kenneally *et al.* in 1988 and used by Butler in his text-book *Mobilization of the Nervous System* in 1991. (Kenneally described the upper limb tension test as the 'straight leg raise of the arm'). Currently the neural tissue provocation test is used as a means of assessing mechanosensitivity of the neural tissue, though Butler demurs on the basis that neurosensitization may play a role and on the recognition that other soft tissues besides the neural tissues are challenged on the upper limb tests. As a consequence Butler prefers the term 'upper limb neurodynamics testing'.

The concept of secondary hyperalgesia as the pathophysiological explanation for referred tenderness (palpatory hyperalgesia) and discomfort on active and passive movements (articular hyperalgesia) has gained much ground. It reflects the increasing awareness of abnormal sensory processing. Cohen *et al.* (1992) can take much credit for their projection of neural dysfunction as the cause of some cases of previously undiagnosed upper limb pain.

Biopsychosocial model

The demand for an alternative to the disease-illness (biomedical) model, which had supported medical practice for centuries and was reinforced by the pathomorphological concepts of Virchow (1858), gathered pace through the 1980s. The following points became recognized:

- Contrary to the cartesian theory of pain, (subsequently – though somewhat unfairly with respect to René Descartes – described as the 'duality of pain'), pain perception, and pain behaviour very enormously from person to person.

- Pain does not equate to tissue 'injury' in most cases of back pain.

- Chronicity of back pain, also neck pain arising from whiplash, and some upper limb pain syndromes, correlates poorly with tissue injury or structural disorder.

- Psychosocial factors are better predictors of recovery or chronicity than pathomorphological considerations.

- Disability is distinct from somatic dysfunction. Although impairment of function is a component in the development of disability, there are often significant psychological, social, and iatrogenic factors.

The biopsychosocial model of pain, health care, and disability, for which much credit should go to Waddell and colleagues (1984, 1987), addresses these and other issues. In effect this model is an extension of Waddell's views on the distinction between distress, disability and dysfunction (with which I entirely concur). The psychosocial factors are explored further elsewhere in the text. A useful synopsis is the recognition that:

- Acute pain is a complex sensory and emotional experience, often associated with distress. Although pain is distinct from disability, both are subjective phenomena.

- The chronicity and severity of pain, particularly (but not exclusively) spinal pain, correlate well with psychosocial factors that include premorbid psychological profile, environmental stresses, misattributions and beliefs, iatrogenesis, and litigation.

Pragmatism and complexity

Patients' expectations in the twenty-first century are increasing. Across the spectrum of health issues, patients are very likely to have and to declare values and preferences. They expect to be involved in decision-making, seeking quality of treatment that is predicated upon their individual circumstances. In parallel with patients' 'New Age' views, there have been significant societal anxieties and cultural changes in recent years. Accordingly, clinicians need to be increasingly flexible to address the complexity of health-related problems. Herein lies an enigma. Evidence-based medicine is virtually *de rigueur* in the current decade, demanded by health authorities and viewed as an essential component of 'governance' (the medical profession's all-encompassing self-regulating mechanism). However, individual tailor-made treatment programmes providing value, and independent of meta-analytical medical judgements, are demanded by patients. A multidisciplinary approach is often required. Can we square the circle? To do so we must understand the application to science of modernism, postmodernism, and complex adaptive systems ('postnormal science').

Based on the science of Galileo and Newton *inter alia*, and the philosophy of thinkers such as René Descartes and Hume in the Age of the Enlightenment, the fundamental principles of modernism were (and remain) logic, reason, rationalism, and reductionism. Theories about disease and illness are based on measurements, thereby explaining reality. If theories have no measurable components, they are essentially invalid. Much of medical practice since the eighteenth century, and continuing to this day, adopts modernist principles based on a biomedical model. Orthopaedic surgery is a prime example.

Postmodernism, on the other hand, is essentially anarchic and eclectic. It rejects dogma, rejects the concept of universal truth, and rejects modernism. Friedrich Nietzsche developed some of these principles, but there have been many subsequent advocates, in particular Lyotard and Fourcault. Specifically, postmodernism rejects the (modernist) mantra that objectivity is possible in scientific work. Objectivity is often compromised by the quest for, or the achievement of, power. Postmodernism espouses non-conformity and diversity. Such principles are congruent with complementary and alternative medicine, and to some extent with manual therapy (in its broadest sense).

Postnormal science has adopted some postmodern ideas (Laugharne 2002). However, its essential principle is that uncertainty and unpredictability are inevitable in complex systems. This often applies for instance to health care. The search for absolute truth is viewed with grave suspicion. In postnormal science, science itself is not rejected. However its boundaries should be expanded to allow discourse regarding sociocultural implications with all interested parties (of which there are many). There are numerous applications of postnormal science. In the so-called 'civilized' countries, issues such as genetically modified foods, stem cell research, and cloning have implications for society in general, engaging many stakeholders.

The introduction of complexity (in the form of uncertainty, unpredictability, and an expanded peer community), a feature of post-normal science referred to as non-linearity, demands adaptability and flexibility on the part of the physician (Wilson and Holt 2001). This type of health care paradigm is known as a **complex adaptive system**, in which patients' problems vary from the simple (with a high degree of agreement between clinicians and a high degree of certainty of diagnosis) to – at the opposite extreme – 'chaotic' in which there is very low agreement and a very low degree of certainty. Most cases are situated between these two extremes, demanding the need (in many cases) for multiple approaches, creativity, and (above all) pragmatism.

An appropriate problem for the study of the often complex relationships between pathomorphology and pathophysiology, and the pertinence of the complexity theory, is posterior thigh pain, or 'hamstring dysfunction'. A 'tear' or 'pull' of the hamstrings is a common problem in sport. Posterior thigh pain has a high prevalence in the general population. Why is hamstring dysfunction so often a 'pain in the butt' and/or thigh, and how do we explain its frquently recurring nature? The answer perhaps lies in the fact that whichever model or paradigm (pathomorphological, biomechanical, biopsychosocial, and pathophyisological) is chosen, there is underlying neuromusculoskeletal weakness, decompensation, or 'vulnerability'.

In the pathomorphological model, hamstring dysfunction is the consequence of intrinsic muscle deficiency, commonly a tear of the biceps femoris muscle. The severity may be based on the clinician's experience, but tissue injury is more accurately graded by MRI: Grade 1, anatomy preserved, oedema; Grade 2, muscle fibre disruption; Grade 3, haematoma. Inevitably, rehabilitation demands attention to restoration of muscle function.

In the biomechanical model, factors such as muscle fatigue, flexibility, strength, and imbalance are considered. Additionally, aging and muscle function with respect to dynamic stability and range of movements of the hip, spine, and knee are valid issues. Gait analysis is often required in investigation. Other factors involved in aetiology are incomplete rehabilitation, inappropriate warm-up before sport, training errors, and associated issues including those enumerated in the pathophysiological model.

In the biopsychosocial model, the psychological aspects of pain, as portrayed in the chapters by Main and Watson (2.3.2),and Blomberg (4.4) are of considerable relevance.

In many patients, adherence to the pathophysiological model is maximally productive. This model is predicated upon neural dysfunction arising in the lower back or pelvis, and adversely affecting hamstring contraction. A likely cause of hamstring inhibition is 'false' or 'disturbed' proprioceptive input from the lower back and pelvis, particularly the spinal facet (apophyseal) joints and sacroiliac joints, and possibly from the periphery such as ankle or knee following lower limb trauma. Characteristic clinical features are spinal dysfunction, sacroiliac dysfunction, myofascial trigger points, neural dysfunction, and muscle weakness patterns, primarily of the S1 myotome. These patterns of lower limb discomfort in young adults, often sportspeople, are mostly 'pseudoradicular' insofar as there is usually no evidence of nerve root compression, merely disturbed neurodynamics, though intervertebral foraminal neural irritation (as a consequence of recess stenosis) is increasingly the cause of thigh pain in the ageing population.

Management strategies are essentially pragmatic. Treatment is directed towards the identifiable dysfunctions, commonly at the spine and pelvis. Rehabilitation should continue until restoration of full functional capacity is achieved. Treatment options include spinal and paravertebral injections in the form of epidural injections, foraminal blocks, and facet blocks. Other injections and needling techniques, particularly for trigger points, are usually helpful. Controversial treatments that are not yet validated but are gaining popularity include injections of enzymes to 'enhance reabsorption of haematomas', injections that include a homeopathic remedy 'to modulate factor P and oxygen radicals', and injections of protein-free ultrafiltrate of calf's blood 'to increase oxygen uptake, to accelerate the processes of granulation and vascularization, and to improve microcirculation'. Additionally, prolotherapy may be required for refractory or recurrent cases (see Dorman, Chapter 4.3.6, and Blomberg, Chapter 4.4).

Management of sclerotomal or 'pseudoradicular' syndromes is a good example of a complex adaptive system paradigm. Mobilization/manipulation, soft tissue treatment, paravertebral blocks, epidural injections, and sclerosant injections (prolotherapy) may all have a place, and followed by a comprehensive rehabilitation protocol. Diverse treatments may of course be given sequentially, but many clinicians, including myself, prefer combined therapy on the basis that individual treatment modalities may have a 'synergistic' rather than additive effect. The pragmatic approach, based on an antidysfunctional management strategy, is discussed more fully by Blomberg(Chapter 4.4).

References

Barré, J. A. (1926) Sur un syndrome sympathique cervical posterieure et sa cause frequente: l'arthrite cervicale. *Rev. Neurol.*, 33, 1246.

Bogduk, N. (1999) Truth in musculoskeletal medicine; truth in diagnosis – validity. *Australasian Musculoskel. Med.*, **4** (1), 32–9.

Butler, D. S. (1991) *Mobilisation of the nervous system*. Churchill Livingstone, Melbourne.

Butler, D. S. (2000) *The sensitive nervous system*. Noigroup Publications, Australia.

Cohen, M. L., Arroyo, J. F., Champion, G. D., Browne, C. D. (1992) In search of the pathogenesis of refractory cervicobrachial pain syndrome. *Med. J. Aust.*, 156, 432–6.

Cohen, M. L., Quintner, J. L (1996) The derailment of railway spine: a timely lesson for post-traumatic fibromyalgia. *Pain Rev.*, 3, 181–202.

Cyriax, J. (1969) *Textbook of orthopaedic medicine*. Williams and Wilkins, Baltimore.

Dorman, T. A. (1995) Concepts in orthopaedic medicine. *Spine: State of the Art Reviews*, 9(2), 323–31.

Engel, G. E. (1977) The need for a new medical model: a challenge for biomedicine. *Science*, **196**(4286), 129–36.

Elvey, R. L. (1979) Brachial plexus tension tests and the pathoanatomical origin of arm pain. In: Idezak, R. (ed.) *Aspects of manipulative therapy*. Manipulative Physiotherapists Association of Australia, Melbourne.

Gargan, M. F. (1995) What is the evidence for an organic lesion in whiplash injury? *J. Psychosomat. Res.*, 39(6), 777–81.

Hutson, M. A. (2001) *Sports injuries: recognition and management*, 3rd ed. Oxford University Press, Oxford.

Kenneally, M., Rubenach, H., Elvey, R. L. (1988) The upper limb tension test: the SLR of the arm. In: Grant, R. (ed.) *Physical therapy of the cervical and thoracic spine*. Churchill Livingstone, New York.

Khan, K. M., Cook, J. L., Bonar, F. *et al.* (1999) Histopathology of common tendinopathies. Update and implications for clinical management. *Sports Med.*, 27, 393–408.

Khan, K. M., Cook, J., Kannus, P. *et al.* (2002) Time to abandon the 'tendinitis' myth. *BMJ*, **329**, 626–7.

Laugharne, R. (2002) Psychiatry, postmodernism and postnormal science. *J. R. Soc. Med.*, **95**, 207–10.

McDonald, C. J. (1996) Medical heuristics : the silent adjudicators of clinical practice. *Ann. Intern. Med.*, **124**, 1, 56–62.

Neumann, H.-D. (1989) *Introduction to manual medicine.* Springer-Verlag, Berlin.

Pilowsky, I. (1969) Abnormal illness behaviour. *Br. J. Med. Psychol.* **42**, 347–51.

Poore, G. V. (1887) Clinical lecture on certain conditions of the hand and arm which interfere with performance of professional arts, especially piano playing. *Br. Med. J.*, **1**, 441–4.

Popper, K. R. (1959) *The logic of scientific discovery.* Harper and Rowe, New York.

Sackett, D. L. (1998) Editorial: evidence-based medicine. *Spine*, **23**(10), 1085–6.

Schrader, H. *et al.* (1996) Natural evolution of late whiplash syndrome outside the medicolegal context. *Lancet*, **347**, 1207–11.

Suarez-Almazor, M. E., Russell, A. S. (1998) The art versus the science of medicine. Are clinical guidelines the answer? *Ann. Rheum. Dis.*, **57**, 67–9.

Virchow, R. (1858) *Die cellular pathologie in ihrer begrundurg auf physiologische und pathologische.* A Hirshwald, Berlin

Vleeming, A., Volkers, A. C. W., Snijders, C. J., Stoeckart, R. (1990) Relation between form and function in the sacroiliac joint. 2: Biomechanical aspects. *Spine*, **15**(2), 133–6.

Waddell, G., McCulloch, J. A., Kummell, E. *et al.* (1980) Non-organic physical signs in low back pain. *Spine*, 5, 117–25.

Waddell, G. (1987) A new clinical model for the treatment of low back pain. *Spine*, **12**, 632–44.

Waddell, G. *et al.* (1984) Chronic low back pain, psychologic distress and illness behaviour. *Spine*, 9, 209–13.

Wilson, T., Holt, T. (2001) Complexity and clinical care. *BMJ*, **323**, 685–8.

Wulff, H. (1999) The two cultures of medicine: objective facts versus subjectivity and values. *J. Royal Soc. Med.*, **92**, 11, 549–552.

Zohn, D. A., Mennell, J. McM. (1976) *Musculoskeletal pain: diagnosis and physical treatment.* Little, Brown, Boston.

1.2 Evidence-based medicine

Jacob Patijn

The value of evidence-based medicine

'Evidence-based medicine' (EBM) is a recent trend in the medical world, in which the current best evidence is used in making decisions about the care of the patient in the broadest sense.

Up to now, many therapeutic and diagnostic approaches taught in universities have been based more on historical traditions than on solid scientific research. If a hypothesis in medicine survived long enough, in the end it would be integrated into medical textbooks and become the 'truth' for medical students and professionals.

Nowadays, the medical practitioner is confronted with numerous meta-analyses of the lack of therapeutic efficacy of their commonly used therapies. Studies on reproducibility, validity, specificity, and sensitivity of their familiar diagnostic procedures sometimes reveal the absence of any diagnostic value. As might be expected, this can lead to insecurity of the medical practitioner in daily practice. The medical certainties taught at university now appear to be obsolete. There are two different reactions to this: one practitioner will state that 'everyone has been doing it for a long time' and 'my patients benefit from my therapy'. The other practitioner will wholeheartedly adopt the EBM concept, which can lead to diagnostic and therapeutic nihilism. For instance, a general practitioner will be guided by the evidence that 90% patients with acute low back pain will recover in 6 weeks, no therapy is effective, and no diagnostic test is valid. The consequence may be that the patient is hardly examined physically, and is sent away with analgesics only.

Although understandable, both reactions are inadequate. The first practitioner will stick to his beliefs, and is moving towards diagnostic and therapeutic automatism. Such a lack of critical attitude will never provide in-depth information about routine diagnostic and therapeutic approaches. Furthermore, he will feel that his clinical freedom has been restricted. The second practitioner uses EBM as 'cookery-book medicine'. He forgets that external clinical evidence can never replace his individual clinical experience. In simply following EBM protocols, he too will not acquire in-depth information about his diagnostic and therapeutic approaches in his patients. Both this individual clinical experience and external clinical evidence are essential. If no account is to be taken of an individual's unique clinical situation, the concept of a medical profession could become superfluous: doctors would be 'out of date'. External clinical evidence without individual clinical experience would evolve to a practice tyrannized by evidence, making evidence-based decision-making in the single patient impossible. Individual clinical experience without external clinical evidence can never lead to a development of a healthy medical profession.

The sometimes shocking results of EBM must therefore not frighten us into unthinkingly accepting the EBM concept; they must be used as a stimulus to urge medical practitioners to develop a more critical attitude towards our practice. The statistical teachings of EBM never fully reflect our daily medical reality. Statistics are always an approximation of our medical reality, with many unknown factors that can influence the outcome. As long as the precise aetiology of a clinical syndrome remains unknown, because the extrinsic and intrinsic factors influencing the individual course or clinical expression are obscure, the population with the syndrome is by definition heterogeneous. Results of efficacy studies with heterogeneous study populations must be interpreted with caution. As a logical consequence, health insurance companies, health care managers, and purchasers should never use EBM as an excuse to cut the costs of patient care.

Currently, if EBM were to be used as the standard criterion for the cost-effectiveness of the entire medical profession, it is probable that many hospital departments would have to be closed. This would also reflect a fundamental misunderstanding by health insurance companies of the financial consequences of EBM results. The primary goal of EBM is not cutting costs, but providing medical practitioners, in combination with their clinical expertise, the best tools for decision-making about the care of individual patients. And EBM helps practitioners to develop a critical attitude towards the medical profession itself, which can lead to better insight of the aetiologies of the patients' diagnoses. In this way, the development of the medical profession is assured.

We have also to realize that external clinical evidence has a temporary value. Scientific work in EBM is a continuous process, in which previously published results may be refuted by newer developments. What may appear to be correct today can indeed be wrong tomorrow. Doctors integrating EBM will identify and apply the most efficacious therapies and choose the best-validated diagnostics, to maximize the quality of their individual patients. Therefore, as a side effect, EBM can sometimes result in a lowering of health care costs, but sometimes in rising costs when more accurate analysis leads to more expensive effective therapies and/or validated diagnostic procedures.

Application to manual/musculoskeletal medicine

All aspects of EBM can be fully applied to manual/musculoskeletal medicine. From a historical point of view, we have seen the development of many different schools of manual/musculoskeletal medicine. Each school created its own philosophy, so that its own diagnostic and therapeutic approaches became integrated into its educational system. Numerous textbooks were written and reprinted. Finally, statements and hypotheses became 'the truth' for our students and professionals in manual/musculoskeletal medicine, despite the lack of scientific evidence. Although this may sound negative, it was the reality in the era when most emphasis and attention was paid to propagation of manual/musculoskeletal medicine by means of educational courses. At that time, it was important to develop hypotheses and theories for our profession, and to teach our students the diagnostic and therapeutic procedures that fitted these educational systems. This period has all the characteristics of a pioneer phase of a medical profession. Nowadays, EBM urges manual/musculoskeletal medicine to change over to the phase of greater professionalism. It also remains true that both individual clinical experience and external clinical evidence are essential for our daily practice. External evidence is important, but not all-important. Individual clinical experience without external clinical evidence will never allow robust development of manual/musculoskeletal medicine. Indeed, our profession could become out of date.

In the literature, much attention has been paid to the efficacy of manual/musculoskeletal medicine, in particular with respect to patients with low back pain. Meta-analyses demonstrate contradicting results for the efficacy of manual/musculoskeletal treatments in acute and chronic low back pain. This is probably due to the fact that patients with low back pain, by definition, comprise a heterogeneous population. Negative as well as positive outcomes of randomized controlled trials may be due to subpopulations within the heterogeneous study population, which are then responsible for the final outcome of a particular trial.

The literature also reflects the current lack of reproducible diagnostic procedures in manual/musculoskeletal medicine to define more homogeneous study populations. This lack of reproducibility is reinforced by the fact that different schools of manual/musculoskeletal medicine have developed different diagnostic tests for the same joint. Table 1.2.1 illustrates this problem with respect to a list of diagnostic tests for the sacroiliac joint. Most of these sacroiliac tests are supposed to diagnose an involvement of the sacroiliac joint in the sense of a hypomobility or as a primary source of the patients' pain. The table illustrates a fundamental problem: there are too many different schools in manual/musculoskeletal medicine in many different countries of the world, with too many different diagnostic procedures and too many different therapeutic approaches. The consequence is five-fold.

- First, most schools within manual/musculoskeletal medicine have not yet validated their own diagnostic procedures in the different regions of the locomotor system, so these diagnostic procedures are still lacking in reproducibility, validity, sensitivity, and specificity.

- Secondly, all the different schools within manual/musculoskeletal medicine still coexist. Because of lack of good reproducibility, validity, sensitivity, and specificity studies, mutual comparison of diagnostic procedures is completely impossible. Scientific information exchange and fundamental discussions between these different schools, based on solid scientific methods, is hardly possible in the present situation.

- Thirdly, the absence of validated diagnostic procedures leads to heterogeneously defined populations in efficacy trials. Therefore, comparison of efficacy trials with the same therapeutic approach (manipulation, for instance) is impossible.

- Fourthly, if the present situation continues, it will lead to a slowing down of the badly needed process of professionalism, and manual/musculoskeletal medicine will become out of date.

- Fifthly, lack of validated diagnostic procedures of different schools, ill-defined therapeutic approaches, and low-quality study designs are the main causes for the weak evidence of a proven therapeutic effect of manual/musculoskeletal medicine.

Reproducibility and validity of diagnostic procedures in manual/musculoskeletal medicine

Many diagnostic procedures have been developed in the different schools of manual/musculoskeletal medicine over recent decades. In the vast majority of these tests, reproducibility is lacking.

Most diagnostic procedures are based on a particular hypothesis and/or philosophy. For instance, various tests are developed to test the mobility of the sacroiliac joint. Reduced mobility of this joint is supposed to be one of the aetiologies of low back pain. However, the value

Table 1.2.1. Diagnostic tests of the sacroiliac joint from different schools of manual/musculoskeletal medicine

Prone position	Supine position	Neutral sitting position	Dynamic upright position
Midline sacral thrust test sacroiliac joint play	Patrick test Flexion adduction test	Flexion test sitting sacroiliac joint PSIS inequality	Standing flexion test Spine test
Prone knee flexion test	Sacroiliac translation test		Retroflexion/ lateral flexion test
Cranial shear sacroiliac compression	Gaelen's test Sacroiliac thigh trust test		Gillet test Pelvic distortion with cervical rotation
Ischial tuberosity level prone	Supine long sitting test		
Four-point sacral motion prone	Iliac crest height Supine leg length Hip rotation		

Reproducibility

Reproducibility evaluates whether two observers find the same result of a diagnostic procedure in the same patient population, or whether a single observer finds the same result of a diagnostic procedure in the same patient population at two separate moments in time.

of all these tests for sacroiliac hypomobility (see Table 1.2.1) remains questionable. Certainly, cadaver studies have shown the existence of mobility of the sacroiliac joint: even in older people there is still a considerable amount of sacroiliac range of motion. These movements, however, are too small for manual detection of sacroiliac asymmetries, even for clinicians with keen palpation and observational skills.

For many tests, the question arises if they really test what they are supposed to test. This illustrates the lack of validity of these tests. This absence of gold standards forms a major problem in manual/musculoskeletal medicine. Gold standards are essential for manual/musculoskeletal medicine just as in general medicine, to provide a scientific base for hypotheses and their associated diagnostic procedures.

Before undertaking validity studies, the most important task for manual/musculoskeletal medicine is first to make the diagnostic tests reproducible, independent of the theory behind the procedures. In reproducibility studies, the kappa value is the most accepted statistical method to measure intra-observer and inter-observer agreement. Dependent on the prevalence, the kappa value can be negative or positive. Kappa values greater than 0.6 are of practical importance. Figure 1.2.1 shows an example of a reproducibility study of two observers (A and B), who performed the same test in the same population of 40 patients. The 2×2 contingency table demonstrates that in 39 of the patients (38 + 1) the observers agreed (overall agreement of 0.98). The frequency of the positive test (index condition) is illustrated

Validity

Validity is determined by measuring how well a test performs against the gold or criterion standard. For a particular clinical test, the criterion standard could be a radiological or surgical finding.

by the prevalence of 0.96. The relation between kappa value and prevalence is seen in the curve on the right. The large dot is the actual kappa value. When prevalence figures are very high or very low, the corresponding kappa values are low. The consequence of this observation is that, when judging the kappa value, the prevalence figure must always be mentioned. A low kappa value in reproducibility studies of a diagnostic procedure does not necessarily mean the procedure has a low diagnostic value, if prevalence figures are too low or too high.

For practitioners in manual/musculoskeletal medicine, these kinds of reproducibility studies are easy and cheap to perform. Reproducible diagnostic procedures are essential for validity as well as for defining clinical syndromes. At this point, individual clinical experience meets external clinical evidence. The experience of the practitioner in recognizing clinical syndromes is necessary in order to define those syndromes based on reproducible diagnostic procedures. Standardized clinical syndromes, for their part, enable us to look for the corresponding gold standard, such as imaging techniques. They also enable us to estimate the specificity and sensitivity of diagnostic procedures.

Randomized controlled trials in manual/musculoskeletal medicine

Homogeneous populations are required for efficacy studies on recognized clinical syndromes. As stated earlier, meta-analyses demonstrate contradictory results for efficacy studies. This is probably because most study populations are heterogeneous: positive as well as negative outcomes of randomized controlled trials may be due to subpopulations in the study population. Furthermore, previously published trials had many methodological flaws, making a definite conclusion about a positive or negative therapeutic effect difficult. This is even more so because many randomized controlled trials in manual/musculoskeletal medicine are dealing only with the effect of a single therapeutic modality: manipulation. The routine practice of manual/musculoskeletal medicine typically comprises a combination of different therapeutic approaches. The lack of specific clinical syndromes in manual/musculoskeletal medicine has so far made it impossible to perform 'fastidious trials', i.e. randomized controlled trials in which a single therapeutic modality is tested on a homogeneous population with a specific diagnosis. In the future, however, when reproducible and evaluated diagnostic procedures in manual/musculoskeletal medicine are at our disposal, fastidious trials will become possible. For the time being, with heterogeneous populations, pragmatic trials are the best format for low back pain.

Conclusion

Including a chapter on EBM in a textbook of manual/musculoskeletal medicine is not meant to disqualify the contents of the other chapters because of any lack of scientific evidence. The present trend towards EBM must stimulate practitioners in manual/musculoskeletal medicine to become more critical about their practice. By integrating external evidence with personal experience, more in-depth information can be acquired about the aetiology of patients' complaints. By defining clinical syndromes on the basis of reproducible diagnostic procedures, effective treatment can be chosen and administered, allowing some prediction of the outcome of therapy.

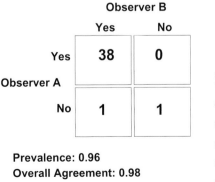

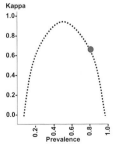

Prevalence: 0.96
Overall Agreement: 0.98
Kappa Value: 0.7

Figure 1.2.1 Kappa values.

At the same time, it is the task of scientists in schools in manual/musculoskeletal medicine to perform reproducibility, validity, specificity and sensitivity studies. The schools must transfer this information to their students by integrating it into their educational systems.

Using EBM in manual/musculoskeletal medicine in the right way, and not simply as a perceived cost-cutting exercise, will lead to further development of our specialty. Validated diagnostic procedures will become interchangeable between the different schools in manual/musculoskeletal medicine. Efficacy trials based on homogeneous populations will become mutual comparable. Good doctors in manual/musculoskeletal medicine will use both their indispensable expertise and the best scientific evidence currently available to provide their patients with optimum care.

Part 2

Morphology; dysfunction; pain

2.1 Structural abnormalities

Richard Ellis

Although there are some structural abnormalities which have not been shown to have any clinical importance, nor functional effect, such as spina bifida occulta, the majority cause some change in how that area of the body copes with normal and abnormal demands.

Because the musculoskeletal system is particularly adapted to compensating for varying stress, the overall functional effect of a structural abnormality, whether coming from normal or abnormal forces, is not easily predictable. A study of osteoarthritis of the knee showed that the symptoms could not be predicted from the radiological appearance.[1] And in the spine, while it is possible to measure the increased stress on a lumbar facet joint when an intervertebral disc becomes damaged, the clinical consequences of that stress will vary in one individual to another.[2] While it might seem attractive to be able to scrutinize a radiograph or scan, and plan a reliable method of treatment, experience, audit and scientific trial have shown us that such an approach will not lead to reliable results. Many of the functional effects will be discussed in detail in Chapter 2.3, but when faced with a structural abnormality one should consider:

- the dynamic results of the change; for example, inequality in leg length results in increased strain on the hip joint and premature osteoarthritis[3]

- associated dysfunction in adjacent areas; for example, inequality in leg length causes increased lumbar strain and episodes of back pain[3]

- the effects of chemical mediators of inflammation or neuro-endocrine factors, especially in the spine; thus lumbar disc injury without anatomical displacement can cause pain.[4]

Some general principles arise from certain structural changes and they are discussed in the following sections.

Intervertebral discs

Disc changes and mechanical derangement in the spine

There are many variations of how the ageing process in intervertebral discs can proceed, with or without more obvious traumatic strains applied to the spine, but whether this is a gradual reduction in water content, protrusion of the margin of the disc, prolapse, sequestration of a fragment, or entirely internal derangement of the disc, changes in function will occur in that segment of the spine. Sometimes the segment will cope adequately: one can question a 70-year old with narrowed disc spaces on the radiograph and hear that he has never had a back pain: more often, the segment will have been causing symptoms, at least for an episode during that process.

Anatomical changes

The central nucleus pulposus of the disc is 70–90% water in the healthy young disc, maintained by the water-holding properties of the proteoglycan aggregates, with the tougher collagen fibres composing only 15–20% of the dry weight of the disc.[5] The water content is already reducing in the third decade. The annulus fibrosus is, however, predominantly type 1 collagen, with 10–12 concentric layers arranged in alternating, oblique directions,[6] giving greater resistance to rotational strain.[2]

Torsion of the trunk, in particular, leads to weakening of the fibres of the annulus fibrosus, and eventually to the development of radial tears, most frequently in the posterolateral direction, i.e. towards the lateral recess of the spinal canal and the exit foramina. Tears of the annulus may themselves cause pain, but when a fissure has appeared through the full thickness of the annulus, the potential for protrusion of the central nuclear material is great. This will typically occur when intradiscal pressure is at its greatest, i.e. during flexion of the trunk, further increased by weightbearing.[7]

Correlation of structural change and effect

In some respects, disc lesions are an excellent demonstration of how variations in structural anatomy will have a predictable effect. This is shown with disc prolapse: a central lumbar disc prolapse will cause predominantly low back pain without neurological change until there is a massive prolapse, compromising the canal and producing a cauda equina lesion; whereas a laterally placed weakness of the lumbar disc will bulge towards the exiting nerve root, so that the pain will develop predominantly in the leg, and progressive neurological change will result in the function of that one nerve root alone. The outer layers of the disc are innervated and sensitive,[8,9] so that pain can result without any pressure on adjacent structures. Frequently the adjacent structures do suffer pressure from bulging of the disc; studies show that the posterior longitudinal ligament, the dura, and the nerve root are sensitive to this.[9]

Directions of disc bulge or prolapse

Superior

The 'Schmorl's node', appearing on plain radiograph as a cyst-shaped deficiency in the vertebral body, results from prolapse of some of the nucleus pulposus through the vertebral endplate. The majority of cases are non-symptomatic, appearing in the first two decades, and are seen as a chance finding in later life.

Anterosuperior

At the ring epiphysis of the thoracolumbar vertebrae, before these epiphyses fuse in later teenage years, damage can occur from pressure of disc material, resulting in lack of further growth of the vertebra, and either a separated fragment occurs at the anterior angle of the vertebra (a 'limbus' vertebra) or a more general effect may occur, so that the vertebrae in this region develop an anteriorly wedged shape with rounded anterior margins and thus some possible kyphosis of that segment (Scheuermann's osteochondrosis).[10] Some stiffness of that portion of the spine can result, with an increase in symptomatic episodes of low back pain, arising from the disadvantaged lower lumbar segments.[11]

Anterior

Anterior to the thoracolumbar discs lie the anterior longitudinal ligament and the aorta. Some low back pain may result, but whether the mechanism of this is similar to internal disc derangement is not known.

Posterocentral

Progressive bulging or prolapse of the disc centrally into the spinal canal puts pressure on the posterior longitudinal ligament and the posterior aspect of the dural tube: both these structures, as well as the outer layers of the annulus fibrosus of the disc, are innervated by the sinuvertebral (recurrent meningeal) nerve.[8] This nerve is anatomically part of an anastomotic network which covers several segments of the spine and pain is typically poorly localized to the low back generally rather than to the specific segment (the multisegmental pain).[12] Most of these disc lesions either regress or, if they increase, are restrained by the midline longitudinal ligament sufficiently to cause them to bulge posterolaterally, so that radicular pain supervenes, with or without neurological compromise. If the longitudinal ligament becomes attenuated or ruptures, central canal compromise occurs, on the cord in the cervical and thoracic segments, and the cauda equina in the lumbar segments.

Posterolateral

A common pattern of disc lesion in the lumbar region is for a posterolateral disc prolapse to have developed from a more central position, with the familiar symptomatic sequence of change in symptoms: the initial back ache or pain develops radiation into the leg. In the cervical spine, the posterolateral corner of the disc deteriorates by the second or third decade, with the formation of the accessory joints of Luschka, so that posterolateral prolapse is the usual primary event, and this occurs quite frequently in other areas of the spine. As the pain may all be in the peripheral distribution of the nerve (whether arm, rib, or leg) and none in the spinal area, diagnostic mistakes can easily be made if the spine is not recognized as a possible source.

Anatomical consequence of disc prolapse

In central and lateral posterior disc prolapse, pressure can develop on the dural tube or the nerve root with its dural sleeve.

Dural impingement results in pain (multisegmental in the spine and adjacent areas when central, and segmental in the limb when on the nerve root sleeve), and positive dural tension tests. The **straight leg raise** (Lasègue) test tautens the nerve root and the attached dura in the lumbar lesions: this can be further progressed by neck flexion, tautening the dura from the neck.[13] Once again the anatomical pattern is preserved: midline disc prolapse is associated with more back pain on straight leg raise, lateral prolapse with provocation of leg pain.[14] The **crossed straight leg raise** sign, where the movement of the non-symptomatic leg provokes the sciatic pain on the opposite side, correlates with disc prolapse in over 90% of cases.[15] The **upper limb tension test** does the same for the cervical segments;[16] in upper thoracic lesions approximation of the scapulae aims to tauten the thoracic dura.

Progressive pressure on the nerve root results in increasing pain until function of the nerve may be lost, and weakness and numbness result: before this there may have been a gradual change of sensory function with paraesthesia, and increasing motor and reflex loss in that segmental nerve peripherally.

The final proof that structural abnormality is the important factor came with the results of discectomy: the normal result of discectomy is dramatic relief of pain.[17,18]

Natural history of disc prolapse

There is a gradually increasing incidence of disc prolapse up to age 40. In the lumbar area after the fourth decade, the incidence of discectomies carried out falls substantially.[19] It is thought that this reflects the higher osmotic pressure associated with the degeneration of the proteoglycan aggregates in the 30–50 age group[20] with the later, more advanced degeneration leading to reduced intradiscal pressure. The capacity of an episode of disc prolapse to resolve spontaneously is indeed quite striking, and the long-term results of conservative management of lumbar disc prolapses is similar to surgical treatment.[21] Pathoanatomical studies using sequential scans shows that regression of a disc prolapse towards its original confines is the norm rather than the exception. In 111 cases of sciatic pain with disc bulge or prolapse, re-scanned after one year, 64% had partial or complete retraction of the disc: prolapse fared much better than bulge of the disc, 75% compared to 25% showing retraction.[22] Saal and Saal[23] showed that prediction of the need for (eventual) surgery was confined to those cases where stenosis was demonstrated.

The only absolute indications for disc surgery have therefore remained cord or cauda equina compression. Permanent neurological damage is not affected by surgery: in Weber's series, over 90% of cases with motor deficit had recovered normal strength at follow-up, although 35% had some residual sensory change.[21]

Dynamic behaviour of the disc

The finding that disc prolapses normally regress emphasizes the dynamic nature of many disc abnormalities. The appearance on plain radiograph is not a reliable sign of current disc symptoms.

Nachemson's studies on intradiscal pressure gave useful insights to disc behaviour, and allow us to correlate symptomatic patterns to mechanical function of the disc. The outcome of his studies, predominantly on the third lumbar disc,[7] is shown in Table 2.1.1. Imaging studies have confirmed the change in disc morphology with load, showing that a disc which looks normal in the lying position can bulge and impinge on sensitive structures with the stimulus of position, or weightbearing.[24] If dye is injected at discography, the capacity of pressure to simulate the symptoms is found.[25]

Inflammatory change with disc lesions

Imaging studies, while confirming many of the dynamic changes which correlate with symptom change, have also shown the frequent lack of symptoms where there is a clear disc bulge or prolapse present.[26] Mean figures for two radiologists' readings are shown in Table 2.1.2. Indeed, this has called into question how disc appearance on MR scans should be classified, as the apparent inflammatory activity of a posteriorly placed high-intensity zone is more predictive of pain than protrusions are.[4]

A proportion of disc prolapse cases do not proceed in the expected way, for spontaneous resolution, and the search for the cause of this variation and its management is ongoing. It is clear that an inflammatory change develops in the area of disc prolapse, at least in a proportion of cases: the inflammation is macroscopic at spinoscopy or operation, and inflammatory mediators are detectable.[27] Cases can proceed to epidural fibrosis or arachnoiditis with or without surgery,[28] but at present we cannot predict which cases these will be.

The term **intradiscal derangement** is given to those symptomatic cases where there is no bulge or prolapse present on imaging, but discography or scan shows that the disc is incompetent, in that injected dye leaks into the epidural space, and that the disc tissue has altered water content.[29] Most 'aged' discs are non-symptomatic, but these ones are associated with persistent pain and varying disability.

Table 2.1.1 Load (kg) on disc, for 70-kg man

Static postures		Activity	
Sitting	100	Twisting	90
Standing	70	Lifting	210
Lying	30	Cough	110
Bending forward 20°	120	Straining	120
		Sit-up exercise	175

Table 2.1.2 MR findings in asymptomatic subjects (from Jensen et al.[26])

Age	Bulge present	Prolapse present
30–39	35	21
40–49	61	32
50–59	79	29

Psychological aspects

The landmark research by Wiltse and Rocchio showed that the results of a procedure for prolapsed disc could be better predicted by preoperative psychological tests than by size of disc prolapse, or neurological deficit.[30] There are various factors which may influence this, such as premorbid personality and the severity of symptoms and their duration. It is a mistake, however, to think that all cases of chronic back pain or poor results from surgery have a psychological origin.[31]

Nerve root and peripheral nerve entrapment

The symptoms of pressure on different parts of the nervous system allow us, when listening to the patient's history, to form an early prediction of the likely diagnosis. In the examination the distinction between upper motor neurone and lower motor neurone can be made, together with exact delineation of any motor, sensory, or reflex change.

Cord pressure

Paraesthesia is a more striking symptom than pain, which may be entirely absent. The distribution of symptoms is typically wide, and sometimes most prominent distally. A cervical cord lesion, while it may cause upper limb paraesthesia, will frequently cause bilateral leg tingling, dysesthesia, and numbness, as well as ataxia and disturbance of other tracts. In the limb, the patient cannot distinguish that the symptoms belong to one aspect, e.g. anterior, rather than another.

Nerve root pressure

Nerve root pressure is normally the most painful of nerve lesions, and this is attributed to the dural sleeve's nerve supply: the nerve root, lying in the intervertebral foramen, is in a confined space between the disc, the vertebral body margin, and the zygapophysial joint and pedicle. Paraesthesia will develop, as will motor and reflex change, in the peripheral distribution of the nerve: it will affect one aspect of the limb, but its margins will be indistinct, because of the overlap of the dermatomes of the different segments.

Nerve trunks

The trunks of the brachial plexus, for example, react differently from the nerve roots. There is no dural sleeve, and any pain is dull, and more likely to be described as discomfort: by contrast, the paraesthesia can be intense and disturbing. The reaction can be delayed from the time of pressure or stretch to the nerve trunk, and the release phenomenon has been described, where the symptoms become more intense after the pressure is relieved, for example on lying down at night relieving the daytime traction of the arms. Waking in the morning with numbness in the arms, where persistent tightness of the scalenes raises the first rib and stretching the trunks, is a form of the thoracic outlet syndrome. Aspect of the symptom is present, typically on the medial side of the arm and forearm, but there is no clear margin.

Peripheral (sensory or mixed) nerve

Paraesthesia is the predominant symptom, with a well-defined aspect and margin corresponding to the distribution of the nerve. Some

Table 2.1.3 Distribution of paraesthesia in cases of carpal tunnel[32]

	Percentage of cases
5th finger 'definitely affected'	31
Whole hand affected	21
Thumb not affected	20

discomfort can be felt, but may not be volunteered by the patient. Carpal tunnel compression of the median nerve at the wrist is an example of this, where proximal discomfort in the forearm occurs: to what extent this may result from concurrent dysfunction in the cervical spine is not known. Although clear-cut lesions predominate, variations occur and must be accepted as possibilities in diagnosis. In 103 patients shown to have electrical evidence of median nerve compression in the carpal tunnel, only 53% had that diagnosis originally assigned to them: and in these cases the distribution of paraesthesia was often not typical (see Table 2.1.3).[32]

Tendonopathies

Tendons undergo deterioration with rupture of small numbers of fibres up to complete tear and, in some areas, it becomes more common to have insufficiency rather than an intact structure, with age. The rotator cuff of tendons shows a macroscopic tear in most older people.[33] Some factors other than age and duration of strain may be present in symptomatic cases:

- **Repetitive stress:** The common extensor origin of the forearm extensors is the commonest site of symptoms at the elbow, and overuse can be a factor in the 'tennis elbow' syndrome. For the Achilles tendon, increased valgus of the calcaneum after heelstrike whips the tendon into excessive strain at each pace. Tendons with sheaths become subject to tenosynovitis in the same way, the swelling causing tension and typical creaking on movement.

- **Triggering:** The finger flexors can, with more chronic strain, and with other factors such as an inflammatory arthropathy or diabetes, develop nodule formation on the tendon, causing triggering when the thickened tendon cannot easily pass the pulleys supporting the tendon sheaths.[34]

- **Anatomical factors of the tendon itself:** The arterial supply to a tendon is sparse relative to such structures as muscles, and sometimes is arranged as end-arteries, some from the bone insertion and some from the muscle: particularly where this place corresponds with habitual pressure, as in the supraspinatus tendon over the humeral head, premature deterioration is more likely.[35]

- **Inflammatory processes:** Rheumatoid arthritis and its variants can cause tendinitis. In the case of spondylarthropathies such as ankylosing spondylitis, the inflammation is an enthesopathy, at the tendon/bone insertion: at the Achilles tendon, this insertional tendonitis contrasts with the degenerative type which is typically 2 cm proximal to the calcaneum. Gout and pseudogout can both be involved in inflammatory actions of tendons.

- **Calcification:** Some calcium deposit is relatively frequently seen on radiographs of tendons (and in the shoulder the reported rate varies from 7.5 to 20%), but the factors causing it are not known, nor the factors which cause the area to become symptomatic. Asymptomatic calcium deposits should be left *in situ*. An acute attack of calcific tendonitis can be severely painful: calcium hydoxyapatite crystals may be found in the surrounding joint or bursa, as in the rotator cuff,[36] and demand steroid injection with adequate analgesia. The calcium deposits may disperse with or without treatment.[37]

- **Dysfunction:** In some cases of pain which appears localized to tendons, and where provocative testing causes increased pain, further investigation for example by magnetic scan, does not reveal a structural lesion. This occurs relatively frequently in the rotator cuff area. The cause of pain would appear to be other than a true inflammatory process, and may result more from abnormal tension on the tendon from its muscle: abnormal muscle balance and tone has long been thought to be a relatively common cause of pain.[38]

Inflammatory disorders

Galen knew the features of an inflamed joint: pain, redness, swelling and heat are typical, and the joint loses some of its function. These remain the hallmarks of diagnosis, despite the investigative techniques available to us. Where an inflamed joint is found, the underlying condition is sought, but in some cases that diagnosis cannot be definitely made at the first visit, without further time showing the course of the disease, and in some cases, no underlying cause of the joint inflammation is ever found. Many cases of postinfective arthritis (e.g. rubella, slapped-cheek virus, etc.) are self-limiting, and in the absence of other evidence, standard symptomatic treatment should be given while awaiting the natural history of the syndrome.

Rheumatoid arthritis

This is the commonest inflammatory arthritis, affecting 2–3% of the population, and in its most typical form with a rapid onset affecting the joints of the limbs including the fingers and toes symmetrically, it does not pose a diagnostic challenge. With more insidious onset, and if only one or two joints are initially affected, confusion with the affects of recent or old trauma, or overuse can result. In the upper half of the body early rheumatoid arthritis can mimic:

- **Neck strain:** A middle-aged person, maybe who works in an office all day, develops increasing neck stiffness and pain worst in the mornings. The restriction of movement will typically be symmetrical, rather than with the typical non-symmetrical pattern of joint dysfunction, and all the cervical levels will often be affected, rather than one.

- **Shoulder pain mimicking a frozen shoulder (adhesive capsulitis):** With hindsight, the onset will have been more gradual with rheumatoid arthritis than with idiopathic capsulitis, but that may not be clear until the second shoulder, or other joints, become involved. If there is doubt, a trial of standard anti-inflammatory treatment with oral drugs or intra-articular injection is appropriate.

Investigations

The diagnosis of rheumatoid arthritis depends on a number of criteria, rather than a single test (see Table 2.1.4). Rheumatoid factor is an unreliable test, present in 10–15% of the normal population and not

Table 2.1.4 Criteria for the diagnosis of rheumatoid arthritis[39]

Criterion	Details
1 Morning stiffness	Lasting around the joints for at least 1 hour
2 Swelling of joints in three or more areas	Simultaneous swelling in right or left limb joints, including digital joints
3 Swelling of hand joints	At least one wrist, MCP or PIP joint
4 Symmetrical arthritis	Simultaneous involvement of the paired joints, such as elbows, MCP joints
5 Rheumatoid nodules	
6 Serum rheumatoid factor	
7 Radiographic changes	Changes on wrist or hand x-rays typical of rheumatoid arthritis, most usually erosions at the joint margin

For the diagnosis of rheumatoid arthritis, the person must have at least four of the seven criteria, and items 1–4, where present, must have been persistent for 6 weeks.

present in 30% of cases of rheumatoid arthritis. The ESR, or plasma viscosity, is not raised in a proportion of cases of active arthritis, and the C-reactive protein, though more sensitive, is non-specific also. But with weight given to the clinical pattern, these tests are nevertheless useful in most cases.

Importance of treatment of rheumatoid arthritis

Apart from being able to give the patient some prognosis and useful guidance on self-help for the limitations caused by the disease, active treatment reduces the progression of joint destruction.[40] Greater concentrations of inflammatory mediators and enzymes in joint cavities, produced by the pannus of inflamed synovium, lead to the destructive erosion of articular cartilage and weakening of the capsular supports to the joint. Good control of the disease is therefore important in the long term, by one or more of the means available: oral anti-inflammatories, intra-articular steroid injections, oral steroids, or disease-modifying drugs such as intramuscular gold, oral methotrexate, sulfasalazine, D-penicillamine, etc., despite their risks.

Temporary splinting for inflamed or weak joints can be beneficial, and occupational therapists play a major role in care of the person by means of education, help with tasks of daily living, and adaptations.

Benefits and dangers of physical treatment

Maintenance of range of movement, or to improve range of movement after a flare-up of the disease, is important; warm water is useful, whether in a basin or in a hydrotherapy pool. The patients usually have limited stamina for physical therapy, however, and this may be a limiting factor. Knowledge of the pattern of joint and ligamentous weakness should inform the therapist in using suitably gentle techniques. In the cervical spine there is concern for atlantoaxial subluxation through ligamentous laxity, threatening the cervical cord; and subluxation can occur even more frequently at the midcervical levels.[41] In mild cases however, where the inflammatory features are well suppressed, and where radiographs (with laterals taken in the flexed and extended positions) reveal no instability, incidental mechanical dysfunctions and pain may respond well to manual mobilization.

Rheumatoid variants

Other chronic inflammatory arthritides, as associated with psoriasis, enteropathic disease such as ulcerative colitis or Crohn's, reactive arthritis, or Reiter's syndrome, vary in joint pattern involvement but have in common that the rheumatoid factor is never present, and the disease is usually less destructive than rheumatoid arthritis. The spine becomes involved in the inflammatory process in a proportion of these cases.

Spondylarthropathy

In a young person under the age of 40 with persistent spinal problems, an inflammatory cause should be considered. Usually the disease starts at the base of the spine with an insidious onset, and causes inflammation in the spinal joints, with or without the sacroiliac joints, and also involves the ligaments with enthesitis. The classical features of the symptoms which are more useful in making the diagnosis of ankylosing spondylitis than investigations are:[42]

- onset under age 40
- gradual onset
- symptoms persistent over 3 months
- morning stiffness
- better with exercise.

Often suspicions are aroused by night pain with the need to get up and walk around, or by midback pain with a feeling of tightness around the lower ribs.

Definitive diagnosis is most easily made, but after an interval, with radiological change in the sacroiliac joints. Clinically the diagnosis is made by matching the symptoms with signs of symmetrical limitation of spinal movement, with or without clinical signs of sacroiliitis. The B27 tissue type, although present in 95% of cases of ankylosing spondylitis,[43] is present in 8% of the normal population in developed countries, and is therefore not a reliable indicator of the diagnosis: the variant spondylarthropathies, such as psoriatic, enteropathic, and Reiter's have lower percentages of the B27 tissue type than ankylosing spondylitis.

Treatment for the spondylarthropathies is important in order to minimize the loss of spinal flexibility.[44] This depends on regular exercises, but the patient may not be able to do this effectively without the help of anti-inflammatory drugs. Phenylbutazone is still regularly used when safer drugs are ineffective, despite the very small danger of blood dyscrasia. Anti-inflammatories are not useful except as a symptomatic measure, however, and disease-modifying drugs such as sulfasalazine are only effective for peripheral joint involvement:[45] Nevertheless, poor prognosis with ankylosing spondylitis is almost all accounted for by the incapacity caused by involvement of the hip or other limb joint.[46]

Monoarthritis: differential diagnosis

A frequent dilemma in diagnosis of inflammatory joint disease is the single inflamed joint without other features. In an audit of efficiency of diagnosis of the acute swollen joint, the importance of previous history is certainly important: general practitioners scored very highly, but most of their cases were of gout. Causes of sudden onset arthritis are:

Clinical investigation of the acute hot joint

- Microscopy of synovial fluid, including polarizing microscopy for crystals
- Gram stain and culture of synovial fluid
- Blood culture and urate
- Full blood count
- Measure of acute-phase reaction (ESR and/or C-reactive protein)
- Joint X-ray

- septic arthritis

- gout

- pseudogout

- haemarthrosis, either from trauma, blood dyscrasia, or rarely villonodular synovitis.

Onset of swelling over a few days or slower provides other possibilities:

- chronic infective arthritis, e.g. tuberculous

- chronic inflammatory arthritis, especially the seronegative variants such as psoriatic or reactive

- osteoarthritis, with or without a loose body

- internal derangement of the joint, as by a displaced or torn meniscus.

For full investigation, a scheme has been published (see box),[47] but aspiration with culture and microscopy where possible, and a blood sample for full blood count, ESR and urate are the most desirable.

Diagnostic routine for structural abnormality

The concept of selective tissue tension

Even using the precise imaging techniques now available, objective diagnosis of structural abnormalities in the soft tissues continues to elude us, with frequent problems in interpretation. The functional methods available to us at the time of physical examination remain our mainstay. The reproduction of the patient's complaint is the linch-pin of this approach. Initially the approach was similar to that in abdominal diagnosis: palpating the site of maximum tenderness. But in the musculoskeletal system, very many lesions cause referred pain. With referred pain, there is frequently associated tenderness, and this can confuse the examiner into thinking that the site of tenderness is the site of the lesion.

The new contribution that Cyriax made[48] was to strain the various soft tissues which might be the cause of pain, in turn, and as selectively as possible. When stretch or compression of that structure caused pain identical to the complaint, it became the prime suspect.

The examination falls into two main categories, of testing the inert tissues (the joint capsules, the discs of the spine, the ligaments, and the bursae) by passive movement of the patient's limb or spine: a second part examines the contractile unit of muscle and tendon, by having the patient contract the unit against resistance without movement occurring – thus placing tension on those tissues but not the inert (and then immobile) ones. For example, if resisted flexion of the elbow hurts, the flexor muscles, biceps or brachialis, or their tendons must be at fault. At that point palpation is the best guide to the exact site of the lesion within those structures.

In testing the inert tissues at each joint, three possibilities arise: that no pain results, exonerating those tissues; that one or some of the movements hurt; or that all of the movements hurt. Using this system, it was found that in cases of known arthritis, all the passive movements were usually painful, in contrast to non-arthritic conditions where one, or a few of the movements were painful. The non-arthritic conditions were:

- internal derangement of the joint

- ligamentous strain

- accessory structure lesions, e.g. bursitis.

The most sensitive part of the joint is the capsule, and the 'arthritic' response was called the **capsular** pattern: short-lived affections of the joint, such as post-traumatic capsulitis, or adhesive capsulitis of the shoulder, will give this pattern. Any other pattern of pain with passive movements is termed **non-capsular** (see Table 2.1.5).

Thus the primary distinction in diagnosis is made on the pain-reaction with selective strain. But a number of other useful findings commonly add to the diagnostic process:

- **Range of movement:** In an early or mild case of arthritis there may be no loss of movement at the joint – but the diagnosis of the type of condition can already be made. If there is a loss of range of movement at the joint, a most useful capsular ratio of movement restriction develops. Each joint of the body has a characteristic ratio of loss of movement, which may result from relative laxity of different parts of the capsule. Every knee, for example, will lose much range

Table 2.1.5 Examination by selective tissue tension

Passive movements
Pain occurs on which movements?

All (capsular pattern)	Some (non-capsular pattern)	None
Capsulitis	Internal derangement	Test resisted movements
Arthrosis	Ligament strain	Test other structures
Arthritis	Accessory structures	

Resisted movements
An isometric contraction results in:

Pain positive: lesions of muscle, tendon or attachment

Weak response: musculoskeletal or neurological lesion (see below)

Result of test	Interpretation
Pain	Strain or partial tear of muscle/tendon
Pain and weakness	Greater strain or partial tear of muscle/tendon
Weakness (painless)	Rupture of muscle/tendon, or neurological lesion

of flexion before extension becomes lost:[49] whereas at the shoulder external rotation is always the most restricted movement, and at the hip internal rotation is always the most restricted.

- **End-feel:** The quality of restraint at the end of range of movement gives further information about the state of the joint (see Chapter 3.1.1).

The spine

Is the selective tissue tension concept useful for the spine? In some respects it fits well: on passive movement examination (often more easily carried out actively, with gravity, rather than their own muscles, assisting the patient) the arthrosis of age (spondylosis) produces discomfort and loss of range in all directions, the ratio of loss of movement characteristically showing that extension range is most affected: the same pattern is found in inflammatory spondylitis. In contrast, internal derangement in the form of intervertebral disc disruption, causes a strongly non-symmetrical pattern in most cases, even to the extent that pain is relieved by some directions of movement. But this asymmetric pattern is also found with mechanical affections of the zygapophysial, facet joints (proven by local anaesthetic injection).[50] Thus the asymmetrical pattern, when found in the spine, is not well termed 'non-capsular'. It is most frequently referred to as a 'mechanical pattern'. Whatever the terms used, the selective tissue tension approach remains most useful as a starting point in physical diagnosis of the spine, as in the limb joints.

References

1. Claessens, A. A., Schouten, J. S., van der Ouweland, F. A. (1990) Do clinical findings associate with radiographic osteoarthritis of the knee? *Ann. Rheum. Dis.*, **49**, 771–4.
2. Krismer, A., Haid, C., Rabl, W. (1996) The contribution of anulus fibres to torque resistance. *Spine*, **21**, 2551–7.
3. Friberg, O. (1983) Clinical symptoms and biomechanics of the lumbar spine and hip joint in leg length inequality. *Spine*, **8**, 643–5.
4. Milette, P. C., Fontaine, S., Lepanto, L., *et al.* (1999) Differentiating lumbar disc protrusions, disc bulges and discs with normal contour but abnormal signal intensity. *Spine*, **24**, 44–53.
5. Beard, H. K., Stevens, F. C. (1980) Biochemical changes in the intervertebral disc. In: Jayson M. I. V (ed.), *The lumbar spine and backache,*. 2nd edn. Pitman, London, pp. 407–36.
6. Hickey, D. S., Hukins S. W. L. (1980) Relation between the structure of the annulus fibrosus and the function and failure of the intervertebral disc. *Spine*, **5**, 100–16.
7. Nachemson, A. (1975) Towards a better understanding of low back pain. *Rheumatol. Rehab.*, **14**, 129–43.
8. Wiberg, G. (1948) Back pain in relation to the nerve supply of the intervertebral disc. *Acta Orthopaed. Scand.*, **19**, 211–21.
9. Kuslich, S. D. (1991) The tissue origin of low back pain and sciatica. *Orthop. Clin. N. Amer.*, **22**, 181–7.
10. Taylor, J. R., Twomey, L. T. (1985) Vertebral column development and its relation to adult pathology. *Aust. J. Physiotherapy*, **31**, 83–8.
11. Stoddard, A., Osborn, J. F. (1979) Scheuermann's disease or spinal osteochondrosis. *J. Bone Jt. Surg.*, **61B**, 56–9.
12. Kesson, M., Atkins, E. (1998) *Orthopaedic medicine: a practical approach.* Butterworth Heinemann, Oxford, p. 15.
13. Breig, A., Troup, J. D. G. (1979) Biomechanical considerations in the straight leg raise test. *Spine*, **4**, 242–50.
14. Edgar, M. A., Park, W. M. (1974) Induced pain patterns on passive straight leg raise in lower lumbar disc protrusions. *J. Bone Jt Surg.*, **56B**, 658–67.
15. Kosteljanetz, M., Bang, F., Schmidt-Olsen, S. (1988) The clinical significance of straight leg raise (Lasegue's sign) in the diagnosis of prolapsed lumbar discs. *Spine*, **13**, 393–5.
16. Elvey, R. L. (1986) The investigation of arm pain. In: Grieve, G. P. (ed.) *Modern manual therapy of the vertebral column.* Churchill Livingstone, Edinburgh, pp. 520–5.
17. Falconer, M. A., McGeorge, M., Begg, A. C. (1948) Observations on the cause and mechanism of symptom production in sciatica and low back pain. *J. Neurol. Neurosurg. Psych.*, **11**, 13.
18. McCulloch, J. A. (1996) Focus issue on lumbar disc herniation: macro- and micro-discectomy. *Spine*, **21** (suppl 42), 445–56S.
19. Kelsey, J. L. (1975) An epidemiological study of acute herniated lumbar intervertebral discs. *Rheumatol. Rehab.*, **14**, 144–59.
20. Kramer, J. (1973) Biomechanische Veranderungen im lumbalen Bewegungssegment. In: *Die Wirbelsaule in Forschung und Praxis*, Bd.58, hrsg. von H.Junghanns. Hippokrates, Stuttgart. Also in: Kramer, J., *Intervertebral disk diseases.* Georg Thieme, Stuttgart 1981.
21. Weber, H. (1983) Lumbar disc herniation. A controlled prospective study with ten years of observation. *Spine*, **8**, 131–40.
22. Bush, K., Cowan, N., Katz, D. E., *et al.* (1992) The natural history of sciatica associated with disc pathology. *Spine*, **17**, 1205–12.
23. Saal, J. A., Saal, J. S. (1989) Non-operative treatment of herniated lumbar intervertebral discs with radiculopathy. *Spine*, **14**, 431–7.
24. ??.
25. Schellhas, K. P., Pollei, S. R., Gundry, C. R., *et al.* (1996) Lumbar disc high-intensity zone: correlation of MRI and discography. *Spine*, **21**, 79–86.
26. Jensen, M. C., Brant-Zawadzki, M. N., Obuchowski, N., *et al.* (1994) Magnetic resonance imaging of the lumbar spine in people without back pain. *New Engl. J. Med.*, **331**, 69–73.
27. Saal, J. S., Franson, R. C., Dobrow, R., *et al.* (1990) High levels of inflammatory phospholipase A2 activity in lumbar disc herniations. *Spine*, **15**, 674–8.
28. Ransford, A. O., Harries, B. J. (1972) Localised archnoiditis complicating lumbar disc lesions. *J. Bone Jt Surg.*, **54B**, 656–65.
29. Schwarzer, A. C., Aprill, C. N., Derby, R., *et al.* (1995) The prevalence and features of internal disc derangement in patients with low back pain. *Spine*, **20**, 1878–83.
30. Wiltse, L. L., Rocchio, P. D. (1975) Preoperative psychological tests as predictors of success of chemonucleolysis in the treatment of the low back syndrome. *J. Bone Jt Surg.*, **57A**, 478–83.
31. Merskey, H., Lau, C. L., Russell, E. S., *et al.* (1987) Screening for psychiatric morbidity. The pattern of psychological illness and premorbid characteristics in four chronic pain populations. *Pain*, **30**, 141–57.
32. Keenan, J. (1991) Carpal tunnel syndrome. *J. Orthop. Med.*, **13**, 43–5.
33. Cotton, R. E., Rideout, D. F. (1964) Tears of the humeral rotator cuff. *J. Bone Jt Surg.*, **46B**, 314–18.
34. Lloyd Davies, A. (1998) Adult trigger finger. *J. Orthop. Med.*, **20**, 7–12.
35. Rathbun, J. B., Macnab, I. (1970) The microvascular pattern of the rotator cuff. *J. Bone Jt Surg.*, **52B**, 540–53.
36. Speed, C. A., Hazleman, B. L. (1999) Calcific tendonitis. *New Engl. J. Med.*, **340**, 1582–4.
37. Ebenbichler, G. R., Erdogmus, C. B., Resch, K. L., *et al.* (1999) Ultrasound therapy for calcific tendinitis of the shoulder. *New Engl. J. Med.*, **340**, 1533–8.
38. Brugger, A.. *Das sternale syndrom.* Huber, Bern.
39. Arnett, F. C., Edworthy, S. M., Bloch, D. A., *et al.* The American Rheumatism Association 1987 revised criteria for the classification of rheumatoid arthritis. *Arthr. Rheum.*, **31**, 315–24.
40. van der Heide, A., Jacobs J. W. G., Bijlsma, J. W. J., *et al.* (1996) The effectiveness of early treatment with 'second-line' anti-rheumatic drugs. *Ann. Int. Med.*, **124**, 699–707.

41. Crockard, H. A., Essigman, W. K., Stevens, J. M., *et al.* (1985) Surgical treatment of cervical cord compression in rheumatoid arthritis. *Ann. Rheum. Dis.*, **44**, 809–16.

42. Calin, A., Porta, J., Fries, J. (1977) Clinical history as a screening test for ankylosing spondylitis. *JAMA*, **237**, 2613–14.

43. Khan, M. A. (1990) Ankylosing spondylitis and related spondylarthropathies. In: *Spine: state of the art review.* Hanley and Belfus, Philadelphia.

44. O'Driscoll, S. L., Jayson M. I. V., Baddeley, H. (1978) Neck movements in ankylosing spondylitis. *Ann. Rheum. Dis.*, **37**, 64.

45. Kirwan, J., Edwards, A., Huitfeldt, B., *et al.* (1993) The course of established ankylosing spondylitis and the effects of sulphasalazine over 3 years. *Br. J. Rheumatol.*, **32**, 729–33.

46. Carette, S., Graham, D., Little, H., *et al.* (1983) The natural disease course of ankylosing spondylitis. *Arthr. Rheum.*, **26**, 186–90.

47. Joint working group of the British Society for Rheumatology (1992) Guidelines and a proposed audit protocol for the initial management of an acute hot joint. *J. Roy. Coll. Phys. Lond.*, **26**, 83–5.

48. Cyriax, J. (1978) *Textbook of orthopaedic medicine.* Baillière Tindall, London.

49. Hayes, K. W., Petersen, C., Falconer, J. (1994) An examination of Cyriax's passive motion tests with patients having osteoarthritis of the knee. *Phys. Ther.*, **74**, 697–709.

50. Aprill, C., Dwyer, A., Bogduk, N. (1990) Cervical zygapophyseal joint pain patterns I: a clinical evaluation. *Spine*, **15**, 458–61.

2.2 Dysfunction

2.2.1 Somatic dysfunction
Michael L. Kuchera

Definition and underlying concepts

Somatic dysfunction is formally defined as 'impaired or altered function of related components of the somatic (body framework) system: skeletal, arthrodial, and myofascial structures, and related vascular, lymphatic and neural elements'.[1,2] This diagnostic term thus embraces a wide range of relevant clinical findings and conditions. The term broadly encompasses Maigne's 'minor intervertebral derangements',[3] Travell and Simons' 'myofascial trigger points',[4] Jones' 'tender points',[5] Maitland's 'locked joint',[6] and various generic 'manipulable lesions', 'fixations', 'chiropractic subluxations', and 'blockages'. The term 'somatic dysfunction', first coined in 1961 by the Educational Council on Osteopathic Principles (ECOP), replaced the provincial term 'osteopathic lesion'. Somatic dysfunction is now recognized as a valid and codable diagnostic term in the *International Classification of Diseases*.[2]

The palpable characteristics of somatic dysfunction may be caused by structural or architectural changes (often associated with a loss of range of motion) or by functional aberrations in various somatic tissues associated with recognized physiologic and pathophysiologic processes. These palpable characteristics are interpreted by various health care practitioners to be associated through their anatomic, central nervous system (CNS), or autonomic connections with a particular joint or joints, myofascial structure, subcutaneous tissue or fascia, viscera, or condition.[7] Myofascial trigger points, facet syndromes, and somatovisceral reflex phenomena are all examples of somatic dysfunction discussed in this text on musculoskeletal medicine. In this subchapter, however, these specific conditions are not discussed in diagnostic isolation. Instead, a broad conceptual understanding of somatic dysfunction is presented to expand diagnostic and therapeutic options, integrating otherwise disparate approaches to patient complaints.

Certain generalizations apply to somatic dysfunction, its diagnosis and its treatment. This subchapter will address the most important of these generalizations:

- Somatic dysfunction reflects a summation of peripheral and central physiological mechanisms underlying a condition that interferes with maximal health and function.

- Diagnostic testing for somatic dysfunction consists of simple, reproducible palpatory and provocative examinations.

- The four diagnostic criteria for somatic dysfunction are <u>s</u>ensory change, <u>t</u>issue texture change, <u>a</u>symmetry, and <u>r</u>estriction of motion. These objective findings are summarized by the mnemonic, 'S.T.A.R.'.

- Somatic dysfunction can be subdivided into its physiologic characteristics (e.g. acute, chronic); its anatomic location (e.g. cervical, lumbosacral); and/or the specific constellation or pattern of anatomic and physiologic characteristics (e.g. acute psoas syndrome, latent sternocleidomastoid myofascial trigger point).

- The severity of somatic dysfunction can be differentiated; graded 'mild,' 'moderate,' or 'severe'; and recorded to separate background levels of somatic dysfunction from significant 'key' dysfunction.

- **Primary somatic dysfunction** typically responds well to various manipulative medicine approaches, whereas **secondary somatic dysfunction** may respond but recur, respond less well, or fail to respond when addressed by these approaches alone.

- Failure to consider somatic dysfunction in diagnosis and treatment overlooks an important underlying pathophysiologic process that may limit optimum health and performance and that plays a role in a significant number of patient complaints.

- A manual medicine prescription, if indicated, considers individual characteristics of the somatic dysfunction, the patient-as-a-whole, and the skills of the treating physician.

- A number of precipitating and/or perpetuating factors warrant consideration in the diagnosis and treatment of patients with somatic dysfunction.

- Despite the quality of care initially given, recurrent patterns of somatic dysfunction require patient re-evaluation and reconsideration of the patient's present management.

Other chapters will address the significance of somatic dysfunction in specific regional disorders (3.3) and physician management strategies (4.3.1 and 4.4).

Physiological basis

Physicians in neuromusculoskeletal medicine fields distinguish between peripheral stimuli that can produce pain and the experience of pain itself. The central transmission of noxious stimuli is referred to as **nociception**, the patient's experience as **pain**, and the neuromusculoskeletal reflexes elicited by the nociceptors as being **nocifensive** or **nociautonomic**.[7] The importance of pain itself is variable in the diagnosis and treatment of somatic dysfunction and is often dependent upon the model used by the neuromusculoskeletal practitioner.

Several physiological principles implicated in the production and maintenance of pain and somatic dysfunction require an understanding of both peripheral and central mechanisms. For example, nociception results in local (peripheral) vasodilation and tissue edema; over time, the central nocifensive and nociautonomic reflexes result in peripheral vasoconstriction, tissue ischemia, altered sweat gland activity and other different, but predictable, tissue responses. Thus, local palpatory findings will depend upon the physiologic summation of peripheral and central influences.

Substance P plays a role in both peripheral and central processes. Peripherally, up to 90% of substance P produced by sensory neurons is stored and released (as in a paracrine gland) from terminal branches.[8] It is pro-inflammatory, and results in vasodilation, hyperalgesia, and edema (Figure 2.2.1). Centrally, substance P, performing as a slow-acting neuromodulator, is co-released in the dorsal horn along with other neurotransmitters that are fast acting.[9] These neurotransmitters, in concert, influence the neural plasticity of the dorsal horn leading to segmental spinal facilitation and a shift from acute to chronic pain patterns.[10]

Ultimately, even though the initiating event may have been traumatic, it appears that nociceptive stimuli from local tissues play a major role in initiating the cord-level reflexes that, in turn, alter muscle length, tone, and balance. Other somatic reflexes then play a role in maintaining and organizing these aberrant reflexes. Finally, because of 'cross-talk' by the cord-level segmental circuitry controlling autonomic and visceral functions, the local somatic findings of altered muscle length, tone, and balance are frequently accompanied by segmentally related autonomic and visceral aberrations, completing the symptom complex of somatic dysfunction.

In this manner, the CNS functions both as an 'integrator' that senses and analyzes the environment, generating command signals along the motor pathways to muscles and other effectors,[11] and as an 'organizer' useful in interpreting segmentally related patterns of pain and dysfunction.[12] (Figure 2.2.2). The CNS is able to interpret and

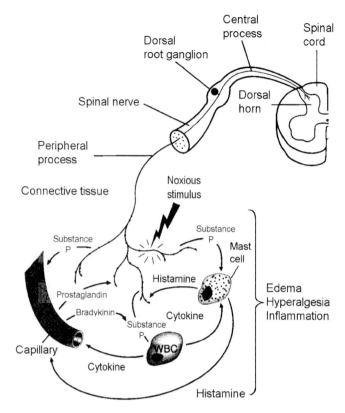

Figure 2.2.1 Interaction of afferent impulses and immune system. Noxious stimulant initiates secretion of neuropeptides such as substance P from primary afferent fiber. The result is a feedforward cascade of inflammatory events producing edema and hyperalgesia. (From Willard.[10])

assign differing priorities to afferent nociceptive stimuli[13] with subsequent automatic nocireflexive changes and adaptations largely occurring without conscious awareness.[14] Because not all signals from the peripheral nociceptors reach conscious pain, there is a wide variability in pain thresholds and perceived pain intensity, even with the same stimulus in the same person.[15] Nonetheless, the barrage of nociceptive stimuli has significant physiological (nociflexive and nociautonomic) ramifications that are capable of manifesting centrally organized peripheral tissue texture abnormalities. At the spinal cord level, these segmental and suprasegmental circuits maintain muscle length and tone and guide reflexes. Ultimately, short-term and chronic alterations in sensory input to the CNS can result in enduring changes in central processing[16] and recurrent somatic dysfunction.[17]

The physiologic impact of somatic dysfunction is not limited to pain and peripheral palpatory changes. In addition to initiating protective reflexes and providing the CNS with warning signs, noxious somatic stimuli influence the release of extracellular messengers from the endocrine–immune axis (Figure 2.2.3).[10] Subsequent increased activity in the hypothalamic–pituitary–adrenal axis results in alteration of levels of adrenal cortical hormones, norepinephrine, and other modulators of homeostasis and immune function. This additional emphasis on the role of somatic dysfunction in disrupting and modulating homeostasis is a major consideration for physicians in neuromusculoskeletal medicine fields who chose to integrate osteopathic concepts.

After differential diagnostic concerns, the primary objective in applying the principles of neuromusculoskeletal medicine is to restore local tissue function while simultaneously promoting central integra-

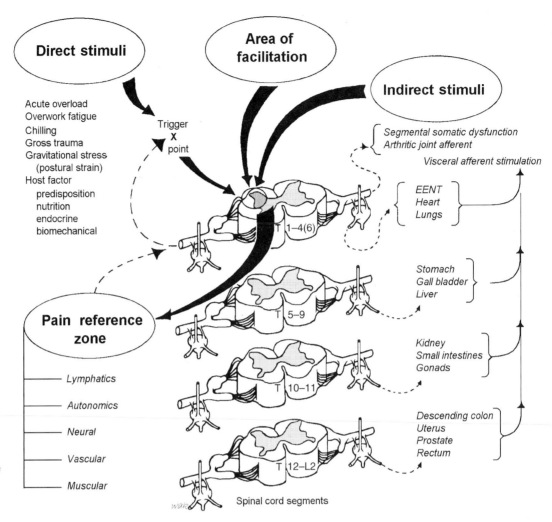

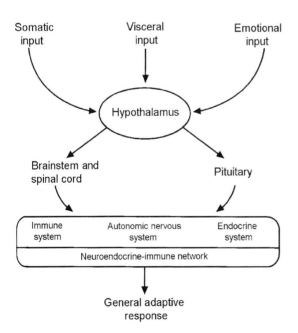

Figure 2.2.2 Pain reference regions for spinal pain afferent impulses. (From Kuchera.[17])

Figure 2.2.3 Response of neuroimmune network to signals emanating from somatic, visceral or emotional dysfunction. (From Willard.[10])

tion of the resultant afferent stimuli from the region. This is intended to bring about optimal biomechanical alignment and function for the individual. Long-term objectives seek to optimize tissue level health and to identify and reduce sources of chronic nociception.

Examination and diagnosis

Diagnostic testing for somatic dysfunction consists of simple, reproducible palpatory and provocative examinations. Developing the art of palpation is an asset for any physician, regardless of specialty, but is paramount for physicians specializing in the field of neuromusculoskeletal medicine. Diagnostic palpation is an acquired skill requiring time, patience, and practice. It may be defined as 'the application of variable manual pressure to the surface of the body for the purpose of determining the shape, size, consistency, position, inherent motility, and health of the tissues beneath'.[1] The art of interpreting diagnostic palpation also requires an extensive knowledge base of normal anatomy and physiology, as well as recognition of host variability and pathophysiologic connections and manifestations. Early palpatory evidence of underlying pathophysiologic change requires a higher level of palpatory skill than that required in palpation of a frank pathologic state such as a tumor.[18]

Diagnostic, time-efficient palpation for somatic dysfunction combines screening and scanning surveys of the entire body framework and those specific region(s) indicated by historical and physical findings or the need for a differential diagnosis. Focused layer palpation is then directed at any suspected or identified sites of significance. Rather than going into details about surveying and specific diagnostic palpatory examinations in this subchapter, they will be described in other appropriate sections of this text including Chapter 3.3.

The use of **layer palpation** to identify neuromusculoskeletal diagnostic clues in cutaneous, subcutaneous, fascial, muscular, ligamentous, bony, and arthrodial structures has a long history. This process begins with critical palpation of successively deeper body anatomic layers and the physiologic interpretation of the findings.

In examining patient complaints, the sites and the scope of palpation are selected according to the physician's knowledge of pain and referred pain mechanisms, structural interconnectedness (including tensegrity – see Chapter 2.2.5), and the differential diagnosis that is progressively developed. At each of these sites, physicians trained in neuromusculoskeletal evaluation are initially guided by **S.T.A.R. findings** (see above). These findings can be interpreted as a diagnosis of local or regional 'somatic dysfunction' and may alert the astute clinician to also evaluate for the presence or absence of other underlying pathophysiologic diagnoses within the neuromusculoskeletal and/or visceral systems.

Additional screening and specific tests are often suggested by initial palpatory examination findings. These additional tests should supplement evaluation of the functional ability of potentially significant somatic and visceral structures. The choices of tests are those consistent with accepted professional standards of care and with respect to the neuromusculoskeletal model selected. Deviation from normal structure and function at this level of palpatory evaluation warrants further testing of that structure or expanding testing to other related structures. Additional evaluations include neurologic or orthopedic tests or even laboratory, radiographic, and/or electrophysiologic testing.

Integration of historical symptoms with the physical examination results in a presumptive diagnosis. The palpatory portion of the physical examination specifically augments differential diagnosis and provides data for guiding decisions regarding the indications, contraindications, and other factors for considering the medical, surgical, and/or manipulative prescription.

S.T.A.R. testing

Sensory change

Sensory change, including neuresthesia, paresthesia, or anesthesia, can be objectively elicited and evaluated in a number of ways. Subjective perception of pain and other sensation should also be integrated with these findings. However, pain is a subjective symptom and its presence alone is not an indication of somatic dysfunction. Findings can be quantified in several manners, as can patterns of perceived sensory change and pain. These include progressive layer palpation and provocative testing to elicit pain or altered sensory change in a dermatomal pattern; pain or hyperreactivity of muscles in isolation or in a myotomal pattern; and sclerotomal sensitivity elicited by applying pressure or stress over ligaments or bony sites. Sensitivity perceived as pain with 4 kg or less of pressure (quantified by the use of a 'dolorimeter') in certain sites (see Chapter 2.2.3), can be interpreted as consistent with a fibromyalgia picture.[19]

Sensitivity accompanied by a referred pattern of pain or dysesthesia may also match a radicular, sclerotomal, neural, or trigger point pattern. Sensitivity accompanied by different types of tissue texture change is

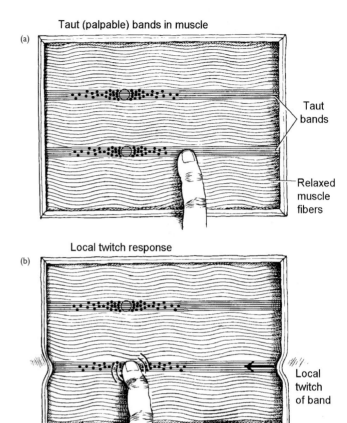

Figure 2.2.4 Trigger point palpation: (a) taut band, (b) 'twitch' of taut band.

common in tender point systems,[20,21] and trigger point diagnosis[22] (see Chapter 4.3.9) and other local and regional somatic dysfunction diagnoses. The trigger point pattern is especially likely if the point of sensitivity lies in a taut band that jumps with snapping palpation (Figure 2.2.4).

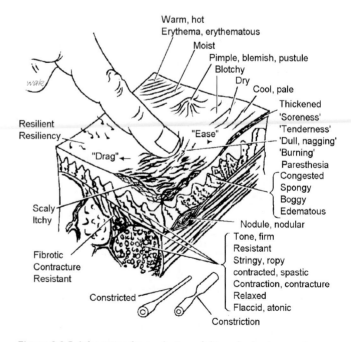

Figure 2.2.5 Information from palpation of skin and subcutaneous tissues.

Tissue texture change

This includes appreciation of moisture (cutaneous humidity), oiliness, dryness, heat or coolness, roughness, as well as the presence or absence of blemishes seen or noted with light palpation (Figure 2.2.5). Palpation of deeper layers may reveal changes described as subcutaneous swelling, edema, emphysema, fibrosis, spasm, hypertonicity, flaccidity, atrophy, myofascial points, tumor, nodularity, etc. – each type of tissue texture change having its own different diagnostic consideration. The best way to assess tissue changes is by comparing adjacent tissues or the same tissues on the contralateral side. Furthermore, provocative tests for tissue texture change include skin stroking to observe variations in the red reflex (Figure 2.2.6) and skin rolling (Figure 2.2.7).

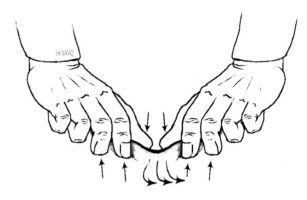

Figure 2.2.7 Skin rolling.

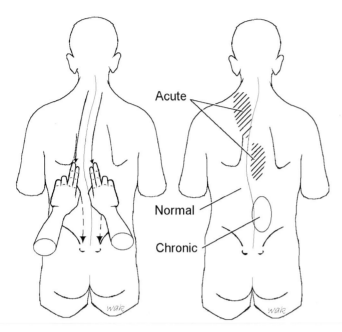

Figure 2.2.6 Red reflex. Prolonged reddening indicates acute physiology; rapid blanching indicates chronic physiology.

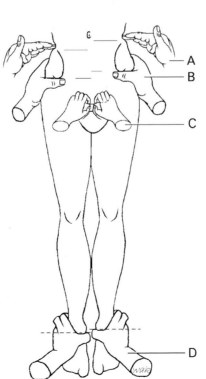

Figure 2.2.8 Anterior and posterior palpation of horizontal planes. A = iliac crests; B = anterior superior iliac spines; C = pubic rami; D= medial malleoli; E = mastoid processes; F = acromioclavicular joints; G = inferior scapular angles; H = iliac crests; I = greater trochanters; J = posterior superior iliac spines.

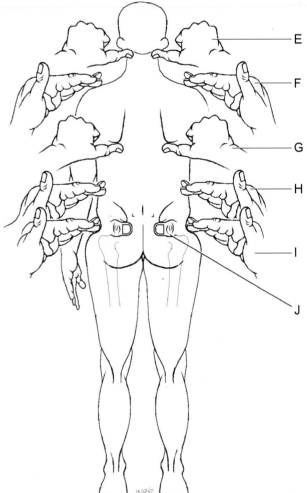

Asymmetry

This alone is rarely sufficient for making a specific diagnosis of somatic dysfunction, because true perfect symmetry is rare in humans. Nonetheless, asymmetry of paired structures increases sensitivity for recognition of minor dysfunction or change. Asymmetry of bony landmarks (Figure 2.2.8) as a screening procedure often provides an early finding suggesting subsequent motion testing.

Restriction of motion

This may be assessed and described in many meaningful, albeit different, ways. The method selected to assess restricted motion and the number of directions tested depends on the structure studied, the patient's condition, and the model used by the examining physician. Restriction of motion can be grossly quantified by total range of motion in degrees (Table 2.2.1) and compared to established normal ranges or to a corresponding joint in the same individual. Gross motion asymmetry is more often associated with pathologic, diseased, or orthopedic problems in the joint. Somatic dysfunction usually manifests as asymmetry of the minor or gliding motions of the joint and can range from subtle to gross.

Most neuromusculoskeletal medicine physicians will also assess the quality of motion at the barrier to motion – this is called the 'end feel'. The end feel of an anatomic, a physiologic, a pathologic or a dysfunctional barrier (Figure 2.2.9) will have different palpatory characteristics, warranting different descriptors. Absence of any barrier may indicate pathologic change of the restraining structures as occurs in a third-degree ligamentous tear; whereas an abrupt restriction without any normal physiologic 'springiness' at the end of motion may indicate differential possibilities ranging from arthrodial somatic dysfunction to osteoarthritis.

Motion restriction in a single plane may be assessed, but combinations of motion restrictions often provide greater diagnostic insights. Combinations of barriers created by certain pathophysiologic processes (such as inflammation) create '**capsular patterns**' of restricted motion that are unique to each joint (Table 2.2.2).[25]

Both active and passive motion testing provide valuable information. Because different anatomic and/or physiologic components may be tested using these different methods, active and passive motion testing may provide different motion information in some joints (Figure 2.2.10). This is also the case in some joints when tested with postural load as opposed to a non-weightbearing supine or prone position. For these reasons, if reproducibility is desired, it is best to describe the position and form of motion testing used. When the palpatory characteristics and tests used in identifying somatic dysfunction are delineated in this fashion and calibration-training sessions are conducted, reproducibility increases with kappa values (see Chapter 1.2) in the good to excellent range.[26–29]

Sensory changes, asymmetry, restricted motion, and tissue texture abnormalities are objective and reliable findings in manual medicine diagnostics. They reflect dysfunction in the anatomic–physiologic axis and carry clinical relevance warranting further investigation and consideration of appropriate treatment. Neuromusculoskeletal medicine physicians therefore often use varying combinations of these characteristics to name and/or classify somatic dysfunction in their notes or in the literature.

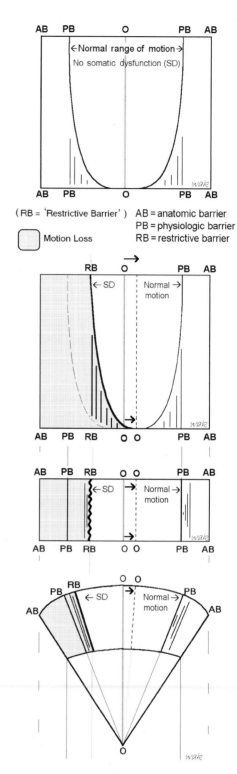

(RB = 'Restrictive Barrier')   AB = anatomic barrier
                                  PB = physiologic barrier
☐ Motion Loss   RB = restrictive barrier

Figure 2.2.9 Concepts of joint motion in a single plane: end-feel of motion in a normal joint and a joint with somatic dysfunction.

Anatomic and physiologic classification systems

Somatic dysfunction is often subdivided by its anatomic location (e.g. cervical, lumbosacral); by its physiologic characteristics (e.g. acute,

Table 2.2.1. Spinal gross and vertebral unit motion[23,24]

Craniocervical junction/superior cervical segment

Physiologic motion: OA SxRy regardless of sagittal plane; AA limited to discussion of Rx or Ry

Vertebral unit	Flexion/extension	Sidebending	Rotation
C0 (OA)	10° flex and 25° extension	3–8° left and 3–8° right	4–6° left and 4–6° right
C1 (AA)	10° total but not typically involved in somatic dysfunction	0–4° but not typically involved in somatic dysfunction	25° left and 25° right

Typical cervical spine

Minimal norms for C0–C7: flexion (60°), extension (75°), SB (45° ea), rotation (80° ea)

Physiologic motion: RxSx regardless of sagittal plane

Vertebral unit	Flexion/Extension		Sidebending		Rotation	
	Range	Mean	Range	Mean	Range	Mean
C2	5–23	8	11–20	10	6–28	9
C3	7–38	13	9–15	11	10–28	11
C4	8–39	12	0–16	11	10–26	12
C5	3–34	17	0–16	8	8–34	10
C6	1–29	16	0–17	7	6–15	9
C7	4–17	9	0–17	4	5–13	8

Thoracic spine

Minimum norms: flexion (50°), rotation (30° ea)

Physiologic motion: Type I = SxRy with neutral sagittal; Type II = RxSx in extremes of F or E

Vertebral unit	Flexion/extension		Sidebending		Rotation	
	Range	Mean	Range	Mean	Range	Mean
T1	3–5	4	5	6	5–14	9
T2	3–5	4	5–7	6	4–12	8
T3	2–5	4	3–7	6	5–11	8
T4	2–5	4	5–6	6	4–11	8
T5	3–5	4	5–6	6	5–11	8
T6	2–7	5	6	6	4–11	8
T7	3–8	6	3–8	6	4–11	8
T8	3–8	6	4–7	6	6–7	7
T9	3–8	6	4–7	6	3–5	4
T10	4–14	9	3–10	7	2–3	2
T11	6–20	12	4–13	9	2–3	2
T12	6–20	12	5–10	8	2–3	2

Lumbar spine

Minimum norms: flexion (60°), extension (25°); SB (25° ea)

Physiologic motion: Type I = SxRy within neutral sagittal; Type II = RxSx in extremes of F or E

Vertebral unit	Flexion/extension		Sidebending	Rotation		
	Range	Mean	Range	Mean	Range	Mean
L1	9–16	12	3–9	6	1–3	2
L2	11–18	14	3–9	6	1–3	2
L3	12–18	15	5–10	8	1–3	2
L4	14–21	17	5–7	6	1–3	2
L5	18–22	20	2–3	3	3–6	5

Table 2.2.2. Somatic dysfunction vs pathology: comparison of palpatory patterns in selected joints (somatic dysfunction vs capsular pattern)

Joint(s)	Somatic dysfunctional pattern	Capsular (pathologic) pattern
Cervical spine (C2–C7)	Sidebending–rotation limitation to same side; free in opposite directions	Flexion usually spared; equal limitation in all other directions
Thoracic spine	Limitation in one direction, freedom in opposite direction (3 planes linked)	Limitation of extension, sidebending and rotation; less limitation of flexion
Lumbar spine	Limitation in one direction, freedom in opposite direction (3 planes linked)	Marked and equal limitation of sidebending; limitation of flexion–extension
Shoulder	Minor motions limited before major motions; minor motions affect quality of major motions; in each pattern of motion, one direction is limited while the opposite direction shows complete freedom of motion	Great limitation of abduction > external rotation limitation > internal rotation limitation
Elbow	Same description as shoulder	Flexion limitation > extension limitation (rotations full and painless except in advanced cases)
Wrist	Same description as shoulder	Flexion limitation = extension limitation; others minimal restriction
Hip	Same description as shoulder	Marked flexion and internal rotation limitations; typically spares adduction and external rotation
Knee	Same description as shoulder	Flexion markedly limited >> extension limitation
Ankle	Same description as shoulder	Plantar flexion limitation > dorsiflexion limitation
Talocalcaneal joint	Same description as shoulder	Varus limitation progresses until fixation in valgus position
Big toe (1st MTP)	Same description as shoulder	Extension markedly limited >> Flexion limitation

chronic); by the specific constellation or pattern of anatomic-physiologic characteristics (e.g. chronic psoas syndrome, latent sternocleidomastoid myofascial trigger point); and/or by its order of onset (e.g. primary, secondary). Sometimes it is subdivided by its apparent reflex relationship (e.g. viscerosomatic, somatovisceral, or somatosomatic).

The most obvious system of classifying somatic dysfunction is by its anatomic location. This form of classification names the specific skeletal, arthrodial, or myofascial structure or region where the somatic dysfunction is located. Although simple in its naming, differential diagnosis for anatomically named dysfunction requires a thor-

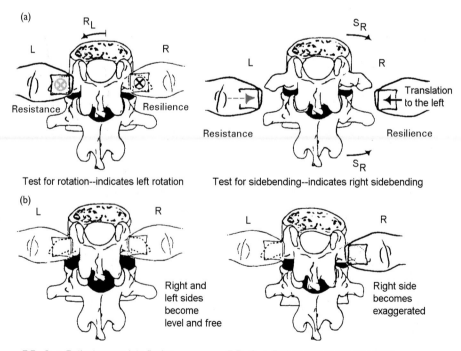

Figure 2.2.10 Motion testing: (a) passive motion indicates vertebral unit $R_L S_R$, (b) active motion indicates $FR_R S_R$. (From Kuchera.[17])

ough understanding of the functional characteristics and innervation of each of these skeletal, arthrodial, and myofascial structures. Joint inflammation and pathology produce different palpatory findings in different joints (see Table 2.2.2) and spinal physiologic motion mechanics are different in different anatomic regions (Chapter 3.3).

Pain referral patterns are different for different muscles (Figure 2.2.11), for different ligaments (Figure 2.2.12), and for different spondylogenic/sclerotomal reflexes (Figure 2.2.13). In addition, each of these structures influences motion characteristics; often in a distinctive manner that provides palpatory clues to the source of dysfunction. Somatic dysfunction associated with various regional disorders and their management is subdivided in this manner and presented in Chapters 3.3 and 4.3.

Anatomic classification delineating positional and motion aspects may also be used in describing somatic dysfunction. According to the 'Glossary of Osteopathic Terminology',[1] the positional and motion aspects of somatic dysfunction are best described using at least one of three parameters:

- position of the body part as determined by palpation and referenced to its adjacent defined structure

- directions in which motions are freer

- directions in which motions are restricted.

This form of classification provides descriptors that can be used to formulate specific treatment to correct the specific somatic dysfunction named. For example, somatic dysfunction in which the 5th thoracic vertebrae permits freer motion towards extension, rotation and sidebending to the right on the 6th thoracic vertebrae could be represented by the standard formula for motion present as T5 ER_RS_R. This formula could be used to set up indirect method manual treatment – for example, stacking the joint in the direction it prefers to a point of ligamentous balance.[30] This nomenclature for somatic dysfunction also denotes that the T5 vertebra on T6 *is restricted* in flexion, rotating left and sidebending left. In the Mitchell muscle energy system,[31] T5 ER_RS_R might be reversed with a direct method manipulative technique designed to create sidebending and rotation to the left along with flexion thereby reestablishing the lost or restricted motion characteristics. For this same somatic dysfunction, the Maigne star diagram records motion freedom and restriction as shown in Figure 2.2.14. In Maigne's system, the directions in which the motion is freer are combined with patient subjective responses to constitute his therapeutic 'rule of no pain and free movement'.[3]

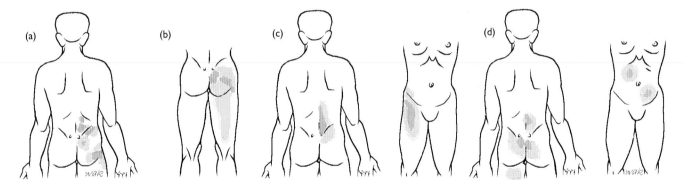

Figure 2.2.11 Pain referral regions of muscles: (a) quadratus lumborum, (b) piriformis, (c) iliopsoas, (d) rotatores and multifidi muscles.

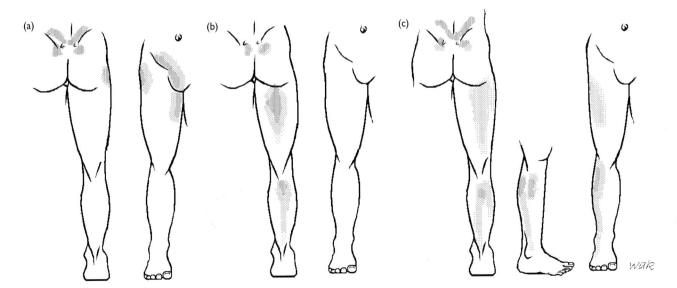

Figure 2.2.12 Pain referral regions of ligaments: (a) iliolumbar ligament, (b) sacrospinous and sacrotuberous ligaments, (c) posterior sacroiliac ligament.

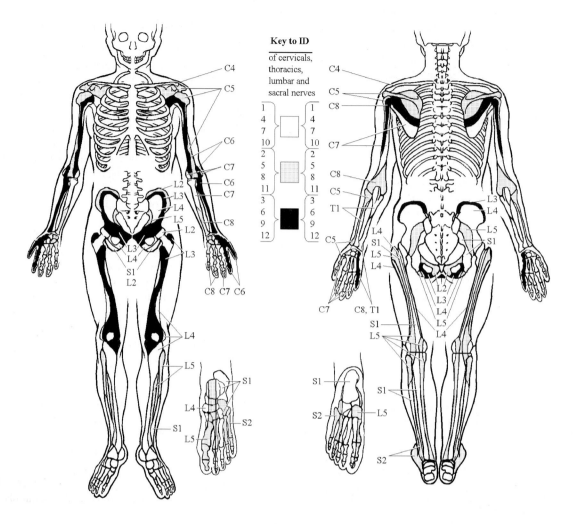

Figure 2.2.13 Sclerotome pain regions.

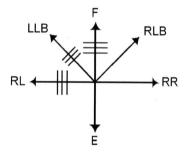

Figure 2.2.14 Star diagram of Maigne, illustrating the direction in which the patient feels pain. The bars indicate the grade of pain: three bars indicate significant pain, which will correlate with direction of restricted motion. Key: F, flexion; E, extension; RL, rotate left; RR, rotate right; LLB, left lateral bend; RLB, right lateral bend. Somatic dysfunction diagnosis: E R$_R$S$_R$. In Maigne's system, manipulation should be considered only when three directions are free of pain when motion is introduced.

Clinically relevant classification systems should also assist in making diagnostic and/or management choices. Keeping this perspective in mind, underlying physiologic characteristics, reflected by tissue texture abnormalities, contribute to an especially valuable system of classification. Tissue texture abnormalities are defined as 'palpable changes in tissues from skin to periarticular structures that represent any combination of the following signs: vasodilation, edema, flaccid-ity, hypertonicity, contracture, fibrosis; and the following symptoms: itching, pain, tenderness'.[1] Thoroughly understanding the pathophysiologic mechanisms associated with each tissue texture abnormality leads to a physiologic classification of somatic dysfunction as 'acute' or 'chronic'.

Understanding the different conditions in which somatic dysfunction is acute or chronic is vital to selecting effective treatment strategies ranging from the choice of medication to the choice of a manipulative activating force. Specific acute and chronic characteristics used in the physiologic classification of somatic dysfunction appear in Table 2.2.3.[32] Management strategies based on this classification system may be found in Chapter 4.3.1.

Yet another classification system used for somatic dysfunction integrates constellations of signs and symptoms recognized as common patterns of dysfunction seen in clinical practice. With time, every practitioner of neuromusculoskeletal medicine will come to recognize common, recurrent patterns that, in turn, increase the efficacy and efficiency of patient management. The most commonly seen and clinically significant group patterns are designated by syndrome names. Such inter- and intraprofessional classifications permit common combinations of signs and symptoms to be discussed quickly and conveniently. In neuromusculoskeletal medicine, common examples include tennis elbow syndrome,[33] psoas syndrome,[34] theatre (cocktail party) syndrome,[35] spondylogenic (non-radicular) syndrome,[36] and others that will be individually addressed as examples throughout this text.

Table 2.2.3. Physiologic classification of acute and chronic somatic dysfunction

	Acute	Chronic
History	Recent, often an injury	Long-standing
Pain descriptors	Acute, severe, cutting, sharp	Dull, achy; paresthesias (crawling, itching, burning, gnawing)
Vascular	Vessels injured, release of endogenous peptides = chemical vasodilation, inflammation	Vessels constricted because of increased sympathetic tone
Skin	Warm, moist, red, inflamed (via vascular and chemical changes)	Cool, pale (via chronic sympathetic vascular tone increase)
Sympathetics	Systemically increased sympathetic activity contributes some local vasoconstriction (but local effect overpowered by bradykinins resulting in overall local vasodilation due to chemical effect)	Has vasoconstriction due to hypersympathetic tone. Regional sympathetic hyperactivity. Systemic sympathetic tone may be reduced toward normal
Musculature	Local increase in muscle tone, muscle contraction, hypertonicity and reactivity, increased tone of the muscle spindle	Decreased muscle tone, flaccid, mushy, limited range of motion because of contracture
Mobility	Range often normal, quality is sluggish	Limited range, with normal quality in the motion that remains
Tissues	Boggy edema, acute congestion, fluids from vessels and from chemical reactions in tissues	Chronic congestion, doughy, stringy, fibrotic, ropy, thickened, increased resistance, contracted, contractures
Adnexa	Moist skin, no trophic changes	Pimples, scaly, dry, folliculitis, pigmentation (trophic changes)
Visceral	Minimal somatovisceral effects	Somatovisceral effects are common

Source: Kuchera, W. A., Kuchera, M. L. *Osteopathic principles in practice*, 2nd edn. Greyden Press Columbus, Ohio, 1994, p. 25.

Finally, it should be stated that systems of classification are often mixed as in discussing the 'acute, viscerosomatic L2 FR_LS_L' vertebral unit somatic dysfunction typically found as part of a 'left psoas syndrome' that is secondary to a left ureteral calculus.

Recording severity and significance

Individual S.T.A.R. components can be quantified and recorded. For example, sensory characteristics can be objectively quantified by measuring the amount of pressure needed to elicit pain (using a dolorimeter) or by measuring the distance between stimuli as in a two-point discrimination. These measurements can then be respectively expressed in kilograms or millimeters or clinically interpreted relative to established normative data. In like manner, tissue texture abnormalities, asymmetries, and restriction in motion can also be individually qualified.

Each S.T.A.R. component can be numerically scaled and expressed as a number or informally designated as mild, moderate or severe. Common scales used by musculoskeletal practitioners may combine component evaluations, as in the Krauss–Weber grading of flexibility, strength, and endurance. (Table 2.2.4).

It is also possible to differentiate and record variable grades of severity with respect to somatic dysfunction itself. This is valuable in separating background levels of somatic dysfunction from significant 'key' dysfunction. It is also vital in following treatment outcomes in which somatic dysfunction is specifically or reflexly treated.

Simple method of recording severity using S.T.A.R. characteristics

A simple system using S.T.A.R. characteristics and recording severity from 0 to 3 was defined by the Educational Council on Osteopathic Principles and adopted as a standard by the Bureau on Health Care Facilities Accreditation of the American Osteopathic Association (AOA) (Figure 2.2.15 and Table 2.2.5). The scale shown in Table 2.2.5 has been adopted by the osteopathic profession in the USA for recording somatic dysfunction severity. As part of their admitting history and physical examination, every patient admitted by a doctor of osteopathy (DO) into an AOA-accredited hospital in the USA is required to have an osteopathic musculoskeletal structural examination recorded in the fashion shown in Figure 2.2.15 or in a specified narrative form.

Background levels of somatic dysfunction exist in almost every individual. Its presence is universal, resulting in few subjects totally free of minimal dysfunction in all anatomic regions. This 'background' level is rarely of clinical significance and is recorded with a '0' on this 0–3 scale as is the absence of somatic dysfunction. A severity of '1' indicates 'minimal' somatic dysfunction with minor (S.T.A.R.) palpatory findings. At the other end of the scale, a highly significant somatic dysfunction representing extensive and impressive (S.T.A.R.) characteristics, especially involving tissue texture abnormalities and restriction of motion, would be designated 'severe' and documented as a '3'. Severe somatic dysfunction is typically significant and/or symptomatic. The remaining designation of '2' would be more than 'minimal' but less than 'severe.' Typically clinically relevant, moderate (level 2) somatic dysfunction may or may not be symptomatic.

Primary versus secondary somatic dysfunction

Somatic dysfunction is interpreted and managed consistent with its origin and maintaining factors. If somatic dysfunction originated from direct tissue injury or a somatic stressor, palpable S.T.A.R. characteristics would be consistent with a diagnostic classification of **primary somatic dysfunction**. Somatic dysfunction arising from a vis-

Table 2.2.4. Modified Krauss–Weber muscle testing

Muscles tested	Patient position	Physician action	Instructions	Interpretation
Test 1: Strength Upper abdominal muscles with psoas action	Supine – hands folded across chest and legs fully extended	At foot of table holding patient feet down	'Curl your head and body off the table.'	Success – 30° plus = upper abdominal muscles adequate. 60° to upright = psoas adequate
Test 2: Strength Abdominal muscles without psoas action	Supine – hands folded across chest. Flexed hips and knees; feet flat on the table	At foot of table holding patient feet down	'Curl your body up to the sitting position.'	1. unable – poor muscle strength 2. able with effort – moderate strength 3. without difficulty – strong
Test 3: Strength Lower abdominal muscles	Supine – hands behind the neck and both legs extended	At head of table holding patient shoulders to the table. (Count the 10 seconds during patient effort)	'With your legs straight, lift your feet 10 inches off the table and hold them there for 10 seconds.'	1. unable – poor muscle strength 2. able with effort – moderate strength 3. without difficulty – strong
Test 4: Strength Upper back muscles	Prone – pillow under the abdomen. Legs fully extended; hands clasped behind back.	At foot of the table holding patient hips and legs down. (Count the 10 seconds during patient effort)	'Raise your chest and abdomen off the table and hold that position for 10 seconds.'	1. unable – poor muscle strength 2. able with effort – moderate strength 3. without difficulty – strong
Test 5: Strength Lower back muscles	Prone – pillow under the abdomen. Legs fully extended; hands clasped behind neck	At head of the table holding patient hips and legs down. (Count the 10 seconds during patient effort)	'Without bending your knees, lift both legs off the table and hold that position for 10 seconds.'	1. unable – poor muscle strength 2. able with effort – moderate strength 3. without difficulty – strong
Test 6: Strength Spinal flexion and hamstring extensibility	Standing completely upright with feet together and hands to the sides	Stand by the patient and measure distance of patient's fingertips to the floor	'Without bending your knees, bend forward and try to touch the floor.'	<45° = stiff spine. Not to floor = poor hamstring extensibility. Touches floor = good spinal flexion and good hamstring extensibility.
Test 7: Strength Hamstring extensibility	Supine with legs fully extended	Stand by the patient on the side that is to be tested	'Do not use your muscles. Let me raise your legs without your help.'	<60 ° = loss of hamstring extensibility 80–90 ° = good extensibility of gluteus maximus >90 ° = good erector spinae mass extensibility

Source: DiGiovanna, E. L., Schiowitz, S., Dowling, D.: *An osteopathic approach to diagnosis and treatment*, 2nd edn. Lippincott-Raven, Philadelphia, 1997, pp. 96–8.

cerosomatic or somatosomatic reflex may be classified **secondary somatic dysfunction**. These classifications are parallel to Travell and Simons' classification of trigger points (primary dysfunction) arising from direct somatic stress including trauma, overuse, and chilling and those myofascial points that arise secondary to cardiac, gallbladder, or other visceral indirect stimulus.

Several mechanisms have been proposed and/or documented to explain various aspects of the tissue texture abnormalities and other somatic, visceral, vascular, lymphatic, immune, and neural responses seen in primary and secondary somatic dysfunction.[36–39] Nociceptive levels of somatic dysfunction, especially in severe somatic dysfunction, create segmental spinal facilitation and significant peripheral

Table 2.2.5. Standardized severity rating for somatic dysfunction

S.T.A.R.		Severity scale	
S	Sensitivity of tissue – i.e. tenderness	0	No SD; or only background level changes
T	Tissue texture changes	1	Minor S.T.A.R.; more than background levels
A	Asymmetry	2	S.T.A.R. is obvious (esp. R and T); ± symptoms
R	Restriction of motion	3	Symptomatic; R and T very easily found; this is the 'key lesion'

Source: Kuchera, M. L., Kuchera, W. A., *Osteopathic musculoskeletal examination of the hospitalized patient*. American Osteopathic Association, 1998.

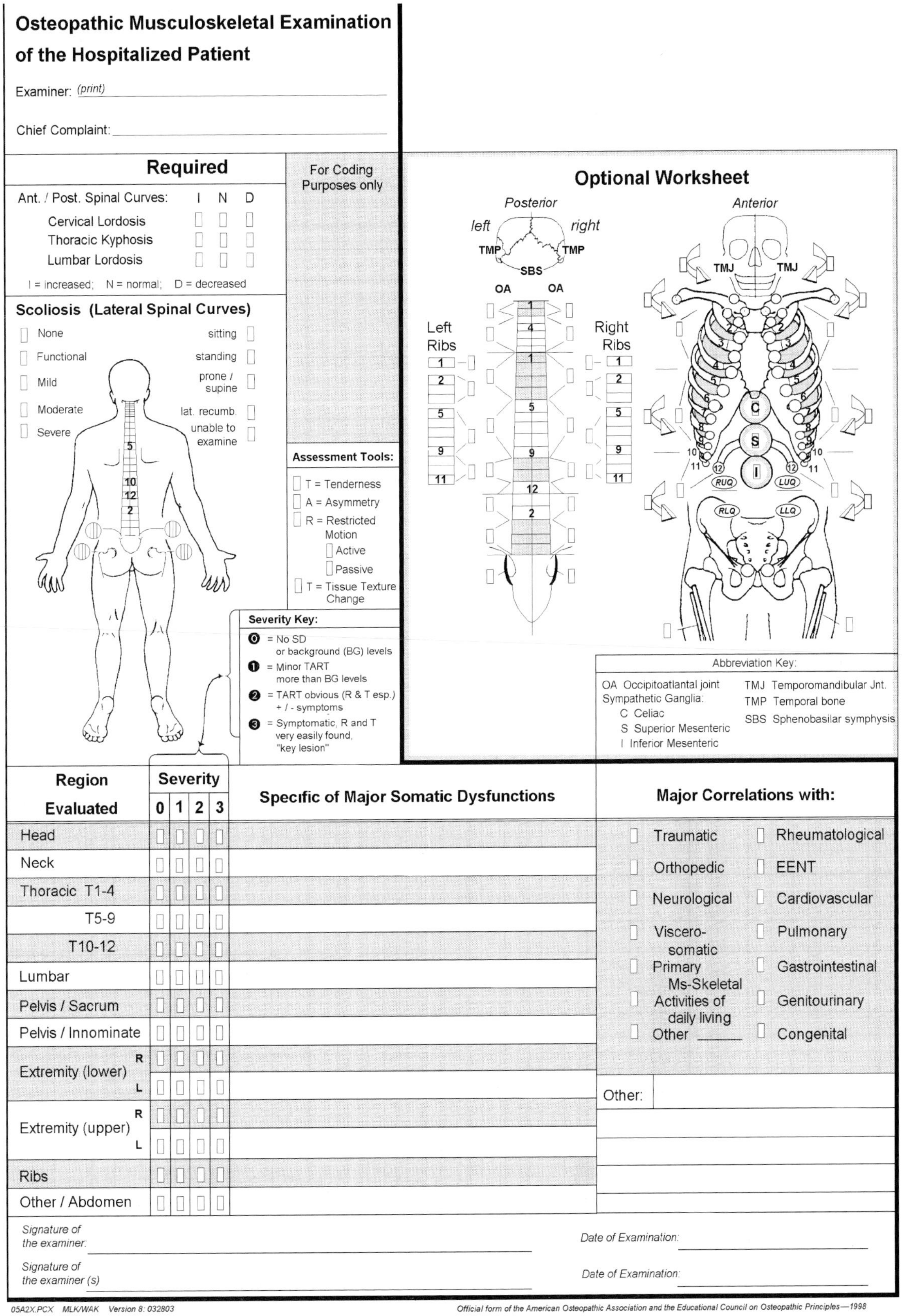

Osteopathic Musculoskeletal Examination of the Hospitalized Patient

Examiner: (print) _____

Chief Complaint: _____

Required

For Coding Purposes only

Ant. / Post. Spinal Curves: I   N   D

	I	N	D
Cervical Lordosis	☐	☐	☐
Thoracic Kyphosis	☐	☐	☐
Lumbar Lordosis	☐	☐	☐

I = increased;   N = normal;   D = decreased

Scoliosis (Lateral Spinal Curves)

☐ None   sitting ☐
☐ Functional   standing ☐
☐ Mild   prone / supine ☐
☐ Moderate   lat. recumb. ☐
☐ Severe   unable to examine ☐

Assessment Tools:

☐ T = Tenderness
☐ A = Asymmetry
☐ R = Restricted Motion
   ☐ Active
   ☐ Passive
☐ T = Tissue Texture Change

Severity Key:

❶ = No SD or background (BG) levels
❶ = Minor TART more than BG levels
❷ = TART obvious (R & T esp.) + / - symptoms
❸ = Symptomatic, R and T very easily found, "key lesion"

Optional Worksheet

Posterior

left   right

TMP   TMP
SBS
OA   OA

Left Ribs   Right Ribs

Anterior

TMJ   TMJ

C
S
I
RUQ   LUQ
RLQ   LLQ

Abbreviation Key:

OA Occipitoatlantal joint   TMJ Temporomandibular Jnt.
Sympathetic Ganglia: TMP Temporal bone
  C Celiac   SBS Sphenobasilar symphysis
  S Superior Mesenteric
  I Inferior Mesenteric

Region Evaluated	Severity 0	1	2	3	Specific of Major Somatic Dysfunctions
Head	☐	☐	☐	☐	
Neck	☐	☐	☐	☐	
Thoracic T1-4	☐	☐	☐	☐	
T5-9	☐	☐	☐	☐	
T10-12	☐	☐	☐	☐	
Lumbar	☐	☐	☐	☐	
Pelvis / Sacrum	☐	☐	☐	☐	
Pelvis / Innominate	☐	☐	☐	☐	
Extremity (lower) R	☐	☐	☐	☐	
L	☐	☐	☐	☐	
Extremity (upper) R	☐	☐	☐	☐	
L	☐	☐	☐	☐	
Ribs	☐	☐	☐	☐	
Other / Abdomen	☐	☐	☐	☐	

Major Correlations with:

☐ Traumatic   ☐ Rheumatological
☐ Orthopedic   ☐ EENT
☐ Neurological   ☐ Cardiovascular
☐ Viscero-somatic   ☐ Pulmonary
☐ Primary Ms-Skeletal ☐ Gastrointestinal
☐ Activities of daily living ☐ Genitourinary
☐ Other _____   ☐ Congenital

Other: _____

Signature of the examiner: _____   Date of Examination: _____

Signature of the examiner (s) _____   Date of Examination: _____

05A2X.PCX   MLK/WAK   Version 8: 032803

Official form of the American Osteopathic Association and the Educational Council on Osteopathic Principles—1998

Figure 2.2.15 Chart for recording musculoskeletal examination of a hospitalized patient. (From Kuchera, M. L., Kuchera, W. A. (1998) *Osteopathic musculoskeletal examination of the hospitalized patient.* American Osteopathic Association.)

pathophysiologic change[40,41] resulting in significant tissue texture abnormalities. Similarly, many primary visceral afferent fibers affecting the spinal cord have the characteristics of nociceptive fibers. They produce neuropeptides such as substance P and calcitonin gene-related polypeptide and respond to nociceptive stimuli. Some are even capable of eliciting a neurogenic inflammatory response in the surrounding tissue.[7,42] Thus both somatic and visceral conditions are capable of creating musculoskeletal clues palpable as somatic dysfunction.

Again, primary somatic dysfunction typically responds well to the various management strategies discussed in this text (Part 4)[43,44] whereas secondary somatic dysfunction responds variably and often recurs[4,45] when addressed by these approaches alone.

Significance of somatic dysfunction in health and 'dis-ease'

Failure to consider somatic dysfunction limits the differential diagnosis and overlooks an important underlying pathophysiologic process that may limit optimum health and performance or play a role in patient complaints. The presence of moderate to severe somatic dysfunction in particular spinal patterns correlates with and thereby augments the differential diagnosis of a wide range of visceral conditions.[45–48] Indeed, irritation of upper thoracic spinal joint receptors simultaneously evokes numerous reflex alterations, including paravertebral muscle spasm and alterations in endocrine, respiratory and cardiovascular functions.[49]

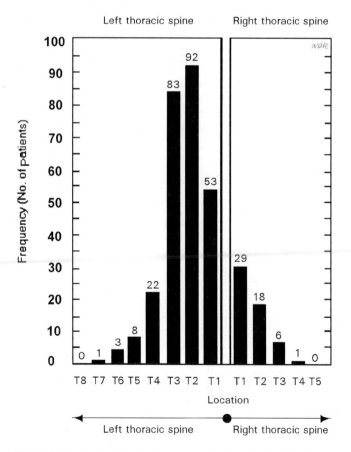

Figure 2.2.16 Spinal referral pattern for cardiac disorders (n = 94) that correlates well with angiography (From Kuchera[45], p. 59.)

The cardiovascular system is perhaps the most documented system in which the clinical recognition of somatic dysfunction in health and 'dis-ease' has been demonstrated. Specific palpatory findings of upper thoracic somatic dysfunction (especially affecting left upper thoracic paraspinal tissues) were reported in the *British Medical Journal* as being consistently found in myocardial infarction.[50] Beal[47] reported 79% specificity of thoracic palpatory findings compared to angiography in coronary artery patients (Figure 2.2.16). Similarly, Travell and Simons report the palpatory finding of trigger points in the pectoralis major muscles in 61% of 72 patients with cardiac disease.[51] These palpatory findings of somatic dysfunction have a completely different pattern than secondary somatic dysfunction associated with patients with gastrointestinal problems.[47] (Figure 2.2.16)

Conversely, evidence of somatovisceral reflexes is cited by Travell and Simons. Removal of primary myofascial somatic dysfunction in the pectoralis major muscle on the right in patients with some forms of supraventricular tachyarrhythmia 'promptly restores normal sinus rhythm … and also can eliminate recurrences of the paroxysmal arrhythmia … for a long period of time'.[51] Other somatovisceral reflexes are implicated in functional gastrointestinal disorders and from systemic symptoms ranging from asthma to duodenal ulcers to dysmenorrhea.

In response to a variety of stimuli, homeostatic functions are defensively altered through a series of complex feedback loops that monitor conditions in the peripheral tissues and make local and systemic adjustments as needed. Excessive driving stimuli or dysfunction of the feedback circuits themselves results in decreased compensatory reserve, 'dis-ease', and increased susceptibility to disease. The three primary driving stimuli (stressors) initiating the cascade of chemical messengers first described in Selye's general adaptive response are emotional, somatic, and visceral dysfunction.[52] These and other stressors create an allostatic load capable of disturbing the individual's normal homeostatic set point.[53–55] Their role and the role of somatic dysfunction specifically plays in disturbing homeostasis through reflex[56] and neuroendocrine–immune[57] responses to the inflammation, edema, and nociceptive biochemical mediators of somatic dysfunction[40] have been extensively documented and elegantly discussed.[57,58]

Neuromusculoskeletal medicine physicians are capable of assisting the body in maintaining homeostasis by recognizing and modifying any or all of the driving stimuli (stressors). Thus the education of these practitioners now emphasizes the importance of integrating biopsychosocial, anatomical, and pathophysiological models.[59,60] Previously challenged by some musculoskeletal practitioners,[61] this aspect of neuromusculoskeletal care has most widely been championed by osteopathic physicians of the American school.

Somatic dysfunction and the manual medicine prescription

A knowledgeable physician capable of fully assessing risk–benefit ratios and cost-effectiveness is best equipped to direct a manual medicine prescription, if indicated, and its implementation. This is also extremely important for selecting the type of manual method, activating force, frequency, and duration of this form of treatment and its place in the total management of the patient. Individual characteristics of the somatic dysfunction, the biopsychosocial aspects of the patient as a whole, any other underlying pathophysiological processes, and the skills of the treating physician dictate many of these choices.

The neuromusculoskeletal physician specifically ponders the following:

- **Goal:** What area or physiologic process would benefit from a manual medicine approach? Is there an acceptable risk-to-benefit ratio to consider such an approach?

- **Method:** What forms or techniques of manual medicine are indicated and contraindicated?

- **Dose:** What are the underlying homeostatic reserves of the patient and what duration of treatment administration would provide maximal benefit?

- **Frequency:** How frequently should the manipulation be repeated within the parameters of patient response and cost-efficacy?

The manual medicine prescription[62] takes form after appropriate evaluation and establishment of a working diagnosis by a knowledgeable and skilled physician who then seeks to accomplish a definable therapeutic goal. As with most prescriptive care, in subsequent visits the patient is re-assessed for symptomatic and physiologic change including a re-examination for somatic dysfunction before making a decision to re-initiate any subsequent manipulative treatment. Clinical outcomes, patient response to the previous treatment, and visit-specific findings of somatic dysfunction influence the goals, methods, and dose used in follow-up visits and to adjust manipulative frequency decisions.

Limiting factors[63] considered in the formulation of a manual medicine prescription and its delivery include:

- **Patient-centered factors** including the knowledge or concern of the patient's ability to respond because of age, sex, size, occupation, dietary or life-activity risk factors, allostatic load (including biopsychosocial stressors), support system, allergies to potential treatment alternatives, and response to similar treatments or modalities given in the past.

- **Disease-centered factors** especially those accompanied by osteoporotic, rheumatologic, orthopedic, neurologic, cardiovascular or oncologic change. Even without specific diagnosis, signs or symptoms of other acute or chronic pathophysiologic processes affecting the neuromusculoskeletal or related systems must be considered. These conditions often dictate treatment position, the manual medicine method or activation employed, and treatment duration and frequency.

- **Physician-centered factors** including the ability of the physician to accomplish the treatment or to appropriately refer the patient for that form of care. Other factors might include personal stature, training, specialization background, license limitations, and ability to maintain advances made in the manual medicine field through continuing medical education.

For these reasons, the International Federation of Manual/Musculoskeletal Medicine (FIMM) and the AOA advocate that only practitioners fully trained in all diagnostic and therapeutic modalities have the total perspective required to make proper manual medicine management decisions in neuromusculoskeletal medicine fields. These management decisions require weighing relative risk-to-benefit ratios as well as the choice and frequency of technique, duration of care, and its potential for integration with other modalities. In workman's compensation cases in the USA, physician-level education with core manual medicine training appears to be more cost-effective than management by those employing manual approaches without physician training or physician training without core training in palpatory diagnosis and manual techniques (Figure 2.2.17).[64]

While fully licensed physicians with additional training in the skills of manual medicine diagnosis and treatment are arguably better equipped to take responsibility for the formulation and delivery of the manual medicine prescription, other health care providers must continue to be involved. Though they lack the manual medicine physician's perspective to fully identify and weigh risk–benefit ratios, physical therapists and non-physician manipulative practitioners are typically regulated by licensing and other regulating bodies and may play a role in interdisciplinary management teams. Likewise, although physicians without manual medicine education cannot fully consider relative efficacy or cost-effectiveness of manual intervention, they are

Average Cost of Treatment per patient in Dollars

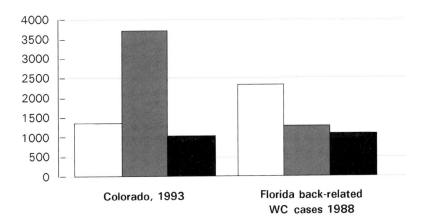

Figure 2.2.17 Average cost of treatment per patient in US dollars for workman's compensation cases treated with and without manual medicine techniques. White bars, nonsurgical MD; gray bars, chiropractor; black bars, doctor of osteopathy. Data compiled by Labor and Industry computers in Florida (FCER 1988, Arlington, Virginia) and Colorado (Tillinghast 1993, Denver, Colorado).

valuable in interdisciplinary management teams to provide specialty perspectives, consultation, or appropriate referral to those who have additional education in the neuromusculoskeletal medicine field.

Precipitating and perpetuating factors in somatic dysfunction

A number of precipitating and/or perpetuating factors warrant diagnostic and treatment consideration in patients with somatic dysfunction. Musculoskeletal physicians[44,65] subclassify precipitating and perpetuating host factors to include mechanical stressors; nutritional, metabolic and endocrine inadequacies; co-existing radiculopathies, plexopathies, and neuropathies; psychologic factors; and chronic infections and infestations.

Mechanical stressors

These are a major consideration in a neuromusculoskeletal practice. Gravitational stress is magnified in a number of postural and structural disorders such as leg length inequality, small hemipelvis, obesity, and accentuation of sagittal plane postural curves.[17] Acute overload or overwork fatigue[67] can be aggravated by prolonged exposure to ill-fitting furniture, poor and/or excessive habitual body mechanics, obesity, immobility, repetitive occupational motions, or inappropriate gait mechanics due to pronated or Morton's foot deformity. Direct muscular constriction or trauma as well as joint micro- and macrotrauma are precipitating and perpetuating factors for somatic dysfunction. Assessing whole-body postural alignment, analysis of standing postural radiographs, or assessing ergonomic factors in the home or workplace may augment diagnosis. Treatment may require adjunctive use of foot or pelvic orthotics, postural and/or proprioceptive reeducation, use of assistive devices, and modification of activities of daily living.

Nutritional, metabolic and endocrine inadequacies

These preclude the body from using nutritive building blocks, or impair physiologic pathways necessary for neuromusculoskeletal function. Travell and Simons note the importance and balance of vitamins B_1, B_6, and B_{12} as well as folic acid, vitamin C, calcium, iron, and potassium in the health of myofascial tissues.[66] They also note the clinical relevance of conditions such as hypothyroidism and hypoglycemia that interfere with muscular energy metabolism. Cigarette smoking interferes with myofascial tissue oxygenation and metabolism and is therefore a perpetuating factor for somatic dysfunction and soft tissue healing.[67,68] Tests for thyroid function, fasting blood sugar, serum vitamin levels, or other blood chemistry profiles may therefore be helpful in diagnosis. Treatment may require pharmacologic or dietary strategies as well as patient education. Orthopedic medicine physicians have empirically seen benefit in nutritionally supplementing patients with the myofascial tissue building blocks, glucosamine and chondroitin sulfate.[69]

Radiculopathy or proximal neural entrapment neuropathies

Coexisting radiculopathy or proximal neural entrapment neuropathies have further been implicated in decreasing axoplasmic flow needed to provide trophic factors required in the periphery. This is the mechanism proposed in the so-called 'double-crush' phenomenon,[70] leading to increased incidence and symptomatology from more distal somatic dysfunction and neural entrapments. This could also account, in part, for the 10% of patients with carpal tunnel syndrome who are found to have a primary cervical radiculopathy.[71] Such diagnoses can usually be made clinically but may require special imaging or neuro-electrodiagnostic studies to localize an anatomic cause or physiologic consequence. Treatment may require integration of pharmacologic, physical therapeutic, and/or surgical elements.

Psychologic factors

As well as arising from chronic pain and dysfunction, these factors perpetuate pain and somatic dysfunction, Thus suspicion and special questioning may be required to identify those factors interfering with optimum function of the individual. Treatment of underlying anxiety or depression may be required before complete resolution of somatic dysfunction can be accomplished.

Infections and infestations

A variety of viral infections as well as underlying occult infections and infestations[72] (e.g. *Diphyllobothrium latum, Giardia lamblia, Entamoeba histolytica*) are capable of causing muscle ache and perpetuating myofascial somatic dysfunction. Such a diagnosis might be initiated by the presence of eosinophilia or an elevated white count. Antibiotics, dental care, or other pharmacologic intervention for chronic infection may be required before the musculoskeletal findings can be addressed satisfactorily.

The coexistence of many precipitating and perpetuating factors requiring diagnosis and treatment is yet another reason that a broad knowledge base and the capability of ordering and interpreting laboratory, radiographic, nuclear, and neuroelectrophysiologic examinations is needed for successful management of neuromusculoskeletal medicine conditions. Treatment requiring integration of pharmacologic, physical therapeutic, orthotic, exercise prescription, and surgical approaches is also best coordinated by a physician educated to recognize the indications, contraindications, and relative efficacy of each. Manual diagnostic and treatment techniques alone are rarely sufficient to successfully practice neuromusculoskeletal medicine.

Recurrent patterns of somatic dysfunction

The presence of recurrent patterns of somatic dysfunction despite quality care indicates the need for re-evaluation and reconsideration of the existing patient management. Most commonly, recurrent patterns arise from one (or more) of three causes:

- postural compensation
- viscerosomatic referral
- repetitious habitual or occupational posturing and/or motions.

Postural compensation

Patterns of postural compensation occur when gravitational force, acting on individual structures, is biomechanically amplified[73] in patients who possess a less than ideal postural alignment. Musculo-ligamentous structures associated with maintenance of posture are, in this manner, subjected to increased strain. When there is viscoelastic deformation of muscle, restraining ligaments, and other connective tissues are unable to resist the stress, neuromuscular reflex activity is automatically and subconsciously initiated to maintain postural equilibrium. Continuous gravitational stress results in various combinations of predictable pathophysiologic change,[17] which begins in the connective tissues. It is accentuated and perpetuated by inadequate compensatory mechanisms, including peripheral and central reflexes.

Postural muscles, adapted structurally to function in the presence of prolonged gravitational stress, generally resist fatigue. When their capacity to resist stress is overwhelmed, they become irritable, tight, and shortened. Both structural (anatomic) and functional (physiologic and biochemical) changes occur in myofascial structures. They undergo sustained changes in length, and studies[74] suggest that deleterious change is most pronounced in shortened rather than lengthened muscles. New collagen, with a half-life of 10–12 months, realigns the connective tissues in response to stress vectors, thus perpetuating the resultant posture and maintaining biomechanical amplification of gravitational stress. Abnormal stresses, chronically applied to connective tissues, modify their structure and function until they are no longer capable of compensating for the effects of gravitational strain. In an extension of Wolff's law that calcium is laid down along lines of stress, the discovery of bony exostoses and ligamentous calcification may provide radiographic evidence of the stress placed on these soft tissue structures and the fibro-osseous junction.

Thus when host mechanisms are overwhelmed, signs of gravitational stress appear, including recurrent somatic dysfunction, recurrent myofascial trigger points, postural decompensation, chronic or recurrent strains and sprains, pseudoparesis, and ligamentous laxity. The patient's symptoms include recurrent low back pain, pain referred to extremities, headache, fatigue, weakness, dysfunctional symptoms from various viscera, and other sequelae of neural, vascular, and lymphatic dysfunction resulting from somatic stress. Treatment of the neuromusculoskeletal findings in isolation is often beneficial for short periods of time, but they recur typically with the same underlying patterns of somatic dysfunction.

In general, gravitational stress and the resultant postural effects are most likely to be related to anatomic, histologic, physiologic, and dysfunctional changes at transitional (junctional) areas of the spine, as these sites are already predisposed to injury and somatic dysfunction. Thus, key patterns of spinal somatic dysfunction commonly occur at the craniocervical, cervicothoracic, thoracolumbar, lumbopelvic, and sacroiliac junctions.[17,75] The histologic junctional zones created by connective tissue attachments of ligaments, tendons, and joint capsules are also vulnerable to the biomechanical stress of postural decompensation, especially at the site of the fibro-osseous junction of restraining ligaments. The key to efficient diagnosis is to recognize such signs and symptoms as pathophysiologic elements of a common musculoligamentous strain pattern caused by gravitational stress.

Viscerosomatic reflex patterns

A second common cause of recurrent patterns of somatic dysfunction may be found in patients with underlying visceral disease or dysfunction. Some of these viscerosomatic reflex patterns, such as those associated with acute appendicitis and gallstones, are widely known and described in a number of texts. Other patterns are less generally known and are described in surgical[48] or pain[76] texts written for specialists in those fields. Osteopathic primary care practitioners and specialists in osteopathic manipulative medicine employ these patterns regularly in their practice of neuromusculoskeletal medicine. Regardless of practice type or degree, the finding of specific recurrent patterns of somatic dysfunction in the distribution or combination, as shown in Figure 2.2.18, should prompt the astute neuromusculo-skeletal medicine practitioner to consider visceral dysfunction as part of the complete differential diagnosis. A compilation describing the specific role of somatic dysfunction in visceral problems is found in *Osteopathic considerations in systemic dysfunction*.[45]

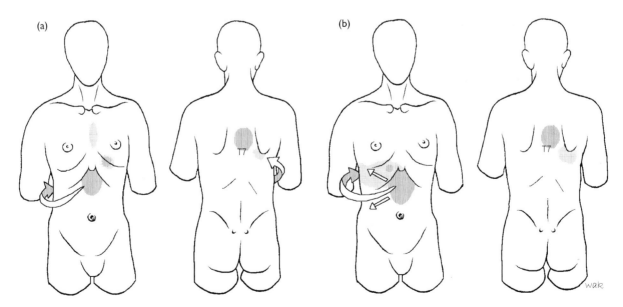

Figure 2.2.18 Pain patterns: (a) cholelithiasis, (b) gastric ulcer. (From Kuchera, M. L., Kuchera, W. A. (1994) *Osteopathic considerations in systemic dysfunction*, 2nd edn, revised. Greyden Press, Columbus, OH.)

Recurrent posturing or repetitive motions

A final cause of recurrent patterns of somatic dysfunction arises from recurrent posturing or repetitive motions associated with habit or occupation. With this in mind, history and an ergonomic evaluation often provide insights to diagnosis and treatment.

Conclusion

Concepts associated with somatic dysfunction pragmatically permit consolidation of many clinically relevant models used in neuromusculo-skeletal and manual medicine fields. Building upon anatomic and pathophysiologic scientific bases, these concepts can be discussed, explored, and tested. Perhaps even more importantly, neuromusculo-skeletal physicians can use 'somatic dysfunction' and associated concepts to communicate with one another. In both situations, palpatory diagnosis and treatment of patients with somatic dysfunction expands the physician's ability to assist patients in their pursuit of function and/or pain relief.

References

1. Education Council on Osteopathic Principles. Glossary of osteopathic terminology. In Ward, R. C. (ed.). *Foundations for osteopathic medicine*, 2nd edn (2002). Lippincott, Williams & Wilkins, Baltimore, MD.

2. *International classification of diseases, 9th revision, clinical modification* (ICD-9-CM). 3rd edn (1979). World Health Organization, Geneva.

3. Maigne, R., Liberson, W. T. *Orthopedic medicine: a new approach to vertebral manipulations* (1972). C. C. Thomas, Springfield, IL.

4. Simons, D. G., Travell, J. G., Simons, L. S. *Travell and Simons' myofascial pain and dysfunction: the trigger point manual, volume 1. Upper half of body* (1999). Williams & Wilkins, Baltimore, MD.

5. Jones, L. H. *Strain and counterstrain* (1981). American Academy of Osteopathy, Newark, OH.

6. Maitland, G. D. Acute locking of the cervical spine. *Australian Journal of Physiotherapy* 1978, **24**, 103–9.

7. Gilliar, W. G., Kuchera, M. L., Giulianetti, D. A. Neurologic basis of manual medicine. *Physical Medicine and Rehabilitation Clinics of North America.* November 1996, **7**(4), 693–714.

8. Pernow, B. Substance P. *Pharmacol Rev* 1983, **35**, 85–141.

9. Battaglia, G., Rustioni, A. Coexistence of glutamate and substance P in dorsal root ganglion neurons of the rat and monkey. *J Comp Neurol* 1988, **227**, 302–12.

10. Willard, F. H., Mokler, D. J., Morgane, P. J. Chapter 9. Neuroendocrine-immune system and homeostasis. In Ward, R. C. (ed.). *Foundations for osteopathic medicine* (1997). Williams & Wilkins, Baltimore, MD, pp. 107–35.

11. Konnitinen, Y. T., Koski, H., Santavirta, S., *et al.* Nociception, proprioception, and neurotransmitters. In Bland, J. H. (ed.). *Disorders of the Cervical Spine*, 2nd edn (1994). W. B. Saunders, Philadelphia, pp. 319–38.

12. Korr, I. M. Hyperactivity of sympathetic innervation: a common factor in disease. In Greenman P. E. (ed.). *Concepts and mechanisms of neuromuscular functions* (1984). Springer-Verlag, Berlin, , pp 1–8; and Korr, I. M. The spinal cord as organizer of disease processes: the peripheral autonomic nervous system. *J Am Osteopath Assoc* 1979, **79**, 82–90.

13. Dubner, R., Bennett, G. J. Spinal and trigeminal mechanisms of nociception. *Annu Rev Neurosci* 1983, **6**, 381–418.

14. Mitchell, F. L., Mitchell, P. K. *The muscle energy manual* (1995). MET Press, East Lansing, MI, p. 33.

15. Cervero, F. Mechanisms of acute visceral pain. *Br Med Bull* 1991, **47**, 549–560.

16. Patterson, M. M., Steinmetz, J. E. Long-lasting alterations of spinal reflexes: a potential basis for somatic dysfunction. *Manual Med* 1986, **2**, 38–45.

17. Kuchera, M. L. Gravitational stress, musculoligamentous strain, and postural alignment. *Spine: State of the Art Reviews* 1995, **9**(2), 463–90.

18. Mitchell, F Jr. The training and measurement of sensory literacy in relation to osteopathic structural and palpatory diagnosis. *J Am Osteopath Assoc* 1976, **75**, 881.

19. Wolfe, F., Smythe, H. A., Yunus, M. B. *et al.* The American College of Rheumatology 1990 criteria for the classification of fibromyalgia. Report of the Multicenter Committee. *Arthritis Rheum* 1990, **33**, 160–72.

20. Jones, L., Kusunose, R., Goering, E. *Jones' strain-counterstrain.* (1995). Jones Strain-Counterstrain, Inc.

21. Owens, C. *An endocrine interpretation of Chapman's reflexes.* (1963 reprint). American Academy of Osteopathy, Indianapolis, IN.

22. Kuchera, M. L., McPartland, J. Myofascial trigger points as somatic dysfunction. In Ward, R. C. (ed.). *Foundations for osteopathic medicine*, 2nd edn (2002). Lippincott, Williams & Wilkins, Baltimore, MD, pp. 1034–50.

23. *AMA guidelines to the evaluation of permanent impairment*, 3rd edn, revised (1990). AMA, Chicago, IL.

24. White, A. A., Panjabi, M. M. The basic kinematics of the human spine: a review of past and current knowledge. *Spine* 1978, **3**, 12.

25. Cyriax, J. H., Cyriax, P. J. *Cyriax's illustrated manual of orthopaedic medicine*, 2nd edn (1993). Butterworth-Heinemann, Oxford.

26. Sciotti, V. M., Mittak, V. L., DiMarco, L. Clinical precision of myofascial trigger point location in the trapezius muscle. *Pain* 2001, **93**, 259–66.

27. Degenhardt, B. F., Snider, K. T., Johnson, J. C., Snider E. J. Interexaminer reliability of osteopathic palpatory evaluation of the lumbar spine. *J Am Osteopath Assoc* 2002, **102**(8), 442.

28. Degenhardt, B. F., Snider, K. T., Johnson, J. C., Snider E. J. Retention of interexaminer reliability in palpatory evaluation of the lumbar spine. *J Am Osteopath Assoc* 2002, **102**(8), 439.

29. Mense, S., Simons, D. *Muscle pain, understanding its nature, diagnosis, and treatment.* (2001). Lippincott Williams and Wilkins, Philadelphia, PA.

30. Speece, C. A., Crow, W. T., Simmon, S. L. *Ligamentous articular strain: osteopathic manipulative techniques for the body* (2001). Eastland Press.

31. Mitchell, F. L. *The Muscle Energy Manual: Vol I.* (1995). Vol II (1998). Vol III (1999). MET Press, East Lansing, MI.

32. Kuchera, W. A., Kuchera, M. L. *Osteopathic principles in practice*, 2nd edn, revised (1994). Greyden Press, Columbus, OH. p. 25.

33. Simons, D. G., Travell, J. G., Simons, L. S. *Travell and Simons' myofascial pain and dysfunction: the trigger point manual, volume 1. Upper half of body* (1999). Williams & Wilkins, Baltimore, MD, pp. 728–42.

34. Kappler, R. E. Role of psoas mechanism in low back complaints. *1973 Academy Yearbook,* 1973, AAO Press, Indianapolis, IN, p. 130.

35. Dorman, T. A., Ravin, T. H. *Diagnosis and injection techniques in orthopedic medicine* (1991). Williams & Wilkins, Baltimore, MD.

36. Dvorak, J., Dvorak, V., Drobny, T. *Manual medicine: diagnostics* (1984). Georg Thieme Verlag, Stuttgart, pp. 30–45.

37. Korr, I. M. (ed.). *The neurobiologic mechanisms in manipulative therapy* (1978). Plenum Press, New York.

38. Greenman, P. E. (ed.). *Concepts and mechanisms of neuromuscular function* (1984). Springer-Verlag, Berlin.

39. Patterson, M. M., Howell, J. N. (eds). *The central connection: somato-visceral/viscerosomatic interaction* (1989). University Classics, Athens, OH.

40. Willard, F. H., Patterson M. M. (eds). *Nociception and the neuroendocrine-immune connection* (1991). University Classics, Athens, OH.

41. Van Buskirk, R. L. Nociceptive reflexes and somatic dysfunction: a model. *J Am Osteopath Assoc* 1990, **90**, 792–809.

42. Dockray, G. J., Sharkey, K. A. Neurochemistry of visceral afferent neurones. *Prog Brain Res.* 1986, **67**, 133–48.

43. Schott, G. D. Visceral afferent: their contribution to 'sympathetic dependent' pain. *Brain* 1994, **117**, 397–413.

44. Ward, R. C. (ed.). *Foundations for osteopathic medicine* (1997). Williams & Wilkins, Baltimore, MD.

45. Kuchera, M. L., Kuchera, W. A. *Osteopathic considerations in systemic dysfunction*, 2nd edition, revised (1994). Greyden Press, Columbus, OH.

46. Steele, K. M. Treatment of the acutely ill hospitalized patient. Chapter 75 in: Ward, R. C. (ed.) *Foundations for osteopathic medicine* (1997). Williams & Wilkins, Baltimore, MD, pp. 1037–48.

47. Beal, M. C. Viscerosomatic reflexes: a review. *J Am Osteopath Assoc* 1985, **85**(12), 53–68; Beal M. C. Palpatory testing for somatic dysfunction in patients with cardiovascular disease. *JADA* 1983, **82**, 73-82.

48. Smith, L. A. (ed.). *An atlas of pain patterns: sites and behavior of pain in certain common disease of the upper abdomen* (1961). C. C. Thomas, Springfield, IL.

49. Wyke, B. D. The neurologic basis of thoracic spinal pain. *Rheum Phys Med* 1970, **10**, 356.

50. Nicholas, A. S., DeBias, D. A., Ehrenfeuchter, W., *et al.* A somatic component to myocardial infarction. *Br Med J.* 1985, **291**, 13–17.

51. Simons, D. G., Travell, J. G., Simons, L. S. *Travell and Simons' myofascial pain and dysfunction: the trigger point manual – volume 1. Upper half of body* (1999). Williams & Wilkins, Baltimore, MD, pp. 832–33.

52. Willard, F. H. Neuroendocrine-immune network, nociceptive stress, and the general adaptive response. In Everett, T., Dennis, M., Ricketts, E (eds). *Physiotherapy in mental health: a practical approach* (1995). Butterworth-Heinemann: Oxford, pp. 102–26.

53. Sterling, P., Eyer, J. Allostasis: a new paradigm to explain arousal pathology. In Fisher, S. Reason, J. (eds) *Handbook of life stress, cognition and health* (1988). Wiley, New York, pp. 629–49.

54. Seeman, T. E., Singer, B. H., Rowe, J. W., Horwitz, R. I., McEwen, B. S. Price of adaptation – allostatic load and its health consequences: McArthur studies of successful aging. *J Clin Endocrinol Metab* 1997, **157**, 2259–68.

55. McEwen, B. S. Protective and damaging effects of stress mediators. *New Engl J Med* 1998. **338**, 178–9.

56. Denslow J. S. Pathophysiologic evidence for the osteopathic lesion: the known, unknown, and controversial. *J Am Osteopath Assoc* 1975, **74**, 315–421.

57. Willard, F. H., Mokler, D. J., Morgane, P. J. Chapter 9. Neuroendocrine-immune system and homeostasis. In Ward, R. C. (ed.). *Foundations for osteopathic medicine* (1997). Williams & Wilkins, Baltimore, MD, pp. 107–35.

58. Peterson, B (ed.). *The Collected Papers of Irvin M. Korr* (1979). American Academy of Osteopathy, Newark, OH.

59. Core Education Documents, International Federation of Musculoskeletal/Manual Medicine (FIMM) (1999).

60. Core Educational Documents, Educational Council on Osteopathic Principles of the American Association of Colleges of Osteopathic Medicine (1999).

61. Cyriax, J., Russell, G. *Textbook of orthopaedic medicine: volume 2, treatment by manipulation, massage, and injection*, 10th edn (1980). Baillière Tindall: London, pp. 60–9.

62. Kimberly, P. E. Formulating a prescription of osteopathic manipulative treatment. In Beal, M. C. (ed.). *The principles of palpatory diagnosis and manipulative technique* (1992). American Academy of Osteopathy: Newark, OH, pp. 146–52.

63. Kuchera, W. A., Kuchera, M. L. *Osteopathic Principles in Practice*, 2nd edn, revised (1994). Greyden Press, Columbus, OH, pp. 297–302.

64. Data compiled by Labor and Industry computers in Florida (FCER, 1988, Arlington, Virginia) and Colorado (Tillinghast, 1993, Denver, Colorado).

65. Simons, D. G., Travell, J. G., Simons, L. S. *Travell and Simons' myofascial pain and dysfunction: the trigger point manual – volume 1. Upper half of body* (1999). Williams & Wilkins, Baltimore, MD, pp. 178–235.

66. Simons, D. G., Travell, J. G., Simons, L. S. *Travell and Simons' myofascial pain and dysfunction: the trigger point manual – volume 1. Upper half of body* (1999). Williams & Wilkins, Baltimore, MD, pp. 186–220.

67. Amoronso, P. J. *et al.* Tobacco and injuries: an annotated bibliography. U.S. Army Research Laboratory Technical Report ARL-TR-1333 (1997); Naus, A *et al.* Work injuries and smoking. *Industrial Med Surg* 1966, **35**, 880–1; Reynolds, K. L. *et al.* Cigarette smoking, physical fitness, and injuries in infantry soldiers. *Am J Preventive Med* 1994, **19**, 145–50.

68. Treiman, G. S., Oderich, G. S., Ashrafi, A., Schneider, P. A. Management of ischemic heal ulceration and gangrene: an evaluation of factors associated with successful healing. *J Vasc Surg* 2000, **31**(6), 1110–18.

69. Deal, C. L., Moskowitz, R. W. Nutraceuticals as therapeutic agents in osteoarthritis. The role of glucosamine, chondrotin sulfate, and collagen hydrosalt. *Rheum Dis Clin North Am* 2000, **25**(2), 75–95.

70. Hurst, L. C., Weissberg, D., Carroll, R. E. The relationship of the double crush to carpal tunnel syndrome (an analysis of 1000 cases of carpal tunnel syndrome). *J Hand Surg* 1995, **10B**(2), 202–204.

71. Upton, A. R., McComas, A. J. The double crush in nerve entrapment syndromes. *Lancet* 1973, **ii**, 359–362.

72. Simons, D. G., Travell, J. G., Simons L. S. *Travell and Simons' myofascial pain and dysfunction: the trigger point manual – volume 1. Upper half of body* (1999). Williams & Wilkins, Baltimore, MD, pp. 223–5.

73. Kapandji, I. A. *Physiology of the joints: volume 3* (1974). Churchill Livingstone, New York.

74. Gossman, M. R., Sahrmann, S. A., Rose, S. J. Review of length-associated changes in muscle. *Phys Ther* 1982, **62**, 1799–807.

75. Zink, J. G., Lawson, W. B. An osteopathic structural examination and functional interpretation of the soma. *Osteopath Ann* 1979, **7**, 12–19.

76. Cousins, M. J. Visceral pain. In Andersson, S., Bond, M., Mehta, M., Swerdlow M (eds). *Chronic non-cancer pain: assessment and practical management* (1987). MTP Press, Lancaster.

2.2.2 Muscles in the pathogenesis of musculoskeletal disorders

Vladimír Janda

Although muscles represent the only active tissue that protects the joints, and joints and muscles together form a functional unit, the importance of muscle–joint correlation remains widely underestimated or misunderstood in clinical practice. Even in musculoskeletal medicine, muscles are not considered as an essential factor in the pathogenesis of pain of the musculoskeletal system. These facts are mirrored in the insufficiently precise evaluation of muscle function and in too many unproven treatment programs. Ironically, active muscle is commonly viewed from a passive aspect, such as various myofascial syndromes and/or trigger points.

One of the first who systematically stressed the importance of muscles in the pathogenesis of low back pain was Hans Kraus. In the 1950s and early 1960s, he noticed that some weakness of the trunk muscles could be demonstrated in about 80% of patients with low back pain (Kraus 1970). Kraus was also one of the first, if not the first, who stressed not only muscle weakness but also muscle tightness in an era when the concept of muscle imbalances was not yet known. Kraus also noticed that dysfunction of the musculoskeletal system starts to develop during childhood. To elucidate this situation he introduced the **Kraus–Weber test** for screening muscle dysfunction (both weakness and tightness) in children. Although more than 50 years old, this test is still valuable.

The role of muscles in pain syndromes of the musculoskeletal system can be considered from several aspects:

- the role of muscles in an acute pain syndrome, both in the pathogenesis as well as in treatment
- the role of muscles in development of chronic pain syndromes
- the role of muscles as a predisposing cause for joint dysfunction
- the role of muscles in prevention of recurrences of acute pain syndromes
- the improvement of muscle function as a basis for a rational treatment program
- alteration of muscle function in reaction to joint dysfunction, and vice versa.

Muscles in acute pain syndromes

Probably the most important factor that contributes to an acute pain syndrome is the increased tone in a muscle which has anatomical or functional relation to the joint in dysfunction (joint blockage). Generally speaking, the joint blockage is in itself painless. It is commonly the added presence of increased muscle tone to the joint dysfunction that leads to a noticeably painful condition. This fact is often ignored, as detailed evaluation of muscle tone is too rarely carried out. This is indeed surprising, as most (if not all) therapeutic techniques used to treat acute pain syndromes are designed to normalize the increased muscle tone.

Muscle tone or hypertonicity are still obscure clinical entities. Although muscle tone changes can be found in almost every patient, there is no accepted consensus of definition either of muscle tone or of its increase. This is true even for a clinical syndrome such as spasticity.

In musculoskeletal medicine, we have to deal with increased muscle tone that develops as a result of dysfunction (but not a structural lesion) of different levels of the nervous system. These types of hypertonicity are usually described as muscle spasm, although the terminology is not unified and different authors use different terminology for the same phenomenon. Certainly the term 'spasm' should not be confused with 'spasticity'.

From the clinical point of view, muscle tone is a combination of at least two phenomena: shortening of contractile muscle fibers and changes of viscoelasticity, i.e. of the connective tissue of the muscle. Both changes are closely associated with alteration of the irritability threshold of motor units. In musculoskeletal disorders we have to deal with both types of increased muscle tone, although under different conditions.

Clinical assessment

The clinical assessment of muscle tone is poorly validated and almost always subjective, as all evaluation techniques are non-specific and measure not only the tension of muscle fibers but of all tissue including the skin and subcutaneous tissue. Practical evaluation of muscle tone is currently by deep layer palpation using the examiner's proprioceptive perception.

At least five types of pathologically increased muscle tone can be clinically differentiated in the functional pathology of the motor system. Each can appear separately or in combination. The differential diagnosis is of a paramount importance as this may influence the therapeutic result.

These five types of increased muscle tone (Janda 1990) may occur due to:

- dysfunction of the limbic system
- dysfunction on the spinal cord segmental level, evidently due to altered function of the interneurons
- impaired coordination of motor unit activation which may finally result in trigger points
- irritation through pain from the musculoskeletal system as well as from the viscera
- muscle tightness (which however is more a result of altered elasticity and will be discussed later in description of muscle imbalance).

The evaluation of muscles can be performed in several ways:

- Evaluation of individual muscles in relation to the joint in dysfunction. This concerns mainly palpation and assessment of muscle spasm and inhibition (muscle pattern), trigger points, and other myofascial syndromes.

- Evaluation of tight and weakened muscles within the framework of muscle imbalance which results in altered biomechanics of the joints, faulty transmission of load across the joint, faulty afferentation from the joint receptors, and ultimately impaired function of joints with pain as a consequence.
- Evaluation of simple movement patterns in which the main interest is concerned with fine muscle coordination and the sequence in which the main muscles are activated.

Whereas evaluation of muscle spasm should be as a rule part of examination of an acute pain syndrome, evaluation of muscle imbalance and movement patterns is reliable only when the acute episode has subsided and the patient is pain free or almost so.

Treatments

To decrease muscle hypertonicity due to limbic dysfunction, a locally oriented treatment is generally fruitless. The treatments of choice are techniques oriented to psychological status, such as the autogenic training of Schulze, Alexander technique, some yoga techniques, or even the Feldenkreis approach. Various techniques are available to decrease the other types of hypertonicity, most of them based on principles of postfacilitation inhibition, muscle relaxation, and finally muscle release. However, the details of the treatment technique vary according to the type of hypertonicity. A detailed description is beyond the scope of this chapter, although the differences in technical performance of the therapeutic procedures are quite substantial and may greatly influence the therapeutic effect.

The length of the effect of postfacilitation inhibition techniques varies. It should therefore be considered as an initial treatment that should be followed by an attempt to improve the function of the whole motor system, such as muscle balance or movement patterns.

Muscle imbalance

Muscle imbalance should be considered as one of the principal factors that adversely influence the biomechanics of a joint and contribute to the deterioration of joint function. Muscle imbalance describes the situation in which some muscles become inhibited and weak, while others become tight, lose their extensibility, and become overactive. Moderately tight muscles are usually stronger than normal; however, in the case of pronounced tightness, a decrease of muscle strength occurs. This decrease of muscle strength is called **tightness weakness** (Janda 1993). The principal problem of a tight muscle is not so much the shortening of contractile muscle fibers but rather the altered elastic properties of the connective tissue within the myofascial unit and the decreased irritability threshold of the tight muscle.

The tendency for some muscles to develop weakness or tightness does not occur randomly. Instead, typical patterns of muscle imbalance can be described. The important point is that the development of muscle imbalance follows typical rules that vary individually by degree, but not which muscle will develop tightness or inhibition. Therefore these patterns can be predicted clinically, and this enables the introduction of preventative measures.

Muscles that are tightness-prone are: triceps surae, rectus femoris, hamstrings, thigh adductors, iliopsoas, tensor fasciae latae, quadratus lumborum, pectoralis major and minor, paraspinal extensors, upper trapezius and levator scapulae, and sternocleidomastoid. Less evident tightness-prone muscles are the suprahyoids, in particular the digastric, masseter, and temporalis. In the upper extremity, the flexor muscles are tightness prone.

On the other hand, muscles that are basically inhibition- or weakness-prone are the dorsiflexors of the foot, vastus medialis, gluteus maximus, medius and minimus, some abdominal muscles, lower stabilizers of the scapula, deep neck flexors (scaleni, longus colli), and deltoid. In the upper extremity, the extensor muscles are inhibition prone.

Although muscle imbalance as a systemic response of different muscle groups has been recognized for several decades, there are still some controversies and some muscles are almost ignored. Thus, for example, we do not have enough knowledge about the differentiation between the abdominal muscles. Evidently the recti are more inhibition prone whereas the obliqui often have a tendency to become overactivated. Another muscle which escaped attention for a long time is the transversus abdominis, which is now considered as an important postural muscle (Richardson et al. 1999). Similarly, the importance of the latissimus dorsi is often underestimated and its postural role is uncertain.

Although muscle imbalance involves the whole body, it develops gradually and predictably either in the pelvic region, where we speak of the pelvic or distal crossed syndrome, or in the shoulder girdle/neck region, where we speak of the proximal or shoulder girdle crossed syndrome (Janda 1979)

If it starts to develop in the pelvic/hip region and spreads out to the upper part of the body, we speak of the **distoproximal development** of muscle imbalance. If it starts to develop in the shoulder/neck area first and gradually spreads out into the distal part of the body, we speak of the **proximodistal generalization** of muscle imbalance.

There is a correlation between the type of generalization of muscle imbalance and clinical symptoms. Patients with proximodistal generalization suffer first from shoulder–neck problems, whereas those with distoproximal development suffer more from back pain. It is interesting that if the muscle imbalance starts to develop in children, it usually follows the proximodistal direction. This corresponds with clinical experience, as symptoms of neck origin such as school headache are much more frequent in children than low back pain (Gutmann 1984).

Proximal crossed syndrome

The proximal crossed syndrome is characterized by development of tightness of the upper trapezius, levator scapulae, sternocleidomastoid, and pectorals and, on the other hand, inhibition of the deep neck flexors (scaleni) and lower stabilizers of the scapula (serratus anterior, rhomboids, middle and lower trapezius). Topographically, when the inhibited and tight muscles are connected, they form a cross. This type of muscle imbalance results in an altered posture of the upper body. A typical forward position of the head can be found, which results in overstress of three critical segments, i.e. the cervicocranial junction, the cervicocervical transition, i.e. the segments C4 and C5 and finally T4 where neck flexion starts. The shoulders are elevated and protracted, altering the resting position of the scapula. This results in an altered position of the axis of the glenoid fossa, which runs more perpendicularly. This increases stresses on the joint capsule and decreases the stability of the joint. As a consequence, altered movement patterns in the shoulder neck region will develop. This situation can be considered as a predisposing factor for development of typical pain syndromes arising from this region (Janda 1994).

All these changes are not only mirrored in an altered posture but also influence the quality of movements of the whole body, most importantly of gait.

Distal crossed syndrome

Tightness of the hip flexors and trunk erectors and inhibition and weakness of the gluteal and abdominal muscles characterize the distal crossed syndrome. Again, a connection of tight and inhibited muscles forms a cross. This imbalance results in an anterior pelvic tilt, increased flexion of the hips and a compensatory hyperlordosis. Again, the result is overstress not only of the hips but of the low back as well.

Layers syndrome

In addition to these two syndromes a layers (stratification) syndrome can be recognized. This syndrome is in principle a combination of the two previous syndromes and can be considered as a response of the muscular system to a long-lasting dysfunction. This development generally means a poor prognosis, and less satisfactory therapeutic results can be expected (Janda 1979). The diagnosis of this syndrome is quick and easy, but important. When the standing patient is observed from the back, the shape of the body looks as if it is composed of layers of bricks. From the bottom, the hamstrings are as a rule hypertrophied and tight, the gluteal muscles hypotonic and loosely hanging and often even atrophied. The paraspinal extensors in the low back area may be atrophied forming a typical groove in the level of lumbar segments, in particular L5–S1. This seems to be paradoxical, as these muscles are usually tightness prone. Although not confirmed experimentally, this groove may be a result of atrophy of the multifidus, as described by Richardson *et al.* (1999). This hypotrophied layer is followed by a hypertrophied layer of muscles in the thoracolumbar junction. This hypertrophy is usually associated with segmental hypomobility at the same level. The interscapular area usually shows a marked hypotrophy which can be recognized as flattening of this region. This hypotrophy is frequently associated with shoulder protraction as a result of imbalance between weakened lower stabilizers of the scapula on one hand and shortened pectorals on the other hand. The most proximal layer is formed by a hypertrophied upper trapezius and levator, mostly together with shortened deep neck extensors. Altogether the result is an altered shape of this area, clinically described as **gothic shoulders**.

From the front this syndrome is less pronounced. The most striking appearance is hypotonic abdominal rectis, whereas the obliques are shortened. This can be seen as a deepening along the lateral edge of the recti.

Evaluation of movement patterns

Evaluation of movement patterns is of a paramount importance, as it gives important information about the quality of function of the motor system and in particular of central nervous system (CNS) motor regulation. The more it is understood that function and dysfunction of joints depends on the quality of motor control, the clearer it becomes that movement pattern evaluation is important.

The term 'movement pattern' describes a chain of conditioned and unconditioned motor reflexes that become fixed. Repetition of movement causes this chain to become fixed. Once fixed, the patterns are difficult to change. Borrowing computer language, the patterning process can be compared to the software, whereas the anatomical pathways are the hardware.

Evaluating movement patterns helps us to estimate the degree of inhibition of muscles that are inhibition prone. Rather than estimating individual muscle strength or weakness, our focus is to determine to what extent, if at all, the particular muscle is included in a specific functional chain.

Basic movement patterns

For diagnostic purposes, in musculoskeletal medicine, six basic movement patterns are used, which cover the main segments of the body (Janda 1996).

The first three movement patterns are related to gait (hip extension, hip abduction, curl-up (sit-up) from the supine position); the others relate to the movements of the shoulder girdle and head (head flexion, prone push up, and shoulder abduction).

Hip extension

This is an important part of the gait cycle. Full hip extension allows minimum anterior tilt of the pelvis in walking and thus reduces the demands and stresses of the low back. The pattern is tested in a prone position. Only the last 10–15° are examined. The most important muscles observed are hamstrings, gluteus maximus, and lumbar and thoracic spinal erectors. The ideal sequence of muscle activation in this chain is: ipsilateral hamstrings, followed by activation of the ipsilateral gluteus and then contralateral lumbar and thoracolumbar erectors. A first sign of an impaired pattern is when the ipsilateral spine erectors precede the activation of the contralateral side. This results in decreased stability of the pelvis and increased anterior pelvic tilt, with overstress of the low back as a consequence. The next step in development of pathology is an increased activity of the thoracolumbar spine erectors and delay of activation of the gluteus maximus, which may in extreme cases even result in its inhibition and inactivity. In patients with chronic low back pain this inhibition (pseudoparesis) is one of the most frequent pathological findings of the muscle system (Janda 1985).

Hip abduction

Hip abduction and the estimation of the quality of function of the hip abductors is another important evaluation as it gives important information about the stabilization of the pelvis in one leg stance and thus about the degree of lateral shift of the pelvis and overstress on the low back segments in the frontal plane. Tested in a side lying position, the patient abducts the leg and the sequence of three major muscles is estimated. The ideal sequence is gluteus medius, followed by activation of the tensor fascia lata and the stabilizing role of the quadratus lumborum. The pathological pattern shows the prevalence of the tensor fascia lata, whereas the activity of the gluteus medius is delayed or even absent. In this situation instead of pure hip abduction a combined movement composed of hip abduction, flexion and external rotation, and usually pelvic rotation produces the movement. This mechanism is described as a tensor mechanism of hip abduction. A worse scenario occurs when the movement is initiated by phasic activity of the quadratus lumborum. In this case instead of stabilizing the pelvis, the pelvis is shifted up and overstresses the low back.

Curl-up from the supine position

This is used to estimate the interplay between the abdominal muscles and the iliopsoas. The estimation of this relationship is important as the tendency is for the abdominal muscles to weaken whereas the iliopsoas is usually strong and tight. The more active the iliopsoas is, the weaker the abdominals become, which again results in an unwanted overstress of the lumbar segments. The psoas paradox is a situation whereby the functional axis of the tight iliopsoas is shifted beyond the axis of the spine and the muscle by bilateral action instead of functioning as a flexor of the spine becomes an extensor of the spine, increasing the lumbar lordosis and the pressures on the lumbar segments.

The test is performed from the supine position. The subject performs an active plantar flexion against the operator's resistance, slight knee flexion pressing the heels toward the plinth. In addition, contraction of the buttocks can be added. During curl-up the range of motion is stopped when the pelvis starts to tilt forward. The normal range is elevation of the thoracic area (at the level of the inferior angle of the scapula) about 5 cm (2 inches) from the plinth.

Push-up

This gives valuable information about the stabilization of the scapula. Stabilization of the scapula is essential for performance of all movements of the upper extremity. The dysfunctional movements indirectly overstress the cervical spine. Under ideal conditions, the stabilization of the scapula during the push-up should be perfect, i.e. the scapula should not move except at the end of the range of movement, when scapula protraction and abduction normally occurs. Under pathological conditions the scapula is shifted into adduction or elevation (or both), and in the most severe situation scapula winging occurs.

When considering muscle function and/or dysfunction in relation to musculoskeletal disorders we mainly think in terms of muscle weakness of some muscle groups or of muscle shortening in a muscle imbalance syndrome. It has gradually become clear that a chronic pain syndrome is a result of impaired programming of movement or impaired central nervous motor control which has caused impaired coordination between various muscle groups.

As already mentioned, muscles represent the only active tissue which can protect the joints. The question remains, however, as to what are the mechanisms which enable the muscles to protect the joint. It is evident now that the strength of the muscle does not give protection to the joint. Strengthening programs do not influence the frequency of recurrences of acute pain, so it is necessary to look at other possibilities. Muscle imbalance is definitely one of them. Ekstrand (1982) has shown convincingly in a series of studies on a group of soccer players that those who were imbalance-prone suffered almost 10 times more frequently from soft issue injuries than those who maintained a reasonably good muscle balance. When he introduced a training program oriented toward reducing muscle imbalance, the frequency of soft issue injuries dropped to average. As a result of these observations, Ekstrand concluded that the best way to prevent soft tissue sport injuries is to restore a reasonably good muscle balance. Similarly, much back pain can be compared to a soft tissue injury and one can make a similar conclusion about treatment.

Muscle balance is not, however, to be considered as the only protective factor. Probably the greatest danger for a joint injury is an uncontrolled or poorly controlled movement in a joint beyond its physiological movement barrier. In such cases the protective function of the muscles is to prevent an excessive range of movement. This depends on the ability of the central nervous system to activate the necessary number of motor units quickly. In other words, one of the important protective function of muscles is an improvement of the motor unit firing pattern. The ability of the muscle to activate its motor units fast, and thus to achieve the required intensity of muscle contraction, seems to be the most essential process. Achieving such a fast activation of motor units is a substantial part of a rational exercise program and seems to be the most effective way to prevent recurrences of acute pain syndromes.

Speed of motor unit firing is thus considered as an important aspect of the role of muscles, not only in treatment but also in the pathogenesis of many pain syndromes.

Muscle patterns

The concept of muscle patterns in relation to joint dysfunction is rather new, although it has been known for a long time that a dysfunction or a structural lesion of a joint is associated with changes in muscles that cross the particular joint. These changes, however, were considered to be a reaction of an isolated muscle. Probably the best known example is a vastus medialis wasting associated with knee pathology. Today it is known, however, that these muscle reactions do not just occur in an isolated muscle but involve a group of muscles in a typical pattern. The muscular reaction is not only inhibition, atrophy and weakness but also muscle spasm. This is true not only for the peripheral joints but for the spinal joints as well. Thus in a joint movement restriction (blockage) we can find that some intrinsic muscles develop spasm whereas others develop inhibition. As these muscles are small and positioned deeply, it is difficult to estimate exactly which muscles respond in which way. This knowledge would facilitate in particular the treatment of segmental instability and improve long-term results of mobilization/manipulation of the segment.

In musculoskeletal medicine probably the most important pattern is that associated with the dysfunction of the sacroiliac joint. On the blocked side there is spasm in the piriformis and iliopsoas and inhibition of the gluteus maximus. The contralateral side develops inhibition of the gluteus medius and minimus. As a sacroiliac dysfunction is in principal a pelvic torsion, a concurrent shearing tension in the pubic symphysis occurs, evidently resulting in irritation of the lower quadrants of the abdominal recti and thus their spasm and tenderness.

The question remains as to which comes first – the muscle or the joint dysfunction. However, improvement of the muscle pattern may – although there are exceptions – correct the joint dysfunction. More investigation in this area is necessary, but improvement of the muscle pattern often can lead to the correction of the joint dysfunction.

Conclusion

The purpose of this chapter is to highlight the enormous importance of muscles in the pathogenesis of musculoskeletal conditions and the need to analyze muscles in much greater detail. This is the case not only in relation to trigger points but also in terms of function. The analysis of function/dysfunction of a single muscle is important, but the coordinated activity of the whole muscle system is in many situations more critical. Any change of position of a joint, active or passive, normal or pathological, is immediately followed by changes within the muscular system. Any change in the CNS is also associated with changes in the muscle system. Muscles can thus be considered as being at a crossroad where any function, either in the periphery or in the CNS, is mirrored. Muscles therefore belong one of the most overstressed systems of the body. We are not always aware that even a mental activity is associated with changes in the muscle system.

In addition, muscles should not be understood only as effectors but as an important source of kinesthetic information. This information regulates the function of the CNS which in turn works out the movement patterns and our motor behavior in general. This fact should be reflected in the treatment of musculoskeletal disorders such as improvement of proprioception and activation of structures that regulate posture and equilibrium (such as cerebellar and vestibular system), as well as activation of the brain stem structures (using primitive locomotion).

References

Ekstrand, J. (1982) *Soccer injuries.* Medical Dissertation No 130, Linkoping, Sweden.

Gutmann, G. (1984) *Die Halswirbelsäule.* G. Fischer Verlag, Stuttgart.

Janda, V. (1979) Die muskulären Hauptsyndrome bei vertebragenen Beschwerden. In: Neumann, H. D., Wolff H. D. (eds) *Theoretische Fortschritte und praktische Erfahrungen der manuellen Medizin.* Konkordia Verlag, Bühl-Baden.

Janda, V. (1985) Pain in the locomotor system – a broad approach. In: Glasgow, E. F., Twomey, L. T., Scull, E. R., Kleyhans, A. M., Idzak R. M. (eds) *Aspects of manipulative therapy.* Churchill Livingstone, Melbourne.

Janda, V. (1990) Differential diagnosis of muscle tone in respect of inhibitory techniques. In: Paterson, J. K., Burn, L., *Back pain.* Kluwer, Dordrecht.

Janda, V. (1993) Muscle strength in relation to muscle length, pain and muscle imbalance. In: Harms-Ringdahl, K. (ed) *Muscle strength.* Churchill Livingstone, Edinburgh.

Janda, V. (1994) Muscles and motor control in cervicogenic disorders' assessment and management. In: Grant, R., *Physical therapy of the cervical and thoracic spine,* 2nd edn. Churchill Livingstone, New York.

Janda, V. (1996) Evaluation of muscle imbalance. In: Liebenson C (Ed). *Rehabilitation of the spine.* Williams and Wilkins, Baltimore, MD.

Kraus, H. (1970) *Clinical treatment of back and neck pain.* Mc Graw-Hill, New York.

Richardson, C., Jull, G., Hodges, P., Hides, J. (1999) *Therapeutic exercise for spinal segmental stabilization in low back pain.* Churchill Livingstone, Edinburgh.

2.2.3 Fibromyalgia: mechanisms and treatment
Hugh Smythe

Overview

More than a decade has passed since the publication of the American College of Rheumatology 1990 Criteria for the Classification of Fibromyalgia (Figure 2.2.19).[1] It should be emphasized that these criteria were designed to identify groups of subjects suitable for research studies. They embodied no theory of causation, so that studies of pathogenesis could proceed without inbuilt bias. Many thousands of studies have been published citing the 1990 Criteria, yielding so much valuable information that they are not likely to be abandoned.

However, the criteria were not optimized for the diagnosis or evaluation of individual patients. Without additional information, they can not form a basis for evaluations of relative severity, or usefully address issues of medicolegal interest. They have helped show that treatment strategies still in common use do not give sustained benefit. Worse, long-term studies from major centers have shown no treatment benefit, by any measure of outcome, at any of the reporting centers.

Why is diagnosis so difficult?

It really becomes quite straightforward, if one obstacle is overcome. We humans are unable to feel deep structures in the body, because they are not represented in our cerebral cortex or in consciousness. A large area in our cerebral cortex is dedicated to our hand. This is needed for the uniquely human skills that involve eye–hand coordination. Any time we wish, we can think of our hand, and its position in space. If we touch a hot stove, we feel at once the site and nature of the injury, and react appropriately. In other words:

- awareness of injury is almost instant
- we accurately recognize the quality of a burn as distinguished from a cut
- the localization is very precise
- the appropriate response is obvious and immediate.

None of this is true of structures that lie deeply in our body. We are unable to feel the fifth bone in the neck or low back. (I choose these, because they are common sites of damage, and sources of pain.) When pain arises in these structures, the brain feels pain, often hours or days later, and cannot identify the site of the injury. The pain must be **referred**; that is, misinterpreted as arising in some other, innocent tissue that shares the same nerve supply. Worse, there may be changes in quality, specific to the area of reference. What is felt as pain in one region, may be a burning, swelling, tingling, or numbness elsewhere. The quality of the sensation is no guide to the nature of the injury. In the absence of timely, anatomically and qualitatively reliable information, the patient has no clues as to the cause and nature of the symptoms.

Many health professionals are just as badly off. It is normal for them to direct their efforts at diagnosis and treatment to the area of complaint; that is, to the normal tissues that – like innocent bystanders – are blamed for symptoms that arise in deep structures of which the patient is unaware. Misdiagnoses are common. If a careful examiner recognizes that the painful 'shoulder', 'hip', or 'knee' is anatomically normal, the persistent complainer may be thought to have coping or neurotic problems, requiring behavioral or psychological therapy. The distraught patient may even agree.

Fibromyalgia: a clinical definition

The location of the symptoms, and quite separate locations of the characteristic sites of tenderness, are best explained by mechanical factors, with pain referred from the spine, specifically from the lower cervical and lower lumbar spine.

In addition, the severity and persistence of the pain, and the presence of a variety of other symptoms such as fatigue, are further influenced by amplifying factors. There are many of these, but most attention is given to nonrestorative sleep and physical deconditioning.

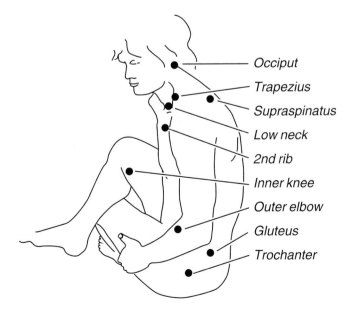

Figure 2.2.19 Sites specified in the ACR criteria.

Occiput

Trapezius

Supraspinatus

Low neck

2nd rib

Inner knee

Outer elbow

Gluteus

Trochanter

Evidence base for referred pain

Classic period – Kellgren and others

Kellgren and his colleagues showed that experimental pain of deep origin is referred, interpreted as arising from structures remote from the stimulus. It must be so:

> The adult has a . . . body image. Though the skin and the more obvious deep structures, such as the peripheral limb joints, are clearly represented within the body image, structures lying deeply inside the trunk and limb girdles are not represented at all.[2]

It follows that

> in every case it is well to preserve an open mind at the outset and to examine carefully all the structures which, by virtue of their segmental innervation, could give rise to the pain under consideration.[3]

One should suspect that a mysterious pain may be referred from some deep structure, but how to proceed? The key is the finding of unexpected localized marked tenderness at anatomically constant sites. Deep and skin tenderness within regions of referred pain had been described by Kellgren and others. The most helpful sites lie in deep structures outside of the distribution of pain, therefore unknown to the patient. To quote Kellgren again,

> The deep tender spot, on the other hand, frequently lies outside the distribution of pain, and the patient is unaware of its existence until it is discovered by the physician. Firm pressure on the deep tender spot produces the steep rise in pain which is characteristic.[3]

Later it was found that there are many such sites, constant in location.[4] These have become the defining criteria for fibromyalgia. With other such sites, they should equally be recognized as markers of referred pain from the spine. They are much more commonly found, in localized distributions, in regional pain syndromes of spinal origin.

Recent studies: evidence of spinal origin

It is well documented that the muscles are normal in fibromyalgia, except for the effects of deconditioning. Similarly, there is no pathology adequate to account for the severity of the tenderness at the 'deep tender spots'. Elevations of concentrations of substance P[5] in the cerebrospinal fluid have been confirmed in at least three other independent studies,[6–8] and elevated levels of other pain neurotransmitters in the cerebrospinal fluid have been found.[9] Blocking studies confirmed that the (pain) stimulus for the release of substance P originated peripheral to the central nervous system. Epidural anesthetic completely abolished resting pain and tender points.[10]

Additionally, three clinical studies may be grouped to make a common point. Buskila and others described increased rates of fibromyalgia following cervical spine injury;[11] all of the extra points required to meet the criteria were in the upper body. With treatment, patients with the C6–7 syndrome[12] had lost all tenderness in the upper body sites defined in the ACR criteria, but remained symptomatic, with a specific but different pattern of upper body tender points. In patients with chronic low back pain studied by Griep and others,[13] the extra points were predominately in the lower body in those meeting criteria for fibromyalgia. Together, these three papers point to specific regions of the spine as the site of origin of the referred pain in fibromyalgia.

Experimentally induced pain

The patterns of referred pain described earlier by Kellgren have been replicated by a variety of experimental studies. Pain produced by distending facet joints in the cervical spine,[14] and by discography of cervical discs,[15] produced similar patterns. Similar symptoms, including frontal headache, were produced by carefully controlled, low-speed rear-end automobile collisions.[16] Discography in the lumbar spine had earlier demonstrated the pain patterns referred from the lower spine.[17] The most common areas of reference were to the low lumbar and trochanteric regions. Spread of pain to the lower extremity, even as far as the foot, occurred following injection of any of the three lower spaces, but was twice as common at L5 as at L3. A less common but important area of reference was to the lower lumbar and inguinal regions, common sites of pain in patients with fibromyalgia.[18]

Role of the nervous system

The nervous system acts as a communications network, and also like the amplifier in a sound system, increasing or modifying the response to a given input. Below the level of consciousness, activation of thalamic nuclei and the cingulate cortex has been shown in chronic pain patients,[19,20] including those with fibromyalgia.[21] Stimulation of thalamic nuclei in turn can produce peripheral symptoms, most strikingly studied in subjects with missing limbs.[22] Neural phenomena also produce long-lasting pain memories, analogous to those responsible for phantom limb pain. (This is too brief an introduction to a rapidly developing area of highly relevant research.)

Treatment strategies

General remarks

In the last decade the concepts of referred pain have vanished from the fibromyalgia literature. The phrase 'we don't know the cause, and there is no cure' is often used or implied. The results of therapy in patients with fibromyalgia have been dismal – and these aspects may be linked. Kellgren's message has been lost; so the nature of the pain in fibromyalgia has become literally inconceivable, unknown to health professionals and to patients. Therapy has been directed to the innocent sites to which pain is referred, or to symptomatic relief, or to coping strategies; and these therapies have been ineffective.[23,24]

Rheumatologists are not comfortable with neck and back problems. The details of the strategies needed are all extremely important, and not intuitively obvious. The literature indicates that our colleagues in other disciplines equally fail to help those with chronic neck and back problems; so that referral is not yet a useful option. Rheumatologists may prefer to avoid fibromyalgia, but they must not. It will remain a major confounder in many of their patients presenting with other conditions. Tender point counts correlate well not just with pain, but with measures of quality of life in other diseases: lupus,[25–27] rheumatoid arthritis,[28] psoriatic arthritis,[29] osteoarthritis,[30] familial Mediterranean fever,[31] AIDS,[32] and other conditions.[33–37]

The ultimate goal of therapy is to restore a high degree of comfort, fitness, and function. However, fibromyalgia patients cannot begin a meaningfully aggressive fitness program until they have a safe neck and a safe back. The treatment program requires two phases. In the first the mechanical factors in the spine must be identified, and specific remedial strategies implemented. The second phase restores fitness and endurance.

Detailed strategies

The details of strategies needed to correct neck and back problems are all extremely important, but not intuitively obvious. The patient can perceive neither the location nor the quality of the problems deep in the spine. In this summary, I can only introduce the level of detail needed. Let us begin with the neck.

Figure 2.2.20 shows the most common pain described by patients with a neck (cervical) problem; at the side and back. When one suggests that upper body pain has its origin in the neck, patients will accept this possibility. If asked where in the neck, they will point to the side and back, where they feel the pain. But massage of this area 'feels good'. It hurts to massage a broken bone, and this characteristic, relief with massage, indicates that the pain is referred from elsewhere. On examination, extreme tenderness, unsuspected by the patient, is found in the bones and attached structures adjacent to the C5–6 and C6–7 disks anterolaterally. All awareness of this tenderness vanishes when the examiner's thumb is removed, and palpation 2 cm above or lateral to this site reveals no comparable tenderness. This precise localization defines both the treatment opportunity and the challenge.

The shoulder problem

When we sleep on our side, the top shoulder is in a natural position, strutted well to the side with our uniquely human, long collar-bone. However, in adapting to the flat surface of our bed, the lower shoulder rises up and forward to the level of the jaw. The attached collar bone and muscle also rise, and block access to the low neck for pillow support (Figure 2.2.21). This is the shoulder/jaw problem. (Sleeping face-down or on the back presents other difficulties.) The unsupported lower neck sags and locks, with tight ligaments and compressed bone.

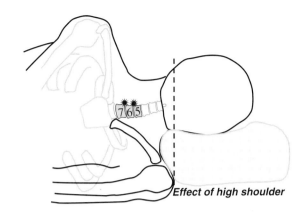

Effect of high shoulder

Figure 2.2.21 During sleep, the high lower shoulder blocks access to the low neck.

Solutions to the shoulder/jaw problem

Delivery of reliable support to the lowest levels of the neck may be difficult. Access to the lowest levels of the front of neck can be obtained by rolling the upper body forward, opening a large space between the jaw and shoulder. For most, all of this works best if the lower arm is behind the back (Figure 2.2.22). This assures smooth support to the lower neck, and to the bones of the upper chest, without uncomfortable pressure on the throat. Breathing is better because the tongue falls forward – a cure for snoring.

To avoid pressure on the lower shoulder and arm, the patient may collapse into a belly-down position, causing the neck to twist. It may help to place a supportive 'arch support' pillow under the rib cage and waist, lifting the trunk enough to take pressure off the hip and shoulder. Finish off with a pillow between the bent knees, and we have a

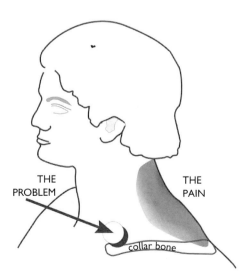

THE PROBLEM

THE PAIN

collar bone

Figure 2.2.20 The key site, the location of marked tenderness deep in the front of the low cervical spine, is free of local symptoms. The pain is felt at the side and back of the neck.

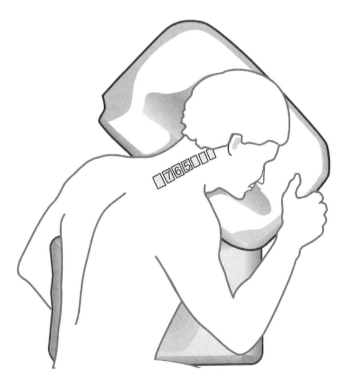

Figure 2.2.22 Rolling the upper body forward.

three-pillow solution. Both knees should be kept well bent to maintain the pelvis, shoulders, and neck in a neutral position.

What to expect?

It is hard to change the habits of a lifetime, so it may take a few weeks for the patient to feel comfortable with neck support. Even if everything is done perfectly, the symptoms may persist for some time. The nervous system is sensitized by chronic pain, and long-standing sensations may continue. Typically, diagnostic tenderness fades before the referred pain. So if symptoms remain, the situation should be reviewed. Perhaps the tenderness is easing as expected, but it may be that the treatment strategy needs refinement.

Back problems

Evolution of the human spine

Unlike other animals, we walk upright. Our ancestors assumed the upright posture 4 million years ago, before the evolution of the modern brain, or hand. Indeed, the upright posture allowed the development of the special skills of our arms and hands, which in turn required the evolution of our brain for integration and control. This freedom was obtained at the cost of developing a hollow curve in our low back, a curve unique to humans.

Figure 2.2.23 shows our spine at birth; comparable to that of all other mammals. There is only one curve, in the chest region, to accommodate our heart and lungs. The low back is straight until we reach 1 year of age, and begin to walk. But babies don't have s trong abdominal muscles. Their cute bellies hang out in front, and their bottoms behind. So their low back becomes hyperextended (Figure 2.2.24).

The strong position for our back is the position of an athlete, with knees, hips, and back partly flexed.

Avoiding locked lumbar hyperextension; role of lower abdominal muscles

If the abdominal muscles are weak, locked lumbar hyperextension is inevitable. Assessment of abdominal muscle strength is therefore an essential part of the evaluation of a patient with recurring or chronic

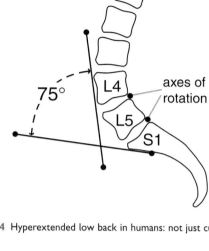

Figure 2.2.24 Hyperextended low back in humans: not just curved, but locked.

low back pain (in the absence of nerve root pressure or severe osteoporosis).

If abdominal muscles are weak, they must be rebuilt, with carefully designed exercises, which must be tough, safe, and pain-free. For safety, make sure that that back is well flexed (like the baby's spine), with knees, hips, trunk, and neck all well bent, and feet held (Figure 2.2.25). The exercise should begin with a pelvic tilt, to make sure the vulnerable low back is curled before the real load is applied. Then the patient should put the chin to the chest, and curl up, keeping the tummy sucked in tight! Especially, the tight muscles and curved lower spinal posture should be maintained while easing back down.

When done properly, this exercise can be (must be) pain-free. The forces through the back are strong, but painless because the spine is in the safe position – not locked in hyperextension. There are three victories. First, the patient has done their first sit-up, and must do it every day for the rest of their life. Secondly, they have learned that there is a safe position for the back, and can carry this information into their postural strategies. Finally, they learn by contrast that there are dangerous positions for their back.

Once patients have developed strong abdominal muscles, we must learn to use them. There is a tremendous cultural prejudice in favor of the erect posture; aristocrats stand upright, and only peasants stand with a bent, but strong back. We teach patients power walking as a simple exercise, with tummy tight and knees bent; but it takes an effort

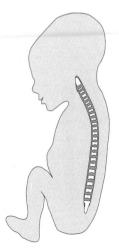

Figure 2.2.23 Babies have no lumbar curve.

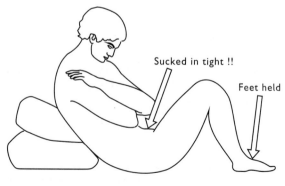

Figure 2.2.25 Abdominal exercise.

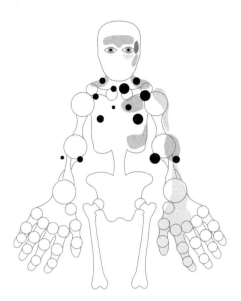

Figure 2.2.26 Pain patterns (shaded) with neck problems. The black dots mark the tender sites.

to overcome the ghostly voice of their parents telling them to 'stand up straight!'

Other causes of lumbar hyperextension may be identified, such as flexed hips, due either to joint disease or to tight surrounding ligaments. A pelvic tilt, due to unequal leg length or spinal problems, may be a correctable factor.

Pain patterns

'Widespread pain' in fibromyalgia is often summarized as 'pain all over', perhaps by the patient. However, if they list or draw their sites of pain carefully, a pattern emerges which is different from but just as characteristic as the pattern of tender sites. This may be incomplete and variable. The pattern is not segmental, and involves regions served by trigeminal nerves, especially the first division, the spinal accessory nerves, as well as cervical nerves. The organizing principle is the neurology of eye–hand coordination. (Figure 2.2.26). No one has yet come complaining of pain in their tongue, although this is very well represented in cortex and body image.

Regional and local pain syndromes

Local or regional pain distributions are far more common than the pattern required in the criteria for fibromyalgia. In these patients regional patterns of tenderness will often point to a spinal origin with referred pain. Let me repeat Kellgren's dictum that

> in every case it is well to preserve an open mind at the outset and to examine carefully all the structures which, by virtue of their segmental innervation, could give rise to the pain under consideration.[3]

If tender points are not assessed, misdiagnoses will certainly occur.

Other 'active' sites

Extra sites are particularly useful in the assessment of patients with regional pain syndromes. The lateral pectoral and inner elbow points

were included in the 1990 Fibromyalgia study and performed well. They were excluded from the ACR Criteria as redundant, providing no information not available from included sites. Their value became apparent later, when they remained tender in treated but still symptomatic patients after the other upper body sites became nontender. They are related to the C6–7 level in the very lowest level of the anterior cervical spine; thus defining both the treatment opportunity and the treatment essentials.[12] In the lower body two additional sites can be very helpful. Tenderness in that medial fat pad about 7 cm distal to the knee joint line performs as well as the specified site proximal to the knee joint. It is commonly attributed to 'anserine bursitis' but extends posterior to the tibia, and its tissue location is better defined by a pinch technique than by pressure against bone. The tenderness here will be in striking contrast to the lack of tenderness at a 'control' site laterally, overlying the neck of the fibula.

A further characteristic site of referred tenderness from the low back is in the instep, very specifically in the origin of the short flexor to the big toe. As is usual, the active site is not central to the area of referred pain, which may be in the nontender forefoot or ankle region.

'Control' sites

Modest deep tenderness, skin tenderness, and reactive hyperemia in sites to which pain was referred were described by Kellgren, and studied extensively by Littlejohn.[38] Lower pain thresholds (assessed by dolorimetry) are found at 'control' sites in groups of patients with fibromyalgia.[39] However, the contrast between the marked tenderness to digital palpation at 'active' sites in regions without local pain, and the lack of tenderness with firmer palpation 2 cm distant is extremely striking. Other 'control' sites have been sought in areas that generally remain nontender, even when they lie in regions to which pain is commonly referred. These sites must be prespecifed. The lower forearm (junction of mid and lower thirds, usually extensor surface), the thumbnail, and the muscles above or below the outer knee, are common such sites. Perhaps the best site is the heel pad, which strikes the ground with the full force of body weight with each step. This topic has been insufficiently studied. Perhaps the best target group would recruit patients with clearly asymmetric pain, rather than patients with fibromyalgia.

Assessment of pain and pain exaggeration

Is the patient exaggerating pain for psychological reasons, wilful or unconscious? The ACR Criteria do not address this issue, which can be very important. We conducted two studies, using experienced but blinded observers, given the task of identifying normal responses or modest, deliberate exaggeration.[40] Sensitivity to deliberate exaggeration was improved from 60 to 90% by adding a prestructured assessment of pain behaviors, to assessments of 'active' and 'control' site tenderness. In discriminating between 'honest' and 'exaggerated' responses, the control sites gave most information, and dolorimetry was much more effective than manual palpation.

Waddell's criteria[41] have often been used, but lack face validity, sensitivity, and interobserver reproducibility.[42]

More unfortunate is the misapplication of techniques developed by committees of the US National Institute of Occupational Safety and Health (NIOSH) to define safe limits for manual lifting in the workplace. These were not designed to be applied to subjects with neck and back pain, and an inability to perform the defined tasks because of pain was never intended to be a measure of inappropriate pain behavior.

Conclusion

The symptom patterns in a patient with fibromyalgia are as characteristic as the patterns of tenderness. Within a short time an examiner can make reasonably accurate guesses about the likely findings on physical examination, and the treatment strategies that are likely to be appropriate.

But it is not enough that the examiner understands the problem. The patient must become equally knowledgeable, a difficult, time-consuming task, given that there will be no intuitive feedback to remind the patient of all of these details. The good news is that they can be much better. The bad news is that only they can implement the necessary strategies. Relief of pain and fatigue does not occur quickly; and then they must fight to improve fitness and endurance. But the victory is theirs.

References

1. Wolfe, F., Smythe, H. A., Yunus, M. B., *et al.* The American College of Rheumatology 1990 Criteria for the classification of fibromyalgia, report of the multicenter trial committee. *Arthritis Rheum*, 1990, **33**, 160–72.

2. Kellgren, J. H. Deep pain sensibility. *Lancet*, 1949, **i**, 943–949.

3. Kellgren, J. H. Pain. Chapter 3 in: Copeman W. S. C. (ed) *Textbook of the rheumatic diseases*, 3rd edn, 1964, E&S Livingstone, Edinburgh, pp. 28–30.

4. Smythe, H. A., Moldofsky, H. Two contributions to understanding of the 'fibrositis' syndrome. *Bull Rheum Dis* 1977, **28**, 928–31.

5. Vaeroy, H., Helle, R., Forre, O., Kass, E., Terenius, L. Elevated CSF levels of substance P and high incidence of Raynaud phenomenon in patients with fibromyalgia: new features for diagnosis. *Pain*, 1988, **32**, 21–26.

6. Russell, I. J., Orr, M. D., Littman, B. *et al.* Elevated cerebrospinal fluid levels of substance P in patients with the fibromyalgia syndrome. *Arthritis Rheum*, 1994, **37**, 1593–601.

7. Bradley, L., Alarcón, G. S., Sotolongo, A *et al.* Cerebrospinal fluid (CSF) levels of substance P (SP) are abnormal in patients with fibromyalgia (FM) regardless of traumatic or insidious pain onset. *Arthritis Rheum*, 1998, **41** (supplement 9) S256, Abstract 1341.

8. Welin, M., Bragee, B., Nyber, F., Kritansson, M. Elevated substance P levels are contrasted by a decrease in met-enkephalin-arg-phe levels in CSF from fibromyalgia patients. *J Musculoskel Pain*, 1995, **3**(suppl #1) 4, (abstract).

9. Giovengo, S. L., Russell, I. J., Larson, A. A. Increased concentrations of nerve growth factor in cerebrospinal fluid of patients with fibromyalgia. *J Rheumatol*, 1999, **26**, 1564–9.

10. Bengtsson, M., Bengtsson, A., Jorfeldt, L. Diagnostic epidural opioid blockade in primary fibromyalgia at rest and during exercise. *Pain*, 1989, **39**, 171–80.

11. Buskila, D., Neumann, L., Vaisberg, G., Alkalay, D., Wolfe, F. Increased rates of fibromyalgia following cervical spine injury. *Arthritis Rheum*, 1997, **40**, 446–52.

12. Smythe, H. A. The C6–7 syndrome – clinical features and treatment response. *J Rheumatol*, 1994, **21**, 1520–6.

13. Griep, E. N., Boersma, J. W., Eef, G. W. M., Lentjes, A., de Kloet, E. R. Function of the hypothalamic-pituitary-adrenal axis in patients with fibromyalgia and low back pain. *J Rheumatol*, 1998, **25**, 1374–81.

14. Dwyer, A., Aprill, C., Bogduk, N. Cervical zygapophyseal joint pain patterns. I: a study in normal volunteers. *Spine*, 1990, **15**, 453–7.

15. Schellhas, K. P., Smith, M. D., Gundry, C. R., Pollei, S. R. Cervical discogenic pain. *Spine*, 1996, **21**, 300–12.

16. Brault, J. R., Wheeler, J. B., Siegmund, G. P., Brault, E. J. Clinical response of human subjects to rear-end automobile collisions. *Arch Phys Med Rehabil*, 1998, **79**, 72–80.

17. Fernström, U. A discographical study of ruptured lumbar intervertebral discs. *Acta Chir Scand*, 1960, Suppl 258.

18. Katz, R. S., Ruderman, E. M., Fraser, J., Soltes, B. Pelvic tenderness in women with chronic pelvic pain correlates with fibromyalgia syndrome (FMS) tenderness. *Arthritis Rheum*, 1999, **42**, No.9 (suppl). S150, Abstract 480.

19. Hutchison, W. D., Davis, K. D., Lozano, A. M., Tasker, R., Dostrosky, J. O. Pain-related neurones in the human cingulate cortex. *Nature Neurosci*, 1999, **2**, 403–5.

20. Davis, K. D., Taub, E., Duffner, F. *et al.* Activation of the anterior cingulate cortex by thalamic stimulation in patients with chronic pain: a positron emission tomography study. *J Neurosurg*, 2000, **92**, 64–9.

21. Bradley, L. A., Sotolongo, A., Alarcon, G. S. *et al.* Dolorimeter stimulation elicits abnormal pain sensitivity and regional cerebral blood flow (rCBF) in the right cingulate cortex (CC) as well as passive coping strategies in non-depressed patients with fibromyalgia (FM). *Arthritis Rheum*, 1999, **42**, No.9 (suppl).S343, Abstract 1625.

22. Davis, K. D., Kiss Z. H. T., Luo, L., Tasker, R., Lozano, A. M., Dostrosky, J. O. Phantom sensations generated by thalamic stimulation. *Nature*, 1988, **391**, 385–7.

23. Wolfe, F., Anderson, J., Harkness, D. *et al.* Health status and severity in fibromyalgia: results of a six-center longitudinal study. *Arthritis Rheum*, 1997, **40**, 1571–9.

24. Carette, S., Bell, M., Reynolds, J., *et al.* Comparison of amitriptyline, cyclobenzaprine, and placebo in the treatment of fibromyalgia. A randomized, double-blind clinical trial *Arthritis Rheum*, 1994, **37**, 32–40.

25. Urowitz, M., Gladman, D., Gough, J., MacKinnon, A. Fibromyalgia is a major contributor to quality of life in lupus. *J Rheumatol*, 1997, **24**, 2145–8.

26. Smythe, H. A., Lee, D., Rush, P., Buskila, D. Tender shins and steroid therapy. *J Rheumatol*, 1991, **18**, 1568–72.

27. Abu-Shakra, M., Mader, R., Langevitz, P., Codish, S., Neumann, L., Buskila, D. Quality of life in systemic lupus erythematosus: a controlled study. *J Rheumatol*, 1999, **26**, 306–9.

28. Moldofsky, H., Chester, W. J. Pain and mood patterns in patients with rheumatoid arthritis. *Psychosomat Med*, 1970, **32**, 309–318.

29. Blackmore, M. G., Gladman, D. D., Husted, J., Long, J. A., Farewell, V. T. Measuring health status in PsA: the Health Assessment Questionnaire and its modification. *J Rheumatol*, 1995, **22**, 886–93.

30. Moldofsky, H., Lue, F. A., Saskin, P. Sleep and morning pain in primary osteoarthritis. *J Rheumatol*, 1987, **14**, 124–128.

31 Langevitz, P., Buskila, D., Finkelstein, R., Zaks, N., Smythe, H. A., Pras, M. Fibromyalgia in familial Mediterranean fever. *J Rheumatol*, 1994, **21**, 1335–7.

32. Buskila, D., Gladman, D. D., Langevitz, P., Urowitz, S., Smythe, H. A. Fibromyalgia in Human Immunodeficiency Virus infection. *J Rheumatol*, 1990, **17**, 1202–6.

33. Goldenberg, D. L., Simms, R. W., Geiger, A., Komaroff, A. L. High frequency of fibromyalgia in patients with chronic fatigue seen in a primary care practice. *Arthritis Rheum*, 1990, **33**, 381–7.

34. Buskila, D., Press, J., Gedalia, A., *et al.* Assessment of nonarticular tenderness and prevalence of FS in children. *J Rheumatol*, 1993, **20**, 368–70.

35. Olschewski, E., Zangger, P., Mahomed, N., Smythe, H. A., Bogoch, E. R. Tender points are associated with unexplained pain in patients with technically satisfactory total hip arthroplasty. *J Bone Joint Surg*, 1997, **79B**, suppl 1 (abstract). 77.

36. Fallon, J., Bujak, D. I., Guardino, S. D., Weinstein, A. The Fibromyalgia Impact Questionnaire is useful to evaluate physical impairment in patients with post Lyme syndrome. *Arthritis Rheum*, 1996, **39** (no. 9, supplement), S316, abstract 1730.

37. Crook, J., Moldofsky, H. The clinical course of musculoskeletal pain in empirically derived groupings of injured workers. *Pain*, 1996, 67, 427–33.

38. Littlejohn, G. O., Weinstein, C., Helme, R. D. Increased neurogenic inflammation in fibrositis syndrome. *J Rheumatol*, 1987, **14**, 1022–5.

39. Smythe, H. A., Buskila, D., Urowitz, S., Langevitz, P. Control and 'fibrositic' tenderness, comparison of two dolorimeters. *J Rheumatol*, 1992, **19**, 768–71.

40. Smythe, H. A., Gladman, A., Mader, R., Peloso, P., Abu-Shakra, M. Strategies for assessing pain and pain exaggeration, controlled studies. *J Rheumatol*, 1997, **24**, 1622–29.

41. Waddell, G., Pilowsky, I., Bond, M. R. Clinical assessment and interpretation of abnormal illness behaviour in low back pain. *Pain*, 1989, **39**, 41–53.

42 McCombe, P. F., Fairbank J. C. T., Cockersole, B. C., Pynsent, P. B. Reproducibility of physical signs in low-back pain. *Spine*, 1989, **14**, 908–18.

2.2.4 **Neurodynamics**

David Butler

Optimal communication and response in all situations are the main functions of the nervous system. The complexity of electrochemical communication is remarkable enough, but the fact that it must be achieved in a sensitive, reactive, and plastic structure which is continually sliding, stretching, rubbing, and angulating during movement is still poorly acknowledged. This concept of mechanical aspects of the nervous system, or **neurodynamics** (Shacklock 1995) is relatively new, and has only recently been incorporated into medicine and physiotherapy, although by no means universally (e.g. Breig 1978, Elvey 1986, Maitland 1986, Butler 1989, 1991, Rydevik *et al.* 1989, Selvaratnam *et al.* 1994, Shacklock 1995, Gifford 1998a). Orthopaedic and neurology texts and reviews frequently recommend a basic examination of the physical abilities of the nervous system (e.g. Maitland 1986, Brukner and Khan 1993, Goldner and Hall 1997, Klein and Garfin 1997, Magee 1997); however, skilled clinicians can take a neurodynamic examination further and include it in management.

Clinicians and patients can easily visualize the mechanical actions of muscles and joints, but not of the nervous system. This chapter is an introduction to the physical aspects of the nervous system. It also provides an anatomical and biological foundation for a clinical evaluation of the nervous system.

Gross movements: the nervous system must adapt

Although the nervous system biologically controls movement, it must also physically adapt during movement and perhaps mechanically contribute to the limitation of some movements. For example, from spinal extension to flexion, the spinal canal of a healthy individual may increase in length by up to 7–9 cm (Inman and Saunders 1942, Louis 1981). During a straight leg raise of 90°, the sciatic nerve must somehow adapt to change in length of tissues around the nerve of at least 12% (Beith *et al.* 1995). When you lift your arm up from your side, the tissues encircling the median nerve could be nearly 20% longer (Zoech *et al.* 1991). Somehow the nervous system must physically adapt to these movements with minimal inference to electrochemical conduction.

Yoga, tai chi, athletic and dance stretching, and martial arts all involve varying degrees of adaptation of the nervous system as well as of other tissues. Neurodynamics is certainly not new. It is the attempt to include it in manual therapy models that is.

An operating definition of a neurodynamic test such as the straight leg raise is 'a movement which aims to test the mechanics and sensitivity of a portion of the nervous system'. It is therefore a test of the dynamic anatomy of the nervous system, thus of neural structures, relationships to surrounding structures, and the sensitivity of the peripheral and central nervous systems.

Neuroanatomical basis for neurodynamics

There are revealing design features in the nervous system which point to significant mechanical abilities. Design features have been detailed elsewhere (e.g. Sunderland 1978, Lundborg 1988, Butler 1991, 2000, Rossitti 1993, Rempel *et al.* 1999). A summary follows.

Neural connective tissues – design for movement

The connective tissues of the nervous system provide the neurones, supporting tissues, and fluids with protection from undesired forces and chemicals. The neural connective tissues form the basis of a continuous tissue tract from peripheral nerves to the spinal and cranial dura mater.

Central nervous system connective tissues

The dura mater, forming a continuous enclosed tube, is the toughest and strongest of the meninges. It consists primarily of collagen fibres and some elastin fibres aligned in the longitudinal axis, but also obliquely and in layers (Rogers and Payne 1961, Tunturi 1977, Patin *et al.* 1993). There is twice as much elastin in the posterior dura as in the anterior (Nagakawa *et al.* 1994), thus allowing for the greater loads on posterior dura during spinal flexion. Spinal dura mater has considerable strength in the longitudinal axis, more than in the transverse axis (Haupt and Stoept 1978, Zarzur 1996). If dura mater tears, for example from trauma or durotomy, it may tear in the longitudinal axis.

The arachnoid and pia mater, far more delicate than the dura, are comprised of a mesh or lattice of collagen fibres. This structure allows some 'telescoping' during elongation and compressive movements (Breig 1978), thus providing some protection to the neural tissues they surround. The pia mater is a continuous bilayered tissue enveloping the cord and brain, providing a barrier control between neural tissue and the cerebrospinal fluid. The arachnoid mater lines the inner dural theca. The many 'tight cell' junctions in the arachnoid and pia mater point to their role as a controlling barrier to fluid and ion movement (Haines *et al.* 1993).

Between the arachnoid and the pia mater is the subarachnoid space, filled with flowing cerebrospinal fluid (CSF). In addition to its nutritive role, CSF also cushions the central nervous system (CNS) by providing shock absorption during rapid movements and by allowing some mechanical buoyancy (Louis 1981). The CSF cushion is sometimes lost during dural puncture and consequently traction forces on cranial dura and blood vessels increase and may cause headache (Spielman 1982, Vandam 1992).

Peripheral nervous system connective tissues

Peripheral nerves are tough, strong, and by necessity mobile. The tissues of the connective tissue sheath (epineurium, perineurium, and endoneurium) guide and protect the conducting tissues during movement. Approximately half of a peripheral nerve is connective tissue sheath, but the range is broad: from 21% in the ulnar nerve at the elbow to 81% in the sciatic nerve at the buttocks. (Sunderland 1978). This variation is probably an adaptive protective mechanism, as the ulnar nerve is well protected from mechanical forces in the ulnar groove, whereas the sciatic nerve needs some protection, given the time humans spend sitting on it.

The epineurium is the outermost structure of the sheath, embedding and cushioning the fascicles. It surrounds bundles of nerve fibres which are in turn surrounded by the perineurium. Interfascicular gliding is necessary when a nerve has to bend (Millesi 1986) which the ulnar nerve does to a great extent during flexion of the elbow. Thus peripheral nerve has an extraneural (nerve and surrounding tissue) and an intraneural (fascicle on fascicle) gliding surface. A well-developed lymphatic network exists in the epineurium, but not in the perineurium and the endoneurium, meaning that oedema which gains access to the perineurium is difficult to disperse (Sunderland 1978).

The perineurium is the connective tissue sheath surrounding bundles of nerve fibres, thus forming fascicles. It is multilayered, with no basal lamina between perineurial cells, thus there are overlapping cells and 'tight junctions' (Thomas and Olsson 1984) similar to those seen in the arachnoid mater. Perineurium also has a very important role as a diffusion barrier, controlling fluids and ions which come in contact with the neural tissues (Lundborg 1988). Myelinated fibres or groups of unmyelinated fibres are surrounded by the endoneurium. This is a distensible elastic structure made up of closely packed collagen tissue. It maintains a constant environment for the nerve fibres, including constant pressure and content of the endoneurial fluid, all necessary for health (Sunderland 1978, Lundborg 1988).

Surrounding the entire nerve is a loose connective sheath, the mesoneurium. This tissue allows a nerve to glide alongside adjacent tissues, as well as contracting in an 'accordion like arrangement' (Smith 1966). This gliding layer obviously facilitates movement. It is probably the tissue responsible for the hard 'cordlike' feel of a nerve slipping away when palpated. Early movement after surgery or trauma would seem essential to keep these tissues moving and minimize scar formation (Mackinnon and Dellon 1988, Nathan et al. 1995).

Innervation

It would be a healthy advantage for an organ with such mechanical abilities as the nervous system to be sensitive to movement and not reliant on the neighbouring tissues to alert the body to the presence of potential injury. In addition, a tissue that is injured requires adaptable sensitivity to allow the most appropriate behaviour for healing. The innervated connective tissues of the nervous system partly fulfil this role.

The meninges, especially the dura, are richly innervated. The dura of the posterior cranial fossa and the spinal canal is innervated by the sinuvertebral nerve which passes via the foramen magnum from the upper three cervical segments. Sinuvertebral nerves are tiny, hardly visible to the unaided eye. They emerge distal to the dorsal root ganglion from a union of a somatic root off the ventral ramus and a sympathetic root from the grey rami communicantes, or a sympathetic ganglion. The nerve then returns into the spinal canal through the intervertebral foramen (Hovelaque 1927, Bridge 1959, Kimmel 1961, Edgar and Nundy 1966, Edgar and Ghadially 1976, Bogduk

1983, Cuatico et al. 1988, Groen et al. 1988). The sinuvertebral nerve also innervates the nerve root sheath, periosteum, epidural tissues, and spinal canal.

Sinuvertebral nerves are designed for movement. The nerve fibres in the dura are in coiled bundles allowing significant forces to be placed through the dura before the nerve endings are excited (Groen et al. 1988).

There are some reports of pain produced from noxious stimuli to the dura mater (Penfield and McNaughton 1940, Wirth and van Buren 1971). A recent immunohistochemical study demonstrated populations of substance P, calcitonin gene-related peptide (CGRP), and tyrosine hydroxylase reactive nerve fibres in dura and the longitudinal ligaments in rabbits, providing more evidence of the dura as a pain source (Kallakuri et al. 1998). While nociceptive fibres seem likely, the dura also contains sympathetic fibres (Cavallotti et al. 1998, Kallakuri et al. 1998) which, in the right circumstances, may also enhance nociceptive activity.

Less well studied than the larger dura is the innervation of the leptomeninges. Bridge (1959) noted nerves running longitudinally in the pia mater though not the arachnoid. Janig and Koltzenburg (1990) also described pial innervation. There are mechanoreceptors of unknown function in the pial ligaments (Parke and Whalen 1993), the small ligaments that attach the anterior spinal artery to the linea splendens.

Sunderland (1978) commented that the innervation of the connective tissue sheath of peripheral nerve was an area worthy of greater experimental attention, and recently more attention has been given to it. These tissues have an intrinsic innervation, the nervi nervorum which arises from local axonal branching. There is also an extrinsic vasomotor innervation by autonomic fibres from approximating perivascular plexuses (Hromada 1963, Thomas and Olsson 1984, Dhital et al. 1986, Lincoln et al. 1993). The findings from Hromada's original work using silver staining have been confirmed by modern immunoreactivity techniques. Bove and Light (1995) demonstrated that the epineurium and perineurium contain a plexus of fine unmyelinated nerve fibres containing the neuropeptides CGRP and peripherin.

The connective tissues of the dorsal roots and dorsal root ganglia are innervated by fibres originating in the dorsal root ganglia (Pedersen et al. 1956, Hromada 1963, Edgar and Nundy 1966, Parke and Watanabe 1990). The unmistakable and simple message is that, like any innervated connective tissue, they may initiate impulses that may lead to the perception of pain when given adequate mechanical and or chemical stimulation. However, the exact clinical presentations and circumstances of pain perception can only be hypothesized.

Neural attachments to surrounding structures

The nervous system has a variable anatomical relationship with surrounding tissues. There is variability in the kind of tissue, amount of movement, and space around the neural tissue. With pathological changes in surrounding tissues, for example the chemical and mechanical consequences of disc degeneration or fluid in a nerve bed, neural tissue may be influenced.

The cranial dura mater adheres tightly to the suture levels at the foramen magnum (Murzin and Goriunov 1979), and at the caudal end the external filum terminale, which is very thin and elastic, attaches the dural theca to the coccyx. The dura mater is also anchored along its anterior aspect to the anterior and anterolateral aspect of the spinal canal by meningovertebral ligaments, sometimes referred to as Hoffman's ligamants or dural ligaments (Hofmann 1898, Spencer *et al.* 1983, Tencer *et al.* 1985, Wiltse *et al.* 1993, Bashline *et al.* 1996).

A connection exists between the rectus capitis posterior muscle and the dura mater, between the occiput and the atlas. This connection may assist in limiting dural infolding during extension (Hack *et al.* 1995, Rutten *et al.* 1997) or could also act to provide static and dynamic proprioceptive feedback to the CNS, particularly since this muscle contains a large number of proprioceptors (Rutten *et al.* 1997). There is also a continuous connection between the posterior dura mater and the ligamentum flavum (Blomberg 1986).

Neural/non-neural connections in the peripheral nervous system have not had as much experimental attention. It appears that there are variations in the strength of connections. For example, the common peroneal nerve is quite firmly attached at the head of the fibula, more so than in neighbouring areas.

The vasa nervorum moves and stretches to support the nervous system

Neurones are particularly bloodthirsty cells. Anatomical adaptations in the vasa nervorum allow blood supply in most postures and during most movements, usually by feeder vessel length reserve or compensatory intraneural and extraneural back-up systems. Further details of the mechanical design of the circulatory supply to the nervous system may be found elsewhere (Breig 1978, Parke and Watanabe 1986, Lundborg 1988, Dommisse 1994).

The vascular system is not immune to elongation forces. Arrest of blood flow will begin when a peripheral nerve is elongated approximately 8%, and complete arrest will occur at around 15% (Lundborg and Rydevik 1973, Ogata and Naito 1986); this induced hypoxia may cause pain. The dynamism of the system means that a shunting of blood and variations in supply occurs with every movement.

Neurones unfold, unravel, and stretch

Neurophysiology texts usually portray neurones and the tracts of the spinal cord as a straight lines to and from the brain, but this does not do justice to neuronal cytomechanics.

Neurones in the spinal cord are arranged in folds and spirals which straighten as the spinal cord elongates and refolds as the cord shortens. This mechanism, along with some movement in relation to the spinal canal, protects the cord during movement (Breig 1978). Similar adaptive mechanisms have been reported in the feline spinal cord (Transfeldt and Simmons 1982). There is a similar folding in the peripheral nervous system, though not as marked (Sunderland 1978). Peripheral nerves also have an internal plexiform arrangement of fascicles which allows some force dissipation. In addition, a structure such as the brachial plexus could also be viewed as allowing force dissipation. A tensile force on the ulnar nerve, for example, may be transmitted to five or six roots.

Excursion and strain in the nervous system

Most of the research on the mechanics of the nervous system has been obtained from cadavers (e.g. Gelberman *et al.* 1998, Kleinrensink *et al.* 2000), in animals (e.g. Lew *et al.* 1994) and novel *in vitro* experiments in humans (e.g. McLellan and Swash 1976). There have also been recent contributions from MRI (e.g. Greening *et al.* 1999, Muhle *et al.* 1998), myelography, and surgical observations. The major methodological difficulty is that it is rare for any researcher to state the starting position for experimentation. For example, if carpal tunnel neurodynamics is studied, the position of the rest of the body should be controlled and recorded. For a full summary of research on neurodynamics in specific body areas, see Butler (2000)

Brieg's work on the neurodynamics of the central nervous system is unsurpassed (Breig 1960, 1978, Breig *et al.* 1966); see also a review by Rossitti (1993). Because of the continuous nature of the nervous system, cervical movements have a significant mechanical effect on brain structures. When the head and spine are moved, the shape of the brain stem, ventricles, and spinal cord changes (Breig 1960, 1978). The variation in the length of the brain stem between flexion and extension is between 0.8 cm and 1.4 cm, and the cranial nerves are pulled tight to their exit zones in the base of the skull (Breig 1960).

The spinomedullary angle of the cord undergoes considerable change during flexion and extension, ranging from 1 to 32° (mean 14°) in asymptomatic subjects (Doursounian *et al.* 1989). The cervical cord flattens on the skeleton of the spinal canal. The centrode of the spinal motion segment is close to the middle of the disc (Gertzbein *et al.* 1985). With the spinal canal approximately 7 cm longer in flexion than in extension, it is obvious that spinal flexion, by elongating the canal, will place a strain on the contained cord, roots, and meninges. These tissues follow the path of least resistance and will move anteriorly in the spinal canal.

The transmission of forces is quite remarkable. Cervical flexion will cause mechanical changes in the lumbar spine and further (Breig 1978). Spinal lateral flexion leads to a shorter spinal canal and cord on the concave side and elongation on the convex side.

Peripheral nervous system adaptations can be quite dramatic. For example, the median nerve can slide up to 2 cm in relation to surrounding tissues in the upper arm (McLellan and Swash 1976, Wright *et al.* 1996). Pressures in nerves during movement will double, even quadruple (e.g. Pechan and Julis 1975), often slowing or stopping blood flow to segments of neural tissue. The most dramatic neural movement occurs when the ulnar nerve subluxes during elbow flexion, something that occurs in approximately 15% of the population (Childress 1975, Rayan *et al.* 1992).

The ulnar nerve in the cubital tunnel provides an example for the rest of the body. During elbow flexion, the nerve will be tractioned, flattened, and change in area by up to 50% (Gelberman *et al.* 1998). The cubital tunnel is also up to 50% smaller in flexion than in extension (Apfelberg and Larson 1973, Gelberman *et al.* 1998). The physical challenges to the nerve are not only on elbow flexion. On extension, the ulnar nerve may buckle a little when the elbow is in full extension (Gelberman *et al.* 1998). This may be more of a problem if the nerve is anteriorly transposed. Not only must a nerve be physically healthy, it must be able to adapt to dynamic surroundings.

Nerve roots, like the spinal cord, receive much of their nutrition from the CSF. Like the rest of the nervous system, nerve roots are not static. They move within the CSF and in relation to surrounding tissues despite variable dural ligaments. As Weinstein (1997) suggests, it is this 'micromotion' that allows the root to keep its mechanical properties and receive nutrition, something lost with tissue irritation and resultant fibrosis from disc pathology or stenosis.

Some roots may go to the sympathetic nervous system, particularly where the trunk is separate from the somatic nervous system. Interested readers are referred to cadaveric studies by Nathan (1987) and Giles (1992) and associated hypotheses (Butler and Slater 1994, Slater *et al.* 1994).

Sensitivity

So far, mechanical aspects of the nervous system have dominated the chapter. A neurodynamic test, like any physical test, evaluates mechanics and sensitivity related to the test. The issue of sensitivity to movement is complex, not least because people may have quite marked pathological changes in neural tissues yet experience no pain (e.g. Neary and Eames 1975). The computation of whether an input hurts or not and which pain behaviours are selected is extremely complex, although answers are beginning to come from the rapidly growing field of neurobiology. Sensitivity to neurodynamic tests can be explored in terms of peripheral and central sensitivity and the links between them.

Peripheral sensitivity

Any structure with a nerve supply is a candidate for a pain source. Therefore, sensitivity to physical distortion may occur from the innervated connective tissue sheaths of the nervous system. The nature of this sensitivity is unknown, although there are suggestions that symptoms would be similar to any other innervated connective tissue (Sunderland 1978, Asbury and Fields 1984, Butler 1991). Damage and changes to the long conducting fibres are more likely to cause persistent and troublesome neuropathic pain.

When a peripheral nerve is partially injured, a process of sensitization, evoked pain, and sometime spontaneous activity in nociceptive and other afferent fibres can occur. This process is well summarized by Devor and Seltzer (1999). Nerve trunks usually conduct impulses, not generate them, but damaged and regenerating nerve trunks and ganglia may initiate impulses. The injured or structurally altered sites are known as abnormal impulse generating sites (AIGS) or ectopia. Known stimuli which can fire an AIGS include mechanical, metabolic, noradrenaline, and temperature stimuli. The biological changes that allow this are at the axolemma and seem to be related to changes in kind, number, and activity of sodium channels. Pathological processes where this occurs could include sprouting neurites, neuroma development and demyelination. Ion channels are usually inserted into the axolemma at the nodes of Ranvier and it appears that loss of myelin, as in injury or regenerating axons, creates available space for ion channel insertion. Many of these sites will be sensitive to mechanical forces such as Tinel's test, neurodynamic tests, or movements which close down and pinch on nerve (Devor and Seltzer 1999).

Alpha-adrenoreceptor expression on injured axolemma may also occur after injury, allowing noradrenaline to contribute to depolarization or raise the generator potential (Chung *et al.* 1993, McLachlan *et al.* 1993). The dorsal root ganglion needs special consideration here. It has an inherent mechanosensitivity and great potential for adrenosensitivity and will respond with injury elsewhere along the nerve trunk. Much research remains to be done in this area (Devor 1999). These processes are what must underlie the sensitivity to movement during loading or compressions on nerves, and should allow explanations of many pain and movement behaviours.

There are clear messages here for clinicians. First, the connective tissues and particularly the receptor upregulation in the long fibres provides an anatomical substrate for symptoms on a neurodynamic test. The most common scenario would be pain on movement or antalgic postures (e.g. elevated shoulder, ipsilateral lists) as patients attempt to unload pressures on nerve. Peripheral neuropathies such as carpal tunnel syndrome often behave with a clear on/off behaviour, but this is not always the case. The dorsal root ganglia may be the culprits here, contributing to ongoing pain, and afterdischarging from small movements, sustained postures, or the presence of stress-related chemicals (Devor 1999). All aware clinicians must have noted the clinical link between depression/anxiety and neuropathic pain. The recent work on adrenoreceptor upregulation provides an anatomical base for that. Given that the half-life of ion channel turnover is 1–3 days (Schmidt and Catterall 1986), a reasonable proposal is that peripheral sensitivity may be decreased by removing the reasons for elevated blood and tissue noradrenaline levels and also environmental forces upon nuclear machinery to manufacture adrenoreceptors. This may be as simple as skilled interaction which reduces fear by providing accurate diagnoses, goals, prognoses, and a good physical examination.

Central sensitivity

After cerebrovascular accident and trauma, the CNS is usually more sensitive to input (Bowsher 1996). However, there is a growing awareness that pathological changes in the peripheral nervous system, such as ectopia, are likely to have consequences for the sensitivity of CNS pain transmission neurones (Hardy *et al.* 1952, Koltzenburg *et al.* 1992, LaMotte *et al.* 1991, Woolf 1991, Torebjörk *et al.* 1992, Coderre *et al.* 1993). See Doubell *et al.* (1999) or Dubner and Basbaum (1994) for a summary.

An afferent barrage, especially in the more glandular-like C fibres, causes the release of excitatory amino acids such as glutamate and neuropeptides such as substance P into the dorsal horn. Second-order cells respond by increasing sensitivity (reducing firing threshold and increasing responsiveness) and also expanding their receptive fields, all dependent on internal controls such as the descending endogenous pain control systems. This is a potentially dangerous state. If altered afferent input persists – and particularly, it seems, if the existing neural architecture is sensitive as could occur from various external and internal stressors – long-lasting morphological changes could occur. This includes inhibitory interneurone death by amino acid toxicity, permanently upregulated CNS neurones, persistence of excitatory neurotransmitters at synaptic clefts, inappropriate dendritic sprouting, and synaptic uncoupling. The net effect is exaggeration of inputs. See Doubell *et al.* (1999) for a summary. The persistence of this central sensitization appears to be dependent on continued nociceptor input (LaMotte *et al.* 1992) such as that provided from ectopic or persistent inflammation. It appears that the greater the severity of afferent input, the greater the CNS changes (Svendsen *et al.* 1998).

Note that changes in CNS sensitivity are normal. The CNS becomes sensitive after any injury, and this is a normal process to assist healing. However, when the injury and circumstances improve, the CNS sensitivity level slowly reverts, although some CNS memories of the injury and the modes of responses which seemed best are probably left for future reference. The clinical links to neurodynamics are discussed below.

Integrating neurodynamic concepts into the clinic

The continuum of the nervous system

Neck movements will move neural tissue in the lumbar spine (Breig 1978), hand movements pull and slide neural tissue in the upper arm (McLellan and Swash 1976). Neural tissue continuity is a basic premise of a neurodynamic assessment. Consider a person who has hamstring area pain in the slumped position with knee extension. (The slump test is described in Chapter 4.3.7.) As many clinicians may have noted by now, cervical extension (often minimal) usually relieves the posterior knee leg pain, and the subject or patient is able to extend the knee further. This process is frequently more dramatic for patients with spinal/hamstring area problems. The physiological and anatomical mechanisms behind this remotely derived pain relief are not known, but it seems to be due to a combination of neural movement, pressure-induced ischaemic neurones, and altered input into the CNS. The implication of the continuity is that mechanical, electrical, and chemical changes in one part of the nervous system may have far-reaching effects on other parts and that the mechanical, electrical, and chemical events are related.

Relationship to joint axes

Because of the varying relationship of the nervous system to the joint axes, it is self-evident that all limb and trunk movements will place mechanical forces upon neural tissues. There are three main clinical consequences of this:

- First, when listening to a patient's history, particularly of the mechanics of injury and movements that ease or aggravate, give some thoughts to forces on neural tissues. For example, complaints of lumbar pain from a patient who reported symptoms getting into a car, especially when the neck was flexed, should initiate a clinical decision to perform the slump test.

- Secondly, it should therefore not be difficult for clinicians with good handling skills to derive tests for various nerves. For example, a review of the anatomy of the lateral femoral cutaneous nerve makes it obvious that hip extension and adduction may challenge the nerve. In addition it is widely reported that activities which require hip extension aggravate the symptoms of 'meralgia paraesthetica' (e.g. Mumenthaler and Schliack 1991). Peripheral neuropathy texts (such as Sunderland 1978, Mumenthaler and Schliack 1991, Stewart 1993) have many similar examples of certain movements aggravating symptoms related to a particular nerve trunk.

- Thirdly, since the neighbouring joint has so much effect on the nervous system, its health should also be evaluated. The attachments to surrounding tissues and the nature of surrounding tissues must also dictate the loading on the tissue. For example, pathological changes relating to disc injury are likely to affect neural tissue.

Relationship to surrounding tissues

The concept of 'neural container' (Shacklock 1995) or 'mechanical interface' (Butler 1991) is useful. It is clear that not only does the nervous system strain and move during loading, the tissues around the system also move and change shape, creating a dynamic relationship.

For example, during wrist and finger flexion and extension, the tendon excursion in the carpal tunnel is three times as much as that of the median nerve (Szabo et al. 1994). When the foot is everted from a neutral position, the tarsal tunnel intracompartment pressures are significantly higher (Trepman et al. 1999). The clinical implication is that when a patient has a sensitive test, sources of sensitivity may come from anywhere along the nervous system. For example if an upper limb neurodynamic test is sensitive and appears related to a carpal tunnel syndrome, contributing sources could be tissue changes in the wrist, the pectoralis minor muscle, or the neck. Thinking of 'what else is along the track' may also create an awareness that instability around the shoulder girdle area may also need attention for optimal performance of the wrist.

Spinal canal movements such as flexion and lateral flexion away from the test side demand considerable nervous system adaptation (Inman and Saunders 1942, Breig 1978, Louis 1981). Analysis of the clinical implications of these movements should take into account the variations in cross-sectional dimensions of the spinal canal. The cervicothoracic spine is quite spacious, though less so around the C5–6 level, and the upper cervical spinal canal is quite large. A narrow zone exists at the T4–9 vertebral levels, referred to as a critical vascular zone, where minimum space reduction may compromise the spinal cord and meninges (Dommisse 1994).

The roominess of an intervertebral foramina also changes dramatically. In general, spinal flexion increases the size of intervertebral foramina in the spine and spinal extension will decrease it. Lateral flexion and rotation towards the test side will decrease foraminal size (Penning and Wilmink 1987, Yoo et al. 1992, Inufusa et al. 1996). With healthy joints this will not be a problem. However degenerative joints and resultant narrowed intervertebral foramina may allow nerve root pinching on extension.

Order of movement

The sequences of movements involved in a soccer kick are different to those in a kung fu kick. Knee extension comes before hip flexion in soccer, and vice versa in a kung fu kick. The sequence of hip/knee movements during slump testing is different to a straight leg raise. The sequence of joint movements used in a neurodynamic test, or any movement, appears to affect the responses. This may relate in part to Breig's (1978) 'tissue borrowing' phenomenon; that is, the first movement tested 'borrows' the neural tissue first and thus allows a better examination of it. It appears that the sequence of movement influences the neural mechanics involved in gliding. Breig and Marions (1963) showed that in the lumbar region, neural structures slid rostrally when cervical flexion was performed. This contrasts with the finding of Louis (1981), who noted that lumbar neural movements were in a caudal direction when the whole spine was flexed. In physical examination it may be worthwhile applying different sequences of testing. The key principle is that the greatest challenge to a segment of neural tissue will occur when the adjacent joint to the nerve is loaded first in a sequence of testing (Shacklock 1995). Thus the most vigorous challenge to the terminal branches of the peroneal nerve would occur when ankle plantar flexion was performed first, then the straight leg raise performed. These features could well be researched further, but are well worth utilizing clinically when there appears to be peripheral neurogenic pain. They are of less use in more complex pain states or where the central nervous system is sensitized. The principle makes for safer testing. For example, if a patient had an acute disorder, say at the shoulder, the neurodynamic tests could be performed beginning at the wrist first. This requires some handling skills, further discussed by Butler (2000).

Judgements of sensitivity are necessary

A straight leg raise or any physical test is also a test of the state of the CNS at the time and environment of being tested. The straight leg raise provides a barrage of inputs into the CNS and if the CNS is upregulated, then inputs which may not have hurt or only evoked minor pain now hurt or hurt a lot more (hyperalgesia). Reasoning strategies will therefore require some consideration to mechanisms of symptoms (e.g. peripheral, central) as well as sources (e.g. joint, nerve) (Gifford and Butler 1997, Butler 1998, Gifford 1998b, Woolf et al. 1998). In management strategies, the unhealthy tissues involved in a straight leg raise could well be exercised, but reasons for the maintained elevated CNS threshold control will also need identifying and addressing. This may well be fear, anger, or beliefs that are inappropriate for healing. Exposure to sensitive movements may need some pacing, not only for restoration of tissue health, but also to teach the CNS to accept the input as non-threatening and thus avoid potentially damaging stress responses.

Conclusion

The nervous system is a physically complex structure made up of tissues with varying mechanical abilities, but which combine to allow the nervous system to slide, stretch, and angulate during movements. The extent of movement and strain is remarkable and worthy of consideration in manual therapy strategies. With injury the nervous system may become mechanosensitive from combined peripheral and central mechanisms and lose some of its physical abilities.

References

Apfelberg, D. B., Larson, S. J. (1973) Dynamic anatomy of the ulnar nerve at the elbow. *Plastic and Reconstructive Surgery*, 51, 76–81.

Asbury, A. K., Fields, H. L. (1984) Pain due to peripheral nerve damage: an hypothesis. *Neurology*, 34, 1587–1590.

Bashline, S. D., Bilott, J. R., Ellis, J. P. (1996) Meningovertebral ligaments and their putative significance in low back pain. *Journal of Manipulative and Physiological Therapeutics*, 19, 592–596.

Beith, I. D., Robins, E. J., Richards, P. R. (1995) An assessment of the adaptive mechanisms within and surrounding the peripheral nervous system, during changes in nerve bed length resulting from underlying joint movement. In: *Moving in on pain*, M. O. Shacklock, ed., Butterworth-Heinemann, Australia, pp. 194–203.

Blomberg, R. (1986) The dorsomedian connective tissue band in the lumbar epidural space of humans. An anatomical study using epiduroscopy in autopsy cases. *Anesthesia and Analgesia*, 65, 747–752.

Bogduk, N. (1983) The innervation of the lumbar spine. *Spine*, 8, 286–292.

Bove, G. M., Light, A. R. (1995) Calcitonin gene-related peptide and peripherin immunoreactivity in nerve sheaths. *Somatosensory and Motor Research*, 12, 49–57.

Bowsher, D. (1996) Central pain: clinical and physiological charateristics. *Journal of Neurology, Neurosurgery and Psychiatry*, 61, 62–69.

Breig, A. (1960) *Biomechanics of the central nervous system*. Almqvist and Wiksell, Stockholm.

Breig, A. (1978) *Adverse mechanical tension in the central nervous system*. Almqvist and Wiksell, Stockholm.

Breig, A., Marions, O. (1963) Biomechanics of the lumbosacral nerve roots. *Acta Radiologica*, 1, 1141–1159.

Breig, A., Turnbull, I., Hassler, O. (1966) Effects of mechanical stresses on the spinal cord in cervical spondylosis: a study on fresh cadaver material. *Journal of Neurosurgery*, 25, 45–56.

Bridge, C. J. (1959) Innervation of spinal meninges and epidural structures. *Anatomical Record*, 133, 533–561.

Brukner, P., Khan, K. (1993) *Clinical sports medicine*. McGraw-Hill, New York.

Butler, D. S. (1989) Adverse mechanical tension in the nervous system: a model for assessment and treatment. *Australian Journal of Physiotherapy*, 35(4), 227–238.

Butler, D. S. (1991) *Mobilisation of the nervous system*. Churchill Livingstone, Melbourne.

Butler, D. S. (1998) Integrating pain awareness into physiotherapy – wise action for the future. In: *Topical issues in pain*, L. S. Gifford, ed., NOI Press, Falmouth.

Butler, D. S. (2000) *The sensitive nervous system*. Noigroup, Adelaide.

Butler, D. S., Slater, H. (1994) Neural injury in the thoracic spine: a conceptual basis for manual therapy. In: *Physical therapy of the cervical and thoracic spine*, R. Grant, ed., Churchill Livingstone, New York.

Cavallotti, D., Artico, M., De Santis. S., Iannetti, G., Cavallotti, C. (1998) Catacholaminergic innervation of the human dura mater involved in headache. *Headache*, 38, 352–355.

Childress, H. M. (1975) Recurrrent ulnar-nerve dislocation at the elbow. *Journal of Bone and Joint Surgery*, 38A, 978–984.

Chung, K., Kim, H. J., Na, H. S., *et al.* (1993) Abnormalities of sympathetic innervation in the area of an injured peripheral nerve in a rat model of neuropathic pain. *Neuroscience Letters*, 162, 85–88.

Coderre, R. J., Katz, J., Vaccarino, A. L., Melzack, R. (1993) Contribution of central neuroplasticity to pathological pain: review of clinical and experimental evidence. *Pain*, 52, 259–285.

Cuatico, W., Parker, J. C., Pappert, E., Pilsl, S. (1988) An anatomical and clinical investigation of spinal meningeal nerves. *Acta Neurochirurgica*, 90, 139–143.

Devor, M. (1999) Unexplained peculiarities of the dorsal root ganglion. *Pain*, Supplement 6, S27–36.

Devor, M., Seltzer, Z. (1999) Pathophysiology of damaged nerves in relation to chronic pain. In: *Textbook of pain*, P. D. Wall and R. Melzack, eds., Churchill Livingstone, Edinburgh.

Dhital, K. J., Lincoln, J., Appenzeller, O., Burnstock, G. (1986) Adrenergic innervation of vasa and nervi nervorum of optic, sciatic, vagus and sympathetic nerve trunks in normal and steptozotocin-diabetic rats. *Brain Research*, 367, 39–44.

Dommisse, G. F. (1994) The blood supply of the spinal cord and the consequences of failure. In: *Grieve's modern manual therapy*, J. D. Boyling and N. Palastanga, eds., Churchill Livingstone, Edinburgh.

Doubell, T. P., Mannion, R. J., Woolf, C. J. (1999) The dorsal horn: state dependent sensory processing, plasticity and the generation of pain. In: *Textbook of pain*, P. D. Wall and R. Melzack, eds., Churchill Livingstone, Edinburgh.

Doursounian, L., Alfonso, J. M., Iba-Zizen, M. T., Roger, B. (1989) Dynamics of the junction between the medulla and the cervical spinal cord: an in vivo study in the sagittal plane by magnetic resonance imaging. *Surgical and Radiologic Anatomy*, 11, 313–322.

Dubner, R., Basbaum, A. I. (1994) Spinal dorsal horn plasticity following tissue or nerve injury. In: *Textbook of pain*, P. D. Wall and R. Melzack, eds., Churchill Livingstone, Edinburgh.

Edgar, M. A., Ghadially, J. A. (1976) Innervation of the lumbar spine. *Clinical Orthopaedics and Related Research*, 115, 35–41.

Edgar, M. A., Nundy, S. (1966) Innervation of the spinal dura mater. *Journal of Neurology, Neurosurgery, and Psychiatry*, 29, 530–534.

Elvey, R. L. (1986) Treatment of arm pain associated with abnormal brachial plexus tension. *Australian Journal of Physiotherapy*, 32, 225–230.

Gelberman, R. H., Yamaguchi, K., Hollstein, S. B. (1998) Changes in interstitial pressure and cross-sectional area of the cubital tunnel and of the ulnar nerve with flexion of the elbow. *Journal of Bone and Joint Surgery*, **80A**, 492–501.

Gertzbein, S., Seligman, J., Holtby, R. (1985) Centrode patterns and segmental instability. *Spine*, **10**, 257–261.

Gifford, L. S. (1998a). Factors influencing movement – neurodynamics. In: *Rehabilitation of movement*, J. Pitt-Brooke *et al.*, eds, Saunders, London.

Gifford, L. S. (1998b). *Topical issues in pain*. NOI Press, Falmouth.

Gifford, L., and Butler, D. (1997) The integration of pain sciences into clinical practice. *Journal of Hand Therapy*, **10**, 86–95.

Giles, L. G. F. (1992) Paraspinal autonomic ganglion distortion due to vertebral body osteophytosis: a cause of vertebrogenic autonomic syndromes? *J Manipulative Physiol Ther*, **15**(9), 551–555.

Goldner, J. L., Hall, R. L. (1997) Nerve entrapment syndromes of the lower back and lower extremities. In: *Management of peripheral nerve problems*, G. E. Omer, M. Spinner, and A. L. Van Beek, eds., W.B. Saunders, Philadelphia.

Greening, J., Smart, S., Leary, R., Hall-Craggs, M. (1999) Reduced movement of the median nerve in carpal tunnel during wrist flexion in patients with non-specific arm pain. *Lancet*, **354**(9174), 217–218.

Groen, G. J., Baljet, B., Drukker, J. (1988) The innervation of the spinal dura mater: Anatomy and clinical implications. *Acta Neurochirurgica*, **92**, 39–46.

Hack, G. D., Koritzer, R. T., Robinson, W. L. (1995) Anatomic relation between the rectus capitis posterior minor muscle and the dura mater. *Spine*, **20**, 2484–2486.

Haines, D. E., Harkey, H. L., al-Mefty, O. (1993) The subdural space: a new look at an outdated concept. *Neurosurgery*, **32**, 111–120.

Hardy, J. D., Wolff, H. G., Goodell, H. (1952) *Pain sensations and reactions*. Haffner Publishing, New York.

Haupt, W., Stoept, E. (1978) Uber die Dehnbarkeit und Reißfestigkeit der Dura mater spinalis des Menschen. *Verhandlungen Anatomische Gesellschaft*, **72**, 139–144.

Hofmann, M. (1898) Die befestigung der dura mater im wirbelcanal. *Archives of Anatomy and Physiology*, 403–412.

Hovelaque, A. (1927) *Anatomie des nerfs craniens et rachidiens et du système grand sympathetique chez l'homme*. Gaston Doin et Cie, Paris.

Hromada, J. (1963) On the nerve supply of the connective tissue of some peripheral nervous system components. *Acta Anatomica*, **55**, 343–351.

Inman, V. T., Saunders, J. B. d. C. (1942) The clinico-anatomical aspects of the lumbosacral region. *Journal of Radiology*, **38**, 669–678.

Inufusa, A., An, H. S., and Lim, T. (1996) Anatomic changes of the spinal canal and intervertebral foramen association with flexion-extension movements. *Spine*, **21**, 2412–2420.

Janig, W., Koltzenburg, M. (1990) Receptive properties of pial afferents. *Pain*, **45**, 300–306.

Kallakuri, S., Cavanaugh, J. M., Blagoev, D. C. (1998) An immunohistochemical study of innervation of lumbar spinal dura and longitudinal ligaments. *Spine*, **23**, 403–411.

Kimmel, D. L. (1961) Innervation of spinal dura mater and dura mater of the posterior cranial fossa. *Neurology*, 800–809.

Klein, J. D., Garfin, S. R. (1997) Clinical evaluation of patients with suspected spine problems. In: *The adult spine: principles and practice*, J. W. Frymoyer, ed., Lippincott-Raven, Philadelphia.

Kleinrensink, G. J., Stoeckart, R., Mulder, P. G. H., Hoek, G. v. d. (2000) Upper limb tension tests as tools in the diagnosis of nerve and plexus lesions. *Clinical Biomechanics*, **15**, 9–14.

Koltzenburg, M., Lundberg, L. E. R., Torebjörk, H. E. (1992) Dynamic and static components of mechanical hyperalgesia in human hairy skin. *Pain*, **51**, 207–220.

LaMotte, R. H., Shain, C. N., Simone, D. A. (1991) Neurogenic hyperalgesia: psychophysical studies of underlying mechanisms. *Journal of Neurophysiology*, **66**, 190–211.

LaMotte, R. H., Lundberg, L. E. R., Torebjörk, H. E. (1992) Pain, hyperalgesia and activity in nociceptive C units in humans after intradermal injection of capsaicin. *Journal of Neurophysiology*, **448**, 74.

Lew, P. C., Morrow, C. J., Lew, A. M. (1994) The effect of neck and leg flexion and their sequence on the lumbar spinal cord. *Spine*, **19**, 2421–2425.

Lincoln, J., Milner, P., Appenzeller, O., Burnstock, G., Qualls, C. (1993) Innervation of normal human sural and optic nerves by noradrenaline- and peptide-containing nervi vasorum and nervorum: effect of diabetes and alcoholism. *Brain Research*, **632**, 48–56.

Louis, R. (1981) Vertebroradicular and vertebromedullar dynamics. *Anatomia Clinica*, **3**, 1–11.

Lundborg, G. (1988) *Nerve injury and repair*. Churchill Livingstone, Edinburgh.

Lundborg, G., Rydevik, B. (1973) Effects of stretching the tibial nerve of the rabbit. A preliminary study of the intraneural circulation and barrier function of the perineurium. *Journal of Bone and Joint Surgery*, **55B**, 390–401.

Mackinnon, S. E., Dellon, A. L. (1988) *Surgery of the peripheral nerve*. Thieme, New York.

Magee, D. (1997) *Orthopedic physical assessment*. W.B. Saunders, Philadelphia.

Maitland, G. D. (1986) *Vertebral manipulation*. Butterworths, London.

McLachlan, E. M., Janig, W., Devor, M., *et al.* (1993) Peripheral nerve injury triggers noradrenergic sprouting within dorsal root ganglia. *Nature*, **363**, 534–536.

McLellan, D. L., Swash, M. (1976) Longitudinal sliding of the median nerve during movements of the upper limb. *Journal of Neurology, Neurosurgery, and Psychiatry*, **39**, 566–570.

Millesi, H. (1986) The nerve gap: theory and clinical practice. *Hand Clinics*, **2**(4, November), 651–663.

Muhle, C., Wiskirchen, J., Weinert, D. *et al.* (1998) Biomechanical aspects of the subarachnoid space and cervical cord in healthy individuals examined with kinematic magnetic resonance imaging. *Spine*, **23**, 556–567.

Mumenthaler, M., Schliack, H. (1991) *Peripheral nerve lesions*. Thieme, New York.

Murzin, V. E., Goriunov, V. N. (1979) Study of strength of fixation of dura mater to the cranial bones. *Zh Vopr Neirokhir*, **4**, 43–47.

Nagakawa, H., Mikawa, Y., Watanabe, R. (1994) Elastin in the human posterior longitudinal ligament and spinal dura. A histologic and biochemical study. *Spine*, **19**, 2164–2169.

Nathan, H. (1987) Osteophytes of the spine compressing the sympathetic trunk and splanchnic nerves in the thorax. *Spine*, **12**(6), 527–532.

Nathan, P. A., Keniston, R. C., Meadows, K. D. (1995) Outcome study of ulnar nerve decompression at the elbow treated with simple decompression and an early programme of physical therapy. *Journal of Hand Surgery*, **20B**, 628–637.

Neary, D., Eames, R. A. (1975) The pathology of ulnar nerve compression in Man. *Neuropathology and Applied Neurobiology*, **1**, 69–88.

Ogata, K., Naito, M. (1986) Blood flow of peripheral nerve effects of dissection, stretching and compression. *Journal of Hand Surgery*, **11B**, 10–14.

Parke, W. W., Watanabe, R. (1986) The intrinsic vasculature of the lumbosacral spinal nerve roots. *Spine*, **10**, 508–515.

Parke, W. W., and Watanabe, R. (1990) Adhesions of the ventral lumbar dura: an adjunct source of discogenic pain? *Spine*, **15**, 300–303.

Parke, W. W., Whalen, J. L. (1993) The pial ligaments of the anterior spinal artery and their stretch receptors. *Spine*, **18**, 1542–1549.

Patin, D. J., Eckstein, E. C., Harum, K., Pallares, V. S. (1993) Anatomic and biomechanical properties of human lumbar dura mater. *Anesthesia and Analgesia*, **76**, 535–540.

Pechan, J., Julis, F. (1975) The pressure measurement in the ulnar nerve: a contribution to the pathophysiology of cubital tunnel syndrome. *Journal of Biomechanics*, **8**, 75–79.

Pedersen, H., Blunck, C., Gardner, E. (1956) The anatomy of lumbosacral posterior rami and meningeal branches of spinal nerves (sinuvertebral nerves). *Journal of Bone and Joint Surgery*, **38A**, 377–391.

Penfield, W., McNaughton, F. (1940) Dural headache and the innervation of the dura mater. *Archives of Neurology and Psychiatry*, **44**, 43–75.

Penning, L., Wilmink, J. T. (1987) Posture-dependent bilateal compression of L4 or L5 nerve roots in facet hypertrophy. *Spine*, **12**, 488–500.

Rayan, G. M., Jensen, C., Duke, J. (1992) Elbow flexion test in the normal population. *Journal of Hand Surgery*, **17A**, 86–89.

Rempel, D., Dahlin, L., Lundborg, G. (1999) Pathophysiology of nerve compression syndromes: response of peripheral nerves to loading. *Journal of Bone and Joint Surgery*, **81A**, 1600–1610.

Rogers, L. C., Payne, E. E. (1961) The dura mater at the cranio-cervical junction. *Journal of Anatomy*, **95**, 586–588.

Rossitti, S. (1993) Biomechanics of the pons-cord tract and its enveloping structures: an overview. *Acta Neurochirurgica*, **124**, 144–152.

Rutten, H. P., Szpak, K., van Mameren, H. (1997) Letters. *Spine*, **22**, 924–928.

Rydevik, B., Lundborg, G., Skalak, R. (1989) Biomechanics of peripheral nerves. In: *Basic biomechanics of the musculoskeletal system*, M. Nordin and V. H. Frankel, eds., Lea and Febiger, Philadelphia, 75–87.

Schmidt, J. W., Catterall, W. A. (1986) Biosynthesis and processing of the alpha subunit of the voltage-sensitive sodium channel in rat brain neurons. *Cell*, **46**, 437–445.

Selvaratnam, P. J., Matyas, T. A., Glasgow, E. F. (1994) Noninvasive discrimination of brachial plexus involvement in upper limb pain. *Spine*, **19**, 26–33.

Shacklock, M. (1995) Neurodynamics. *Physiotherapy*, **81**, 9–16.

Slater, H., Vincenzino, B., Wright, A. (1994) Sympathetic slump. The effect of a novel manual therapy technique on peripheral sympathetic nervous system function. *Journal of Manual and Manipulative Therapy*, **2**, 156–162.

Smith, J. W. (1966) Factors influencing nerve repair. *Archives of Surgery*, **93**, 335–341.

Spencer, D. L., Irwin, G. S., Miller, J. A. A. (1983) Anatomy and significance of fixation of the lumbosacral nerve roots in sciatica. *Spine*, **8**, 672–679.

Spielman, F. J. (1982) Post lumbar puncture headache. *Headache*, **22**, 280–283.

Stewart, J. D. (1993) *Focal peripheral neuropathies*. Raven Press, New York.

Sunderland, S. (1978) *Nerves and nerve injuries*. Churchill Livingstone, Melbourne.

Svendsen, F., Tjolsen, A., Hole, K. (1998) AMPA and NMDA receptor-dependent spinal LTP after nociceptive tetanic stimulation. *NeuroReport*, **9**, 1185–1190.

Szabo, R. M., Bay, B. K., Sharkey, N. A., Gaut, C. (1994) Median nerve displacement through the carpal canal. *Journal of Hand Surgery*, **19A**, 901–906.

Tencer, A. F., Allen Jnr, B. L., Ferguson, R. L. (1985) A biomechanical study of thoracolumbar spine fractures with bone in the spinal canal: part III. Mechanical properties of the dura and its tethering ligaments. *Spine*, **10**, 741–747.

Thomas, P. K., Olsson, Y. (1984) Microscopic anatomy and function of the connective tissue components of peripheral nerve. In: *Peripheral neuropathy*, P. J. Dyck, P. K. Thomas, E. H. Lambert, and R. Bunge, eds., Saunders, Philadelphia.

Torebjörk, H. E., Lundberg, L. E. R., LaMotte, R. H. (1992) Central changes in processing of mechanoreceptive input in capsaicin-induced secondary hyperalgesia in humans. *Journal of Physiology*, **448**, 765–780.

Transfeldt, E. E., Simmons, E. H. (1982) Functional and pathological biomechanics of the spinal cord: an in vivo study. *Scoliosis Research Society*.

Trepman, E., Kadel, N. J., Chisholm, K., *et al.* (1999) Effect of foot and ankle position on tarsal tunnel compartment pressure. *Foot & Ankle International*, **20**, 721–726.

Tunturi, A. R. (1977) Elasticity of the spinal cord dura in the dog. *Journal of Neurosurgery*, **47**, 391–395.

Vandam, L. D. (1992) Symptoms following lumbar puncture may be related to decreased cerebrospinal fluid pressure and/or venous dilation. *Anesthesiology*, **76**, 321.

Weinstein, J. N. (1997) Pain. In: *The adult spine: principles and practice*, J. W. Frymoyer, ed., Lippincott-Raven, Philadelphia.

Wiltse, L. L., Fonseca, A. S., Amster, J., Dimartino, P., Bavessoud, F. A. (1993) Relationship of the dura, Hofmann's ligaments, Batson's plexus and a fibrovascular membrane lying on the posterior surface of the vertebral bodies and attaching to the deep layer of the posterior longitudinal ligament. *Spine*, **18**, 1030–1043.

Wirth, F. P., van Buren, J. M. (1971) Referral of pain from dural stimulation in man. *Journal of Neurosurgery*, **34**, 630–642.

Woolf, C. J. (1991) Generation of acute pain: central mechanisms. *British Medical Bulletin*, **47**, 523–533.

Woolf, C. J., Bennett, G. J., Doherty, M. (1998) Towards a mechanism-based classification of pain. *Pain*, **77**, 227–229.

Wright, T. W., Glowczewski, F., Wheeler, D., Miller, G., Cowin, D. (1996) Excursion and strain of the median nerve. *Journal of Bone and Joint Surgery*, **78A**, 1897–1903.

Yoo, J. U., Zou, D., Edwards, W. T. (1992) Effect of cervical spine motion on the neuroforaminal dimensions of human cervical spine. *Spine*, **17**, 1131–1136.

Zarzur, E. (1996) Mechanical properties of the human lumbar dura mater. *Arquivos de Neuropsiquiatria*, **54**, 455–460.

Zoech, G., Reihsner, R., Beer, R., Millesi, H. (1991) Stress and strain in peripheral nerves. *Neuro-Orthopedics*, **10**, 73–82.

2.2.5 Tensegrity: the new biomechanics

Stephen Levin

> The 'design' of plants and animals and of traditional artifacts did not just happen. As a rule both the shape and materials of any structure which has evolved over a long period of time in a competitive world represent an optimization with regard to the loads which it has to carry and to the financial or metabolic cost. (Gordon 1978, p. 303)

The anomalies

If we accept the precepts of most present day biomechanical engineers, a 100-kg weight lifted by your average competitive weightlifter will tear his erector spinae muscle, rupture his discs, crush his vertebra and burst his blood vessels (Gracovetsky 1988). Even the less daring sportsperson is at risk: a 2-kg fish dangling at the end of a 3-m fly rod exerts a compressive load of at least 120 kg on the lumbosacral junction. If we include the weight of the rod and the weight of the torso, arms, and head, the calculated load on the spine would easily exceed the critical load that would fracture the lumbar vertebrae of the average man. This would make fly fishing an exceedingly dangerous activity. Pounded by the forces of the runner striking the ground, with the first metatarsal head acting as the hammer and the ground as the anvil, the soft sesamoids would crush. A batter striking a baseball traveling at 100 mph (160 km/h), will be sheared from the ground, spikes and all. A hockey player striking a puck will be propelled backwards on the near-frictionless ice, as for every action there is an equal and opposite reaction.

There is more to ponder. The brittleness of bones is about the same in a mouse as it is in an elephant, as the strength and stiffness of bones is about the same in all animals. Animals larger than lions, for example horses, jumping on their slender limbs, would smash their bones with any leap (Gordon 1988). According to the linear mechanical laws that dominate biomechanical thinking, the mass of an animal must be cubed as its surface area is squared, so an animal as large as an elephant will be crushed by its own weight. The large dinosaurs could never have existed, let alone be a dominant species for millions of years. Biologic tissues work elastically at strains that are about a thousand times higher than strains that ordinary technological solids can withstand. If they behaved as most non-biologic materials do, with each heartbeat the skull should explode as the blood vessels expand and crowd out the brain, and urinary bladders should thin and burst as they fill. The pregnant uterus should burst with the contractions of delivery.

Not only mechanical but also physiologic processes would be inconsistent with linear physics. Pressure within a balloon decreases as it empties. Following the same physics, the systolic pressure should decrease as the heart empties – but, of course, it increases. We could never get the air out of our lungs or empty our bladders or bowels. If we functioned as columns and levers, our center of gravity is too high and our base is too small and weak for ordinary activities. When swinging an ax, sledgehammer, golf club or fishing rod our center of gravity would fall outside our base and topple us over. We could not lift a shovel full of dirt. The os calci is a very soft bone. Our heels should crush from the superincumbent load and could not sustain the load of a gymnast dismounting a high bar. The 'iron cross' position (Figure 2.2.27) attainable by any competent gymnast, would tear him limb from limb unless he defied the cosine law taught in every basic physics course which, in effect, states that the forces pulling on a rope strung between two poles become infinite as the rope becomes straight.

When confronted by these anomalies, biomechanical engineers either ignore the problem or go to great and circuitous lengths to try to justify the results. However, these explanations rarely stand the test

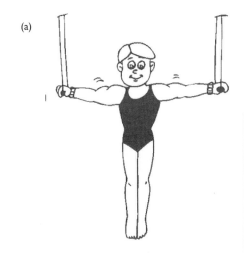

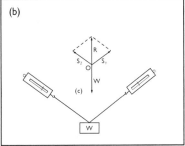

Figure 2.2.27 Gymnast's 'iron cross' position.

Newtonian mechanics

Hooke's law: For any given material that obeys Hooke's law, the slope of the graph, or the ratio of stress to strain, will be constant. Biologic tissues are non-Hookian and get stiffer and stronger as they load. The strength and stiffness of bone is the same in all animals. Their brittleness is such that they should fracture easily once an animal reaches the size of a human or lion, if Hookian theory is applicable. Since larger animals exist, it is obvious that Hookian theory cannot apply to biologic tissues.

Euler's formula: $P = {}_{,,}{}^2E/L^2$, where P is the load at which a column will buckle and E is the Young's modulus of the material. The taller the column, the weaker and less stable it is. Very tall columns will bend of their own weight. If the Empire State Building had the same proportions as a stalk of wheat, it would be less than 2 m wide at its base. The spinal ligament should buckle under a load of only 2 kg, which is less than the weight of a person's head.

Galileo's square–cube law: As the surface area of a structure squares, its volume cubes. Eventually it will crush of its own weight. If we use calculations based on Newtonian mechanics and known tissue strengths, the maximum size of a land-based animal can be no more than a modern elephant. Many dinosaurs far exceeded these weights, which leads to the conclusion that either large dinosaurs did not exist, or their tissues were much stronger, or Galileo's law does not apply to large animals.

Poisson's ratio: If you stretch an elastic material, it gets thinner. If you compress the material, it bulges out. The ratio of these changes in material is Poisson's ratio, which is a constant in most building materials. For engineering materials, the ratio lies between 0.25 and 0.5 and cannot exceed 0.5. However, biologic materials usually have a ratio greater than 0.5 and may approach unity.

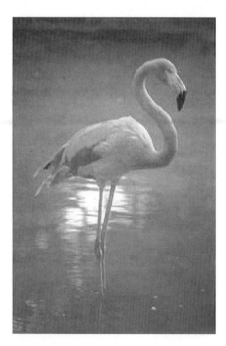

Figure 2.2.28 The slender leg of a flamingo.

of scientific scrutiny or even good sense. According to bioengineers, living organisms are modeled like skyscrapers (Schultz 1983). There are serious inconsistencies that test this model. The base of a skyscraper is always stronger than its top. It is dependent on gravity to hold it together. It cannot be flipped over or even tilted very far as the internal shear created would tear it apart. Its joints must be rigidly welded. Biologic hinges are freely moving, not rigidly welded. We are not constructed like skyscrapers with our base firmly and forever rooted to the ground and held in place by the force of gravity. Animals balance on flimsy supports. How does a flamingo leg, a long, thin strut, with a near frictionless hinge in the middle, hold up a flamingo (Figure 2.2.28)? Most biologic organisms that are upright, including plants, have their top half heavier than their base. Stonewalls and skyscrapers, but not flamingos, are, necessarily, thicker at their base. If our center of gravity falls outside our base we are not torn apart by internal shear forces, as happens to columns of stone. Biologic structures exist independent of gravity. They are omnidirectional structures that can exist and adapt to water, land, air, and space.

The evolution of structure

Certainly, no natural laws are broken. It is just that bioengineers usually consider only Newtonian mechanics as their basis for calculations. Biologic materials are non-Hookian and non-Newtonian behaving physical structures and we cannot use Hookian and Newtonian laws to understand the material behavior of biologic organisms. Hookian and Newtonian materials behave in a linear, additive fashion. Biologic materials behave nonlinearly or nonadditively, and are not predictable using Hookian and Newtonian mechanics (Gordon 1978). As pointed out by Gould (1989), the combined action of any of the parts yields something other than the sum of the parts and new properties or synergies emerge. What is clearly needed is a new model to replace the post and beam, column and lever, Hookian and Newtonian model that now dominates the thinking of biomechanics.

The military maxim of 'never stand when you can sit, never sit when you can lie down, never stay awake when you can be asleep' applies to nature's ways. Evolution is an exercise in optimization. The solution requiring the least energy will eventually happen, and once it happens that solution will become the norm. Nature has a predilection for using and reusing whatever works, and works with the least amount of energy expenditure. Patterns and shapes in nature will evolve to their fittest form (Stevens 1974) with the tightest fit, and least energy expenditure. Nature also functions in a 'minimum inventory, maximum diversity' mode, trying to make do with the least amount of basic material to gain the maximum effect (Pearce 1978). DNA is constructed with just four nucleic acids and most of the DNA material of a lowly worm is repeated in the human genome. These genes are then used as templates to construct larger proteins, larger proteins add to other proteins and so on.

The development of biological structure, whether organelles packed in a cell, cells packed in tissues, tissues packed in organs, or organs packed in organisms is always in a 'closest packed' environment (Figure 2.2.29). The same is true of fish eggs in water, bee eggs in a hive, embryos in eggs, and fetuses *in utero*. Structural evolution of biologic organisms will therefore obey the physical laws of 'triangulation' and 'closest packing' that apply to structures filling space such as soap bubbles, grains of sand on a beech, oranges in a crate (Figure 2.2.30),

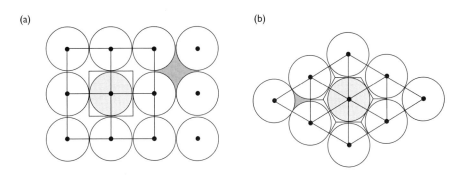

Figure 2.2.29 'Closest packed' environment.

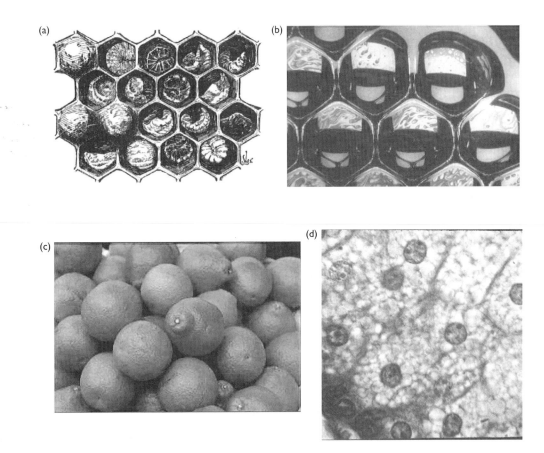

Figure 2.2.30 Physical laws of triangulation and closest packing.

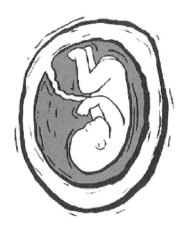

Figure 2.2.31 In the uterus, the fetus adapts to compressive forces.

molecules of water in a drop, or boulders on a mountain. In closest packing there is a balance of the external forces of molecules, sand grains, droplets, cells, or whatever crowding each other and the internal forces of the structure being crowded pushing out to keep from being crushed. This balance of forces assumes the least energy-consuming relationships.

The developing mammalian fetus is initially adapting to the closest-packed compressive forces *in utero* (Figure 2.2.31). Biologic tissue adapts to the forces applied by getting stronger and developing specialized structures and tissues to resist those forces (Wolff 1892, Carter 1991). It is remarkable that the fetus, developing to resist the omnidirectional pressure within the uterus, can then resist the asymmetrical and very high compressive forces of delivery through the birth canal and then instantly adapt to a completely new environment.

Initially adapting to and balancing compressive forces from without so as not to get crushed, it now has to resist the expanding forces from within without exploding. With each heartbeat and breath, the newborn should blow up like a balloon. The newborn is not a wineskin taking its shape from the unconstrained and unorganized fluid within, and neither are any cells that maintain their shape, closest packed, within the structure or completely removed to an open space environment. The outer container, the skin, does not contain the contents like the walls of a cylinder; the restraint of the explosive forces within comes from deep within the structure itself. The same is true of cells, tissues, and organs. The chondrocyte has to balance the internal pressures with its external loads; otherwise, it would crush or explode. The chondrocytes in the knee joint must be contained when unloaded but instantly able to withstand the crushing loads of a fullback running down the field. Cartilage tensile strength is 30 times weaker than bone, muscle tensile strength 1000 times weaker than tendon. Cartilage should shear right off the bone and muscles should tear with only minimal tendon pulls, unless the loads are distributed through the tissues. We know, from Darwinian theory and Wolff's law, that cartilage and muscle are as strong as they need be. There must be some distribution and dispersing of loads in biologic structures. There is a hierarchy of individual closest-packed structures, from subcellular to cellular to tissue to organ to organism, that are interdependent of and, at the same time, independent of one another. These structures must evolve consistent with Darwinian concepts and must be self-generating, omnidirectional, independent of gravity, and least-energy-consuming structures.

To understand the evolution of biologic structures we must understand how nature fills space. Two-dimensional space filling is an exercise in triangulation. The triangle is the simplest, most stable, and least energy-requiring polygon. It will not deform even with flexible corners (vertices) as long as the sides remain connected, straight, and at the same length. Square-frame constructs are unstable and will deform into a parallelogram and eventually flatten to a pancake (Figure 2.2.32). They require rigidly fixed corners to maintain themselves. If a structure exists with all its joints flexible, then it must be fully triangulated. When we pack six equilateral triangles arranged around a point in a plane, they form a hexagon. Closest-packed hierarchical arrays of triangles in self-generating hexagons fill a planar space (Figure 2.2.33). If we pack equal-sized discs, such as coins, in a planar space, their centers form equilateral triangles and assume the same relationship. This is the least-energy-requiring arrangement of structure in two-dimensional space, familiar as the cross section of a

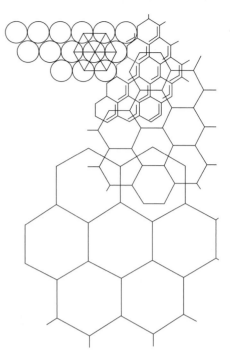

Figure 2.2.33 Closest-packed hierarchical arrays of triangles in self-generating hexagons fill a planar space.

beehive. Hexagons, however, will not enclose three-dimensional space. In the three-dimensional world in which we live, pentagons and hexagons are mathematical concepts with only two dimensions. In three dimensions they can only exist as part of some stable three-dimensional structure: a tetrahedron, octahedron, or icosahedron, which are the only fully triangulated regular polyhedra (Figure 2.2.34). To do that, the geometry changes a bit. Five equilateral triangles will form a bowl with its perimeter a pentagon. When you continue to add triangles in a closest-packed environment, they curve back on it and become a hollow closed space. Twenty planar triangles fit together as an icosahedron, perfectly enclosing the space. This configuration, too, has self-generating properties (Figure 2.2.35). This is one of the Platonic regular convex polyhedra, of which there are only five, which were known to the Greeks and other early mathematicians. All convex polyhedrons are some combination, permutation, or higher frequency of these five basic polyhedrons. Only three of the five are fully triangulated and, therefore, least-energy structures. They are the tetrahedron with four sides, the octahedron with eight sides, and the

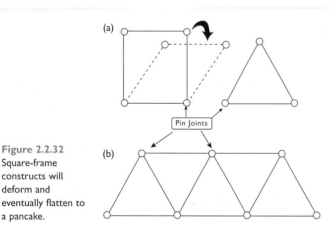

Figure 2.2.32 Square-frame constructs will deform and eventually flatten to a pancake.

Pin Joints

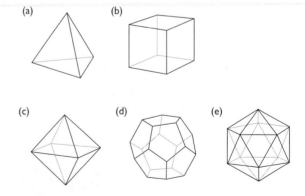

Figure 2.2.34 Tetrahedrons, octahedrons, and icosahedrons are the only fully triangulated regular polyhedrons.

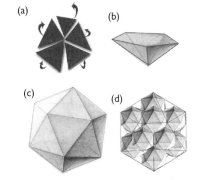

Figure 2.2.35 An icosahedron has self-generating properties.

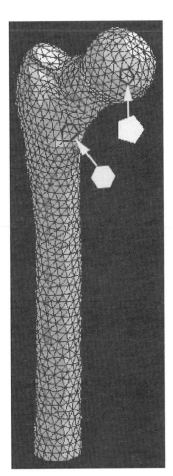

Figure 2.2.36 Tetrahedral modeling is consistent with biologic structure.

smaller, icosahedral-shaped vacuole. As fractals (Mandelbrot 1983), sharing faces and edges and intersecting one another, just as soap bubbles do, they will form an infinite array of interlinked, hierarchical, stable structures functioning as a whole or as subsets of icosahedrons.

Biotensegrity

The icosahedron has many things going for it. In addition to its self-generating properties and its ability to enclose three-dimensional space, it is mathematically the most symmetrical structure and is omnidirectional in form and function. It has the largest volume for surface area of the regular polyhedra, and larger structures are only higher-frequency icosahedrons. The icosahedron has 30 edges and 12 vertices with 20 sides. If the edges are rigid, then pressure at any point transmits around the 30 edges, putting some under pressure and others under tension, in a regular pattern. The 12 vertices each have 3 edges that come together at that corner. Some of these edges are under tension and some under compression, depending on the vector of force applied to the structure. The compression load can be transferred away from the outside of the structure by connecting the vertices opposite to one another by rigid, compression-bearing rods. These rods do not pass through the center of the icosahedron but are slightly eccentric and pass each other without touching (Figure 2.2.37). These compression rods are now joined at the icosahedral vertices by a continuous tension shell with all the edges on the outside of the icosahedron under tension, the 'tensegrity' icosahedron. These, too, can form infinite arrays and the tensegrity icosahedron can be a fractal generator (Mandelbrot 1983) (Figure 2.2.38).

Tensegrity, a word coined by Buckminster Fuller (1975) to describe continuous tension discontinuous compression structures, was applied to constructs designed by Kenneth Snelson (Snelson 2002) and Fuller. Examples of these structures are Snelson's Needle sculpture at the Hirshhorn Museum, Washington DC (Figure 2.2.39), Fuller's now

icosahedron with twenty sides. Water molecules, silicone molecules, carbon molecules, and methane molecules are all tetrahedrons. Twelve pentagon faces will enclose space as a duodecahedron. However, a duodecahedrons is an unstable frames structurally, as is the cube. Using the commonly utilized hexagonal (cube) modeling for finite-element analysis would not reflect the structural integrity of the tissue: tetrahedral modeling is more consistent with the way biologic structure forms and behaves (Figure 2.2.36). Filling the interiors of the hollow polyhedrons must follow the same closest packing laws. Closest packing twenty tetrahedrons around a point in three-dimensional space will create an icosahedron, just as six triangles created a two-dimensional hexagon (Figure 2.2.35D). Twelve equal-sized icosahedrons closest pack to form another icosahedron, joining at their fivefold symmetry (pentagon) edges. The center is a hollow, somewhat

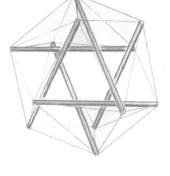

Figure 2.2.37 The rods do not pass through the center of the icosahedron but are slightly eccentric and pass each other without touching (see text).

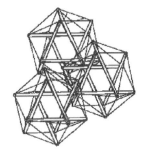

Figure 2.2.38 The tensegrity icosahedron as a fractal generator.

ubiquitous geodesic domes (Figure 2.2.40), and the wire-spoke bicycle wheel. Biotensegrity is the application of tensegrity principles to biologic structures. The tension or tensegrity icosahedron, is a pre-stressed, semi-rigid structure constructed of tension and compression members where none of the compression units compressing each other. They 'float' within the tension outer skin. Just as the single icosahedron can have either an exo- or endoskeleton, the linked, hierarchical structure can internalize its compression components and the whole structure can behave as a single icosahedron. As you can see, what happens is that a hierarchy of icosahedrons creates itself, balancing the external forces and internal forces as a self-generating structure.

The dandelion puffball (Figure 2.2.41), is easily recognized as a tensegrity structure. The bicycle wheel is the most common easily recognizable non-biologic tensegrity structure. The mechanics of a wagon wheel and a bicycle wheel are completely different (Figure 2.2.42). A wagon wheel transmits the wagonload to the ground through the axial compressing the spoke between it and the ground. The spoke has to be strong enough to withstand the full weight of the wagon; it gets no help from the other spokes, which, at that moment, sustain no load. Besides the compressive loads, internal shear is created within the spoke. The intervening rim acts as the

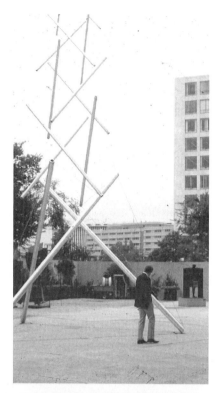

Figure 2.2.39 Snelson's Needle sculpture, Hirshhorn Museum, Washington, DC.

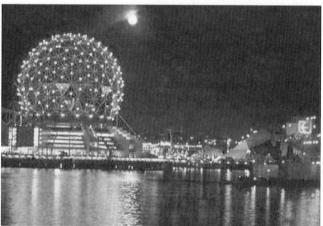

Figure 2.2.40 Fuller's geodesic domes.

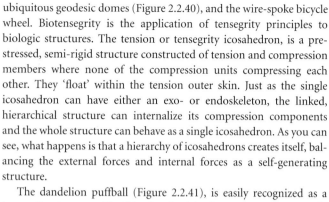

Figure 2.2.41 Dandelion puffball.

(a) (b)

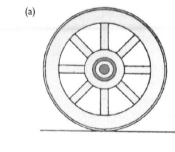

(c)

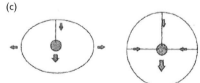

Figure 2.2.42 The mechanics of a wagon wheel and a bicycle wheel.

pedestal of the columnar spoke and has to be equal to the task of being crushed by the full weight of the wagonload. As the wheel rotates, it vaults from spoke to spoke. Halfway through the transfer of compressive load from one spoke to the next the rigid rim acts as a lever, creates bending moments, and has to be strong enough to withstand the additional loads. At any one moment in time, the structures are locally loaded and the remaining elements can be stripped away without seriously compromising the structural integrity. (The wheel just could not roll on.) In a bicycle wheel, the hub is suspended, hanging from the topmost spoke. This would cause the thin, weak rim to buckle. It is kept from buckling by the other wire spokes constantly pulling in on the rim to keep it round. All the spokes are under constant and equal tension. The tensions are preset, and do not vary with the load. The wheel is an integrated structure, with each spoke depending on every other to share the load at all times. The compression of the ground to the rim is distributed through the tension spokes to the hub. Therefore, there is no direct compression link between the load on the bicycle frame and the ground reaction force. The bicycle is suspended off the ground in a tension spoke network, hanging like a hammock, and the same system works equally well in a unicycle as a bicycle or tricycle. In a cycle wheel, the hub and rim are compression elements kept apart by tension spokes. There are no bending moments in the tension spokes, which are prestressed, under constant tension. The cycle wheel exists only as an integrated structure. One spoke will not hold up under the weight of the load.

Once constructed this way the tension elements remain in tension and compression elements remain under compression, no matter the direction of force or point of application of the load. It makes no difference where you compress the rim of the cycle wheel; the load is equally distributed through the spokes to the hub. The rim of the bicycle is a geodesic, connecting the many points of the spoke attachments: the more spokes, the rounder it gets. If the narrow rim is expanded to a sphere by creating great circle bands around the hub then the outer, exoskeleton of the geodesic-sphere is rigidly fixed to the central hub and transmits load to or away from that hub by the tension spokes.

As already noted, in some tensegrity structures the compression elements can be internalized and the tension elements externalized to create an endoskeleton using the same mechanics with the outer skin under tension and the inner skeleton intertwined in the tension network. The structure is truly omnidirectional. It never has to change tension elements to compression elements, or vice versa, to resist the compressive forces from without or the explosive forces from within, no matter from which direction the load is applied. Loads applied to the surface of linear, Hookian structures create a dimple right under it. Loads applied to a point on the skin of a tensegrity icosahedron are distributed evenly around all the edges in tension and across the floating rods under compression. Since load applied to the surface is distributed uniformly over the entire surface, instead of flattening and spreading out, the whole structure starts to compress and the tension icosahedron uniformly becomes smaller and more compact with the compression rods approximating each other more closely. The internal pressure of the icosahedron increases as it becomes more compressed, and it does so as a factor of the square of the radius. The graph of this relationship is a J-shaped curve that represents a nonlinear stress–strain relationship. This is radically different from the Hookian, linear behavior of most non-biologic materials and structures (Figure 2.2.43). In Hookian structures, for each increment of stress, there is a proportional strain until the point of elastic deformation just before it breaks. Hookian structures weaken under load. In the tensegrity structures, there is rapid deformation with the initial load but then the structure stiffens and becomes more rigid and stronger. This J-shaped nonlinear curve is also a characteristic response of biologic tissues from cells to spines. Tug on your lip and you will note that as you tug the skin is loose at first and then becomes stiffer and effects larger and larger areas of skin. The cells under the heel could not sustain crushing loads of the runner without this type of elasticity, as they would burst. This behavior not only is of the skin, it also then connects deeper eventually reaching right down to the bone. The process is reversed when any pressure is applied to the skin, as through the sole of the foot, with the soft tissues resisting the compressive force by tension, just as does the wire spoke, and then distributing through the compressive bearing bones.

The importance of the J-shaped nonlinear response of biologic tissue and the difference between the soft tissue mechanics of biologic materials and structures cannot be overemphasized. The rigid materials used in non-biologic constructs generally operate at elastic strains in the region of 0.1%. Rarely they may strain, that is deform to the point to which they can fully recover, 10 times that amount. Conceivably, they can go to elastic strains of 20%, but at that level, Hookian material reaches the level when its chemical bonds would explode. Biologic tissues commonly operate at strains of 50–100% or more, often 1000 times greater than those of conventional engineering materials do. Neither does it behave like rubber, which has an

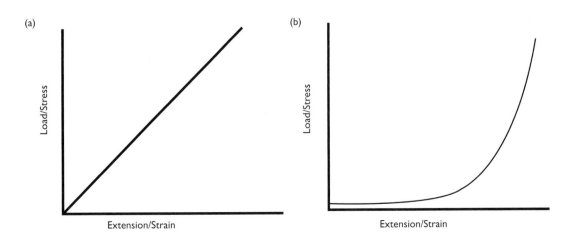

(a)

(b)

Figure 2.2.43 J-shaped curve representing a nonlinear stress–strain relationship.

Load/Stress

Extension/Strain

Load/Stress

Extension/Strain

S-shaped stress–strain curve and is characterized by bursting at its elastic limit and aneurysm formation that would not do well in arteries. The elastic behavior of biologic tissue when initially stressed behaves almost like the surface of a liquid at low and moderate strains. It then rises in its very characteristic, non-Hookian, J-shaped response. Mathematically this is the only sort of elasticity that is completely stable under the fluid pressures at high strains found in blood vessels, alveoli, bladders, bowels, muscles, uteri, and most other biologic soft tissues (Gordon 1978). The properties imparted by this curve are flexible and tough. With this configuration, biologic tissue is unlikely to fracture, explode, or be prone to aneurysm formation. Tendons and bone can store large amounts of energy and return it like a spring in leaps and bounds. The model usually used to approximate this type of behavior is the so-called 'viscoelastic' behavior of biologic tissues. This is a complicated and rather contrived behavior that puts the response of a Hookian elastic material (see box) parallel with the response of a Newtonian-behaving fluid like water and those, then, in series with another Hookian body. Modeling life's behavior would be simplified if there were a naturally occurring structure, such as the tensegrity icosahedron, that nature can use for its constructs.

Biologic tissues are prestressed, with the J-curve never zeroing out, so that there is always a balance of dynamical forces acting on the structure. Often compression and tension roles can be reversed in these types of structure but the sum function may remain the same. To appreciate these qualities consider a pneumatic tire or a balloon, which are also prestressed structures. The walls of the pneumatic structures are prevented from collapsing by the collision of molecules of gas within it pushing on all surfaces equally. The pressure in a tire is the same whether the car is up on a lift or sitting on the ground. Sitting there, the tire seems a little flat. To get a more efficient roll you can put in more air or heat up the gas inside the tire, creating more energy in the tire and more collisions of molecules on the walls. The friction on the road does just that. It is the balance of the internal energy of the gas and the external elastic energy of the tire wall, which is under tension that defines its functional capabilities. It reacts to its load but is not dependent on it. In a wire spoke wheel, the spokes pull the rim toward the center. Until an adequate number of spokes are properly placed, the spokes cannot be tightened. Once at that point (the minimum number is 12), the wire wheel behaves as the pneumatic tire does, only in reverse. Instead of the gas molecules pushing out, the spokes pull the rim toward the center, the tension is inside and the compression is outside. This shows how the tension and compression elements can be reversed, but still perform similar functions.

Over the years, I (Levin 1982, 1986, 1995, 1997) and others (Wildy and Home 1963, Ingber and Jamieson 1985, Wang *et al.*, 1993, 2001, Stamenovic *et al.* 1996, Ingber 1997, 2000) have proposed a new model for biologic structures based on the concept of tensegrity. In vertebrates the skeleton would be compression elements within a highly organized soft tissue construct, rather than the frame supporting an amorphous soft tissue mass. The same organization occurs at the cellular level with the cytoskeleton and the, anything but amorphous, cytoplasm. Tensegrity structures are omnidirectional, independent of gravity, load distributing and energy efficient, hierarchical, and self-generating. They are also ubiquitous in nature, once you know what to look for. They can be used to model biologic structures, from viruses to vertebrates and their systems and subsystems. They are fully triangulated and therefore, least-energy systems, that are stable even with flexible hinges. The tensegrity icosahedron can be linked in an infinite array in hierarchical systems and fractal constructs that can function together in unison acting as an icosahedron no matter what its shape. It can be considered the finite structural element and used as a building block for all biologic structures. Its nonlinear stress–strain curve is a characteristic, and even defines biologic tissues (Gordon 1988). The tensegrity model is now gaining wide acceptance as a model for biologic mechanics (Ingber 1998) and is very useful in understanding the mechanisms of action in orthopedic medicine.

The shoulder modeled as a biotensegrity structure

The principal of tensegrity modeling can be well demonstrated in the shoulder, which is the joint complex least successfully modeled using Newtonian mechanics. In multisegmented mathematical shoulder models, rigid beams (the bones) act as a series of columns or levers to transmit forces or loads to the axial skeleton. Forces passing through the almost frictionless joints must, somehow, always be directed perfectly perpendicular to the joints, as only loads directed at right angles to the surfaces could transfer across frictionless joints. Loads transmitted to the axial skeleton would have to pass through the moving ribs or the weak jointed clavicle and then through the ribs. As the arm circumducts in any plane, it inscribes the rim of an imaginary wheel (Figure 2.2.44). The arm becomes the spoke that transfers the load at the hand to the axial skeleton. Present models conceptualize the upper extremity as the spoke of a wagon wheel (Figure 2.2.42). This is a classic Newtonian construction with columns, beams, levers, and fulcrums, with resulting bending moments and torque. The bones of the arm are envisioned as the rigid spokes but, although there is a bony articulation at the glenohumeral joint that might be able to transfer compressive loads from the arm to the scapula, there is no rigid, compressive load-bearing structure between the scapula and the axial skeleton, nor is there a suitable fulcrum. In a linked lever system a seamless continuum of compression elements is necessary. Bone must compress bone. The almost frictionless joints would require forces to be always directed at right angles to the joint; otherwise, the bone would slide right out of the joint. The scapula is not anatomically situated to transfer loads through the ribs to the spine. Even if it were, the ribs could not take these loads and act as levers to connect to the spine.

The ribs themselves, by shape, position, and connection, are not structurally capable of transferring these loads. The clavicle is in no shape to transfer loads, either. It is a crank-shaped beam that connects

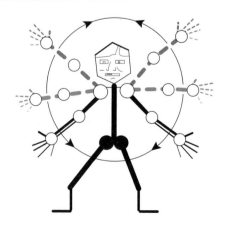

Figure 2.2.44 As the arm circumducts, it inscribes the rim of an imaginary wheel.

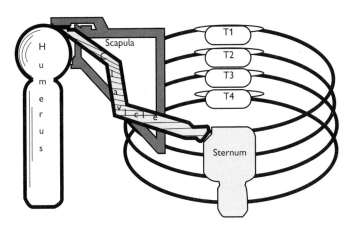

Figure 2.2.45 The clavicle connects the scapula to the sternum by a small, mobile joint.

the scapula to the sternum by a small, mobile joint that could not transfer compressive loads of any significant magnitude (Figure 2.2.45). Cats do not have articulating clavicles, but they can run and climb with the best of us creatures. The scapula of quadrupeds and bipeds hangs on the thorax by a network of muscles, and all the moment and compression forces generated in the arm must be transferred to the axial skeleton through these soft tissues A rope cannot withstand compressive loads, nor can it function as a lever, and neither can muscle or tendon. A wagon wheel, which depends on rigid, compressive load-bearing spokes to transfer loads, is not a suitable analogy for shoulder girdle mechanics. If we use a wire cycle wheel tensegrity structure as our model, the shoulder is readily modeled and takes into account all the necessary factors in joint modeling. If we consider the scapula functioning as the hub of a tensegrity structure, then the forces coming from the spoke-like arm could be transferred to the axial skeleton through the soft tissues rather than the circuitous and imposing linked levers of the bones.

A bicycle wheel–tensegrity model is mechanically more efficient than a spoked wagon wheel model. In a wagon wheel, only one or two spokes are sustaining loads at any one time. The spoke must be rigid and strong enough to withstand the entire weight thrust upon it. It gets no help from its neighbors. The rim of the wagon wheel must also be strong enough to withstand these crushing loads directly at the point of contact with the road. In a wire wheel, forces are distributed, all the elements act in concert and all the spokes contribute all the time. The rim is part of the system and the compressive load, directed at a point, is taken by the entire rim. Tensegrity structures are fully triangulated and, therefore, there are no bending moments in these structures, just tension and compression, and therefore significantly less loads to be reckoned with. Tensegrity structures are omnidirectional load distributors. The tension elements always remain in tension and the compression elements always remain in tension, no matter in what direction the loads are applied. This is not so in a column or a lever which is rigidly oriented to resist a load from a specific direction. Because the loads in tensegrity structure are distributed all the time, each structural element can be lighter.

Grant (1952) used a tension model to suspend the body, hammock like, when it hangs between gymnastic parallel bars (Figure 2.2.46). However, hammock-like suspension is unidirectional. Turn the hammock or suspension bridge over and not only does everything fall out of the hammock or off the roadbed, the hammock or roadbed also

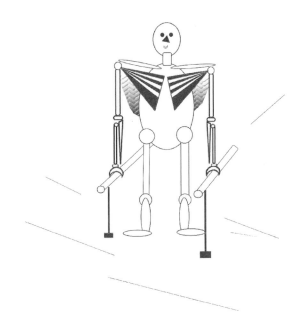

Figure 2.2.46 Grant's tension model.

collapses. A tensegrity structure is omnidirectional in form and function and can be used right side up, upside down, or any position in between and still maintain its form, its structural integrity, and its ability to transmit loads. When modeling a shoulder as a tensegrity structure the bones that 'float' in the tension network of soft tissue are only being compressed. There are no moments at the joints because the structure is fully triangulated. In this model the shoulder becomes inherently stable and changes position only when one of the elements of the triangle is shortened or lengthened, just as changing the tension in a wire spoke will distort the wheel. The continuous tension present in the soft tissues stabilizes the joints at each moment. Therefore, considerably less energy is needed to 'stabilize' the joints.

The scapula, suspended in the 'spokes' of the attached muscles and soft tissue, could function as a stable base for the arm. It could also transfer loads to the 'rim' of vertebrae through these same spokes. With the scapula as a hub in a tensegrity system, loads are transferred from the arm to the spine through the large amount of available muscle and ligaments through a stable yet easily mobilized, omnidirectional, low-energy-requiring system that would utilize lighter, less bulky parts and accommodates global motion and stability. This contrasts with a multisegmented articulated column model that is inherently unstable and has high energy requirements. In multisegmented systems, with each change of direction of load, new mechanics must be established. The tensegrity model is readily visualized when modeling scapular mechanics, since there are really no suitable compressive load-bearing joints that can connect the scapula to the spine.

Muscles, as well as all other soft tissue elements in the body, are always under some tension – they are prestressed. It is the tone of the muscle that holds us upright, keeps our jaw from dropping, and our scapulas from sliding off our chest wall, as we do these things when the EMG is electrically silent (Basmajian 1962), meaning there is no active contraction of the muscles. The tone of the muscles and the stored elastic energy in the soft tissues must be reckoned with as stabilizers and as motors to understand the forces that control stability and mobility in the body. The transfer of forces in the body could possibly be through these already tense soft tissue elements.

The glenohumeral articulation may appear, at first, to be a more traditional compressive loadbearing joint. But, for the joint to be stable forces must be directed at right angles (normal) to the joint since the cartilaginous surfaces are essentially frictionless. The glenohumeral joint is a multiaxial ball-and-socket joint. The head of the humerus is larger than the glenoid fossa and the surfaces are incongruous ovals and not true spheres. There is no bony structural stability and the joint is loosely packed, with a great deal of play between the surfaces. There are very few positions of the arm in which the humeral head directs its compressive forces normal to the glenoid fossa. Usually the forces are directed almost parallel to the joint surface. Since there is a change in direction of forces, in order to transfer forces to the scapula, the glenohumeral joint must function much like the universal joint of an automobile drive shaft. As Fuller (1975) points out, the universal joint is analogous to the wire wheel as a basic tensegrity system. It relies on the differentiation of tension and compression for its effectiveness. The soft tissues, the capsule, ligaments and muscles act as the connecting pins of a universal joint. Both the scapulothoracic and the glenohumeral joints may be modeled, efficiently and easily, as tensegrity-structured joints. Modeling the shoulder as a rigid, multisegmented lever is a struggle.

Motion

Movement is an integral part of animal life, and even the strongest trees sway in the wind. A multilinked Hookian mechanical structure would move just as you would expect a machine to move, with robotic jerkiness, because of the very nature of Hookian elastic materials. Hookian material has very abrupt transition from stress to unstressed, lending itself to jerky movements, hence the need for dampening springs with shock absorbers on automobiles. Tensegrity structures restore their full elastic energy more slowly; for example, bent grass returning to its normal, upright stance. Tensegrity structures move as a unit. Tighten one tension member and a ripple of movement runs through the entire structure, be it one cell or billions. The highly integrated flowing movement of the simplest and smallest to the most complex and largest organism is not possible with Hookian systems. Whales and walruses leave no wake, ships and submarines do. The free-flowing integrated movement of a bee buzzing; a bat on the wing, a baboon swinging, a ballet dancer *en pointe*, and a basketball player doing a lay-up cannot be matched by any mechanical device. Flemons (2002) and others have modeled sculptures from tensegrity units (Figure 2.2.47) that demonstrate how these structures move in a flowing transition from one configuration to the next.

Elastic structures store energy when deformed, and the energy is released as they return to their original shape. Much of the movement is with stored elastic energy. Stress, and the resultant strain, stores energy within the system. In bone and tendons, this energy can be quite large and when modeled as tensegrity structures even more impressive because of its nonlinearity and the resulting initial explosive force that automatically smoothes out as it reaches its resting state. Once an icosahedron reaches its resting point, which, unlike Hookian material, is prestressed, it will nonlinearly resist the overreach recoil. This makes for smooth, flowing movements like a pendulum swinging back and forth. Because of its collagen matrix, live bone has the springiness of a vaulter's pole and when the icosahedrons are compressed and released, they put bounce in each step but do not skip him along.

The linkages of icosahedrons are similar to organic chemical linkages. There can be one, two, or three bonds between linked icosahedrons, and this imparts varying stability between the links. The joints would be very rigid with three-bond linkage and less so with fewer links. A tree most likely has triple bonding. The double tiebar hinge arrangement in the knee is an example of a typical two-bar link, with the crossed cruciate ligaments under tension imparting rotations and translations and the stored energy of the ligaments assisting in knee flexion and extension. If the spine were linked in such a system, movement would cascade up and down the structure like a toy 'Jacob's ladder' (Figure 2.2.48).

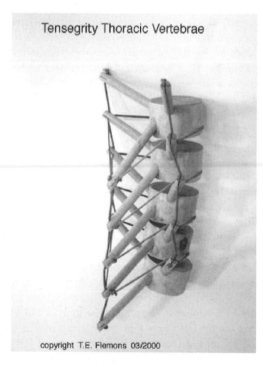

Tensegrity Thoracic Vertebrae

copyright T.E. Flemons 03/2000

Figure 2.2.47 Sculptures modeled from tensegrity units.

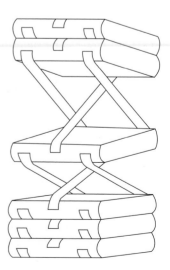

Figure 2.2.48 The spine modeled as a toy 'Jacob's ladder'.

Conclusion

It is an engineer's job to understand, simplify and offer predictability when dealing with structures. Imprecise natural processes can only be subjected to approximate descriptions. As Toffler (1984) says,

> While some parts of the universe may operate like machines, these are closed systems, and closed systems, at best, form only a small part of the physical universe. Most phenomena of interest to us are, in fact, open systems, exchanging energy or matter, (and, one might add, information), with their environment. Surely biologic and social systems are open, which means that the attempt to understand them in mechanistic terms is doomed to failure.

Biologic structures are chaotic, nonlinear, complex, and unpredictable by their very nature. The new sciences of chaos (Prigogine and Stengers 1984, Gleick 1988) and complexity (Waldrop 1992) are needed to explain and understand biologic structural mechanics.

Tensegrity structures have unique characteristics that parallel the structural requirements of biology. The giant leap from Newtonian to tensegrity models in biologic modeling can be taken in small hops. Cells are tensegrity structures. Ingber, in a series of experiments, has proved that the cytoskeleton is a tensegrity structure and it is connected to the nucleus hub, which is also a tensegrity structure. Pulling on the cell wall, distorting its skin, has a direct effect on the nucleus and shows that they are structurally connected through the cytoskeleton. Clathrins (subcellular structures) are geodesic domes, and geodesic domes are tensegrity structures. Actin, the contractile element of muscle, and leukocytes are arranged as geodesic domes. Viruses are icosahedra, which are the lowest-frequency geodesic dome. *Radiolaria*, *Volvox*, insect eyes, pith, dandelion puffballs, and blowfish are all geodesic domes. Carbon-60, ubiquitous in the universe, is a self-generating geodesic dome (Kroto 1988). Unlike Hookian structures, the mechanics of geodesic domes are nonlinear. As the structure is compressed, it uniformly shrinks, increasing its internal pressure nonlinearly. The heart, alveoli, bladder, arteries, and all other hollow vesicles within the body do the same. Bone, discs, muscles, and ligaments individually and as composites, behave nonlinearly. In terms of mechanics and physiology, biologic tissues behave the same way as tensegrity structures.

As already noted, from the physicalist and biomechanics viewpoint, as well as Darwinian theory, the evolution of structure is an optimization problem (Pearce 1978). At each step of development, the evolving structure optimizes so that it exists with the least amount of energy expenditure. At the cellular level the internal structure of the cells, the microtubules, together with the cell wall, must resist the crushing forces of the surrounding milieu and the exploding forces of its internal metabolism. Following Wolff's law, the internal skeleton of the cell aligns itself in the most efficient way to resist those forces. A hierarchical construction of an organism would use the same mechanical laws that build the most basic biologic structure and use it to generate the more complex organism. Not only is the beehive an icosahedron, so also is the bee's eye.

Of the known tensegrity structures the tension icosahedron has particular attributes that make it the most suitable for biologic musculoskeletal modeling (Levin 1986). Icosahedral tensegrity structures are self-organizing space frames that are hierarchical and evolutionary (Kroto 1988). They will build themselves, conforming to the laws of triangulation, close packing, and, in biologic constructs, Wolff's law

and Darwinian evolutionary concepts. In the model we have used, the scapula, fixed in space by the tension of its muscles, ligaments, and fascial envelope, functions as the connecting link between the spine and the upper arm, ontogenetically directed not only by phylogenetic forces but also by the physical forces of embryologic development. Wolff and Thompson state that the structure of the body is essentially a blueprint of the forces applied to these structures. Carter theorizes that the mechanical forces *in utero* are the determinants of embryologic structure that, in turn, evolve to fetal and then newborn structure. What is obvious in the shoulder joint is equally efficient and functional in all other joints of the body, from the cellular level on up. In makes no evolutionary sense to create different mechanical models for each species, or for each cell, each tissue, each joint, each position in space, or for each activity from swimming in the water to walking on land, swinging from trees or flying in the air, when there is one mechanical model that does it all, efficiently and with the least energy expenditure. The biotensegrity model does all this, in any direction and under any conditions.

References

Basmajian, J. V. (1962) *Muscles alive – their function revealed by electromyography*. Williams & Wilkins, Baltimore, MD.

Carter, D. R. (1991) Musculoskeletal otogeny, phylogeny, and functional adaptation. *Journal of Biomechanics*, 24, 3–16.

Flemons, T. (2002) http://intensiondesigns.com.

Fuller, R. B. (1975) *Synergetics*. Macmillan, New York.

Gleick, J. (1988) *Chaos*. Penguin, New York.

Gordon, J. E. (1978) *Structures: or why things don't fall down*. De Capa Press, New York.

Gordon, J. E. (1988) *The science of structures and materials*. W. H. Freeman, New York.

Gould, S. J. (1989) Gratuitous battle. *Civilization*, **87**.

Gracovetsky, S. (1988) *The spinal engine*. Springer-Verlag, New York.

Grant, J. C. B. (1952) *A method of anatomy*. Williams and Wilkins, Baltimore, MD.

Ingber, D. E. (1997) Tensegrity: the architectural basis of cellular mechanotransduction. *Annual Review of Physiology*, **59**, 575–99.

Ingber, D. (1998) The architecture of life. *Scientific American*, **278**, 48–57.

Ingber, D. E. (2000) The origin of cellular life. *Bioessays*, **22**, 1160–70.

Ingber, D. E., Jamieson, J. (1985) Cells as tensegrity structures. Architectural regulation of histodiferentiation by phsical forces trasduced over basement membrane. Academic Press, New York.

Kroto, H. (1988) Space, stars, C60, and soot. *Science*, **242**, 1139–45.

Levin, S. M. (1982) Continuous tension, discontinuous compression, a model for biomechanical support of the body. *Bulletin of Structural Integration*. Rolf Institute, Boulder, CO, pp. 31–3.

Levin, S. M. (1986) The icosahedron as the three-dimensional finite element in biomechanical support. *Proceedings of the Society of General Systems Research Symposium on Mental Images, Values and Reality. International Conference on Mental Images, Values, and Reality, SGSR 30th Annual Meeting, Philadelphia*, **I**, G14–26.

Levin, S. M. (1995) *The importance of soft tissues for structural support of the body*. Hanley & Belfus, Philadelphia, PA.

Levin, S. M. (1997) Putting the shoulder to the wheel: a new biomechanical model for the shoulder girdle. *Biomedical Sciences Instrumentation*, **33**, 412–17.

Mandelbrot, B. B. (1983) *The fractal geometry of nature*. W. H. Freeman, New York.

Pearce, P. (1978) *Structure in nature as a strategy for design*. MIT Press, Cambridge.

Prigogine, I., Stengers, I. (1984) *Order out of chaos: man's new dialogue with nature.* Bantam Books, London.

Schultz, A. B. (1983) Biomechanics of the spine. Low back pain and industrial and social disablement. Back Pain Association, London: 20–25.

Snelson, K. (2002) http://www.kennethsnelson.net/.

Stamenovic, D., Fredberg, J. J., Wang, N., Butler, J. P., Ingber, D. E. (1996) A microstructural approach to cytoskeletal mechanics based on tensegrity. *Journal of Theoretical Biology,* **181,** 125–36.

Stevens, P. S. (1974) *Patterns in nature.* Little, Brown, Boston.

Toffler, A. (1984) Science and change. In: I. Prigogine and I. Stengers (eds.) *Order out of chaos: man's new dialogue with nature.* Bantam Books, London, pp. xi–xxxi.

Waldrop, M. M. (1992) *Complexity.* Penguin, London.

Wang, N., Butler, J. P., Ingber, D. E. (1993) Mechanotransduction across the cell surface and through the cytoskeleton. *Science,* **260,** 1124–7.

Wang, N., Naruse, K., Stamenovic, D., *et al.* (2001) Mechanical behavior in living cells consistent with the tensegrity model. *Proceedings of the National Academy of Sciences of the USA,* **98,** 7765–70.

Wildy, P., Home, R. W. (1963) Structure of animal virus particles. *Progressive Medical Virology,* 5, 1–42.

Wolff, J. (1892) *Das Gesetz der Transformation der Knocchen.* Hirschwald, Berlin.

2.2.6 The fascioligamentous organ

Thomas Dorman

An understanding of the dynamic function of the fascioligamentous organ is a most important conceptual requirement in musculoskeletal medicine. Clinicians who understand the function of the organ they are about to treat are self-evidently much more likely to plan treatment well.

Most soft tissue injuries presenting with pain, such as back pain, neck pain after a whiplash accident, tennis elbow, sprains of the knees, etc., are due to a localized failure of the **fascioligamentous organ**. This organ encompasses the whole body and constitutes approximately 6% of its makeup. Concentrations of connective tissue in certain areas were given specific names by the early anatomists. Examples include the ligamentum nuchae in the posterior part of the neck, or the posterior sacroiliac ligaments (about which much more later) in the low back. We should maintain in our minds, however, an image of the fascioligamentous organ **as a whole**. It is a continuous structure, and no amount of emphasis is redundant in making this point. Much of the present book deals with specific 'lesions' in specific areas – a reductionist approach. No criticism of this approach is implied in this section; it is essential in analyzing specific problems. Contrariwise, a holistic view of the fascioligamentous organ of our bodies is also necessary. It is particularly important when a reductionist approach, such as treating a somatic dysfunction in one location repeatedly, or failing to correct an area of recurrent sprain and inflammation by repeated topical steroid injection. It is in this context that a holistic point of view is likely to yield a fresh analysis and thence a fresh therapeutic approach.

Recent research has demonstrated the unique qualities of the human pelvis as a major anatomical device for the purpose of walking. This perspective has shed much light on the role of ligaments as organs for the storage and release of elastic energy. The fascioligamentous organ transfers the forces of tension through the whole body. It is best thought of as a tensegrity system. For psychological reasons which are not entirely clear to me, it is a characteristic of the human mind that it can easily visualize the transfer of forces through columns, beams, lintels and cantilevers, but we have difficulty in visualizing the transfer of forces diffusely through a tensegrity model (see Chapter 2.2.5). Nevertheless, experience teaches us that the concepts of the tensegrity model are not only germane to understanding the function of our own bodies, but indispensable when analyzing its dysfunction. To help with this psychological difficulty I will use a single example. Automobiles travel reliably on soft material. The air and the rubber constituting the tire and the inner tube of a wheel are each insufficient to support our vehicles, but the integrated function is something we have come to take for granted. This is a simple model

because it is nonhierarchical. A multitude of subdivisions or septa between the compartments in an hierarchical tensegrity system provides certain integrated qualities to what are inherently weak structures, giving them combined strength. This is how organic systems work, and certainly how our own bodies function. From the point of view of the orthopedic physician, training oneself to think in these terms is invaluable. It affords the tools that allow the practitioner to analyze clinical problems in orthopedic medicine effectively, and hence make productive therapeutic plans.

Role of elastic tissue in the human pelvis

Fishes and snakes advance by waves of lateral contraction and relaxation of groups of muscles within metamers. Reptiles with four legs maintain this mode of locomotion. Their body weight is supported directly on the ground. Quadruped walking of mammals is more complex. The organism alternately supports body quadrants over the swing leg, requiring greatly increased coordination and balance because the body is no longer on the ground. The complexity of the nervous system and the size of the brain parallel the increased intricacy of locomotion and coordination.

Though passive dynamic walking calls for little action from the nervous system (McGeer 1990), biped walking represents another increment in complexity. The static support of any structure on legs calls for at least three points of support, a possibility in the quadruped stance. Biped locomotion, on the other hand, is predicated on balance and coordination with continuous movement. Perhaps this is the reason for the additional increase in size of the human brain (Sinclair and Leakey 1986).

Evolutionary consideration

Since Charles Darwin's (1871) proposal of a common ancestral origin for *Homo sapiens* and humanoids, it has been assumed that the human biped posture is an evolutionary development from a more primitive quadruped one. The absence of a confirmatory paleontological link after 140 years of research should now raise the consideration that bipedal locomotion and the upright stance represent an earlier, or intrinsic, characteristic of *Homo sapiens* (Brown *et al.* 1985, Berge 1986, Hasegawa *et al.* 1987). Though it might appear heretical to some contemporary readers, the suggestion that mechanical and gravitational influences have contributed to morphological ontogeny and by implication to phylogeny is neither new (Thompson 1917, Berg 1922), nor passé (Carter 1987). In this context it might be interesting to consider the anatomy, comparative anatomy, and physiology of walking in the human frame as not necessarily closely analogous to quadruped walking.

The physiology of walking

Studies on the efficiency of locomotion have recorded a paradox (Alexander and Jayes 1983). Oxygen consumption in human running is substantially less than calculated from the work done. (It has also been shown that various forms of terrestrial locomotion have similar energy economics; Cavagna *et al.* 1977). Although a large bibliography has accumulated on gait, the 'research front' (Vaughn 1982) has been on instrumentation based on electromyography and the use of dynamic imaging modalities for comparison of normal and abnormal gait in various conditions. Just as there has been little interest in the anatomy of the pelvic ring in general and the sacrum in particular, so has there has been a deficiency in analysis of the role of these structures in locomotion (Gracovetsky 1988). There has been an interesting suggestion recently that the anatomy of the human pelvis has evolved, teleologically speaking, to accommodate efficient walking rather than parturition (Abitbol 1987, 1988a). The width of the pelvis in the oldest humanoid skeleton has also been given this significance (Rak 1991).

It is 'advantageous' for the bipedal organism to conserve energy during locomotion. Conservation can take several forms.

Walking: a pendulum

A pendulum conserves energy. The analogy of a large pendulum in a grandfather clock might serve as a first approximation. The kinetic energy is stored in the upswing, as gravitational energy, to be released after the pendulum momentarily stops at the inertia point. A small amount of energy is imparted to the pendulum with each swing, the additional push being just sufficient to compensate for the loss by friction. By this means, the clock (with its pendulum) re-uses the swing energy time and again, kinetic and gravitational energy alternating, recycling. On observing a walking man, the analogy acquires flesh (Alexander 1975), and this contrasts with the relative inefficiency of quadruped walking (Abitbol 1988b). The efficiency of stride length and speed of walking have been evaluated by means of studying oxygen consumption (Inman et al. 1981). There is an optimal speed of walking for each individual, which can be predicted by physical measurements (Holt et al. 1991). It is suggested here that these observations support the analogy with a pendulum. First, walking begins as a controlled fall, then, as the pelvis hitches up on the stance leg and the

swing leg departs from the ground, the leg gains momentum at first and decelerates before heel contact. The first acceleration occurs from the controlled forward fall forward and the deceleration occurs at the end of the swing. Was the decelerating energy dissipated as heat? We now know from some previous studies that at least in human running there is some storage or reutilization of energy (Alexander 1975). It is my impression that the kinetic energy of the decelerating leg is transferred in part into forward locomotion (every force is opposed by an equal and opposite force; Newton's third law of motion). The upper end of the swing leg, being attached to the pelvis and thence to the trunk, transmits forward locomotion to the body with deceleration. This can be observed in gait-analysis studies as there is uneven acceleration of the trunk during forward progression.

The body wobbles backwards and forwards during forward walking. In order to appreciate this wobble, which is superimposed on the overall advancement, it is advantageous to subtract the average forward movement. The easiest way to appreciate this is to watch a person walking on a treadmill. This wobble is thought to represent the cyclic intake and dissipation of kinetic energy in synchrony with the pendular movement of the legs.

We know that walking is more efficient than running (Cavagna 1978, Pierrynowski et al. 1980).

Trunk bobbing

During normal walking, the head (and body) move up and down in the equivalent of a sinusoid wave. What is the fate of the gravitational energy dissipated on the down-slope? It is proposed that this energy is, by and large, not converted to heat, and thus lost, but stored in the 'walking machine'. Part of it is transmitted to forward locomotion, a fall off the stance leg. Part is transmitted into elastic tissues such as, for instance, the collagen of the ligaments reinforcing the anterior aspect of the hip joint. In long strides, just before the rear leg is converted from a stance to a swing leg, tension can be sensed in the front of the hip. This stretch – elastic energy – is, of course, promptly released again as the stance leg begins to swing. In fact, it contributes to the acceleration of the swing leg together with the gravitational contribution mentioned earlier.

In this context it is interesting to note that it is more efficient to carry a weight on the head than in a back pack (Maloiy et al. 1986): presumably the weight on the head does not interfere with the vertical 'clockwork mechanism' we are discussing here.

Elastic energy

The storage of elastic energy has been recognized and taken for granted by the keepers of physiologic knowledge within the medico-scientific establishment since the turn of the century.

Respiration

Inspiration is the result of active contraction of intercostal muscles and the diaphragm; the chest expands. The initial phase of expiration is passive, the elastic chest wall collapsing to a smaller volume. Forced expiration calls for muscle action contracting the chest to a smaller volume. The neutral position is known in fact to represent a dynamic neutrality because the lungs, when observed outside the rib cage, collapse to an even smaller volume. The vacuum in the pleural space

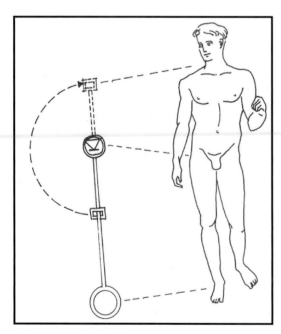

Figure 2.2.49 Walking: a pendulum.

(sometimes called negative pressure, erroneously) stops them from collapse. So the neutral position of the chest in the intact organism represents a greater degree of pulmonary expansion than would be spontaneous for the lungs alone. On the contrary, the chest wall itself is pulled inwards by the elasticity of the lungs proper, so its resting posture is more contracted than would be the case without the inward pull of the lungs. The balance, therefore, is a dynamic equilibrium. In this instance, the elasticity of the rib cage is balanced by the elasticity of the lungs. The breathing organism needs only shift the balance to and fro a little for the bellows to work. The analogy with a pendulum comes to mind, but a better analogy is that of the coiled balance spring of a watch escapement. It was the invention of Christiaan Huygens (1629–1695), a Dutch watchmaker, who was first able to store elastic energy in a spring where formerly clockmakers could only use the gravity pendulum. So it is that as we advance our understanding of the walking machine, another analogy from the clockmaker's trade is brought into service. Where else in the body, we might ask, is elastic energy stored in each step? It would, speaking teleologically again, be advantageous for the walking machine to use the spring-storage model as extensively as possible.

Joint capsules as stores of elastic energy

Anyone can confirm the storage of elastic energy in the ventral ligaments of his interdigital joint capsule by stretching a finger backwards and releasing it. From watching the cycle of walking, it seems that elastic energy is stored (as mentioned earlier) in the anterior part of the hip capsule (not only by extension but also by internal rotation of the femur). In this context, note the alignment of the main collagenous fibers in the anterior portion of the hip joint: they are stretched by this movement. Next, the posterior ligaments of the knee, the so-called ligament of Valois; in the foot, the plantar aponeurosis, as well as the ligaments of the deep arches of the foot are all stretched at the end of the stance phase and all release energy as the limb begins its swing.

Fasciae

I use the term fasciae to describe the sheets of connective tissue made up predominantly of woven collagen fibers which in a previous generation were referred to as surgical fasciae and intermuscular septae. Ligaments are connective tissue structures which bind bone to bone. Tendons are connective tissue structures which bind muscle to bone (and occasionally muscle to muscle, as in the digastric or omohyoid muscles). Fasciae are flat sheets of collagenous material which bind other elements of the musculoskeletal system to each other and traverse the body widely (Macintosh and Bogduk 1990). The aphorism of old anatomists that 'the fascia is continuous' is worth repeating.

Storage of elastic energy

A ballerina in the fifth position winds up each leg in external rotation, so tension is created between them. Each is wound up, so to speak, in an opposite direction on the pelvis. When the ballerina initiates the pirouette with a slight muscle-induced knee extension she releases the stored energy which is converted to a vertical jump. In dancing circles this force has been recognized since before the days of Diaghilev. In this example, where is the elastic energy stored? It is quite plain that some of it is stored in the foot (as in the case of the posterior stance leg

discussed earlier), some is stored in the medial collateral ligaments of the knee, some in the anterior ligaments of the hip joint. But anyone who assumes this position, to test it, will sense the tension in the enveloping fasciae of calf and thigh. A crouched runner in a start position similarly stores energy in his calf, although a lot of this elasticity is stored in the triceps surae. Hitherto, conventional wisdom has ascribed the functions of wrapping and compartmentalization to fascia. We now know that fascia has the additional function of the **storage of elastic energy** (Vleeming *et al.* 1989).

Locus of energy storage

As far as I have been able to understand, it seems that the storage of elastic energy has been imputed to the muscles since early research on locomotion (Cavagna *et al.* 1964, Thys *et al.* 1972), and even recent authoritative researchers have accepted a role in elastic storage merely to the tendons of muscles (Alexander 1991). It seems, however, that this ascription has been arbitrary. The contractile elements of muscles, i.e. the actin and myosin, are not inherently elastic; the storage is therefore much more suitably ascribed to collagen and elastin, i.e. the fascial component of the myofascial structures, and to ligaments proper.

In the case of the spring ligament of the foot, it is easy to understand how the talus is supported by elastic tension between calcaneum and navicular. The weight of the body transmitted via the talus stretches the spring ligament, which releases its energy to the uprising foot. In the final analysis, it can be reasonably assumed that the energy is stored in electrostatic forces in the outer electron shells of the stretched atoms making up the collagen molecules and strands, right inside the spring ligament (Nimni 1997).

As a final example, contemplate a discus thrower who has wound up his torso just before starting the swing that will eventually transmit all his elastic, muscular, and kinetic energy into the flying discus. Can an analysis be made of the exact locus of the stored elastic energy at that moment? For that matter, in the case of the coiled watch spring in the mechanical wristwatch escapement, can an analysis be made of where in the spring the elastic energy is stored? In both cases the answer has to be that the energy is stored diffusely in the whole structure. (It is intuitively understandable that it is not rational to ascribe the storage of a small amount of energy in the spring to a group of molecules at one end of it, and it is proposed here that to a certain extent this analogy can be taken into the body's fascia.) Just as the fascia is anatomically continuous, it is proposed here that so it is with the stored energy. The storage is diffuse. We should start thinking of the connective tissue as an organ for energy storage.

Torque

The arms swing alternately and synchronously with walking. In fact, the upper girdle rotates back and forth with each step. The angular momentum and acceleration are proportionate to the speed of walking. An horological analogy is available. The store of energy in a horizontal circular (so-called) pendulum, which is really a flywheel torqued on a suspensory spring, was invented in the Black Forest in 1881 and serves as the basis for the famous 400-day clock. Though not suspended, the upper girdle functions the same way. Torque is stored in the spine (and a little gravitational energy in the rising and falling arms). It is a common experience that with the arms bound, or the upper girdle restrained with a haversack frame, walking is fatiguing, chaffing, and inefficient. Measurements of oxygen consumption when

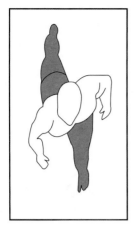

Figure 2.2.50 Elastic energy: alternating synchrony.

the torso is in a brace have confirmed this impression (Inman 1966). It is also apparent that the pelvic girdle swivels with each step in time with the swing leg and in alternating synchrony with the upper girdle. We now know that elastic energy is stored in the pelvic girdle itself.

The spinal engine

Gracovetsky (1988) has summarized and explained the mechanisms by which the small muscles of the spine convert their contractions into locomotion, and his text is an invaluable reference. Side bending is converted to torque through the 'gearbox' of the zygoapophyseal joints. Finally, pelvic rotation activates the legs. Immobilization of the trunk retards the efficiency of walking (Ralston 1965), as judged by oxygen utilization. Does this represent an interference with the action of the spinal muscles in the 'spinal engine', or does it mean that there is interference with the storage and release of elastic energy (torque) which might enhance the pendular (flywheel) efficiency of the 'walking machine'?

Pelvic dynamics

The opinion once held by scientists that the three pelvic bones are immobile warrants no further comment, except as a reminder that widely held views are not always correct (Weisl 1953, 1955). The relative movement of the ilia versus the sacrum and each other in space, in time, and with the activity of walking in health and disease have been the subject of active study in recent years, and a number of relative movements, axes of rotations, and other dynamics have been suggested. The little research so far available points to variation and differences (Fryette 1954). The presence of movement and the presence of asymmetry are emerging as the norm. All these measurements are based on anatomic observations of the bony parts. The problem is confounded by the complexity of bony geometry, the extraordinary degree of variation, and the extreme difficulty in defining a reference point. Are we perhaps asking the wrong questions? Perhaps we would be better asking questions about the storage capacity of the elastic structures and about hysteresis. In contemporary podiatry, the role of ligaments in the storage of elastic energy with stepping is gaining acceptance (Dananberg 1992). It can, however, be stated with confidence that the iliac bones move with respect to each other and the

sacrum with each step. Asymmetry of the inclination of the pelvis is common (normal in allopathic terminology). It is enhanced in dysfunction and painful conditions and restored towards symmetry with effective healing, whether manual or other (LaCourse *et al.* 1990).

The relationship of torque at the sacrum to weightbearing with the alternation of stepping in walking has been demonstrated (Stevens 1990), and probably represents the first step in understanding the connection between the passive dynamic walking model of McGeer (1990) and the synchronous flywheel (or rotary pendulum) of the upper trunk, shoulders, and arms, sprung on the elastic spine.

An elastic landscape

If we can allow ourselves, therefore, to look at ligaments and fasciae for a moment only from the perspective of the storage of energy, we should note that ligament tissue is most plentiful in the pelvis. The posterior sacroiliac ligaments are by far the heftiest ligaments in the body. For a while, this observation was dismissed as a pique of nature. Later it was recognized, by analogy (which may have been false analogy) with the quadruped position, that the sacrum is suspended from the ilia and hence the whole weight of the organism is suspended by these ligaments. The strength was attributed to this function. It might be, however, that the function is that of an hierarchical icosahedron, functioning as a whole, so the local concentration of ligament tissue may not necessarily have a role in suspension, after all (Levin 1986a, 1986b). As we now recognize that torque occurs through the sacroiliac joints with each step, perhaps we should regard these massive posterior sacroiliac ligaments as analogous to the mainspring of a clock (the horological analogies are not quite exhausted). There is no reason why a very short but very strong spring should not store a great deal of energy in a small moment. It is, of course, a very small amount of movement that can occur at the sacroiliac joints.

Asymlocation

A universal link in machinery is a unit which transmits forces or torque while allowing free movement in several directions through a series of couplings. As the body has the same requirement, there are connections in the body, consisting of two or more joints usually

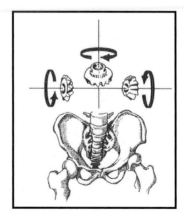

Figure 2.2.51 Asymlocation of the pelvis.

around one 'universal link' bone, which approximate these models. There are only a few instances in human anatomy where an intervening bone has no muscular or tendinous attachments at all (an example is the lunate at the wrist or the talus at the ankle). In the axial skeleton there are, however, a few instances where one of the bones is almost free of ligament and muscle attachments and is prone to asymlocation, like a universal link. The best examples are the atlas and the sacrum, although the lower lumbar vertebrae (usually the fifth, of course) are also prone to this phenomenon. When asymmetric tensions of the surrounding retaining part, for instance, the lumbodorsal fascia, is present, the universal links are apt to be situated with a degree of asymmetry that exceeds the usual or normal and can be a source of dysfunction and pain. I have coined the term **asymlocation** to describe this phenomenon.

It seems obvious that the sacrum is suspended from the ilia in the quadruped position. This can be appreciated by viewing the skeleton of any quadruped mammal, or viewing the arrangement in the human model in the quadruped position. What is the function of the sacrum in biped standing? The word 'function' is used here rather broadly to discuss the forces controlling it. As we know, the sacrum has been compared to the keystone of an arch. The architectural arch is a uniquely stable arrangement. The vertical forces enhance the stability of the masonry. The greater the weight on the arch, the more stable it is. This is so because the adherence of the high-friction surfaces between the stones cut into trapezoid forms is enhanced. Does the sacrum indeed function as a keystone in any circumstance at all?

It is a commonplace observation that humans are a little asymmetric. Not only are the internal organs distributed this way, but some asymmetry seems to be common (normal in allopathic terminology, in the sense that it is usual) in what has been loosely termed the **soma**. For instance, a recent survey of the inclination of the pelvis in healthy athletes has demonstrated that the right ilium is rotated forward in osteopathic terminology normally in right-handed individuals versus the left in left-footed ones. Anyone taking a class in osteopathic manipulation will have observed other class members, who may be seemingly healthy, to have multiple asymmetries in the pelvis and spine which are currently termed **somatic dysfunction** (although I am reluctant to using the term 'dysfunction' for what is usual or normal). It is also a common observation in osteopathic and chiropractic circles that when these asymmetries are abolished by manual methods in symptomatic individuals, the dysfunction is often corrected. In this context dysfunction and disease bear a proximity. What about the 'dysfunction' in the asymptomatic individual? The term 'asymlocation' (Dorman and Ravin 1991) is very helpful here. It seems best suited to describe this circumstance, and it is proposed that when asymlocation is marked the propensity to pain (dysfunction) is increased. Contrariwise, as the dysfunction of the retaining structures (that is to say, ligaments and fasciae) is healed, asymlocation diminishes.

Perhaps this framework will help bridge the unnecessary gap between osteopathy and allopathic medicine.

The sacroiliac joints as friction absorbers

The irregularities of the auricular surfaces were recognized by early anatomists, and the relation to age defined precisely (Lovejoy *et al.* 1985), but it is only in recent times that the qualities of the two opposing cartilaginous surfaces of this joint have been demonstrated to function as friction devices. This has been demonstrated in gross

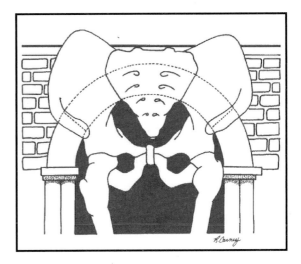

(a)

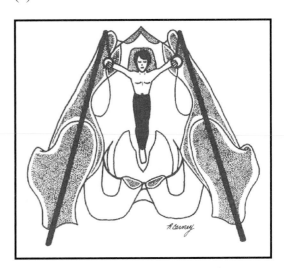

(b)

Figure 2.2.52 Stability of the sacrum in the pelvis (a) as the keystone of an arch and (b) by form and force closure.

anatomy as well as microscopically. These surfaces of the sacroiliac joints can be said, therefore, to function in a manner which is different from that of other synovial joints. They absorb movement by gliding with friction. They encourage stability rather than free movement (Vleeming *et al.* 1990). It can be easily understood that when forces are acting across these joints in a direction other than pure shear they are apt to offer a high resistance.

Form and force closure

The importance of friction in the function of the sacroiliac joints has been conveyed through the introduction of the contrasting concepts of **form closure** and **force closure** (Snijders *et al.* 1992). Form closure refers to a stable situation with closely fitting joint surfaces. In an idealized model of form closure, weightbearing (and the transfer of other forces) would be achieved through snugly fitting geometrical forms alone. Functional analysis of living joints shows that various mechanical refinements are usually present in each. In the case of the sacroiliac joints, the additional factors are distinct. On first inspection the sacrum appears to be wedged between the ilia. It has, however, been shown that on standing, the closed kinematic chain is predicated on lateral pressures through the rough surfaces of these joints. This has been termed **force closure**. In the sacroiliac joints both a compressive lateral force and friction are needed to withstand vertical loads. Shear at the sacroiliac joints is prevented by a combination of the specific anatomical features (form closure) and the compression generated by ligaments and muscles acting across the high friction surfaces (force closure).

Movement and governance of the sacroiliac articulation

A recognition that buttock and leg pain may arise from hypermobility of the joint was raised by Goldthwait and Osgood (1905). Movement of these joints has been accepted since then. Weisl's (1953) work reinforced this understanding. Movement in living humans has been demonstrated stereophotogrammetically (Sturesson *et al.* 1989) with radiology by the placement of Kirschner wires in sacrum and ilium (Colachis *et al.* 1963) and observing the external movement, and through actual measurements of iliac positions with calipers (LaCourse *et al.* 1990, Pitkin and Pheasant 1936). Motion at the sacroiliac joints is maintained even in advanced age. Movement of these joints has been recognized in manual medical circles through methods of palpation throughout the history of osteopathy (Greenman 1989) and well established in physiotherapy circles as well (DonTigny 1993, Hesch 1994).The main controlling soft tissue seems to be by the several periarticular ligaments such as the sacroiliac and sacrotuberous ligaments. The capsule of the sacroiliac joint has been shown radiologically to be incomplete in some cases with back pain (Aprill 1992). An analysis of movement at either sacroiliac articulation calls into question movement at the other two joints of the pelvic ring. Although interconnected through the soft tissues, the relative movement of each of the bones versus the others in the three directions of space, let alone the interaction with the fascial tube of the whole organism, creates a three-dimensional puzzle of great complexity. That manual treatment can be beneficial is now official (Schekelle *et al.* 1991), though the *modus operandi* of the various therapies remains empirical.

What can be said regarding the attendant ligaments and other soft tissue structures surrounding this joint? What role do any of them have in the governance of function? Interestingly, recent research has shown that the large ligamentous bands, recognized of old in the pelvis, play substantial roles in the governance of the sacrum. Finally, to the extent that there is a modal, i.e., most typical pattern of movement round an hypothetical 'axis', it turns out that the deep posterior interosseous ligaments of the sacroiliac joints play that role (Egund *et al.* 1978, Sturesson *et al.* 1989).

Self-bracing

The forces acting in the pelvis in the upright biped position are self-bracing. The keystone of the arch, the sacrum, being wider superiorly, trends downward from the weight of the body and the traction this applies to the ilia – through the posterior sacroiliac ligaments – tends to bring the ilia into adduction. The wedge shape of the sacrum overall being wider in front tends to displace it anteriorly (into the pelvis). A balance occurs between the forward vector and the downward vector. Regardless of the balance, the adducting forces are enhanced through both these vectors. It is plain that the sacrum does not descend into the standing pelvis because of the bracing mechanism and the posterior sacroiliac ligaments. Self-bracing, therefore, is a unique characteristic of the biped human pelvis.

Intuitively it is understandable that self-bracing applies while we are standing on both legs. Walking, however, consists of one leg support alternating continuously. Hence self-bracing is switched on and off normally in gait. Each sacroiliac joint is locked and unlocked with each step alternately. The joint on the stance side is braced. The demonstration of the production of torque at the sacroiliac articulations with one-legged weightbearing (Stevens 1990) can also be taken to imply the reverse, i.e. the dissipation of the stored (torque) energy into the swing leg with step off. There is a regular transmission of energy back and forth with locomotion, contributing to the efficiency of the 'walking machine'.

Clinical patterns and approach to treatment

The use of hypothesis

Assuming then that asymlocation and self-bracing are commonly the cause of dysfunction and chronic back pain (recurrent and later becoming continuous), and seeing that objective confirmation from the laboratory is not forthcoming, what can the clinician do about it? From the above discussion, the question is rhetorical: (1) put it back; (2) keep it back. Hence, the idea that appropriate manipulation to restore symmetry to the pelvis might be followed by ligament refurbishment – **prolotherapy**. This working hypothesis served as the model for the clinical trial of Ongley's technique (Ongley *et al.* 1987). It is to his clarity of thought that we owe not only an understanding of the mechanisms discussed above, but also the development of the combined technique for treatment. This is perhaps a suitable place to reemphasize the importance of meticulous diagnosis in orthopedic medicine. The simple application of a technique of treatment to all comers with back pain, though it will be effective in many, is neither rational nor wise. Not all back pain has one cause.

Points of weakness

A sailor will tell you that in a frayed halyard the concentration of strain always occurs at the weak point. The weak point itself is always where the rope was damaged first. It is not surprising that clinicians have observed the same phenomenon in the inner lining, the fascia. Just as there are characteristic points of wear for a halyard, so it is that strains in the moving part of the body tend to concentrate and eventually lead to injuries at internal sites which have patterns. The patterns have mechanical origins which we may or may not be able to analyze mathematically, intellectually, or intuitively. Nonetheless, the clinician recognizes patterns.

Tensegrity

The form of the body is maintained (in part) by tensegrity, as discussed by Steven Levin in Chapter 2.2.5. This concept explains how variation in the tension of one component of the system affects the whole. We have discussed above how the pelvic girdle serves as a transmission and differential in locomotion, and how the initiating energy arises in muscles but the transmission is through fasciae and ligaments. The transfer of energy from glycogen to distance in walking is modulated by an escapement analogous to that of a clock in several regards. A major component of the efficient mechanism is in the elastic storage of energy in ligaments and fasciae proportionate to their abundance.

Fault propagation

An example of a typical case might consist of a middle-aged or elderly person who walks typically slightly stooped forward and to the right. There is slight compensatory lumbar or thoracolumbar scoliosis to the left. The right ilium is anterior and the right leg slightly externally rotated. On supine examination, one might find a pseudo leg-length discrepancy, the left side being slightly longer, although this is usually easily corrected. There might be a tendency to valgus deformity of the right knee with early osteoarthritic changes and a sprain of the medial coronary and perhaps the medial collateral ligaments. Subsequently, a degree of laxity of the posterior and anterior cruciate ligaments, in that order, will appear. The foot is a little bit flat and the navicular prominent, i.e. there is pronation of the foot. If such an individual is inspected while standing on a glass platform with an illuminated mirror below, unequal distribution of the weight is seen with the person standing. The usual footprint might be maintained on the left, but on the right pronation is observed and the big toe may not press fully on the glass. When the person walks, the medial step-off syndrome is observed. This will have a tendency to produce a degree of hallux valgus on that side and a hammertoe on the second and perhaps third toes. The foot will become painful on walking. Partial avulsion of the plantar fascia might develop and a 'spur' detected if a lateral foot radiograph is taken. If this leads to unwise podiatric surgery, the tendency for the fascial strain will be aggravated. If orthotics are used, this will give temporary relief but aggravate the long-term dysfunction of the fascial windlass operating from the dorsolumbar fascia through the whole fascial sleeve of the lower limb, the surgical fascia of the leg onto the foot. This typical scenario might also arise from an exaggerated forward rotation of the right ilium, asymlocation. The back may or may not be symptomatic at present, and back pain may or may not have been present in the past. The patient may present with a foot problem, a knee problem, or even a problem in the right hip. As the 'walking machine' deteriorates with inefficiency in walking, with increased strain and pressure exerted on the fascial tube, fault propagation might begin to affect the second side. After hip replacement on the first (in this case right) side the left may be involved, and typically a decade might pass before the same phenomenon appear on the other side. It goes without saying that early correction of the fault is more productive than an attempted late correction. When permanent stretches occur in the fascia and ligament, as in the example given, restoring the 'walking machine' to a pristine condition is a hopeless proposition. Nonetheless, many of these patients benefit if the primary dysfunction is corrected, and that is more often than not in the pelvis. It must be acknowledged, however, that a dysfunction in the foot can induce the phenomenon of fault propagation retrograde. In other words, the process is interactive. In conclusion, one should note that the most characteristic and common example of fault propagation in the tensegrity system of the axial skeleton is the phenomenon of pain at the other end of the spine appearing 3–6 months after an injury at the first. I phrase it this way because the initial injury may be in the neck from a whiplash occurrence, or in the low back from a fall on the buttock, or an awkward instance of stooping and lifting with rotation provoking an exaggerated asymlocation – amounting to somatic dysfunction in the pelvis. It is an extraordinarily common observation that individuals suffering from a dysfunction at one end of the spine in due course develop a dysfunction at the other end. Fault propagation through the fascioligamentous tensegrity system is the likely cause.

References

Abitbol, M. (1987) Evolution of the lumbosacral angle. *Am J Physical Anthropol*, **72**, 361–372.

Abitbol, M. (1988a) Evolution of the ischial spine and the pelvic floor in the hominoidea. *Am J Physical Anthropol*, **75**, 53–67.

Abitbol, M. (1988b) Effect of posture and locomotion on energy expenditure. *Am J Physical Anthropol*, **77**, 191–199.

Alexander, R. M. (1975) *Biomechanics*. Chapman & Hall, London.

Alexander, R. M. (1991) Energy-saving mechanisms in walking and running. *J Exp Biol*, **160**, 55–69.

Alexander, R. M., Jayes A. S. (1983) A dynamic similarity hypothesis for the gaits of quadrupedal mammals. *J Zool A*, **207**, 467–482.

Aprill, C. N. (1992) The role of anatomically specific injections into the sacroiliac joint in low back pain and its relation to the sacroiliac joint. Symposium, November 1992, San Diego, CA.

Berg, L. S. (1969) *Nomogenesis or evolution determined by law*. MIT Press, Cambridge, MA. (Originally published in Russian in 1922.)

Berge, C., Kasmierczak J. B. (1986) Effects of size and locomotor adaptations on the hominid pelvis: Evaluation of Australopithecine bipedality with a new multivariate method. *Folia Primatol*, **46**, 185–204.

Brown, F., Harris, J., Leakey, R., Walker A. (1985) Early *Homo erectus* skeleton from west lake Turkana, Kenya. *Nature*, **316**, 788–792.

Carter, R. D. (1987) Mechanical loading history and skeletal biology. *J Biomechanics*, **20**(11), 1095–1109.

Cavagna, G. (1978) Aspects of efficiency and inefficiency of terrestrial locomotion. In: *Biomechanics VI-A*. University Park Press, Baltimore, MD, pp. 3–22.

Cavagna, G. A., Saibene, F. P., Margaria R. (1964) Mechanical work in running. *J Appl Physiol*, **19/20**, 249–256.

Cavagna, G. A., Heglund, N. C., Taylor R. C. (1977) Mechanical work in terrestrial locomotion: two basic mechanisms for minimizing energy expenditure. *Am J Physiol*, **233**, R243–261.

Colachis, S. C., Worden, R. E., Bechtol C. O. *et al.* (1963) Movement of the sacro-iliac joint in the adult male: A preliminary report. *Archiv Phys Med Rehabil*, 44, 490–498.

Dananberg, H. J. (1992) Subtle gait malfunction and chronic musculoskeletal pain. *J Orthop Med*, **14**(1), 18–25.

Darwin, C. (1871) *The descent of man and selection in relation to sex*. 6th edn., London.

DonTigny, R. L. (1993) Mechanics and treatment of the sacroiliac joint. *J Manual Manipulative Ther*, 1(1), 3–12.

Dorman, T., Ravin T. (1991) *Diagnosis and injection techniques in orthopedic medicine*. Williams & Wilkins. Baltimore.

Egund, N., Olson, T. H., Schmid, H., Selvik, G. (1978) Movement in the sacroiliac joints demonstrated with roentgen stereophotogrammetry. *Acta Radiol Diag*, **19**, 833–846.

Fryette, H. H. (1954) *Principles of osteopathic technic.* Academy of Applied Osteopathy, Carmel.

Goldthwait, J. E., Osgood R. B. (1905) Essential of body mechanics in health and disease. *Med Surg J*, **152**, 593–634.

Gracovetsky, S. (1988) *The spinal engine.* Springer-Verlag, New York.

Greenman, P. E. 1989 Principles of manual medicine. Williams & Wilkins, Baltimore, MD.

Hasegawa, M., Kishino, H., Yano, T. (1987) Man's place in hominoidae as inferred from molecular clocks of DNA. *J Mol Evol*, **26**, 132–147.

Hesch, J (1994) *The Hesch method of treating sacroiliac joint dysfunction.* 14117 Grand Ave, N. E., Albuquerque, NM.

Holt, K. G., Hamill, J., Andres, R. O. (1991) Prediccting the minimal energy costs of human walking. *Med Sci Sports Exer*, **23**(4), 491–498.

Inman, V. T. (1966) Human locomotion. *Can Med Assoc J*, **94**, 1047–1057.

Inman, V. T., Ralston, J. H., Todd F. (1981) *Human walking.* Williams & Wilkins. Baltimore, MD, pp. 62–69.

LaCourse, M., Moore, K., Davis, K., Fune, M., Dorman, T. (1990) A report on the asymmetry of iliac inclination: A study comparing normal, laterality and change in a patient population with painful sacro-iliac dysfunction treated with prolotherapy. *J Orthop Med*, **12**, 69–72.

Levin, S. M. (1986a) Proceedings of the 30th annual meeting of the Society of General Systems Research, Philadelphia, PA, 1, G14–26.

Levin, S. M. (1986b) The ichosahedron as the three dimensional finite element in biomechanical support. A natural hierarchical system. Presented at the NAAM Annual Meeting, Philadelphia.

Lovejoy, C. O., Meindl, R. S., Pryzbeck, T. R., Mensforth, R. P. (1985) Chronological metamorphosis of the auricular surface of the ilium: A new method for the determination of adult skeletal age at death. *Am J Phys Anthropol*, **68**, 15–28.

Macintosh, J. E., Bogduk, N. (1990) Basic biomechanics pertinent to the study of the lumbar disc. *J Man Med*, **5**, 52–7.

Maloiy, G. M. O., Heglund, N. C., Prager, L. M., Cavagna, G. A., Taylor, R. C. (1986) Energetic costs of carrying loads: have African women discovered an economic way? *Nature*, **319**, 68–9.

McGeer, T. (1990) Passive dynamic walking. *Int J Robotics Res*, **9**, 2.

Nimni M. E. (1997) Collagen, structure and function. In: *Encyclopedia of human biology*, 2nd edn, 2, 559–574. Academic Press, New York

Ongley, M. J., Klein, R. G., Dorman, T. A. *et al.* (1987) A new approach to the treatment of chronic back pain. *Lancet*, ii, 143–146.

Pierrynowski, M., Winter, D., Norman, R. (1980) Transfers of mechanical energy within the total body and mechanical efficiency during treadmill walking. *Ergonomics*, **23**, 147–156.

Pitkin, H. C., Pheasant, H. (1936) Sacrarthrogenic telalgia. A study of sacral mobility. *J Bone Jt Surg*, **18**, 365–74.

Rak, Y. (1991) Lucy's pelvic anatomy: its role in bipedal gait. *J Human Evol*, **20**, 283–290.

Ralston, H. J. (1965) Effects of immobilization of various body segments on the energy cost of human locomotion. *Proc 2nd IEA Conference Dortmund, 1964.* Supplement to *Ergonomics*, p. 53.

Schekelle, P. G., Adams, A. H., Chassin, M. R., Hurwitz, E. L., Phillips, R. B., Brook, R. H. (1991) *The appropriateness of spinal manipulation for low-back pain.* Rand, 1700 Main Street, Santa Monica, CA.

Sinclair A. R. E., Leakey, M. D. (1986) Migration and hominid bipedalism. *Nature*, **324**(27), 307–8.

Snijders, C. J., Vleeming, A., Stoeckart, R. (1997) Movement, stability, and low back pain: the central role of the pelvis. Churchill Livingstone, p. 103–13.

Stevens, A. (1990) Side bending and axial rotation of the sacrum inside the pelvic girdle. Proceedings of the First International Congress on Low Back Pain and the Sacro-Iliac Joint, San Diego, November.

Sturesson, B., Selvik, G., Udèn, A. (1989) Movement of the sacroiliac joints: a roentgen stereophotogrammetic analysis. *Spine*, **14**(2), 162–165.

Thompson, D. W. (1961) *On growth and form.* Cambridge University Press, Cambridge. (First published in 1917.)

Thys, H., Faraggiana, T., Margaria, R. (1972) Utilization of muscle elasticity in exercise. *J Appl Physiol*, **32**, 491–4.

Vaughn, K. (1982) *Biomechanics of human gait: An annotated bibliography.* Dept Biomedical Engineering, University of Cape Town.

Vleeming, A., Stoeckart, R., Snijders, C. J. (1989) The sacrotuberous ligament: A conceptual approach to its dynamic role in stabilizing the sacro-iliac joint. *Clin Biomech*, **4**, 201–203.

Vleeming, A., Stoeckart, R., Volkers A. C. W., Snijders, C. J. (1990) Relation between form and function in the sacro-iliac joint. *Spine*, **15**(2), 133–136.

Vleeming, A., Van Wingerden, J. P., Dijkstra, P. F., *et al.* (1992) Mobility in the sacro-iliac joints at high age. In: *The sacroiliac joint: a clinical, biomechanical and radiological study.* Erasmus University, Rotterdam.

Weisl, H. (1953) The relation of movement to structure in the sacro-iliac joint. Ph.D. thesis, University of Manchester.

Weisl, H. (1955) The movement of the sacro-iliac joint. *Acta Anat*, **23**, 80–91.

2.3   Pain

2.3.1   Pain concepts: chronic pain

Bruce L. Kidd

Pain is a disabling symptom that is associated with costs to the individual and to society. Although it has undoubtedly evolved as a protective response, pain may also have less benign effects on physical and psychological well-being that require recognition if effective treatment is to be given.

One of the cardinal features of musculoskeletal disease is that normally innocuous stimuli produce pain. Since the publication of the gate control theory by Melzack and Wall (1965) it has been apparent that the nervous system is not fixed or rigid, but rather is capable of a range of responses according to different conditions (neural 'plasticity'). Subsequent research has characterized the mechanisms by which these changes occur as well as highlighting the importance of environmental factors on perception of pain.

This chapter describes the mechanisms that encode and transmit noxious information from the periphery to the brain. This physiological process is contrasted with the perceptual one that results in experience of pain at higher levels. The peripheral and central mechanisms underlying neural plasticity that lead to the development of hypersensitivity are discussed, together with a short review of the assessment of chronic pain.

Definitions

Pain

Even casual reflection results in the conclusion that pain is a complex and varied phenomenon. To ancient Greeks, pain was pure emotion, at the opposite end of a continuum with pleasure. In contrast, more recent descriptions have focused largely on the sensory aspects of pain, in part as a result of the availability of quantitative sensory testing methods developed in the early twentieth century.

A reconciliation of these two perspectives occurred in the late 1960s when the existence of separate sensory–discriminative and affective–motivational pain components was first proposed by Melzack and Casey (1968). This approach has since gained broad acceptance and has had a profound impact on subsequent research. Contemporary opinion recognizes the multidimensional character of pain by distinguishing both sensory and emotional components (Merskey and Bogduk 1994) (see box).

Although the 'unpleasant' character of pain is emphasized in most current definitions, it is accepted that there are a number of unpleasant somatic sensations that are not intrinsically painful. Itch, for example, is unpleasant but not painful. In addressing this problem Fields (1999) has suggested that the term 'algosity' be applied to the property of an unpleasant sensation that allows an individual to identify it as pain. Thus itch, for example, would have unpleasantness with zero algosity, whereas pain would have both unpleasantness and algosity. Whether this approach will prove fruitful in leading to new concepts and new definitions of pain remains to be seen.

Hypersensitivity

Further problems are encountered with words used to describe the clinical features of pain. Many terms in current use were introduced to describe the clinical features of neurological lesions and have less value when describing the features of other diseases. For example, hyperalgesia (see box) refers to enhanced pain in response to a noxious stimulus, whereas allodynia refers to pain following a normally innocuous stimuli. This distinction is helpful when using such discrete stimuli as light touch and pinprick, but it becomes less meaningful when a graded stimulus such as increasing pressure is applied.

Some useful definitions

Pain: An unpleasant sensory and emotional experience associated with actual or potential tissue damage, or described in terms of such damage

Hyperaesthesia (hypersensitivity): Increased sensitivity to stimulation, excluding the special senses

Hyperalgesia: Increased pain in response to a noxious stimulus

Allodynia: Pain due to a stimulus that does not normally produce pain

From the International Association for the Study of Pain (IASP) definitions (Merskey, and Bogduk 1994)

Strictly speaking, joint disease is characterized by mechanical allodynia as symptoms generally arise following movement within the normal (usually innocuous) range. Similarly, the discomfort experienced when pressure is applied to a so-called 'tender point' might also be termed mechanical allodynia for the same reasons. In practice, when applied to musculoskeletal disease the terms hyperalgesia and allodynia tend to be used interchangeably and the more general term **hypersensitivity** (or hyperaesthesia) is to be preferred. Whatever term is used, however, it should be remembered that symptoms and signs may not necessarily specify the underlying pathophysiology for, as will be discussed later, similar clinical features may be produced by a number of different mechanisms.

The process of pain

A comprehensive understanding of pain requires an appreciation not only of neural pathways and the mechanisms by which pain occurs, but also of the consequences of pain to the individual. At the physiological level pain leads to a stress response involving activation of neuroendocrine and autonomic systems as well as behavioural change. Although during acute pain these effects are generally short lived and relatively benign, in chronic situations they may include fatigue, dysphoria, myalgia, and impaired mental and physical performance (see Chapman and Gavrin 1999 for review).

In clinical settings it may be useful to identify four broad processes as being associated with pain: nociception, pain perception, suffering, and pain behaviours (Loeser and Melzack 1999).

- **Nociception:** This may be defined as the detection of noxious stimuli or tissue damage and the subsequent transmission of encoded information to the brain In this process tissue injury is followed by activation of receptors (transduction), relay of information from the periphery to the central nervous system (CNS) (transmission), and neural activity controlling the pain management pathway (modulation).

- **Pain perception:** In essence, whereas nociception is a physiological process, pain is a perceptual one that involves higher CNS mechanisms (Turk and Okifuji 1999). Although it is usually triggered by a noxious stimulus, pain can also arise in the absence of nociceptive activity. All too often this important fact is overlooked. The view that underlying pathology correlates directly with pain perception remains prevalent in both clinicians and patients alike, and leads inevitably to the misapprehension that pain is either organic (i.e. 'real') or psychogenic (i.e. somehow 'made up').

- **Suffering:** Pain and suffering are not identical. Although pain and suffering may coexist, they are distinct phenomena. Suffering is a state of distress that is often present in patients with chronic pain, but may also accompany other experiences such as fear or anxiety. Defining suffering is difficult but it may be regarded as the 'perception of serious threat or damage to oneself', and often develops when a discrepancy develops between expectations and functional abilities (Cassell 1982). Such discrepancies often arise following either physical or psychological stress, with resultant neuroendocrine activity triggering adaptive responses that a person experiences as sickness.

- **Pain behaviours:** Following an acute injury, pain behaviours serve a protective function and include simple verbal and motor responses.

In chronic situations pain behaviours become more complex and are often maintained as a result of environmental reinforcement. Whilst pain perception and suffering are private, subjective experiences such as pain behaviours are overt expressions that communicate pain and distress to others. These can be recorded and form a useful component of the clinical assessment.

Nociception

Nociception is not the same as pain. Nevertheless, knowledge of underlying nociceptive mechanisms is helpful in identifying both the likely cause and the best treatment for a particular symptom or sign.

Cutaneous and deep somatic tissues, including joints and muscles, are innervated by primary afferent neurones that synapse with second-order neurones in the dorsal horn of the spinal cord. Sensory information is then relayed via spinothalamic and spinoreticular tracts to supraspinal structures including the thalamus and the brain stem. Powerful internal controls are present at all levels, as exemplified by descending modulatory systems.

The periphery

The primary sensory neurones have three functions with respect to their role in nociception: transduction, or detection of the stimulus; conduction of action potentials to the CNS; and transmission to central neurones (Woolf and Costigan 1999).

Transduction

The musculoskeletal system is abundantly supplied with encapsulated receptors and free nerve endings that detect and encode environmental stimuli. More specialized encapsulated receptors are found mainly in fibrous periarticular structures, but free nerve endings are more widely distributed in fibrous capsules, adipose tissues, ligaments, menisci and periosteum (Mapp *et al.* 1990).

The properties of receptors that detect either normal low intensity stimuli or intense noxious stimuli differ in many important respects. Receptors for everyday non-painful stimuli (such as light touch or movement) are characterized by specificity to a particular stimulus, a high degree of gain to amplify weak signals, and rapid adaptation to increasing signal intensities (Cesare and McNaughton 1997). In contrast, the primary imperative following a noxious or damaging stimulus is to withdraw the affected area as quickly as possible. Under these conditions receptor specificity is not so important. Therefore it is not surprising that most high-threshold nociceptors respond to a variety of thermal, chemical, and mechanical stimuli.

A further and clinically relevant characteristic of nociceptors is that far from adapting to an activating stimulus, they actually increase their sensitivity by a process termed **sensitization** (see below). Although sensitization will obviously serve a protective function in the acute stages of injury it often has deleterious consequences when the stimulus is prolonged as in, for example, inflammatory arthritis.

The detailed molecular and cellular mechanisms underlying the detection of painful stimuli are being revealed as new technologies become available. It is apparent that many specialized receptors are present on sensory terminals. These include a series of ion-channel-linked receptors such as the heat sensitive vanilloid receptor 1 (VR1), and others sensitive to protons and intense mechanical deformation of the membrane. A series of receptors sensitive to chemical stimuli alone, including kinins and various cytokines, have also been described (Woolf and Costigan 1999).

Conduction

Sensory, or 'afferent' neurones within nerves arising from musculo-skeletal structures can be classified in a number of different ways. Morphologically, three groups of afferent neurones can be distinguished: heavily myelinated A beta fibres, thinly myelinated A delta fibres and unmyelinated C fibres. Articular nerves also contain unmyelinated sympathetic postganglionic fibres. It is notable that the vast majority of articular neurones are unmyelinated, comprising sensory C fibres and sympathetic efferent fibres in nearly equal numbers (Langford and Schmidt 1983).

Myelinated A beta fibres are rapidly conducting (conduction velocities greater than 30 m/s) and within the musculoskeletal system are mainly concerned with conveying proprioceptive information from their encapsulated receptors. In contrast, thinly myelinated A delta fibres (conduction velocities 2.5–30 m/s) and unmyelinated C fibres (conduction velocities less than 2.5 m/s) have free nerve endings. Although most of these neurones are nociceptors, others are activated by non-noxious stimuli but then increase their activity as the intensity of the stimulus increases (for a review see Schaible and Grubb 1993).

One interesting group of nociceptors cannot normally be activated and become excitable only under pathological conditions such as inflammation. These 'silent' or 'sleeping' nociceptors were first found in joint tissue but have subsequently been described in other tissues as well (Schaible and Grubb 1993, Besson 1999).

Two major classes of C fibres have recently been characterized on the basis of biochemical and anatomical differences (Snider and McMahon 1998). Like all peripheral neurones, sensory nerves require connections with their target tissues and a source of nerve growth factors, neurotrophins, for their survival during development. By adulthood this requirement is lost, but around 40% of dorsal root ganglion cells continue to express the nerve growth factor (NGF) TrkA receptor. These cells project to areas associated with nociceptive transmission and also produce and transport a variety of neuropeptides that are involved in neuromodulation and peripheral neurogenic inflammation. A further 30% lose TrkA developmentally and become responsive to a second neurotrophic factor, glial cell line-derived neurotrophic factor (GDNF), although their function remains unclear.

Ion channels, including sodium and potassium channels, mediate conduction in nociceptors from peripheral receptors to the spinal cord. Neuronal voltage-gated sodium channels can be classified into two types: those sensitive to the puffer fish toxin, tetrodotoxin (tetrodotoxin-sensitive, TTXs) and those resistant to it (tetrodotoxin-resistant, TTXr). Large-diameter neurones only express a TTXs sodium current, whereas small-diameter nociceptor neurones express both TTXs and TTXr currents. Two sensory neuron-specific TTXr sodium channels have been recently been cloned – SNS/PN3 and SNS2/NaN (Woolf and Costigan 1999). Although the exact significance of these observations remains to be established, blocking TTXr receptors presents an attractive therapeutic strategy for analgesia.

The spinal cord

Small-diameter afferent neurones passing within peripheral nerves have their cell bodies in the posterior (dorsal) root ganglia and enter

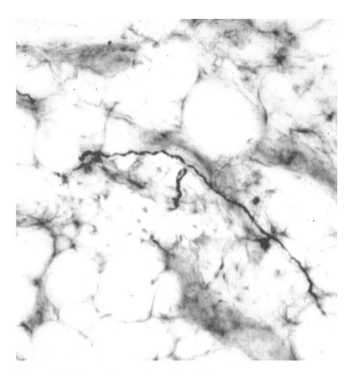

Figure 2.3.1 Photomicrograph: peripheral fibre.

the spinal cord through posterior roots to synapse in the dorsal horn (Figure 2.3.1). Unlike other neurones, the cell bodies of these neurones have no synaptic connections and probably play no role in instantaneous signal processing.

The grey matter of the spinal cord has been divided into 10 laminae on the basis of the neuronal architecture (Rexed 1952). Small-diameter afferents project to the more superficial laminae (I and II) of the dorsal horn whereas the larger diameter A beta afferents terminate in the deeper laminae (III or deeper). Within these laminae, three major classes of neurones have been identified: projection neurones, excitatory interneurones, and inhibitory interneurones (Fields 1987). Projections neurones relay nociceptive information to higher brain centres; interneurones relay information to either projection neurones or other interneurones. Cells responding only to primary nociceptive afferents are called 'nociceptive specific' or 'high threshold', whereas 'wide dynamic range' cells respond to input from both nociceptive and non-nociceptive afferents.

A delta fibres terminate mainly in lamina I where they synapse with rapidly conducting nociceptive projection neurones. Unmyelinated C fibres, on the other hand, are concentrated in lamina II (the substantia gelatinosa) and generally synapse with the more slowly conducting interneurones (Cervero and Iggo 1980). Nociceptive projection neurones arise mainly in laminae I and V and cross the midline to ascend in the contralateral anterolateral cord which is the major pathway for ascending nociceptive transmission to brainstem and thalamus (Fields 1987).

The brain stem and beyond

Spinothalamic tract neurones divide into lateral and medial branches as they approach the thalamus. Fibres in the lateral branch terminate in the lateral nuclei of the thalamus (ventrobasal nucleus and the 'posterior group' nuclei) in a somatotopically arranged fashion (i.e. the projections are arranged in a body map) (Jones and Derbyshire 1996). Nociceptive signals then pass relatively rapidly to the somatosensory cortex. Together this constitutes the 'lateral pain system' that was initially considered to be concerned with processing acute pain. More recent studies have lent support to the alternative hypothesis that the lateral system is dealing primarily with the sensory-discriminative aspects of pain including the localization and identification of noxious stimuli (Jones and Derbyshire 1996).

The more medial thalamic projections from the spinothalamic tracts terminate most densely in the medially situated intralaminar nuclei of the thalamus and subserve the 'medial pain system'. This area also receives input from the brainstem reticular formation, supplied by spinoreticular axons arising from the spinal dorsal horn (Fields 1987). Transmission within the medial pain system is slower than in the lateral system with neurones having large and often bilateral receptive fields with a non-somatotopic organization. Inputs from deep, musculoskeletal receptors are common (Peschanski *et al.* 1981).

Medial thalamic nuclei project widely within the ipsilateral cortex. Projections have been noted to terminate in the anterior cingulate sections of the limbic cortex (involved in integration of cognition, affect and response selection) as well as to the prefrontal cortex. Deafferentation of the anterior cingulate does not abolish chronic pain but reduces the unpleasantness of it (Jones and Derbyshire 1996). This and other data has led to the suggestion that the medial pain system is concerned mainly with motivational-affective components of the pain response.

Accumulating experimental evidence and the failure of any single cortical lesion to consistently abolish pain suggests that there is no single or 'ultimate' pain centre. In keeping with other sensory modalities, such as vision, pain sensations appear to be processed in parallel networks or matrices (Figure 2.3.2) distributed within cortical and subcortical structures (Loeser and Melzac 1999).

Plasticity

Plasticity may be regarded as the property of the nervous system that enables it to modify its function according to different conditions

(Coderre *et al.* 1993) and is pivotal to the development of hypersensitivity.

Under normal circumstances pain is only generated following a noxious or damaging stimulus and results from activation of high threshold nociceptors. It is, however, apparent that after tissue injury, pain can arise spontaneously or after the application of normally innocuous stimuli. Pain on movement and tissue tenderness are two such examples. This mechanical hypersensitivity is an expression of neural plasticity and arises as a result of mechanisms operating at multiple levels within both the CNS and the peripheral nervous system.

Peripheral sensitization

Tissue injury is followed by the release of mediators from damaged cells, the recruitment of inflammatory cells and the release of further inflammatory mediators including cytokines and growth factors (Figure 2.3.3). These factors include ions (K^+, H^+), histamine, bradykinin, prostaglandins, ATP, nitric oxide, cytokines (IL-1, TNFα, IL-6), and growth factors (leukaemia inhibitory growth factor, NGF). Some of these mediators activate peripheral nociceptors directly and lead to spontaneous pain. The majority, however, act by changing the response properties of the sensory neuron (peripheral sensitization) rather than activating it directly.

Peripheral sensitization arises as a result of changes within the receptor molecules or in sodium channels on the terminals of the nociceptor neurones. For example, inflammation upregulates both VR1 (a transducer molecule for thermal stimuli) and SNS (a sodium channel) by a number of different mechanisms including phosphorylation (for a review see Woolf and Costigan 1999).

Neurophysiological studies have confirmed that joint inflammation is followed by enhanced responsiveness of both small- and large-diameter sensory neurones (Grigg *et al.* 1986). Firstly, the high-threshold nociceptors become sensitized to movements in the normal range and may have resting activity in the absence of mechanical stimulation. Secondly, a proportion of the initially mechano-insensitive sensory fibres develop responsiveness to mechanical stimuli. Activity with large-diameter sensory neurones is also increased. It is relevant that the time course of these changes mirrors the development of

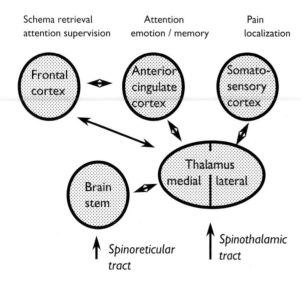

Figure 2.3.2 Schematic diagram of some of the main anatomical components of the 'pain matrix' and their functional significance.

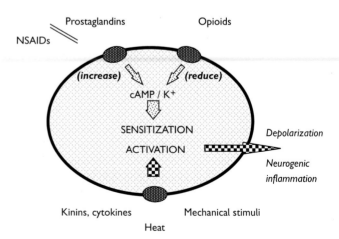

Figure 2.3.3 The peripheral nociceptor: sensitization and activation after inflammation.

pain-related behaviours arising in consequence of acute inflammation (Schaible and Grubb 1993).

Modulation

Different mediators released either by inflammatory cells or from sympathetic nerve terminals will produce varying effects on sensory receptors and may contribute to the diverse clinical features seen in different disorders (Dray 1994). Prostaglandins act to sensitize primary sensory neurones to mechanical and other chemical stimuli, probably via a stimulatory G protein and the cAMP second-messenger pathway. Opioids, on the other hand, induce formation of inhibitory G proteins and act to inhibit this pathway, thereby providing a theoretical basis for the analgesic synergy that is observed clinically between NSAIDs and opioids such as codeine or morphine. The recently described cannabinoid receptor is believed to act via a similar mechanism.

Central sensitization

Whilst pain hypersensitivity following an inflammatory stimulus is, in part, a consequence of peripheral sensitization, other mechanisms are also involved. Sustained or repetitive activation of peripheral sensory nerves produces substantial changes to the function and activity of central neurogenic pathways.

In the first instance, spinal nociceptive responses to non-tissue-damaging noxious stimuli are mediated by the excitatory amino acid glutamate acting on AMPA (α-amino-3-hydroxy-5-methylisoxazole) receptors. Importantly, repetitive stimulation or higher stimulus intensities, such as those associated with tissue damage, are associated with the functional expression of a second glutamate-responsive receptor, the NMDA (N-methyl-D-aspartate) receptor (Dickenson and Sullivan 1987). Activation of this receptor produces a sequence of events leading to increased excitability of dorsal horn neurones. This facilitated state of neurotransmission within the spinal cord has been termed 'central sensitization' (Woolf 1983).

Higher stimulus intensities are associated with the release from dense core vesicles of neuropeptides, including substance P, from central terminals of C fibres. Substance P, acting via neurokinin (NK-1) receptors located on dorsal horn neurones, enhances the activity of NMDA receptors (Thompson *et al.* 1994). This interaction takes place through the activation of protein kinase C that can phosphorylate the NMDA receptor, thereby changing its responsiveness to subsequent stimuli. Under normal circumstances magnesium ion binding blocks the NMDA receptor but the alteration of magnesium binding kinetics allows its release from the receptor and permits glutamate-induced activation and subsequent depolarization of the cell membrane.

Central sensitization results only from C fibre input and is dependent on co-release of both neurotransmitters (glutamate) and neuromodulators (including substance P and brain-derived neurotrophic factor, BDNF). The consequences are increased intracellular calcium levels and activation of kinases that act to change the response properties of membrane-bound receptors and ion channels. The net result is that the responsiveness of dorsal horn cells are increased, both to existing inputs and to previously sub-threshold inputs producing: (1) exaggerated responses to normal stimuli, (2) expansion of receptive field size, and (3) reduction of the threshold for activation by novel inputs (e.g. from mechanoceptive A beta fibres) (Figure 2.3.4) (Woolf and Costigan 1999).

Modulation

A number of endogenous mediators, including prostaglandins, nitric oxide, opioids, and adrenergic agonists have also been shown to influence the excitability of spinal neurones. Whereas prostaglandins and nitric oxide appear to facilitate spinal excitability, alpha$_2$ adrenergic and mu opioid receptor agonists produce analgesia by presynaptic inhibition of C-fibre neurotransmitter release and postsynaptic hyperpolarization

Neurobiology	**Clinical consequences**
Increase magnitude and duration of response to noxious stimuli	Enhanced primary hyperalgesia
Expansion of receptive field size to noxious stimuli	Secondary hyperalgesia
Reduced threshold for activation by large diameter (e.g. proprioceptive) inputs	Mechanical and thermal allodynia

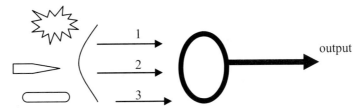

Figure 2.3.4 Consequences of central sensitization.

of second-order neurones (Besson 1999). Co-administration of intrathecal morphine and selected alpha$_2$ agonists or non-steroidal anti-inflammatories (NSAIDs) results in substantial analgesic synergy (Malmberg and Yaksh 1992) and highlights a role for combination therapy in clinical settings.

Assessment

Classification of pain

Musculoskeletal diseases characteristically have clinical symptoms and signs that arise both over sites of tissue injury and over apparently normal tissues. Although it would be wrong to claim that the basic science observations described in the previous section explain all clinical features they do allow for a basic appreciation of likely mechanisms and provide a means for novel mechanism-based classification schemes.

In 1950, Hardy proposed two types of hyperalgesia, primary and secondary. Primary hyperalgesia was defined as increased sensitivity to noxious stimuli **at the site** of an injury, while secondary hyperalgesia was defined as increased sensitivity extending **beyond the site** of injury, sometimes to remote sites distant from the site of injury (Coderre *et al.* 1993). Peripheral sensitization undoubtedly makes the major contribution to primary hyperalgesia and is therefore responsible for the increased pain and tenderness observed over the site of injured or inflamed tissues. This might be conveniently termed 'level 1' or 'primary' pain and with the major contribution arising in response to changes in peripheral tissues (see Table 2.3.1). An important implication is that there is a reasonable correlation between the initiating stimulus and the resultant symptoms and signs. Level 1 pain is most likely to occur immediately after injury or as a result of relatively minor tissue injury and treatment measures directed against the injury (i.e. rest, ice, topical or systemic anti-inflammatories, etc.) are usually effective.

Although peripheral sensitization makes an important contribution to acute and chronic pain states, it is not the sole determinant. Changes within spinal pathways (i.e. central sensitization) also contribute to pain perception and tenderness at the site of injury and are responsible for development of pain and tenderness in normal tissues both adjacent to and removed from the primary site. Increased numbers of muscle tender points or the presence of trigger points may all indicate the presence of spinal hyperexcitability. Such symptoms, reflecting the presence of changes within spinal pathways, might be termed **level 2** or 'secondary' pain and are likely to respond to measures that influence spinal processing (e.g. acupuncture, TENS, low-dose opioids, etc.). Given that spinal hyperexcitability is contingent to a large degree on ongoing input from peripheral nociceptors, therapies directed towards abnormal peripheral tissues are also likely to be

effective. Disappearance of referred knee pain following hip surgery for osteoarthritis provides a convenient example.

Psychosocial factors also make an important contribution to pain, particularly in more chronic conditions. Although exact mechanisms are unclear, it is probable that sensitization of pain pathways occurs at cortical levels in a similar fashion to that observed within the dorsal horn of the spine. Such cortical sensitization appears to produce a state of hypervigilance resulting in more diffuse symptomatology including a history of altered and often bizarre symptoms, such as peripheral parasthesiae in the absence of peripheral nerve injury. These symptoms can be regarded as **level 3** or tertiary pain and may respond to centrally acting therapeutic modalities (e.g. cognitive behavioural therapy, tricyclic antidepressants, etc.). Importantly, level 3 pain can become dissociated from the initiating injury such that peripheral therapies may prove ineffective.

Methods of assessment

Any objective assessment of pain must take into account psychosocial, behavioural, and organic factors. It should be recognized at the outset that the patient's self-report of pain reflects multiple contributing factors of which disease or tissue injury is but one. Other factors such as cultural conditioning, expectations, mood state and perception of control, may equally affect the experience of pain and should be determined as part of the overall review (see Turk and Okifugi 1999, for a review).

Rating scales

The simplest form of measurement is a qualitative scale where the patient simply reports whether pain is absent or present. More sensitive assessments can be performed using simple self-reporting rating scales such as numeric scales, descriptive rating scales, visual analogue scales, and box scales. For example, a verbal analogue scale grades pain as none, mild, or severe. A visual analogue scale presents a pictorial representation of pain as a 10-cm line with two 'anchors' at either end. Usually, such a scale is designed to assess pain intensity so that the anchors might include no pain, or worst possible pain.

McGill pain questionnaire

Rating scales are generally used to measure pain intensity although modified instructions can also be used to assess other pain components including unpleasantness or distress. An alternative approach to measuring these latter components was developed by Melzack (1975) who asked patients to specify pain in terms of sensory, affective, and evaluative descriptors. The resultant McGill pain questionnaire has three parts including a descriptive scale of present pain intensity, a human figure on which patients can indicate the location and quality of their pain, and a third part that requires patients to select words from a list that best reflect their pain.

Tables 2.3.1. Types of pain

	Underlying mechanism	Clinical feature	Treatment options
Level 1 (primary) pain	Peripheral sensitization	Local pain and tenderness	Rest, ice, topical NSAIDs
Level 2 (secondary) pain	Spinal sensitization	Referred pain and tenderness	Acupuncture, TENS, low-dose opioids
Level 3 (tertiary) pain	Cortical sensitization	Hypervigilance and enhanced somatic sensations	Cognitive behavioural therapy, tricyclic antidepressants

The words employed by the McGill pain questionnaire are designed to reflect the sensory, affective, and cognitive components of pain. The sensory words relate to pain as it is experienced in the body (e.g. throbbing, aching, shooting, etc.) whereas the affective words describe generally negative feelings (e.g. frightful, vicious). Regular use of the questionnaire during treatment may enable more accurate assessments to be made of patients' progress, although it is mainly used in experimental settings. Melzack has suggested that clinicians develop their own short form of the scale which incorporates 15 common descriptors representing sensory and affective components of pain, each of which is rated from 1 (none) to 3 (severe). This may be a more practical proposition for the clinician in general (i.e. non-research) settings.

Functional activities

Commonly used physical tests such as range of joint movement correlate poorly with the actual behaviour of the patient. Measures to assess a patient's functional status can quantify symptoms, function and behaviour more directly (Turk and Okifuji 1999). Self-report measures include walking up stairs, lifting specific weights, performing activities of daily living. There are also various functional assessment scales such as the Roland–Morris disability scale, functional status index, and Oswestry disability scale. For direct examination of patients the sickness impact profile is a more comprehensive instrument, but takes longer to perform.

Pain behaviours

Acute pain is often accompanied by both somatic and autonomic responses. Common pain behaviours are listed in the box. Learned pain behaviours are not the same as malingering. Such behaviours generally result from either nociceptive input or environmental reinforcement.

Pain behaviours

Verbal/localization

Sighs, moans
Complaints

Motor

Facial grimacing
Distorted gait (limping)
Rigid or unstable posture
Excessively slow or laboured movement

Seek help/reduce pain

Take medication
Use of protective device (stick, cervical collar)
Visit doctor

Functional limitation

Resting
Reduced activity

From Turk and Okifuji (1999)

Psychological indices

It is generally accepted that there is a relationship between pain, depression, and anxiety and it has been estimated that about 50% of people with chronic pain are clinically depressed (Romano and Turner 1985). Many scales have been developed to measure depression, including the Beck depression inventory and the Hospital Anxiety and Depression scale. The latter is easy to use, but as with all such instruments care must be taken in interpretation. Detailed assessment of psychological factors generally requires specialist referral.

References

Besson,, J. M. (1999) The neurobiology of pain. *Lancet*, 353, 1610–15.

Cassell, E. J. (1982) The nature of suffering and the goals of medicine. *New England Journal of Medicine*, 306, 639–45.

Cervero, F., Iggo A. (1980) The substantia gelatinosa of the spinal cord. A critical review. *Brain*, 103, 717–72.

Cesare, P., McNaughton, P. (1997) Peripheral pain mechanisms. *Current Opinion in Neurobiology*, 7, 493–9.

Chapman, C. R., Gavrin, J. (1999) Suffering: contributions of persistent pain. *Lancet*, 353, 2233–7.

Coderre, T. J., Katz, J., Vaccarino, A. L., Melzack R. (1993) Contribution of central neuroplasticity to pathological pain: review of clinical and experimental evidence. *Pain*, 52, 259–85.

Dickenson, A. H., Sullivan, A. F. (1987) Evidence for a role of the NMDA receptor in the frequency dependent potentiation of deep rat dorsal horn nociceptive neurones following C-fibre stimulation. *Neuropharmacology*, 26, 1235–8.

Dray, A. (1994)Tasting the inflammatory soup: the role of peripheral neurones. *Pain Reviews*, 1, 153–71.

Fields, H. L. (1999) Pain: an unpleasant topic. *Pain*, S6, 61–9.

Fields, H. L. (1987) *Pain*. McGraw-Hill , New York, pp. 41–79.

Grigg, P., Schaible, H., Schmidt, R. F. (1986) Mechanical sensitivity of group III and IV afferents from posterior articular nerve in normal and inflamed cat knee. *Journal of Neurophysiology*, 55(4), 635–43.

Jones, A. K. P., Derbyshire, S. W. G. (1996) Cerebral mechanisms operating in the presence and absence of inflammatory pain. *Annals of the Rheumatic Diseases*, 55, 411–20.

Langford, L. A., Schmidt, R. F. (1983) Afferent and efferent axons in the medial and posterior articular nerves of the cat. *Anatomical Record*, 206, 71–78.

Loeser, J. D., Melzack, R. (1999) Pain: an overview. *Lancet*, 353, 1607–9.

Malmberg, A.B., Yaksh, T.L (1992) Antinociceptive actions of spinal non-steroidal anti-inflammatory agents on the formalin test in the rat. *Journal of Pharmacology and Experimental Therapeutics*, 263(1), 136–46.

Mapp, P. I., Kidd, B. L., Gibson, S. J., *et al.* (1990) Substance P- calcitonin-related peptide- and C-flanking peptide of neuropeptide Y-immunoreactive fibres are present in normal synovium but depleted in patients with rheumatoid arthritis. *Neuroscience*, 37, 143–53.

Melzack, R. (1975)The McGill pain questionnaire: major properties and scoring methods. *Pain*, 7, 277–99.

Melzack, R., Casey, K. L. (1968) Sensory, motivational and central control determinants of pain. In: Kenshalo, D. (ed.), *The skin senses*, C. C. Thomas, Springfield, IL, pp. 423–39.

Melzack, R., Wall, P. D. (1965) Pain mechanisms: a new theory. *Science*, 150, 971–9.

Merskey, H., Bogduk, N. (1994) *Classification of chronic pain*. IASP Press, Seattle, pp. 209–13.

Peschanski, M., Guilbaud, G., Gautron, M. (1981) Posterior intralaminar region in rat: neuronal responses to noxious and non-noxious cutaneous stimuli. *Experimental Neurology*, 72, 226–38.

Rexed, B. (1952) A cytoarchitectonic atlas of the spinal cord in the cat. *Journal of Comparative Neurology*, **96**, 415–95.

Romano, J. M., Turner, J. A. (1985) Chronic pain and depression. Does the evidence support a relationship? *Psychological Bulletin*, **97**, 18–34.

Schaible, H., Grubb, B. D. (1993) Afferent and spinal mechanisms of joint pain. *Pain*, **55**, 5–54.

Snider, W. D., McMahon, S. B. (1998) Tackling pain at the source: new ideas about nociceptors. *Neuron*, **20**, 629–32.

Thompson, S. W. N., Dray, A., Urban, L. (1994) Injury-induced plasticity of spinal reflex activity, NK1 neurokinin receptor activation and enhanced A- and C-fiber mediated responses in the rat spinal cord in vitro. *Journal of Neuroscience*, **14**, 3672–87.

Turk, D. C., Okifuji, A. (1999) Assessment of patient's reporting of pain: an integrated perspective. *Lancet*, **353**, 1784–8.

Woolf, C. J. (1983) Evidence for a central component of post-injury pain hypersensitivity. *Nature*, **306**, 686–8.

Woolf, C. J. (1996) Windup and central sensitization are not equivalent. *Pain*, **66**, 105–8..

Woolf, C. J., Costigan, M. (1999) Transcriptional and posttranslational plasticity and the generation of inflammatory pain. *Proceedings of the National Academy of Sciences of the USA*, **96**, 7723–30.

2.3.2 Psychological aspects of musculoskeletal pain

Chris J. Main and Paul J. Watson

This chapter is based on an article in *Manual Therapy*, 1999, 4, 203–15.

Research into the factors that make musculoskeletal pain likely to become chronic has continued to highlight psychosocial factors. Although the original research related to low back pain, similar research for other areas of the spine has revealed that similar factors operate there; and there are indications that peripheral areas such as the shoulder are subject to prolongation of pain with adverse psychological and social factors.

Pain is the most common presenting complaint in people seeking the help of a manual therapist. A manual therapist typically attempts to identify the cause of the pain at initial examination. During the clinical interview, the therapist will attempt to establish the mode of onset, the specific characteristics of the pain, and a range of possible precipitating or easing factors including the reported influence of movement. This interview will be followed typically by a physical examination, including palpation and observation of movement. Reproduction of the pain sensation and/or the identification of abnormality of motion may help to suggest possible pain mechanisms.

The cause of the pain can, however, be elusive, and even when the therapist feels that the probable cause has been identified, there is no guarantee the treatment will be successful. The relationship between pain, physical impairment, and the level of disability is remarkably variable. Research has shown that although these factors are related, the relationships are relatively modest and vary according to the duration of symptoms and clinical subgroups (Turk *et al.* 1996). In chronic back pain in particular there is frequently little relationship between demonstrable physical impairment and the accompanying degree of functional incapacity or psychological distress (Waddell and Main 1984).

The nature of pain

Although contemporary models of pain include psychological factors, early theories of pain were very different. In the seventeenth century,

Descartes (1664) had developed the concept of a pain pathway linking the periphery of the body with higher centres in the brain. It led to the specificity theory, in which pain was considered to be a specific sensation independent of the other sensations. The sensory system responsible for mediating pain has, in the recent past, been regarded as relatively rigid and straightforward in that any tissue damage was assumed to initiate a sequence of neural events that inevitably produced pain. However, this approach is unable to explain either pain in the absence of tissue damage or variation in pain across individuals with (apparently) the same amount of tissue damage. Individual variation in the perception of pain is frequently attributed to psychological factors, although the nature of such psychological factors is seldom specified.

Therapists may attribute poor outcomes of treatment to incomplete or inadequate assessment, although limitation in therapeutic treatment skills may also be admitted. Possible explanations for the failure of treatment, however, will usually be restricted to those which lie within the boundaries of the therapist's preferred therapeutic model. Much medical and therapeutic education is based on a biomedical model of illness and a specificity theory of pain. This requires that the signs and symptoms are assessed and interpreted in terms of pathology. Once the exact pathology is determined, then a treatment approach is indicated. While such an approach is essential, particularly in the acute stages of the condition, an over-zealous application of this model can lead to the inappropriate classification of patients' problems as physical or psychological. This can lead to suboptimal treatment, the denial of treatment, or referral for psychological or psychiatric intervention. As will be discussed below, if patients have previously endured painful assessment and treatment they may be apprehensive about therapy and display guarded movements or apparently exaggerated responses to examination such as palpation or movement. It is important to realize, however, that reaction with a degree of distress to a painful and limiting condition, especially if previous treatment has not been successful, is a normal not an abnormal reaction. Patients presenting with painful conditions and associated loss of function are very rarely psychiatrically ill, and inappropriate referral may simply magnify their distress. In offering a biopsychosocial framework within which to understand therapeutic intervention (Waddell *et al.* 1984), it is appropriate first to consider the nature of pain.

The multidimensional nature of pain

According to the gate control theory (Melzack and Wall 1965) and its later derivatives (Melzack and Casey 1968), pain perception depends on complex neural interactions in the nervous system where impulses generated by tissue damage are modified both by ascending pathways to the brain and by descending pain suppressing systems activated by various environmental and psychological factors. Pain is thus not merely the end product of a passive transmission of nociceptive impulses from receptor organ to an area of interpretation: it is the result of a dynamic process of perception and interpretation of a wide range of incoming stimuli, some of which are associated with actual or potential harm and some of which are benign but interpreted and described in terms of damage.

The gate control theory has generated a wide range of research (Melzack 1996) but its importance from the psychological point of view has been that it produced a testable model of how psychological factors could activate descending pain inhibitory systems, modulate nociceptive processing, and thereby modulate pain. It has offered a way of integrating concepts of pain behaviour, both as a response to pain and as behaviour that could come under environmental

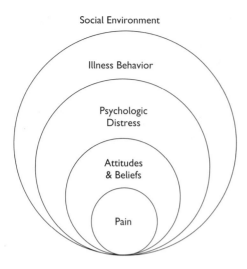

Figure 2.3.5 The biopsychosocial model of low back pain and disability (adapted from Waddell 1998, p. 228).

influences and control. The gate control theory has stimulated interest in the role of beliefs about pain, attention to pain, appraisal of its significance, fears about pain and pain-related coping strategies. The theory has encouraged the investigation of the nature of pain-associated disability and led to the development of biopsychosocial models (Waddell and Main 1998a) that have attempted a wide integration of physical, psychological, and social perspectives (Figure 2.3.5).

Models of pain, illness, and disability

A complex chain of events links perception of part of the body as painful and the development of chronic disability. Although the process is multifactorial and not fully understood, a number of key processes seem to be involved. Manual therapy is based on a biomedical understanding of incapacity. The patient's report of pain leads to a pain-focused clinical history with a clinical examination. It has long been considered that chronic pain can only be understood within a biopsychosocial framework (Loeser 1980), but it is now clear that psychological factors are important at an early stage.

The biopsychosocial model of pain and disability

Pain is a symptom, not a sign, and therefore is multiply determined. In specific instances there may be a clear and specific indication for manipulation, but the dysfunction needs to be understood within a wider model such as the biopsychosocial model of pain and disability (Waddell *et al.* 1984, Turk 1996, Waddell and Main 1998a).

At the heart of the biopsychosocial model is the assumption of an ongoing sensation that is nociceptive in nature or which is perceived by the sufferer as being painful. The patient's cognitions, i.e. what they think and understand about this sensation, will influence their emotional reaction to it. The behaviour demonstrated by an individual at any point in time will be a product of their beliefs and the emotional

response to the pain and may in turn be influenced (reinforced or modulated) by the social environment in which the behaviour takes place. The model offers a radically different way of understanding the nature of pain-associated incapacity. In understanding manual therapy it is important to be familiar with the elements from which the biopsychosocial model has been constructed.

The nature of psychological influences on pain

Fundamental mechanisms

Psychological factors have a wide-ranging effect on the perception of pain and its effects. There is now convincing evidence that central mechanisms can influence the perception of nociceptive signals from the periphery of the body (Woolf 1996). The perception of pain is influenced both by sensory qualities and by the emotional impact (Price *et al.* 1997). Recent research into experimental pain using PET scanning suggests that individuals may differ in how the brain first reacts to incoming pain signals and leads to the perception of pain (Roland 1993). Perceptual differences in terms of both intensity and aversive response may occur and, as a result, different parts of the brain become 'energized'. It is commonly observed clinically that pain 'feels worse' when patients are feeling tired or depressed. Pain often seems to feel worse during the night when the brain has 'less to do'.

The role of attention and memory

Factors relating to attention are important (Eccleston 1995). Some patients can be taught to distract themselves quite successfully from pain. Research has also shown that individuals differ not only in pain threshold but also in their ability to discriminate pain of different qualities and intensities. The reasons for this are not fully understood. Research into memory of pain suggests, however, that aversive pain memories may have a powerful influence on the perception of new pain stimuli (Price *et al.* 1997). Psychobiological investigations have demonstrated a wide range of conditioned peripheral and central responses to pain involving both physiological and biochemical events (Flor and Birbaumer 1994). It would appear that the significance of fundamental psychological mechanisms to the perception of clinical pain may be of much more importance than has hitherto been recognized.

Pain, learning, and neuroplastic change

The perception of painful stimuli has been shown to respond to learning (Crombez *et al.* 1997) and is subject to neuroplastic change (Dubner 1997). Experimental evidence has demonstrated that the brain's response to a painful stimulus as measured by electroencephalography, and the accompanying report of that pain, can be conditioned in some subjects by the offering of a financial reward. Cross-sectional studies have also demonstrated that the magnitude of response to painful stimuli changes with the duration of chronic pain conditions and may be mediated by attention (Eccleston 1995). In a series of experiments, Flor *et al.* (1997) demonstrated that patients with chronic low back pain had a significantly greater cortical evoked magnetic field response to pain than normal controls and the difference was greatest when the low back was stimulated. They interpreted this increase in the magnitude of the response as more widespread cortical assembly activation and psychophysiological hyper-reactivity as a result of neuroplastic change.

Muscle pain, muscle activity, and perception

In a recent study of patients suffering from shoulder pain (Vassiljen and Westgaard 1996), it was suggested that the perception of pain may be better explained by the subjects' perception of muscle tension than by the actual electromyographic activity in the muscle itself. They found, furthermore, that psychologically stressful working conditions and psychological characteristics of individual office workers were significant determinants of whether they reported the perception of muscle tension and pain. In another study of a group of office workers (Vassiljen et al. 1995), a reduction in reported pain was highly correlated with reported reduction in perceived muscle tension, although the reduction in perceived tension was independent of actual electromyographic activity.

In conclusion, therefore, it appears that the perception of pain bears a complex relationship to nociception. A full understanding of this relationship requires consideration of central physiological mechanisms involved in coding the information in the brain, as well as secondary psychological processes affecting perception.

The role of emotion

Anxiety, fear, depression, and anger are the four emotions which best characterize the distress of chronic pain sufferers. These features frequently overlap in the individual patient. Many of these features can be identified from the behaviour that the patient displays or expresses during assessment and treatment. Manual therapists often deal with patients with significant pain problems that are inextricably linked with anxiety, fears about their condition (and the future), depression about their current pain-associated limitations, and anger at previous failed management or the attitudes of others to their condition.

Anxiety and fear

Generalized anxiety

Specific anxieties and fears are a common feature of pain patients, particularly when they have not been given a clear explanation for their pain or its likelihood to respond to treatment. Such specific concerns should be distinguished from global or generalized anxiety in which there is no clear focus to the patient's concerns. Widespread long-standing anxiety is sometimes seen in general musculoskeletal practice and may require treatment in its own right. The physician or therapist may treat this, or refer to an appropriate service (see Chapter 4.3.12). The presence of generalized anxiety does not mean, however, that the specific fears and concerns about local musculoskeletal pain and pain-associated incapacity should not be addressed at the first port of call.

Somatic awareness

A subgroup of patients does nor seem to be particularly anxious or fearful but may demonstrate heightened awareness of all sorts of symptoms (Main 1983). This heightened somatic awareness can be indicative of somatic anxiety. Such patients tend to have difficulty in coping with treatment and its side effects. If sufficiently marked, such preoccupation may need to be understood as a form of hypochondri-asis or a somatization disorder for which there are DSM-IV criteria (American Psychiatric Association 1994), and may require psychologically oriented treatment in its own right. Symptoms of such severity are rare, and concern about symptoms is perhaps best understood as a normal phenomenon rather than a psychopathological one (Sullivan and Katon 1993). If such concern is long-standing or marked it may be considered as a cognitive distortion or misperception. Patients may become preoccupied with bodily sensation of all kinds and this inevitably focuses attention to painful events. If such specific concerns are accompanied by other features of distress or displays of pain behaviour, the patient may require more psychologically oriented treatment such as a pain management programme (Flor et al. 1992a, Main et al. 1992). In treating patients with heightened somatic awareness, it is important for us to offer repeated explanation and reassurance to our patients about the nature of their pain.

Fears

Patients differ in their interpretation of symptoms. The meaning patients assign to physical symptoms is profoundly influenced by their beliefs, assumptions, and so called 'commonsense explanations' that they may have 'inherited' from influential individuals (whether family, friends, or health care professionals) (Coiffi 1991). Amongst the most disabling of such concerns are specific beliefs about hurting and harming (see below). These beliefs should always be addressed during assessment and treatment.

Conclusion

In summary, in terms of clinical management, it is important to consider whether heightened somatic concern or fear may have led to misinterpretation of the patient's symptoms and have led to a labelling of relatively normal sensations as abnormal if not pathological (Weir et al. 1994). Frequently, apparently unfocused anxiety is based on specific fears of hurting/harming, distorted ideas about the nature of pain and illness, or that the pain will become uncontrollable with progressive and increasing pain-associated incapacity. Individuals high in somatic anxiety have a strong propensity for catastrophizing ('fearing the worst'), and while post-treatment report of catastrophizing is significantly diminished, levels of somatic anxiety are little changed. It may be that in individuals who are somatically focused, it is the degree of catastrophizing that governs emotional and physiological arousal which in turn alters pain sensitivity and response to treatment. It is imperative, therefore, that these issues are addressed.

The nature of depression

The term depression can be misleading. In common parlance it is used to refer to a wide spectrum of emotion ranging from the slightly demoralized or fed-up to the suicidal. Pain patients certainly frequently seem to be demoralized or depressed. The similarities between chronic pain patients and depressed patients have led to a debate about the nature of 'depression' in pain patients (Averill et al. 1996). It is therefore important to distinguish dysphoric mood from depressive illness for which there are clear diagnostic criteria such as DSM-IV (American Psychiatric Association 1994).

Influence of the passage of time

The initial reaction to a painful injury is usually recognized in terms of anxiety, shock, and fear rather than depression (Geisser et al. 1996).

With the passage of time, and the failure of treatment, however, a patient's coping skills can become exhausted and depression or anger can become evident. If it is possible to avoid painful activities or compensate successfully by changing activities and routines, then patients are unlikely to become depressed (even with persistence of pain). If, however, the pain is sufficiently severe, cannot be controlled, and as such has a widespread effect on a patient's life, then depression is much more likely (Rudy *et al.* 1988).

Learned helplessness

Pain-associated depression is often best viewed as a form of 'learned helplessness' that can develop after many different types of chronic unresolved stress, including health-related problems. In the context of chronic pain it is best understood as a psychological consequence of the persistence of pain and its incapacitating effects. If sufficiently severe it may merit pharmacological treatment in its own right, but can usually best be treated using a cognitive-behavioural approach (Turk *et al.* 1983, Gatchell and Turk 1996), returning a measure of control to the patient over their pain and pain-associated incapacity, and re-establishing their self-confidence.

The influence of anger and frustration

Patients express anger in a number of ways. Anger is often self-evident from the manner and content of the patient's communication. Patients may be disaffected with many aspects of their situation (DeGood and Kiernan 1996). They may be angry about how they have been treated in the past, or may believe that referral for physical treatment may have been undertaken simply because the referring doctor could think of no alternative. Emotional intensity may range from mild annoyance to hostility or even frank aggression.

Patients may be angry about a range of features such as the severity or persistence of their pain, the effect of their pain on daily activities, sleep, sexual functioning, and ability to work. They may also be disaffected by their previous treatment or the socioeconomic consequences of their pain-associated incapacity.

This complex relationship between anger/hostility and adjustment is as yet not well understood. Anger has physiological effects, and persistent anger clouds judgement. It would seem to merit much further investigation, particularly in its influence on compliance and response to treatment (Fernandez and Turk 1995).

Beliefs and coping strategies

Beliefs about pain and outcome of treatment have been identified as key determinants of response to treatment (Waddell and Main 1998c). The term 'cognitive' is frequently taken as synonymous with 'beliefs', but in fact has a wider application and has come to refer to a range of factors influencing the perception of pain and response to treatment. It is therefore perhaps helpful to distinguish three distinct fields of enquiry (DeGood and Shutty 1992):

- specific beliefs about pain and treatment
- the thought processes involved in judgment or appraisal
- coping styles or strategies.

Each patient is characterized by an individual combination of cognitive features which underpins the appraisal of pain and the response to treatment. The complexity of these interrelationships is indicated in the following quotation:

> Patients who believe they can control their pain, who avoid catastrophizing about their condition, and who believe they are not severely disabled appear to function better than those who do not. Such beliefs may mediate some of the relationships between pain severity and adjustment. (Jensen *et al.* 1991, p. 249)

Specific beliefs about pain and treatment

Clinically, pessimistic or negative beliefs regarding pain and outcome of treatment are easily recognized. Amongst the most commonly found beliefs are that hurt is synonymous with harm, that pain uniquely determines physical functioning, and that future structural and/or physiological decline is inevitable. Such beliefs not only lead to significant demoralization but also to establishing dysfunctional patterns of behaviour and deconditioning. Such beliefs can also compromise response to therapy and lead to chronic incapacity. Indeed, research has shown that beliefs about the extent to which pain can be controlled appear to be one of the most powerful determinants of adjustment to pain and the development of incapacity (Crisson and Keefe 1988).

Beliefs about control

A recurrent finding in research is the importance of beliefs about the controllability of pain. A number of 'pain locus of control' scales have been developed (Crisson and Keefe 1988, Main and Waddell 1991). In one study, the role of perceived self-control as a factor that mediates pain and depression was explored by Rudy *et al.* (1988). Although the direct association between pain and depression was minimal, depression developed principally when pain significantly interfered with family, work, and social interactions, and/or existed in conjunction with pessimism about being able to control pain. The issue of 'controllability' may be even more important in relationship to adjustment to pain and incapacity. Optimal adaptation to a chronic condition thus seems to depend on the patient's ability to come to terms with what they can and cannot control.

> Pain patients who perceive themselves lacking the capacity to acquire self-management skills might be less persistent, more prone to frustration, and more apt to be non-compliant with treatment recommendations. Hence, some patients might demonstrate adequate understanding of a particular treatment rationale, yet be non-compliant due to their perceived inability to produce the behaviour necessary to follow treatment recommendations. (DeGood and Shutty 1992, p. 221)

This perspective has two major implications in musculoskeletal medicine:

- First, exercise prescriptions, advice on posture, and graded increase in activity are given to patients to enhance the effectiveness of specific manipulative treatments. The degree to which the patient complies and persists with the recommendations will be determined by the patient's belief in how much personal control they have over their condition.

- Secondly, manual treatment may unwittingly reinforce the patient's perception of lack of control. During 'hands-on' therapies such as manipulation, mobilization, and massage, the doctor or therapist is in control and accepts responsibility for the management of the condition. The patient's role is one of passive acceptance of the therapy. In susceptible individuals this may foster the belief that they do not have a role in the management of their condition. Recovery is seen as the responsibility entirely of the professional. Over-directing the patient in the resumption of activities, or strict advice to perform only very specific activities and exclude others, may encourage an over-reliance on the therapist. Such a therapeutic relationship may make it extremely difficult if not impossible to foster the patient's own self-management skills as part of the therapeutic process. See Chapter 4.2.

Beliefs about self-efficacy (or successful implementation)

Patients may believe that they will be unsuccessful in gaining control over pain or re-establishing function. Such beliefs are frequently called **self-efficacy beliefs** (Bandura 1977, Nicholas *et al.* 1992). Clinical and experimental investigations suggest that perceived coping inefficacy may lead to preoccupation with distressing thoughts and concomitant physiological arousal, thereby increasing pain, decreasing pain tolerance and leading to increased use of medication, lower levels of functioning, poorer exercise tolerance, and increased invalidism.

A careful line must be drawn between giving good advice and creating a dependent patient. The most useful strategy is to encourage the patient to identify specific activities and goals for increased exercise and incorporate these into a self-management plan.

Mistaken beliefs about hurting and harming

Perhaps the most powerful, yet least acknowledged, cognitive factors are mistaken beliefs about hurting and harming. It is crucial to recognize the role of fear and avoidance as obstacles to rehabilitation after injury (Asmundson *et al.* 1997). As might be expected, the construct of 'fear-avoidance' has both a behavioural and a cognitive component. Behavioural theorists such as Fordyce (1976) explained the development of 'avoidance learning' where successful avoidance of pain established a behavioural pattern which was successful in reducing pain but with the cost of maintaining the disability. Vlaeyen *et al.* (1995) found that fear of movement and re-injury were more related to depressive symptoms and catastrophizing (fearing an inevitable poor outcome) than to pain itself. His model linking fear, catastrophizing, and avoid-

ance in the development of chronic disability following painful injury has been widely influential. It is illustrated in Figure 2.3.6.

A number of new instruments for the assessment of fear and avoidance such as the FABQ (Waddell *et al.* 1993) and the TSK (Kori *et al.* 1990) have been developed. Evidence from experimental studies in chronic pain patients has demonstrated a close relationship between experimental pain (pressure algometry) and fear of injury. Interestingly, this relationship appears to be independent of the current level of clinical pain (Watson *et al.* 1996). This has important implications because it suggests that although patients' perception of pain is closely associated with fear in experimental pain situations, there may be much wider influences on patients' rating of clinical pain once it has become chronic. For a manual therapist evaluating a patient, therefore, it is important not be over-reliant on the report of pain intensity without taking the issues of fear and avoidance into account.

Coping styles and strategies

Active and passive coping strategies

It is also important to consider how people cope with pain. How people react to pain is an important determinant of its future course. Patterns of fear-mediated avoidance behaviour have already been described, but in fact patients use a wide range of behavioural and coping strategies in order to limit the effects of pain. Choice of strategies will depend on patients' beliefs about pain, on their confidence in being able to influence events, and of course on their repertoire of coping behaviours. Brown and Nicassio (1987) made the distinction between active and passive coping strategies. Active strategies (e.g. taking exercise), require the individual to take a degree of responsibility for pain management by either attempting to control pain or attempting to function despite pain. Passive strategies (e.g. resting), involve either withdrawal or the passing on of responsibility for the control of pain to someone else (for example, the therapist). This distinction is of major importance and key to understanding patients' responses to therapy (Snow-Turek *et al.* 1996).

Appropriate (effective) and inappropriate (ineffective) coping strategies

In the research literature, perhaps the most important distinction is between effective (or appropriate) coping strategies and ineffective (or inappropriate) coping strategies, as assessed for example by the Coping Strategies Questionnaire (CSQ) (Rosenstiel and Keefe 1983). This questionnaire identifies both positive (or adaptive) and negative (or maladaptive) coping strategies. Several studies have shown that negative or ineffective coping strategies such as catastrophizing ('fearing the worst') are associated with higher levels of self-reported disability or adjustment (Keefe *et al.* 1989, Jensen *et al.* 1991, Main and Waddell 1991). The catastrophizing scale has also shown impressive predictive value for outcome of treatment, particularly in patients with acute low back pain. Burton *et al.* (1995) and Main and Burton (1995) found that passive coping and in particular catastrophizing were highly predictive of disability and pain report at 1 year in a group of subjects with acute low back pain (less than 4 weeks' duration).

Coping strategies and adjustment

The relationship between the use of these strategies and psychological adjustment is complex (Jensen *et al.* 1994). Keefe *et al.* (1997) demon-

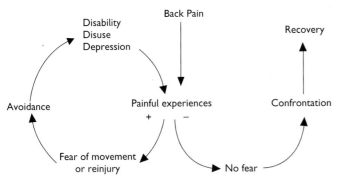

Figure 2.3.6 Vlaeyen's model of fear of movement and reinjury on back pain (adapted from Waddell 1998, p. 234).

strated that perceived daily coping efficacy was associated with greater use of relaxation, redefining of pain, spiritual support seeking with a consequent reduction in pain, negative affect, and enhancement of positive mood. Furthermore, individual judgement of coping effectiveness resulted in lower pain levels on the following day; improvement in mood the following day was also attributed to use of relaxation strategies. As Turner (1991) points out, however, specific coping strategies are not inherently adaptive or maladaptive. A strategy that is useful at one point in time may be of little value at another and some strategies may be of benefit if used in moderation, but not if used to the exclusion of others. Furthermore, the overall efficacy of coping techniques appears to be moderated by levels of pain intensity and appraisals of perceived pain control abilities (Jensen and Karoly 1992).

Recently, there has been further clarification of the psychological mechanisms involved. It appears that pain-related coping strategies lead to a reduction of disability only when a high degree of flexibility in goal adjustment was possible (Schmitz et al. 1996).

Finally, there has been recent interest in the distinction between emotion-focused coping strategies (which aim to control stress) and problem-focused coping strategies (e.g. reducing maladaptive coping) which are aimed at attempting to relieve or solve the problem more directly. Such strategies are a core component of teaching in most pain management programmes, but are rarely used in acute or subchronic pain situations.

In attempting to maximize patient adherence to treatment recommendations, it is important to consider the sorts of coping strategies that individual patients actually use.

Pain behaviour

Range and complexity

There are many different examples of pain behaviour, ranging from the simple to the complex. The classical definition of pain behaviour is

> any and all outputs of the individual that a reasonable observer would characterize as suggesting pain, such as (but not limited to) posture, facial expression, verbalizing, lying down, taking medicines, seeking medical assistance and receiving compensation (Loeser and Fordyce 1983).

Many such behaviours are crucial in the interaction between patients and those treating them. Patients may communicate pain both verbally and non-verbally. Their expressions of pain may in turn produce a range of reactions from the person treating them.

Behavioural mechanisms

Most therapists understand pain behaviour (of whatever sort) simply as a response to pain and treat it as such. But, since the 1970s, behavioural theorists have investigated the behavioural mechanisms involved in such treatment contexts and it appears that the situation can be much more complex. There are two major perspectives concerning pain behaviour.

Classical conditioning

Within the classical conditioning paradigm (of which Pavlov's experiments with his dogs are perhaps best known), pain behaviour can be viewed simply as an unconditioned response to a pain stimulus (noci-

ception). Through learning, however, conditioning can occur so that fearful patients may begin to show similar responses to situations in which they were injured (the development of fear of hurting and harming can be understood within this paradigm). Not only secondary pain behaviour, but also pain itself, can become conditioned. High-intensity pain can be re-experienced during flashbacks of traumatizing painful injuries. No new injury is occurring, but memory of the circumstances surrounding the injury can reproduce the pain.

Experimental work has demonstrated the conditioning of muscular responses to painful stimuli and to the expectation of a painful stimulus in healthy controls. Flor and Birbaumer (1994) gave electric shocks, paired with an audible tone, to a group of students. The students demonstrated an increase in muscle tension in response to the shock. After a series of trials, the tone alone could elicit the muscular response. The muscular responses were even more pronounced if paired with slides associated with negative emotional states. They also report that the responses were more easily conditioned and took longer to extinguish in those students who reported frequent episodes of neck and shoulder pain, suggesting a susceptibility to conditioned muscular responses.

Operant conditioning

Persistence of pain behaviour can also be understood in terms of its consequences. If the pain behaviour is successful in reducing pain, or leads to pleasant consequences (such as increased attention from a spouse (Romano et al. 1996), absence from a stressful job, or financial compensation), it is likely that the pain behaviour will increase in frequency. The change has been brought about by operant conditioning. Such pain behaviour may have only a small respondent component. Pain behaviours that initially produced an escape from the painful stimulus can produce patterns of complete avoidance. As has been stated elsewhere, 'fear of pain can become more disabling than pain itself' (Waddell et al. 1993). Many such influences can be observed during the course of manual therapy. Successful avoidance of painful activity (such as a painful exercise programme) can inhibit therapeutic progress. Interestingly, patients are often unaware of the mechanisms underpinning their behaviour.

Assessment of pain behaviour

A number of different measures have been developed specifically for the assessment of pain behaviour.

Behavioural rating scales

Behaviourally based interventions require careful assessment, and a number of observation schedules have been developed. Typically, the rater is asked to observe the patient and indicate when certain behaviours occur on a behavioural rating scale devised for the purpose (Richards et al. 1982). Such scales are used to rate the videotaped observations described above, but can also be used to code naturally occurring behaviours. These scales are merely adaptations of observational scales that can be used for many other purposes. The 'diary' format enables the accurate recording of the incidence of such behaviours and their relationships with other events. The information can therefore be used for a 'functional analysis'. Vlaeyen et al. (1987) also used an observational method in which patients were observed over a long period (e.g. during an inpatient rehabilitation programme) and a wide range of pain behaviours were recorded. Although sometimes highly informative, such methods are not practicable in typical outpatient clinical practice. A number of more clinically based instruments have been developed.

The following section of the paper is abstracted from a recent review of more commonly used pain behaviour measures in clinical practice (Waddell and Main 1998b). All these tests offer patients an opportunity to communicate about their pain and therefore can be viewed as pain behaviour measures.

Pain drawing test

Pain drawings (manikins) are frequently used in clinics. Patients usually show no reluctance to complete them, and indeed sometimes do so with relish. The drawing indicates where the patient reports pain and other altered sensations. Ransford *et al.* (1976) originally attempted to distinguish 'non-organic' from 'psychogenic' pain on the basis of drawings. The drawings are evaluated for the extent to which they appear to correspond to a clear anatomic pathway. Widespread patterns, with non-anatomical distributions and use of all sorts of additional emphasis, are considered indicative of 'psychological overlay' or distress. They should not be over-interpreted. A clearly abnormal pain drawing is almost always indicative of pain-associated distress, and should alert the clinician to the need for a more careful psychosocial assessment. However, 50% of distressed patients produce pain drawings with absolutely no indications of distress (Parker *et al.* 1995) and so the test is insufficiently sensitive to be recommended as a single screening procedure to identify distress.

Overt pain behaviour

Keefe and Block (1982) developed the behavioural observation rating test, a 10-minute videotaped analysis of a 10-minute observation of patients going through a series of movements. Although useful as a research tool, it has been found that clinicians cannot make such ratings reliably without careful training (Waddell and Richardson 1992).

It has also been suggested that naturalistic observation may not allow observation of tasks sufficiently strenuous to precipitate pain behaviour. A task-oriented measure of pain behaviour requiring the patient to perform a series of tasks (such as lifting, carrying, and stair-climbing), has, however, been devised (Watson and Poulter 1997). This measure has proved reliable in a pain management setting and seems to address some of the limitations of the other methods.

Behavioural (non-organic) signs

In clinical practice the most widely used measure of pain behaviour in patients with chronic back pain is the behaviour (non-organic) signs test (Waddell *et al.* 1980). The test was devised originally to identify 'non-organic' components in the patient's presentation. The original research led to the development and standardization of seven such behavioural signs:

- superficial tenderness
- non-anatomical tenderness
- simulated axial loading
- simulated rotation
- straight leg raise (under conditions of distraction)
- regional weakness
- regional sensory disturbance.

The method of assessment was carefully standardized. The signs were found to be clearly separable from other physical signs and to correlate highly with measures of psychological distress. They were conceptualized originally as psychological screeners, with the caveat (as with the behavioural symptoms) that isolated signs should not be overinterpreted. The fact that they have been misused and misinterpreted as indicators of malingering has prompted a reappraisal of their use (Main and Waddell 1998a).

Behavioural symptoms

The behavioural symptoms test (Waddell *et al.* 1984) includes the assessment of five specific symptoms and two clinical history items suggestive of a marked emotional reaction to pain. The five symptoms are:

- pain at the tip of the tailbone
- whole leg pain
- whole leg numbness
- whole leg giving way
- complete absence of spells with very little pain in the previous year.

The two clinical history items are:
- intolerance (or adverse reaction) to many previous treatments
- emergency admission to hospital with simple backache.

As with the pain drawing test, the behavioural symptoms test should not be over-interpreted. Only if the clinician finds three or more such 'symptoms' should the presence of a pain behaviour syndrome be investigated.

Chronic pain (or pain behaviour syndrome)

The persistence of pain can produce wide-ranging and devastating effects on patients (Main and Spanswick 1995). They may display marked and seemingly inappropriate pain behaviour, indicate high levels of distress, and yet have been offered a significant amount of treatment. Such patients frequently require a comprehensive pain management programme (Flor *et al.* 1992a), although not all can be helped. Such patients are characterized not by isolated or specific indicators of pain behaviour, but by an entire pattern of invalidism. Such presentations are frequently observed in patients involved in litigation (although by no means confined to such situations). Repeated evaluations in an essentially adversarial medicolegal system seem to exacerbate their distress and make assessment even more difficult. We should be aware, therefore, of our patient's economic and occupational contexts lest there is a significant disincentive for the patient to recover.

Conclusion

In summary, pain behaviour has to be understood in terms of its context. Indeed, pain has been defined as 'an interesting social communication the meaning of which has still to be determined' (Fordyce 1976). This perspective offers a radically different approach to the understanding of the therapeutic mechanisms during therapy compared to the traditional medical model. For the practising therapist, the most useful aspects of pain behaviour seems to be the observation of guarded movements, the identification of fear-related responses to examination, and the communication of distress.

The role of expectation and influence of previous treatment

The role of patient expectation

Psychological factors influencing response to treatment include patient's expectation, non-specific (placebo) responses to treatment, compliance with treatment (including adherence to treatment protocols), and acceptance of appropriate responsibility for the management of their symptomatology. Patients who have been in pain for a long period of time or who have a recurrent pain problem may have seen several other professionals and received a range of treatments which have proved ineffective.

The adverse influence of failed treatment

Failed treatment can have a profoundly demoralizing effect. The patient may have lost confidence in the likely benefit of any further treatment. They may be concerned that 'something has been missed' (e.g. cancer). They may be significantly disaffected with health care professionals, particularly if they feel they have been misled in terms of likely benefit from treatment, if they feel that they have not been believed, or it has been implied that the problem is 'all in their mind'. Such iatrogenic factors can have a significant influence on a patient's decision to accept treatment or to comply with it (Waddell and Main 1998b).

Implications for the relationship between patient and therapist

The adverse influences of repeated ineffective treatment, and differences in diagnosis (as offered by different specialists) have been highlighted. It can lead to significant apprehension about further consultations and demonstrations of pain behaviour in the form of distress and anger (Main and Waddell 1998b). It should be recognized, therefore, that the behaviour demonstrated at initial consultation may have been influenced significantly by previous experiences. This perspective is not just of theoretical importance. Consider a patient presenting with acute low back pain who may have had repeated periods of severe pain on movement in the days before consulting. They may also have had a painful examination by another practitioner (e.g. their GP) and this in turn may influence their willingness to move. They may demonstrate muscle guarding (which may be misidentified as involuntary muscle spasm) and appear to be responding excessively to further physical examination. If litigation is involved, unsympathetic assessors attempting to raise doubts about the genuineness of their difficulties may have further confounded the distress.

Psychophysiological responses to pain

Psychophysiological researchers have examined the interaction between mental and physical events in a number of disorders (Turpin 1989), including pain, in which the genesis and maintenance of pain in terms of both central and peripheral mechanisms has been discussed (Flor et al. 1990, 1997). Underlying the theory of psychophysiological reactivity is the development of a fundamental hyperarousal of the sympathetic nervous system in response to stimuli or stressors. Abnormal psychophysiological reactions to stress and pain have been found in a number of painful conditions. Whether these reactions are

the antecedents of the painful condition or merely reactions to it is still unclear, but may be helpful to attempt to differentiate non-specific or generalized responses from more specific reactions that may serve to maintain or exacerbate the pain (Flor et al. 1992b). Non-specific reactions to pain are heightened responses in skin sweating, heart rate, and general physiological arousal during painful or stressful conditions. These reactions per se are not normally painful but may serve to increase the perception of pain from a specific source. They may cause pain in conditions where pain is sympathetically maintained such as complex regional pain syndrome. Specific reactions are themselves algogenic (pain-producing) and serve as a source of nociception in susceptible individuals. For example, site-specific muscle hyper-reactivity has been identified in patients with chronic low back pain and tension headaches, and alterations in vascular flow have been found in some migraine sufferers. The role of muscle activity should be of particular interest to those working in musculoskeletal medicine.

Specific investigations of muscle activity

Flor et al. (1985) identified site-specific hyper-reactivity in patients with chronic low back pain. Increases in surface electromyography readings were demonstrated during a personally relevant stressor. These responses were not demonstrated during an arithmetical control stressor and they did not generalize to other non-painful areas. They concluded that increases in site muscle activity may contribute to pain through increased muscle tension. Site-specific increase in lumbar paraspinal muscle activity in patients with low back pain in response to a tonic pain stressor, the cold pressor test, has been demonstrated by Watson et al. (1998). However, the change in paraspinal activity was not accompanied by a change in back pain report and so the precise relationship between increases in static muscle activity and a possible myogenic mechanism for pain requires further investigation.

The nature of pain-associated movement abnormalities

The evidence for abnormalities of movement in chronic pain conditions is much more convincing than that for elevated resting baselines. With careful methodology, electromyographic recording of standardized movements can be repeatable and reliable. Patients with chronic low back pain demonstrate different patterns of activity when compared with pain-free controls during movement. Not only that, but the differences in movement can discriminate the patient with back pain from the healthy control with a good degree of sensitivity (Watson et al. 1997a). Changes in these abnormalities have been demonstrated to be more closely related to change in fear of activity and pain self-efficacy beliefs (the relative confidence that one will be able to perform a movement despite the pain) than the level of clinical pain (Watson et al. 1997b). The clinical significance of these abnormalities prospectively still needs to be examined.

Clinical implications: the development of guarded movements

After an injury, there is a natural tendency to guard the injured area to allow for rest and recovery. The development of guarded movements can be understood from both behavioural and cognitive perspectives (as discussed above). Thus, if a patient experiences pain on the performance of an activity, with repeated pain on activity, the muscular guarding responses can become conditioned not only to the performance of the movement but also to the anticipation of the performance of that movement as the patients anticipate the learned outcome – pain. This respondent conditioning can result in abnormalities of muscle activity which themselves may be implicated in the generation of pain. Guarded movements may become further established through operant conditioning (if the guarded activity is followed by reinforcing events such as displays of increasing concern or sympathy from a spouse or clinician; 'escape' from a painful situation following an invitation to rest; or a financial circumstance which is dependent on continued demonstrations of pain or incapacity). The aforementioned cognitive factors such as fear of further injury or pessimism about being able to achieve increase in function may also contribute to the development of guarded movements (Main and Watson 1996).

Implications for clinical management

- Musculoskeletal assessment places considerable reliance on the patient's report of pain and, in arriving at a diagnosis and treatment plan, reported pain intensity is assumed to bear a close relationship to underlying nociception. Perception of pain in experimental situations is influenced by fear, perception of control, and predictability, and it may be more helpful to consider acute pain (or indeed recurrent flare-ups) as a fear-mediated phenomenon.

- The rating of chronic clinical pain, however, appears to be influenced by a number of other influences and therefore its validity as a measure of response to nociception is unclear.

- During the course of a clinical examination, the assessor may attempt to arrive at a clinical diagnosis through replication of the patient's pain by palpation of the induction of mechanical stress. There are two problems with this approach: first, response to pain provocation (whether palpation or induction of biomechanical stress) can be affected by fear of an adverse outcome (such as pain) and fear of injury. Secondly, a patient's global rating of their pain may be widely influenced by factors in addition to nociception.

- The musculoskeletal assessment must therefore be placed within a biopsychosocial framework. In appraising the patient's response, it may be helpful to incorporate specific assessment of subjectively reported fear or behavioural indicators of fear such as guarded movements or behavioural signs. In manual and musculoskeletal treatments we are frequently managing the patients' pain behaviour and distress, rather than simply the nociceptive component of their pain.

- Where musculoskeletal pain has become chronic it is necessary to rely on the principles of chronic pain management (which are discussed in Chapter 4.3.12).

References

American Psychiatric Association (1994) *Diagnostic and Statistical Manual of Mental Disorders (DSM-IV)*, 4th edn. American Psychiatric Association, Washington.

Asmundson, G. G., Norton, G. R., Allerdings, M. D. (1997) Fear and avoidance in dysfunctional back pain patients. *Pain*, **69**, 231–6.

Averill, P. M., Novy, D. M., Nelson, D. V., Berry, L. A. (1996) Correlates of depression in chronic pain patients: a comprehensive examination. *Pain*, **65**, 93–100.

Bandura, A. (1977) Self-efficacy: towards a unifying theory of behavioral change. *Psychological Review*, **84**, 191–215.

Brown, G. K., Nicassio, P. M. (1987) The development of a questionnaire for the assessment of active and passive coping strategies in chronic pain patients. *Pain*, **31**, 53–65.

Burton, A. K., Tillotson, K. M., Main, C. J., Hollis, S. (1995) Psychosocial predictors of outcome in acute and subchronic low back trouble. *Spine*, **20**, 722–8.

Cioffi, D. (1991) Beyond attentional strategies: a cognitive-perceptual model of somatic interpretation. *Psychological Bulletin*, **109**, 25–41.

Crisson, J. E., Keefe, F. J. (1988) The relationship of locus of control to pain coping strategies and psychological distress in chronic pain patients. *Pain*, **35**, 147–54.

Crombez, G., Eccleston C. Baeyens, F., Eelen, P. (1997) Habituation and the interference of pain with task performance. *Pain*, **70**, 149–54.

DeGood, D. E., Kiernan, B. (1996) Perception of fault in patients with chronic pain. *Pain*, **64**, 153–9.

DeGood, D. E., Shutty, M. S. Jr (1992) Assessment of pain beliefs, coping and self-efficacy. In: Turk, D. C., Melzack R (eds) *Handbook of pain assessment*. Guilford Press, New York, pp. 214–34.

Descartes, R. (1664) *L'homme*. E. Angot, Paris.

Dubner, R. (1997) Neural basis of persistent pain: sensory specialisation. sensory modulation and neuronal plasticity. In: Jensen, T. S., Turner, J. A., Wiesenfeld-Hallin, Z. (eds) *Progress in pain research and management (Proceedings of the 8th World Congress on Pain)*. IASP Press, Seattle, **8**, 243–57.

Eccleston, C. (1995) The attentional control of pain: methodological and theoretical concerns. *Pain*, **63**, 3–10.

Fernandez, F., Turk, D. C. (1995) The scope and significance of anger in chronic pain. *Pain*, **61**, 165–75.

Flor, H., Birbaumer, N. (1994) Acquisition of chronic pain: psychophysiological mechanisms. *American Pain Society Journal*, **3**, 119–27.

Flor, H., Turk, D. C., Birbaumer, N. (1985) Assessment of stress-related psychophysiological stress reactions in chronic back pain patients. *Journal of Consulting and Clinical Psychology*, **53**, 354–64.

Flor, H., Birbaumer, N., Turk D. C. (1990) The psychobiology of chronic pain. *Advances in Behaviour Research and Therapy*, **12**, 47–87.

Flor, H., Fydrich, T., Turk, D. C. (1992) Efficacy of multidisciplinary pain treatment centers: a meta-analytic review. *Pain*, **49**, 221–30.

Flor, H., Braun, C., Elbert, T., Birbaumer, N. (1997) Extensive reorganization of primary somatosensory cortex in chronic back pain patients. *Neuroscience Letters*, **224**, 5–8.

Fordyce, W. E. (1976) *Behavioural methods for chronic pain and illness*. Mosby. St Louis.

Gatchell, R., Turk, D. C. (1996) (eds) *Psychological approaches to pain management: a practitioner's handbook*. Guilford Press. New York.

Geisser, M. E., Roth, R. S., Bachman, J. E., Eckert, T. A. (1996) The relationship between symptoms of post-traumatic stress disorder and pain. affective disturbance and disability among patients with accident and non-accident related pain. *Pain*, **66**, 207–14.

Jensen, M. P., Karoly, P. (1992) Pain-specific beliefs, perceived symptom severity and adjustment to chronic pain. *Clinical Journal of Pain*, **8**, 123–30.

Jensen, M. P., Turner, J. A., Romano, J. M., Karoldy, P. (1991) Coping with chronic pain: a critical review of the literature. *Pain*, **47**, 249–83.

Jensen, M. P., Turner, J. A., Romano, J. M., Lawler, B. K. (1994) Relationship of pain-specific beliefs to chronic pain adjustment. *Pain*, **57**, 301–9.

Keefe, F. J., Block A. R. (1982) Development of an observational method for assessing pain behavior in chronic low back pain patients. *Behavior Therapy*, **13**, 363–75.

Keefe, F. J., Brown, G. K., Wallston, K. A., Caidwell. D. S. (1989) Coping with rheumatoid arthritis pain: catastrophising as a maladaptive strategy. *Pain*, 37, 51–6.

Keefe, F. J., Affleck, G., Lefebvre, J., Starr, K., Caldwell, D. S., Tennen, H. (1997) Pain coping strategies and pain efficacy in rheumatoid arthritis: a daily process analysis. *Pain*, 69, 35–42.

Kori, S. H., Miller, R. P., Todd, D. D. (1990) Kinisophobia: a new view of chronic pain behaviour. *Pain Management*, Jan/Feb, 35–43.

Loeser J. D. (1980) Perspectives on pain. In: Turner, P. (ed.) *Clinical pharmacy and therapeutics*. Macmillan, London, pp. 313–16.

Loeser, I. D., Fordyce, W. E. (1983) Chronic pain. In: Carr, J. E., Dengerik, H. A. (eds) *Behavioural science in the practice of medicine*. Elsevier, Amsterdam.

Main, C. J. (1983) The modified somatic perception questionnaire. *Journal of Psychosomatic Research*, 27, 503–14.

Main, C. J., Burton A. K. (1995) The patient with low back pain: who or what are we assessing? An experimental investigation of a pain puzzle. Pain Reviews 2: 203–209.

Main, C. J., Spanswick, C. C. (1995) Functional overlay and illness behaviour in chronic pain: distress or malingering? Conceptual difficulties in medico-legal assessment of personal injury claims. *Journal of Psychosomatic Research*, 39, 737–53.

Main, C. J., Waddell, G. (1991) Cognitive measures in pain. *Pain*, 46, 287–98.

Main, C. J., Waddell, G. (1998a) Spine update: Behavioural responses to examination: a re-examination: a reappraisal of the interpretation of 'nonorganic signs'. *Spine*, 23, 2367–71.

Main, C. J., Waddell, G. (1998b) Psychologic distress. In: Waddell, G. (ed.) *The back pain revolution*. Churchill Livingstone, Edinburgh, pp. 173–86.

Main, C. J., Watson, P. J. (1996) Guarded movements: development of chronicity. *Journal of Musculoskeletal Pain*, 4, 163–70.

Main, C. J., Wood, P. L. R., Hollis, S., Spanswick, C. C., Waddell, G. (1992) The distress assessment method: a simple patient classification to identify distress and evaluate risk of poor outcome. *Spine*, 17, 42–50.

Melzack, R. (1996) Gate control theory: on the evolution of pain concepts. *Pain Forum*, 5, 128–38.

Melzack, R., Casey, K. L. (1968) Sensory, motivational and central control determinants of pain. In: Kenshalo, D. R. (ed.) *The skin senses*. Charles C. Thomas, Springfield, IL, pp. 423–39.

Melzack, R., Wall, P. (1965) Pain mechanisms: a new theory. *Science*, 150, 971–9.

Nicholas, M. K., Wilson, P. H., Goyen, I. (1992) Comparison of cognitive behavioural group treatment and an alternative non-psychological treatment for chronic low back pain. *Pain*, 48, 339–347.

Parker, H., Wood, P. L. R., Main, C. J. (1995) The use of the pain drawing as a screening measure to predict psychological distress in chronic low back pain. *Spine*, 20, 236–43.

Price, D. D., Mao, J., Mayer, D. J. (1997) Central consequences of persistent pain states In : Jensen, T. S., Turner, J, A. Weisenfeld-Hallin, Z, (eds) *Progress in pain research and management (Proceedings of the 8th World Congress on Pain)*. IASP Press, Seattle, 8, 155–84.

Ransford, A. O., Cairns, D., Mooney, V. (1976) The pain drawing as an aid to the psychological evaluation of patients with low back pain. *Spine*, 1, 127–34.

Richards, J. S., Nepomuceno, I. A., Riles, M., Suer, Z. (1982) Assessing pain behaviour: the U A B pain behaviour scale. *Pain*, 14, 393–8.

Roland, P. E. (1993) *Brain activation*. Wiley Liss, New York.

Romano, I. M., Turner, J. A., Jensen, M. P., *et al.* (1996) Chronic pain patient–spouse behavioral interactions predict patient disability. *Pain*, 63, 353–61.

Rosenstiel, A. K., Keefe, F. J. (1983) The use of coping-strategies in chronic low back pain pa tients: relationship to patient characteristics and current adjustments. *Pain*, 17, 33–4.

Rudy, T. E., Kerns, R. D., Turk, D. C. (1988) Chronic pain and depression: toward a cognitive–behavioral mediation model. *Pain*, 35, 129–40.

Schmitz, U., Saile, H., Nilees, P. (1996) Coping with chronic pain: flexible goal adjustment as an interactive buffer against pain-related distress. *Pain*, 67, 41–51.

Snow-Turek, A. L., Norris, M. P., Tan, G. (1996) Active and passive coping strategies in chronic pain patients. *Pain*, 64, 455–62.

Sullivan, M., Katon, W. (1993) Focus article: somatization: the path between distress and somatic symptoms. *American Pain Society Journal*, 2, 141–9.

Turk, D. C. (1996) Biopsychosocial perspective on chronic pain. In: Gatchel, R., Turk, D. C. (eds) *Psychological approaches to pain management: a practitioner's handbook*. Guilford Press, New York, pp. 3–32.

Turk, D. C., Meichenbaum, D. H., Genest, M. (1983) *Pain and behavioral medicine: a cognitive-behavioral perspective*. Guilford Press, New York.

Turk, D. C., Okifuji, A. Sinclair, I. D., Starz, T. W. (1996) Pain, disability and physical functioning in subgroups of patients with fibromyalgia. *Journal of Rheumatology*, 23(7), 1255–62.

Turner, J. A. (1991) Coping and chronic pain. In: Bond, M. R., Charlton, J. E., Woolf, C. (eds) *Proceedings of the VIth World Congress on Pain*. Elsevier, New York, pp 219–27.

Turpin, G. (ed.) (1989) *Handbook of clinical psychophysiology*. Wiley, Chichester.

Vassiljen, J. O., Johansen, B. M., Westgaard, R. H. (1995) The effect of pain reduction on perceived tension and E. M.G recorded trapezius muscle activity in workers with shoulder and neck pain. *Scandinavian Journal of Rehabilitation Medicine*, 27, 243–52.

Vassiljen, J. O., Westgaard, R. H. (1996) Can stress-related shoulder pain develop independently of muscle activity? *Pain*, 64, 221–30.

Vlaeyen, J. W. S., Kole-Snidjers, A. M. J., Boeren, R. G. B., van Fek, H. (1995) Fear of movement and (re)-injury in chronic low back pain and its relation to behavioural performance. *Pain*, 62, 363–72.

Vlaeyen, J. W. S., van Eek, H., Groenman, N. H., Schuerman, J. A. (1987) Dimensions and components of observed chronic pain behaviour. *Pain*, 31, 65–75.

Waddell, G., Main, C. (1984) Assessment of severity in low back disorders. *Spine*, 9, 204–8.

Waddell, G., Main, C. J. (1998a) A new clinical model of low back pain and disability. In: Waddell, G. (ed.) *The back pain revolution*. Churchill Livingstone, Edinburgh, pp. 223–40.

Waddell, G., Main, C. J. (1998b) Illness behaviour. In: Waddell, G. (ed.) *The back pain revolution*. Churchill Livingston, Edinburgh, pp. 155–72.

Waddell G. Main C. J. 1998c Beliefs about back pain. In: Waddell, G. (ed.) *The back pain revolution*. Churchill Livingstone, Edinburgh, pp. 187–202.

Waddell, G., Bircher, M., Finlayson, D., Main, C. J. (1984) Symptoms and signs: physical disease or illness behaviour? *British Medical Journal*, 289, 739–41.

Waddell, G. McCulloch, J. A., Kummell, E. Venner, R. M. (1980) Nonorganic physical signs in low back pain. *Spine*, 5, 117–25.

Waddell, G., Richardson, J. (1992) Clinical assessment of overt pain behaviour during routine clinical examination. *Journal of Psychosomatic Research*, 36, 77–87.

Waddell, G., Somerville, D., Henderson, I., Newton, M., Main, C. J. (1993) A fear avoidance beliefs questionnaire (FABQ) and the role of fear avoidance beliefs in chronic low back pain and disability. *Pain*, 52, 157–68.

Watson, P. J., Johnson, T. W., Main, C. J. (1996) Low back tenderness in CLBP: the influence of pain report and psychological factors. Paper presented at the 8th World Congress on Pain, Vancouver, Canada.

Watson, P. J., Booker, C. K., Main, C. J., Chen, A. C. N. (1997a) Surface electromyography in the identification of chronic low back pain patients: the development of the flexion relaxation ratio. *Clinical Biomechanics*, 12, 165–71.

Watson, P. J., Booker, C. K., Main, C. J. (1997b) Evidence for the role of psychological factors in abnormal paraspinal activity in patients with chronic low back pain. *Journal of Musculoskeletal Pain*, 5, 41–56.

Watson, P. J., Chen, A. C. N., Booker, C. K., Main, C. J., Jones, A. K. P. (1998) Differential electromyographic response to experimental cold pressor test in chronic low back pain patients and normal controls. *Journal of Musculoskeletal Pain*, **6**(2), 51–64.

Watson, P. J., Poulter, M. (1997) The development of a functional task-oriented measure of pain behaviour in chronic low back pain patients. *Journal of Back and Musculoskeletal Rehabilitation*, **9**, 57–9.

Weir, R., Browne, G., Roberts, J., Tunks, E., Gafni, A. (1994) The meaning of illness questionnaire: further evidence for its reliability and validity. *Pain*, **58**, 377–86.

Woolf, C. J. (1996) Windup and central sensitization are not equivalent. *Pain*, **66**, 105–8.

2.3.3 Placebo theory

Milton L. Cohen

Why discuss placebos? It has been said that the placebo phenomenon '. . . seems to shake our belief in the reliability of our sensory experience' (Wall 1992). Perhaps this arises out of the unpredictability of individual responses to therapy, especially in chronic illness; or perhaps from the recognition that therapies which could not possibly be influencing a known mechanism of disease are nonetheless effective. Mention of placebo tends to evoke images of charlatanism in practice or of nuisance in research. Sporadic reviews have appeared over the last decade (Peck and Coleman 1991, Richardson 1994, Turner *et al.* 1994, Harrington 1997) but no textbook devoted to the subject has appeared since that of White *et al.* (1985). Although the phenomena attached to the placebo concept are recognized commonly and universally, their study is confounded by problems of definition, by myths, and by elusiveness of mechanism.

Definitions

The enormous literature on placebos has been dominated by debate, dilemma and difficulty regarding definition. Gøtzsche (1994) concluded that '. . . the placebo concept as presently used cannot be defined in a logically consistent way and leads to contradictions' and '. . . Because of the logical problems, and since placebos may be powerful interventions, the focus of interest should switch from whether or not an intervention is a placebo towards the magnitude of the effect and the choice of effect variable. This shift would help to bridge the gap between scientific and unscientific medicine.' Gøtzsche also noted that, while placebos are deliberately used in scientific trials to allow inference of specific effect of an intervention, the opposite occurs in clinical practice where an attempt is made to maximize **placebo effect**. Although a fair reflection, this statement raises the problem of the semantic confusion which permeates the field. To resolve this confusion is the task of this section.

Responses to therapy are attributed to three main processes:

- Natural history and regression to the mean, which identify the self-limiting nature of some illnesses or the typical fluctuations of others (Whitney and Von Korff 1992). Thus apparent responses to treatment may reflect random variations in illness expression. Measurement error may also contribute to such observations.

- Specific effects attributable to the characteristic content of the intervention (Turner *et al.* 1994).

- The so-called **nonspecific effects of treatment**, those that may be associated with the sociocultural context in which a treatment is delivered. These are referred to as **placebo effects** (Brody 1985).

This leads to two considerations. First is Grünbaum's (1985) definition, tying the definition of placebo effect to the theory being investigated: whether a given positive effect of a treatment on a target disorder is or is not a placebo effect depends on whether it is produced by treatment factors that are incidental to the theory or those that are characteristic according to the theory. Thus, the status of being a placebo is related both to a theory of therapy and to a specific disorder (Richardson 1994). This allows factors other than the purely pharmacological to be considered as characteristic or incidental, and raises the possibility that a particular factor, such as patient expectation, may be characteristic in one therapy but incidental in another (Peck and Coleman 1991). This approach avoids the use of the term 'nonspecific', as it is possible that, although currently unknown, placebo effects may be mediated by specific mechanisms (Grünbaum 1985). It also acknowledges that the phenomenon of placebo effect(s) has been universally recognized.

The second issue is to distinguish between placebo effect, as defined above, and **placebo response**, a major cause of conceptual confusion. A placebo is an inert substance or treatment. Placebo response is, literally, a response to the administration of a known inert treatment, or placebo. A placebo response is therefore likely to be observed in an experimental trial situation where a known placebo is administered as a 'control' intervention. That known placebos can exert therapeutic effect is itself a remarkable phenomenon, balanced by the observation that in certain circumstances, known nonplacebo treatments may fail to exert their characteristic effect (see 'placebo sag', below). Placebos appear to have their own 'pharmacology' (Lasagna *et al.* 1958) with dose–response, time-effect and side-effect profiles not unlike those of nonplacebos and indeed often related to the comparison nonplacebo (Ross and Olson 1982).

The result of administration of a placebo may be detrimental or negative: this is referred to as a 'nocebo' response. In a review of 109 double-blind drug trials, the incidence of adverse events in healthy subjects in response to the administration of placebo was 19% (Rosenzweig *et al.* 1993). Placebos can be associated with worsening of existing symptoms and can produce pain in normal subjects (Schweiger and Parducci 1981). Analogously, negative effects incidental to the theory of therapy for a given disorder could be referred to as 'nocebo effect'.

However, so long as the terms 'placebo response' and 'placebo effect' are used together, the potential for confusion will be sustained. For that reason the term 'contextual effect' will be used in this chapter as synonymous with 'placebo/nocebo effect', as defined. It follows that a nonplacebo treatment will elicit both a characteristic effect and a placebo (now called contextual) effect. It follows also that a placebo (contextual) effect does not require a placebo.

Myths and their refutation

Two major sets of misconceptions permeate the literature on the placebo phenomenon: the fixed-fraction myth and the special mentality myth.

Fixed-fraction myth

The fixed-fraction myth has two lobes: that approximately one-third of the population responds to placebos, and that the extent of that response is also approximately one-third of the response to the active comparison drug (Wall 1992). This myth has been perpetuated following a misrepresentation of the pioneer work of Beecher (1955), whose figure of about 35% was the average proportion of placebo responders from 11 studies, among which there was a very large variation.

This issue of variation of the placebo response was examined by McQuay *et al.* (1995) in a review of five randomized double-blind parallel-group trials of analgesics in postoperative pain. Individual patients' scores with placebo varied from 0 to 100% of the maximum possible pain relief. Between 7 and 37% of patients given placebo achieved more than 50% pain reduction, reflecting the results obtained by Beecher (1955) in five acute pain studies where that degree of pain reduction was achieved by 15–53% of patients.

It had been claimed by Evans (1974) that the placebo response was about 55% of the response to the active treatment, irrespective of the strength of the active treatment. That is, the stronger the drug, the stronger the placebo response. In the study by McQuay *et al.* (1995), comparison of the mean placebo response with the mean active drug response did produce a regression line with a slope of 0.54 – essentially the same result as Evans' – but with 95% confidence intervals of 0.03–1.08. However, the latter study noted that patient responses were not normally distributed. If median rather than mean responses were used for descriptive purposes, the range of median placebo responses in the five trials surveyed became 2–14%. On average the median placebo score was less than 10% of the median active score, with the slope of the regression line 0.12, with 95% confidence interval of –0.24 to 0.48. This is the expected result if there is no bias in the studies, and dispels the myth that there is a constant relationship between effective analgesic and placebo responses. These fixed-fraction myths can now be seen to have arisen as artefacts of an inappropriate statistical description.

Special mentality myth

The special mentality myth also has two lobes: that placebo responders have nothing wrong with them (or, more bluntly, that their apparent response is an hallucination) and that placebo responders suffer some personality defect, such as being 'neurotic', 'suggestible' or 'willing to please' (Wall 1993). Not only are these contentions quite unsupported by the literature (Richardson 1994) but also it has been shown that under appropriate circumstances, any person can become a placebo responder (Voudouris *et al.* 1989, 1990). Furthermore, placebo responsiveness itself may not be a consistent characteristic, varying according to time and context (Liberman 1964) Placebo response is not due to psychological pathology in the patient and does not indicate absence of organic pathology.

Mechanisms of placebo response and contextual (placebo) effect

Here again the literature is confusing, as most of the experimental work deals with placebo response. However, it may be possible to extrapolate from this to possible mechanisms of contextual (placebo) effect. The main theories address the role of anxiety, of endogenous opioid production, of conditioning, and of expectancy.

Anxiety reduction

Reduction in anxiety as a mechanism was proposed by Evans (1974), but there is little empirical evidence to support this. Not only is there no consistent finding of trait anxiety in placebo responders, but also state anxiety bore a variable relationship to pain tolerance in a study of placebo analgesia (Richardson 1994). The anxiety reduction hypothesis in the context of pain is complicated by the relationship between pain and anxiety, especially when physiological indices are measured (Gross and Collins 1980). Another consideration is the relationship between anxiety and stress on the one hand and the phenomenon of stress-induced analgesia on the other. It might be expected that (stress-induced) anxiety may in fact reduce pain (Richardson 1994). The relationship of changes in anxiety to placebo phenomena awaits clarification.

Endogenous opioids

The proposition that activation of endogenous opioids may mediate placebo phenomena arose out of the use of the opioid antagonist naloxone administered in double-blind design in association with placebo analgesic (Levine *et al.* 1978). However, the methodological problems which confound that study have not been solved in attempts to replicate or refute it, leading to contradictory results (Grevert and Goldstein 1985). This hypothesis, also, remains open.

Conditioning

The conditioning theory for the explanation of placebo phenomena arises out of the observation of learning through association. The classical animal experiments of Pavlov (1927) included the demonstration of an anticipatory action when his dogs who had previously received morphine were placed in the same experimental environment – a conditioned placebo (contextual) effect.

The conditioned placebo model has been articulated by Wickramasekera (1985). The principle is the linking of an unconditioned stimulus (UCS), such as an effective drug which evokes an unconditioned response (UCR), with features of the treatment setting, including persons, places or things, such that those neutral features themselves alone may elicit a component of the UCR. Thus those neutral stimuli become conditioned stimuli (CS) and elicit and a conditioned response (CR). Diagrammatically:

(i)   UCS   →   UCR
(ii) UCS + CS   →   UCR (conditioning step)
(iii) CS   →   CR

Placebo *responses* can be conditioned in humans. Voudouris *et al.* (1985, 1989, 1990) performed conditioning trials in which a neutral cream was associated with reduction in experimental iontophoretically-induced cutaneous pain. When the same levels of experimental pain were then administered with and without the cream, subjects who had received the conditioning reported a lower response with the cream than control subjects. That is,

(i)   experimental stimulus   →   pain
(ii) lowered stimulus + neutral   →   less pain
      cream   (conditioning step)
(iii) experimental stimulus +   →   less pain
      neutral cream

As responses to a placebo can be conditioned by pairing with an experimental stimulus, it follows that responses to a nonplacebo may also be modfied by pairing with neutral stimuli; that is, a contextual response may be conditioned.

(i) nonplacebo analgesic in clinical pain $\rightarrow$ reduction in pain

(ii) nonplacebo analgesic + white uniform $\rightarrow$ reduction in pain (conditioning step)

(iii) white uniform $\rightarrow$ some reduction in pain

This model posits that environmental settings (therapists, uniforms, syringes, pills, rituals) which have been associated with ameliorative effects may thereby become conditioned stimuli for the alleviation of symptoms. Similarly the association of neutral stimuli with aversive stimuli could condition negative or nocebo effects.

The implications of this model are profound (Peck and Coleman 1991). Given that learning (or conditioning) is inevitable, the response to, for example, a drug will comprise an UCR (nonplacebo response) and a CR (placebo or contextual effect). This provides one basis for understanding variability in responses between and within subjects: individual learning differences arising out of having experienced particular forms of treatment in particular contexts. Through response generalization, positive and negative CRs may potentiate or attenuate responses to subsequent treatments. It follows that to maintain a strong contextual effect (CR), the treatment environment must be associated regularly with effective treatment. The use of powerful nonplacebos will enhance the contextual component of effect; the use of weak nonplacebos or of placebos will attenuate the nonplacebo (UCR) component of effect. This is particularly relevant in chronic conditions, where negative contextual effects (nocebo effect) from ineffective therapy may generalize, attenuating responses to a subsequent potent unconditioned stimulus, be that a treatment or a treatment provider. This is the phenomenon of 'placebo sag' (Wickramasekera 1985).

Expectancy

It is almost axiomatic that the expectations of subject, clinician, and researcher will influence outcome of clinical or experimental therapy. Expectation here is synonymous with faith, hope, belief, confidence (Wall 1993, Chaput de Saintonge and Herxheimer 1994). In this situation it is important to avoid teleological reasoning: that placebo (contextual) effect occurred because it was expected by the patient. Like conditioning, expectation is a learned phenomenon, and indeed any distinction between the two may be artificial. There appears to be a reciprocal relationship between expectancy and conditioning, as expectancies may be formed through conditioning and conditioning may be expressed as expectancy. If there is in fact a difference between them, it may be related to (classical) conditioning being attributed to unconscious passive learning of relatively trivial behaviours, whereas expectations are held to arise from conscious cognitive learning. However, examination of conditioned (or, more correctly, conditional) learning suggests that simple stimulus–response associations are an insufficient explanation (Dickenson 1987).

The question arises as to whether expectancies can be formed in the absence of direct experience, that is, through observation, information, or persuasion (Bootzin 1985, Evans 1985, Kirsh 1985). Studies of alcohol ingestion have found that when individuals have expectan-cies that are contrary to the drug's pharmacological effect, their expectancies prevail (Kirsch 1985). By contrast, in their studies of conditioned placebo analgesia, Voudouris et al. (1989, 1990) found that the direct experience of conditioning was more powerful than expectancy through verbal persuasion. In replicating these experiments, however, Montgomery and Kirsch (1997) added the modification of informing one group of subjects that stimulus intensity would be lowered during the 'conditioning' period and thereby eliminated the development of placebo analgesia.

The mechanism of expectancies remains unclear. One proposal suggests that, given that pain and illness are appreciated as aversive events beyond one's control, an expectancy that treatment may exert some control over those events may reduce anxiety, stress, and feelings of being unable to cope. Consistent with that view would be the observations that placebos may be most effective in anxious patients (Evans 1985) and of a larger proportion of placebo responders in clinical pain states than in experimental pain (Beecher 1959). Another proposal links changes in expectancy to changes in behaviour, through either the adoption of coping beliefs or the resumption of physical activity (Bootzin 1985).

Rapprochement

In this discussion it should be noted that authors have made inferences of phenomenon, if not mechanism, from the experimental manipulation of placebo response to the clinical observation of contextual (placebo/nocebo) effect. In the former situation the 'treatment' is the neutral partner in the pairing; in the latter the environment plays that role. Montgomery and Kirsch (1997) argued that conditioning trials themselves can be viewed as expectancy manipulations. They claimed that (classical) conditioning is not sufficient, and that expectation of therapeutic effect is necessary for placebo *responses*. Given that it is unlikely that classical (that is, noncognitive) conditioning occurs in humans (Dickensen 1987), it seems probable that the learning-by-association proposed by the conditioned placebo model to explain clinical contextual *effects* is mediated by expectancy. This was supported by Price et al. (1999) who found that, although classical conditioning may occur, expectancy – whether subtly or overtly induced – was the proximal mediator of placebo analgesic responses. A role for desire for pain relief as a contributor to those responses was not supported. The neurobiological bases for these proposals are yet to be established.

Implications of placebo theory for musculoskeletal medicine

For practice

The conditioning/expectancy models of placebo effect suggest that it is the context of a treatment rather than the patient or the treatment itself which determines the degree of the nonspecific component of any patient's response. Given that under the right circumstances anyone might become a placebo responder, the model predicts that every interaction with medical or other therapeutic professionals plays a role in determining the contextual (or nonspecific or placebo) component of a person's future response to treatment (Peck and Coleman 1991). Expectations or faith or hope are largely learned through experience with the medical system: the challenge is how these effects can be harnessed (Chaput de Saintonge and Herxheimer 1994). These divide into enhancing positive contextual (placebo) effects and limiting negative contextual (nocebo) effects.

Exploitation of positive contextual effects does not extend to the use of known inert treatments (placebos). Indeed, the continued use of inert remedies may lead to 'placebo sag' (Wickramasekera 1985). By contrast, conditioning theory predicts that placebos may be of most effect when paired with powerful nonplacebos; that is, drug **and** placebo rather than drug **or** placebo (Ader 1985). An example is the use of the pain cocktail, where the unconditioned stimulus (the powerful nonplacebo) is paired with a neutral conditioning stimulus (the placebo) and then gradually withdrawn. Ethical principles are not violated: patients are informed about the withdrawal but remain unaware of its timing. Thus it may be possible to achieve the same effect at a lower dosage of the powerful nonplacebo.

However, it is not necessary to use a placebo to enhance a contextual (placebo) effect: as a component of the latter is involved in every nonplacebo treatment, enhancement of that component should improve outcome. Choice of size, colour, or route of administration of nonplacebo treatments may manipulate response, as may pairing with specific suggestions (Chaput de Saintonge and Herxheimer 1994). Expectancies related to the context of treatment may be enhancing factors. These include the credibility of the therapist, of the therapeutic setting, and of the specific treatment itself, including the credibility of the ritual of administration (Wickramasekera 1985).

Expectancies related to the nature of the patient–therapist interaction itself may be the most important in this area (Shapiro and Morris 1978). Factors include aspects of doctor or therapist's behaviour such as friendliness; consideration of patients' concerns; provision of time; clear explanations of diagnosis, prognosis and treatment; enthusiasm for treatment; and the choice of words, gestures, or other nonverbal forms of communication. Consideration of these interactional skills follows from expectancy theory, and it has been argued that they should be accorded as much priority in training as the attaining of medical knowledge (Friedman and DiMatteo 1982).

Lastly in this arena of enhancing contextual (placebo) effects is the importance of assessing treatment history, including past experiences of treatments and expectations, as the contextual component of such past interactions may have had a positive or negative effect on the nonplacebo component (Voudouris et al. 1985). The high rate of noncompliance suggests that therapists need to assess directly their patients' expectations of the effectiveness of treatment and be prepared to receive and discuss feedback (Peck and King 1986).

The other side of this coin is to limit negative contextual (nocebo) effects. In the context of musculoskeletal medicine, chronic pain conditions are unsuccessfully treated pain problems. Conditioning/expectancy theory predicts that the experience of many and varied unsuccessful treatments may contribute to extinction of the contextual component which in turn may attenuate the effectiveness of even powerful nonplacebos (Peck and Coleman 1991). This consideration implies that therapists should be aware of the effects of overservicing patients with chronic pain, especially when the treatments used have questionable efficacy and may in fact be pure placebos. As well as contributing to the phenomenon of extinction, the failure of placebo treatments which are believed by the patient to be nonplacebo treatments may lead to anxiety out of concern that the underlying condition is worse than appreciated (Ross and Olson 1981). It follows that the use of known placebos for 'diagnostic' purposes is fundamentally flawed.

In research

The expectancy and conditioning models take into account the experience of the individual and the consequent potential for modifying both the contextual effect of nonplacebo treatments and the response to known placebos themselves. In musculoskeletal medicine, with its major pain component, a major factor in research design is the choice of appropriate controls. (Peck and Coleman 1991, Kleijnen et al. 1994). In pharmacotherapeutic studies, the usual comparison of parallel groups under double-blind conditions fails to control for expectancy and conditioning. To counter this, a 'balanced placebo' design has been suggested by Marlatt and Roshenow (1980). In this, half the subjects are told that they will receive the drug and the other half that they will not. Within each of these two groups, half actually receive the drug and the other half do not. This design generates four groups, to cater for all combinations of drug and expectancies.

The complicated interaction between expectancy and efficacy may also apply to within-subject designs. It has been shown that there is an order effect: placebos administered after effective nonplacebos were rated as more effective than when administered before effective nonplacebos (Kantor et al. 1966). Modifications of the balanced placebo design have been proposed, to control for such order effects (Koch et al. 1989) and for the expectancy of the administrators of the trial as well as those of the subjects (Rosenthal 1985).

Meta-analysis has added new caveats contingent upon placebo phenomena. In a study of nonsteroidal anti-inflammatory drugs (NSAID) trials, Gøtzsche (1993) found no significant difference in response between patients receiving an NSAID in comparative studies and those receiving the same NSAID in placebo-controlled studies. By contrast, Rochon et al. (1999) found that the same NSAID was likely to be rated as less efficacious and associated with fewer withdrawals due to adverse effect when administered in a placebo trial than when administered in a comparative trial. These findings were attributed to subjects' knowledge of the type of trial in which they were involved, as predicted by placebo theory. This led to the suggestion that placebo-controlled trials may be more appropriate for evaluation of efficacy and comparative trials may be more appropriate for assessment of adverse effects.

To some extent in pharmacotherapeutic research, the introduction of the number-needed-to-treat (NNT) technique in reporting trial results has acknowledged the pervasiveness of contextual effects. Rather than quote a response rate of subjects to a drug, NNT focuses on the number of patients who need to be treated in order for one of them to achieve a successful outcome who would not have done so with placebo (Cook and Sackett 1995). Mathematically, NNT is the reciprocal of the difference between the experimental response rate and the control response rate. A NNT of less than 4 is considered to reflect an effective therapy.

It must be conceded that extension of these principles to physical therapy (Gam et al. 1993), to invasive techniques including surgery (Johnson 1994), and indeed to psychotherapy (Horvath 1988) poses particular difficulty. The often-quoted double-blind study of internal mammary artery ligation for angina pectoris (Cobb et al. 1959) raises the question of the contextual effect in all invasive procedures, whilst the effect of sham ultrasound on the pain – and swelling – following wisdom-tooth extraction (Hashish et al. 1988) suggests that noninvasive technology cannot escape these considerations either. In the context of musculoskeletal medicine, there is an onus on researchers seeking to demonstrate the specific effects of physical therapies to be especially mindful of these implications of placebo theory.

Conclusion

The phenomenon of placebo or contextual effect pervades all forms of therapy. Placebo phenomena have to date been more comprehensively appreciated through sociobiological than neurobiological approaches. A combination of conditioning and expectancy models provides the most explanatory power for these phenomena in the current state of knowledge. Although much remains to be established in terms of mechanism, both the practitioner and researcher in musculoskeletal medicine must be aware of the complex interactions that constitute the healing process and strive to distinguish interpretations of aetiology of disease from recognition of contextual factors.

References

Ader, R. (1985) Conditioned immunopharmacological effects in animals: implications for a conditioning model of pharmacotherapy. In *Placebo: theory, research, and mechanisms*, ed. L. White, B. Tursky, and G. E. Schwartz, Guildford Press, New York, pp. 306–323.

Beecher, H. K. (1955). The powerful placebo. *Journal of the American Medical Association*, **159**, 1602–6.

Beecher, H. K. (1959) *Measurement of subjective responses*. Oxford University Press, New York.

Bootzin, R. R. (1985) The role of expectancy in behaviour change. In *Placebo: theory, research, and mechanisms*, ed. L. White, B. Tursky, and G. E. Schwartz, Guildford Press, New York, pp. 196–210.

Brody, H. (1985) Placebo effect: an examination of Grünbaum's definition. In *Placebo: theory, research, and mechanisms*, ed. L. White, B. Tursky, and G. E. Schwartz, Guildford Press, New York, pp. pp. 37–58.

Chaput de Saintonge, D. M., Herxheimer, A. (1994) Harnessing placebo effects in health care. *Lancet*, **344**, 995–8.

Cobb, L. A., Thomas, G. I., Dillard, D. H., Merendino, K. A., Bruce, R. A. (1959) An evaluation of internal mammary artery ligation by a double-blind technic. *New England Journal of Medicine*, **20**, 1115–18.

Cook, R. J., Sackett, D. L. (1995) The number needed to treat: a clinically useful measure of treatment effect. *British Medical Journal*, **310**, 452–4.

Dickenson, A. (1987) Conditioning. In *The Oxford companion to the mind*, ed. R. L. Gregory, Oxford University Press, Oxford, pp. 159–60.

Evans, F. J. (1974) The placebo response and pain reduction. In *Advances in neurology* Vol. 4, ed J. J. Bonica, Raven Press, New York, pp 289–96.

Evans, F. J. (1985) Expectancy, therapeutic instructions and the placebo response. In *Placebo: theory, research, and mechanisms*, ed. L. White, B. Tursky, and G. E. Schwartz, Guildford Press, New York, pp. 215–28.

Friedman, H. S., DiMatteo, M. R. (eds.) (1982) *Interpersonal issues in health care*. Academic Press, New York.

Gam, A. N., Thorsen, H. and Lønnberg, F. (1993) The effect of low level laser therapy on musculokeletal pain: a meta-analysis. *Pain*, **52**, 63–6.

Gøtzsche, P. C. (1993) Meta-analysis of NSAIDs: Contribution of drugs, doses, trial design and meta-analytic techniques. *Scandinavian Journal of Rheumatology*, **22**, 255–60.

Gøtzsche, P. C. (1994) Is there logic in the placebo? *Lancet*, **344**, 925–6.

Grevert, P., Goldstein, A. (1985) Placebo analgesia, naloxone and the role of endogenous opioids. In: *Placebo: theory, research, and mechanisms*, ed. L. White, B. Tursky, and G. E. Schwartz), Guildford Press, New York, pp. 332–50.

Gross, R. T., Collins, F. L (1980) On the relationship between anxiety and pain: a methodological confounding. *Clinical Psychology Reviews*, **1**, 375–86.

Grünbaum, A. (1985) Explication and implications of the placebo concept. In: *Placebo: theory, research, and mechanisms*, ed. L. White, B. Tursky and G. E. Schwartz, Guildford Press, New York, pp. 9–36.

Harrington, A. (ed.) (1997) *Placebo: Probing the self-healing brain*. Harvard University Press, Boston.

Hashish, I., Feinman, C., Harvey, W. (1988) Reduction of post-operative pain and swelling by ultrasound: a placebo effect. *Pain*, **83**, 303–11.

Horvath, P. (1988) Placebos and common factors in two decades of psychotherapy research. *Psychological Bulletin*, **104**, 214–25.

Johnson, A. G. (1994) Surgery as a placebo. *Lancet*, **344**, 1140–2.

Kantor, T. G., Sunshine, A., Laska, E., Meisner, M., Hopper, M. (1966) Oral analgesic studies: pentazocine hydrochloride, codeine, aspirin and placebo and their influence on response to placebo. *Clinical Pharmacology and Therapeutics*, **7**, 447–54.

Kleijnen, J., de Craen, A. J. M., van Everdingen, J., Krol, L. (1994) Placebo effect in double-blind clinical trials: a review of interactions with medications. *Lancet*, **344**, 1347–9.

Kirsch, I. (1985) Response expectancy as a determinant of experience and behaviour. *American Psychologist*, **40**, 1189–202.

Koch, G. G., Amara, I. M., Brown, B. W., Colton, T., Gillings, D.B. (1989) A two-period cross-over design for the comparison of two active treatments and placebo. *Statistical Medicine*, **8**, 487–504.

Lasagna, L., Laties, V. G., Dohan, J. L. (1958) Further studies on the "pharmacology" of placebo administration. *Journal of Clinical Investigation*, **37**, 533–7.

Levine, J. D., Gordon, N. C., Fields, H. L. (1978) The mechanism of placebo analgesia. *Lancet*, **3**, 654–7.

Liberman, R. (1964) An experimental study of the placebo response under three different situations of pain. *Journal of Psychiatric Research*, **2**, 233–46.

Marlatt, G. A., Roshenow, D. J. (1980) Cognitive processes in alcohol use: expectancy and the balanced placebo design. In *Advances in substance abuse: behavioural and biological research*, ed. N. K. Mello, JAI Press, Greenwich, CT, pp. 150–9.

McQuay, H. Carroll, D., Moore A. (1995) Variation in the placebo effect in randomised controlled trials: all is as blind as it seems. *Pain*, **64**, 331–5.

Montgomery, G. H., Kirsch, I. (1997) Classical conditioning and the placebo effect. *Pain*, **72**, 107–13.

Pavlov, I. (1927) *Conditioned reflexes*. Oxford University Press, London.

Peck, C., King, N. J. (1986) Medical compliance. In *Health care: a behavioural approach*, ed. N. J. King, A. Remenyi), Grune & Stratton, New York, pp. 185–92.

Peck, C., Coleman, G. (1991) Implications of placebo theory for clinical research and practice in pain management. *Theoretical Medicine*, **12**, 247–70.

Price, D. D., Milling, L. S., Kirsch, I., Duff, A., Montgomery, G. H., Nicholls, S. S. (1999) An analysis of factors that contribute to the magnitude of placebo analgesia in an experimental paradigm. *Pain*, **83**, 147–56.

Richardson, P. H. (1994) Placebo effects in pain management. *Pain Reviews*, **1**, 15–32.

Rochon, P. A., Binns, M. A., Litner, J. A., *et al.* (1999) Are randomized controlled trial outcomes influenced by the inclusion of a placebo group? A systematic review of nonsteroidal antiinflammatory drug trials for arthritis treatment. *Journal of Clinical Epidemiology*, **52**, 113–22.

Rosenthal, R. (1985) Designing, analyzing, interpreting and summarizing placebo studies. In *Placebo: theory, research, and mechanisms*, ed. L. White, B. Tursky, and G. E. Schwartz, Guildford Press, New York, pp. 110–36.

Rosenzweig, P., Bohier, S., Zipfel, A. (1993) The placebo effect in healthy volunteers: influence of experimental conditions on the adverse effects profile during phase I studies. *Clinical Pharmacology and Therapeutics*, **54**, 578–83.

Ross, M., Olson, J. M. (1981) An expectancy-attribution model of the effects of placebos. *Psychological Reviews*, **88**, 408–37.

Ross, M., Olson, J. M. (1982) Placebo effects in medical research and practice. In *Social psychology and behavioural medicine*, ed J. R. Eiser, John Wiley, New York, pp. 441–58

Schweiger, A., Parducci, A. (1981) Nocebo: the psychologic induction of pain. *Pavlovian Journal of Biological Science*, **16**, 140–3.

Shapiro, A. K., Morris, L. A. (1978) The placebo effect in medical and psychological therapies. In *Handbook of psychotherapy and behavioural change*, 2nd edn, ed. A. E. Bergin and S. Garfield, John Wiley, New York, pp. 369–410.

Turner, J. A., Deyo, R. A., Loeser, J. D., Von Korff, M., Fordyce, W. E. (1994) The importance of placebo effects in pain treatment and research. *Journal of the American Medical Association*, **271**, 1609–14.

Voudouris, N. J., Peck, C. L., Coleman, G. (1985) Conditioned placebo responses. *Journal of Personal and Social Psychology*, **48**, 47–53.

Voudouris, N. J., Peck, C. L., Coleman, G. (1989) Conditioned response models of placebo phenomena. *Pain*, **38**, 109–16.

Voudouris, N. J., Peck, C. L., Coleman, G. (1990) The role of conditioning and verbal expectancy in the placebo response. *Pain*, **43**, 121–8.

Wall, P. D. (1992) The placebo effect: an unpopular topic. *Pain*, **51**, 1–3.

Wall, P. D. (1993) Pain and the placebo response. *1993 Experimental and theoretical studies of consciousness* (Ciba Foundation Symposium), Wiley, Chichester, pp. 187–216.

White, L., Tursky, B., and Schwartz, G. E. (eds) (1985) *Placebo: theory, research, and mechanisms*. Guildford Press, New York.

Whitney, C. W., Von Korff, M. (1992) Regression to the mean in treated versus untreated chronic pain. *Pain*, **50**, 281–5.

Wickramasekera, I. (1985) A conditioned response model of the placebo effect: predictions from the model. In *Placebo: theory, research, and mechanisms*, ed. L. White, B. Tursky, and G. E. Schwatrz), Guildford Press, New York, pp. 255–287.

Part 3

Regional disorders

The development of a clinical diagnostic routine

Every reader of this page uses a method of making a diagnosis, whether this is by physical examination or by looking at a radiograph or other imaging data. How reliable is our method? In many areas of musculoskeletal medicine we do not know, because we do not have enough data to support our method, and it has not been researched. In this chapter we later itemize currently accepted routines that the authors use routinely. But improvements in our diagnostic methods may be possible, by studying the performance of our current routine in the various respects of reliability, which are:

- the **validity** of the routine for identifying that diagnosis accurately, in two aspects:

  - the **sensitivity**, so that all cases of that type are recognized (giving no false negative results), and
  - the **specificity**, so that only cases of that particular type are identified (giving no false positives)

- the **repeatability** of the routine, so that the same result is reliably obtained each time the routine is used
  - by the same examiner (the within-observer repeatability) and
  - by different examiners (the inter-observer repeatability)

An exercise in developing the best routine of reliable diagnosis was carried out by ourselves for common upper limb musculoskeletal disorders[2]. The stages of the project were as follows.

Choice of examination routine to be tested

Currently in musculoskeletal medicine diagnosis is made from a number of subjective features, such as the history of the condition, and a number of physical examination findings (only sometimes are investigations such as radiographs used). There is enormous potential for variability in the method and application of such criteria. The first step to a 'best examination' in this case was the formation of consensus criteria by a 'Delphi' technique workshop of ergonomists, epidemiologists, occupational physicians, orthopaedic surgeons, rheumatologists, and physiotherapists.

Clarification of definitions

Features of the consensus criteria for each diagnosis then needed better definition, such as anatomical boundaries of the 'neck' and 'shoulder' and what comprises 'restriction' and 'tenderness'. Methods of obtaining physical signs were defined, such as posture of examiner and patient in range of movement assessment, and techniques for tests such as Tinel's test for carpal tunnel syndrome.

Reference standard

For some conditions the 'true' diagnosis can be determined by easily recognized features, such as appearance at surgery, imaging techniques, histology, or blood tests. This is a rarity in musculoskeletal medicine, and in this exercise the reference standard was the diagnosis made by an experienced (independent) rheumatologist.

Training of examiners

So that the routine can be fairly tested, the examiners must receive appropriate training. For this exercise, a rheumatologist and research nurse studied the examination protocol and practised it in 12 sessions over 6 weeks, to obtain familiarity with the tests and uniformity in their application.

Inter-observer and within-observer repeatability

Consecutive cases from hospital outpatient clinics were examined either by the nurse and then the rheumatologist (or vice versa), or by the nurse on two occasions, always with 10 minutes between the separate examinations. The differences in results of the paired examinations were then calculated statistically.

Validity test

The diagnosis that resulted from the test routine was compared with the reference standard (in this case the diagnosis of the independent rheumatologist). The results were separately analysed for each examiner, the nurse, and the doctor.

Upper limb conditions and the MRC schedule of examination

Examples of conditions considered by the consensus group[1] and the criteria for the diagnoses are shown in Table 3.1.1.

Analysis

The results of the exercise[2] showed that within-observer repeatability was excellent (kappa coefficient = 1) and that interobserver repeatability was generally good or excellent. There was most variation in the range-of-movement examinations, not surprisingly, but the actual differences were small (up to 11°). The most reliable measurement in the neck was extension, and in the shoulder both active and passive external rotation (these latter are particularly useful in monitoring progress of such conditions as adhesive capsulitis, inflammatory arthritis of the shoulder, etc.).

The validity tests showed sensitivity to be generally good. Medial epicondylitis was not picked up by the test examiners using the criteria chosen. If the consensus criteria were reduced to a requirement of medial elbow pain and **either** local tenderness **or** pain on resisted wrist flexion, sensitivity would increase to 67%, specificity remaining good at 98% (Table 3.1.2).

The main difference in frequency of diagnostic agreement between reference standard (the independent doctor) and the routine being tested was for rotator cuff tendinitis. In all cases of adhesive capsulitis, the routine also diagnosed rotator cuff tendinitis. This is likely to be

Table 3.1.1. Diagnostic criteria from the Delphi consensus workshop[1]

Disorder	Diagnostic criteria
Rotator cuff tendinitis	History of pain in the deltoid region and pain on resisted active movement (abduction, external and internal rotation)
Bicipital tendinitis	History of anterior shoulder pain and pain on resisted active flexion or supination of forearm
Shoulder capsulitis	History of pain in the deltoid area and equal restriction of active and passive glenohumeral movement with capsular pattern (external rotation > abduction > internal rotation)
Lateral epicondylitis	Epicondylar pain and epicondylar tenderness and pain on resisted extension of the wrist
Medial epicondylitis	Epicondylar tenderness and pain on resisted flexion of the wrist
De Quervain's disease of the wrist	Pain over the radial styloid and tender swelling of first extensor compartment and either pain reproduced by resisted thumb extension or positive Finkelstein's test
Tenosynovitis of wrist	Pain on movement localized to the tendon sheaths in the wrist and reproduction of pain by resisted active movement
Carpal tunnel syndrome	Pain or paraesthesia or sensory loss in the median nerve distribution, and one of Tinel's sign positive, Phalen's test positive, nocturnal exacerbation of symptoms, motor loss with wasting of abductor pollicis brevis, abnormal nerve conduction time

Table 3.1.2. The sensitivity and specificity of the consensus examination under test

Disorder	Standard diagnosis	Diagnosis by test	Diagnosed by both	Sensitivity (%)	Specificity (%)
Adhesive capsulitis	15	20	13	87	90
Bicipital tendinitis	1	3	1	100	98
Rotator tendinitis	12	19	7	58	84
Lateral epicondylitis	11	10	8	73	97
Medial epicondylitis	3	0	0	0	100
Carpal tunnel syndrome	15	10	10	67	100
De Quervain's syndrome	7	5	5	71	100
Tenosynovitis	1	4	1	100	97

because of some pain occurring with the resisted movements of the shoulder in these cases, thus requiring the diagnosis of rotator cuff tendinitis concurrently. But the routine suggests that the two conditions may be truly coexistent, and further study is required to decide where the truth lies.

Summary

From this exercise, it is clear that examinations can be improved to give a certain, measured degree of reliability. The requirements will change constantly, according to the development of new techniques of examination, and through increased knowledge of the conditions being studied, for example by investigative tests (as has occurred for the carpal tunnel syndrome with neurophysiology).

Technique of examination

Musculoskeletal conditions are often the easiest and simplest to diagnose. A short history of the complaint followed by a physical examination will often give a clear answer, so that management can start without the delay of investigations which would require time, travel-

Examination: essential features

The history (often termed the subjective examination)

The pain (or other complaint)

Onset: The time and the circumstances, including
- external forces on the area of the body (if pulled, pushed, hit, pressed, etc.)
- internal strains, e.g. twisting of the trunk, stretching the shoulder

Nature: The quality of the pain, its severity, and whether it is continuous or intermittent.

Spread: Any change in position or extent, since the onset.

Variation: Does the symptom change with:
- time of day
- posture
- activity, or other feature

Associated symptoms
- Paraesthesia or numbness, for example, are useful clues that neural elements are involved in the complaint
- Other joint or muscular pains, possibly indicating a systemic condition

Previous pains or symptoms of this nature
- To indicate conditions with a tendency to recurrence, and their duration and reaction to treatment

Global view
- The person's age, occupation, and family members
- Other musculoskeletal complaints or conditions, other illnesses, medications taken
- The person's mood and any understanding or anxiety about the possible nature of the current symptoms

ling, and expense. Care must be taken not to leave out essential features of the examination (see box).

The history may or may not be contributory to the diagnosis, but should never be left out. As an example, and as discussed in the first section, it may not be possible to distinguish between shoulder capsulitis and rotator cuff strain on physical examination alone, but the history will point to differences in duration, intermittency, and reaction to activity which are typical of the conditions, and may allow the distinction to be made.

Physical examination

Musculoskeletal symptoms can arise from (a) structural conditions, e.g. fracture or arthritis, or (b) dysfunction of anatomically normal structures, e.g. from strain. Two systems are commonly used in the physical diagnosis.

Selective tissue tension

This system was developed by Cyriax.[3] The examiner puts strain sequentially on the possible structures at fault: when the person's pain is reproduced, the structure under test is identified as the likely cause.

The advantage of this system is that it can be focused to one area of the body, giving speed and simplicity to the examination. The disadvantage is that the area tested must be extensive enough to include potential distant sources of referred pain (especially the spine). Also, if there is generalized sensitivity of the tissues, a local condition may be diagnosed where a general condition exists (e.g. fibromyalgia or hypothyroidism).

Functional examination

This method was developed particularly by the osteopathic schools, and in this book is described masterfully by Kuchera in Chapter 3.3. The site of pain may not be used as the focus for the examination, but the whole musculoskeletal system is scanned for evidence of any disturbance of function in the spinal segments and limbs, or of posture and gait.[4]

The advantage of this system is that when the cause of a complaint is distant from the symptom, that cause will not be missed: the associated symptoms will not be mistaken for the main problem. The disadvantage is that it is more time-consuming and that abnormalities will be identified which may not be relevant to the person's complaint (and may be treated).

The most effective approach is likely to be a fusion of elements of both disciplines, and these will be found in the following sections. There is no evidence at present to guide us more to one system than another.

How objective is the physical examination?

While the history is termed the subjective part, and the physical examination is termed the objective part, there are many subjective features to the examination, and repeatability and validity studies of diagnosis depend on adequate care being taken to follow the examination protocol. The examiner can easily put greater strain or pressure on a structure that is presupposed to be the cause of the complaint. By all means structure your examination to follow the clues given by the history, but keep an open mind to the diagnosis.

The system presented here puts initial emphasis on the selective tissue tension routines originally developed by Cyriax, in order to diagnose the structural conditions (Chapter 2.2) of the spine, joints, nerves, muscles, tendons, and bursae. Thence sometimes by the absence, as well as the presence, of features on that examination, the likelihood of a non-structural dysfunction may be raised, requiring appropriate further steps. Alternatively, the nature of the possible structural problem may require investigations.

Active movements

The patient is asked to move the trunk or limb in a particular way. It is often quickest to demonstrate this to the patient. Watch for:

- reproduction of pain
- range of movement
- quality of the movement, e.g. hesitation or antalgic compensation.

The active movements demonstrate the willingness of the patient. For example, the active range of movement may be poor compared to that obtained in the subsequent passive examination . Other features will give clues as to where there are physical or psychological factors at play.

Passive movements

The examiner carries out the movement on the spine or limb, while the patient relaxes. This examination is most useful for testing the inert structures, i.e. the joints' capsules, and ligaments and bursae, and for internal derangements.

The purpose of passive movement examination is

- to reproduce pain
- to show the range of movement
- to appreciate the end-feel of the movement

When a pain is produced by the passive movement, ensure that it is the patient's complaint that is being reproduced, and that it is not another, incidental strain reaction that occurs. For the range of movement, always consider comparing it with the opposite side of the body, where there is doubt on normality: in some areas the two sides can be tested simultaneously. For end-feel, approach the full range of the joint with care, and gauge the elasticity, springiness, or hardness of the restraint, as well as the reaction of the patient: comparison with the other side is often useful.

The result of the passive movement examination reveals whether a capsular or non-capsular pattern is present (see Chapter 2.2.6).

Resisted movements

The examiner asks the patient to hold a certain position of the limb or spine and applies a force which is then resisted, actuating the contractile structures and their attachments, the muscles, tendons and insertions to bone. Weakness on the resisted movement can have a number of causes:

- **pain** may inhibit a good contraction
- **neurological deficit** may prevent muscular action.

Thus on the resisted movements the possible findings are:

- **pain only:** a muscle or tendon partial tear or inflammation is present

- **pain and weakness:** a more severe muscle or tendon partial tear/inflammation
- **weakness with no, or little, pain:** a rupture of the unit (tendon or muscle); or a neurological lesion (whether peripheral nerve, nerve root, cord, or brain).

Examining the 'whole patient'

In any consultation, a doctor is faced with the dilemma of how extensive the examination should be: at a follow-up visit, the examination will almost always be limited to the parts affected (in a one-system condition). In musculoskeletal medicine, there are special concerns at the initial consultation for two possibilities: systemic disease and psychological factors.

From the moment that the patient walks into the consultation, his or her gait, posture, mood and manner are under scrutiny for features of psychological or general ill health. In the physical examination one should be equally alert to:

- **features of general ill health:** The face, hands and skin, and tendon reflexes provide valuable clues.

- **discrepancies and over-reactivity:** Sensitivity to palpation and examination may be the direct result of wind-up of the nervous system, but the often-associated abnormal levels of anxiety may require treatment in their own right. Discrepancies revealed by observation, or found on separate parts of the examination, should alert the examiner. For example, a person who can flex the spine to take off shoes, but is severely restricted when scrutinizing lumbar movements, is signalling something other than a straight relationship between handicap and disability. The person's perception about ability to work and prognosis is worth exploring. The Waddell tests (originally described as being for 'non-organic' pain) are an attempt to measure such factors.[5]

Cervical spine

The cervical spine, like all parts of the spine, can produce both local and referred pains. Its examination (Table 3.1.3) is therefore relevant to many cases of upper limb pain or dysfunction and many cases of thoracic pain. The referral patterns of the cervical nerve roots were the first to be established,[6] followed by the work of Lewis[7] on the ligaments, and then the demonstrations of zygapophysial joint referrals by Dwyer et al.[8,9] The cervical spine may be implicated also in leg symptoms, such as ataxia due to cord compression, or disease, in the cervical area. Hence evaluation of function of the cervical spine is necessary in most cases of upper limb or upper trunk pain, unless there are striking abnormalities peripherally that can explain all the patient's complaints. But symptoms are sometimes the summation of central and peripheral lesions; it is wise never to forget the spine.

The greatest challenges often occur with occupational or overuse syndromes. While in some of these there are generalized findings, in themselves often difficult to assess (see Chapter 3.5), often there appear to be no abnormal findings on examination. The examination can, however, be made more sensitive with manoeuvres such as the upper limb tension test, and studying trigger or tender points in the muscles associated with postural stress, such as the suboccipital,

Table 3.1.3. Examination of cervical spine

Focus of examination	Fig	Procedure	Typical findings/ interpretation
General	T1.1	Gait Posture Muscle bulk Standing or sitting 'Point to your pain' 'Does the movement change your pain?'	Postural or structural abnormality
Gross movement exam	Cervical spine T1.2, T1.3	**Active movements** Rotations	Capsular/non-capsular pattern
	T1.4, T1.5	Side flexions	

Table 3.1.3. Examination of cervical spine (*continued*)

Focus of examination	Fig	Procedure	Typical findings/ interpretation
	T1.6	Extension	
	T1.7	Flexion	
	T1.8, T1.9	**(Passive movements as above)**	End-feel

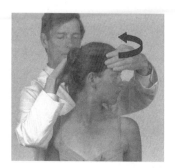

Table 3.1.3. Examination of cervical spine (*continued*)

Focus of examination	Fig	Procedure	Typical findings/ interpretation
		(Resisted movements)	Muscular/bone lesions
	T1.10		
		If there are shoulder or arm symptoms:	
Exclusion of alternative cause of pain	T1.11	**Upper limb Active** Shoulder elevation	Shoulder pathology
Neurological	T1.12	**Resisted** Shoulder shrugging	C2,3,4

Table 3.1.3. Examination of cervical spine (*continued*)

Focus of examination	Fig		Procedure	Typical findings/ interpretation
			Resisted shoulder	
	T1.13		Abduction	C5
	T1.14		Resisted adduction	C7
	T1.15		Resisted external rotation	C5
	T1.16		Resisted internal rotation	C6

Table 3.1.3. Examination of cervical spine (*continued*)

Focus of examination	Fig	Procedure	Typical findings/ interpretation
		Elbow	
	T1.17	Resisted flexion	C5,6
	T1.18	Resisted extension	C7
		Wrist	
	T1.19	Resisted extension	C6
	T1.20	Resisted flexion	C7

Table 3.1.3. Examination of cervical spine (*continued*)

Focus of examination	Fig		Procedure	Typical findings/ interpretation
			Thumb	
	T1.21	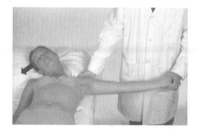	Resisted abduction	C8
			Finger	
			Resisted abduction/adduction	T1
			Sensory examination	
			Reflexes – upper limb	
			Plantar response	Cord compromise
Specific articular examination	T1.22		Specific joint assessment and of myofascial tender points/triggers	Segment affected
Neural sensitization	T1.23, T1.24		Upper limb tension test – see text	Overuse, increased neural sensitivity

Table 3.1.3. Examination of cervical spine (*continued*)

Focus of examination	Fig	Procedure	Typical findings/interpretation
	T1.25, T1.26	Fibromyalgia trigger points (see box, 'Points for palpation' below)	Generalized sensitivity

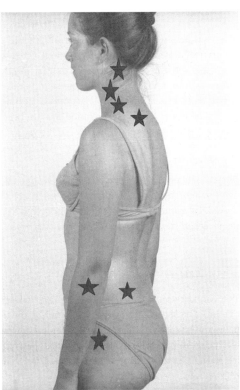

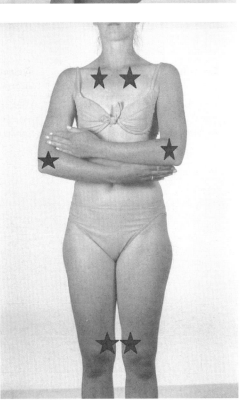

Points for palpation

- *Suboccipital*: under the nuchal line, halfway between the midline and the mastoid process
- *Lower cervical spine*: laterally at C5-7 levels
- *Anterior trapezius*: at the midpoint between occiput and acromion
- *Supraspinatus*: near its origin at the medial border of the scapula
- *Second rib*: just lateral to the costo-chondral
- *Lateral epicondyle*: 2 cm distal to the epicondyle over the radial head/neck
- *Gluteal*: below the iliac crest at the postero-lateral gluteal origin (maximus/medius)
- *Greater trochanter*: posterior to the trochanter
- *Knee*: superior to the medial joint line, on fat pad.

The upper limb tension test[11],[12]

The patient lies on the couch, the examiner standing at the side of the patient's head . The examiner uses his inner hand to keep the shoulder depressed (stretching the brachial plexus): his outer hand takes the patient's hand to maintain the fingers and wrist in extension with the forearm supinated, and, keeping the elbow flexed, takes the shoulder into abduction and 90° of external rotation. The test is positive if the elbow cannot be extended, because of pain and/or tingling in the limb. A comparison is made with the other side, and the effect of contralateral sidebending of the neck can be studied, implicating the neck as a source of the upper limb symptoms.

trapezius, levator scapulae, and scapular muscles. The history takes on a more important role in these cases, and observation of the individual at work may be invaluable.

Routine of the examination

After the initial postural assessment, the patient is asked to point to the pain, and to let the examiner know if the pain changes during the various manoeuvres. The active movements of the cervical spine will usually give a clear indication whether any or all of them alter the pain. If none alters the pain, or the patient appears timid, passive movements can be used, to ensure that the full range of motion is tested, with the added bonus of giving the examiner the end-feel, possibly revealing muscle spasm or bony block to a movement. Resisted movements are rarely helpful in everyday diagnosis in the cervical spine, but

in a case of psychological overlay, the striking lack of effort made by the patient can be revealing. Resisted movements will certainly be painful in cases of bone compromise such as fracture and metastasis. Following the examination of the cervical movements, the shoulder is briefly tested, in case it is an additional cause of pain, and the neurological examination follows. Detailed information on the function of the cervical segments can be obtained by passive, specific examination, a manual skill which must be learnt by practice under supervision. Accurate assessment of which segment is at fault is possible.[10] Abnormal sensitivity of the neural tissues, whether from structural causes such as disc prolapse or from neuroplasticity ('wind-up') can be assessed by the upper limb tension test. Although variations of the test are described their interpretation has not been validated, and the generic one is most used.

Fibromyalgia

The chosen points, of which 11 of a possible 18 (9 pairs) must be painful, are palpated with a thumb or fingertip. The distal fingernail should just blanch with the pressure applied. A 'control' point such as the forehead should give a negative response.[13]

Shoulder

The cervical spine screening examination (of cervical movements) (Table 3.1.4) should always be carried out before the shoulder examination, as so many pains at the shoulder are referred from the spine.

The examination contrasts the effects of passive movements, where the strain is maximized on the inert structures, against the effect of the resisted movements, which reveals the effect on the musculotendinous

Table 3.1.4. Examination of shoulder

Focus of examination	Fig	Procedure	Typical findings/ interpretation
General		Observe posture and muscle bulk	Wasting: tendon rupture or neurogenic origin
Alternative causes of pain		Cervical spine active movements	Cervical origin of pain
Overall shoulder function		**Active shoulder movement**	
	T2.1 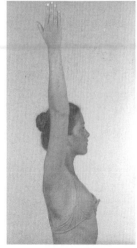	Elevation of arm through flexion	

Table 3.1.4. Examination of shoulder (*continued*)

Focus of examination	Fig	Procedure	Typical findings/ interpretation
		Passive	
	T2.2	Elevation to end-feel	Abnormal end-feel, restriction (or pain) – acromioclavicular joint
		Active	
	T2.3	Abduction	Painful arc
Glenohumeral capsule		**Passive glenohumeral**	
	T2.4	Abduction	Capsular/non-capsular pattern
	T2.5	External rotation	

Table 3.1.4. Examination of shoulder (*continued*)

Focus of examination	Fig	Procedure	Typical findings/interpretation
	T2.6	Internal rotation	
Muscles and tendons		**Resisted**	Pain = strain
	T2.7	Abduction	Supraspinatus
		Resisted Shoulder	
	T2.8	Adduction	Pectoralis major, etc.
	T2.9	External rotation	Infraspinatus
	T2.10	Internal rotation	Subscapularis

Table 3.1.4. Examination of shoulder (*continued*)

Focus of examination	Fig		Procedure	Typical findings/ interpretation
	T2.11		**Elbow** flexion	Biceps
	T2.12		Elbow extension	Triceps/bursitis
Acromioclavicular joint			**If the above tests are negative or equivocal:**	
	T2.13		Passive adduction in flexion	Joint/ligament strain
For laxity/subluxation			**If above tests are negative:** For anterior laxity:	
	T2.14		Patient lies: shoulder is abducted to 90°, and slowly externally rotated	Watch for apprehension and pain. Compare to other side
	T2.15		Relocation: Anterior pressure on upper humerus	Does it clear symptoms?

Table 3.1.4. Examination of shoulder (*continued*)

Focus of examination	Fig	Procedure	Typical findings/ interpretation
	T2.16 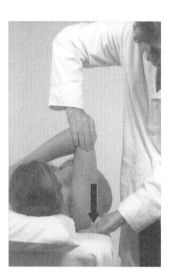	For posterior laxity: Patient lies: with arm in 90° flexion, internally rotated 90°, and elbow flexed, give axial pressure to sublux humeral head posteriorly. Other hand monitors humeral head	
	T2.17, T2.18 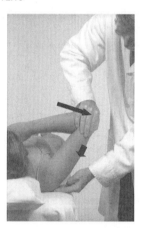 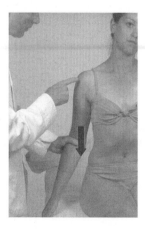	Relocation: Maintaining the axial pressure, gradually abduct the humerus: a subluxed head will clunk back into position.	

Table 3.1.4. Examination of shoulder (*continued*)

Focus of examination	Fig	Procedure	Typical findings/ interpretation
For rotator cuff ruptures		Standing	
	T2.19, T2.20	External rotation lag sign (supraspinatus and infraspinatus): Passively abduct the humerus 20° and support it. Passively externally rotate the humerus to 5° less than maximum.	Can the patient maintain the external rotation?
		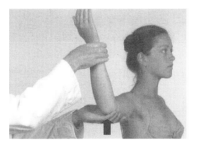	
Rotator cuff ruptures	T2.21, T2.22	Drop sign (infraspinatus): Support the elbow with the shoulder in 90° abduction, and almost full external rotation, and the elbow flexed.	Release the wrist: can the patient maintain the external rotation or does the forearm 'drop'?
		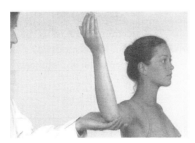	

Table 3.1.4. Examination of shoulder (*continued*)

Focus of examination	Fig	Procedure	Typical findings/ interpretation
	T2.23, T2.24 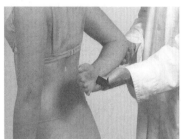 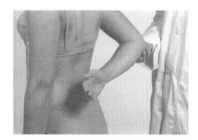	Internal rotation lag sign (subscapularis): The humerus is extended behind the back 20° and is 20° abducted. Get near-maximum passive internal rotation.	Can the patient maintain the rotation?

structures, the rotator cuff being a frequent source of tendinous lesions.

The 'ratio of pains'

Sometimes many movements will be painful, for example all the passive and resisted movements. This would seem to indicate that both the capsule of the joint and the rotator cuff are affected, which may indeed be the case. However, determine which of the two types of movement is the more painful, the passive or the resisted. If the passive range of movement is restricted and more painful, it is generally beneficial to treat the capsule first, as the resisted movement pain may clear at the same time as the capsular features.

The acromioclavicular test is reliable[14] only if the glenohumeral joint has full range: it is therefore carried out last as the movement also stretches the posterior glenohumeral capsule, and the posterior rotator cuff.

Accessory tests

Laxity/subluxation

Anterior[15] (Figures T2.14 and T2.15)

The patient lies with the arm abducted to 90°, and elbow flexed also to 90°. Watch for apprehension and pain with increasing passive external rotation and extension, and compare to the other side.

Relocation

Press downwards on the upper humerus: this will clear the symptoms of anterior capsular stretch.

Posterior[16] (Figures T2.16)

The patient lies with the upper arm vertical and internally rotated, the elbow flexed at 90°. While the examiner's one hand monitors the joint line posteriorly, the other applies axial pressure through the humerus to sublux the head posteriorly. The movement and apprehension should be clear: the examiner should use caution not to dislocate a very lax joint.

Relocation

Maintaining the axial pressure, gradually abduct the humerus: a subluxed head will clunk back into position.

Inferior[17] (Figures T2.17)

Axial traction is applied to the humerus in the anatomical position, and inferior ligamentous laxity will allow a sulcus to become apparent between acromion and humeral head anterolaterally.

Rotator cuff ruptures[18]

External rotation lag sign (supraspinatus and infraspinatus) (Figures T2.19 and T2.20)

The humerus is abducted 20° and supported under the elbow. External rotation is taken passively to 5° less than maximum. Can the patient maintain the position?

Drop sign (infraspinatus) (Figures T2.21 and T2.22)

Support the elbow at 90° shoulder abduction, and almost full external rotation, with the elbow flexed 90°. Release the wrist: can the patient maintain the external rotation, or does the forearm 'drop'?

Elbow

Internal rotation lag sign (subscapularis) (Figures T2.23 and T2.24)
The humerus is 20° extended and 20° abducted, with the elbow flexed behind the back. Passive internal rotation is taken to near maximum. Can the patient maintain the internal rotation?

See Table 3.1.5. When examining for strain at the common flexor and extensor origins of the forearm, it is important for the patient to maintain full extension of the elbow, as otherwise a false negative result for tennis elbow, etc. will result.

Table 3.1.5. Examination of the elbow

Focus of examination	Fig		Procedure	Typical findings/interpretation
General			Observation	Valgus deformity, swelling
			Palpation for heat, swelling	Synovitis, bursa
Elbow joint			**Passive elbow/forearm movements**	
	T3.1	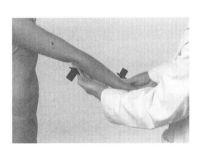	Flexion	Capsular/non-capsular pattern
	T3.2		Extension	End-feel

Table 3.1.5. Examination of the elbow (*continued*)

Focus of examination	Fig		Procedure	Typical findings/ interpretation
Radioulnar joints	T3.3	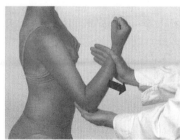	Pronation	
	T3.4		Supination	
Upper arm muscles and tendons	T3.5		**Resisted** Elbow flexion	Biceps, brachialis
	T3.6		Extension	

Table 3.1.5. Examination of the elbow (*continued*)

Focus of examination	Fig		Procedure	Typical findings/ interpretation
Forearm muscles				
	T3.7		Pronation	Pronators, common flexor origin
	T3.8		Supination	Supinator, biceps
	T3.9		Wrist extension	Common extensor origin
	T3.10		Wrist flexion	Common flexor origin

Wrist and hand

Following the examination indicated (Table 3.1.6), or if the patient has specific complaints in the fingers, local palpation of the joints in the affected area, for swelling, restriction of movement, or crepitus during movement is indicated. A search for flexor tenosynovitis, with or without triggering, is made by local palpation, and passive flexion/ extension of the finger while monitoring the tendon around the level of the metacarpophalangeal joint.

Table 3.1.6. Examination of the wrist and hand

Focus of examination	Fig		Procedure	Typical findings/ interpretation
General			Observation	
			Palpation	Heat
Inferior radioulnar joint			**Passive forearm movements**	
	T4.1		Pronation	
	T4.2		Supination	
			Passive	
Wrist and carpal joints	T4.3		Extension	Intercarpal joint problem
	T4.4		Flexion	Wrist joint, capsular/ collateral ligament strain

Table 3.1.6. Examination of the wrist and hand (*continued*)

Focus of examination	Fig		Procedure	Typical findings/ interpretation
	T4.5		Ulnar deviation	
	T4.6		Radial deviation	
Muscles and tendons			**Resisted**	
	T4.7		Extension	Tendonitis
			Resisted wrist	
	T4.8		Flexion	Tendonitis
	T4.9		Ulnar deviation	

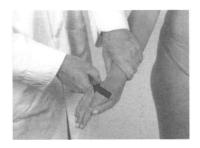

Table 3.1.6. Examination of the wrist and hand (*continued*)

Focus of examination	Fig	Procedure	Typical findings/ interpretation
	T4.10	Radial deviation	
Basal thumb joint	T4.11	Passive thumb movement Adduction/extension	Arthrosis/arthritis
Tendon function	T4.12	Resisted thumb Extension	De Quervain's
	T4.13	**Resisted thumb** Flexion	Tenosynovitis/trigger
	T4.14	Abduction	Weak = median nerve/C8/T1

Table 3.1.6. Examination of the wrist and hand (*continued*)

Focus of examination	Fig		Procedure	Typical findings/ interpretation
	T4.15		Adduction	Weak = ulnar nerve/T1
Interossei			Finger abduction/adduction	Pain = strain, tendonitis Weakness = neurological
			If triggering/tendon symptoms: Active finger flexion and palpation	Trigger finger
Peripheral nerve function			Sensory examination Tinel's test/wrist flexion	Compression of median nerve

Thoracic spine

Scapular pain and interscapular pain, as well as anterior upper chest pain, is frequently due to cervical lesions, so that the cervical spine must be examined at the start of examination for thoracic spine pain (Table 3.1.7).

The examination moves from the overall, gross movements to the movements of each segment. While postural conditions will be highlighted by the general examination, as will general structural conditions such as ankylosing spondylitis, the localized dysfunctions become apparent on the segmental examination.

Rib movement abnormalities may be the cause or result of dysfunction or pain at their joints, the costovertebral and costochondral joints, as well as at the vertebral joints. Mobility and position can be assessed both posteriorly, and (for the upper ribs with their 'pump-handle' action) anteriorly, and (for 'bucket-handle' action of the lower ribs) laterally.

As with the cervical spine, where no clear localized dysfunction or structural problem is apparent, but there is generalized hypersensitivity, fibromyalgia or neural sensitization should be considered possible diagnoses.

Table 3.1.7. Examination of thoracic spine

Focus of examination	Fig		Procedure	Typical findings/ interpretation
General			**Standing**	
			Gait	Posture, deformity
			Posture in standing	Kyphosis, scoliosis
			Posture in flexion	To emphasize scoliosis
Gross movements			**Sitting**	
			Cervical active movements	Identify cervical lesion referral
	T5.1, T5.2		Thoracic spine: active and passive rotations	Symmetrical/asymmetrical

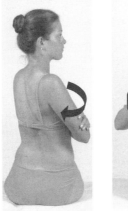 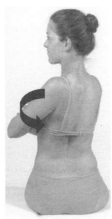

Table 3.1.7. Examination of thoracic spine (continued)

Focus of examination	Fig		Procedure	Typical findings/ interpretation
Trauma	T5.3		Compression of ribs	Rib fractures
Specific segmental exam	T5.4		Skin drag Passive movements Flexion/extension	Level and type of lesion
	T5.5		Rotation Active/passive range of 1st and 2nd ribs Lying	Costovertebral joint function
	T5.6		Vertebral springing	Level of lesion, flexibility, severity
	T5.7		Individual rib movement	Costovertebral joint function
Neurological			Sensory examination Plantar response	If symptoms present Cord lesion/pressure

Lower back

With experience the doctor modifies the examination according to the situation and the presentation of the patient (Table 3.1.8). Thus a neurosurgeon, often being referred cases of possible cauda equina compression, will always test for sensation in the perineum and for anal tone, but will not usually examine for sacroiliac strain or inflammation: whereas a doctor who undertakes manual treatments, in a case with no sciatica or paraesthesia, will omit the sensory examination and examine sacroiliac and lumbar segmental function in detail.

Provocative tests

The McKenzie school has developed provocative tests for disc-related pain, causing centralization or peripheralization of pain. The tests study change of pain during standing extension and flexion, side-gliding with and without overpressure, lying extension and flexion,

Table 3.1.8. Examination of lower back

Position	Fig	Action	Observe
Standing		History and general appraisal	
		(Waddell 5, see box, p. 149)	Manner, sighing
		Posture	Scoliosis, antalgic
	T6.1	Leg length	Discrepancy

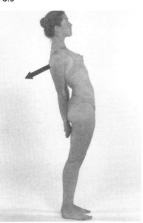

| | T6.2, T6.3 | Articular movements | Extension, side flexion |

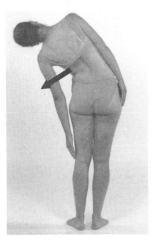

Table 3.1.8. Examination of lower back (*continued*)

Position	Fig	Action	Observe
	T6.4, T6.5	Articular movements	Side flexion, flexion

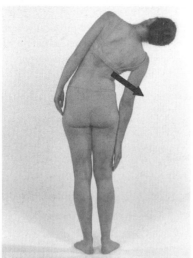

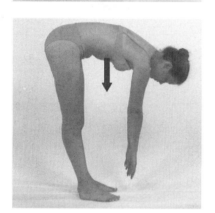

Position	Fig	Action	Observe
	T6.6	Rotation	
		Axial loading (not illustrated)	(Waddell 2, see box, p. 149)	Simulation

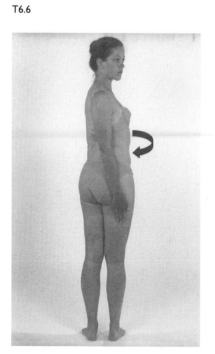

Table 3.1.8. Examination of lower back (*continued*)

Position	Fig		Action	Observe
	T6.7		Forwards flex for PSIS locking sign	Asymmetry of movement
Sitting	T6.8		Tip toe for soleus, gastrocnemius strength	S1, S2 weakness
	T6.9		Sacroiliac position – PSIS	Asymmetry at rest
	T6.10		Sacroiliac locking sign (forwards flex)	Asymmetry of movement

Table 3.1.8. Examination of lower back (*continued*)

Position	Fig		Action		Observe
	T6.11		Straight leg raise	(Waddell 3, see box, p.149)	Distraction
	T6.12		Slump test		Dural/neural sensitivity
Supine	T6.13		ASIS position		Asymmetry at rest
	T6.14–16		Hip flexion and rotations		Exclude hip as pain source

Table 3.1.8. Examination of lower back (*continued*)

Position	Fig	Action	Observe
	T6.17	Sacroiliac strain – axial femoral pressure in flexion and adduction	Sacroiliac strain/inflammation
	T6.18, T6.19	Straight leg raise and add neck flexion	Dural/neural sensitivity
	T6.20–22	Muscle tests L2 (3) 4 5 S1 (Waddell 4, see box, p.149)	Motor problem/non-anatomic L2
			L3, 4
			L5, S1

Table 3.1.8. Examination of lower back (*continued*)

Position	Fig	Action		Observe
	T6.23–25	Muscle tests	(Waddell 4, see box, p. 149)	Motor problem/non-anatomic
				L4
				L5
				S1
		Sensory testing, reflexes		Nerve root compromise
Prone	T6.26	Femoral nerve stretch		Midlumbar nerve root/muscle hypertonus
	T6.27	Contrast with hip extension		

Table 3.1.8. Examination of lower back (*continued*)

Position	Fig	Action		Observe
	T6.28	Muscle test: glutei		S1, 2
	T6.29	Palpation of lumbar spine	Waddell 1 (see box below)	Localized/generalized
	T6.30	(Assessment of segmental motion)		Segmental function

Non-organic signs in back pain (Waddell)

Four out of five of these features are taken as evidence of significant abnormal illness behaviour.[5]

1. Widespread tenderness	- skin and superficial tissues, non-anatomic distribution
2. Simulation of 'strain'	- axial loading, by pressing on the head when standing
	- rotation, holding the hands to the side, giving no strain to the lumbar segments
3. Distraction, repeating a test differently	- straight leg raise, in the sitting position
4. Regional neurological features	- motor testing producing weakness in many of the leg muscle groups
	- sensory changes in the whole limb or a non-anatomic pattern
5. Overreaction	- disproportionate verbal or facial reaction, muscle tension, or juddering response to testing, etc.

---

and flexion/rotation with overpressure. Correlation with disc lesions identified by discography is good.[19] If such tests are negative, but sacroiliac strain tests are positive, there is greater certainty of identifying cases where the sacroiliac joint is generating pain.

Sacroiliac tests

While hip flexion and adduction has been validated as a test for sacroiliac pain due to sacroiliitis,[20] controversy continues about the validity of any of the tests proposed for mechanical sacroiliac pain,[21] with no tests showing good concordance with cases responding to differential local anaesthetic blocks of the joint. The hip adduction and flexion, or thigh-thrust test, shows good reliability between observers,[22] and we favour it. But the diagnosis of mechanical strain of the sacroiliac joint continues to rely on a process of deduction and features suggestive of the diagnosis in the history and the examination.

Psychosocial tests

The history should alert the examiner to the psychosocial factors that are relevant, and the physical examination can usefully include tests that correlate with psychological variables. The Waddell tests for non-organic pain have been correlated both with psychological tests and with prognosis for return to work (see box above).[23] Some of the

Waddell manoeuvres are part of the 'organic' examination (for example, sensitivity of the spine, and motor and sensory examination), whereas others need to be added, to ensure that the five categories are studied. Further prognostic information can be obtained from psychological test questionnaires such as the Distress Risk Assessment Method,[24] the Coping Strategies Questionnaire[25] or the General Health Questionnaire.[26]

Hip

See Table 3.1.9. The hip most frequently refers pain to the groin (and anterior thigh to the knee), but lesions are often associated also with pain laterally or in the buttock. As both lumbar and sacroiliac lesions are capable of referring pain to these areas, the hip examination should include the lumbar spine. Although pain (and/or restriction of range) on internal rotation is a reliable sign of joint abnormality,[27] loss of extension is also characteristic of capsular lesions. This restriction of range causes Thomas's sign, where flexing the normal hip causes the thigh on the abnormal side to rise, as the pelvis tilts posteriorly and the lack of extension at that hip becomes apparent.

The test for psoas bursa (Figure T7.12) has not been validated. It presupposes normal hip and sacroiliac examination, as the combination of flexion and adduction stresses the hip capsule and the sacroiliac ligaments, as well as pinching the psoas tendon and bursa.

Table 3.1.9. Examination of hip

Focus of examination	Fig		Procedure	Typical findings/ interpretation
General			**Standing/walking**	
Preliminary			Posture	Stiff, weak (Trendelenburg), or disordered muscle function
			Gait	
			Examination of lumbar spine	Referred pain
Hip joint			**Supine**	
			Passive hip movements	
	T7.1		Flexion	Range, Thomas's sign
	T7.2		External rotation	Capsular/non-capsular pattern

Table 3.1.9. Examination of hip (*continued*)

Focus of examination	Fig		Procedure	Typical findings/ interpretation
	T7.3		Internal rotation	
	T7.4		Adduction	
	T7.5		Abduction	
Muscles	T7.6		**Resisted** Flexion	Sprain, weakness
	T7.7		Abduction	Trochanteric bursitis

Table 3.1.9. Examination of hip (*continued*)

Focus of examination	Fig		Procedure	Typical findings/ interpretation
	T7.8		Adduction	Adductor strain
Hip capsular range			**Prone** **Passive**	
	T7.9		Extension	End-feel, range
	T7.10		Internal rotation	Bilaterally, compare range
Muscles			**Resisted**	
	T7.11		Knee flexion	Hamstring strain, bursa
			If above tests are negative,	
Psoas bursa			**Supine**	
	T7.12		**Passive** flexion/adduction	Groin pain = bursa; posterior = ?sacroi

Knee

Knee examination (Table 3.1.10) is valuable in the initial assessment of all knee pains, but the knee is an area where investigative techniques have greatly enhanced accuracy of diagnosis. A suspicion of meniscal injury will be raised by the history (e.g. locking and recurrent effusion) and features such as the McMurray test, but investigations such as MR scan, arthroscopy, and arthrography have been shown to be more accurate than clinical examination.

Following the functional examination, sites of pain and tenderness can be examined, as the extensor mechanism and accessory structures are frequent sources of symptoms. The margins of the patella where the retinaculum and quadriceps insert, the patellar ligament, and its attachments, and the tibial tubercle should be examined. Medially the infrapatellar fat pad and the medial synovial plica can be assessed, and laterally the iliotibial band may give symptoms. The superior tibiofibular joint may be affected by ankle injuries as well as direct trauma. It can be assessed for tenderness, pain on movement, and range of movement.

Table 3.1.10 Examination of knee (consider preliminary examination of the lumbar spine and hip for referred pain)

Focus of examination	Fig	Procedure	Typical findings/ interpretation
General and alignment		Posture	Varus/valgus, patellar squint, foot pronation
		Gait	Knee/foot alignment
	T8.1	Squat	Extensor mechanism/ meniscus
Inflammation		Palpation	Heat, bursa
		Test for fluid	Effusion, haemarthrosis
Knee capsule		**Passive knee movements**	
	T8.2	Flexion	Capsular/non-capsular pattern

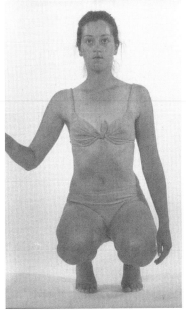

Table 3.1.10 Examination of knee (consider preliminary examination of the lumbar spine and hip for referred pain) (*continued*)

Focus of examination	Fig		Procedure	Typical findings/ interpretation
	T8.3		Extension	
Ligaments	T8.4		Varus	In 30° flexion
	T8.5		Valgus	For collateral ligaments
	T8.6		Anterior drawer	Cruciate ligaments
	T8.7		Posterior drawer	

Table 3.1.10 Examination of knee (consider preliminary examination of the lumbar spine and hip for referred pain) (*continued*)

Focus of examination	Fig		Procedure	Typical findings/ interpretation
	T8.8		Lachmann's test	
	T8.9		Pivot shift test	Anterolateral instability (cruciate)
Menisci	T8.10		Internal rotation	Lateral coronary (menisco-tibial ligt.)
	T8.11		External rotation	Medial coronary
	T8.12		McMurray test	Menisci

Table 3.1.10 Examination of knee (consider preliminary examination of the lumbar spine and hip for referred pain) *(continued)*

Focus of examination	Fig		Procedure	Typical findings/ interpretation
Musculotendinous lesions			**Resisted**	
	T8.13		Flexion	Hamstrings
	T8.14		Extension	Extensor mechanism
If positive,			**Palpate** hamstring or extensor mechanism	Site of tendonitis, rupture, patellar pathology or ligament strain
If negative,			**Palpate** for	
			Joint margin	Cysts
			Patellar margins	Chondromalacia, patellar attachment
	T8.15		Apprehension test	Patellar subluxability
			Fat pad	Haematoma
			Plica	Trauma
			Iliotibial band	Iliotibial band friction
			Superior tibiofibular joint	Dysfunction

Ankle and foot

The standard examination (Table 3.1.11) will usually reveal the structures that are suffering from strains, but the mechanism of the strain may not be apparent without studying the dynamics of gait. Thus, looking at the individual's gait and ankle and foot alignment is the part of the examination which may reveal the type of treatment required in many cases of foot and ankle pain, and this can be enhanced further by videorecording, for example on a treadmill.

Following the standard examination, palpation of painful structures will further aid diagnosis, both for conditions such as Achilles tendonitis, plantar fasciitis, and, especially in the forefoot, for intermetatarsal neuroma, metatarsal or distal joint swelling, inflammation, or deformity.

Table 3.1.11. Examination of ankle and foot

Focus of examination	Fig		Procedure	Typical findings/ interpretation
General	T9.1	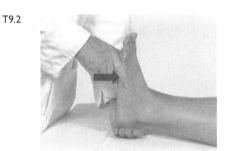	Gait	Antalgic patterns, alignment
			Alignment of foot	Calcaneal angle, pronation
			Weightbearing	
			Shoes	Uneven wear
			Palpation	Heat, swelling, colour change
Ankle joint			**Passive**	
	T9.2		Ankle dorsiflexion	Capsular/non-capsular pattern
	T9.3	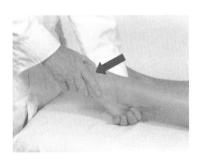	Plantarflexion	

Table 3.1.11. Examination of ankle and foot (*continued*)

Focus of examination	Fig		Procedure	Typical findings/ interpretation
Ankle ligaments	T9.4		Plantarflexion with inversion	Lateral ligaments
	T9.5		Plantarflexion with eversion	Medial ligament
If ankle instability suspected	T9.6		Ankle(tibiotalar) drawer test	Instability with ligament rupture
Subtalar joint	T9.7		Varus	Pain/restriction = arthrosis/itis
	T9.8		Valgus	Clunk/laxity = interosseous diastasis or talar dome pathology

Table 3.1.11. Examination of ankle and foot (*continued*)

Focus of examination	Fig		Procedure	Typical findings/ interpretation
Midtarsal joints	T9.9		Inversion	Pain/range
	T9.10		Eversion	mid-tarsal and adjacent joints
	T9.11		Dorsiflexion	
	T9.12		Plantarflexion	
Muscles, tendons			**Resisted**	
	9.13		Dorsiflexion	Tibialis anterior

Table 3.1.11. Examination of ankle and foot (*continued*)

Focus of examination	Fig		Procedure	Typical findings/ interpretation
	T9.14		Resisted inversion	Tibialis posterior
	T9.15		Eversion	Peronei
	T9.16		Plantarflexion	Achilles tendon
Other lesions If tests negative:			Palpate area of pain, e.g. Plantar fascia Achilles tendon	Arthritis, strain, or neuroma
	T9.17		Metatarsal joints Metatarsal neuroma	

Acknowledgement

The assistance of Professor David Coggan, Dr Keith Palmer and Dr Karen Walker-Bone in preparing the section on the examination schedule, and of the Arthritis Research Council in supporting the underlying research, is gratefully acknowledged.

References

1. Harrington, J. M., Carter, J. T., Birrell, L., Gompertz, D. Surveillance case definitions for work-related upper limb pain syndromes. *Occup Environ Med*, 1998, **55**, 264–271.

2. Palmer, K., Walker-Bone, K., Linaker, C. *et al.* The Southampton examination schedule for the diagnosis of musculoskeletal disorders of the upper limb. *Ann Rheum Dis* 2000, **59**, 5–11.

3. Cyriax, J. *Rheumatism and soft tissue injuries.* Hamilton, London, 1947.

4. Neumann, H-D. *Introduction to manual medicine.* Springer-Verlag, Berlin, 1989.

5. Waddell, G., McCulloch, J. A., Kummel, E., Venner, R. M. Non-organic signs in low back pain. *Spine*, 1980, **5**, 117–25.

6. Foerster, O. Dermatomes in man. *Brain*, 1933, **56**, 1.

7. Lewis, T., Kellgren J. H. Observations relating to referred pain. *Clin Sci*, 1939, **4**, 478–71.

8. Dwyer, A., Aprill, C., Bogduk N. Cervical zygapophyseal joint pain patterns I: a study in normal volunteers. *Spine*, 1990, **15**, 453–7.

9. Aprill, C., Dwyer, A., Bogduk, N. Cervical zygapophyseal joint pain patterns II: a clinical evaluation. *Spine*, 1990, **15**, 458–61.

10. Jull, G., Bogduk, N., Marsland, A. The accuracy of manual diagnosis for cervical zygapophyseal joint pain syndrome. *Med J Australia*, 1988, **148**, 233–6.

11. Elvey, R. L. The investigation of arm pain. In: Grieve, G. P., ed., *Modern manual therapy of the vertebral column.* Churchill Livingstone, Edinburgh, 1986, pp. 530–5.

12. Quintner, J. L. A study of upper limb pain and paraesthesiae following neck injury in motor-vehicle accidents: assessment of the brachial plexus tension test of Elvey. *Br J Rheumatol*, 1989, **28**, 528–33.

13. Wolfe, F., Smythe, H. A., Yunus, A. B. The American College of Rheumatology 1990 criteria for the classification of fibromyalgia. *Arthritis Rheum*, 1990, **33**, 160–72.

14. Patijn, J., Jonquiere, M., Brouwer, R., Kingma, H. () The whiplash-associated acromioclavicular syndrome. *J Orthop Med*, 1998, **20**, 10–12.

15. Jobe, F. W. Painful athletic injuries of the shoulder. *Clin Orthop Rel Res*, 1983, **173**, 117.

16. Gerber, C., Ganz, R. Clinical assessment of instability of the shoulder. *J Bone Joint Surg*, 1984, **66B**, 551–6.

17. Neer, C. S., Foster, C. R. Inferior capsular shift for involuntary inferior and multidirectional instability of the shoulder. *J Bone Joint Surg*, 1980, **62A**, 897–908.

18. Hertel, R., Ballmer, F. T., Lambert, S. M., Gerber, C. Lag signs in the diagnosis of rotator cuff ruptures. *J Shoulder Elbow Surg*, 1996, **5**, 307–13.

19. Donelson, R., Aprill, C., Medcalf, R., Grant, W. A prospective study of centralization of lumbar and referred pain. *Spine*, 1997, **22**, 1115–22.

20. Rudge, S. The clinical assessment of sacro-iliac joint involvement in ankylosing spondylitis. *Rheumatol Rehabil*, 1982, **21**, 15–20.

21. Dreyfuss, P., Michaelsen, M., Pauza, K., *et al.* The value of medical history and physical examination in diagnosing sacroiliac joint pain. *Spine*, 1996, **21**, 2594–602.

22. Laslett, M., Williams, M. The reliability of selected pain provocation tests for sacroiliac joint pathology. *Spine*, 1994, **11**, 1243–9.

23. Kummel, B. M. Non-organic signs of significance in low back pain. *Spine*, 1996, **21**, 1077–81.

24. Main, C. J., Wood, P. L., Hollis, S., Spanswick, C. C., Waddell, G. The distress and risk assessment method. *Spine*, 1992, **17**, 42–52.

25. Burton, A. K., Tillotson, K. M., Main, C. J., Hollis, S. Psychosocial predictors of outcome in acute and subchronic low back trouble. *Spine*, 1995, **20**, 722–8.

26. Croft, P. R., Nahit, E. S., Macfarlane, G. J., *et al.* Interobserver reliability in measuring flexion, internal rotation and external rotation of the hip using a plurimeter. *Ann Rheum Dis*, 1996, **55**, 320–23.

27. Thijn, C. J. P. Accuracy of double contrast arthrography and arthroscopy of the knee joint. *Skeletal Radiol*, 1982, **163**, 731–5.

3.1.2 Investigative techniques

Richard M. Ellis and Cyrus Cooper

Investigations

Bad habits can develop during a doctor's years of training. In the typical hierarchical system of medical training, the trainee may be responsible for arranging the patient's investigations, so that these can be presented to the senior doctor when complete, but the trainee may not be responsible for any active direction in the treatment. Thus the idea that investigation is more important than treatment, or that investigation is all that is required, or that it precludes treatment, can arise. What is certain is that investigations can delay treatment, for good or bad reasons. Remember that one of the patient's most important concerns is pain relief. Can you start some treatment that is safe and will not complicate subsequent management?

Blood tests

Systemic abnormalities frequently cause musculoskeletal symptoms, but mechanical causes are far more common, and routine investigations for all cases of musculoskeletal pain are not justifiable. In a survey of cervical spine X-rays, it was calculated of over 1200 X-rays taken, only one caused a change in management of the case.[1]

The doctor is alerted to the need for X-rays by:

- unexplained features in the history and/or examination
- a previous history of systemic disease such as cancer, immunosuppression, infection, or haemoglobinopathy
- generalized symptoms
- failure to progress with normal management.

Table 3.1.12. Tests for systemic disorders giving generalized musculoskeletal pain

Condition	Suggested tests
Cancer, leukaemia	Full blood count, bone metabolism
Lung cancer	Chest radiograph
Thyroid dysfunction	TSH, T4
Diabetes mellitus	Urinalysis
Hyperparathyroidism	Bone metabolism
Inflammatory arthritis	ESR or plasma viscosity (also consider C-reactive protein: rheumatoid factor is present in 15% of normals)
Polymyositis	ESR, creatine kinase

Some of the commonest systemic diseases that may be associated with musculoskeletal symptoms, and suitable blood tests, are shown in Table 3.1.12.

Imaging techniques

Each successive advance in medical imaging has helped the ease and accuracy of identification of structural abnormalities. The disadvantage of these techniques is that they do not quantify the degree, if any, of functional disturbance caused. Many examples of structural change, such as spondylolisthesis, spondylosis, or even osteoarthritis, may not change function or comfort. Imaging, like other investigations, must be given its correct importance in reaching a diagnosis – neither too high nor too low.

We would rate the particular uses of imaging in musculoskeletal medicine to be:

- to identify cancer, whether primary or metastatic, at the earliest possible stage
- to clarify technical factors in cases where surgery appears indicated
- to clarify the assessment where first-line treatment has failed.

Although a case could be made for imaging every case attending for diagnosis, taking factors of cost-effectiveness into account, as well as safety, opinion is strongly in favour of managing typical cases on lines indicated by clinical assessment in the first instance.[2]

Radiography

Where a person has been subject to significant trauma, a radiograph should be considered, and with increasing age the threshold should be lowered, as bone density and strength inevitably decrease, both in the spine and in the limbs. If clinical suspicion of a fracture remains despite a negative report, consider repeating the test. In some cases, most notoriously with march fractures of the metatarsals, the fracture becomes apparent only later because of callus formation. Radionuclide bone scan can show the abnormality also (and in stress fractures), and is useful where the urgency of the case demands an early definitive diagnosis e.g. with a spondylolysis, or spinal neural arch fracture. In other cases the problem is well recognized, such as with scaphoid fractures, or subcapital fractures of the femoral neck, so that clinical management can be carried out on an agreed protocol, entirely on the clinical examination findings. CT scan will often reveal the changes soon after injury, but the expense and time delay may not be justified in simple cases.

CT scan

Although superseded by MRI in spinal pain diagnosis for most abnormalities, certain CT techniques remain the best available. Because CT shows bone cortex distinctly, fractures are well shown: loose bodies in joints, and defects in articular cartilage (e.g. osteitis dissecans or effects of trauma) are often best shown by CT arthrograms.

MRI

Fine resolution obtainable in different planes has allowed greater diagnostic accuracy in spinal diagnosis, especially with nerve root pressure, whether by spinal stenosis, by disc prolapse centrally or laterally inside or beyond the exit foramen, or by osteophytes or other space-occupying lesions. Disc disruption without change of external contour can also be seen. Inflammatory change associated with annular tears of the disc can be identified. Degeneration of disc substance can be shown, with the loss of water content. Internal disc disruption can be shown on discography: discography tests the disc's competence for holding the injected material, or whether it is ruptured, and whether the patient's pain is reproduced by pressure on that disc at that level.[3] Differentiation of nerve root embarrassment by fibrosis (postoperative, for example) rather than by new disc prolapse can be made by gadolinium enhancement.

Radionucleotide bone scan

Isotopic bone scan is the investigation of choice for detection of bony metastasis, for example causing pain or pathological fracture. An unexpectedly raised alkaline phosphatase can be followed by this investigation. Subsequent radiographs of a single area of increased uptake may, however, show another diagnosis such as osteomyelitis or Paget's disease of bone.

Ultrasonography

Changes in water content occurring with inflammation or degeneration can identify soft tissue lesions on ultrasound scans: these will show in muscle, tendon, or tendon sheaths. Diagnosis can be specific to the one tendon (if several are in the same anatomical area) or to one part of the structure that has been otherwise identified as the source. False positive results can occur with non-symptomatic lesions, and ultrasound will provide the best results when correlated with clinical findings.

Neurophysiology

Some peripheral nerve lesions and root lesions give a clear-cut clinical picture requiring no further confirmation, but neurophysiology offers useful help in some diagnoses and essential help in others. Techniques of most use in musculoskeletal medicine are:

- nerve conduction tests
- electromyography (EMG)
- sensory-evoked potentials

Nerve conduction tests

Nerve entrapment neuropathies can be identified and their severity measured by the increased latency of action potentials across the point of suspected compression, together with any reduction in the size of the action potential.

The frequent clinical problem of limb paraesthesia includes the possibility of lesions at two points, a 'double crush' at a peripheral point such as the carpal tunnel and a proximal one such as a nerve root. If the peripheral point's latency is normal or only slightly reduced, and there are clinical indications of a proximal lesion, that lesion should be treated in the usual way, before any surgical decompression, or other treatment of the peripheral lesion is considered.

As nerve conduction tests have become more detailed, it has been established that subclinical abnormalities exist.[4] Many of these cases do not develop clinical syndromes. As with imaging investigations, the results of tests should not be acted on unless they correlate with clinical features.

In peripheral neuropathy, nerve conduction tests allow distinction to be made between lesions of individual nerves (mononeuritis) several nerves (mononeuritis multiplex), sensory nerves, and motor nerves. The distinction between demyelinating and axonal peripheral neuropathies is important, as the inflammatory demyelinating neuropathies may respond to active treatment with gammaglobulin or corticosteroids. Demyelination of the peripheral nerve causes more delay in conduction, whereas axonal degeneration causes more attenuation of sensory action potentials.

F wave response

Stimulation of a peripheral nerve causes, in addition to the usual distal response, a proximal, antidromic response to the spinal cord, followed by a second response distally. Delay in this secondary response can confirm a proximal compression, e.g. of the nerve root by a disc. With the use of sensory evoked potentials (best for lower limb lesions), and improved imaging, however, the F wave response is less used.

EMG

Electromyographic recordings, from a concentric needle electrode in muscle, will show the size and quality of muscle action potentials with voluntary contraction or after electrical stimulation, as well as any spontaneous electrical activity. Any delay in response to stimulation can be detected. EMG is most useful in the diagnosis of muscle weakness: a lower motor neurone lesion will give, after about 3 weeks duration, a typical pattern of spontaneous discharge (fibrillation). If there is some re-innervation, the large polyphasic units will appear and are easily recognized. The typical finding in myogenic weakness, as opposed to neurogenic problems, is small amplitude, brief potentials: these will be seen both in inflammatory, or hereditary muscle disease, and further differentiation requires correlation with clinical features, and blood tests (as well, sometimes, as muscle biopsy). There are specific features on EMG of other muscle diseases such as myasthenia gravis, and dystrophia myotonica.

Sensory evoked potentials

Electrical stimulation in the peripheral sensory distribution of a nerve creates a response which can be detected by a scalp electrode over the sensory cortex. An abnormally slow response indicates that damage has occurred to the pathway, at some time, but does not identify the site of the damage.

The technique has shown reliable results in the investigation of sciatic symptoms: while the normal latencies for age and sex have been established, unilateral lesions can be identified with confidence and correlated with imaging studies (which on their own may be equivocal).

References

1. Heller, C. A., Stanley, P., Lewis-Jones, B., Heller R. F. Value of X-ray examinations of the cervical spine. *Br Med J*, 1983, **287**, 1276–8.
2. Clinical Standards Advisory Group *Back pain*. HMSO, London, 1994.
3. Donelson, R., Aprill, C., Medcalf, R., Grant, W. A prospective study of centralization of lumbar and referred pain. *Spine*, 1997, **22**, 1115–22.
4. Ferry, S., Pritchard, T., Keenan, J., Croft, P., Silman, A. Estimating the prevalence of delayed median nerve conduction in the general population. *Br J Rheumatol*, 1998, **37**, 630–5.

3.2 Endoscopically determined pain sources in the lumbar spine

Martin T. N. Knight

Endoscopy and aware-state surgery have allowed us to develop a patient-sensitive system for identifying sources of pain in the foramen and epidural zones, termed **viviprudence**. Endoscopy allows us to palpate foraminal and epidural structures under direct vision, with the definition of pain sources by the patient directly.

Patient feedback has taught us that the disc, epidural, foraminal, and extraforaminal structures, once irritated or inflamed, provide readily evoked pain. Endoscopy has shown us that new sites of pain exist, and that these are aggravated by tethering or repetitive microtrauma. These discrete pain sources are associated with persistent and disabling pain. The resolution of symptoms by their specific treatment or ablation confirms the significance of such sources. These hitherto unappreciated sources of pain can be treated by reduction of the irritation by postural stabilization, adjunctive anti-inflammatory injections, or endoscopic surgical ablation in the more recalcitrant cases, without the need for open surgery.

Appreciation of the presence of the 'new' pain sources will assist in the development of precise conservative and minimally invasive treatment techniques in the future. Their presence may account for the persistence of elusive back pain and sciatica following conventional treatment and may provide the focal explanation of 'memory' pain, 'illness behaviour', 'instability syndromes', 'failed back syndromes', and 'failed back surgery syndromes'. The plethora of syndromes built upon indirect methods of examination is a testimonial to our ignorance of the source of axial and referred pain. This admission is endorsed by their absence after the treatment of chronic joint pain precisely treated by prosthetic replacement. Their derivation is an indication that the primary cause of the pain has not been addressed. Endoscopic aware-state surgery has detected many such foci and offers an opportunity to develop specific and discrete low-morbidity methods of detection and treatment.

Background

Since 1990 we have used aware-state surgery to treat spinal disorders as part of the process of viviprudence. Viviprudence is the evaluation cascade of in-depth questionnaires, postural analysis, extended clinical examination, and weightbearing radiographs which underpin initial examination. This is followed by extended postural restabilization and motor reprogramming physiotherapy for 6–12 weeks, after which persistent debilitating symptoms merit MR scanning. This is followed by spinal probing and discography, with spinal probing being the more valuable. Multiple point probing serves to pinpoint pain sites at the facet margin, neural margins, annulus, and safe working zone. The safe working zone is a triangular region bounded by the dura or traversing nerve medially, the medial border of the exiting nerve laterally and the superior endplate margin of the inferior bounding vertebra.

Discography reproduces pain in only 27% of patients with non-compressive radiculopathy, but is valuable in defining the disposition of degeneration within the disc and the integrity of the annulus. Discography defines most leaks and their direction of emission. The acceptance volume of radio-opaque dye defines the degree of degeneration present.

For those cases where pain is either incompletely reproduced or there is overlap in the symptoms reproduced, the **differential discography** is particularly valuable. Differential discography uses the intradiscal instillation of methylprednisolone, Omnipaque 240 or bupivacaine to produce amelioration of symptoms for 6–10 days, 12–18 hours, and 5–8 hours respectively to determine the contribution to a symptom complex from each specific segment.

Our experience with aware-state surgery began in 1990, when we performed percutaneous discectomy. The 12.5% annual recurrence rate led us to explore laser disc decompression as a minimalist alternative to treating compressive and non-compressive radiculopathy. In 1992 we developed biportal endoscopic intradiscal discectomy but found that although this technique could address more significant lesions such as disc extrusion and large focal protrusions, it was extremely susceptible to lateral recess stenosis. This led us to develop a method of foraminal decompression termed endoscopic laser foraminoplasty (ELF) which provides the means to explore the epidural, foraminal, and extraforaminal zones as well as effect intradiscal discectomy, all by the posterolateral route and in the aware state. Clinical implementation of uniportal ELF started in 1994.

The system of viviprudence and aware-state endoscopic examination has been used to address lateral recess stenosis, epidural scarring, osteophytosis, settlement, listhesis, disc extrusion, spondylolytic spondylolisthesis, 'instability', sequestration, 'failed back syndrome', and 'failed back surgery syndrome' in over 775 patients. This experience has demonstrated numerous unsuspected causes of pain arising in degenerative disc disease and include:

- superior foraminal ligament impingement
- superior notch osteophytosis
- dorsal and shoulder osteophytes
- facet joint impaction
- facet joint cysts
- pars interarticularis tethering
- safe working zone and notch engorgement
- ligamentum flavum infolding
- disc pad
- posterior longitudinal ligament irritation
- intertransverse ligament and muscle entrapment
- inferior external pedicular tethering
- annulus
- annular tears
- shoulder osteophytes
- lateral osteophytosis
- paravertebral bone graft tethering
- postfusion discitis
- instrumentation neural tethering
- perineural and neural tethering and irritation.

Surgical protocol

Patients were consented for a staged procedure consisting of:

- Spinal probing and discography at suspected levels approached on the side of maximal symptoms.
- ELF consisting of exploration of extraforaminal, foraminal, and epidural zones with flexible endoscopic intradiscal discectomy, neurolysis, undercutting of facets, and osteophytectomy as required. However, the final decision for the second stage (EFL) was made only after spinal probing and discography had reproduced the pain of type, intensity, and distribution described as that which the patient experienced normally.
- Where symptom reproduction was imperfect then a differential discogram was performed with the instillation of 2 ml of methylprednisolone at the presumed level. If postoperative observation revealed a reduction of symptoms for 5–10 days, then those affected symptoms could be expected to be modified by ELF at that level.

Spinal probing differs from discography in that it relies on specific probing of the anterior margin of the facet joint, perineural structures, and the disc wall at several points. The essential and distinctive step in viviprudence is, therefore, spinal probing and differential discography. Discography defines the distribution of degeneration within the disc and the acceptance volume, and the presence of annular leaks. If discography on a contained disc produces radicular pain, then this further endorses that that disc is the index level for the compressive pain. Similarly, if a leak reproduces the patient's compressive or noncompressive pain then this identifies the targeted disc as a contributor to that evoked pain. Where probing evokes pain then subsequent endo-

scopic aware state examination confirms these structures to be sources of pain. Endoscopy demonstrates the contribution to the pain arising from inflamed disc, disc pad, and foraminal structures.

Operative technique

Neurolept (aware-state) analgesia was performed using 0.03 mg/kg Hypnoval bolus at the onset of the operation, 2–5 µg/kg fentanyl and 30–70 µg/kg droperidol. Patient feedback is essential in these cases where the presence of perineural scarring is often unexpectedly dense and masks the neural structures. A bolus dose of 1.5 g cefuroxime was given at the onset of operation. The skin and subcutis was infiltrated with local anaesthetic (xylocaine 0.25% 0.75–1.5 mg/kg) with 1 : 200 000 adrenaline.

Push-up test

The push-up test consisted of extending the arms, hyperextending the lumbar spine while encouraging the abdomen to sag in the prone position on the operating table before surgery. If this manoeuvre evoked the patient's leg or back pain before surgery, then clearance of the pain at the end of the procedure denoted sufficient clearance of the cause of the pain and a positive push-up test.

Lasing technique

The probe is replaced with a guide wire and, under biplanar radiographic control, a 4.6-mm dilator tube is railroaded to the exit root foramen. During the entire procedure an image intensifier is used at intervals to ensure the correct position of the endoscope and the laser probe. The trocar is removed and a Richard Wolf endoscope with an eccentrically placed 2.5-mm working channel and two irrigation channels inserted. A side-firing 2.1-mm diameter laser probe with internal irrigation is inserted through the endoscope. The extraforaminal zone and margin of the foramen are cleared. The ascending and descending facet joint surfaces are then excavated and undercut to allow admission of the endoscope beyond the isthmus of the foramen into the epidural space. Vertebral body and facet joint osteophytes, ligamentum flavum and superior foraminal ligament, perineural and epidural scarring are ablated and the facet joint undercut until the annulus and epidural space are displayed.

The exiting and transiting nerve roots are mobilized and decompressed medially and laterally until the functional axilla of the root at the apex of the safe working zone are displayed.

The nerve is cleared of perineural fibrosis. The bone margin of the superior notch and the superior foraminal ligament are then addressed. Osteophytes along the ascending facet joint and in the superior notch, dorsum of the vertebral margin and the vertebral shoulder (shoulder osteophytes) are ablated under endoscopic vision. In the presence of a disc protrusion in the epidural or foraminal zone, disc degeneration, annular collection or leaks, the disc is entered and cleared by laser ablation and manual punches.

Anatomy and pathology

Experience of over 775 endoscopic laser foraminoplasties and 173 flexible endoscopic intradiscal discectomies has taught us that new pathological entities lie in the foramen and extraforaminal regions (Figures 3.2.1, 3.2.2) including:

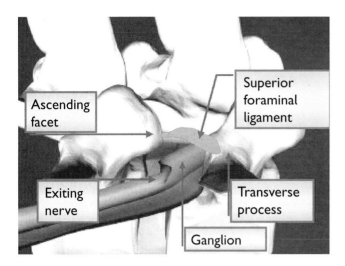

Figure 3.2.1 Foraminal anatomy and superior foraminal ligament and the impacting ascending facet joint margin deforming the nerve and ganglion.

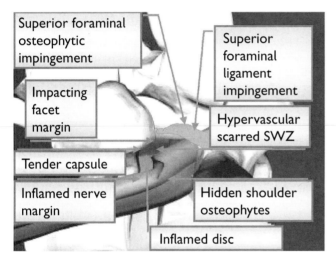

Figure 3.2.2 Some of the foraminal pathologies demonstrated by endoscopic aware state evaluation of the foramen via the posterolateral approach.

- superior foraminal ligament impingement
- superior notch osteophytosis
- dorsal and shoulder osteophytes
- facet joint impaction
- facet joint cysts
- pars interarticularis tethering
- safe working zone and notch engorgement
- ligamentum flavum infolding
- disc pad
- posterior longitudinal ligament irritation
- intertransverse ligament and muscle entrapment
- inferior external pedicular tethering
- annulus

- annular tears
- shoulder osteophytes
- lateral osteophytosis
- paravertebral bone graft tethering
- post fusion discitis
- instrumentation neural tethering
- perineural and neural tethering and irritation.

Superior foraminal ligament impingement

The superior foraminal ligament passes from the ascending facet to the base of the transverse process. As settlement occurs so this ligament bears down on the exiting nerve, which may become tethered, causing local hyperaemia and irritation of the nerve at that point. This irritation is further aggravated by calcification of the ligament. The ligament is often found adherent to the nerve and the nerve inflamed and tender at that point. While normal radicular symptoms may be elicited from quiescent sections of the same nerve, the inflamed nerve may produce atypical dysaesthesiae.

Superior notch osteophytosis

As the superior foraminal ligament is resected so superior notch osteophytes may be displayed in the superior notch adherent to the exiting nerve and producing local inflammation. These osteophytes arise from the superior facet joint margin.

Dorsal and shoulder osteophytes

Osteophytes are covered by a soft tissue cap which increases their compressive effect on adjacent tissues. This effect is worsened by tethering between the osteophyte fibrous cap and the nerve, posterior longitudinal ligament or dura. Shoulder osteophytes can be found as a peripheral extension of dorsal osteophytes or as individual entities. Usually the dorsal osteophyte arises usually from the upper vertebral body margin and produces midline or medial foraminal tethering and inflammation and displacement of the nerve pathway. This tethering or displacement is especially noticeable during flexion. Shoulder osteophytes may also occur on the superior or inferior vertebral margin in the foramen or lateral foramen lying anterior to the nerve and tethering same. These are often hidden from view unless an active search is made on the medial or anterior (deep) surface of the nerve. These appear to lie in the pathway of the abutting impacting ascending facet joint and may indeed arise as a consequence of such impaction. The endoscopy cannula can be used to mobilize and retract the nerve while it is separated from the fibrous cap of the osteophyte and subsequently ablated.

Facet joint impaction

Facet joint impaction arises from the ascending facet joint impacting on the exiting nerve root or the tissues in the safe working zone. The consistent presence of tissues tethering the nerve to the facet margin increases the effect of the impaction as and when disc degeneration leads to overriding of the facet joints during settlement and displacement. The effect is worsened as retrolisthesis and anterior listhesis occurs. Tethering between the facet joint needs to be resected and the facet joint needs to be undercut to remove the dynamic impaction. Such dynamic impaction may be the mechanism underlying many instances of so-called 'instability'.

Facet joint cysts

These can cause compression on exiting and traversing nerves and can increase in size during activity and can be marsupialized after the foraminal isthmus has been enlarged and traversed.

Pars interarticularis tethering

Pars interarticularis defects cause tethering to traversing and exiting nerve roots. The tethering to the fibrous defect and to the bone of the anterior pars fracture site can be resected and the nerve root mobilized and decompressed. In the presence of anterior displacement the disc wall is deformed and causes dorsal displacement of the traversing nerve roots; often in addition a knuckle of disc wall displaces into the foramen, further compromising the exiting nerve root. Each of these elements can be resected under vision with amelioration of symptoms without fusion.

Safe working zone and notch engorgement

Hypervascular tissue consisting of scar, hypervascular veins, and arterioles can be found in the superior and inferior notch and in the safe working zone. This can become engorged, producing stenotic and claudicant symptoms, and may itself be directly tender when inflamed.

Ligamentum flavum infolding

The ligamentum flavum infolds as disc height is reduced. The infolding crowds the exiting nerve root in the superior notch and in the inferior notch if the nerve is displaced. On occasions the ligamentum flavum may be found to blend with the posterior disc pad and posterior longitudinal ligament. Resection of the ligamentum flavum at these sites serves to decompress the exiting and traversing nerve roots and mobilize same from local tethering. The procedure should be combined with anterior mobilization of the nerve at the index level to achieve full mobilization.

The ligamentum flavum may blend with the posterior foraminal ligament which passes from the superior notch, blends with the capsule, and extends to the inferior notch but of itself does not appear to cause compression.

Disc pad

On the posterior aspect of the disc, a pad of tissue may be found which is thick and contains inflammatory blood vessels and nerves which may be locally tender, in contradistinction to the annulus itself which if not injected is often pain-free to probing. Removal may produce immediate relief of local back pain. This may occur in the absence of a posterior collection of dye in the annulus, or a leak, but is more commonly found in association with them.

Posterior longitudinal ligament irritation

The posterior longitudinal ligament may be inflamed and locally tender but is usually found in this state when adjacent tissues such as the disc are inflamed. Local neurolysis and ablation of adjacent inflamed tissues can resolve the inflammation. Probing of the inflamed posterior longitudinal ligament will produce pain arising in territories normally expected to be subtended by both the index and adjacent levels.

Intertransverse ligament and muscle entrapment

The intertransverse ligament and muscle pass on the lateral aspect of the exiting nerve. In the degenerate state the nerve may be tethered on the lateral aspect to the intertransverse ligament and muscle, causing local inflammation. Alternatively, degenerative loss of disc height may lead to crowding of the exiting nerve by the intertransversus muscle and ligament, so preventing the exiting nerve from escaping the impacting ascending facet. Endoscopic neurolysis and division of the ligament and muscle relieves lateral constraint and assists access and mobilization of the nerve root.

Inferior external pedicular tethering

The exiting nerve may be tethered to the external surface of the inferior pedicle especially following previous surgery and prior posterolateral bone grafted fusion. Local endoscopic neurolysis is valuable in mobilizing the nerve root from the pedicle and combined with resection of dorsally placed hypertrophic tethering bone graft.

Annulus

The annulus may be extruded or protruding into the foramen, lateral foraminal zone, or epidural posterolateral or central zones. Discectomy or resection of the central or posterolateral bulging disc may be appropriate and concur with expected clinical findings. However, protrusions in the lateral foramen may impact on the exiting nerve and produce unexpected clinical signs. The disc protrusion in this area may be surprisingly small, even imperceptible on the MR scan, and yet produce significant impact on the nerve, especially where the nerve is tethered to the disc wall.

In situations of degenerate disc height loss, the wall of the disc may be playing only a limited role in the pathogenesis of symptoms and under these circumstances the wall of the disc may be shrunk thermoplastically with the laser, rather than removing and further damaging the degenerate remnants of the disc.

In 68% of cases, intradiscal clearance may be performed without pain. This indicates that in these cases the inosculation of blood vessels and nerves into the annulus had either not been contributory to the symptom complex or was not extensive.

Annular tears

The annulus may be the site of intradiscal tears which may breach the annulus either under the posterior longitudinal ligament (subligamentous) or through it (transligamentous), occasioning symptoms according to the point of liberation of breakdown products. The most symptomatic are those ejecting breakdown products directly on to the nerve in the foramen. Their effect is amplified where the nerve is tethered adjacent to the exit portal of the tear. The reaction to the leakage may be to lay down perineural scarring causing adherence of the nerve to the disc, thus impeding movement of the nerve away from the point of leakage during flexion or rotation. The fibrous response may cause encapsulation of the leakage, resulting in containment and concentration of the breakdown products around the nerve. These effects worsen the symptoms and are found in patients with long-lasting preoperative symptoms.

Clearance of the perineural scarring and mobilization of the nerve should be complemented by opening of the radial tear orifice and removal of debris often holding the tear open. The course of the tear is often serpiginous, so the route of the tear cannot be fully explored. It is recommended that the nucleus be explored and that degenerate material be removed manually and by laser ablation. The wall of the disc is then treated by thermoplastic annealing.

Lateral osteophytosis

Lateral osteophytes displace the exiting nerve root dorsally and into the inferior notch, amplifying compression by the redundant annulus at that point. In addition, the lateral osteophytes cause displacement of the nerve in to the middle section of the foramen, thus placing it in the path of the impacting facet joint. Partial resection of the osteophytes where they displace the nerve is valuable as part of general undercutting and enlargement of the foramen.

Paravertebral bone graft tethering

After instrumented or non-instrumented fusion, paravertebral bone graft causes anterior tethering to exiting nerve roots with profound entrapment often in the presence of a secure and technically correct fusion. Wide neurolysis on the anterior surface of the graft results in nerve root mobilization and resolution of symptoms resulting from tethering from such extraforaminal entrapment.

Postfusion and aseptic discitis

Postfusion and aseptic discitis manifest as a highly inflamed and tender annulus which can be relieved by manual and laser discectomy under endoscopic control. If clinical evidence of infection exists then a fine cannula can be placed intradiscally to insert antibiotics until intravenous conversion is achieved. However, in cases of aseptic discitis, removal of the inflamed disc contents serves to reduce the back pain significantly, with subsequent resolution after short time.

Instrumentation and neural tethering

Pedicle screw instrumentation can produce neural tethering either by direct impingement of the metal work or by tethering of the nerve to misplaced metalwork or microfractures of adjacent pedicles. When identified, the former should be treated by endoscopic mobilization of the nerve and removal of the metalwork and the latter should be treated by mobilization of the nerve only.

Perineural tethering and nerve irritation

Perineural tethering may arise as a consequence of direct irritation from a disc protrusion or facet joint impaction or the release of breakdown products. The nerve may be reddened because it is entrapped by an impacting facet joint, osteophytes, and inflamed engorged hypervascular tissues in the notch. The inflammation may be aggravated by displacement of the nerve by scarring, lateral small knuckles of disc protrusion, and shoulder osteophytes. The nerve may be found adjacent to annular tears which cause inflammation by direct release of intradiscal breakdown products on to the nerve.

The exiting or traversing nerve root will produce normal radicular signs with compression. However, the irritated reddened nerve will often produce dysaesthesiae of unexpected distribution. Interestingly, adjacent sections of the nerve not irritated produce symptoms in expected territories. This may explain the cause of persistent symptoms after conventional surgery using conventional guidelines rather than the results of aware-state feedback which may indicate that the nerve is being irritated at an adjacent and unexpected level.

Outcome of endoscopic laser foraminoplasty

The results of ELF[1] indicate that this technique provides a minimalist means of exploring the extraforaminal zone, the foramen, and the epidural space, and performing discectomy, osteophytectomy, and perineural neurolysis with encouraging results. It incorporates the prophylactic advantage of foraminal undercutting and provides a promising means of identifying and treating the pain of 'failed back surgery' and back pain and sciatica of indeterminate origin and patients with 'instability'. Done in the aware state, ELF serves to identify and localize the source of pain generation at the time of surgery and the relevance of these findings. It avoids the morbidity associated with open spinal surgery and serves as a useful means of effecting 'keyhole' neurolysis without extensive exploration and fusion. Current improvements in equipment promise wider application and more encouraging results in the future.

Discussion

Instability is not a diagnosis but merely a mechanism, the treatment of which requires an understanding of the effects that such micromovement has upon adjacent tissues and structures. This micromovement becomes in effect microtrauma and as such produces inflammation and irritation in these adjacent structures, with consequent symptoms.

The posterolateral approach conducted in the aware state, with the additional benefit of endoscopic evaluation, has confirmed that the foramen and extraforaminal zone is the source of hitherto unknown causes of pain, parasthesiae, and neurological deficit. In the foramen the facet joint is consistently found to be tethered to the nerve and may be tethered to the disc. When there is partial settlement or listhesis, micromovements occur which result in abnormal movements and particular impaction between the facet joint and the nerve or bulging disc. This causes irritation and sensitization of nerve receptors and evoked pain. This nerve compromise arises at the foramen as nerve leaves the spinal canal; the pain distribution matches that normally attributed to segmental disease at the level above. This leads to misdiagnosis and incorrect indications for surgery.

Other features of the foraminal construct provide unfamiliar causes of symptoms. The superior foraminal ligament may contain small osteophytes. Either individually or in combination the superior foraminal ligament or the contained osteophytes may impinge upon the exiting nerve root. This is often seen as reddening at the point of impact. Again, the guillotining action of these structures is aggravated by settlement or short pedicles.

The nerve may be tethered directly to the disc, which, if inflamed or focally weak at the point of tethering, will be distorted and irritated causing pain in the exiting or occasionally the transiting nerve. Again this would be attributed to the superior adjacent disc level, especially as the MR scan will not demonstrate small areas of focal annular weakness nor tethering to the disc.

After prior surgery or trauma, or in the case of settlement or facet joint hypertrophy, the nerve may be displaced medially or occasionally displaced superiorly and laterally. The displacement is then held by perineural scarring. Under these circumstances the nerve cannot deploy normally into the superior or inferior notches during flexion, extension, and rotation and is vulnerable to impact from the facet joint, focally distorted or broad-based bulging disc, or a combination of the two.

Shoulder osteophytes occurring on the shoulder of the vertebral rim lie anterior to the exiting nerve and usually arise from the superior vertebral margin in the plane of the impacting facet. They result in tethering of the exiting nerve, and local irritation and marked sensitivity. This can occur even in the presence of a successful fusion or conventional decompression and may account for persistent symptoms following technically satisfactory surgery and contribute to the 'failed back surgery' syndrome.

Conventional discectomy, decompression or fusion, and height restoration fail to treat, for instance, the nerve tethered to the disc wall or the superior notch and superior foraminal ligament tethering and indeed may aggravate it. Endoscopy would determine the presence of such pathology and specifically treat it without the need for extensive surgery such as a fusion.

Tears and leaks are a common source of elusive pain. The distribution of pain depends upon the direction of the leak and its containment around the exiting or transiting nerve or dispersal along and around the posterior longitudinal ligament. Lumbar leakage may produce global dysthaesthesia, urinary irritation, partial weakness, partial numbness, disproportionate back, buttock, or leg pain individually or in any combination.

These clinical examinations indicate that in cases of non-compressive radiculopathy or mild compressive radiculopathy the textbook guidelines to the source of the pain may be seriously misleading. Elusive back pain and referred pain may arise from a variety of sources which may be difficult to determine from clinical examination, X-rays, and scans alone. Spinal probing and endoscopy, however, do provide a reliable method of identifying pain sources and treating these specifically, accurately, and discretely.

The conventional diagnostician favours an axial diagnosis or a facet joint arthropathy, but ignores the adjacent level foramen and may therefore be addressing the wrong level. In our experience facet joint injections may be misleading because the steroid injection, rather than affecting the joint itself, is in fact influencing the pathology in the foramen on the anterior aspect of the joint.

The failures of conventional treatment may often arise because the pathology is not in or around the midline or epidural space, but surprisingly commonly affecting the same nerve as it exits the subjacent foramen.

We pay lip service to the fact that conventional surgery may fail because the incorrect level has been addressed. In fact it may not just be the wrong level but the wrong structure at that level that has been addressed. Acknowledging the prerequisite to address the correct level, surgeons seem peculiarly reluctant to the pain site accurately before proceeding to intervention. Aware-state surgery and endoscopy provide an ideal solution to identifying the level and the aetiopathology.

The inexplicably elevated severity or persistence of symptoms should not be classed as 'illness behaviour' but rather should spark a quest to further identify the remaining pain source and treat this specifically. After all, after effective hip or knee replacement in patients with long-term pain, surgeons do not need to resort to concepts of 'memory pain', 'centrally perpetuated pain', 'coping courses', or 'psychiatric support', because the source of the pain has been effectively eradicated.

Aware-state surgery offers us the opportunity to learn more about the mechanisms of pain arising in the back and neck and referred pain, and to address these by conservative rehabilitation or minimalist surgical intervention. It has already shown us that there are many extremely sensitive pain sources hitherto unappreciated in and about the foramen. I consider that this technique allows us to step forward from diagnostic guesstimating to precise definition of pain sources and devise specific discrete conservative or minimalist treatment.

References

1 Knight, M. T. N., Goswami, A. K. D., Patko, J. Endoscopic laser foraminoplasty and aware state surgery: a treatment concept and outcome analysis. *Die Arthroscopie*, 1999, **2**, 1–12.

3.3 Regional somatic dysfunction

Michael L. Kuchera

Expertise in the field of neuromusculoskeletal medicine provides unique insights into the performance of a physical examination and the formulation of a differential diagnosis. It presupposes extensive, specific knowledge of the regional and systemic structure (anatomy) and function (physiology and kinesiology), integrated with a comprehensive understanding of the patient as a unique individual. It necessitates highly practiced palpatory skills with the ability to diagnose somatic dysfunction and competence in delivering therapeutic modalities to effectively rectify dysfunctions affecting skeletal, arthrodial, and/or myofascial structures. It requires the perspective of a broadly trained physician to perform the examinations needed to establish a differential diagnosis and to fully weigh the indications, contraindication, and risk-to-benefit ratios of different treatment approaches. At all times, it is tempered by the distinctive patient–physician relationship incorporating the art and compassion of the health care professional with an understanding of biopsychosocial, biomechanical, orthopedic, biophysiological, and neurological models of care.

The knowledge, skill, training, and art of the manual medicine physician are then focused through a unifying model, philosophy, or perspective in a safe, time-efficient, and cost-effective manner. Current practitioners of neuromusculoskeletal medicine may practice under a variety of titles denoting their approach to this field. Some are specialists with certification or other recognition in disciplines termed 'physical medicine and rehabilitation', 'musculoskeletal medicine', 'osteopathic manipulative medicine', 'neuromusculoskeletal medicine', or 'orthopaedic medicine'. The American schools of osteopathic medicine integrate this perspective and core manual medicine skills into the pre-doctoral education of all physicians in training, regardless of their eventual specialty. Other physicians obtain core postgraduate training in manual medicine skills and add these skills to an evolving perspective gained through reading and professional interactions with colleagues in one or more of these disciplines.

Although a specialty or school of training may emphasize a different component of the whole neuromusculoskeletal medicine field or even a different explanatory model, each recognizes the value of:

- diagnostic screening, regional, and local palpatory examinations to identify somatic dysfunction and neuromusculoskeletal pathophysiology
- safe and effective treatment skills including the ability to select and deliver any of a core of manual medicine techniques used in modifying the neuromusculoskeletal system
- a patient-centered approach requiring an individualized neuromusculoskeletal prescription.

In the USA, independent studies of patients receiving workman's compensation in several different states compared the cost of management of different musculoskeletal complaints by different types of health care practitioners (see Figure 2.2.17 in Chapter 2.2.1). These studies included musculoskeletal problems in each anatomic region and care for each provided by surgical MDs and doctors of osteopathy (DOs), nonsurgical MDs and DOs, chiropractors, and physical therapists. Of all practitioners included in this review, only the US-trained DO has an educational combination of core training in manual medicine techniques, unifying philosophy emphasizing the neuromusculoskeletal system, and complete medical training paralleling that of the international musculoskeletal medicine physician. Nonsurgical osteopathic physicians with this educational background were the most cost-effective in every anatomic region.[1] Such studies suggest that physicians with core training in manual techniques and a unifying philosophic approach to neuromusculoskeletal problems will be more cost-effective than nonphysicians employing manual approaches alone. These studies may also suggest the value of a manual medicine education of physicians without such core training to promote cost-effective patient management. Further controlled cost-efficacy studies are warranted.

Applying concepts of somatic dysfunction to regional disorders

This chapter develops the clinical importance of somatic dysfunction in various regions of the body, and approaches for recognizing it.

Somatic dysfunction is an umbrella term embracing impaired or altered function of related components of the somatic system (body framework): skeletal, arthrodial, and myofascial structures, and related vascular, lymphatic, and neural elements.[2,3] Concepts of somatic dysfunction are fully discussed in Chapter 2.2.1, and an understanding of those concepts is essential to the clinical value of this chapter.

In keeping with values previously outlined, this chapter describes screening, regional, and local palpatory examinations for somatic dysfunction, as well as those patient-centered variables that play a role in individualizing the manual medicine prescription.[4–6] For each region, one or more common clinical condition in which somatic dysfunction plays a major role has been chosen to illustrate the application of these values. Specific treatment of somatic dysfunction in various regions, using manual medicine techniques, is more fully discussed in Chapter 4.3.1.

Screening, regional, and local examinations for somatic dysfunction

A palpatory examination for somatic dysfunction is an integral part of the physical examination in this field of medicine. This examination should not be conducted in isolation, nor tacked on as an afterthought. It is individually designed to evaluate various aspects of the neuromusculoskeletal system on the basis of a careful history and other findings in the general physical examination. In moving toward the differential diagnosis of a patient's complaint, the physician's understanding of pathophysiology, pain generators, referred and reflex pain mechanisms, and the interconnectedness of function and structure direct the site and extent of an appropriate palpatory examination.

Time-efficient examination for somatic dysfunction is best performed in stages, culminating in a final site-specific definition based on the S.T.A.R characteristics (sensory changes, tissue texture abnormality, asymmetry, and restriction of motion; see Chapter 2.2.1).[7,8] Within each stage of the examination, any number of specific tests may be integrated, their specific order being related to the manual medicine model adopted and to the experience and preference of the examining physician.

A multistage examination for somatic dysfunction usually progresses from **screening** the patient for initial general impressions, to intermediate **scanning** of body regions identified by the screening process. The scanning process, in turn, identifies specific regions, joints, or tissues to be targeted for the more detailed **local examination** used in differential diagnosis and appropriate for designing an individualized neuromusculoskeletal prescription. Although certain principles apply, each examination is different and evolves from the progressive integration of discovered historical and physical findings unique to the patient being examined. Rarely, if ever, will a physician include all test procedures outlined in this chapter in a single examination.

Neuromusculoskeletal screening, scanning, and local examinations incorporate palpatory test choices according to the musculoskeletal model selected and lead to a peer-accepted standard of care.[9–15] Identification of structure or function that deviates from normal at each level of palpatory evaluation invites a differential diagnosis and leads either to further specific testing of that site or to the expansion of testing to other related structures. Findings may eventually warrant additional neurologic or orthopedic tests or even laboratory, radiographic, and/or electrophysiologic testing to fully establish a differential diagnosis and to safely and effectively reach an appropriate, individualized manual medicine prescription.

Screening examinations

According to Greenman,[16] a relevant screening examination answers the question, 'Is there a problem within the musculoskeletal system that deserves additional evaluation?' Screening examinations of the neuromusculoskeletal system often include observation of general appearance, including general health status, presence of systemic disorders, and structural stressors apparent to observation; posture; gross movements, and gait. General health status, systemic disorders, and structural stressors significantly affect the progression and form of the examination for somatic dysfunction. Screening for these factors also influences the subsequent intent, type, extent, and prognosis expected from treatment of the patient with musculoskeletal medicine techniques. General appearance provides clues to general health status and the possibility of certain systemic diseases.

- In particular, examination of hair, skin, and nails with respect to tissue texture abnormalities may uncover clues to underlying tissue health. Hair texture and distribution often provide clues to metabolic or endocrine disorders, and a number of rheumatologic disorders also present with clues in ectodermal tissues. From a rheumatologic perspective alone, the neuromusculoskeletal physician should especially note alopecia, nail pitting or ridging, skin ulcers, psoriasis, photosensitivity, purpura, malar rash, Raynaud's phenomenon, or tightening of the skin.[17] Skin turgor in patients who abuse nicotine is quite distinctive, empirically suggests poor connective tissue health,[18] and prognosticates a lesser response to otherwise successful strategies for re-establishing neuromusculoskeletal health.

- The patient's general appearance may also suggest certain biomechanical stressors. For example, various types of obesity and pregnancy each alter the distribution of weight with respect to the center of gravity. Likewise, the presence of a foot with an elongated second ray (Dudley J. Morton foot) is capable of altering the biomechanics of gait. Postural observation provides significant insight into patterns of somatic dysfunction and the inherent capability of that individual to compensate to gravitational stress and strain.

Various other external signs provide clues to systemic disease with associated musculoskeletal ramifications as well as underlying skeletal abnormalities and biomechanical disadvantages. Each can be recognized by careful observation of the patient's appearance.

Generalized postural analysis provides screening information about joints, muscles, and supportive connective tissues subjected to biomechanical stress. Clinically, this is correlated with the discovery of recurrent patterns of somatic dysfunction and myofascial trigger points (TrPs).[19] Posture must be examined in the three cardinal planes (Figure 3.3.1) for rotoscoliotic as well as accentuated or flattened sagittal plane curves. Static postural analysis also provides an opportunity to palpate and assess symmetry of paired anatomic landmarks including mastoid processes, acromion processes, inferior angles of the scapulae, iliac crests, posterior superior iliac spines, and greater trochanters of the femur (Figure 3.3.2). The presence of aberrant postural alignment may direct a scanning examination of the junctional areas of the spine and postural crossover sites or a local examination of specifically stressed ligaments and muscles.[20] These characteristic sites are well documented[21–23] and are discussed with relevance to each region later in this chapter.

Detailed observation of impaired or altered gross movements offers significant insight into the location and tissue type of an underlying somatic dysfunction.

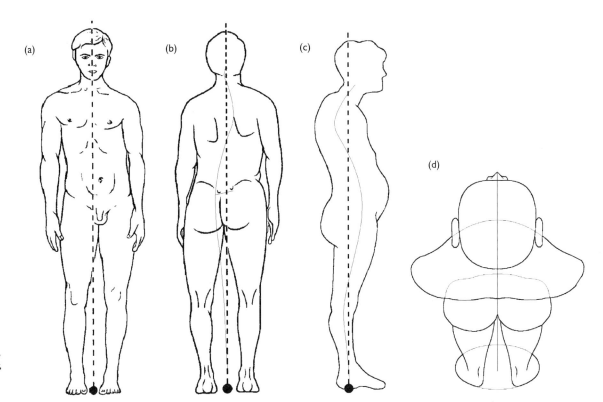

Figure 3.3.1
Observing posture:
(a) anteroposterior,
(b) posteroanterior,
(c) lateral,
(d) cephalocaudad.

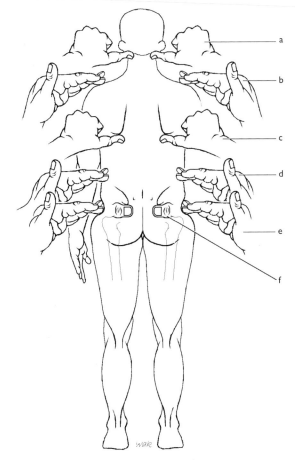

Figure 3.3.2 Posterior horizontal planes: (a) mastoid processes,
(b) acromion processes, (c) inferior angles of the scapulae, (d) iliac crests,
(e) greater trochanters of the femur, (f) posterior superior iliac spines.

● Gross spinal motion observation easily screens total range of motion of the cervical, thoracic, and lumbar regions in flexion, extension, sidebending, and rotation (Figure 3.3.3). It becomes even more informative if, at the end of active regional motion observation, the physician gently continues the passive motion in the direction of the test. This scans for restriction of motion in that particular region and for possible etiologies for the restriction by evaluating and assessing the characteristic quality of the restrictive barrier.

● Comparing side-to-side symmetry during a full respiratory cycle and gently palpating over the anterior upper chest and anterolateral lower rib cage may screen gross motion of the chest cage. In particular, observation of passive respiration provides insight into diaphragmatic and thoracic cage function. Normally, passive inhalation by a supine patient creates visible movement all the way down to the pubic region.

● Fully raising both upper extremities from the anatomic position in the coronal plane and turning the backs of the hands together quickly provides functional motion screening of the upper extremities (especially the shoulder girdle) (Figure 3.3.3).

● Seated and standing flexion tests constitute one style of pelvic screening examination (Figure 3.3.4). Asymmetrical motion during either flexion test indicates dysfunction localized to one side of the body. Comparison of the two tests can assist in determining whether major restrictors involve the pelvic structures or whether function is affected by structures below the pelvis. Test interpretation will be discussed in the pelvic region of this chapter.

● Examination of the lower extremities often includes both a modification of Patrick's FABERE test (Figure 3.3.5) screening for hip or sacroiliac dysfunction/pathology as well as an active deep knee-bend squatting test with heels maintained on the floor

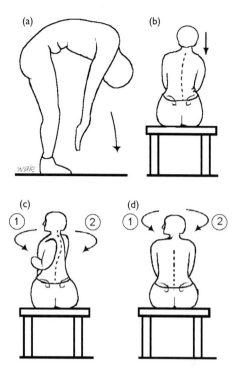

Figure 3.3.3 Active spinal motion testing: (a) flexion, (b) sidebending, (c) thoracolumbar rotation, (d) cervical rotation.

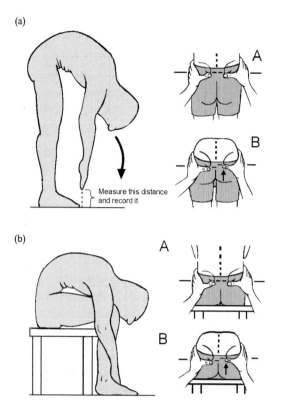

Figure 3.3.4 (a) Standing and (b) seated flexion tests. Each is noted to be positive on the side that moves the farthest or continues to move after the opposite side has stopped.

(Figure 3.3.6) which screens for strength and mobility of hips, knees, ankle, and feet bilaterally.

Any asymmetry or gross restriction of motion in any of these screening tests warrants further study, including more detailed evaluation for regional or local somatic dysfunction.

Beyond recognizing pathologic gaits, the gait analysis portion of the musculoskeletal screening examination provides information about the presence and impact of underlying somatic dysfunction. Gait analysis should assess length, pattern, and symmetry of stride, arm swing, heel strike, toe off, tilting of the pelvis, and shoulder compensatory movements. Additional clues may be obtained by observing the wear patterns of the patient's shoes. Somatic dysfunction is capable of significantly altering the pattern of gait and, over time, may modify central programming enough to maintain the abnormal gait even though there has been a correction or resolution of the somatic dysfunction. Conversely, an improper biomechanical gait, structural change (such as a Dudley J. Morton foot), or anatomically asymmetrical lower extremities will require compensation throughout the body unit. Each subsequently creates recurrent patterns of somatic dysfunction. As the patient walks for you, observe gait for forward head position, a straight lumbar spine, decreased hip flexion during single support phase, flexed knee in midstance, failure of heel lift, and visible foot pronation during the single support phase. Each of these compensatory motions is a screening **gait marker**[24] whose presence warrants further examination.

Those who teach neuromusculoskeletal medicine diagnosis incorporate the above elements in most screening examinations, regardless of the model employed. Their pupils may be taught to approach these elements in a specific order as in standardized '10-step' or '12-step' examinations. This is not so much a requirement as a way of minimizing the number of positional changes made by the patient and pre-

venting the inadvertent omission of one or more of the screening elements. Taught and performed in sequence, most screening examinations are, in fact, quick and efficient diagnostic tools to identify where to look next for neuromusculoskeletal clues, including somatic dysfunction.[25] Nonetheless, the guiding principle that must be addressed in its entirety is the original question, 'Is there a problem within the musculoskeletal system that deserves additional evaluation?' Thus, testing sequence, time needed for the examination, and stated preference of specific tests by teachers of various schools, models, or disciplines are all less important to the neuromusculoskeletal medicine practitioner than answering this question and proceeding to the next diagnostic level.

Somatic dysfunction regional scanning and local examinations: overview

The definition of a **scanning examination** is 'an intermediate detailed examination of specific body regions which have been identified by findings emerging from the initial screen; the scan (for somatic dysfunction) focuses on segmental areas for further definition or diagnosis'.[2] According to Greenman,[26] a scanning examination simply answers the questions, 'What part of the region and what tissues within the region may be significantly dysfunctional?'

All neuromusculoskeletal scanning examinations will seek to identify one or more of the S.T.A.R. findings in the region. Combinations of these findings constitute the objective diagnostic criteria for local or regional somatic dysfunction, but, in isolation, may alert the astute clinician to also evaluate for the presence or absence of other underlying pathophysiologic diagnoses.

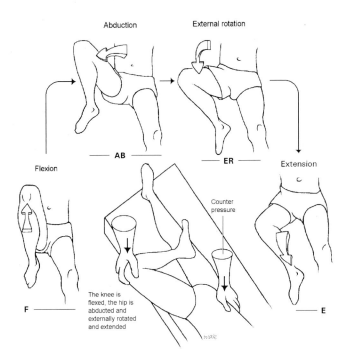

Figure 3.3.5 FABERE hip test with augmented external rotation to test sacroiliac structures.

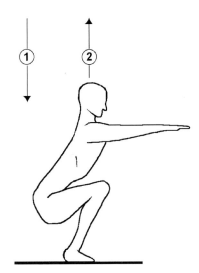

Figure 3.3.6 Squat test for screening flexion of joints of the lower extremity.

Directed by the screening and scanning examinations to significant tissue sites, local diagnostic testing for the remaining S.T.A.R. characteristics should be performed to gather the final information needed to formulate an individualized manual medicine prescription.

Most manual medicine clinicians initially scan regions with a quick survey of tissue texture characteristics (Figure 3.3.7). Typical scanning tests of tissue texture abnormalities include skin drag, red reflex induction, and skin rolling.

- To perform **skin drag** (Figure 3.3.7(a)), the fingers pass over the skin with varying degrees of pressure depending upon the information sought. The lightest pressure is used to sense minor variations in skin temperature or sweat gland activity. In the paraspinal regions, increased resistance to lightly dragging the pads of the fingers along the skin in a stroking fashion denotes relative cutaneous humidity; less resistance denotes dryness.

- Significant changes can also be visually monitored in the friction-induced **red reflex** pattern (Figure 3.3.7(b)) produced by heavier stroking with the finger pads. Positive skin drag testing is demonstrated by asymmetrical responses in temperature, sweat gland activity, hyperesthesia, drag or ease, and/or the reddening-blanching pattern of the skin.

- **Skin rolling** (Figure 3.3.7(c)) is another scanning tool commonly used in the neuromusculoskeletal examination to assess tissue texture abnormalities. A positive finding is the provocation of local tenderness and pain in a dermatomal distribution with tightness of the skin and loss of resiliency in the related subcutaneous structures. Small tender nodules may also be identified in or on the deeper fascia using this test. Generally touted as a scanning test, skin rolling can be very segmentally specific.[12]

Layer palpation involves increasing pressure over muscles, ligaments, vertebral processes, joint lines, or other clinically relevant structures in each region. It is yet another scanning tool for assessing

sensation and tissue texture abnormalities. A positive test involves palpable tissue texture abnormalities, subjective tenderness, and pain provocation over the local structure. Pressure on one site may also elicit a pain referral pattern consistent with that structure. In the case of muscle, contraction or inhibition are palpable reactions to pressure, providing clinically valuable information. In the spinal region, this test, applied to the supraspinal ligaments and over each transverse process, identifies vertebral units requiring further examination

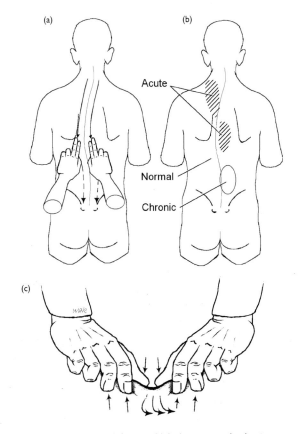

Figure 3.3.7 Scanning spinal regions. (a) Light paraspinal palpation, (b) red reflex, (c) skin rolling.

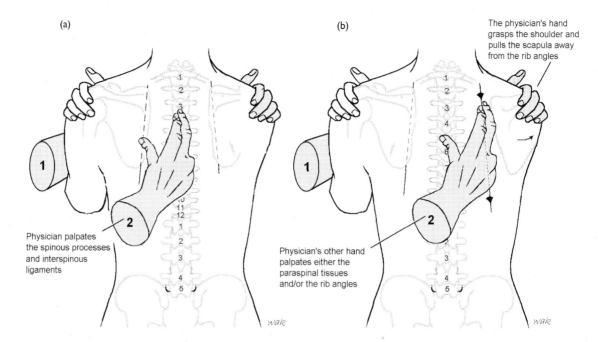

(a)

(b)

The physician's hand grasps the shoulder and pulls the scapula away from the rib angles

Physician palpates the spinous processes and interspinous ligaments

Physician's other hand palpates either the paraspinal tissues and/or the rib angles

Figure 3.3.8
(a) palpating spinal processes;
(b) paraspinal and rib angle palpation.

(Figure 3.3.8). Maigne[27] advocates use of a key instead of a finger to induce pressure over the supraspinal ligaments and therefore refers to this test as the 'key test' or 'key sign'. This is not to be confused with the 'key lesion' or 'key somatic dysfunction'[2] discussed extensively in the osteopathic literature.

Layer palpation is also effective in identifying various myofascial points. Three specific types of myofascial points merit specific mention: myofascial TrPs empirically mapped by Travell and Simons;[28,29] myofascial tender points used in Jones' system of strain–counterstrain;[30] and myofascial reflex points empirically mapped out by Chapman.[31]

● **Myofascial TrPs:** Scanning for TrPs involves adequate pressure in flat muscles and pincer grip in certain other muscles to look for the presence of tenderness and tissue texture changes, including a taut muscle band. The subject typically experiences exquisite tenderness that is most prominent over the TrP nodule found in this palpable taut band of muscle. Quickly drawing the finger across this site perpendicular to the taut band (a 'snapping palpation') typically elicits a local muscular twitch response. Pressure on an active TrP site typically elicits ('triggers') or exacerbates a distant pain pattern and occasionally provokes an autonomic response consistent for that muscular TrP. As with most palpatory findings, interexaminer reliability for TrPs is at its highest when there has been specific training and calibration of the examiners.[32] Kappa values (see Chapter 1.2) have been shown to vary from muscle to muscle, depending on a variety of factors including depth of the muscle palpated and experience of the palpating hand.[33,34]

● **Jones tender points:** These are located near bony attachments of tendons or ligaments, or in muscle bellies. They are also discovered through pressure over these sites. Palpably, they are described as small, tense, edematous, and locally tender areas. Unlike TrPs, they do not trigger pain to some distant site. Careful questioning, however, often uncovers the history of prolonged or awkward shortening of the muscle harboring the tender point. Simons[35] describes

a significant overlap in location between tender points and TrPs. Chaitow[36] also believes their distinction is arbitrary. Nonetheless, the empiric diagnostic and manual treatment system described by Jones is easily learned and applied.

● **Chapman reflex points:** A third myofascial point system of interest is attributed to Chapman.[37] These are correlated with reflex somatic change initiated by dysfunction of viscera.[38,39] These points have many of the same palpatory characteristics and tenderness as Jones points. Therefore, questioning and other physical examination to begin to differentiate between somatic and visceral underlying causes must follow finding a positive tender point in certain locations. Like Jones and Travell points, Chapman reflex point scanning employs pressure over empirically mapped points of the system. The anterior points in the Chapman system (Figure 3.3.9) are generally much more tender to palpation than posterior points and more likely to be used for viscerosomatic diagnosis than posterior points. Unlike Jones and Travell points, Chapman points are secondary forms of somatic dysfunction. Patients with Chapman points are less likely to present with primary musculoskeletal complaints and often present with visceral symptoms.

In all three systems, scanning palpation assesses sensation and tissue texture characteristics. Each system of myofascial points is well mapped out and a physician's knowledge of the common tender points for each speeds the diagnostic evaluation and eventual treatment. Differential scanning of a region for TrPs, tender points, and/or viscerosomatic reflex points follows largely from the screening clinical history, presenting complaints, and elicitable mechanism of injury or overuse (see Table 3.3.1, p. 181).

Alternatively, a myofascial tender point scan may be initiated because the screening examination revealed variations from ideal posture. Both Travell's and Jones' myofascial points have been associated with articular somatic dysfunction,[39,40] and their discovery in a scanning process therefore warrants further specific diagnosis. Chapman reflex points are referred from organ dysfunctions, and each

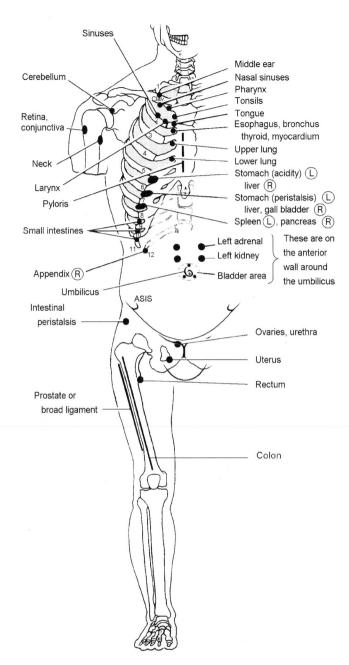

Figure 3.3.9 Anterior Chapman's points. All are bilateral except where indicated as R for right and L for left. (From Kuchera and Kuchera[41].)

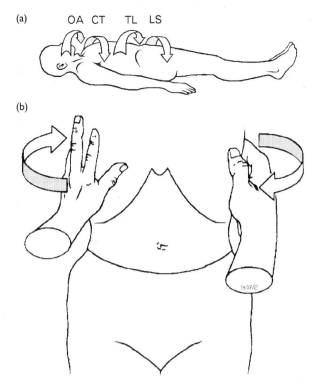

Figure 3.3.10 (a) Total body fascial pattern with common compensatory pattern depicted; (b) testing rotation of the fascias at the thoracolumbar region.

organ or group of organs has a differing but predictable pattern of associated articular and soft tissue dysfunction.[41] Conversely, both Jones tender points and Travell TrPs are specific diagnoses in themselves, constituting branch points for various therapeutic options where identified.

The analysis of the systems of myofascial points and articular dysfunction pioneered by various neuromusculoskeletal practitioners provides significant clinical insight, regardless of their underlying proposed origin. It reinforces the clinical utility of careful observation and palpation of the musculoskeletal system when looking for clues to differential diagnosis. Each system views the body as an interconnected unit with all parts and systems working together. Each expresses a common goal: the identification and treatment of somatic elements to

re-establish normal functional characteristics that promote beneficial changes in the body's homeostatic mechanisms.

Scanning for motion restriction can be quickly and efficiently applied to regions or specific segments. In screening transitional regions of the body (craniocervical junction, cervicothoracic junction, thoracolumbar junction, and lumbopelvic junction), the fascial tissues of each junctional region may be manually engaged (Figure 3.3.10). Each area is rotated and/or translated to the point where the tissues begin to tighten. Fascial drag and ease are noted. Asymmetrical motion characteristics in any region are considered a positive test result. Often the pattern of restriction from region to region provides as much insight into the underlying dysfunction as the individual regional restriction. Alternating fascial patterns are usually compensatory and may be relatively asymptomatic. Fascial patterns whose regional directions of restriction do not alternate from one transition zone to the next are said to be **noncompensated**, and are often traumatically induced and/or symptomatic.[42]

Alternating side-to-side pressures over vertebral transverse processes and/or alternating left–right translational pressures can also be used as a quick scan for segmental restriction of rotation and sidebending motion, respectively (Figure 3.3.11). A positive scan for vertebral somatic dysfunction reveals restriction in one direction and freedom of motion in the opposite direction. Zygopophyseal tenderness is often elicited on the restricted side.[43] Significant regional asymmetrical restriction or tenderness identified in this manner should be examined more completely on a local (segmental) basis.

Another scanning technique for either regional or segmental motion involves springing the test sites. Typically, the heel of the hand or a thumb is gently positioned, depending on the amount of area to

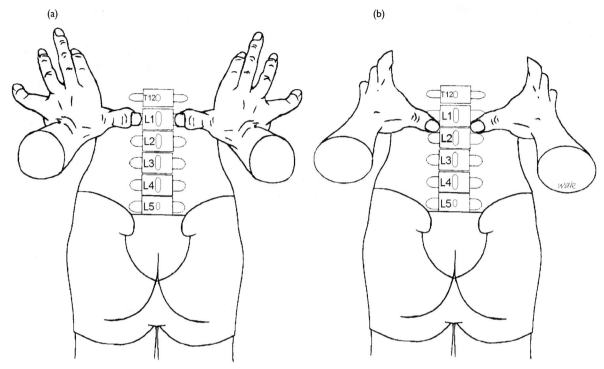

Figure 3.3.11 Scanning or local tests. (a) Testing L1 rotation; (b) testing L1 sidebending.

be tested. Gradual pressure is applied, compressing soft tissues that overly the deeper tissues being evaluated. A springing force is then gently applied seeking to assess the quality of the end-feel barrier. A positive **springing test** is recorded if the tissues have an abrupt rather than a physiologic resilient end-feel. This form of testing is commonly applied over ribs, vertebral spinous processes, poles of the sacrum, and ASIS (Figure 3.3.12). Comparing left to right side, a springing test may provide a **lateralization test** for naming dysfunction. In some manual medicine models, elicited pain rather than restricted motion constitutes a positive scan test for regional or segmental springing.

Common principles and methods govern clinically meaningful segmental examinations of the vertebral column. Because of the anatomic structure of typical vertebral segments and their articulations, segmental motion characteristics in each region of the spine follow certain general physiologic motion parameters.[44] Physiologic motion affecting the typical cervical segments C2–7 has been documented to involve coupled sidebending and rotation to the same side in all cervical positions. Conversely, physiologic motion in the thoracic and lumbar regions has been shown to depend upon sagittal plane position when the patient's motion occurred. Thoracic and lumbar sidebending and rotation occur to the same side when the vertebral unit facets are engaged, as in extreme forward or backward bending. In the 'easy neutral' positions between these two extremes, sidebending to one side in these regions automatically induces rotation to the opposite side.

In the thoracic and lumbar regions, where sagittal plane position modifies the pattern of coupled motion, two types of somatic dysfunction can be differentiated:

- **Type I somatic dysfunction** occurs when the patient is in the easy neutral position and sidebending and rotation occur to opposite sides, usually in groups.

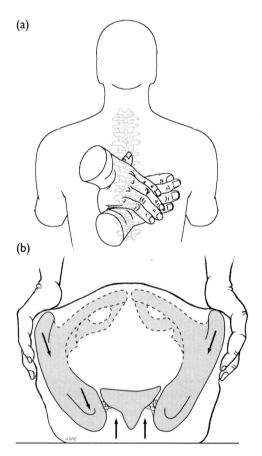

Figure 3.3.12 (a) Spinal compression for extension screening; (b) ASIS compression test. (Alternate left then right pressure into respective SI joint. Test is positive on the restricted side.)

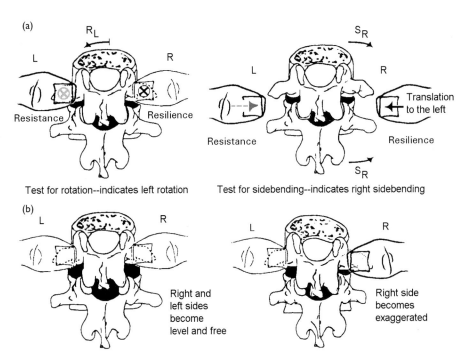

(a)

Test for rotation--indicates left rotation

Test for sidebending--indicates right sidebending

(b)

Right and left sides become level and free

Right side becomes exaggerated

F R$_R$S$_R$: Patient moves into flexion

F R$_R$S$_R$: Patient moves into extension

Figure 3.3.13 Testing for spinal motion: (a) passive testing, (b) active testing.

● In **type II somatic dysfunction**, occurring with significant flexion or extension, rotation and sidebending occur at a single segment and to the same side.

In all regions, somatic dysfunction occurring as restricted spinal motion within the physiologic range of motion will demonstrate the capability of moving further in the direction associated with initiation of somatic dysfunction and be restricted in the direction that was associated with the starting position.

Generally, type II somatic dysfunctions in the thoracic and lumbar regions are more symptomatic and create more physiologic discord by restricting motions associated with normal activities of daily living. For example, consider a situation in which a worker has bent forward enough to significantly engage the facets of his lumbar spine and then tries to move a large box off to the left. If, in the middle of this activity, the box hits a nail in the floor and abruptly arrests the physiologic spinal motion that is taking place, the timing or stress might be sufficient to initiate a somatic dysfunction. When the patient tries to return to an upright position, he is likely to experience pain when the somatic dysfunction barrier is reached. That is because this barrier restricts his further backward bending, sidebending right, or rotation right needed to regain his neutral position. Clinically, this discomfort may be provoked every time the patient tries to function in a neutral position. The somatic dysfunction in this example is a type II, single-segment L3 somatic dysfunction. Motion testing would reveal that it prefers to flex, rotate left, and sidebend left.

As previously noted, rotation and/or lateral translation tests may be performed at each level as a scan or used for specific diagnosis of individual spinal levels. To test for the rotational component of somatic dysfunction, the clinician should place the palpating fingers over the left and right articular pillars in the cervical region or over the transverse processes of the thoracic/lumbar vertebral unit in question. Either the patient's active rotation or the physician's induction of passive rotation is used as the physician palpates and assesses the quality of the

end-feel of any barrier to motion (Figure 3.3.13). Additional palpatory information is gained if this is repeated with the spine in both forward-bent and backward-bent positions. In the lateral translation test, assessing sidebending capabilities, the physician places fingertips over the posterolateral aspects of the articular column in the typical cervical region or in the lateral region of the articular facets in the thoracic or lumbar spine. The force is localized to one segmental level and translation is checked in each direction. (Note: translation to the left creates sidebending to the right.) This test can also be performed with the spine in flexion and then repeated in extension. Restriction in left translation (restricted right sidebending) at C5 on C6, worse in extension and coupled with restriction in right rotation, may be recorded as a C5 flexed, sidebent and rotated left somatic dysfunction. The Fryette formula for C5 F R$_L$S$_L$ somatic dysfunction with pain elicited in the directions where motion is restricted could also be recorded as shown using Maigne's star diagram (Figure 3.3.14).

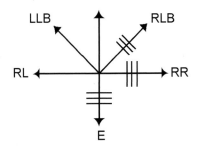

Figure 3.3.14 Star diagram of Maigne, illustrating the direction in which the patient feels pain. The bars indicate the grade of pain: three bars indicate significant pain, which will correlate with direction of restricted motion. Key: F, flexion; E, extension; RL, rotate left; RR, rotate right; LLB, left lateral bend; RLB, right lateral bend. Somatic dysfunction diagnosis: F RLSL. In the Maigne system, manipulation should be considered only when three directions are free of pain when motion is introduced.

Clinicians regularly use several of the regional scanning (and some local) examinations for somatic dysfunction described in this chapter as screening examinations. For example, patients presenting with low back pain may be routinely screened with a hip drop test, pelvic side shift test, stork test, and Trendelenburg test. Conversely, screening tests modified to gather more specific information are more properly classified as scanning examinations. Some regional scanning tests, such as skin rolling or palpation for myofascial tender/TrPs, are easily adapted to provide specific 'local' diagnostic information. The screening, regional scanning, and local tests described in this chapter provide additional insight into the structure and function of various regions or segments of the body.

Appropriately classifying a test as a screening, scanning, or local examination is of little importance compared to properly performing, understanding, and interpreting the information gained. Nonetheless, understanding these artificial classifications helps to shape the eventual patterns of palpatory examination that each manual medicine physician adopts. It also allows physicians and nonphysicians to communicate accurately with each other. In the end, the amount of detail sought, its interpretation, and the level of clinical suspicion will influence the selection of any additional examination procedures that will be needed.

With minor adaptations for patient position and consideration of the distinctive regional anatomic variations, the principles, methods, and nomenclature discussed in this overview are applicable in conducting a segmental palpatory examination in every region.

Somatic dysfunction overview: indications for specific joint examinations

Indications for regional scanning and local palpation of specific somatic regions and their related component parts include the suspicious history, physical, or screening examination findings listed in Table 3.3.1.[41,55] This chapter covers only the spinal and pelvic regions.

Despite the artificial regional grouping of clinical presentations in Table 3.3.1, regions distant from those that are symptomatic should be considered because of tensegrity principles[46] (see Chapter 2.2.5) and the body's physiologic response as a unit. Compensatory, reflex, and central mechanisms dictate that a change in one region creates dysfunction in adjacent regions. Table 3.3.2, for example, depicts common combinations of somatic dysfunction associated with common clinical conditions. A single somatic dysfunction (segmental or regional) is unlikely to be the sole cause or consequence of most clinical presentations.

This chapter introduces additional palpatory diagnostic examinations pertinent to each region or condition and applies the diagnostic principles and considerations discussed thus far to conditions commonly encountered in the clinical arena. Considering the number of specific joints and the wide range of clinically relevant conditions, relatively few conditions in each region were selected for presentation. However, each part of the 'Regional Disorders' section below discusses the role of regional somatic dysfunction and provides examples of a neuromusculoskeletal approach to palpatory diagnosis.

Regional disorders

Head and craniocervical junction areas

Regional somatic dysfunction of the head and craniocervical junction initiate a wide range of presenting signs and symptoms, as indicated previously in Table 3.3.1. Anatomic relationships in this region are capable of significant pain referral as well as autonomic and cranial nerve dysfunction. Furthermore, palpatory diagnostic findings in this section are particularly relevant to common musculoskeletal disorders such as headache and temporomandibular joint dysfunction.

Conversely, examples of reflex relationships between visceral disorders and this region as discussed in conditions such as sinus disorders (trigeminal reflexes) or gastric disturbances (vagal reflexes), reflect the importance of providing complete differential diagnosis in conjunction with the discovery of somatic dysfunction during the palpatory examination. Diagnosis and manipulative treatment of such secondary somatic dysfunction may provide additional symptomatic care or may even play a role in improving physiologic homeostatic mechanisms important in healing.[41]

Certain manual medicine techniques may be inappropriate or contraindicated in some conditions in this region.[47] Therefore, the following should be documented:

- The specific time, mechanism, and extent of head and cervical trauma.

- Prior responses to manual techniques. A history of ataxia or other significant neurologic sequelae to prior manual techniques or cervical trauma may alert the physician to the possibility of a potentially fatal vertebral artery abnormality. (This is discussed further in Chapter 4.3.1.)

- Headaches that wake the patient at night, are progressively more severe, or are accompanied by neurologic change.

- Evidence or absence of physical findings suggestive of Down syndrome and/or severe rheumatoid arthritis, as these conditions influence manual treatment considerations.

Head area

Headache is the most common pain-presenting complaint in the USA and among the most frequent complaints of patients presenting for any problem to both generalists and neurologists.

Many structures of the head are pain-sensitive or are capable of pain referral. Pain in this region of the body can result from afferent referral from eyes, ears, sinuses, temporomandibular joint, teeth, pharynx, respiratory tract, heart, and upper gastrointestinal tract as well as musculoskeletal referral from the cervical region. Pain-sensitive intracranial structures include the venous sinuses, the arteries of both the pia–arachnoid and the dura mater, and the dura itself. There are also a number of extracranial structures that are pain-sensitive, including skin, myofascial structures, regional articulations, arteries, and the cranial periosteum. Nociception from dysfunction, displacement, or encroachment on these structures is transmitted along cranial nerves V, VII, IX, and X as well as cervical nerve roots from C2 and C3. Even when head pain is not of musculoskeletal origin, secondary somatic dysfunction may result from repeated muscular splinting and positional compensations that the patient makes to reduce pain.[48] Differential diagnoses therefore require evaluation of each of these structures.

Differential diagnosis should attempt to separate life-threatening causes from those that limit quality of life, structural from functional causes, and primary from referred causes. The neuromusculoskeletal physician must be expert at this differential, current in management skills, and have the capability of treating functional causes and sequelae while decreasing pain and increasing the patient's quality of life.

Table 3.3.1. Suspicious history, physical, or screening examination findings

Region	History	Physical/screening exam
All regions	Significant trauma (e.g. motor vehicle accident or fall) Recurrent microtrauma (occupational, habitual) General aches and/or pain	Pelvic shear somatic dysfunctions Unlevel sacral base; small hemipelvis and/or short lower extremity Postural asymmetry Gait disorder Dudley J. Morton foot
Head/craniocervical junction	Headaches (any type) Dizziness/vertigo/ataxia Atypical facial pain EENT symptoms (e.g. sinus conditions, tinnitus, baroacusis, recurrent otitis media, strabismus, diplopia) Tooth/jaw symptoms (e.g. tooth pain, bruxism, jaw popping/pain) Asthma Ataxia, especially with concomitant travel sickness	+ Screen/scan tests: Regional S.T.A.R. findings Nonparallel mastoid and occipital planes; head, face, jaw or ear angle asymmetry Forward-head posture Fullness in supraclavicular area Asymmetric or low amplitude CRI Ataxic gait Fullness in supraclavicular area Abnormal cranial nerve testing Sacral somatic dysfunction Eustachian tube dysfunction Strabismus; extraocular muscle weakness Sternocleidomastoid or trapezius TrPs High arch palate and narrow dental arch Dysfunction/disease of EENT, sinuses, heart, respiratory tract and/or upper GI system[49]
Lower cervicals, CT junction, superior thoracic inlet	Headaches (any type) Symptoms of EENT, cardiac, pulmonary, or upper GI disorders Postural dizziness, vertigo, nausea Inertial injury Habitual or occupational accentuated cervical posturing or compression over trapezius muscle(s) Cervical crepitus, esp. with discomfort Significant coughing Recurrent or prolonged singultus (hiccoughs) Upper extremity paresthesias or dysesthesias aggravated by cervical or arm positions Upper extremity vascular or sympathetic-instability symptoms including Raynaud's phenomenon, finger swelling, cold/sweaty palm(s) Ataxia, especially with concomitant travel sickness	+ Screen/scan tests: Regional S.T.A.R. findings Cervical pointe sonnette (cervical doorbell) sign Mandibular skin rolling test Maigne key test Acromion drop test Supine thoracoabdominal passive inhalation observation Ataxic gait Sternocleidomastoid or trapezius TrPs Neurologic findings in upper extremity(ies), esp. aggravated by Valsalva or cervical position +Cervical compression test +Upper extremity deep tendon reflexes Loss of radial pulse with any of several provoking cervical or shoulder positions Signs of ENT, heart, and/or respiratory tract[50] disorder
Thoracics, thoracic cage	History of chest wall trauma or significant motor vehicle accident while wearing a shoulder strap Prolonged use of steroids or NSAIDs Chest wall pain, esp. if aggravated by coughing, sneezing, or sidebending Chest pain in a dermatomal pattern Visceral symptoms (e.g. gastritis, irritable bowel dysfunction, hypertension, cardiac dysrhythmia, dysmenorrhea), esp. if aggravated by stress	+ Screen/scan tests: Regional S.T.A.R. findings Postural asymmetry; flattened or increased thoracic kyphotic curve; rotoscoliosis Maigne key test Asymmetric 'shingle test' of Kuchera[51] Spring test over anterior and lateral rib cage Supine passive inhalation efforts failing to extend to pubic region Anterior intercostal Chapman points Tender fullness over abdominal collateral ganglion sites Pectus excavatum or pectus carinatum Skin eruptions in dermatomal pattern Quadratus lumborum TrP or spasm Puffy fingers or hands Objective findings of cardiovascular, gastrointestinal, kidney, lung, ovarian or uterine disorder

Table 3.3.1. Suspicious history, physical, or screening examination findings (*continued*)

Region	History	Physical/screening exam
Thoracolumbar junction, inferior thoracic outlet, lumbars	History or symptoms of visceral dysfunction originating the lower urinary system, the descending colon, sigmoid colon, rectum, uterus, or prostate Irritable bowel syndrome or a tendency towards constipation when stressed Recurrent or chronic low back pain Inability to stand upright; recurrent psoas posturing Systemic congestive phenomena Pain, dysesthesia, or other symptoms that radiate from the low back into one or both lower extremities	+ Screen/scan tests: Regional S.T.A.R. findings Postural asymmetry; reduced or increased lumbar lordosis; rotoscoliosis; inability to stand upright or pelvic side-shift Supine passive inhalation efforts failing to extend to pubic region Straight lumbar curve on hip drop test + Skin rolling over buttocks[52] +Thomas test for psoas Spondylolisthesis drop-off sign Short leg syndrome or small hemipelvis Palpable quadratus lumborum TrPs, tender iliopsoas points within pelvic brim Spinous process spondylolisthesis drop-off sign or a tuft of hair over lumbars Abnormal neurologic exam or reduced lower extremity (LE) deep tendon reflex + Lasegue's test (straight leg raising) + Trendelenburg test Abnormal LE muscle strength testing Objective findings of lower GI or GU disorder; lower lobe pneumonic signs
Lumbopelvic Junction, pelvis (sacroiliacs, sacrococcygeal, and pubic symphysis)	Low back pain ± lower extremity radiation Postpartum headache, depression or excessive fatigue; other symptom related to pregnancy/postpartum period Pelvic floor complaints (dyspareunia, prostatodynia, menstrual bloating, hemorrhoids, pelvic floor spasm) Enuresis, urinary frequency Buttock trauma and/or pratfalls Auto accident while bracing lower extremity; pelvic bruising by seat belt Lifting injury in an awkward position Twisting movements while weight-bearing Onset of problem after sit-ups or falling asleep in a soft recliner	+ Screen/scan tests: Regional S.T.A.R. findings Seated and/or standing flexion tests Stork test (aka Gillet's or march/stork test) + Pelvic side shift test +Supine long sitting test +SI joint stress/spring tests (thigh thrust, cranial shear, sacral thrust, SI gapping) +Hip rotation test +Thigh thrust SI stress test (aka posterior pelvic pain provocation test) +Yeoman's test +Gaenslen's test +Trendelenburg test Postural asymmetry; reduced or increased lumbar lordosis; rotoscoliosis; inability to stand upright or pelvic side-shift; unlevel iliac crests, greater trochanters, sacral base Spondylolisthesis drop-off sign Supine passive inhalation efforts failing to extend to pubic region Short leg syndrome or small hemipelvis Spinous process spondylolisthesis drop-off sign or a tuft of hair over lumbars Abnormal neurologic exam or reduced lower extremity deep tendon reflex + Lasegue's test (straight leg raising) + Trendelenburg test Abnormal muscle strength testing Objective findings of lower GI or GU disorder; lower lobe pneumonic signs

Table 3.3.1. Suspicious history, physical, or screening examination findings (*continued*)

Region	History	Physical/screening exam
Lower extremities	Lower extremity pain or dysesthesia with or without low back pain 'Buckling knee' Leg cramps 'Restless legs' 'Growing pains' Recurrent ankle sprains Foot drop History of inappropriate footwear	+ Screen/scan tests: Regional S.T.A.R. findings Postural asymmetry Gait disturbance Inability to deep squat and return Tight, ticklish, tender inguinal area; fullness in popliteal area; fullness around Achilles tendon Abnormal sole wear pattern Coxa and/or genu varus/valgus; increased Q angle; pronated or supinated foot Heel spur Patellar grind with compression Foot calluses, hammertoes, bunions Somatic dysfunction T11–L2 Abnormal neurologic exam or reduced lower extremity deep tendon reflex + Lasegue's test (straight leg raising) + Trendelenburg test Lower extremity muscle weakness +Tinel's over fibular head Abnormal orthopedic exam (lower extremity) +Patrick-Fabere (aka Figure 4) test with ligament stress +Drawer, pivot-shift, valgus/varus stress tests of knee +Ant. ankle drawer test
Upper extremities	Upper extremity pain or dysesthesia with or without cervical pain Repetitious habitual or occupational upper extremity motion Reduced grip strength	+ Screen/scan tests: Regional S.T.A.R. findings Postural asymmetry Shoulder girdle ROM screen Elbow spring tests (extension, valgus, and varus) Posterior axillary fold tissue texture abnormalities Abnormal neurologic exam or reduced upper extremity deep tendon reflex +Tinel's at wrist or ulnar groove +Phalen's test T2–8 somatic dysfunction
Abdomen	Visceral symptoms (e.g. gastritis, irritable bowel dysfunction, constipation, dysmenorrhea) esp. if aggravated by stress Inability to stand upright; recurrent psoas posturing Onset of problem after sit-ups or falling asleep in a soft recliner	+ Screen/scan tests: Regional S.T.A.R. findings Postural asymmetry; flattened or increased thoracic kyphotic curve; rotoscoliosis; psoas posturing Supine passive inhalation efforts failing to extend to pubic region Anterior intercostal Chapman points Tender fullness over abdominal collateral ganglion sites Weakness of abdominal muscle testing Recurrent somatic dysfunction of OA-C2, T5–L2, and/or sacroiliac regions Objective findings of cardiovascular, gastrointestinal, kidney, lung, ovarian or uterine disorder

Table 3.3.2. Examples of multiregional somatic dysfunction complexes in common clinical conditions

Common clinical conditions	Examples of possible associated multiregional somatic dysfunction complexes
Common headache	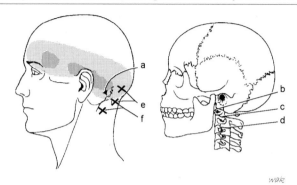
(a) left occipitomastoid suture	
(b) OA = E $S_R R_L$	
(c–d) C2–3 = E $R_R S_R$	
(e) Travell points for upper end of semispinalis muscle	
(f) Travell points for suboccipital muscle	
Sternocleidomastoid headache	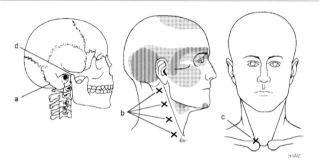
(a) right occipitomastoid suture	
(b) Travell right sternocleidomastoid trigger points	
(c) Jones AC7 point	
(d) temporomandibular joint dysfunction	
Reactive airway	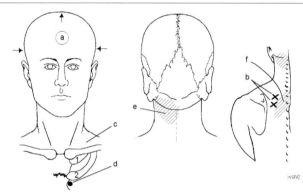
(a) extension-type cranium	
(b, d) left rib 2–3 somatic dysfunction	
(c) fullness of left supraclavicular region	
(d) Chapman's point; tender point reference to the bronchus	
(e) C2 TTC (tissue texture change)	
(f) Left T1–3 TTC	
Gastritis	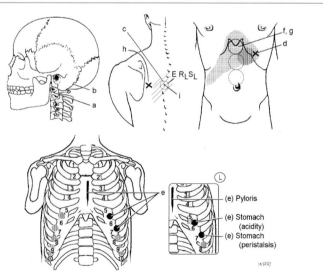
(a) left C2 TTC	
(b) left occipitomastoid suture TTC	
(c) T5 E $R_L S_L$	
(d) Travell external oblique muscle TrP and pain pattern	
(e) Chapman's stomach and pylorus reflex points	
(f) celiac ganglion tension	
(g) epigastric congestion	
(h) left rib 5 SD	
(i) postural crossover at T5	

TTC = tissue texture change; TrP = trigger point; SD = somatic dysfunction

Table 3.3.2. Examples of multiregional somatic dysfunction complexes in common clinical conditions (*continued*)

Common clinical conditions	Examples of possible associated multiregional somatic dysfunction complexes
Irritable bowel dysfunction	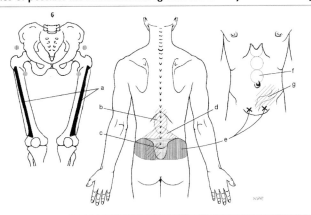

Irritable bowel dysfunction

(a) bilateral iliotibial band tenderness and TTC (Chapman's)

(b) thoracolumbar SD and TTC

(c) left SI TTC

(d) post. Chapman's lumbar TTC (low back pain).

(e) lower rectus abdominis muscle TrP and pain pattern

(f) inferior mesenteric ganglion TTC

(g) sigmoid loop palpable

Right carpal tunnel syndrome

(a) elevated first rib SD

(b) thoracic inlet SD

(c) right supraclavicular congestion

(d) right posterior axillary fold tenderness and TTC

(e) generic elbow SD

(f) generic wrist SD

(g) right paraspinal T2–8 SD

(h) scalene TrP and pain patterns of the right arm

(i) Jones CTS points

(j) Travell trigger points: J1, pronator teres; J2, flexor digitorum; J3, flexor carpi radialis; J4, flexor pollicis longus; J5, opponens pollicis

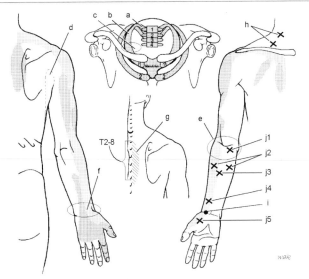

Sprained right ankle

(a) plantar SD of cuboid and navicular bones

(b) posterolateral talus SD

(c) externally rotated tibia

(d) anteromedial glide of the tibia

(e) internally rotated femur

(f) posterior right innominate

(g) L5 $S_R R_L$

(h) sacrum rotated right on right oblique axis

(i) Travell trigger points

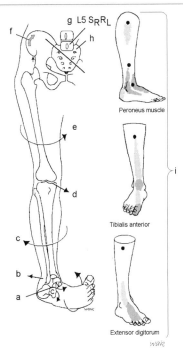

TTC = tissue texture change; TrP = trigger point; SD = somatic dysfunction; CTS = carpal tunnel syndrome

Headache management by physicians trained in neuromusculo-skeletal diagnosis and the value of treating related somatic dysfunction in this condition is well established.[49–51] Other such conditions in this region commonly managed or co-managed by the neuromusculo-skeletal practitioner include:[52]

- temporomandibular joint dysfunction
- atypical facial pain
- malocclusive dental syndromes
- cervical spine syndromes
- cranial neuralgias
- cranial suture syndrome
- nerve encroachment syndrome
- myofascial pain syndromes.

Each of these conditions deserves careful screening, scanning, and where indicated, local diagnosis and management, of regional somatic dysfunction.

Regardless of other diagnoses, myofascial pain due to TrPs is likely to contribute to and complicate management of most chronic pain complaints in the region.[53] Specific tissue texture scanning for myofascial tender points and TrPs is therefore very productive. In patients presenting with headaches, temporomandibular joint pain and/or dysfunction, atypical facial pain, sinus pain and/or dysfunction, toothache, dental occlusal disharmony, eustachian tube dysfunction, difficulty in swallowing, tinnitus, and/or visual disturbances, Travell and Simons advocate searching for TrPs using pressure over specific cranial muscle sites.[54] These authors point out that 'it is important to remember that a systematic and thorough examination of *all* of the head and neck muscles looking for active and latent myofascial TrPs is essential for complete evaluation of any persistent or chronic head and neck pain complaint'.

Greenman also advocates palpating the skull itself, scanning for resiliency in general, noting that normal bone has a characteristic pliability that is lost in the presence of motion restriction.[55] Pressure applied over the supraorbital or infraorbital foramina (Figure 3.3.15) often reveals both tenderness and edematous change when visceral afferents facilitate the trigeminal nerve, as in a case of sinusitis.[41]

Pressure can also be applied to scan regional articulations such as the cranial sutures. Scanning palpation of the head region can begin with the application of pressure over or across sutures looking for ten-

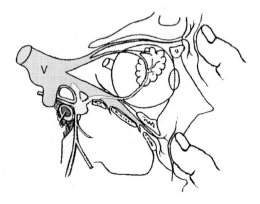

Figure 3.3.15 Palpation of supraorbital and infraorbital branches of trigeminal nerve for tissue texture change or tenderness.

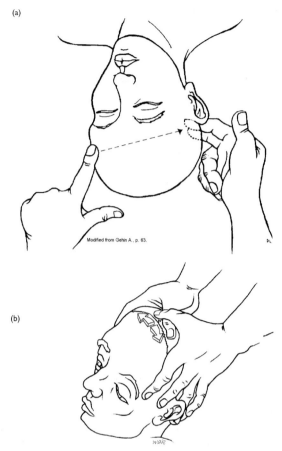

Modified from Gehin A., p. 63.

Figure 3.3.16 (a) Occipitomastoid suture spread with fluid force; (b) V-spread of sagittal suture of skull. (Modified from Gehin, A. Atlas of manipulative techniques for the cranium and face (1985). Eastland Press, Seattle, WA.)

derness and/or tension as well as widening or narrowing of the sutural sites.[55] This is especially useful in planning treatment for patients with dizziness, posterior headaches, or functional symptoms associated with the upper respiratory, cardiac, or upper gastrointestinal systems. In these patients, there is edematous tissue texture change over the occipitomastoid suture and it is frequently tender to palpation.[41] Interparietal sutural somatic dysfunction often extends the typical tension headache pattern to include the vertex along the sagittal suture. Patients scanned by applying pressure across a sagittal suture with somatic dysfunction typically experience a pain of 'ice-pick' intensity at the site of the restriction (Figure 3.3.16).

Examine the temporomandibular joint and the masseter muscles more closely if there is a positive postural screen for anterior head positioning, Dudley J. Morton foot,[56] or short leg syndrome – especially if accompanied by a history of jaw clicking, temporomandibular joint pain, tinnitus, or problems chewing. Asking the patient to open and close the mouth while simultaneously observing and palpating the region may further scan for the etiology of these latter symptoms. Mandibular opening in an adult should be 40–60 mm (normally admitting a tier of two to three knuckles between the incisor teeth)[57] and should be symmetrical. Watch for jaw deviation and listen or palpate for a click emanating from either joint.

Palpate the lateral poles of each temporomandibular joint by applying pressure with fingertips immediately anterior to the tragus of

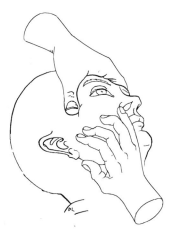

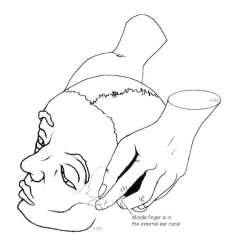

Figure 3.3.17 Palpation of temporomandibular joint with index finger anterior to the tragus. Note any asymmetry of tracking or clicking as mouth opens and closes.

Figure 3.3.18 Temporal lift.

the ear as well as palpating the retrodiscal tissues by placing fifth digits just inside the ear (Figure 3.3.17). In a positive scanning examination for dysfunction or pathology, the jaw will deviate and/or be restricted in its range of motion. Deviation is toward the side of a restriction (pathological or dysfunctional) of the temporomandibular joint itself, toward the side of a temporal bone with external rotation somatic dysfunction, and away from an internally rotated temporal bone.[58] Sphenoid dysfunction also may affect the temporomandibular joint through the influence of the sphenomandibular ligament. If asymmetric jaw deviation goes away when the patient open the mouth with tongue placed high on the hard palate, the lateral pterygoid muscle is often the source of the patient's dysfunction.[59] There are multiple causes for temporomandibular joint dysfunction, and a positive scanning examination of the temporomandibular joint should be followed with local diagnosis for articular somatic dysfunction of the sphenoid, temporal bones, and mandible and for myofascial somatic dysfunction of the posterior temporalis, lateral pterygoid, masseter, digastric, and buccinator muscles.

The temporal bone has justifiably been named 'the troublemaker of the head'[60] because of its structural and functional connections. A more detailed scan or local diagnosis for temporal bone somatic dysfunction is especially indicated with a patient's history of dizziness or vertigo, strabismus, Bell's palsy, trigeminal neuralgia, headache, swallowing or suckling disorders, otitis media, acute torticollis, and temporomandibular joint dysfunction. In my experience, myofascial TrPs in the sternocleidomastoid or trapezius muscles may fail to respond to conventional treatment until dysfunction of the temporal bone (especially at the occipitomastoid suture) is first diagnosed and treated. Magoun claims that functional disorders of the temporal bones may be responsible for affecting 9 of the 12 cranial nerves – excluding only the olfactory, optic, and hypoglossal nerves.

Greenman describes a **temporal lift** scanning examination to assess temporal somatic dysfunction.[55] With the patient supine, each temporal bone is gently grasped with the middle finger in the external auditory meatus, the thumb and index finger on the superior and inferior aspect of the zygomatic process respectively, and the mastoid process between the fourth and fifth digits (Figure 3.3.18). In the scan, each temporal is gently pulled toward the vertex and then allowed to settle back to its neutral position. A positive scan for dysfunction is indi-

cated by restriction in joint play on one or both sides. This same hand position (the temporal hold) is used for specific diagnosis of either internal or external rotation somatic dysfunction of a temporal bone.[61]

Scanning or more detailed palpation of the frontal bone and its membranous attachments is indicated in a variety of conditions. This is especially true when there is a history of a blow to the forehead, headaches (especially sinus and following lumbar puncture), and post-traumatic alteration of smell, including smelling scents that are not present. In the supine patient with the physician seated at the patient's head, a **frontal lift** can be either a scanning examination or can be modified into a treatment modality (discussed in Chapter 4.3.1). For this lift, the frontal bone is gently grasped with the index fingers approximated over the glabella and the ring fingers at the lateral aspect of the brow on the orbital portions of the frontal bone. Thumbs are crossed in such a fashion as to provide a controlled lifting pivot (Figure 3.3.19). The maneuver begins with ring fingers slightly compressing toward the center of the patient's head. The physician then applies a gentle anterior lift (toward the ceiling for a supine patient) of the frontal bone by elevating both ring fingers and pivoting around both thumbs and index fingers. Like the temporal lift, any restriction

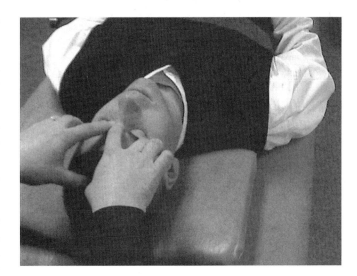

Figure 3.3.19 Frontal lift.

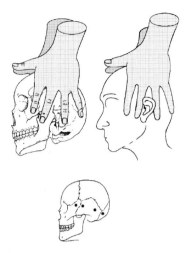

Figure 3.3.20 Vault hold.

in joint play constitutes a positive screen for frontal bone somatic dysfunction. Furthermore, when this lift is held at a point of balanced membranous tension, if the patient experiences relief of headache and/or has a sensation of opening of the sinuses, then further palpatory diagnosis of the cranial bones or reciprocal tension membranes is warranted.

The **vault hold** of the cranium provides an extremely useful scanning examination of the cranial base and vault, and many neuromusculoskeletal physicians use it as a general screening examination. The physician sits comfortably and relaxed at the patient's head with forearms resting on the table and fingers relaxed. Hand placement in the supine patient is specific with index fingers monitoring the sphenoid, fifth digits monitoring the occiput, and the middle two fingers on either side of the ear monitoring the temporal bones (Figure 3.3.20). The palpable motion sensation, termed the **cranial rhythmic impulse** (CRI), normally has an amplitude of 40 μm to 1.5 mm and a rate of 10–14/minute.[62] Altered CRI amplitude, rate and/or asymmetrical motion indicate a positive scan warranting further palpatory diagnosis. Amplitude has traditionally been believed to be a general indicator of a patient's vitality, but has been the focus of less study than rate or symmetry pattern.

Specific palpatory diagnosis of sphenobasilar somatic dysfunction can be accomplished with the same vault hold described above. Both passive palpatory monitoring and active motion test assessments of the position as well as inherent motion of midline bones are possible with this hold. Normal palpatory findings include symmetrical movement into flexion and extension while paired bones move into external and internal rotation respectively. Static and dynamic asymmetry or generalized, severely restricted motion indicates somatic dysfunction of the sphenobasilar synchondrosis; dysfunction patterns are illustrated in Figure 3.3.21).

More detail in diagnosing myofascial somatic dysfunction and TrPs of the head, scanning of facial bone articular dysfunction, or even the specific diagnosis of other cranial bones is beyond the scope of this chapter. Trigger points are covered more completely in Chapter 4.3.9. For more information about the Sutherland approach in this region, the reader is referred to *Osteopathy in the cranial field*[61] and other standard texts.

Craniocervical junction area

The craniocervical junction includes the occipital condyles and squama, the atlas, the axis, and all of the muscular, ligamentous, and other connective tissues, governing the function of these bony structures. Even though each of its component joints is atypical when compared to other cervical vertebral units or even to each other, this superior cervical complex behaves synergistically as a functional unit. Dysfunction here is common, and even 80% of asymptomatic individuals will demonstrate a fascial preference for sidebending and rotating the entire craniocervical complex to the left.[23] Nonetheless, because each of the articulations in this transition area is different in its motion characteristics, a positive palpatory scan of the suboccipital region requires local individual testing of each of these joints.[63]

Scanning of this region is best accomplished by palpating the suboccipital region for S.T.A.R. abnormalities. A positive scan here may indicate somatic dysfunction affecting the occipitoatlantal (C0) vertebral unit, the atlantoaxial (C1) vertebral unit, and/or the C2 on C3 (C2) vertebral unit. Articular and myofascial dysfunction within the suboccipital region typically coexist. Travell and Simons cite TrPs in the splenii capitis muscles commonly found in conjunction with C0 and/or C2 dysfunction as an example of this close interrelationship.[64] Thus, suboccipital joints cannot truly be examined in isolation. It should also be noted that secondary tension and tissue change present in the suboccipital region and initiated by ipsilateral upper thoracic and rib problems will improve significantly after manipulative treatment of the primary problem.[62]

After screening and/or scanning the area, the examination order for skeletal, arthrodial, and myofascial components of somatic dysfunction becomes an individual decision. Different approaches by different expert practitioners appear to have similar outcomes. For example, because soft tissue dysfunction often alters articular motion characteristics in the craniocervical junction, I prefer to diagnose and address any soft tissue dysfunction before attempting a definitive articular diagnosis through specific segmental examination. Others find that treatment of somatic dysfunction associated with the combined motion characteristics addresses both articular and myofascial components at the same time.

Recent attempts to document the interrelationship between articular and myofascial components and to link them to relevant historical and physical findings have expanded our understanding of the diagnosis and treatment of the suboccipital region. For example, *Travell and Simons' myofascial pain and dysfunction* points out the common combination of C0, C1, and/or C2 articular somatic dysfunctions found in patients with semispinalis capitis TrPs (myofascial somatic dysfunction).[65] This combination was very likely in a population of patients with cervicogenic headaches, where 91% of patients had C0 or C1 articular somatic dysfunction and 56% had TrPs in the semispinalis capitis muscle predominantly ipsilateral to the symptomatic side.[66] Likewise, Kappler reports that a referred retro-orbital pain pattern, consistent with Travell's upper semispinalis capitis (location 2) trigger point (Figure 3.3.22), is often found on the palpably anterior portion of a rotated C1 somatic dysfunction.[63]

Our understanding has also been expanded through documentation of patterns of dysfunction found within functional units. With respect to the superior cervical complex and headache, for example, Greenman[67] reports a pattern found in most patients presenting with cervical spine stiffness and associated hemicephalgia running from the

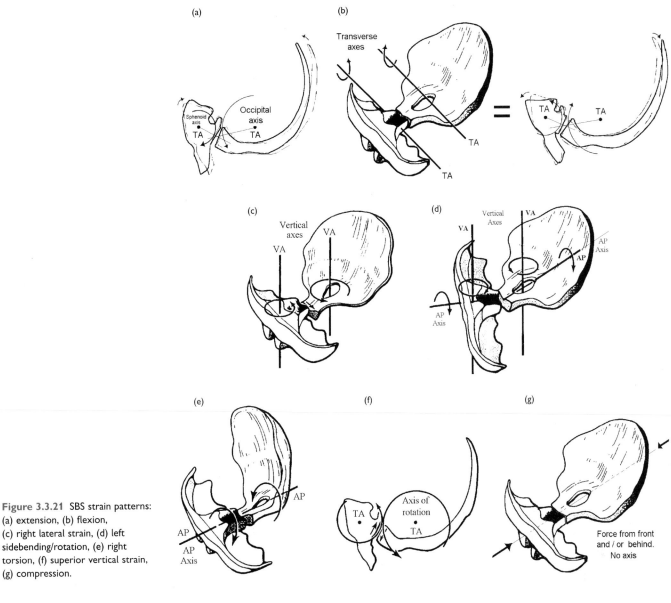

Figure 3.3.21 SBS strain patterns: (a) extension, (b) flexion, (c) right lateral strain, (d) left sidebending/rotation, (e) right torsion, (f) superior vertical strain, (g) compression.

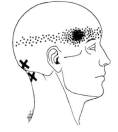

Figure 3.3.22 Retro-orbital pain pattern seen in both upper semispinalis capitis TrP and in C1 somatic dysfunction. (From Simons, Travell, and Simons[65].)

occiput to the retro-orbital area. The most common palpable structural diagnostic findings included this combination were:

- left occipitomastoid suture restriction
- C0 $S_R R_L$
- C1 rotated right
- C2–3 E $R_L S_L$

Restriction of motion segmental scanning for C0 dysfunction is often accomplished passively using a **lateral translation test**. Palpating digits placed in the suboccipital triangle sense the end-feel (freedom or resistance) of translation of the skull to the right and to the left with respect to the atlas. Another active scan at this same level is to ask patients who do not have temporomandibular joint dysfunction to actively open their jaw or to tuck their chin while the physician

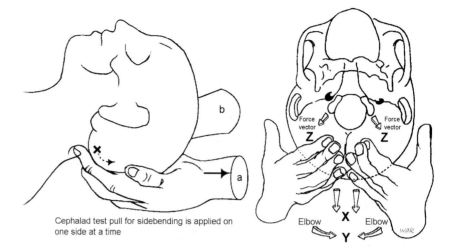

Cephalad test pull for sidebending is applied on
one side at a time

Figure 3.3.23 Easy occipitoatlantal motion test.
Unilateral pull along the facet tests side bending (which
is coupled with rotation in the opposite direction);
bilateral traction along both facets tests flexion and is
sometimes held to relax suboccipital muscles thereby
allowing more accurate articular diagnosis.

observes. This active scan is positive for C0 dysfunction if the chin deviates from the midline to either side. Cradling the head with fingertips of the middle digits contacting the tissues in the suboccipital region permits a supine scan for regional motion restriction. Pulling the physician's own forearms and wrists together while hands and fingers traction cephalically automatically pulls the fascia posteriorly and cephalically along the plane of the occipitoatlantal condylar facets. Enough pressure to reach the point where the suboccipital fascia first begins to resist the drag allows evaluation of resiliency (ease) or resistance (drag) to sidebending the region right or left. Scanning tests for C0 dysfunction are shown in Figure 3.3.23.

Scanning for C1 somatic dysfunction may be accomplished by fully forward bending the entire cervical spine (if tolerated) to physiologically lock out motion below the atlas, followed by rotating the head and atlas on the axis. As rotation is the primary motion allowed between the atlas and the axis, and occipitoatlantal rotation is limited to approximately 3°, asymmetrical motion indicates a positive test. A positive test, or factors prohibiting the performance of this scanning

examination, suggests the need for segmental evaluation of C1 (Figure 3.3.24). C2 will be discussed with the lower cervical complex in the next section.

Scanning tests need not be limited to palpation in the suboccipital region. Maigne describes an effective scanning examination for headache patients with the **eyebrow pinch-roll test** (Figure 3.3.25).[68] This scan is positive when the supraorbital skin fold on the symptomatic side is painful to pinch and feels palpably thickened. According to Maigne, a positive eyebrow pinch-roll test, in conjunction with tenderness in the suboccipital triangle over C2, suggests a headache of cervical origin involving the upper cervical complex.

As in all regional scanning examinations, a positive finding should alert the clinician to the need for local or segmental examination. Classification of acute or chronic somatic dysfunction in this region is largely based on the tissue texture characteristics discussed in Chapter 2.2.1.

Segmental examination for occipitoatlantal somatic dysfunction requires recognition that there are two occipitoatlantal joints, one on

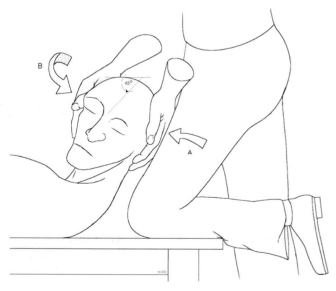

Figure 3.3.24 Easy atlantoaxial motion test. Locking out other cervicals permits testing of the upper cervical unit. A number of cervical conditions preclude this test however.

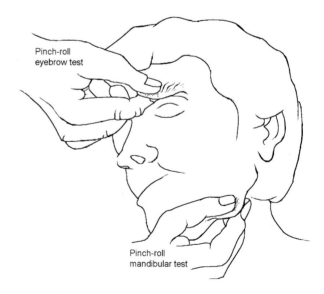

Pinch-roll
eyebrow test

Pinch-roll
mandibular test

Figure 3.3.25 Eyebrow pinch test.

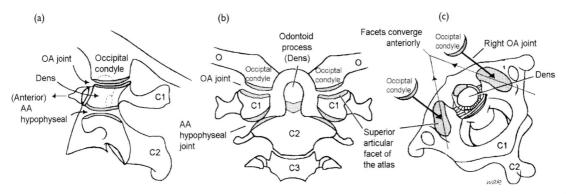

Figure 3.3.26 Occipitoatlantal and atlantoaxial joints illustrated with direction of superior facets of the atlas: (a) sagittal view, (b) coronal view, (c) superior oblique view.

each side. These joints are placed so as to converge anteriorly (Figure 3.3.26). In sagittal plane (forward or backward bent) somatic dysfunction of C0 both occipitoatlantal joints are tender, both demonstrate equal tissue texture changes, and together they typically limit the ability for the joint to sidebend or rotate in either direction. In forward-bent C0 dysfunction, the occiput will allow forward bending but is restricted when backward bending is attempted; the opposite is true for a backward-bent C0 dysfunction. In coupled plane somatic dysfunction at this level, sidebending and rotation occur to opposite sides.[69] In a C0 sidebent left, rotated right somatic dysfunction, the occiput is restricted when sidebending to the right and rotation to the left are attempted. Because of the two condylar joints, motion characteristics of C0 somatic dysfunction can be localized further to the right and/or the left occipitoatlantal articulation according to the dominant sensitivity, tissue texture abnormality, and restriction of motion. Thus in the example of coupled motion above (C0 $S_L R_R$), there may be an anterior left occiput, a posterior right occiput, or both. By changing the focus of attention when specifically testing C0, the anterior occiput exhibits restriction of flexion and there is a sense that the occiput cannot glide posterolaterally on that side; the posterior occiput exhibits restriction of extension and cannot glide anteromedially on that side.

Segmental motion examination of C1 (atlantoaxial joint) is best accomplished by stabilizing the axis with one hand. This is accomplished by grasping the posterior spine of C2 (the axis) between the thumb and index finger of one hand; the occiput is cupped in the other hand with the fingers in the suboccipital groove and resting over the posterior arch of the atlas (Figure 3.3.27). Right and left rotation of the occipitoatlantal unit on C2 is then assessed. Somatic dysfunction in this joint is uniplanar.

The nerve root of C2 has direct anatomic attachments to the vagus and C2 is a common palpatory site of secondary somatic dysfunction. This results from vagal visceral afferent stimuli arising from dysfunction of certain upper respiratory, cardiac, and/or upper gastrointestinal structures. Its own innervation of the posterior scalp and dura of the posterior cranial fossa makes this vertebral segment important when considering diagnosis and treatment of patients with a wide range of problems. Nonetheless, the segmental examination of C2 is conducted in the same manner as all typical cervical vertebral units in the lower cervical area and is discussed below.

In interpreting palpatory findings in this region, a wealth of clinical evidence, including a 5-year double-blind study of 5000 hospitalized patients,[70] suggests that the differential diagnosis of palpatory findings in this region should include secondary somatic dysfunction from sinus, respiratory, cardiac, and gastrointestinal disorders.[41,71] Paterson provides a synopsis of 'bizarre ENT symptoms' resulting from cervical dysfunction and notes that, in the absence of contraindications, manipulation is the treatment of choice.[72] Maigne indicates that when cervical somatic dysfunction is eliminated with manipulation, precipitating visceral factors that are still present will no longer trigger the referred headaches.[73] In isolation, neither cervi-

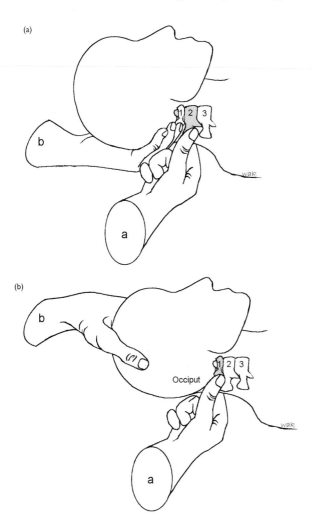

Figure 3.3.27 Two-hand motion tests: (a) for atlantoaxial joint, (b) for occipitoatlantal joint.

cal screening nor suboccipital scanning provides enough diagnostic information to initiate an individualized neuromusculoskeletal prescription. Thus, local cervical diagnosis for specific somatic dysfunction and a physician's diagnostic capability to investigate and/or co-manage those other conditions are required for formulation of a complete differential diagnosis.

Some clinicians advocate for a provocative test of the vertebral artery by positioning the upper cervical complex into hyperextension and rotation for up to 1 minute. This position, referred to as a **postural test**[74] or a **DeKleyns test**,[47] places the artery in its most precarious position and the clinician carefully observes for any posterior headache, vertigo, or eye nystagmus that might alert him or her to vertebral artery dissection or compromise. In the past, some mandated that this position was prerequisite to any cervical manipulation. Today, many authorities feel that the test is more likely to cause an arterial problem in a susceptible patient than the treatments currently advocated for the area. Therefore, if the patient has had no prior history or signs of potential arterial problems, you should avoid hyperextension and rotational activation and carefully proceed with the cervical manual treatment without tests stressing the artery.[47]

Lower cervical, cervicothoracic junction, and superior thoracic inlet

Regional scanning and local palpation of the lower cervical spine, cervicothoracic junction, superior thoracic inlet, and/or any of its component parts are specifically indicated for a patient who has a history and/or the findings on a physical or screening examination that are identified in Table 3.3.2. This region is particularly important in patients with musculoskeletal conditions that are associated with headache, postural imbalance, and upper extremity problems. Because the thoracic lymphatic duct passes through Sibson's fascia of the thoracic inlet twice before emptying into the brachiocephalic vein, dysfunction of this region of anatomy can be a significant obstruction to lymph flow, resulting in congestive phenomena that manifest almost any-

where in the body. Furthermore, cervical chain ganglia locations, as well as the upper thoracic and rib sympathetic anatomic connections, link palpatory findings of somatic dysfunction in this region to a host of eye, ear, nose, and throat (EENT) and cardiopulmonary disturbances (Figure 3.3.28).

In this section, some of the considerations discussed previously in the superior cervical functional segment will be relevant to the discussion of the lower cervical segment. Furthermore, somatic dysfunction in this region also reflects compensation for, or causes compensation in, somatic regions above and below. Therapeutic decision-making in this region also includes patients with:

- history of cervical trauma, especially whiplash (inertial) injury

- response to prior manual techniques in the region, especially historical presence or absence of vertigo, ataxia, or severe posterior headache afterwards or referral to either upper extremity

- evidence or absence of physical findings suggestive of conditions such as osteoporosis, cervical stenosis, cervical ligamentous laxity or spondylolisthesis, severe rheumatoid arthritis, cervical ribs, or mediastinal tumors.

Lower cervical area

The typical cervical spine extends from C2 through C6 or C7. Together with the cervicothoracic junction, this region is responsible for a wide range of functional disorders affecting the head, neck, and upper extremities and contains sympathetic ganglia whose cell bodies originate in the upper thoracic region.

Some clinicians inappropriately suggest that consideration of the cervical spine in the diagnosis and treatment of patients with headaches is 'controversial'. Seasoned neuromusculoskeletal clinicians, however, have experience in differentiating those patients for whom the cervical spine plays a central rather than a secondary or noncontributory role. The International Headache Society (IHS) agrees with the latter group in recognizing that the cervical spine must be

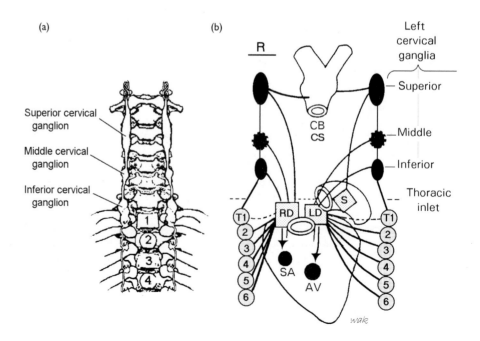

Figure 3.3.28 (a) Cervical chain ganglia; (b) sympathetic innervation of the heart.

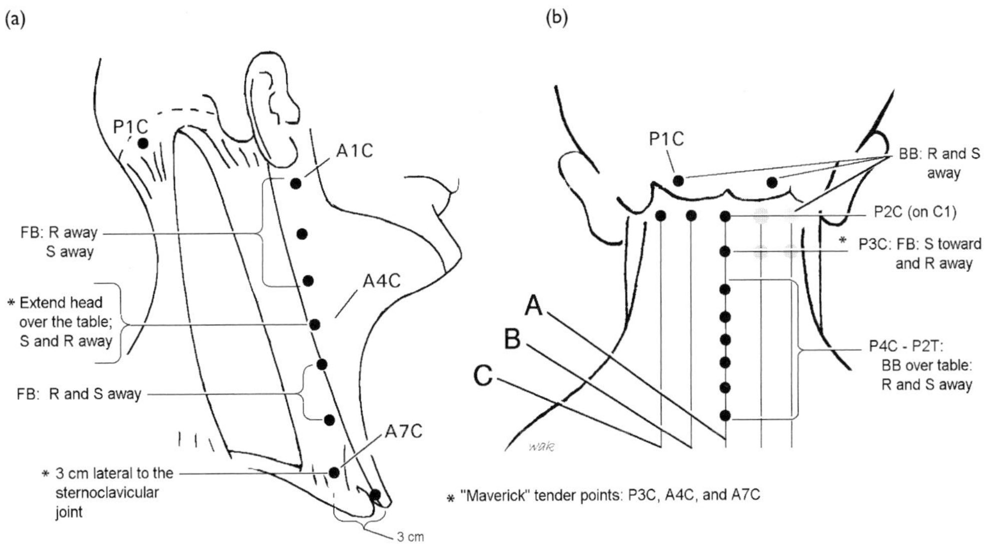

Figure 3.3.29 Jones tender points of the cervical region: (a) anterior: occipitoatlantal point posterior to the mastoid process, occipitoatlantal also between mastoid and angle of jaw, C1–7 along anterior margin of the sternocleidomastoid muscle; (b) posterior: occipitoatlantal point on the occiput; A, C1–7 spinous processes; B, C1–7, also 2.5 cm lateral to the spinous processes; C, C1–7, also 5 cm lateral to the spinous processes.

included in classification schema.[75] According to the IHS, inclusion criteria for the cervical spine includes several of the S.T.A.R. characteristics used to diagnosis cervical somatic dysfunction, including:

- local neck or occipital pain projecting to forehead, orbital region, temples, vertex, or ears
- **either** diminished cervical motion, abnormal cervical contour, texture, tone or response to active and passive stretching and contraction **or** abnormal tenderness of neck muscles
- radiographic evidence of pathology, abnormal posture, **or** reduced range of motion.

Lower cervical region dysfunction has also been implicated in symptoms referred to the upper extremities, upper thoracic region and ribs, diaphragm, and cardiorespiratory systems. Regional dysfunction plays a significant role in acute torticollis, cervical radiculopathies, post-whiplash syndromes, cervical vertigo, carpal tunnel syndrome, and superior thoracic outlet syndrome. From a pathophysiologic perspective, cervical somatic dysfunction has been implicated in reducing the transport of centrally produced trophic substances to the tissues of the upper extremities.[76] This in turn, like the more extreme double crush syndrome, may predispose the upper extremities to increased risk of developing symptomatic entrapment neuropathies and other regional disorders. The area is also subject to secondary somatic dysfunction from disorders of the EENT, cardiopulmonary, and upper gastrointestinal systems.

Both Maigne[77] and Jones[30] advocate use of pressure posteriorly over the cervical spinous processes as a scanning process to identify segmental cervical dysfunction. In their local cervical diagnosis, both of these physicians look for posterior tender points located approximately one finger's breadth from the median line. Jones' nomenclature for these and other body tender points is standardized and used by practitioners of counterstrain manipulative technique (Figure 3.3.29).

Each of these neuromusculoskeletal physicians recognizes the importance of additionally examining the anterior cervical region. Jones recorded a large number of anterior cervical tender points after applying pressure to locations from just under the ear on the posterior ascending ramus of the mandible, down the anterolateral aspect (lateral masses) of the cervical spine to the medial superior end of the sternum. Jones correlated these findings with segmental cervical somatic dysfunction. Maigne describes a very similar location for his cervical *pointe sonnette* (doorbell) sign, elicited by applying a few seconds of moderate thumb pressure in the anterolateral region of the cervical spine. Tenderness and replication of the patient's complaints using Maigne's anterior cervical doorbell (push-button or bell-push) sign is said to indicate the involved or irritated cervical root level. Clinically, he interprets these findings as 'very useful at the level of the middle or lower cervical spine' and notes that this is especially relevant when dealing with atypical upper extremity pain that seems to originate in the cervical region. Both clinical authors note an anterior palpatory finding at the angle of the jaw (whose cutaneous innervation is supplied by anterior branches of C2 and C3). Jones designates two tender points, one just under the ear on the posterior ascending ramus of the mandible and one 2 cm anterior to the angle of the mandible on the medial side of that bone. Maigne uses the skin-rolling method on the mandible to identify dysfunction or pathology associated with either the C2 or C3 level. Note that the differential between cervical region somatic dysfunction and cervical root pathophysiology cannot be made by palpation alone. As pointed out consistently in the work of Simons and Travell, each is capable of creating palpatory change, each is capable of creating neural, vascular and lymphatic dysfunction, and coexistence is common.

More specific tissue texture scanning for myofascial tender points and TrPs in the lower cervical region is productive if the historical, physical, or screening examinations indicate the need for more definitive information about somatic dysfunction. Simons, Travell, and Simons point out that it is common for patients with myofascial points in the trapezii muscles to have somatic dysfunction of C2, C3, and/or C4 as well as hypermobility of C4.[78] They also record that TrPs in the splenii cervicis are commonly found in conjunction with C4 and/or C5 dysfunction[79] and note that articular somatic dysfunction anywhere between C3 and C6 is frequently associated with TrPs in the levator scapulae.[80]

At the segmental level, palpation of C2–7 motion is most easily accomplished by using the passive segmental rotation and lateral translation tests described previously. Because of the anatomic structure of typical cervical vertebrae and orientation of their articulations,

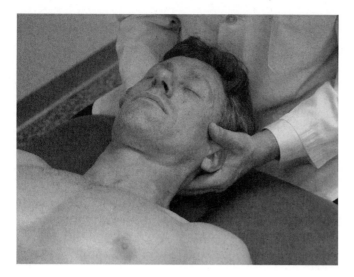

Figure 3.3.30 Rotational testing of cervical spine respects facet facings. Fingers are on the posterior articular pillars.

sidebending and rotation are coupled to allow sidebending and rotation to the same side. To test rotation, support the supine patient's head with fingers contacting the posterior surfaces of the articular pillars (Figure 3.3.30). In the neutral position, rotate each vertebral unit along the plane of its posterior cervical facets (roughly toward the patient's opposite eye) to the right and to the left, assessing the quality of the end-feel in each direction. Additional palpatory information is gained if this is repeated with the cervical spine in both forward-bent and backward-bent positions. In the lateral translation test, the physician contacts the lateral portion of the cervical articular pillars with fingertips while supporting the supine patient's head in his or her hands. Localizing the force to one level, translation is checked in each direction. The test can also be performed with the neck held in flexion and then repeated in extension. The rotation and/or the lateral translation tests may be performed at each level as a scan or used for specific segmental diagnosis of individual levels identified in a scan of the region.

Cervicothoracic junction and superior thoracic inlet areas

While the cervicothoracic junction of the spine literally occurs between C7 and T1, the functional superior thoracic inlet region is made up of:

- the first four thoracic vertebrae
- the first two ribs
- the manubrium of the sternum
- all of the attached connecting and restricting tissues.

This region is extremely important from an autonomic and circulatory perspective. The superior thoracic inlet is in close relationship with the superior thoracic outlet, and dysfunction of one affects the other (Figure 3.3.31). The thoracic duct provides a drainage pathway for lymph from most the body into the brachiocephalic vein and must pass through this region from the chest into the neck and then back through this region from the neck into the chest. Additionally, the lymphaticovenous valve and peristaltic motions of this terminal portion of the thoracic duct are under sympathetic control governed

by lateral horn cell bodies in the spinal cord of this region. These same cell bodies regulate circulation to all the structures of the head and neck, the heart and lungs, and portions of the upper extremities.

Recall that differential diagnostic considerations in this region include viscerosomatic and somatovisceral reflexes. Part of the differential is assisted through palpation of each of the S.T.A.R. characteristics. In primary visceral involvement, the tissue texture abnormalities will often far outweigh the degree of motion restriction and the quality of the restrictive barrier is 'rubbery'. The pattern of the somatic dysfunction sites often is helpful as well. Note that in patients with primary coronary artery/cardiac involvement, somatic patterns include palpable changes most frequently from T2–4 on the left as well as left-sided second rib and pectoralis major TrPs.[81] Upper chest muscle TrPs were reported in 61% of patients with cardiac disease and treatment of this somatic dysfunction is an important factor in reducing reflex coronary artery spasm.[82] Reduction of chest pain in this particular situation, however, does not eliminate the need to clinically assess and treat the underlying cardiac condition.

Regional motion restriction of the entire functional superior thoracic inlet can be scanned on a supine patient by placing hands over the upper trapezius with thumbs placed posteriorly to contact the upper thoracic transverse processes and the fingers anteriorly curled into the infraclavicular region and upper ribs. Use enough pressure to move these tissues to a point where the fascia first begins to resist. Then sense their resiliency (ease) or resistance (drag) to sidebend the region right or left and to rotate the region right or left. Few individuals are perfectly symmetrical and 80% of asymptomatic individuals will demonstrate a fascial preference for sidebending and rotating the superior thoracic inlet complex to the right. This, alternating with the directional fascial preference pattern of left sidebending and rotation most commonly palpated for the craniocervical region above and thoracolumbar region below, is part of the common compensatory pattern of Zink.[23]

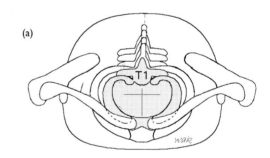

(a)

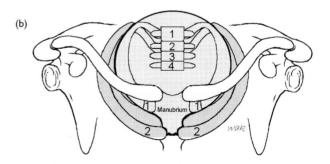

(b)

Figure 3.3.31 Thoracic inlet: (a) anatomical = T1, rib, manubrium, (b) functional = T1–4, rib 1–2, manubrium.

More specific tissue texture scanning for myofascial tender points and TrPs in the cervicothoracic region is warranted if historical, physical, or screening examinations indicate the need for more definitive information about somatic dysfunction. For example, myofascial points in the middle trapezii muscle fibers are commonly accompanied by a palpatory finding of C6, C7, and/or T1 and first rib somatic dysfunction.[77] Another reported association is the presence of any two or more dysfunctional vertebral units between C7 and T5 with rhomboid TrPs.[83] Travell and Simons report that this latter combination often appears as a flattened upper thoracic area centered around T3 with motion characteristics which are extended, sidebent, and rotated to the same side as the involved rhomboid muscle. Interestingly, these authors note that the rhomboid TrP resolves with manipulation of the T3 articular somatic dysfunction. Simple extension somatic dysfunctions of T1, T2, T3, and/or T4 vertebral units are found with bilateral posterior cervical TrPs.[84] Likewise, extended somatic dysfunction at T1 with inability to flex forward and an exquisitely tender T1 spinous process are findings commonly associated with serratus posterior superior TrPs.[85] In yet another example, ipsilateral upper thoracic and rib problems cause secondary suboccipital tension and tissue change that improves significantly after manipulative treatment of the primary problem.[86]

The interrelationship between myofascial dysfunction and articular dysfunction extends to the ribs and adjacent myofascial structures. In this region, Travell and Simons report that rib 1 articular somatic dysfunction often accompanies scalene muscle TrPs[87] and that both resolve with treatment of the TrP. Conversely, Lewit reports that rib 1 'blockage' (somatic dysfunction) is accompanied by reflex scalene muscle spasm that is abolished by manipulative treatment of that rib.[88]

Motion restriction for the first four thoracic vertebrae and the first two ribs may be diagnosed with the patient in a number of positions. In the seated position, screening typically consists of observing and palpating the sidebending curves created by applying vectors of force as shown in the modified acromion drop test (Figure 3.3.32). Asymmetric flattening of the thoracic sidebending curve or palpable resistance indicates the need for further scanning or local palpation.

Scanning and segmental examinations in any position can be accomplished by alternating pressures over upper thoracic transverse processes or through translation at successive levels of the thoracic spine. A sufficient amount of passive head–neck flexion and extension can also be easily introduced, allowing the physician to feel alternating upper thoracic interspinous gapping and approximation, respectively. Palpatory identification of end-barrier restriction to passive motion in any one plane warrants segmental diagnosis of the remaining planes. When placing fingertips to monitor motion characteristics at the same vertebral (segmental) level, the physician should remember that the transverse processes in the region of the upper thoracic spine (T1–3) are anatomically located at approximately the same horizontal level as their spinous processes. An alternative method for both scanning and segmental diagnosis in this region involves palpating the upper thoracic region with fingertips placed 2–3 cm on either side of the spinous process. The patient is directed to nod their head forward and then backwards until motion is induced at the palpated site. The aggravation or reduction of any palpated asymmetry indicates somatic dysfunction that can then be segmentally named. Interexaminer reliability studies demonstrate that different positions and different tests may result in different palpatory responses. Therefore designation of somatic dysfunction by its motion characteristics should include a description of both the patient's position and the test used.

The first two ribs are atypical compared to other ribs. The relatively immobile anterior synchondrosis of the first rib (R1) means that somatic dysfunction is more commonly palpated over the posterior aspect of the rib (dysfunction occurring at the rib head). Gently grasping just anterior to the superior trapezius border and retracting the tissues slightly posteriorly allows direct fingertip pressure over the posterolateral R1 shaft. Ipsilateral tenderness, superior unleveling, and

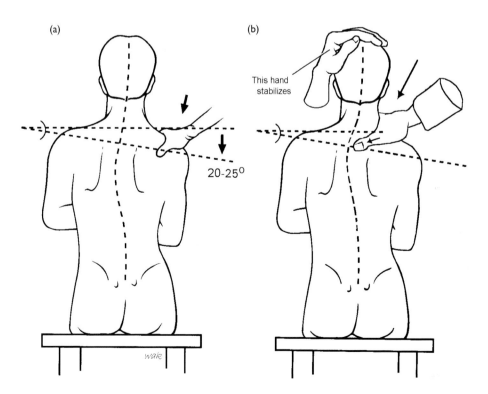

(a)   (b)

This hand stabilizes

20-25°

Figure 3.3.32 (a) Acromion drop test; (b) testing sidebending of the upper thoracic spine, with patient seated adding a translation component.

resistance to inferior compression are apparent in the more commonly found elevated first rib. The scalene muscles, attaching to the first two ribs, play a significant role in the diagnosis and treatment of the superior thoracic inlet region and somatic dysfunction of the first two ribs. Scalene muscle hypertonicity elevates the rib(s) attached to it, but an elevated first rib can cause a reflex contraction of the anterior scalene muscle.

Although much less common, scalene muscle fatigue or prolonged heavy direct pressure on the first rib may result in inferior subluxation of the first rib's posterior aspect. Clinically, this occurs in the respiratory accessory muscle fatigue occurring in patients with severe chronic obstructive pulmonary disease or in those carrying a heavy purse or backpack over one shoulder. With this condition, restriction is indicated when the inferior rib fails to rise with a deep inhalation.

Diagnosis of R1 somatic dysfunction is complicated by the fact that the superior thoracic inlet also manifests first rib asymmetry; however, in the superior thoracic inlet dysfunction the R1–T1 articulations function normally. Thus, coordinating the diagnostic and treatment sequences (discussed in Chapter 4.3.1) becomes very important.

The first and second ribs are both subject to acquiring inhalation and exhalation somatic dysfunction. These dysfunctions can also be initiated by the position of their respective thoracic vertebrae. Each of these can also affect the typical ribs and will be more completely discussed in the thoracic cage section below. Finally, segmental diagnosis of the manubrium, another important component of the functional superior thoracic inlet, is discussed in relationship to the body of the sternum and is presented in the thoracic cage section below.

Thoracic spine and thoracic cage

Specific regional scanning and local palpation for somatic dysfunction in the T5–12 thoracic region, chest cage, and/or any of its component parts (including the ribs and sternum) are indicated if the patient's history, physical, or screening examinations reveal the findings identified in Table 3.3.2. The anatomic relationship of the sympathetic

chain ganglia to the heads of each rib and the wide distribution of sympathetic fibers from cell bodies in the lateral horn of the thoracic region closely link somatic dysfunction of the thoracic cage to visceral and somatic problems throughout the body (Figure 3.3.33). With every respiratory cycle, numerous muscle groups and approximately 146 articulations in the thoracic cage are called upon to move. Thus, somatic dysfunction of component parts of the thoracic cage will have wide-ranging systemic, autonomic, and congestive implications. Therefore, the differential diagnosis must include common somatic problems such as costochondritis, other chest wall syndromes, and a wide range of pathologic and infectious processes.

In addition to thoracic, costal, and sternal somatic dysfunction, the preceding (cervicothoracic junction) and succeeding (thoracolumbar junction) sections present and direct functional connections relevant to this chapter. Likewise, dysfunction in the thoracic cage discussed in this section can be expected to influence function in the cervicothoracic and thoracolumbar junctional areas.

Pathologic change in the thoracic cage or of the viscera referring to the region affects the interpretation of somatic diagnostic clues as well as the choice of a treatment plan. Additional evaluation of the thoracic cage region should therefore include appropriate history and physical examination to rule out these processes.

- Any time diagnosis and treatment of somatic dysfunction in this region might be considered, a trauma and fracture history should be explored. Some forms of osteoporosis affect the anterior portion of the thoracic spine early in the process, increasing the importance of uncovering nutritional, metabolic, pharmacologic, and/or surgical risk factors associated with this pathophysiologic process. Likewise, both osteoporosis and bone metastases can result in spontaneous vertebral or rib fractures when minimal stress is applied to the bone. Thus, these conditions contraindicate most manipulative procedures over the involved site and constitute relative contraindications to certain types of manipulation applied generally.

- Evidence or absence of physical findings suggesting osteoporosis, thoracic kyphosis, or rotoscoliosis should be noted in the neuromusculoskeletal physician's examination, as these conditions affect treatment considerations.

- Visceral disorders stimulate afferents that, in turn, result in progressive and distinctive findings of secondary somatic dysfunction according to the autonomic innervations and sidedness of the involved viscus (Figure 3.3.34). Progression in the early visceral phase tends to be vague, poorly localized, and midline over the appropriate collateral ganglion. As the visceral condition progresses, somatic clues are added in the form of paraspinal tissue texture changes (more so than restricted motion), Chapman's intercostal reflexes, and rib somatic dysfunction. By the time the visceral problem ruptures or irritates adjacent visceral pleura/peritoneum, the peritoneocutaneous reflex localizes over viscus-specific sites (as in the appendix and its McBurney's point). These somatic findings in visceral disturbances have been extensively documented by osteopathic physicians in the USA,[10,41] by surgeons at the Mayo Clinic Foundation,[89] and by pain management specialists[90] worldwide.

Thoracic spinal areas

Segmental diagnosis of thoracic somatic dysfunction is quickly and easily accomplished in those areas identified through historical, physical, and/or screening processes. Segmental motion evaluation

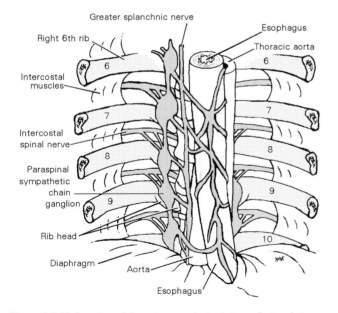

Figure 3.3.33 Location of thoracic sympathetic chain ganglia in relation to the rib heads.

Greater splanchnic nerve

Right 6th rib

Esophagus

Thoracic aorta

Intercostal muscles

Intercostal spinal nerve

Paraspinal sympathetic chain ganglion

Rib head

Diaphragm

Aorta

Esophagus

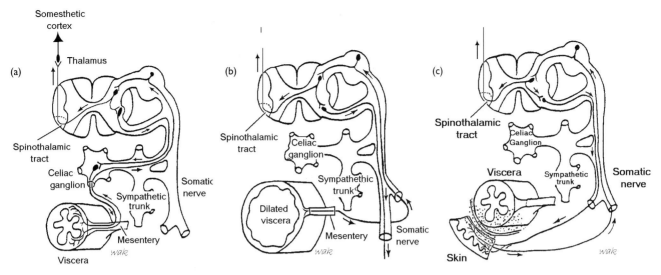

Figure 3.3.34 Visceral pain pathways: (a) visceral, (b) viscerosomatic, (c) pain pattern of Morley. Progression of somatic findings assists in diagnosing visceral disorders and their severity.

requires assessment of the end-feel quality of the barriers to rotation, sidebending, and flexion–extension. Finger placement in making these assessments must be precise and the motion characteristics coordinated for each segment. The 'thoracic rule of threes' is useful in guiding hand placement to corresponding thoracic spinous and transverse processes that progressively change their anatomic relationship from the upper to the lower portion of the thoracic vertebral column. Each group of three thoracic vertebral units demonstrates a different positional relationship (Figure 3.3.35). Once finger placement is assured, segmental motion can be assessed using passive or dynamic methods.

One test unique to the thoracic region is the so-called **shingle test of Kuchera.**[41] It involves placing medial pressure with one thumb on the lateral side of a spinous process at one thoracic level with a counterforce imposed by the other thumb on the spinous process of the thoracic vertebra below. The clinician's thumbs and the pressures are then reversed. Unopposed, pressure on a single spinous process in this manner would typically induce rotation, but in the thoracic region, where the facets lie relatively in a coronal plane, opposite rota-

tions induced at adjacent segments cancel one another. In this manner, only sidebending in the vertebral unit is allowed. Because thoracic spinous processes are situated below the AP axis of lateral flexion, the vertebral unit will attempt to sidebend to the side of the superior thumb (Figure 3.3.36a). In the shingle test of Kuchera, the quality of the end-feel determines the direction of sidebending; named for the freer motion. Similar thumb placement is employed in a **premanipulative test described by Maigne.**[91] In this test, Maigne first checks sidebending at a single thoracic level, seeking pain. When pain is identified, he then assesses for increased pain by adding a counterforce to the spinous process above and below the initial segment. Rather than specifically using this test to determine motion characteristics, Maigne uses the test to reinforce his 'rule of no pain and free motion' as shown in Figure 3.3.36b.

Specific passive motion testing of each of three planes in the thoracic region can be assessed in any position, although for this region it is most easily accomplished with the patient seated or prone. Alternating pressure over the transverse processes of each segment is applied and the end-feel of the barrier to rotation is assessed. Taking into consideration the thoracic rule of threes, translation or passively induced sidebending is applied to assess the quality of that barrier at each thoracic vertebral unit. The third plane of motion is assessed by passively testing interspinous approximation and separation. If there is vertebral unit somatic dysfunction, the quality of each barrier is restrictive in one direction and physiologic in the opposing direction. The combination of restrictive barriers determines whether type I or type II dysfunction is present. Pathologic change affecting spinal motion is the most prominent consideration in the differential diagnosis of somatic dysfunction. Pathologic change in the thoracic region most commonly presents with a capsular pattern of barrier restrictions in which limitation of extension exceeds that of flexion and is combined with varying degrees of restriction of sidebending and rotation in both directions.

In a diagnostic system called **dynamic motion examination** (Figure 2.2.10), the most useful test in this region involves monitoring change in the relationship of transverse process pairs during active forward

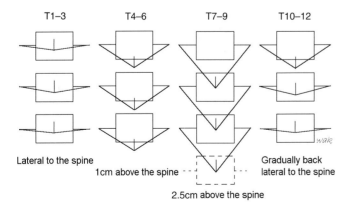

Figure 3.3.35 Location of transverse processes in relation to their spinous processes: 'rule of threes' for the thoracic region.

(a)

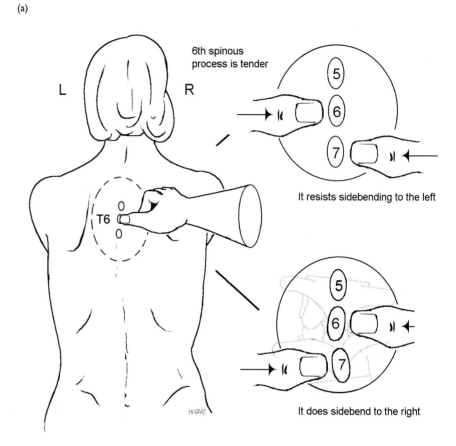

Figure 3.3.36 (a) 'Shingle test' of Kuchera for the thoracic spine. For example, the sixth spinous process is tender to palpation. Simultaneously, medial and opposite pressure is applied to the spinous processes of the sixth vertebral unit (T6 on T7) in one direction and then the other. Ease or resistance to movement is determined. Ease or resistance to rotations is then independently determined by using knowledge of the 'rule of threes' for the thoracic region. A direct method manipulative treatment is then set up to reverse the restriction in sidebending and rotation. The sagittal plane is used to localize the activating force at the dysfunctional vertebral unit. If rotation was also found to be restricted right, set-up would be to take sidebending left to its barrier, apply a fulcrum that will rotate T6 left, localize at T6 in the sagittal plane and apply the activating force. (From Kuchera WA, Kuchera ML. Osteopathic Principles in Practice. Columbus, Ohio: Greyden Press, 1994:532–533. (b) 'Shingle test' of Maigne. Medial pressure on a spinous process in the cervical, thoracic, or lumbar spine is found to be tender to the patient. Simultaneous and opposite pressure to the spinous process above and then to the spinous process below determines the direction for direct manipulation. Direct manipulation is given to the joint that is less tender when the test is applied. In this illustration, direct manipulation would be given to the T6 thoracic segment. (From Maigne R: Orthopedic Medicine, Charles C. Thomas, Springfield, IL, 1972: 97.)

(b)

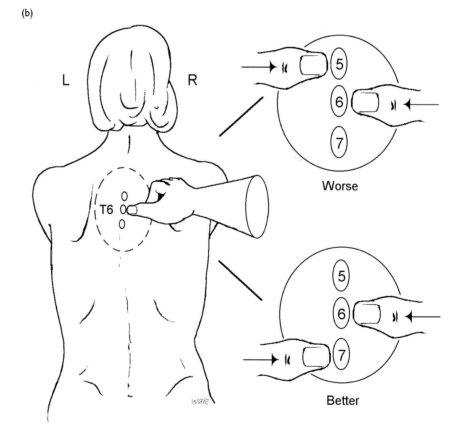

and backward bending motion from a neutral starting point. Two different **type II somatic dysfunction diagnoses** are possible in this region, using this method:

- The **extended, rotated and sidebent (ERS)** somatic dysfunction is diagnosed when the transverse process on one side becomes more prominent with forward bending and more symmetric with backward bending.

- The opposite findings are palpated in a **flexed, rotated and sidebent (FRS)** somatic dysfunction.

Both diagnoses typically involve a single vertebral unit and, in both, the sidebending and rotational restrictions are to the same side. The diagnosis of a **type I somatic dysfunction** typically involves three or more adjacent vertebral units. Dynamic motion testing in type I somatic dysfunction may change the asymmetry of transverse processes slightly, but symmetry is not achieved with either forward or with backward bending.

Specific tissue texture scanning for myofascial tender points and TrPs in the thoracic region is recommended when historical, physical, or screening examinations indicate the need for more definitive information about somatic dysfunction. These points are themselves a specific diagnosis of somatic dysfunction and that they commonly coexist with both thoracic articular and costal somatic dysfunction. As their functional anatomy suggests, the interrelationship between thoracic segmental somatic dysfunction and TrPs in the thoracic paraspinal muscles results in the following clinically observed generalities:[92,93]

- rotatores TrPs commonly induce single segment articular dysfunction at the same level

- multifidi TrPs are commonly seen with dysfunction of two or three adjacent segments

- semispinalis TrPs are often found with group thoracic somatic dysfunction extending over 4–6 vertebral units

- TrPs in the iliocostalis and longissimus muscles are also likely to be associated with group articular thoracic somatic dysfunction.

Greenman goes as far as to state that 'palpable muscle hypertonicity of the deepest muscle layers (of the erector spinae mass), including the multifidi and levator costales, is pathognomonic of vertebral motion segment dysfunction at that level'.[94]

Chest cage and typical costal areas

Diagnosis of this region includes evaluation of both costal and sternal elements of the thoracic cage. Specific diagnosis of ribs is usually delayed until thoracic vertebral somatic dysfunction is removed. Likewise, specific sternal diagnosis is delayed until rib somatic dysfunction is treated. These generalities exist because of the tremendous impact thoracic somatic dysfunction plays on rib function and that rib function plays on sternal function.

Ribs identified in the screening or scanning processes can be individually named according to their structural and respiratory characteristics. (Rib 1 subluxation was fully discussed in the previous section.)

Structural, traumatically induced rib dysfunction diagnoses include:

- **anterior or posterior subluxation:** These ribs exhibit hypermobility and are palpably displaced anteriorly or posteriorly along the axis of motion between the costovertebral and costotransverse articulations. Palpatory findings include a less prominent rib angle with anterior subluxation and a more prominent rib angle with posterior subluxation.

- **torsion:** This characteristic often occurs in conjunction with thoracic rotation (affecting ribs on both sides) and, unless remodeling of the rib shaft takes place over time, should return to normal bilateral symmetry when the thoracic spine returns to a symmetrical position. With T4 rotation to the right on T5, for example, rib 5 on the right would demonstrate external torsion along its long axis resulting in palpable prominence at the superior border of the rib angle and the inferior border of the sternal end. Internal torsion of the left fifth rib would be present with sharper inferior border palpated posteriorly and a sharper superior border palpated anteriorly.

- **anteroposterior or lateral compression:** Trauma from an anteroposterior or a lateral direction may result in sustained deformation. In anteroposterior compression, there is a palpably increased rib shaft prominence in the midaxillary line and decreased prominence anteriorly and posteriorly. In lateral compression of a rib, the palpable prominence is found anteriorly and posteriorly with less prominence in the midaxillary line.

Respiratory characteristics and the location of restricted motion also permit useful diagnostic nomenclature for rib dysfunction. These respiratory dysfunction diagnoses include:

- **Pump-handle or bucket-handle costal somatic dysfunction:** The axis of respiratory motion of ribs 2–10 is influenced by a number of factors including the angle between the body of the thoracic vertebra and the transverse processes (Figure 3.3.37) and the motion of the sternum. In the absence of a true anteroposterior or lateral axis, each of these ribs has a mixture of 'pump-handle' motion (maximally assessed on the anterior chest wall) and 'bucket-handle' motion (maximally assessed on the lateral aspects of the chest wall). By their anatomy, the upper ribs typically have a higher percentage of pump-handle to bucket-handle motion whereas the lower typical ribs have a higher percentage of bucket-handle type motion. In springing the rib cage for restriction, both the anterior and the lateral aspects of the chest cage should be scanned for dysfunction. Likewise in assessing respiratory motion, both anterior and lateral aspects of suspicious ribs should be assessed. Motion loss to either springing or to a portion of the respiratory cycle that is noted anteriorly is described as pump-handle dysfunction; motion loss noted laterally is consistent with bucket-handle dysfunction.

- **Inhalation or exhalation costal somatic dysfunction:** Costal motion with respiration should be assessed both parasternally (pump-handle component of respiration) and along the lateral chest wall (bucket-handle respiratory component). Rib motion of each rib failing the screening or scanning process is compared to its corresponding rib on the other side of the body. Palpating digits straddle each pair of ribs being tested and the patient is instructed to take a full breath in and to let their breath out. During one phase of the respiratory cycle, the rib with restricted motion will stop moving prior to the normal side. The costal dysfunction is named for the respiratory component that is permitted. An inhalation right fifth rib dysfunction, for example, will have palpatory findings in which both fifth ribs rise in inhalation but, during continued exhalation,

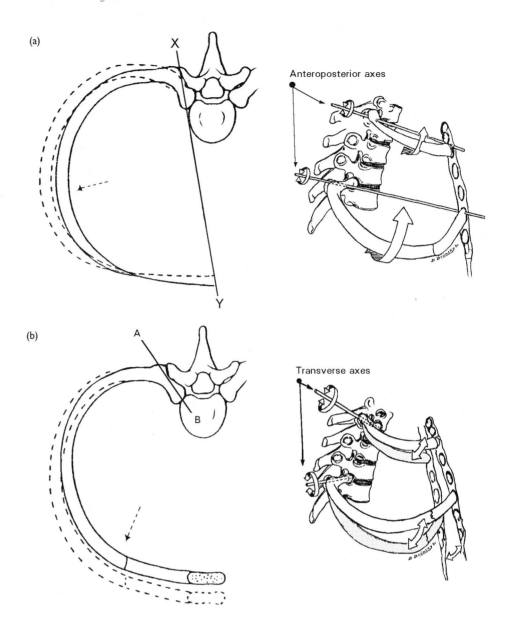

Figure 3.3.37 (a) Bucket-handle rib motion, (b) Pump-handle rib motion.

the right fifth rib stops moving while the left continues inferiorly. Note that the eleventh and twelfth ribs, without an anterior sternal attachment, have more of a pincer or caliper motion, exhibiting a posterolateral motion during inhalation and an anteromedial motion during exhalation. In general, inhalation rib dysfunction often involves several ribs. Conversely, exhalation rib dysfunction often arises in patients with a persistent cough wherein localized spasm of an intercostal muscle typically results in an exhalation dysfunction of a single rib.

The thoracic cage is host to a number of myofascial points which by their location and clinical correlations can be subdivided into Jones' tender points, Travell/Simons TrPs, and Chapman's reflex points (Figures 3.3.9 and 3.3.38). The system described by Lawrence Jones in his strain–counterstrain system[95] is associated with locally tender myofascial points that do not refer pain. The Travell/Simons somatic points trigger empirically mapped musculoskeletal pain or visceral dysfunction. Chapman's points[37,96] appear coincident with visceral problems and are interpreted as secondary viscerosomatic findings.

Jones' system recognizes the coexistence of costal dysfunction and related tenderpoints on the anterior and/or posterior chest wall at specific sites. Simons and Travell also record the common coexistence of TrPs with rib somatic dysfunction:

- pectoralis minor TrPs with inhalation R3, R4, and/or R5 costal somatic dysfunction[97]

- serratus anterior TrPs with pain and palpatory findings anywhere between R2–9, difficult to differentiate from inhalation costal dysfunction[98]

- abdominal TrPs with exhalation somatic dysfunction in the ipsilateral lower half of the rib cage.[99]

Exhalation costal somatic dysfunction at one or two rib levels also responds well to inactivation of the commonly associated TrPs in intercostal muscles attaching to these ribs.[100]

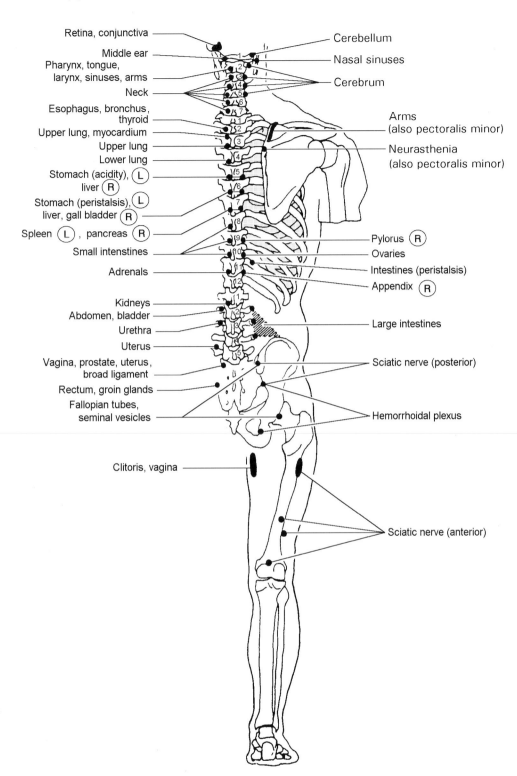

Retina, conjunctiva
Middle ear
Pharynx, tongue, larynx, sinuses, arms
Neck
Esophagus, bronchus, thyroid
Upper lung, myocardium
Upper lung
Lower lung
Stomach (acidity), (L) liver (R)
Stomach (peristalsis), (L) liver, gall bladder (R)
Spleen (L), pancreas (R)
Small intestines
Adrenals
Kidneys
Abdomen, bladder
Urethra
Uterus
Vagina, prostate, uterus, broad ligament
Rectum, groin glands
Fallopian tubes, seminal vesicles
Clitoris, vagina

Cerebellum
Nasal sinuses
Cerebrum
Arms (also pectoralis minor)
Neurasthenia (also pectoralis minor)
Pylorus (R)
Ovaries
Intestines (peristalsis)
Appendix (R)
Large intestines
Sciatic nerve (posterior)
Hemorrhoidal plexus
Sciatic nerve (anterior)

Figure 3.3.38 Posterior Chapman's tender points. All are bilateral except where indicated as R for right and L for left. See also anterior Chapman's diagnostic points (Figure 3.3.9).

Sternal area

The sternum is also subject to somatic dysfunction. This is especially true after a motor vehicle accident in which asymmetrical forces from the shoulder harness portion of the seatbelt are transmitted into the sternum, or in the case of cardiac surgery in which the sternum is wired back together. The manubrium and the sternal body are inde- pendently assessed for their preference to forward or backward bending, sidebending, and rotation. As in other forms of somatic dys- function, restriction in one direction is accompanied by freedom in the opposite direction. Diagnostic testing of various somatic dysfunc- tion combinations of the manubrium, sternal body, and sternal unit is shown in Figures 3.3.39, 3.3.40, and 3.3.41 respectively.

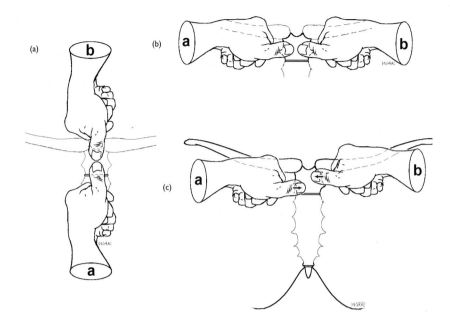

Figure 3.3.39 Diagnosis of manubrium:
(a) flexion or extension, (b) rotation, (c) sidebending.

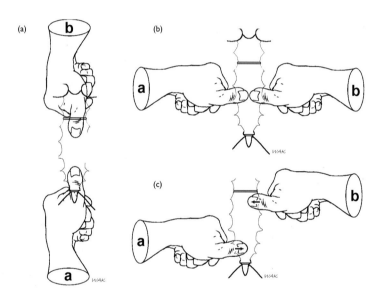

Figure 3.3.40 Diagnosis of gladiolus: (a) flexion or
extension, (b) rotation, (c) sidebending.

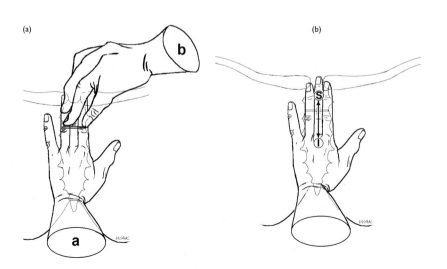

Figure 3.3.41 Diagnosis of the sternum as a whole:
(a) 'plastic hand' method, (b) single hand for F/E,
superior or inferior glide, rotation, sidebending.

Diagnosis of the sternum often is delayed until other components of the thoracic cage are treated as sternal motion is significantly affected by dysfunction of the ribs that are, in turn, significantly influenced by their thoracic vertebral attachments.

Thoracolumbar junction/inferior thoracic outlet and lumbar spine

While the anatomical thoracolumbar junction of the spine occurs between T12 and L1, the functional inferior thoracic outlet includes the lower rib cage as well as several vertebral segments above and below T12–L1. Regional scanning and local palpation for somatic dysfunction in the thoracolumbar junction, the inferior thoracic outlet, and/or any of their component parts are most likely to be indicated if a patient manifests any of the history, physical, or screening examination findings identified in Table 3.3.1. Furthermore, dysfunction or compensation occurring in regions above and below affects this transitional region.

As with the rest of the thoracic cage, pathologic processes including metastasis significantly affect the interpretation of somatic findings and their treatment. Metastasis in this region is a contraindication to several types of manipulation. Batson's valveless venous plexus of veins in the lumbar spinal region drains the pelvic organs and provides a low-pressure area predisposing the region to metastasis of regional cancers, such as those arising in the prostate.[101] Patients with low back pain, especially if it awakens them at night or is accompanied by weight loss or other systemic symptomatology, should therefore have a careful and thorough history and examination of those systems from which metastasis to bone is likely. These additional local and systemic historical and physical examinations are warranted, regardless of the presence or absence of regional somatic dysfunction.

Lumbosacral radiculopathies are not absolute contraindications to any manual technique in this region, but both palpatory and a neurologic examinations are warranted in patients with significant low back pain with or without radiation to one or both lower extremities. Delineation between dermatomal, myotomal, and sclerotomal referral patterns helps the neuromusculoskeletal clinician differentiate between the many causes of low back pain with or without such referral. **Dermatomal** pain is widely recognized, both in distribution and quality. Conversely, **sclerotomal** pain is little known and is characteristically described as a deep, dull toothache or arthritic in quality. **Myotomal** involvement can lead to muscle cramps and/or TrPs; individual muscles may test weak or they may be hypertonic from overuse. Ligamentous pain tends to be sclerotomal; severe myofascial TrPs often demonstrate characteristics of both myotomal and sclerotomal patterns.

Recognize that pain and/or dysesthesia can be caused or referred by either neurologic or somatic structures in patients with lumbar disk disease, spondylolistheses, and severe lumbar degenerative change. To better illustrate the importance of assessing each of the possible somatic structures involved in the differential diagnosis of this region, see Figure 3.3.42. Note the similarity in the distribution of an S1 radiculopathy due to a herniated disk, a gluteus minimus myofascial trigger point due to hip dysfunction, and posterior sacroiliac ligament strain due to sacroiliac shear somatic dysfunction.

Thoracolumbar junction area

Common musculoskeletal and visceral disorders found to have significant somatic dysfunction in this area are:

- quadratus lumborum TrPs and/or iliolumbar ligament strain
- psoas syndrome
- viscerosomatic referral from the kidneys, gonads, intestines, bladder, or uterus
- signs and/or symptoms of hypertension, dysmenorrhea, or constipation.

(a)   (b)   (c)

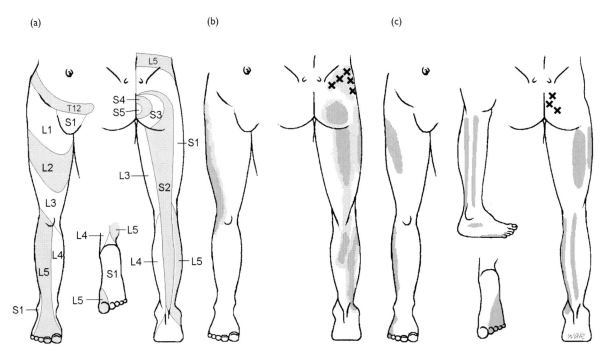

Figure 3.3.42 (a) Radiculopathy (dermatome of LE), (b) gluteus minimus trigger points (Travell), (c) posterior sacroiliac ligament pain (Hackett).

Additionally, the importance of this area through its attachments to the thoracic diaphragm make it a major consideration for somatic dysfunction in the presence of reduced diaphragm motion and in generalized congestive phenomena.

In supine patients, regional thoracolumbar motion is evaluated by exerting rotational and translational pressures over the lower rib cage (Figure 3.3.43) to the point where the fasciae first begin to resist. The physician evaluates for asymmetrical motion characteristics of resiliency (ease) and resistance (drag) in sidebending and rotation, bearing mind that 80% of asymptomatic individuals will demonstrate a fascial preference for sidebending and rotating this inferior thoracic outlet region to the left.[23]

A number of regional screening and scanning examinations identify the need for specific segmental diagnosis of thoracolumbar and lumbar somatic dysfunction. The most commonly used screening tests (Figure 3.3.44), include the hip drop test, trunk sidebending and trunk rotation tests, Schober's test, and the prone lumbar springing test. Infrequently performed tests extend to the observation that a positive skin-rolling test over the buttocks may indicate thoracolumbar dysfunction.[102]

Should historical, physical, or screening examinations indicate the need for more definitive information about the myofascial component of somatic dysfunction, specific tissue texture scanning for posterior myofascial tender points and TrPs in the thoracolumbar junction

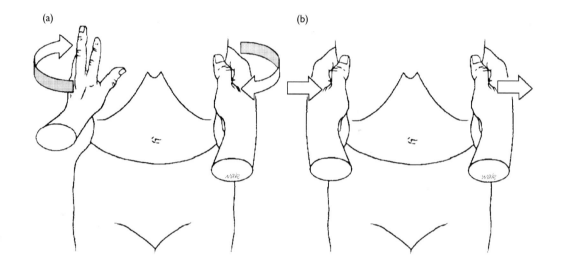

Figure 3.3.43 Inferior thoracic outlet regional motion: (a) right rotational screen, (b) left translation screen (sidebending right). In each case, reverse test and compare end-feel.

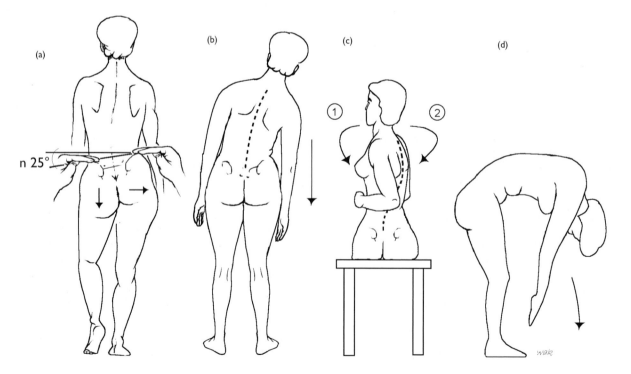

Figure 3.3.44 (a) Hip drop test, (b) sidebending of spine, (c) thoracolumbar rotation, (d) spinal flexion (including Schober's test).

region would provide significant information. Travell and Simons point out that it is common to find articular somatic dysfunction spanning several segments from T7 to L4 in patients with myofascial points in the latissimus dorsi muscles.[103] With these dysfunctions, typically vertebral sidebending occurs toward and rotation occurs away from the involved muscles. Lumbar segmental somatic dysfunction is also commonly seen in patients with myofascial points in the lumbar paraspinal muscles.[104] Here, single-segment articular dysfunction is more likely to be induced by rotators at the same level while multifidi TrPs involve two or three adjacent and semispinalis TrPs involve group lumbar somatic dysfunction extending over 4–6 vertebral units.[105] The authors also note group articular lumbar somatic dysfunction is found with iliocostalis TrPs. The most common articular somatic dysfunctions associated with serratus posterior inferior muscle TrPs are simple T10–L2 dysfunctions that sidebend in one direction and rotate the other. Occasionally TrPs in this muscle will be linked with exhalation somatic dysfunction involving the ipsilateral lower four ribs.[106]

Another extremely common combination of somatic dysfunction findings consists of psoas and quadratus lumborum TrPs in patients with articular somatic dysfunction at the thoracolumbar junction[107] as well as shortened rectus abdominis muscles with palpable TrPs.[107] This is a portion of the total pattern described for gravitational strain pathophysiology[21] and postural decompensation. TrPs in the quadratus lumborum are reportedly the most common and most commonly overlooked cause of myogenic low back pain.[108]

Lumbar area

In those patients identified through historical, physical, and/or screening processes to benefit from a 'low back' examination, segmental lumbar somatic dysfunction is quickly and easily diagnosed. Screening may involve the previously mentioned hip drop test (Figure 3.3.44a) or lumbar spring test.

In lumbar somatic dysfunction, the quality of each barrier is restrictive in one direction and physiologic in the opposing direction. The combination of restrictive barriers determines whether type I or type II dysfunction is present. Pathologic change affecting spinal motion is the most prominent consideration in the differential diagnosis of somatic dysfunction. Pathologic change, such as occurs in degenerative joint disease, most commonly presents with a capsular pattern of barrier restrictions which, in the lumbar region, involves marked but symmetrical limitation of sidebending accompanied by lesser limitation of both flexion and extension. The sagittal plane capsular barriers arising from degenerative and inflammatory processes (such as ankylosing spondylitis) create a positive Schober's test (Figure 3.3.44d).

A number of structural changes predispose to dysfunction in this region. These may be suspected for example with palpation of a drop-off sign between lumbar spinous processes as is common in spondylolisthesis (Figure 3.3.45) or with an isolated midline lumbar tuft of hair as is seen in spina bifida occulta. Spina bifida occulta and isthmic spondylolisthesis have their highest incidence at L5 and S1. Although spina bifida occulta itself is not painful, it is commonly associated with other posterior lumbosacral congenital defects, a higher incidence of acquired isthmic spondylolisthesis, and potential alteration of muscular attachments and function. L5–S1 isthmic spondylolisthesis, affecting 3% of the US population, is associated with extremely high biomechanical risk factors for pathophysiologic stress and strain of posterior lumbosacral support structures.[21,109] Furthermore, patients with the dysplastic form of spondylolisthesis have lumbopelvic articu-

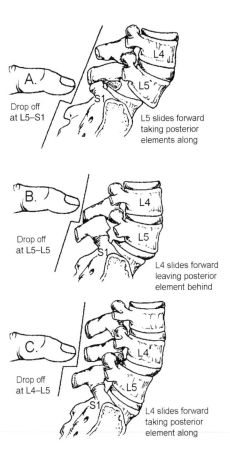

Figure 3.3.45
Drop-off sign.

lar facets that are nearly horizontal and as such, they are poorly designed to support upright postural gravitational stress.

For segmental motion evaluation in somatic dysfunction, the quality of the end-feel of barriers to rotation, sidebending, and flexion–extension is assessed. Finger placement must be precise and the motion characteristics coordinated for each segment. Specific passive triplanar motion testing can be individually assessed in any position, although for this region it is most easily accomplished in the lumbar region with the patient seated or prone. Alternating pressure over the transverse processes of a segment assesses the end-feel of the barrier to rotation at that level. Note that the transverse processes in this region are located essentially in the same horizontal plane as the spinous process of the same vertebra. (In the case of L5, where the anatomy precludes actually palpating transverse processes, the clinician should palpate as far laterally as possible on symmetric portions of the L5 posterior arch.) Translation or passively induced sidebending is applied to assess the quality of that barrier at the same vertebral level. Passively testing interspinous approximation or separation permits assessment of the sagittal plane of motion.

In applying the dynamic motion testing method, patients capable of doing so can change position to permit the clinician to monitor change in the relationship of pairs of lumbar transverse processes. The transverse processes (or lateral posterior arches of L5) are palpated in neutral, extended (sphinx position), and forward bent positions (Figure 3.3.46). As in the thoracic region, two different type II somatic dysfunction diagnoses are possible in this region, ERS or FRS. The ERS somatic dysfunction is diagnosed when the transverse process on one side will become more prominent with forward bending and more

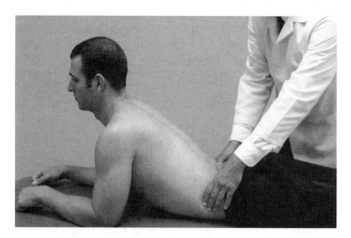

Figure 3.3.46 Prone to sphinx position creates extension in the lumbar spine and sacral nutation (forward bending). Dynamic motion testing may be performed from multiple start positions.

symmetric with backward bending. The opposite findings are palpated in an FRS somatic dysfunction. Both diagnoses typically involve a single vertebral unit and, in both, the sidebending and rotational restrictions are to the same side. The diagnosis of a type I somatic dysfunction typically involves three or more adjacent vertebral units. Dynamic motion testing in type I somatic dysfunction may change the asymmetry of transverse processes slightly, but symmetry is not achieved with either forward or with backward bending.

Pelvis (innominates, pubic symphysis, sacrum, and coccyx) and lumbopelvic junction

This area is strategically located for significant impact on gait, low back function, and postural balance. Therefore, numerous lumbopelvic pain generators have been identified, pain patterns have been mapped, and models have been described to categorize the role of various somatic structures in patient complaints. At the same time, regionally, the pelvis and lumbopelvic junction contain more musculoskeletal congenital anomalies than any other body region. Asymmetry of the lumbar facets (tropism) and sacroiliac joints, important in assessing motion characteristics and the direction of manipulation treatment activation, are ubiquitous. As a consequence of these factors, more variation in lumbopelvic biomechanical models exists amongst different manual medicine schools than perhaps in any other region.

Key differential diagnostic considerations for somatic dysfunction in this region include recognition of hypermobility, structural change due to rheumatologic or degenerative disorders, as well as pain and pathology associated with a malignancy or other severe pathologic condition.

Because certain arthritic, degenerative, or inflammatory processes first become symptomatic in this region (in young men, for instance, ankylosing spondylitis may begin insidiously, resulting in progressive regional motion loss), additional evaluation should therefore include a number of screening palpatory and neurologic tests including tests for stability and mobility as well as screening for possible significant pathologic processes.

● In cases of low back pain of unknown origin, documentation of the presence or absence of pertinent 'red flag' signs and symptoms should appear in the patient record. These include a progressive history of the chief complaint and its response to lying down, movement, or coughing, as well as a detailed description of any neurologic radiation of pain, dysesthesia, or muscle weakness. Record any associated weight loss or disturbance of bowel or bladder function, or functional disturbance such as pain waking the patient at night or limiting the ability to walk more than a short distance. A complete neurologic examination of the low back and lower extremities should also be recorded. Differential diagnostic considerations will often mandate rectal and/or vaginal examinations to rule out primary pathologic sources permitting a simultaneous palpatory examination of coccygeal and pelvic floor S.T.A.R. characteristics.

● Physical findings such as uveitis, urethritis, or pitting of the nails may indicate associated premature sacroiliac fusion or severe rheumatologic disorder, and suggest the need for laboratory or radiographic tests.

● It is a serious sign if the patient experiences more pain when the lower extremity is raised with the hip passively flexed on the trunk and with the knee bent, than when a typical straight leg raising test is performed. This positive 'sign of the buttock' test[110] could indicate iliac metastasis, chronic septic SI arthritis, ischiorectal abscess, sacral fracture, gluteal bursitis, or involvement of the upper femur with neoplasm, bursitis, or osteomyelitis.

Different somatic structures within this region have a significant effect on the function and dysfunction of adjacent structures. For example, sacroiliac articular somatic dysfunction coexists in patients with myofascial points in the quadratus lumborum muscles while both latissimus dorsi and quadratus lumborum TrPs are accompanied by innominate dysfunction.[111] Pubic and innominate dysfunctions are commonly associated with abdominal TrPs.[112] TrPs in the iliocostalis lumborum are associated with pelvic obliquity secondary to the muscle's insertional aponeurosis onto the sacral base that leads to sacroiliac dysfunction.[113] In this latter case, the positive seated flexion test will be worse than the standing flexion test.[114]

Somatic structures in adjacent regions also have a significant effect on lumbopelvic function and dysfunction. This is clearly the synopsis of clinical experts in the interdisciplinary text, *Movement, stability and low back pain: the essential role of the pelvis*,[115] in interpreting the lumbopelvic region. One conclusion is that the ultimate balance between regional stability and mobility (Figure 3.3.47) rests, in part, on form closure contributed by the shape of the sacrum and its angle of nutation/counternutation and, in part, on the proper function of the myofascial *Unterkreuz*[19] in contributing force closure.[116]

Finally, it should be noted upon careful review of Table 3.3.2 that the importance of the sacral base as the foundation upon which the spine sits extends the impact of dysfunction here far beyond the lumbopelvic area. Thus, regional examination of all areas of the musculoskeletal system is warranted in the presence of an unlevel sacral base. Unleveling of the sacral base is well documented to be a precipitating and perpetuating cause of muscle imbalance and myofascial TrPs throughout the entire body[117] as well as a cause of recurrent patterns of somatic dysfunction.[22,118] In addition, segmental facilitated spinal dysfunction arising in compensation for an unlevel sacral base is capable of creating a wide range of visceral and systemic symptomatology.

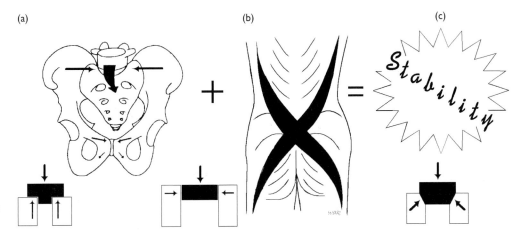

Figure 3.3.47 **(a)** Form closure, (b) force closure, and (c) sacroiliac static–dynamic mechanics. (From Spine: state of the art review, 1995, **9** 463–90.)

Lumbopelvic and sacroiliac (sacrum and/or iliac origin) areas

Patients present to neuromusculoskeletal medicine physicians with low back (lumbopelvic) more so than any other area of the body, with the possible exception of headache. Neuromusculoskeletal physicians have moved significantly beyond the historically unifocal preoccupation with discogenic back pain.[119] Farfan, for example, described the cause of low back pain as mechanical[120] and numerous pain generators are influenced by biomechanical stress and strain. In somatic dysfunction, the lumbar zygopophyseal joints,[121,122] the muscular elements associated with lumbopelvic function and dysfunction,[123] and the sacroiliac joint itself[124,125] are key pain generators. Although the latter component is perhaps the most 'controversial',[126] sacroiliac joint dysfunction is acknowledged to play an 'incontrovertible'[127] role in a number of locally painful spinal disorders. Furthermore, Travell and Simons[128] and others[21] noted the major role of postural imbalance and sacroiliac dysfunction in the perpetuation and precipitation of pain and dysfunction in this region.

Regional scanning and local palpation of the lumbopelvic junction, the pelvic girdle, and its component parts for somatic dysfunction are most likely to be indicated for patients with the presence of the historical, physical, or screening examination findings identified previously in Table 3.3.2. Here different relative symmetry of key structures and their palpatory motion characteristics provide clues to naming dysfunction but, here, diagnosis also depends largely upon the model used for interpretation.

Lumbopelvic regional restriction of motion may be scanned in the supine patient by first gently placing one hand over one anterior superior iliac spine (ASIS) and reaching across to the opposite side to gently grasp the pelvis posterior to the gluteus medius muscle to lift in a manner to rotate the pelvis on the lumbar spine. Alternating palpation of left and right rotation of the region evaluates for resiliency (ease) or resistance (drag). Gently grasping both sides of the pelvis laterally, just below the iliac crests, and translating the pelvis right and left with respect to the lumbar region, assesses the point where the fasciae first begin to resist sidebending. Few individuals are perfectly symmetrical and 80% of asymptomatic individuals will demonstrate a fascial preference for sidebending and rotating of the pelvic complex at the lumbopelvic junction to the right.[23]

Commonly overlooked pain-generating skeletal, arthrodial and myofascial structures include the quadratus lumborum,[128] iliolumbar ligament,[21] and somatic dysfunction originating in this region as a consequence of a half dozen diagnoses[129] including:

- short leg and pelvic tilt syndrome
- type II lumbar somatic dysfunction
- pubic shear somatic dysfunction
- innominate shear somatic dysfunction
- sacral somatic dysfunction restricting nutation (anterior rotation)
- muscle imbalance and dysfunction.

TrPs in the quadratus lumborum (Figure 3.3.48) are noted to be 'one of the most commonly overlooked muscular sources of low back pain' and is often responsible, through satellite gluteus minimus TrPs (Figure 3.3.42b), for the pseudo-disc syndrome and the failed surgical back syndrome.[130] It was also the most commonly involved muscle (32%) in soldiers with musculoskeletal complaints.[131] TrPs in this muscle responded to a variety of manual techniques directed to the muscle itself including massage, tapotement, and postisometric muscle energy manipulative treatment[107,132] (see Chapter 4.3.1). This diagnosis also frequently required correction of underlying muscle imbalance, short leg and pelvic tilt syndrome, sacroiliac somatic dysfunction, and twelfth rib somatic dysfunction to prevent recurrence.

The iliolumbar ligament is positioned to provide stability between the lumbar spine and the pelvis. It is consequently one of the first structures to indicate biomechanical dysfunction in the region. Iliolumbar

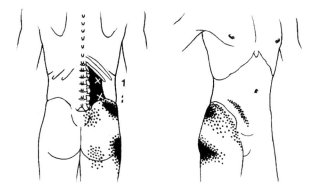

Figure 3.3.48 Quadratus lumborum trigger point pattern.[123]

ligament stress arises from the same biomechanical factors listed for the quadratus lumborum above and has a very similar pain pattern.[133]

The value of diagnosing lumbar and pelvic (sacral, innominate, and pubic) somatic dysfunction is well established in the literature. In a study by Greenman of 183 consecutive patients presenting with disabling low back pain (average duration 30.7 months), three or more of the so-called 'dirty half dozen'[134] somatic dysfunction diagnoses listed above were found in 50% of the population. Correction of the dysfunction through integrated rehabilitative means including manual medicine resulted in restoration of normal activities of daily living (including return to work) in 75% of these patients.

Unfortunately, structure–function interrelationships become especially difficult to evaluate and interpret properly in the presence of anomalies such as sacralization of L5, lumbarization of S1, batwing transverse processes that may or may not have their own articulations with the ilium, and combinations of these and other structural variations at the same spinal level. For these reasons, a significant number of additional screening and scanning examination have been described to assist the clinician in focusing his or her examination. The most commonly used screening and scanning tests have already been described and include:

- **tests for lateralization** including standing flexion test, seated flexion test (also called the Piedallu test or lock sign), and/or ASIS compression test

- direct **dynamic tests** for general restriction of sacroiliac motion including the one-legged stork test (also called the spine test by Dvorak, Gillet's test, and march/stork test) as a variation of the Trendelenburg test or indirect passive examination using long sitting tests (yo-yo sign) and hip rotation tests, and/or the SI gapping test.

- a variety of **pelvic ligamentous stress tests** (Figure 3.3.49) including the cranial shear test, pelvic distraction and compression tests, SI gapping test (also known as the thigh thrust SI stress test, the posterior pelvic pain provocation test, the FADE test and the POSH test), sacral thrust test, Gaenslen's test, Yeoman's test, and/or variations of Patrick's FABERE (or figure 4) test

- generic identification of sacroiliac dysfunction has been shown to be significant if the patient **using a single finger**[135] twice localizes a site (within 1 cm) inferomedial to the PSIS with or without stressing the joint with a Patrick's test – this noting that five other structures attach

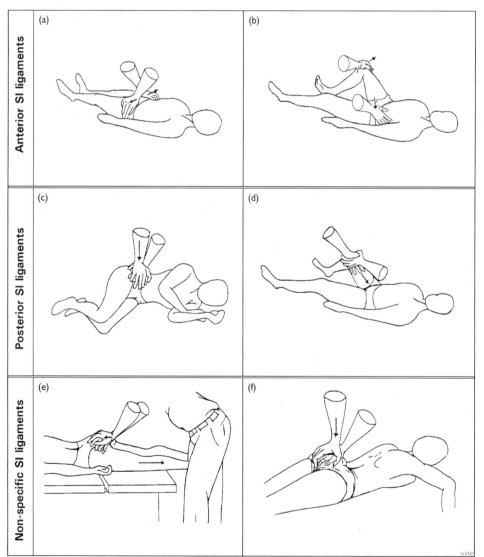

Figure 3.3.49 Tests of pelvic ligaments:
(a) distraction test,
(b) springing during Patrick–FABERE test,
(c) compression test,
(d) sacroiliac gapping (vary thigh angle for S1, S2, S3), (e) cranial shear test, (f) sacral 'thrust' test.

Anterior SI ligaments

Posterior SI ligaments

Non-specific SI ligaments

or are located within 1.5 cm of the PSIS (the L5/S1 facet joint, sacrospinalis, L5/S1 intervertebral disk, gluteus maximus, and SI joint)

- **local motion screening tests** through springing of various areas of the pelvic girdle or through positional changes.

Each of the above tests may be used in screening or scanning the pelvic region for dysfunction. (In this section, dysfunction at the L5–S1 junction will be discussed as part of pelvic somatic dysfunction. Further insights for the lumbopelvic area can also be obtained in the lumbar section above.)

Sacroiliac joint

In the widely adopted osteopathic models, three major systems have had significant impact on the nomenclature now commonly employed. Each of these historic systems examined sacral motion as it related to a different anatomic relationship.

- In the **Strachan (HVLA) model**,[136,137] diagnosis of the sacrum is named largely with respect to its motion, or restriction, relative to the innominates.

- In the **Mitchell (muscle energy) model**,[138] a series of postulated sacral axes is coupled with diagnoses of sacral torsions to reflect sacral motion, or restriction, relative to the lumbar spine and the mechanics of gait.

- In the **Sutherland (craniosacral) model**,[61] motion, or restriction, of the sacrum is described relative to the cranium. Regardless of the model selected, each diagnosis of somatic dysfunction implies freedom in one direction of motion around an axis with restriction in the opposite direction.

Each model has relative benefits depending on the clinical situation, the degree of training of the physician, and the type of manual treatment that will be used to treat the dysfunction. Recognition that differing models exist and that nomenclature is model-specific helps manual medicine physicians greatly in sorting through the literature that would otherwise seem contradictory. For a more complete discussion, refer to the chapter on sacrum and pelvis in the standard text, *Foundations for osteopathic medicine*.[139]

This portion of the chapter limits nomenclature and diagnostic tests to be consistent with the treatment examples presented in Chapter 4.3.1. It considers somatic dysfunction of the sacrum relative to motions around postulated transverse, oblique, and vertical axes as well as one traumatically induced dysfunction (inferior sacral shear) not associated with an axis of motion. A suggested series of local palpatory tests for ascertaining the symmetry of sacral landmarks and the quality of motion available is depicted in Figure 3.3.50. Their interpretation is described more fully in Tables 3.3.3 and 3.3.4.

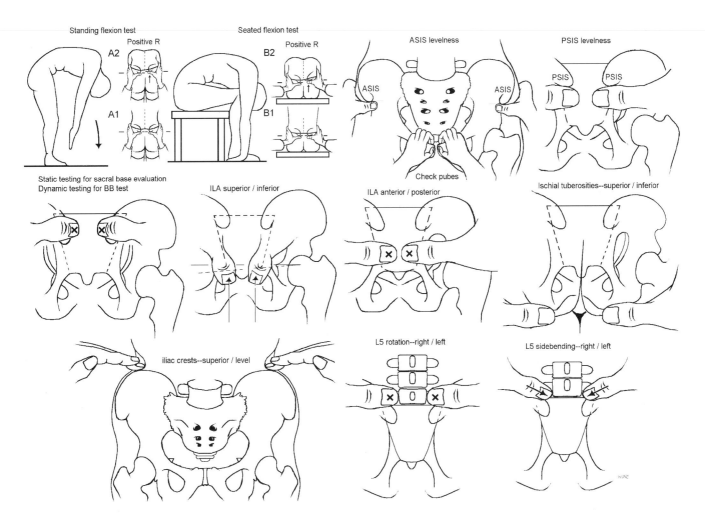

Figure 3.3.50 Palpation series for gathering pelvic somatic dysfunction data.

Table 3.3.3. Examination for somatic dysfunction of the sacroiliac articulation

Step	Patient's position	Examination	Results and postulated interpretation
1	Standing	Evaluate anatomic landmarks, standing flexion test	A positive standing flexion test means dysfunction in the lower extremity an/or pelvis on that side
2	Seated	Perform seated flexion test	Will specifically determine whether there is a sacroiliac dysfunction, and if so, which side (but not which arm) of the sacroiliac joint is dysfunctional
3	Supine	Perform ASIS compression test; positional assessment of ASISs, pubic tubercles, and medial malleoli	Helps determine the etiology of the problem and whether it is purely sacral or a mixed problem, incorporating iliac and pubic dysfunction
4	Prone	Palpate for tissue texture changes, motion testing of the sacrum, motion testing of L5, ligamentous tension testing	Helps the physician discover which axis is involved, find what portion of the SI joint is restricted, determine L5 motion and position, and evaluate pelvic ligamentous tensions

Adapted from Heinking, Jones, and Kappler Pelvis and sacrum In: Ward, R. C., *Foundations for osteopathic medicine*, Williams and Wilkins, Baltimore, 1997.

Table 3.3.4. Sacral somatic dysfunction exemplars

Constellation of static and dynamic findings for common diagnoses of sacral somatic dysfunction	Sacral base anterior (bilateral sacral flexion)	Left rotation on a left oblique axis	Right rotation on left oblique axis	Sacral margin posterior on the left	Left sacral shear (left lateral "uni-lateral" sacral flexion)
Static findigs palpated over sacrum					
Lateralization tests (e.g. restricted side to ASIS springing; longest-last motion in seated flexion test)	NA	Right commonly reported – theoretically either left upper or right lower pole (or both) could be restricted	Right commonly reported – theoretically either left upper or right lower pole (or both) could be restricted	Left	Left
Sphinx test (backward bending test)	N/A Remains symmetrical	More symmetrical than previously	Less symmetrical than previously	Less symmetrical than previously	More symmetrical than previously
Motion testing or "rattle" of the four poles					
Restriction of gapping	N/A	Left upper and lower; right lower	Left upper; right upper and lower	Left upper and lower	Left upper and lower

d, deep; s, shallow; A, anterior; P, posterior; I, inferior.

+, moves; -, restricted; ±, some motion.

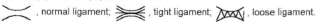 , normal ligament; , tight ligament; , loose ligament.

The goal of local palpatory examination is to compile enough specific information about key landmark asymmetry, sites and characteristics of restricted motion, and evidence of tissue texture change to extrapolate a tentative diagnosis. The guidelines in Table 3.3.3 help with this interpretation.

Consensus on nomenclature used for descriptive findings and their interpretation permits neuromusculoskeletal physicians to communicate their combinations of objective findings in concise, meaningful ways. Because several different models are used in diagnosing and treating this region, exact agreement between all representative schools of thought is difficult. Nonetheless, while various schools may differ on their interpretation, clinical observation and research, consistent nomenclature, and careful consensus permit certain generalizations.

On the basis of lateralization tests and the resulting tentative diagnosis of dysfunction, the manual medicine physician can then initiate treatment designed to re-establish properties needed for motion, stability,[140] and shock absorption.[141] The final goal is to improve function within the pelvis to permit such vital activities of daily living as required for gait or for providing a level foundation for spinal posture.

Sacral somatic dysfunction diagnoses covered in this portion of the chapter (and treatment presented in Chapter 4.3.1) are summarized in Table 3.3.4. They include the following postulated axes and associated somatic dysfunctions:

- **middle transverse axis (S2 level):** sacral base anterior (bilateral sacral flexion) or sacral base posterior (bilateral sacral extension) somatic dysfunctions

- **left oblique axis (upper left S1 to lower right S3):** left or right rotation on a left oblique axis somatic dysfunctions

- **right oblique axis (upper right S1 to lower left S3):** right or left rotation on a right oblique axis somatic dysfunctions

- **sagittal or parasagittal axis:** left or right sacral margin posterior somatic dysfunctions

- **traumatically induced with no axis:** left or right sacral shear (unilateral sacral flexion or extension) somatic dysfunctions.

(The following diagnoses are seen in the literature less frequently and are not fully covered in this chapter: anterior sacrum left or right, superior sacral shear left or right, and posterior sacrum left or right).

Table 3.3.5. Motion testing importance in differential diagnosis of sacral dysfunction (osteopathic model)

'Diagnoses' listed to the right have the same static findings	Left rotation on left oblique axis	Anterior sacrum right	Posterior sacrum left (only in Strachan model)	Left on left forward torsion	Left rotation on right oblique axis
Static findings palpated over sacrum	(Same)			(Same)	
Lateralization tests (e.g. restricted side to ASIS springing; longest-last motion in seated flexion test)	+ Right	+ Right with tissue texture change over right upper pole	+ Left with tissue texture change over left lower pole	+ Right	+ Left
Sphinx test (backward bending test)	More symmetrical	More symmetrical		More symmetrical	Less symmetrical
Motion testing or 'rattle' of the 4 poles					
L5	N/A	N/A	N/A	L5 S$_L$R$_R$	N/A

d, deep; s, shallow; A, anterior; P, posterior; I, inferior.

+, moves; -, restricted; ±, some motion.

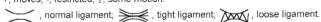, normal ligament; , tight ligament; , loose ligament.

Table 3.3.5 summarizes an example of the importance of moving beyond static landmark assessment and integration of functional tests of motion in making a diagnosis. While each of the five sacral diagnoses has the same static sacral landmarks, variations in the motion characteristics provide different diagnoses and therefore different treatment approaches.

With so much individual host variability and so many models of diagnosis in the pelvic region, it is not surprising that this area, more than many others, evokes disagreement concerning biomechanics and clinical approach to diagnosis and treatment. What is generally agreed upon, however, is the importance of the region as a base of function for many important activities of daily living ranging from sitting and standing postures to ambulation.

With this is mind, greater overall importance might be assigned to screening and lateralization tests that indicate 'if dysfunction exists or not' and, if so, which sites might be monitored to assess return of motion and/or reduction of pain. Local tests leading to a diagnosis specific for a particular model will continue to retain their importance for the individual practitioner in selecting a therapeutic technique but should probably bow to reassessment of the big question concerning treatment; namely, do screening and lateralization tests now indicate stability, mobility, and pain-free function in the region?

Coccyx and pelvic floor

The pelvic girdle is important in congestive phenomena and the respiratory–circulatory model of health described by Zink,[23] in part because of its relationship to the pelvic diaphragm. Specific diagnosis of the pelvic floor is usually undertaken after correction of the bony framework to which the muscles attach.

General assessment of the pelvic floor and related muscles often includes observation of the lower extremities (e.g. external rotation of the lower extremity on the side of increased piriformis tension and direct palpation of the ischiorectal fossa using an external approach (Figure 4.3.62) with fingers directed along the ischial tuberosity).

Specific diagnosis of the coccyx or of certain pelvic floor muscles is often done with a gloved finger inserted in the vagina or rectum. This is most commonly performed as part of the pelvic or rectal examination during a general physical examination or a detailed examination focusing on constructing the complete differential diagnosis of coccygodynia, pelvic floor spasm, incontinence, prostatodynia, and low back pain of unknown origin.

Innominate (iliosacral) and pubic somatic dysfunction

Somatic dysfunction of the innominate bone is often discussed with respect to the lower extremities, but this chapter includes a few relative diagnostic tests related to their impact on regional function of associated joints, myofascial, and ligamentous structures and of the pelvic ring as a whole.

Much of the iliosacral dysfunction transmitted by way of the innominates can be linked with biomechanical imbalance occurring during gait or from the impact of trauma during different components of the gait cycle. Commonly function and dysfunction in this context is associated with the physiologic motions of anterior and posterior rotation of each half of these pelvic bones around a so-called inferior transverse sacroiliac axis.

Trauma transferred up through a lower extremity (or by landing on one ischial tuberosity during a fall) may create nonphysiologic dysfunction (Figure 3.3.51) through forceful gliding of the iliosacral joint (as in a superior innominate shear) or the pubic symphysis (as in a superior pubic shear). Here there is no postulated axis, rather shearing forces following the joint surface(s) are responsible.

The lateralization test most frequently denoting the side of iliosacral or pubic dysfunction is the standing flexion test; however, shifting the direction of force vectors while performing the ASIS compression test is also very helpful in following outcomes return of function here. Local static landmarks used in deriving somatic dysfunction for the innominate are the ASIS, PSIS, and iliac crests. Static local findings used in pubic shear diagnosis are discovery of a 'step' sign rising up or dropping down a few millimeters as the palpating fingers are drawn across the superior and anterior surfaces of the pubic rami on either side of the pubic symphysis.

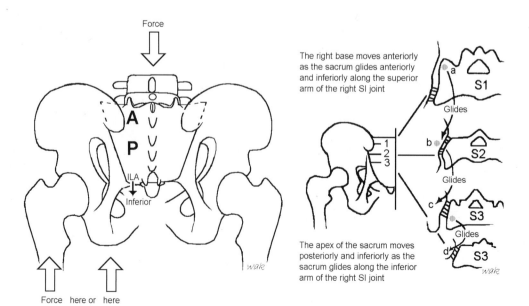

Figure 3.3.51 Left sacral shear.

The right base moves anteriorly as the sacrum glides anteriorly and inferiorly along the superior arm of the right SI joint

The apex of the sacrum moves posteriorly and inferiorly as the sacrum glides along the inferior arm of the right SI joint

Summary: patient-centered approach to somatic dysfunction and diagnosis

Without doubt, somatic dysfunction can be identified in a wide range of patient complaints ranging from local pain and alteration of function to more systemic disturbances. Here it plays a significant role in the differential diagnosis of a broad spectrum of patient complaints. This is the case for each of the many schools of manual medicine: in spite of their many differences in language, emphases on differing tests, and variety of proposed mechanisms, each recognizes the presence of 'somatic dysfunction', the implications of such altered function on local and distant function, and the patient response to removing that dysfunction.

The experience of physicians in various neuromusculoskeletal fields thereby establishes a definitive role for evaluation and treatment of somatic dysfunction. Nonetheless, much additional work needs to be done in standardizing nomenclature, assessing reproducibility and validity of various empirically or theoretically derived clinical–biomechanical models, and expanding the evidence-base for the field of manual medicine.

That said, unfortunately the reductionist approach in identifying and studying an isolated somatic dysfunction in a clinical setting may be ineffective. Radin's experience in this regard led to his remark, 'Functional analysis, be it biological, mechanical or both, of a single tissue will fail to give a realistic functional analysis as, in all complex constructs, the interaction between the various components is a critical part of their behavior'.[142] With these factors in mind (and while researchers continue to explore), physicians engaged in manual medicine will most likely continue to practice a multidimensional, patient-centered, total body approach when assessing somatic dysfunction and the neuromusculoskeletal system. The value of integrating patient-centered and biopsychosocial approaches with diagnosis and treatment of specific anatomic pathophysiology has become standard of care; for example, its current use in predicting orthopedic surgical intervention outcomes in back pain patients.[143,144]

In summary then, the complete neuromusculoskeletal examination begins with looking at function and dysfunction of the whole patient, examining down to smaller and smaller somatic units, and then reassembling the role of these smaller units back into the total body function.

References

1. Data compiled by Labor and Industry computers in Florida (FCER, 1988, Arlington, VA) and Colorado (Tillinghast, 1993, Denver, CO).

2. Education Council on Osteopathic Principles. Glossary of osteopathic terminology. In Ward, R. C. (ed.). *Foundations for osteopathic medicine*, 2nd edn (2002). Lippincott, Williams and Wilkins, Baltimore, MD.

3. *The international classification of diseases, 9th revision, clinical modification (ICD-9-CM)*. 3rd edn (1979). U.S. Government/World Health Organization, Geneva.

4. Dinnar, U. Classification of diagnostic tests used with osteopathic manipulation. *J Am Osteopath Assoc*, 1980, **79**, 451–455.

5. Dinnar, U. Description of fifty diagnostic tests used with osteopathic manipulation. *J Am Osteopath Assoc*, 1982, **81**, 314–321.

6. Kimberly, P. Forming a prescription for osteopathic manipulative treatment. *J Am Osteopath Assoc*, 1980, **79**, 512.

7. Kuchera, W. A., Jones, J. M. III, Kappler, R. E., Goodridge, J. P. Musculoskeletal examination for somatic dysfunction. Chapter 42 in: Ward, R. C. (ed.) *Foundations for osteopathic medicine* (1997). Williams and Wilkins, Baltimore, MD, pp. 489–509.

8. Degenhardt, B. F., Snider, K. T., Johnson, J. C., Snider, E. J. Interexaminer reliability of osteopathic palpatory evaluation of the lumbar spine. *J Am Osteopath Assoc*, 2002, **102**(8), 442; and Degenhardt, B. F., Snider, K. T., Johnson, J. C., Snider, E. J. Retention of interexaminer reliability in palpatory evaluation of the lumbar spine. *J Am Osteopath Assoc*, 2002, **102**(8), 439.

9. Cyriax, J. *Textbook of orthopaedic medicine, volume two: treatment by manipulation, massage and injection*, 10th edn (1980). Bailliére Tindall, London.

10. Ward, R. C. (ed.). *Foundations for osteopathic medicine*, 2nd edn (2002). Lippincott, Williams and Wilkins, Baltimore, MD.

11. Maigne, R. *Orthopedic medicine: a new approach to vertebral manipulations* (1972). C. C. Thomas, Springfield, IL.

12. Greenman, P. E. *Principles of manual medicine* (1996). Williams and Wilkins, Baltimore, MD.

13. Simons, D. G., Travell, J. G., Simons, L. S. *Travell and Simons' myofascial pain and dysfunction: the trigger point manual, volume 1. Upper half of body* (1999). Williams and Wilkins, Baltimore, MD.

14. Lewit, K. *Manipulative therapy in rehabilitation of the motor system* (1985). Butterworth, London.

15. Mennell, J. *Back pain: diagnosis and treatment using manipulative technique* (1960). Brown and Co, Boston.

16. Greenman, P. E. *Principles of manual medicine* (1996). Williams and Wilkins, Baltimore, MD, pp. 18–36.

17. Rubin, B. R. Rheumatology. Chapter 38 in: Ward, R. C. (ed). *Foundations for osteopathic medicine* (1997). Williams and Wilkins, Baltimore, MD, pp. 459–466.

18. Amoronso, P. J. et al. Tobacco and injuries: an annotated bibliography. US Army Research Laboratory Technical Report, ARTR-1333, 1997; Naus A et al. Work injuries and smoking. *Industrial Med Surg*, 1966, **35**, 880–881; Reynolds, K. L. et al. Cigarette smoking, physical fitness, and injuries in infantry soldiers. *Am J Preventive Med*, 1994, **19**, 145–150.

19. Kuchera, M. L. Gravitational strain pathophysiology and 'Unterkreuz' syndrome. *Manuelle Medizin*, 1995, **33**(2), 56.

20. Kuchera, M. L., Kuchera, W. A. General postural considerations. Chapter 69 in: Ward, R. C. (ed.). *Foundations for osteopathic medicine* (1997). Williams and Wilkins, Baltimore, MD, pp. 969–977.

21. Kuchera, M. L. Gravitational stress, musculoligamentous strain, and postural alignment. *Spine: State of the Art Review*, 1995, **9**(2), 463–490.

22. Peterson, B. (ed.). *Postural balance and imbalance. 1983 yearbook of the American Academy of Osteopathy*. AAO Press, Newark, OH, 1983.

23. Zink, J. G., Lawson, W. B. An osteopathic structural examination and functional interpretation of the soma. *Osteopathic Annals*, 1979, **7**, 433–440.

24. Dananberg, H. J. Lower back pain as a gait-related repetitive motion injury. Chapter 21 in Vleeming, A., Mooney, V., Snijders, C. J., Dorman, T. A., Stoeckart R (eds). *Movement, stability and low back pain: the essential role of the pelvis* (1997). Churchill-Livingstone, New York, pp. 253–267.

25. Mitchell, F. L., Moran, P. S., Pruzzo, N. A. *An evaluation and treatment manual of osteopathic muscle energy procedures*. (1979) Private Publishing Firm, Valley Park, MO; Ward, R. C. (ed.) *Foundations for osteopathic medicine*, 2nd edn (2002). Lippincott, Williams and Wilkins, Baltimore, MD.

26. Greenman, P. E. *Principles of manual medicine* (1996). Williams and Wilkins, Baltimore, MD, p 36.

27. Maigne, R. *Orthopedic medicine: a new approach to vertebral manipulations* (1972). C. C. Thomas, Springfield, IL, pp. 84, 268.

28. Travell, J. G., Simons, D. G. *Myofascial pain and dysfunction: the trigger point manual*. Vol. II (1992). Williams and Wilkins, Baltimore, MD.

29. Simons, D. G., Travell, J. G., Simons, L. S. *Travell and Simons' myofascial pain and dysfunction: the trigger point manual, volume 1. Upper half of body* (1999). Williams and Wilkins, Baltimore, MD.

30. Jones, L., Kusunose, R., Goering, E. *Jones' Strain–Counterstrain* (1995). Jones Strain-Counterstrain, Inc.

31. Owens, C. *An endocrine interpretation of Chapman's reflexes* (1963 reprint). American Academy of Osteopathy, Indianapolis, IN.

32. Mense, S., Simons, D. *Muscle pain, understanding its nature, diagnosis, and treatment* (2001). Lippincott Williams and Wilkins, Philadelphia, PA.

33. Gerwin, R., Shannon, S., Hong, C., Hubbard, D., Gervirtz, R. Interrater reliability in myofascial trigger point examination. *Pain*, 1997, **69**, 65–73.

34. Sciotti, V. M., Mittak, V. L., DiMarco, L. Clinical precision of myofascial trigger point location in the trapezius muscle. *Pain*, 2001, **93**, 259–266.

35. Simons, D. G. Muscle pain syndromes. *J Man Med*, 1991, **6**, 3–23.

36. Chaitow, L. *Soft tissue manipulation* (1987). Thorsons, Wellington, UK.

37. Patriquin, D. A. Chapman's reflexes. Chapter 67 in: Ward, R. C. (ed). *Foundations for osteopathic medicine* (1997). Williams and Wilkins, Baltimore, MD, pp. 935–940.

38. Washington, K., Mosiello, R., Venditto, M., *et al*. Presence of Chapman reflex points in hospitalized patients with pneumonia. *J Am Osteopath Assoc*, **103**, 479–83.

39. Adler-Michaelson, P., Jeck, S., Goldstein, F. J. *The reliability of Chapman's reflex points in ovarian pathology* (2003). Submitted and accepted in partial fulfillment of FAAO, American Academy of Osteopathy, Indianapolis, IN.

40. Glover, J. C., Yates, H. A. Strain and counterstrain techniques. Chapter 58 in Ward, R. C. (ed). *Foundations for osteopathic medicine* (1997). Williams and Wilkins, Baltimore, MD, pp. 809–818.

41. Kuchera, M. L., Kuchera, W. A. *Osteopathic considerations in systemic dysfunction*, 2nd edn, revised (1994). Greyden Press, Columbus, OH.

42. Kuchera, M. L. Diagnosis and treatment of gravitational strain patho-physiology: research and clinical correlates (part I and II). In: Vleeming A (ed). *Low back pain: the integrated function of the lumbar spine and sacroiliac joints*. Proceedings of the 2nd Interdisciplinary World Congress, 9–11 November 1995, University of California, San Diego, pp. 659–693.

43. Paterson, J. K., Burn, L. *An introduction to medical manipulation* (1985). MTP Press, Lancaster, UK, p. 144.

44. Kuchera, M. L. Examination and diagnosis: an introduction. Chapter 39 in: Ward, R. C. (ed). *Foundations for osteopathic medicine*, 2nd edn (2002). Lippincott, Williams and Wilkins, Baltimore, MD, pp. 566–573.

45. Paterson, J. K., Burn, L. *An introduction to medical manipulation* (1985). MTP Press, Lancaster, UK, p. 105.

46. Levin, S. M. A different approach to the mechanics of the human pelvis: tensegrity. In: Vleeming, A., Mooney, V., *et al*. (eds) *Movement stability and low back pain: the essential role of the pelvis*. (1997) Churchill-Livingstone, New York.

47. Kuchera, M. L., DiGiovanna, E. L., Greenman, P. E. Efficacy and complications. Chapter 72 in: Ward, R. C. (ed). *Foundations for osteopathic medicine*, 2nd edn (2002). Lippincott, Williams and Wilkins, Baltimore, MD, pp. 1143–1161.

48. Simons, D. G., Travell, J. G., Simons, L. S. *Travell and Simons' Myofascial pain and dysfunction: the trigger point manual, volume 1. Upper half of body* (1999). Williams and Wilkins, Baltimore, MD, p. 254.

49. Kuchera, M. L. Osteopathic principles and practice/osteopathic manipulative treatment considerations for cephalgia. *J Am Osteopath Assoc* Suppl, 1998, **98**(4), S14–19.

50. Paterson, J. K., Burn, L. *An introduction to medical manipulation* (1985). MTP Press, Lancaster, pp. 75–78.

51. Simons, D. G., Travell, J. G., Simons, L. S. *Travell and Simons' myofascial pain and dysfunction: the trigger point manual, volume 1. Upper half of body* (1999). Williams and Wilkins, Baltimore, MD, pp. 237–277.

52. Elkiss, M. L., Rentz, L. E. Neurology. Chapter 34 in Ward, R. C. (ed). *Foundations for osteopathic medicine* (1997). Williams and Wilkins, Baltimore, MD, pp. 401–416.

53. Simons, D. G., Travell, J. G., Simons, L. S. *Travell and Simons' myofascial pain and dysfunction: the trigger point manual, volume 1. Upper half of body* (1999). Williams and Wilkins, Baltimore, MD, p. 256.

54. Simons, D. G., Travell, J. G., Simons, L. S. *Travell and Simons' myofascial pain and dysfunction: the trigger point manual, volume 1. Upper half of body* (1999). Williams and Wilkins, Baltimore, MD, pp. 329–396, 416–431.

55. Greenman, P. E. *Principles of manual medicine* (1996). Williams and Wilkins, Baltimore, MD, p. 166.

56. Simons, D. G., Travell, J. G., Simons, L. S. *Travell and Simons' myofascial pain and dysfunction: the trigger point manual, volume 1. Upper half of body* (1999). Williams and Wilkins, Baltimore, MD, p. 337.

57. Simons, D. G., Travell, J. G., Simons, L. S. *Travell and Simons' myofascial pain and dysfunction: the trigger point manual, volume 1. Upper half of body* (1999). Williams and Wilkins, Baltimore, MD, pp. 256–267, 329–348.

58. Kappler, R. E., Ramey, K. A. Head, diagnosis and treatment. Chapter 44 in: Ward, R. C. (ed). *Foundations for osteopathic medicine* (1997). Williams and Wilkins, Baltimore, MD, pp. 538–539.

59. Simons, D. G., Travell, J. G., Simons, L. S. *Travell and Simons' myofascial pain and dysfunction: the trigger point manual, volume 1. Upper half of body* (1999). Williams and Wilkins, Baltimore, MD.

60. Magoun, H. I. Temporal bone: trouble-maker in the head. *J Am Osteopath Assoc*, 1974, **73**, 825–835.

61. Magoun, H. I. *Osteopathy in the cranial field* (1976). The Cranial Academy, Indianapolis, IN.

62. Kappler, R. E., Ramey, K. A. Head, diagnosis and treatment. Chapter 44 in: Ward, R. C. (ed). *Foundations for osteopathic medicine* (1997). Williams and Wilkins, Baltimore, MD, pp. 515–540.

63. Kappler, R. E. Cervical spine. Chapter 45 in: Ward, R. C. (ed). *Foundations for osteopathic medicine* (1997). Williams and Wilkins, Baltimore, MD, pp. 541–546.

64. Simons, D. G., Travell, J. G., Simons, L. S. *Travell and Simons' myofascial pain and dysfunction: the trigger point manual, volume 1. Upper half of body* (1999). Williams and Wilkins, Baltimore, MD, pp. 432–444.

65. Simons, D. G., Travell, J. G., Simons, L. S. *Travell and Simons' myofascial pain and dysfunction: the trigger point manual, volume 1. Upper half of body* (1999). Williams and Wilkins, Baltimore, MD, pp. 445–471.

66. Jaeger, B. Are 'cervicogenic' headaches due to myofascial pain and cervical spine dysfunction? *Cephalgia*, 1989, **9**(suppl 3), 157–164.

67. Greenman, P. E. *Principles of manual medicine* (1996). Williams and Wilkins, Baltimore, MD, pp. 550–551.

68. Maigne, R. Manipulation of the spine. Chapter 4 in: Basmajian, J. V. (ed). *Manipulation, traction and massage*, 3rd edn. (1985). Williams and Wilkins, Baltimore, MD, pp. 71–134.

69. Kapandji. *The physiology of joints*. (1970). Churchill-Livingstone, New York.

70. Kelso, A. F. A double-blind clinical study of osteopathic findings in hospital patients – progress report. *J Am Osteopath Assoc*, 1971, **70**, 570–592.

71. D'Alonzo, G. E., Krachman, S. L. Respiratory system. Chapter 37 in: Ward, R. C. (ed). *Foundations for osteopathic medicine* (1997). Williams and Wilkins, Baltimore, MD, pp. 441–458.

72. Paterson, J. K., Burn, L. *An introduction to medical manipulation* (1985). MTP Press, Lancaster, UK, p. 77.

73. Maigne, R. Manipulation of the spine. Chapter 4 in: Basmajian, J. V. (ed). *Manipulation, traction and massage*, 3rd edn (1985). Williams and Wilkins, Baltimore, MD, p. 99.

74. Maigne, R. Manipulation of the spine. Chapter 4 in: Basmajian, J. V. (ed). *Manipulation, traction and massage*, 3rd edn (1985). Williams and Wilkins, Baltimore, MD, p. 186.

75. Olesen, J. Classification and diagnostic criteria for headache disorders, cranial neuralgias and facial pain. *Cephalgia*, 1988, **8**(suppl 7).

76. Gilliar, W. G., Kuchera, M. L., Giulianetti, D. A. Neurologic basis of manual medicine. *Phys Med Rehab Clin N Am*, 1996, **7**(4), 693–714; Upton, A. R., McComas, A. J. The double crush in nerve entrapment syndromes. *Lancet*, 1973, **ii**, 359–362.

77. Maigne, R. Manipulation of the spine. Chapter 4 in: Basmajian, J. V. (ed). *Manipulation, traction and massage*, 3rd edn (1985). Williams and Wilkins, Baltimore, MD, p. 82–84.

78. Simons, D. G., Travell, J. G., Simons, L. S. *Travell and Simons' myofascial pain and dysfunction: the trigger point manual, volume 1. Upper half of body* (1999). Williams and Wilkins, Baltimore, MD, pp. 278–307.

79. Simons, D. G., Travell, J. G., Simons, L. S. *Travell and Simons' myofascial pain and dysfunction: the trigger point manual, volume 1. Upper half of body* (1999). Williams and Wilkins, Baltimore, MD, pp. 432–444.

80. Simons, D. G., Travell, J. G., Simons, L. S. *Travell and Simons' myofascial pain and dysfunction: the trigger point manual, volume 1. Upper half of body* (1999). Williams and Wilkins, Baltimore, MD, pp. 491–503.

81. Kuchera, M. L. Travell and Simons' myofascial trigger points. Chapter 66 in: Ward, R. C. (ed). *Foundations for osteopathic medicine* (1997). Williams and Wilkins, Baltimore, MD, pp. 919–933.

82. Simons, D. G., Travell, J. G., Simons, L. S. *Travell and Simons' myofascial pain and dysfunction: the trigger point manual, volume 1. Upper half of body* (1999). Williams and Wilkins, Baltimore, MD, pp. 833, 838.

83. Simons, D. G., Travell, J. G., Simons, L. S. *Travell and Simons' myofascial pain and dysfunction: the trigger point manual, volume 1. Upper half of body* (1999). Williams and Wilkins, Baltimore, MD, pp. 613–622.

84. Simons, D. G., Travell, J. G., Simons, L. S. *Travell and Simons' myofascial pain and dysfunction: the trigger point manual, volume 1. Upper half of body* (1999). Williams and Wilkins, Baltimore, MD, pp. 445–471.

85. Simons, D. G., Travell, J. G., Simons, L. S. *Travell and Simons' myofascial pain and dysfunction: the trigger point manual, volume 1. Upper half of body* (1999). Williams and Wilkins, Baltimore, MD, pp. 900–907.

86. Kappler, R. E., Ramey, K. A. Chapter 44. head, diagnosis and treatment. In Ward, R. C. (ed). *Foundations for osteopathic medicine* (1997). Williams and Wilkins, Baltimore, MD, pp. 545.

87. Simons, D. G., Travell, J. G., Simons, L. S. *Travell and Simons' myofascial pain and dysfunction: the trigger point manual, volume 1. Upper half of body* (1999). Williams and Wilkins, Baltimore, MD, pp. 504–537.

88. Lewit, K. *Manipulative therapy in rehabilitation of the locomotor system*, 2nd edn (1991). Butterworth Heinemann, Oxford, pp. 24, 196–7, 244–5.

89. Smith, L. A. *et al. An atlas of pain patterns: sites and behavior of pain in certain common disease of the upper abdomen* (1961). C. C. Thomas, Springfield, IL.

90. Melzack, R., Wall, P. D. *The challenge of pain: a modern medical classic.* (1989). Penguin, London.

91. Maigne, R. *Orthopedic medicine: a new approach to vertebral manipulations* (1972). C. C. Thomas, Springfield, IL, pp. 97, 144.

92. Simons, D. G., Travell, J. G., Simons, L. S. *Travell and Simons' myofascial pain and dysfunction: the trigger point manual, volume 1. Upper half of body* (1999). Williams and Wilkins, Baltimore, MD, pp. 278–307.

93. Simons, D. G., Travell, J. G., Simons, L. S. *Travell and Simons' myofascial pain and dysfunction: the trigger point manual, volume 1. Upper half of body* (1999). Williams and Wilkins, Baltimore, MD, pp. 913–939.

94. Greenman, P. E. *Principles of manual medicine* (1996). Williams and Wilkins, Baltimore, MD, p. 206.

95. Jones, L. H. *Strain and counterstrain* (1981). American Academy of Osteopathy, Newark, OH.

96. Patriquin, D. A. Viscerosomatic reflexes. In Patterson, M. M., Howell, J. N. (eds). *The central connection: somatovisceral–viscerosomatic interactions*, 1989 International Symposium. (1992). University Classics, Athens, OH, pp. 4–18.

97. Simons, D. G., Travell, J. G., Simons, L. S. *Travell and Simons' myofascial pain and dysfunction: the trigger point manual, volume 1. upper half of body* (1999). Williams and Wilkins, Baltimore, MD, pp. 844–856.

98. Simons, D. G., Travell, J. G., Simons, L. S. *Travell and Simons' myofascial pain and dysfunction: the trigger point manual, volume 1. Upper half of body* (1999). Williams and Wilkins, Baltimore, MD, pp. 887–899.

99. Simons, D. G., Travell, J. G., Simons, L. S. *Travell and Simons' myofascial pain and dysfunction: the trigger point manual, volume 1. Upper half of body* (1999). Williams and Wilkins, Baltimore, MD, pp. 940–970.

100. Simons, D. G., Travell, J. G., Simons, L. S. *Travell and Simons' myofascial pain and dysfunction: the trigger point manual, volume 1. Upper half of body* (1999). Williams and Wilkins, Baltimore, MD, pp. 862–886.

101. Scott, R. A. Orthopaedics. Chapter 28 in: Ward, R. C. (ed). *Foundations for osteopathic medicine* (1997). Williams and Wilkins, Baltimore, MD, pp. 329–347.

102. Paterson, J. K., Burn, L. *An introduction to medical manipulation* (1985). MTP Press, Lancaster, UK, p. 105.

103. Simons, D. G., Travell, J. G., Simons, L. S. *Travell and Simons' myofascial pain and dysfunction: the trigger point manual, volume 1. Upper half of body* (1999). Williams and Wilkins, Baltimore, MD, pp. 572–586.

104. Simons, D. G., Travell, J. G., Simons, L. S. *Travell and Simons' myofascial pain and dysfunction: the trigger point manual, volume 1. Upper half of body* (1999). Williams and Wilkins, Baltimore, MD, pp. 278–307.

105. Simons, D. G., Travell, J. G., Simons, L. S. *Travell and Simons' myofascial pain and dysfunction: the trigger point manual, volume 1. Upper half of body* (1999). Williams and Wilkins, Baltimore, MD, pp. 913–939.

106. Simons, D. G., Travell, J. G., Simons, L. S. *Travell and Simons' myofascial pain and dysfunction: the trigger point manual, volume 1. Upper half of body* (1999). Williams and Wilkins, Baltimore, MD, pp. 908–912.

107. Lewit, K. Muscular pattern in thoraco-lumbar lesions. *Manual Med*, 1986, **2**, 105–107.

108. Simons, D. G., Travell, J. G. Low back pain, part 2: torso muscles. *Postgrad Med*, 1983, **73**(2), 81–92.

109. Kuchera, M. L. Postural considerations in the sagittal plane. Chapter 72 in: Ward, R. C. (ed). *Foundations for osteopathic medicine* (1997). Williams and Wilkins, Baltimore, MD, pp. 999–1014.

110. Cyriax, J. H., Cyriax, P. J. *Cyriax's illustrated manual of orthopaedic medicine*, 2nd edn. (1993). Butterworth-Heinemann, Oxford.

111. Simons, D. G., Travell, J. G., Simons, L. S. *Travell and Simons' myofascial pain and dysfunction: the trigger point manual, volume 1. Upper half of body* (1999). Williams and Wilkins, Baltimore, MD, pp. 572–586.

112. Simons, D. G., Travell, J. G., Simons, L. S. *Travell and Simons' myofascial pain and dysfunction: the trigger point manual, volume 1. upper half of body* (1999). Williams and Wilkins, Baltimore, MD, pp. 940–970.

113. Simons, D. G., Travell, J. G., Simons, L. S. *Travell and Simons' myofascial pain and dysfunction: the trigger point manual, volume 1. upper half of body* (1999). Williams and Wilkins, Baltimore, MD, pp. 913–939.

114. Greenman, P. E. *Principles of manual medicine*, 2nd edn. (1996). Williams and Wilkins, Baltimore, MD, p. 316.

115. Vleeming, A., Mooney, V., Dorman, T., Snijders, C., Stoeckart R (eds). *Movement, stability and low back pain: the essential role of the pelvis* (1997). Churchill Livingstone, New York.

116. Kuchera, M. L. Treatment of gravitational strain pathophysiology. In Vleeming, A., Mooney, V., Dorman, T., Snijders, C., Stoeckart R (eds). *Movement, stability and low back pain: the essential role of the pelvis* (1997). Churchill-Livingstone: New York, pp. 477–499.

117. Simons, D. G., Travell, J. G., Simons, L. S. *Travell and Simons' myofascial pain and dysfunction: the trigger point manual, volume 1. Upper half of body* (1999). Williams and Wilkins, Baltimore, MD; Travell, J. G., Simons, D. G. *Myofascial pain and dysfunction: the trigger point manual*. Vol. II. (1992). Williams and Wilkins , Baltimore, MD.

118. Kuchera, M. L., Kuchera, W. A. Postural considerations in coronal and horizontal planes. Chapter 71 in: Ward, R. C. (ed). *Foundations for osteopathic medicine* (1997). Williams and Wilkins, Baltimore, MD, 983–997.

119. Mixter, W. J., Barr, J. S. Rupture of the intervertebral disc with involvement of the spinal canal. *N Engl J Med*, 1934, **211**, 210–215.

120. Farfan, H. F. The scientific basis of manipulative procedures. *Clin Rheumatol Dis*, 1980, **6**, 159.

121. Mooney, V., Robertson, J. The facet syndrome. *Clin Orthop*, 1976, **115**, 149–156.

122. Fairbank, J. C., T., Park, W. M., McCall, I. W. Apophyseal injection of local anesthetic as a diagnostic aid in primary low-back pain syndromes. *Spine*, 1981, **6**, 598–605.

123. Travell, J. G., Simons, D. G. *Myofascial pain and dysfunction: the trigger point manual*. Vol. II (1992). Williams and Wilkins , Baltimore, MD.

124. Travell, J., Travell, W. Therapy of low back pain by manipulation and of referred pain in the lower extremity by procaine infiltration. *Arch Phys Ther*, 1946, **27**, 537–547.

125. Steinbrocker, O., Isenberg, S. A., Silver, M. *et al*. Observations on pain produced by injection of hypertonic saline into muscles and other supportive tissues. *J Clin Invest*, 1953, **32**, 1045–1051.

126. Greenman, P. E. *Principles of manual medicine* (1996). Williams and Wilkins, Baltimore, MD, pp. 305–311.

127. Mooney, V. Sacroiliac joint dysfunction. In Vleeming, A., Mooney, V., Dorman, T., Snijders, C., Stoeckart R (eds). *Movement, stability and low back pain: the essential role of the pelvis* (1997). Churchill-Livingstone, New York, pp. 37–52.

128. Travell, J. G., Simons, D. G. *Myofascial pain and dysfunction: the trigger point manual*. Vol. II (1992). Williams and Wilkins , Baltimore, MD.

129. Greenman, P. E. Syndromes of the lumbar spine, pelvis, and sacrum. *Phys Med Rehab Clin N Am*, 1996, **7**(4).773–785.

130. Travell, J. G., Simons, D. G. *Myofascial pain and dysfunction: the trigger point manual*. Vol. II (1992). Williams and Wilkins, Baltimore, MD, pp. 28–88.

131. Good, M. G. Diagnosis and treatment of sciatic pain. *Lancet*, 1942, **ii**, 597–598,.

132. Kimberly, P., Funk, S. F. (eds). *Outline of osteopathic manipulative procedures: the Kimberly manual millennium edn* (2000). Walsworth, Marceline, MO.

133. Hackett, G. S. *Ligament and tendon relaxation treated by prolotherapy*, 3rd edn (1958). C. C. Thomas, Springfield, IL.

134. Greenman, P. E. Sacroiliac dysfunction in the failed low back pain syndrome. *First Interdisciplinary World Congress on Low Back Pain and Its Relation to the Sacroiliac Joint, San Diego, 1992*, pp. 329–352.

135. Fortin, J. D., Falco, F. J.E. The Fortin finger test: an indicator of sacroiliac pain. *Am J Orthop*, 1997, **24**(7), 477–480.

136. Strachan, W. F. *et al*. A study of the mechanics of the sacroiliac joint. *J Am Osteopath Assoc*, 1938, **43**(12), 576–578.

137. Walton, W. J. Osteopathic diagnosis and technique. In: *Sacroiliac diagnosis* (1966), Matthews Book Co, St. Louis, MO, pp. 187–197. Reprinted 1970 and distributed by the American Academy of Osteopathy.

138. Mitchell, F. L. Structural pelvic function (1958). In: *American Academy of Osteopathy Yearbook* (1967). American Academy of Osteopathy, Indianapolis, IN.

139. Heinking, K. P., Kappler, R. E. Pelvis and sacrum. Chapter 52 in: Ward, R. C. (ed). *Foundations for osteopathic medicine*, 2nd edn (2002). Lippincott, Williams and Wilkins, Baltimore, MD, pp. 762–783.

140. Vleeming, A., Mooney, V., Dorman, T., Snijders, C., Stoeckart R (eds). *Movement, stability and low back pain: the essential role of the pelvis* (1997). Churchill-Livingstone, New York.

141. Wilder, D. G., Pope, M. H., Frymoyer, J. W. The functional topography of the sacroiliac joint. *Spine*, 1980, **5**, 575–579.

142. Vleeming, A., Snijders, C. J., Stoeckart, R., Mens, J. M. A. The role of the sacroiliac joints in coupling between spine, pelvis, legs and arms. Chapter 3 in: Vleeming, A., Mooney, V., Snijders, C. J., Dorman, T. A., Stoeckart R (eds). *Movement, stability and low back pain: the essential role of the pelvis* (1997). Churchill-Livingstone, New York, pp. 53–71.

143. Waddell, G., Morris, E. W., *et al*. A concept of illness tested as an improved basis for surgical decisions in low-back disorders. *Spine*, 1989, **14**, 838–843.

144. Spinal Surgery Consortium for Outcomes Research (SCORE) bibliography. http://hfhs-cce.org/score/Propbibl.htm; American Academy of Orthopedic Surgeons/Council of Musculoskeletal Specialty Societies/Council of Spine Societies. *Outcomes Data Collection Package: Lumbar Cluster*. AAOS, 1996.

3.4   **Pectoral girdle**

3.4.1   **Thoracic outlet syndrome**

John Tanner

The thoracic outlet syndrome (TOS) comprises a number of syndromes involving the upper quarter and hand that are thought to be caused by compression of the subclavian artery, vein and/or brachial plexus. It is believed that at least one of these structures must be compressed somewhere between the superior opening of the thorax and the axilla to meet this diagnosis.

Anatomy

The thoracic outlet contains many structures in a confined space. The floor of the thoracic outlet is formed by the first rib and fascia of Sibson. This fascia attaches to the transverse process of C7, the pleura, and the first rib. Superiorly lies the subclavius muscle and clavicle, anteriorly the anterior scalene, and posteriorly the middle scalene. The brachial plexus and subclavian artery pass over the first rib between the aforementioned muscles (Figures 3.4.2 and 3.4.3). The lowest part of the nerve plexus lies behind the subclavian artery. According to Pollack (1980), neurovascular compression occurs at any or all of the three levels:

- in the **superior thoracic outlet** bordered posteriorly by the spine, anteriorly by the manubrium, and laterally by the first rib

- more laterally in the **costoscalene hiatus** bordered anteriorly by the anterior scalene muscle, posteriorly by the middle scalene muscle, and caudally by the first rib (Figure 3.4.1)

- most laterally of the three, in the **costoclavicular passage**, bordered laterally by the clavicle, posteriorly by the scapula and medially by the first rib (Figure 3.4.1).

Anatomy of the first rib

The anatomy and function of the first rib, and of a cervical rib if present, are critical to the understanding and therapy of the thoracic outlet syndromes.

The orientation of the first rib is different from the other ribs in that its long axis forms a 45° angle with the horizontal. It articulates with the facet on the first thoracic vertebra (the **costovertebral joint**) and the transverse process of the vertebra (the **costotransverse joint**). This latter joint lacks a superior supporting ligament, making it relatively weaker than those of the other ribs. Furthermore, the muscle attachments to this rib, which function during inspiration and to flex and rotate the cervical part of the spine, impose more stress on the rib and its joints than on any of the other ribs. These stresses are probably greatest at the costotransverse joint. Osteoarthritic changes are found in both these joints, but more frequently in the costotransverse joint. Since the axis of its two articulations lie closer to the coronal plane, elevation of the first rib during respiration increases the anteroposterior diameter, often described as a 'pump-handle' movement.

The posterior segment of the first rib relates to the stellate ganglion, the first thoracic spinal root, and the eighth cervical spinal root. The middle segment of the rib extends from the posterior costal angle to the retroscalenic tubercle, providing insertions for the middle scalene, the first digitation of the serratus anterior, and the intercostal muscles of the first intercostal space. The insertion of the pleura on the periosteum of the first rib is very firm. The anterior segment of the first rib relates to the first thoracic nerve, the subclavian artery and vein, the

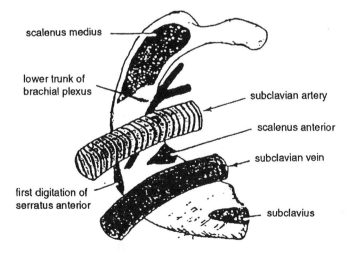

Figure 3.4.1 Structures related to the superior surface of the first rib (taken from Mahran et al. Osteology 1971, University Book Centre Cairo)

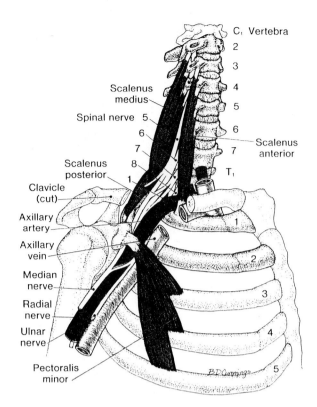

Figure 3.4.2 Thoracic outlet entrapment by the scalene muscles. The neurovascular bundle is spread out to show the relations of its component parts. A portion of the clavicle has been removed. The brachial plexus and axillary artery emerge above the first rib and behind the clavicle, between the scalenus anterior and scalenus medius muscles. The primal nerves are numbered on the left, the vertebrae on the right. The T1 nerve lies dorsal to and beneath the subclavian artery.

pleura, and the lung apex. The anterior scalene muscle inserts into the pre-arterial tubercle of the first rib between the artery posteriorly and the vein anteriorly. The costoclavicular ligaments and the subclavius muscle insert into this portion of the rib (Figures 3.4.1 and 3.4.4).

Developmental anomalies

A **cervical rib** is present in 0.5% of the population, but most remain non-symptomatic. Many anomalous **fibrous bands** (Figures 3.4.5–3.4.6) attaching to the first rib have been described (Roos 1984). A band from the transverse process of C7 will act as a cervical rib (but not appear on a radiograph). In addition, the first rib receives attachments from any cervical rib. The neurovascular bundle slides up on the first rib as on a pulley. Various **congenital anomalies of the first and second ribs** may occur, with anomalous joints of the first rib and asymmetry due to **cervicothoracic scoliosis**. Pathological positions of the first rib have been shown to cause TOS, such as a high first rib and an upward dislocation of the first rib (Figures 3.4.6–9).

Neurology

The first thoracic nerve is at greatest risk of tension as it curves over the first rib, and this will be increased by shoulder girdle depression. The C8 root is similarly embarrassed by a cervical rib or fibrous band. This accounts for the limb symptoms being most prominent on the medial aspect of the upper arm, forearm, and hand.

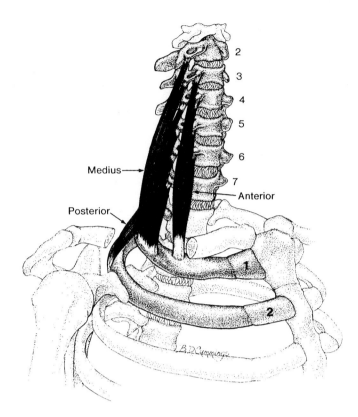

Figure 3.4.3 Oblique view of the attachments of the three major scalene muscles to the cervical vertebrae and to the first and second ribs. The clavicle has been cut and the section that overlies the scalene muscles removed.

Aetiology

The causes most commonly implicated in thoracic outlet syndromes are cervical ribs, structure or function of the first rib, the anterior scalene muscle, and anomalous fibromuscular bands.

Of the 0.5% of the population who possess cervical ribs, only 5–10% ever develop symptoms (Adson and Coffey 1927). The literature cites a cervical rib to be the cause of TOS in 10–100% of cases: American authors favour a higher percentage to be due to fibromuscular bands or scalene muscle abnormalities. A single traumatic episode is reported in

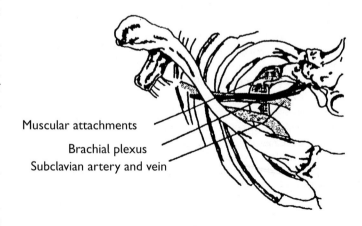

Figure 3.4.4 The costo-clavicular passage.

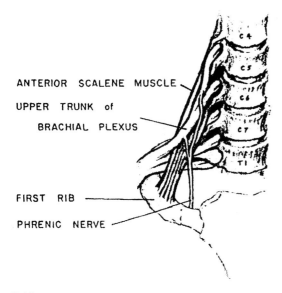

Figure 3.4.5

Table 3.4.1. Aetiological factors in thoracic outlet syndromes

Anatomical factors		Provocative factors
Structural abnormality	Cervical rib	Trauma
	Clavicle malunion	Occupational stresses
	Fibromuscular bands	Shoulder girdle descent
	Pancoast tumour	Overweight conditions
Soft tissue components	Anterior scalene	Pendulous breasts
	Middle scalene	First rib dysfunction
	Pectoralis minor	
	Subclavius	
	Costocoracoid fascia	

21–91% of the patients in several American studies (e.g. Sanders *et al.* 1979, Ellison and Wood 1994) or 10% of cases (UK series, e.g. Sharan *et al.* 1999). Occupational predisposition occurs in over 50% of patients and in these cases musculoskeletal dysfunction is the major factor, aggravated by structural abnormalities when present.

Structural factors are usually present in the vascular types of TOS; they may be present in cases showing neurological features, but the function of the thoracic outlet is of especial importance in occupational cases.

Studies of the normal function of the thoracic outlet are scarce, and the prevalence of neurogenic TOS in the general population is not known. Neurological TOS with objective deficit is a rare lesion with an annual incidence of about 1/1 000 000 (Gilliat 1984): most of the patients are female (9 : 1) and bony anomalies are usually found.

The most elegant studies of first rib function have been performed by Lindgren *et al.* (1990) using a cineradiographic technique. Mobility of the first rib during inspiration and expiration was visualized with the patient lying supine, with a fluoroscopic beam at 30° of caudal angulation. Movement was considered to be restricted if there was no movement along the axis through the costotransverse joint during

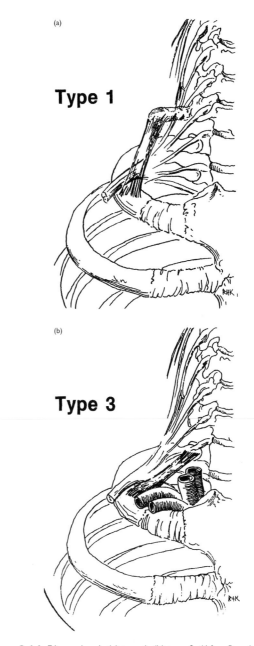

Figure 3.4.6 Fibrous bands (a) type 1, (b) type 3. (After Roos)

expiration and inspiration. The function of the first rib and its stump was studied both clinically and radiologically in unoperated patients with brachialgia and in those whose first rib had been resected. Having visualized abnormal function in a proportion of both conservatively treated and surgically treated cases who continued to have symptoms, Lindgren related these findings to new clinical tests based on the kinesiology of the first rib. These include the expiration-inspiration test and the combined rotation and lateral flexion test (CRLF, Lindgren *et al.* 1992). The interexaminer reliability of the CLRF test was found to be excellent (kappa reliability coefficient $\kappa = 1$). The interreliability between the clinical and radiological tests was also excellent ($\kappa = 0.84$). The sensitivity and specificity of the CRLF test was found to be 92% and 90% respectively as compared with a cineradiographic study.

The CRLF test for first rib function

- Start in neutral position of cervical spine
- Passive rotation away from side to be tested, to maximum
- Gentle passive flexion, moving ear towards chest
  Test negative: 70° flexion with soft end-feel
  Test positive: No movement, or half asymptomatic side range with hard end-feel

Differential diagnosis in TOS

- Cervical nerve root pressure, e.g. disc
- Cervical joint dysfunction
- Apical lung tumour
- Ulnar neuritis
- Carpal tunnel syndrome
- Peripheral neuropathy
- Syringomyelia, multiple sclerosis

Asymmetries of the respiratory movements of the first rib have been shown in association with structural asymmetries of the cervico-thoracic spine (Girout 1983), when an upward dislocation of the first rib has been suggested to be a cause of brachialgia (McGormick *et al.* 1981). As a result of these findings, Lindgren proposes a proper trial of conservative treatment including assessment for impaired first rib mobility and appropriate therapy which may include joint mobilization/manipulation, but in particular long-term self-treatment and maintenance. This aims to restore movements to the first rib by isometric activation of the scalene muscle combined with shoulder girdle exercises. He maintains that if the function is not restored the symptoms continue despite a transaxillary first rib resection.

The diagnosis of arterial TOS is usually made after a severe embolic event involving the arm. Venous TOS is seen in perhaps 1.5% of all patients, manifest as axillary or subclavian thrombosis and they are more frequent than those of arterial insufficiency (Roos 1976).

Clinical presentation

TOS occurs three times more commonly in women, usually around the middle decades. It can present in three ways: neurological, vascular, or combined vascular and neurological.

Symptoms suggesting vascular compression include oedema, heaviness or weakness of the upper extremity and cyanosis, blanching, and erythema similar to Raynaud's phenomenon. Patients may notice that the skin appears blotchy, discoloured, and more often cold. The onset is usually insidious but may follow trauma. The most common complaint is inability to raise or maintain the arm in a static posture for more than short periods without provoking symptoms. The symptoms may also occur with everyday activities, such as cleaning windows, painting a ceiling, or carrying heavy shopping or a briefcase. The symptoms include pain from the neck through the supra-clavicular region into the arm and hand, accompanied by a subjective feeling of easy fatiguability and sometimes swelling. Typical of neurological TOS are paraesthesiae experienced in the inner arm and forearm and the ulnar side of the hand. In a series of 27 cases with cervical ribs, Sharan *et al.* (1999) found symptoms of arm pain, paraesthesia of the lower plexus distribution, pain at the root of the neck, and undue fatigue.

Physical examination

The patient's description of symptoms and their variation with time and activity are often crucial to the diagnosis, particularly in the common case who has few objective signs on examination. Whether symptoms come on with physical activities, or with a sleeping posture (releasing the stretched neural elements over the rib) needs enquiry.

General examination and differential diagnosis

The provocative tests (see below) are carried out in the context of standard examination of the cervical spine, arm, and upper thoracic spine. This examination should exclude cervical disc and nerve root compression, shoulder dysfunction, and peripheral neuropathies. Particular examination for motor deficit in thenar muscles, intrinsic muscles of hand, and triceps should be made, together with provocative manoeuvres for carpal tunnel and ulnar neuritis. Palpation of the supraclavicular fossa may reveal a hard lump (cervical rib), lymphadenopathy, or tumour. Pressure for up to 30 seconds with the thumb over the plexus and first rib may be very tender and elicit familiar symptoms (Spurling's sign). Posture and respiratory pattern should be observed; while soft tissue restriction, and accessory joint motion of all the joints of the shoulder girdle and the rib articulations should be examined.

Examination for vascular features

Auscultation for a bruit above or below the clavicle can be performed (at rest and in the provocative positions) when vascular compromise is suspected. The limb is examined for swelling, discolouration and temperature change, and for evidence of emboli, e.g. splinter haemorrhages in the nail beds.

Postural examination

Observe the patient from all views, both at rest, and if possible when performing tasks which provoke or relieve symptoms.

Poor tone and protraction of the shoulder girdle is often present, while a protracted head position will occur with increased tone in scalenes and sternocleidomastoids. Breathing pattern should be noticed, in particular paradoxical respiration with use of the accessory muscles at rest.

Provocative manoeuvre tests

Anterior scalene or Adson's test (Adson and Coffey 1927)

This evaluates the role of anterior and middle scalene muscles in compressing the subclavian artery which passes between them on its way to the axilla.

The patient hyperextends the neck and rotates the head toward the affected side and takes a deep breath. The examiner monitors the radial pulse which will decrease or become obliterated if the test is positive.

Costoclavicular compression

This is an exaggerated military position designed to narrow the space between the first rib and clavicle thereby compressing the plexus and/or vessels.

The patient sits with arms relaxed at her sides. She retracts and depresses the shoulder girdle while the examiner monitors for a change in the radial pulse.

Wright's hyperabduction manoeuvre (Wright 1945)

This involves passive circumduction of the arm overheard while the examiner monitors the radial pulse. This test is positive if the pulse strength changes and/or symptoms are elicited.

Roos' abduction and external rotation (AER) test or the hands up test (Roos 1976)

This test is performed with the patient sitting, arms abducted 90° and the elbows flexed 90° with the shoulders braced slightly.

The patient is asked to open and close her fingers slowly and steadily for a full 3 minutes. The examiner observes for drooping of the arms, decreased rate of finger flexion, or the onset of typical symptoms.

Cervical rotation lateral flexion test (Lindgren et al. 1992)

The neutrally positioned cervical spine is first passively and maximally rotated away from the side being examined and then in this position gently flexed as far as possible, moving the ear towards the chest. This is done in both directions. Bony restriction blocking the lateral flexion part of the movement partially or totally indicates a positive test; a free movement indicates a negative test.

Expiration–inspiration test (Lindgren et al. 1992)

The movement of the first rib in relation to the clavicle is palpated in the supine position during expiration and inspiration by lightly pressing a finger between the two bones. The right and left sides are compared. In this test the disturbance of the movement of the first rib can be felt as a restriction of the movement during breathing. This test cannot be done on patients who have previously had rib resections, for obvious reasons.

The TOS index

- A history of aggravation of symptoms with the arm in the elevated position.
- A history of paraesthesiae in the segments of C8–T1.
- Tenderness over the brachial plexus supraclavicularly.
- A positive hands-up (AER) test (see text).

Table 3.4.2. Findings in a series of cervical rib cases (Sharan et al. 1999)

Atrophy and weakness of the hand muscles	67%
Positive Roos test (AER)	60%
Palpable lump in the posterior triangle	53%
Supraclavicular tenderness	43%
Supraclavicular bruit	8%

None of the above tests unequivocally establishes the presence or absence of TOS. Ribbe et al. (1986) used a TOS index requiring at least three of four symptoms or signs for the diagnosis. (see box)

Table 3.4.2 lists the findings in Sharan et al.'s (1999) series of cervical rib cases.

Investigations

Diagnostic imaging

Diagnosis of TOS is largely based on history and physical examination, but investigation to identify bony abnormality is appropriate where suspicion of the diagnosis is strong. Cervical spine radiographs will show cervical ribs, abnormally long C7 transverse processes, and the apices of the lungs. If vascular compromise is suggested by the examination, imaging for example by MR or angiography, and/or vascular flow tests by Doppler ultrasound are needed.

Neurophysiology

Claims have been made for the usefulness of ulnar nerve conduction velocity (Urschel and Razzuk 1972), F-wave reflexes (Nishida et al. 1993), and somatosensory evoked potentials (Chodoroff et al. 1985, Machleder et al. 1987) but false positives occur with all tests described, and none can be recommended as reliable (Roos 1976, Wilbourne 1990). When the neural type of TOS is suspected clinically, normal practice is to proceed with conservative treatment and to avoid surgery in most cases.

Treatment

Cases with arterial or venous components to the syndrome must be considered for surgical treatment. In the neurological syndromes, conservative treatment by physical methods is the norm.

Role of physical treatment in conservative management of TOS

There are three phases of treatment:

- demonstration of the ability to control the intensity of the symptoms
- exercises to change the symptom-producing faults
- postural maintenance.

Various regimes have been utilized incorporating shoulder girdle elevation and stabilization exercises, flexibility exercises, exercises for the chest and cervical musculature, and controlled breathing routines. McGough et al. (1979) have extended medical management for as long as 2 years before surgical intervention: 90% of their 1200 patients were successfully relieved without surgery.

Most practitioners blame faulty posture of the cervicothoracic spine and shoulder girdle in the aetiology of TOS, on the basis of the observation that the symptoms of TOS correspond to a loss of muscular support and/or increased muscular tautness in these regions. The question remains whether abnormalities in bony structure, such as a cervical rib, should determine treatment. Peet et al. (1956) included patients with normal and with abnormal cervical radiographs in their treatment regime. After an intensive programme of strengthening and flexibility exercises they concluded that 70% of all patients, regardless of radiographic findings, had the same chance of achieving relief from their symptoms.

Lindgren (1997), with his self-treatment programme to restore function of the first rib, enabled 88% of 119 patients to achieve a satisfactory outcome including 73% returning to work. Radiological screening was found to have normalized in 8 of 10 patients. Lindgren's protocol requires an intensive training for a routine of exercises, which require to be continued at home:

- shoulder girdle active exercises for restoration of mobility
- craniocervical junction nutation for joint mobility and stretching the upper part of the posterior cervical musculature
- scalene muscle activation with active exercise to restore upper rib function
- passive stretching of shoulder girdle muscles, especially upper trapezius, sternocleidomastoids, levator scapulae, and pectoralis minor, using the techniques of Evjenth and Hamberg (1990).

Together with specific exercises customized to the patients particular requirements should be added a general exercise routine, with attention paid to:

- **Posture:** To counteract protracted head position and protraction of the shoulder girdle. Thoracic kyphosis should be minimized.
- **Breathing pattern.**
- **Muscle imbalance and trigger points:** Abnormality with increased tone, trigger points, and shortening may be found in the muscles itemized above (and breathing pattern generally: additional treatment techniques such as postisometric relaxation and trigger point therapy are useful).
- **Joint dysfunction:** Cervical or upper thoracic segmental dysfunction should be corrected, as should first or second rib dysfunction.
- **Ergonomics at home and work:** A change in job or increased workload are common provoking factors for symptoms. Counselling on hours at work, rest periods, posture, and design of workstation is often helpful.

Evaluation of soft tissue restrictions

Recognition of shortened anterior scalene muscle is verified by finding the head position in slight lateral flexion towards the affected side and rotation towards the contralateral side. From the lateral perspective, shortening of this muscle is noted by an increase in lordosis. Spasm of the sternocleidomastoid muscle can be seen from the anterior view and shortening of the upper trapezius will affect the slope of the shoulders seen from the posterior view. Breathing pattern should be noticed in particular paradoxical respiration with use of the accessory muscles at rest. Observation of shoulder girdle posture may reveal protraction of the shoulder girdle with shortening of the pectoralis muscles, exaggeration of thoracic kyphosis, and abducted shoulder position.

Sidebending to the contralateral side may be limited by up to 30° if scalene muscles are shortened. Furthermore, aggravation or provocation of symptoms can occur with overpressure at the extreme of this range. Assessment of shortened pectoralis minor is achieved by lying the patient supine and observing whether the posterior aspect of the shoulder lies in contact with the surface of the table. If the muscle is shortened the shoulder will be in a forward position, as a result of the downward pull on the coracoid process. Passive stretching of the pectoralis minor by pushing the posterior aspect of the shoulder down against the surface of the table may elicit the patient's symptoms. Palpation of the upper trapezius, sternocleidomastoid, and scalene muscles is vital to locate trigger points which may refer symptoms to the upper chest, suprascapular area, and arm. Trigger points may extend to the levator scapulae, pectoralis major, and even subclavius muscle (Howell Wright 1991).

Surgical treatment

The outcome of surgical decompression has been difficult to assess in the absence of satisfactory objective tests for comparing preoperative and postoperative states, in the absence of controlled series, and with most series including those with and without structural abnormalities. Furthermore, some patients who were reported by their surgeons to have benefited have subsequently been described by others on long-term follow-up as not having been helped by surgery (Carroll and Hurst 1982). Sanders *et al.* (1979) reported recurrence of symptoms in 17% of 239 scalenectomy patients and in 17% of the 214 patients who had excision of the first rib. The importance of long term follow up is essential although approximately 60 per cent of recurrences occur within 6 months after surgery. Sharan *et al.* (1999), in a series of 27 cases with cervical ribs, 3 with bilateral symptomatology, classified the syndromes thus: neurogenic type, 24; arterial, 5; venous, 1. In the neurogenic group 3 patients had upper plexus involvement. The mean duration of symptoms was 24 months. Only 3 patients gave a history of injury to the neck, and 2 of the 3 patients with upper plexus symptoms were found to have a double crush syndrome requiring bilateral carpal tunnel decompression subsequently. The structural lesions detected were as follows: 27 cervical ribs (15 complete, 7 incomplete), 5 C7 exostoses, 8 fibromuscular bands, 2 thickened fibrosed anterior scalenes, 1 rudimentary first rib and exostosis of second rib. One patient had an axillary subclavian aneurysm in association with a complete cervical rib which required resection and prosthetic grafting. He chose to resect only the middle third of the cervical rib subperiosteally. A two-surgeon approach was used (an orthopaedic surgeon and a vascular surgeon) with prior assessment by a consultant neurologist. They did not resect the first rib, but division of the omohyoid and anterior scalene were done in all cases while the middle scalene was excised only if the muscle was judged to be abnormal and compressing the neurovascular bundle. Almost all patients were followed up for more than 1 year and some up to 9 years later. In the long term excellent or good results were noted in 87%, with 89% returning to their previous lifestyle or occupation. The only complications reported were hypertrophic scarring in 1 case and 5 patients with infraclavicular anaesthesia.

An earlier series which discusses surgical treatment is that of Sanders *et al.* (1979) who found a recurrence rate of over 15% following first rib resections for TOS. On supraclavicular re-exploration he found the anterior scalene muscle had re-attached to the bed of the first rib. Scalenectomy was successful in each of these cases. This led to the study of anterior scalenectomy as the first operation for all cases of TOS refractory to conservative therapy. Apart from the usual clinical diagnostic tests, Sanders found a scalene muscle block with local anaesthetic was extremely useful. When comparing the results of scalenectomy and rib resection in a prospective study results were almost identical producing 70% good to excellent long-term outcome. He concluded that in patients with a history of neck trauma followed by headache, neck pain, and arm symptoms scalenectomy should be considered. On the other hand, first rib resection is recommended for patients with no history of neck trauma and symptoms limited to the arm and hand, particularly those with signs of vascular insufficiency.

Roos (1976), writing from his personal experience in evaluating more than 2300 patients for TOS and operating on 776 cases of the most severe category who failed to respond to physical therapy and other conservative measures, finds that the most common anomaly is the presence of the fibromuscular band. He maintained that the most effective means of relieving symptoms is a transaxillary approach resecting the entire first thoracic rib from sternum to transverse process, cervical rib if present, and complete excision of all anomalous fibromuscular tissue. The important point about his experience is that resection of the first rib alone cannot be considered adequate decompression. A careful search for the presence of congenital bands must also be made, and these bands must be totally excised for complete neurovascular decompression. He claims a 90% success rate if the correct operation is performed with meticulous technique.

In the present climate of controversy it is right to exercise caution and maintain a relatively high threshold for surgical invasion for neurological TOS, particularly with the improved techniques in manual medicine for treating first rib subluxation, mobilizing the first rib, neuromuscular techniques to relax scalene muscle spasm, and a muscle balance approach for the entire shoulder girdle complex.

References

Adson, A. W., Coffey, J. R. (1927) Cervical rib. *Ann. Surg.*, **85**, 839.

Carroll, R. E. Hurst, L. E. (1982) The relationship of thoracic outlet syndrome and carpal tunnel syndrome. *Clin. Orthop.*, **164**, 149–53.

Chodoroff, G.*et al.* (1985) Dynamic approach in the diagnosis of thoracic outlet syndrome using somatosensory evoked responses. *Arch. Phys. Med. Rehabil.*, **66**, 3–6.

Ellison, D. W., Wood V. C. (1994) Trauma-related thoracic outlet syndrome. *J. Hand Surg.*, **19B**, 424–6.

Evjent, O., Hamberg J. (1990) *Autostretching. The complete manual of specific stretching*. Alfta rehab forlag, Sweden.

Gilliat, R. W. (1984) Thoracic outlet syndromes. In: Dyck, P. J., Thomas, P. K., Lambert, E. H., *et al.* (eds.) *Peripheral neurology*, 2nd edn, pp. 1402-24. W. B. Saunders, Philadelphia.

Girout, J. (1983) Rontgenstudien der dynamik der ersten rippe. *Manuelle Medizine*, **21**, 20–22.

Howell Wright, J. (1991) *Physical therapy of the shoulder*, ed. Robert. A. Donatelli. Churchill Livingstone, Edinburgh.

Lindgren, K. A., Leino, E., Hakola, M., *et al.* (1990) Cervical spine rotation and lateral flexion combined motion in the examination of the thoracic outlet. *Arch. Phys. Med. Rehab.*, **71**, 343–4.

Lindgren, K. A., Leino, E., Manninen, H. (1992) Cervical rotation lateral flexion test in brachialgia. *Arch. Phys. Med. Rehab.*, **73**, 735–7.

Lindgren, K. A. (1997) Conservative treatment fo throacic outlet syndrome: a 2-year follow-up. *Arch. Phys. Med. Rehab.*, **87**, 373–8.

McGormick, C. C. *et al.* (1981) Upward dislocation of the first rib: a rare cause of nerve entrapment producing brachialgia. *Br. J. Radiol.*, **54**, 140–2.

McGough, E. C. *et al.* (1979) Management of thoracic outlet syndrome. *J. Thorac. Cardiovasc. Surg.*, **77**, 169.

Nishida, T. *et al.* (1993) Medial antebrachial cutaneous nerve conduction in true neurogenic thoracic outlet syndrome. *Electromyogr. Clin. Neurophysiol.*, **33**, 285–8.

Peet, R. M. *et al.* (1956) Thoracic outlet syndrome: Evaluation of a therapeutic exercise programme. *Staff Meetings, Mayo Clinic*, **31**, 281.

Pollak, E. (1980) Surgical anatomy of the thoracic outlet syndrome. *Surg. Gynecol. Obstet.*, **150**, 97–103.

Ribbe, E. *et al.* (1986) Clinical diagnosis of thoracic outlet syndrome – evaluation of patients with cervicobrachial symptoms. *Manual Med.*, **2**, 82–5.

Roos, D. B. (1976) Congenital anomalies associated with thoracic outlet syndrome. *Am. J. Surg.*, **132**, 771–7.

Roos, D. B. (1984) Thoracic outlet and carpal tunnel syndromes. In: Rutherford, R. B. (ed.) *Vascular Surgery*. W. B. Saunders, Philadelphia, pp. 708–24.

Sanders, R. J., Monsour, J. W., Gerber, W. F., *et al.* (1979) Scalenectomy versus first rib resection for the treatment of the thoracic outlet syndrome. *Surgery*, **85**, 109–19.

Sharan, D. *et al.* (1999) Two surgeon approach to thoracic outlet syndrome: Long term outcome. *J. Roy. Soc. Med.*, **92**, 239–43.

Urschel, H. C. and Razzuk, M. A. (1972) Management of thoracic outlet syndrome. *N. Engl. J. Med.*, **285**, 1140.

Wilbourne, A. J. (1990) The thoracic outlet syndrome is over-diagnosed. *Arch. Neurol.*, **47**, 328–30.

Wright, I. S. (1945) The neurovascular syndrome produced by hyperabduction of the arms. *Am. Heart. J.*, **29**, 1.

3.4.2 Chest wall pain

John Tanner

Chest pain

Anterior chest pain is a frequent cause of attendance at emergency departments and of admission to hospital, but it has been estimated that about 25–30% of patients admitted with acute anterior chest wall pain remain undiagnosed despite intensive investigation including chest radiograph, ECG, coronary angiography and laboratory tests. Ockene *et al.*(1980) found that 10–30% of cases of chest pain referred for coronary artery imaging had normal investigations. After some time in hospital and these expensive investigations, the patient is told 'we can't find anything wrong with you, it must be musculoskeletal'. Some of these patients are then referred on to a specialist physician or therapist; others are not. In Ockene's series 45% still had pain 1 year later, and over half remained unemployed. In some cases there appears to be dual pathology: Levine and Mascette (1990) evaluated 62 adults referred for coronary arteriography using a systematic physical examination. In 7 patients the chest pain was reproduced on physical examination: 6 of these ultimately received a diagnosis of non-anginal chest pain and 5 had normal coronary arteriograms, although all these patients described their pain in terms often associated with true angina.

Acute chest pain

Obviously the patient in acute distress from chest pain needs careful screening to rule out serious and possibly life-threatening disorders such as angina pectoris, dissecting aneurysm, pneumonia, pleurisy, or pulmonary embolus. Other viscerogenic sources of pain include oesophagitis and reflux symptoms from hiatus hernia. Less common but equally painful may be Bornholm viral myalgia and pancreatitis. Additionally, some conditions refer pain to the posterior chest such as pleurisy and pneumonia, angina pectoris, cholecystitis, dissection of an aneurysm, and eroding peptic ulcers.

Chronic chest pain

Chronic insidious onset of chest wall pain requires careful screening for primary tumours of the lung and breast, metastatic deposits in the rib cage, or metabolic bone diseases such as osteomalacia, rickets, and hyperparathyroidism.

Examination

The clinician should include basic screening of the thoracic spine in the initial examination for chest pain unless the diagnosis is very clearly visceral in origin. This may simply involve asking the patient to perform active trunk movements, particularly observing pain or restriction with thoracic rotation in either direction. This can be followed by springing the thoracic spinal joints and rib joints in sequence. If the pain is in the upper pectoral area or posterior chest wall more closely related to the scapula region, then examination of active and passive cervical spine movements may indicate a cervical source.

When no posterior abnormality is identified as a cause of the pain, possibly referred anteriorly, the anterior structures are individually examined, especially the costochondral and sternal joints, and the muscles and their attachments.

Musculoskeletal chest wall pain

Causes of chest wall pain are summarized in Table 3.4.3.

- **Direct trauma:** Fractures of the sternum or ribs are readily detected clinically and/or by radiography after direct trauma.

- **Indirect trauma** can cause stress fractures of ribs, e.g. in sportsmen such as rowers, and cough fractures are seen in the osteoporotic non-athlete.

- **Cervical spondylosis/strain** may cause pain in the pharynx or upper sternal area. Examination of the cervical spine should reveal the cause: and sometimes imaging, including MRI, is useful, or can be used where a more sinister cause is feared.

- **Thoracic spinal joints:** Anterior chest pain can be referred from dysfunction in the joints of the thoracic spine and ribs. Commonly the patient has developed a pain (possibly also in the posterior chest, but not always) on performing a trivial twisting or bending movement, but it may also follow more vigorous activities from sport or manual work. The patient may describe pain only on deep inspiration. Sometimes paraesthesiae develop, following the course of an intercostal nerve. These pains can also be referred from costovertebral joint dysfunction as well as from the zygapophyseal joints, and from thoracic disc lesions.

- Thoracic disc syndromes are rare, but with the advent of new imaging techniques such as MRI, asymptomatic disc bulges or protrusions are found in as many as 30% of individuals. The symptomatic thoracic disc herniation may produce back pain which radiates either in a girdle-like distribution around one side or directly through the chest towards the sternum or upper abdomen. Careful examination for restricted trunk movements, dural signs

Table 3.4.3. Musculoskeletal causes of chest wall pain

Posterior origin	Anterior origin
Systemic disorders	
Ankylosing spondylitis	Spondylitis or other chronic inflammatory arthritis
	Fibromyalgia
	Hyperventilation syndrome
Local disorders	
Spinal joint dysfunction	Trauma
Disc lesions	Infection
Other spinal pathology	Costochondritis
	Tietze's syndrome

and neurological examination of the lower limbs will allow correlation with any imaging findings.

Bruckner *et al.* (1987) reported on 73 patients with mid dorsal and/or unilateral chest pain seen consecutively in a rheumatology clinic over a 3-year period. Visceral disease was excluded. The majority of sufferers were young women with a continuous, dull pain aggravated by coughing and sneezing and relieved by rest. Frequently tenderness over the thoracic spine and adjacent rib was found with pain at extremes of thoracic spinal movement. In 16% cutaneous hyperaesthesia in a radicular distribution was found, but without other neurological abnormalities. Bruckner initially ascribed this clinical picture to a thoracic disc prolapse, but 10 cases were submitted to MR imaging and no prolapse was seen. However, thoracic intervertebral disc dehydration without associated prolapse was seen in 90% of a later series of patients (and 13% of the controls) and the disc abnormalities corresponded to the symptomatic levels and the clinical examination findings (Bruckner *et al.* 1989). The condition settled in most of the patients following manipulative therapy and advice on back care. Bruckner concludes that this is a common benign condition which deserves wider recognition. He called it the 'benign thoracic pain syndrome': it fits a syndrome of somatic dysfunction in association with disc change. In cases with disc features but no neural compromise, it is our practice to recommend manual treatment with or without manipulation.

Ankylosing spondylitis

Symmetrical aching in the chest wall, in association with discomfort and possible restriction of movement on examination (in a symmetrical pattern also) should raise a suspicion of inflammatory arthritis of the spine. If the classical features of sleep interruption, morning stiffness, and easing with exercise are added, a trial of anti-inflammatory medication should be made, and further investigation arranged (see Chapter 3.1). The same pathology can cause synovitis of individual joints in the chest wall, most commonly the manubriosternal joint. Dawes *et al.* (1988) studied 45 patients with ankylosing spondylitis together with an age- and sex-matched group of normals for the incidence, nature, and frequency of chest pain. They found 25 of the spondylitic group had experienced recurrent chest pain compared to 3 normals, and had a significantly reduced chest expansion. The pain was anterior or posterior, sometimes sharp and intermittent, rather than continuous. They concluded that the presence of chest pain in ankylosing spondylitis can be an early presenting feature of the disease (8 patients had chest pain before spinal symptoms) and is associated with more severe disease.

Fibromyalgia

One of the nine pairs of classical tender points of fibromyalgia is adjacent to the second costochondral junction. The examination should then be extended to test the other points, to settle the differential diagnosis between local and more widespread pathology (see Chapter 2.2.3).

Hyperventilation syndrome

Patients in acute emotional distress may present with difficulty in breathing, a feeling of suffocation, and a variety of chest pains with paraesthesiae in the upper body including face and head. These patients may be observed to sigh frequently and/or breathe rapidly with predominantly upper chest movement, which characterizes the hyperventilation syndrome. Instruction in correct diaphragmatic breathing to eliminate the paradoxical respiration, or the paper bag rebreathing technique, will help normalize blood gases and reduce symptoms within minutes.

Costochondral joints

Specific conditions

The costochondral joints are sometimes subject to the inflammatory changes of ankylosing spondylitis and other spondylarthropathies (see above); as also are the manubriosternal and sternoclavicular joints. Local tenderness occurs with fibromyalgia (see above). Infection of a costochondral or sternal joint has been reported rarely, usually in intravenous drug abusers. The rare autoimmune condition relapsing polychondritis can give a more extensive inflammation and softening of the costal cartilages: inflammatory markers such as the ESR will be raised.

Costochondritis and Tietze's syndrome

There is no evidence that these two conditions of unknown cause, giving pain at one or more of the costochondral joints, do not share the same pathology. The conditions are most common in women aged between 20 and 40 (Calabro 1977). Possible precipitating factors include trauma such as a blow to the chest, undue physical exertion, and upper respiratory tract infection, but many cases appear to have a spontaneous onset. Symptoms from particularly tender or painful joints such as the sternoclavicular or other costochondral joints may be treated by local corticosteroid infiltration. This may have to be repeated more than once, since the relief may not last more than 2–3 months.

In **costochondritis** there is localized pain at the costochondral joints, which are tender on examination, but not swollen. It may affect any of the costochondral junctions and more than one site is affected in 90% of cases. The second to fifth costochondral junctions are most commonly involved. The prognosis is excellent. After 1 year about one half may continue with some discomfort, but only one third report tenderness with palpation.

In **Tietze's syndrome**, which is less common, there is swelling as well as local tenderness of the joints of the chest wall: 80% of cases involve a single joint. It is rarely bilateral, tending to affect neighbouring articulations on the same side of the sternum.

Unless the swelling presents quite obvious deformity it may only be possible to distinguish between Tietze's syndrome and costochondritis by performing a CT or MR scan to reveal the enlargement of the chondral junction.

References

Bruckner, F. E., *et al.* (1987). Benign thoracic pain. *J. Roy. Soc. Med.*, **80**, 286–9.

Bruckner, F. E., *et al.* (1989). Benign thoracic pain syndrome: Role of magnetic resonance imaging in the detection and localisation of thoracic disc disease. *J. Roy. Soc. Med.*, **82**, 81–3.

Calabro, J. J. (1977). Costochondritis. *N. Engl. J. Med.*, **296**, 946–7.

Dawes, P. T., *et al.* (1988). Chest pain a common feature of ankylosing spondylitis. *Postgrad. Med. J.*, **64**, 27–9.

Levine, B. R., Mascette, A. M. (1990). Musculoskeletal chest pain in patients with angina: A prospective study. *South. Med. J.*, **83**(2), 262–3.

Ockene, I. S., Shay, M. J., Weiner, B. J., Daler, J. E. (1980) Unexplained chest pain in patients with normal arteriograms: a follow-up study. *N. Engl. J. Med.*, **303**, 1249–52.

3.4.3 The joints of the shoulder girdle

John Tanner

Acromioclavicular joint dysfunction and injury

The acromioclavicular joint is as prone to develop degenerative changes as other weightbearing joints. In most patients osteoarthrosis does not cause symptoms, but an injury such as a fall on the outstretched hand, or repetitive trauma such as is involved in sports as weightlifting, may cause the joint to become symptomatic. People who report a high exposure to physical workload and/or intense sporting activity are more prone to develop osteoarthritis of this joint.

The patient will usually point to the top of the shoulder joint, almost directly over the acromioclavicular joint, as a source of their pain. On examination, passive adduction of the arm in 90° flexion across the chest (Scarf sign) will provoke the pain, which does not radiate down the arm. Direct pressure applied digitally over the joint will also locate tenderness.

If the symptoms are mild, reduction of workload and/or aggravating sporting activity together with the use of topical non-specific anti-inflammatory (NSAID) gels or oral NSAIDs may settle the problem. If the symptoms are more severe, restricting every day activity, then a local joint injection with a small dose of corticosteroid settles the pain very effectively.

Occasionally inferior osteophytes on the joint will encroach on the subacromial space, resulting in signs of impingement of the rotator cuff and subacromial bursa. If refractory, these osteophytes can be treated by surgical excision. If the osteoarthritis is advanced with gross osteophytosis, removal of the joint by resection of the distal segment of the clavicle is usually curative. Only 5 mm of the distal clavicle needs to be resected to ensure that there is no bone-to-bone abutment.

Osteolysis of the distal clavicle

This is an uncommon condition which tends to occur following trauma or repetitive strain, as in weightlifters and sportsman performing overhead activities. Patients typically present in the second to fourth decade of life with pain localized to the acromioclavicular joint with overhead lifting activity. Radiographs demonstrate osteoporosis, cystic changes, and loss of subchondral bony detail in the distal clavicle. Occasional cystic changes in the acromion may also be found. Radioisotope scan typically shows increased uptake in the distal clavicle and occasionally in the acromion. This can be managed by conservative treatment which includes maintaining range of motion in the shoulder, strengthening and avoidance of activities inducing pain. If patients do not respond to this regime or are unwilling or unable to modify their activities, surgical excision of the distal end of the clavicle is warranted. Cahill (1982) reviewed 46 patients, all male athletes and all but one weightlifters. The surgically treated cases (19) obtained relief, whereas the others only improved by cessation or change of sporting activity and avoidance of weight training.

The cause of osteolysis of the distal clavicle remains obscure. Various proposals for aetiology include autonomic nervous system dysfunction with secondary alterations in blood supply, synovial pathogenesis with invasion of local bone tissue, and subchondral stress fractures due to repetitive trauma. There is a high rate of bilateral involvement of the shoulders.

Acromioclavicular joint injury

The function of the acromioclavicular joint and surrounding ligaments includes suspending the scapula from the clavicle and supporting the weight of the upper extremity. Once the ligaments are destroyed, the stability of the joint must be maintained by the muscles. The loss of suspension can lead to muscle fatigue, encroachment of the acromion on the supraspinatus tendon, and neurologic symptoms secondary to traction on the brachial plexus. Strain or dislocation of the acromioclavicular joint is a common injury seen in athletes and in nonathletes who have fallen heavily on the outstretched arm or on the side of the shoulder. The injury can be classified into three grades:

- **Grade I:** Sprain of the acromioclavicular joint without ligament injury or instability; treated conservatively.

- **Grade II:** Disruption of the acromioclavicular joint with tear of the acromioclavicular ligament and upward displacement of the clavicle of up to half the thickness of the shaft; also usually treated conservatively.

- **Grade III:** Complete disruption of the acromioclavicular joint with tear of the acromioclavicular and coracoclavicular ligaments and dislocation of the clavicle by more than half of the shaft thickness (Figure 3.4.9); best managed surgically.

A variety of surgical procedures have been described, and can be divided into three kinds:

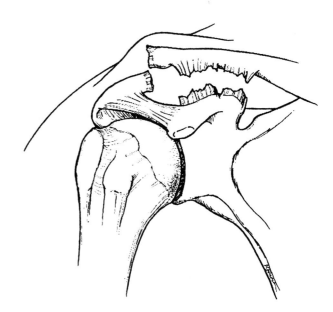

Figure 3.4.9 Complete acromioclavicular dislocation: there is a complete rupture of the acromioclavicular and and coracoclavicular ligaments, damage to the trapezius and deltoid muscle attachments, and tenting of the skin.

- **direct procedure** with sole repair of the acromioclavicular joint and its ligaments.

- **indirect procedure** with sole repair of the coracoclavicular ligaments.

- combined procedures.

In patients whose injury appears to be intermediate between grades II and III, radiological stress views can be obtained. This involves a standard anteroposterior view (usually with a 25° shoot-up angle) followed by asking the subject to hold a 10-kg weight in the affected arm by his side for 5 minutes before repeating the radiograph. In some cases patients who appear to have a grade II injury are shown in fact to have a grade III injury under weightbearing stress. Opinion is divided as to the need for surgical fixation in all cases of complete acromioclavicular separation. Some clinicians recommend conservative management in patients over 45 years of age because of a higher rate of poor results following surgery. However, other authors (Krueger and Frank 1993) obtained good results in older adults who were athletically active. Glick (1987) found that an anatomical reduction was not necessary to obtain a good functional result, although the risk of posttraumatic arthritis in nonsurgically treated individuals is somewhat higher. This does not influence clinical symptoms. There is little information in the literature as to whether better functional results can be obtained with early rather than late operative repair. Weinstein *et al.* (1995) note a trend towards better results in the group of patients undergoing earlier repair, 96% satisfactory results being obtained with a modified Weaver–Dunn technique with only 77% satisfactory results in those undergoing late repair. They advocate surgery for athletes and manual labourers requiring use of a strong arm, and that operative repair should ideally be made before 3 months after injury.

I find that symptomatic grade I and grade II strains usually respond to ligament sclerosant injections (prolotherapy) directed to the acromioclavicular joint, ligament and capsule, and the coracoclavicular ligaments. The efficacy of this form of injection therapy has been shown in treating chronic ligamentous insufficiency in the lumbar and sacroiliac region but has not been studied in any form of controlled trial in peripheral joints (see Chapter 4.3.5). The effectiveness of this treatment obviously depends on at least partial integrity of the involved ligaments.

Sternoclavicular dysfunction and injury

The sternoclavicular joint may undergo primary osteoarthrotic change which produces some mild tenderness, crepitus, and bony deformity. The symptoms are rarely severe enough to require any local treatment. However, trauma such as a fall on the outstretched arm or a heavy fall on the side of the shoulder, as in a rugby tackle, may strain the capsuloligamentous structures in this joint, producing some degree of synovial swelling and laxity of the anterior joint structures. The patient reports local pain and swelling, often radiating along the length of the clavicle, and this is usually associated with symptoms arising from the acromioclavicular joint, upper trapezius, and cervical spine. The patient reports pain on abduction and elevation of the shoulder together with the presence of swelling, deformity, and tenderness over the joint. Mild symptoms respond to conservative therapy including physiotherapy, and anti-inflammatory drugs topically or orally. More severe symptoms may require local joint injec-

tion. Injection of this joint should be performed with great caution using a 25-gauge needle perpendicular to the plane of the joint, taking care to penetrate no further than the anterior joint capsule to avoid puncture of mediastinal structures.

Rarely, the sternoclavicular joint can be dislocated either anteriorly or posteriorly. The posterior dislocation is less common than anterior dislocation because the anterior ligamentous structures are relatively weak. Most of the reported cases occur in young people, mainly men, who have experienced trauma to the shoulder girdle. The patient may present with the neck flexed towards the injured side, supporting the flexed elbow with the opposite hand and complaining of local pain. With an anterior dislocation the obvious swelling and deformity can be seen and in most cases can be managed conservatively since it rarely causes any long-term dysfunction. With posterior dislocation the depression may be seen and palpated if swelling has not yet obscured the picture. To confirm the diagnosis in either case, oblique radiographs are recommended since a routine anteroposterior view often does not show the condition. Because of the close relation of the posteriorly displaced medial clavicle to several vital structures, serious complications have been reported which include pneumothorax, haemothorax, and even compression or laceration of the great vessels or trachea. Where the condition has gone unrecognized, the thoracic outlet syndrome (see Chapter 3.4.1) has been described. In posterior dislocation further investigations are therefore important: chest radiograph, CT, and angiography if any vascular involvement is suspected. In posterior dislocation closed reduction can be obtained by posterolateral traction of the upper arm and digital traction of the medial clavicle forwards. However, open reduction is sometimes necessary. In late diagnosis, which remains symptomatic, resection of the medial part of the clavicle may be the best option. Conservative management consists of a figure-of-eight bandage for 6 weeks followed by maintenance of active shoulder movement and muscle strength.

Adhesive capsulitis (frozen shoulder)

Pathology

Historically, Duplay in 1872 first described this condition of a painful, stiff shoulder, referring to it as humeroscapular periarthritis. In 1934 Codman coined the term 'frozen shoulder', attributing the symptoms to a short rotator tendinitis. In 1945 Neviaser surgically explored 10 cases of frozen shoulder, finding absence of the glenohumeral synovial fluid and the redundant axillary fold of the capsule as well as thickening and contraction of the capsule which had become adherent to the humeral head. Thus he used the term 'adhesive capsulitis'. In the 10 cases he explored, microscopic examinations revealed reparative inflammatory changes in the capsule. However, McLoughlin (1938) reported no evidence of inflammation histologically in the frozen shoulders that he explored. He consistently found that the rotator cuff tendon was contracted and shrunken, which he postulated was due to collagen stiffening. Simmonds (1949) and McNab (1973) proposed that the diffuse capsulitis was caused by a degenerative inflammatory process in the supraspinatus tendon. Lippmann (1943) confirmed both Schrager and Pasteur's theory that bicipital tenosynovitis preceded frozen shoulder. In examining 12 surgical cases of frozen shoulder he found tenosynovitis of the long head of the biceps tendon. DePalma (1983) stated that the pathologic process of frozen shoulder primarily involves the fibrous capsule. He noted that the normally flexible capsule becomes inelastic and shrunken. The mechanism responsible for these changes is unknown. He also observed involvement of the periarticular structures in the various stages of frozen shoulder. In the early stages the capsule contracts with loss of the inferior capsular fold. In later phases increased capsular fibrosis occurs. The synovial membrane becomes thickened and hypervascular. The coracohumeral ligament becomes a thick, contracted cord and the subscapularis tendon also becomes fibrotic.

Cyriax (1978) documented the clinical examination findings of restriction of active and passive movements in characteristic proportions – which he called the **capsular pattern**. This has most limitation in external rotation followed by abduction and then by internal rotation. Both Neviaser (1945) and Kozin (1983) confirmed these findings. Reeves (1975) substantiated the capsular pattern in arthrograms of 17 patients with frozen shoulder. He noticed more contrast dye deposited posteriorly than in any other areas of the joint capsule (implying that adhesions, if present, were anterior), reduction of intracapsular volume, and loss of the inferior capsular fold with obliteration of the subscapularis bursa and biceps sheath. Since then, most research and clinical observation has pointed to capsular adhesions as the cause of glenohumeral stiffness in frozen shoulder.

Aetiology

The pathogenesis of capsulitis or true frozen shoulder remains unknown. Cyriax proposed that a history of trauma, such as a fall on the shoulder or on the outstretched hand, may precede the onset of capsulitis by as much as 6 months, but many patients cannot recall such injuries if they appear relatively minor at the time. Most authors consider the onset to be insidious. It usually occurs in people over 40 years old, affecting both sexes but women rather more commonly. Adhesive capsulitis occurs more commonly in association with hemiparesis, ischaemic heart disease, thyroid disease, pulmonary tuberculosis, chronic bronchitis, and diabetes. Capsulitis is five times more common in diabetics, usually involving the nondominant side, but occurring bilaterally in up to 50%.

Course and clinical features

The natural history of adhesive capsulitis is self-limiting, with an average length of time to recovery of approximately 2 years but varying from 1 to 4 years. Most patients recover full function, but a minority remain with some functional deficit and up to half do not regain full shoulder motion (Shaffer *et al.* 1992). Patients are most likely to require intervention during the painful phase, which may last 2–9 months. Reeves noted that the length of the painful period corresponded to the length of the recovery period in that a shorter period of pain was associated with a shorter recovery period.

Reeves (1975) emphasizes three features which assist in describing phases of the condition: pain, stiffness, and recovery. However, stiffness develops while pain is present, as shown in Figure 3.4.10.

- **Pain** remains from the onset for 2–6 months during which the capsule contracts. Arthrography, although not necessary for diagnosis, when performed at this stage will show decreased joint volume, usually less than 10 ml, sometimes as little as 2 ml, with obliteration of the subscapularis bursa and biceps sheath.

- **Stiffness** remains unchanged for 4–12 months.

- The final stage of spontaneous **recovery** lasts from 5 months to 26 months, during which there is a gradual return of external rotation coinciding with the arthrographic reappearance of the subscapular bursa. During this phase there is a gradual return of abduction and internal rotation.

Symptoms

The typical patient presents with some pain of weeks' or months' duration and insidious onset, and stiffness in the shoulder. They will usually point to the upper arm around the deltoid. The patient will complain of pain produced by attempted movements overhead or behind their back, such as reaching to put on a coat or for the seatbelt in their car. They may complain of spontaneous aching even at rest, but most commonly patients will describe pain when lying on the affected side at night which may radiate to a varying degree down the arm to the elbow and sometimes to the forearm, wrist and hand.

Physical examination

In the painful phase the patient will present with signs of anxiety due to pain and loss of sleep. Arm swing during gait may be reduced and the patient will be restricted while undressing. Sometimes the affected side is elevated because of shortening of the trapezius and levator scapulae. As a consequence, there may be referred pain towards the neck and scapular region. Diagnosis is usually clear-cut, using the routine described in Chapter 3.1.1.

The cervical spine may show a pattern of strain with features of segmental dysfunction. At the shoulder, active elevation is reduced in all but the earliest cases: the striking findings are of pain and restriction of passive glenohumeral movement; i.e. most marked for external

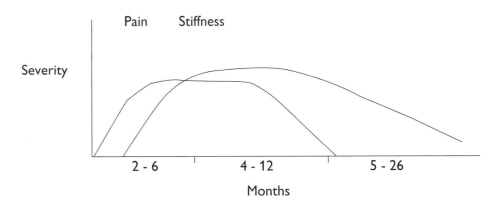

Figure 3.4.10 Resolution of pain and stiffness: adhesive capsulitis.

rotation, less so for abduction, and less still for internal rotation. There may be pain on resisted movements, suggestive of concurrent rotator cuff strain, but in typical cases (1) the resisted movements are less painful than the passive ones, and (2) all the resisted movements are painful, not giving the differential pattern typical of trauma to part of the rotator cuff. Specific examination of accessory movements of the glenohumeral joint shows loss of joint-play.

In cases that follow trauma there may be coexistent rotator cuff tendonitis and/or subacromial bursitis which will require treating independently. Urinalysis is useful to detect diabetic cases, who do not have such a good prognosis for early relief.

Plain radiographs are usually normal apart from occasionally showing some osteoporosis, and arthrography shows reduced joint volume with obliteration of the subscapularis bursa, bicipital tendon sheath, and inferior capsular fold.

Differential diagnosis

Any patient presenting with an acute onset of pain and stiffness in the shoulder with a capsular pattern on examination should be adequately screened to exclude other diseases that may present with monoarthritis (Table 3.4.4). The presence of swelling and warmth to the touch should alert one to the possibility of an inflammatory synovitis or septic arthritis. A brief review of the hands and other joints looking for evidence of nodules, tenosynovitis, or, in the case of seronegative arthritis, rashes and asymmetric articular involvement, should lead to appropriate investigation and the correct diagnosis.

Treatment

The aims of treatment are pain relief and restoration of normal shoulder movement. Treatment should consist of one or more of the following:

- education and reassurance of the patient about the natural history of the condition and support with the use of analgesics or anti-inflammatories
- physiotherapy with the use of mobilization techniques or other modalities
- the use of injection techniques with corticosteroid
- manipulation under anaesthesia.

The choice of treatment depends on the severity of the condition and the stage of the condition. In terms of severity, a mild case will not merit corticosteroid injection.

In terms of stage, we use the criteria developed by Cyriax for gauging whether the case will be sensitive to a steroid injection. We ask the following questions:

- Does pain extend below the elbow?

Table 3.4.4. Other diseases that may present with monoarthritis

Acute onset	Subacute or chronic onset
Septic arthritis	Crystal deposition, e.g. hydroxyapatite
Gout	Rheumatoid arthritis and variants
Pseudogout	Avascular necrosis

- Is pain felt at rest?
- Is the patient unable to sleep on that shoulder?

When these questions are answered yes, manual treatment other than accessory movements is likely to increase pain, and not to achieve better range: if active treatment is required, injection is the treatment of choice.

Injection therapy

The trials of Bulgen *et al.* (1984), Jacobs *et al.* (1991), and Rizk *et al.* (1991) all found conclusive benefit for the use of steroids given intra-articularly to the glenohumeral joint, with the best results found in those patients injected early in the course of the illness. Pain relief was the main benefit, although Jacobs also showed an improvement in long-term outcome.

Multiple-injection techniques

A further trial by Winters *et al.* (1997) was conducted in a primary care setting and this trial reported significant differences between the treatments. In this study treatment was considered successful after 5 weeks for 35 out of 47 patients (75%) treated with injections and for 7 out of 35 (20%) treated with physiotherapy. The corticosteroid treatment consisted of multiple injections administered by the general practitioners. For the purposes of the research study, passive mobilization was not permitted for patients allocated to the physiotherapy group.

Steinbrocker and Argyros (1974) used a triple injection technique into the joint, bursa, and long head of biceps tendon and found that 95% of patients were dramatically better or cured after 1–3 treatment sessions. Another similar study (Roy 1976) used the same entry criteria and a paired injection technique, joint and bursa, with similarly spectacular results. The authors of this latter study comment that an injection into the subacromial bursa or joint cavity alone carries a very low rate of success compared to a paired approach. It is interesting to compare this comment with Hazleman's findings of combined intracapsular and intrabursal inflammatory change during early arthroscopy (Hazleman 1990).

Accuracy of injection technique

The use of 2–3 different injection techniques in one treatment may have advantages when one considers a rather uncertain 'hit rate' when performing the technique blind, i.e. without the benefit of radiographic control. Inaccurate placement of intra-articular injections is reported to occur often, even among trained rheumatologists (Jones *et al.* 1993, Eustace *et al.* 1997, White *et al.* 1996): there is a better response to accurately placed injections. The subacromial bursa is known to be in continuity with the joint space in as much as 25% of the individuals and therefore a paired injection technique may allow more drug to reach the intended target. Most radiologists, when performing shoulder arthrograms in adhesive capsulitis, prefer the posterior approach since so often the anterior capsular structures are retracted. The technique of the posterior approach to shoulder joint injection is shown in Figure 3.4.11.

Jacobs' study used capsular distension with volumes exceeding 25 ml in his study and this could explain the enhanced therapeutic affect in his trial. This may reduce the need for a series of 2–3 injec-

Shoulder Joint

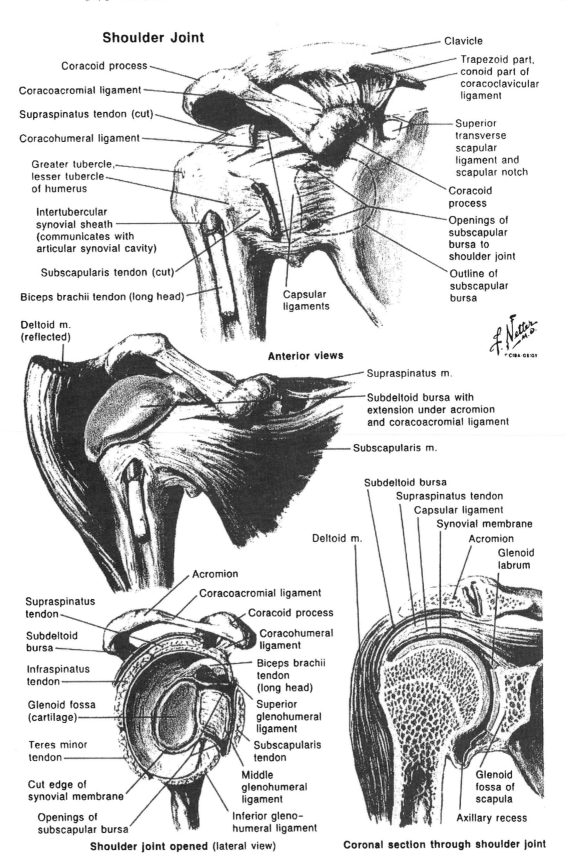

Coracoid process

Coracoacromial ligament

Supraspinatus tendon (cut)

Coracohumeral ligament

Greater tubercle, lesser tubercle of humerus

Intertubercular synovial sheath (communicates with articular synovial cavity)

Subscapularis tendon (cut)

Biceps brachii tendon (long head)

Clavicle

Trapezoid part, conoid part of coracoclavicular ligament

Superior transverse scapular ligament and scapular notch

Coracoid process

Openings of subscapular bursa to shoulder joint

Outline of subscapular bursa

Capsular ligaments

Anterior views

Deltoid m. (reflected)

Supraspinatus m.

Subdeltoid bursa with extension under acromion and coracoacromial ligament

Subscapularis m.

Supraspinatus tendon

Subdeltoid bursa

Infraspinatus tendon

Glenoid fossa (cartilage)

Teres minor tendon

Cut edge of synovial membrane

Openings of subscapular bursa

Acromion

Coracoacromial ligament

Coracoid process

Coracohumeral ligament

Biceps brachii tendon (long head)

Superior glenohumeral ligament

Subscapularis tendon

Middle glenohumeral ligament

Inferior gleno-humeral ligament

Shoulder joint opened (lateral view)

Deltoid m.

Subdeltoid bursa

Supraspinatus tendon

Capsular ligament

Synovial membrane

Acromion

Glenoid labrum

Glenoid fossa of scapula

Axillary recess

Coronal section through shoulder joint

Figure 3.4.11 Anatomical relations of bursae, biceps tendon, and subacromial space to the joint capsule and associated ligaments.

tions, which I find in clinical practice is often required to cover the most painful period of the acute phase.

Injection routine

Appropriate treatment by steroid injection for capsulitis would be initial injection using a single or combined technique as discussed above followed by review in approximately 3 weeks. The dose I recommend is 20 mg of triamcinolone. Some studies have used up to 40 mg and injected this as many as 3 times in 6 weeks. This increases the risk of systemic side effects and therefore the minimum dose necessary to achieve the therapeutic result is recommended. Very few patients complain of soreness after the injection. By following up the patient at 3–4-week intervals the acute phase can be managed by a further booster steroid injection until the most painful phase of the condition has settled. The patient can be reassured that the range of movement will gradually recover with time, although this may take up to 12–18 months. Active and passive exercises can be recommended at this stage, with the caution that over-vigorous mobilization may result in a flare-up of symptoms and therefore require further injection treatment. In my experience most patients find this approach to management satisfactory. Occasionally the shoulder will remain stiff and restricted in the absence of pain beyond the average 2-year period, and then referral for manipulation under anaesthesia might be indicated.

In hospital practice, if two consecutive shoulder joint injections have failed to obtain therapeutic relief we recommend a third attempt under radiographic control. The posterior approach is optimal and with the use of contrast medium the abnormal arthrogram can be visualized. Placement of 5–10 ml of local anaesthetic with 20 mg of triamcinolone intra-articularly will very often produce the desired response.

Physiotherapy

A variety of modalities including heat, ice, diathermy, ultrasound, and infrared have traditionally been used in physiotherapy departments. There is no evidence that any of this is effective except for very short-term relief of symptoms, or perhaps warming of the joint structures before stretching. Mueller (1954) studied the benefit of ultrasound in a placebo control study for periarthritis. Using a power of 2 W/cm^2 he found that this modality was of no value in treating subacute frozen shoulder. Quinn in 1967 found no difference in groups receiving ultrasound at 0.5 W/cm^2 and exercises and those receiving diathermy and exercises.

Active mobilization

In the early, steroid-sensitive phase as described above, all active treatment is contraindicated and treatment should be directed at pain relief, i.e. joint injection. If this is not available, however, the use of ice, analgesics, NSAIDs and TENS may help. In the later stages exercise may be cautiously initiated, with close attention to the patient's response. The timing and degree of exercise can be based on the end-feel and point at which pain develops during passive movement. If pain develops before the therapist reaches the end of range, the joint is too irritable to initiate active or passive mobilization. If, however, pain is only experienced at the end of range, exercises may be attempted but if there is undue exacerbation such as increased pain lasting more than 2 hours after exercise they should be delayed. Some investigators have concluded that of all the treatments available, active exercise is the

most useful (Lee *et al.* 1974). This study showed that both groups receiving exercises did significantly better than patients receiving analgesics alone.

Active mobilization with the use of mechanical exercise such as shoulder wheels, pulleys, and wands has been the traditional mainstay of treatment in the past. Unfortunately it has a major drawback because there is no stabilization of the scapula, no force to depress the humeral head, and the patient tends to extend the spine to decrease demands on glenohumeral motion. Exactly the same criticisms can be levelled at the use of the shoulder wheel and the finger ladder. These techniques should probably be used only when normal gliding is present, since they involve movement only in the cardinal planes of the joint and do not increase joint play. Similarly, Codman or pendulum exercises performed with gravity are pain-free but exercise the joint only in the cardinal planes of movement. These and other exercises may be useful in maintaining flexibility in the joint once it has been obtained through other means.

Passive mobilization

There are a variety of forms of passive mobilization, based on the methods of Maitland (1977), Kaltenborn (1980), and Mennell (1964), but few controlled studies of this method have been undertaken. Bulgen *et al.* (1984) found no superiority of Maitland mobilization over treatment with ice, steroid injections, or no treatment in patients with more than 1 month's symptoms of frozen shoulder. In fact, after 6 weeks of treatment he found the group receiving mobilization had greater loss of motion than the other groups. We therefore avoid mobilization when the joint is 'irritable'. After the inflammatory phase a variety of manual techniques can be tried, if the patient is sufficiently handicapped, using the principles of capsular distraction and improvement of joint-play (accessory movements).

Manipulation under anaesthesia

The literature on this subject is controversial, and various manipulative procedures are described. Some authors state that manipulation under anaesthesia only works by rupturing the capsule, usually the adherent inferior fold of the capsule; and indeed contrast medium can be seen to escape from the capsule during this manoeuvre. Furthermore, long-lever techniques may run the risk of fracturing the humerus, particularly in osteoporotic individuals, and some investigators report tears of the rotator cuff. Despite claims of greatly increasing the range of motion, many physical therapists providing postoperative care find it is common for a patient to have less motion following manipulation, presumably as a result of an acute inflammatory action with muscle spasm. Pain is certainly likely to increase for several days, and modalities such as ice or TENS may be useful.

Thomas (1980) performed a randomized controlled trial on 30 cases with a frozen shoulder of more than 2 months' duration. Both groups received 20 mg of intravenous valium and an injection of 50 mg of hydrocortisone into the shoulder via the posterior approach. One group was manipulated using forced abduction to 90° accompanied by full internal and external rotation. At 1-month follow up only 2 patients had completely recovered, both in the manipulation group. At 3 months 7 patients in the manipulated group (47%) and only 2 patients in the injected group (13%) had completely recovered. Several authors confirm that capsular rupture is an invariable recurrence during manipulation, although Samilson *et al.* (1961) suggests that rupture of the rotator cuff is also a frequent complication. This did not occur in any case of 103 manipulations performed with simultaneous arthrography reported by Lundberg (1969).

A promising study by Placzek *et al.* (1998) using a short-lever translational manipulation on 31 patients under interscalene brachial plexus block has shown significant increases in range of motion both immediately following manipulation and at long-term follow-up (up to 14 months). The average duration of symptoms was over 7 months and all patients were significantly disabled before treatment. Unfortunately, however, all patients also received a 6-day course of 4 mg of prednisolone daily starting the day before manipulation, and no control group was used. Furthermore, after the manipulation all patients received a fairly intensive program of physical therapy. However, the immediate increases in passive range of motion following manipulation obtained in all cases are impressive and there was no tendency to relapse throughout the follow-up period.

Arthroscopic capsular release has been described (Warner *et al.* 1996) as an alternative for the management of patients who have failed to respond to physical therapy or closed manipulation under anaesthesia, but no controlled studies have been reported.

References

Binder, A. I. *et al.* (1984) Frozen shoulder: A long term prospective study. *Annals of the Rheumatic Diseases*, **43**, 361.

Bulgen, D. Y. *et al.* (1984) Frozen shoulder. A prospective clinical study with an evaluation of three treatment regimes. *Annals of the Rheumatic Diseases*, **43**, 353–60.

Cahill, B. R. (1982) Osteolysis of the distal part of the clavicle in male athletes. *Journal of Bone and Joint Surgery*, **64A**, 1053–8.

Codman, E. A. (1934) *The shoulder.* Robert E. Kreiger Publishing Company, Malibar, FL.

Cyriax, J. (1978) *Textbook of orthopaedic medicine*, 7th edn, Vol. 1. Bailliére Tindall, London.

DePalma, A. F. (1983) *Surgery of the shoulder.* J. B. Lippincott, Philadelphia.

Eustace, J. A. *et al.* (1997) Comparison of the accuracy of steroid placement with clinical outcome in patients with shoulder symptoms. *Annals of the Rheumatic Diseases*, **56**, 59–63.

Glick, J.M. (1987) Dislocated acromioclavicular joint: follow up study of 35 unreduced acromioclavicular dislocations. *American Journal of Sports Medicine*, **5**, 264–72.

Hazleman, B. L. (1990) Why is a frozen shoulder frozen? *British Journal of Rheumatology*, **29**(2), 130.

Jacobs, L. G. H. *et al.* (1991) Intra-articular distension and steroids in the management of capsulitis of the shoulder. *BMJ*, **302**, 1494–501.

Jones, A. *et al.* (1993). Importance of placement of intra-articular steroid injection. *BMJ*, **307**, 1329–30.

Kaltenborn, F. M. (1980). *Mobilization of the extremity joints. Examination and basic treatment techniques.* Olaf Bokhandel, Oslo.

Kozin, F. (1983) Two unique shoulder disorders. Adhesive capsulitis and reflex sympathetic dystrophy syndrome. *Postgraduate Medicine*, **73**, 207.

Krueger, M. and Frank, E. (1993) Surgical treatment of dislocations of the acromioclavicular joint in the athlete. *British Journal of Sports Medicine*, **27**, 2.

Lee, P. N. *et al.* (1974) Periarthritis of the shoulder. Trial of treatments investigated by multivariant analysis. *Annals of the Rheumatic Diseases*, **33**, 116–19.

Lippmann, R. K. (1943) Frozen shoulder peri-arthritis bicipital tenosynovitis. Archives of Surgery, **47**, 283.

Lundberg, B. J. (1969). The frozen shoulder. *Acta Orthopaedica Scandinavica Supplement*, **119**, 55–91.

Maitland, G. D. (1977) *Peripheral manipulation*, 2nd edn. Butterworths, Boston.

Mennell, J. (1964) *Joint pain. Diagnosis, treatment using manipulative techniques.* Little Brown Boston.

McLoughlin, H. L. (1961) The frozen shoulder. *Clinical Orthopedics*, **20**, 126.

McNab, I. (1973) Rotator cuff tendonitis. *Annals of the Royal College of Surgeons of England*, **53**, 271.

Mueller, E. E., *et al.* (1954) A placebo-controlled study of ultrasound treatment for periarthritis. *Am J Phys Med*, **33**, 31.

Neviaser, J. S. (1945) Adhesive capsulitis of the shoulder: study of pathological findings in peri-arthritis of the shoulder. *Journal of Bone and Joint Surgery*, **27**, 211.

Placzek, J. D. *et al.* (1998) Long term effectiveness of translational manipulation for adhesive capsulitis. *Clinical Orthopedics and Related Research*, **356**, 181–91.

Quinn, C. E. (1967) Humeroscapular periarthritis. Observation on effects of x-ray therapy and ultrasonic therapy in cases of frozen shoulder. *Ann Phys Med*, **10**, 64.

Reeves, B. (1975) The natural history of the frozen shoulder syndrome. *Scandinavian Journal of Rheumatology*, **4**, 193.

Rizk, T. E. *et al.* (1991) Corticosteroid injections in adhesive capsulitis, an investigation into their value and site. *Archives of Physical Medicine and Rehabilitation*, **72**, 20–22.

Roy, S., *et al.* (1982) Frozen shoulder. *BMJ*, **284**, 117-18.

Samilson, R. L. *et al.* (1961) Arthrography of the shoulder joint. *Clinical Orthopedics*, **20**, 21–23.

Shaffer, B., Tibone, J. E., Kerlan, R. K. (1992) Frozen shoulder – a long-term follow-up. *Journal of Bone and Joint Surgery*, **74A**, 738–46.

Simmonds, F. A. (1949) Shoulder pain with particular reference to the frozen shoulder. *Journal of Bone and Joint Surgery*, **31B**, 426.

Steinbrocker, O., Argyros, T. G. A. (1974) Study on adhesive capsulitis of the shoulder *Archives of Physical Medicine and Rehabilitation*, **55**, 209.

Thomas, D. *et al.* (1980) The frozen shoulder: a review of manipulative treatment. *Rheumatology and Rehabilitation*, **19**, 173–9.

Warner, J. J. *et al.* (1996) Arthroscopic release for chronic refractory adhesive capsulitis of the shoulder. *Journal of Bone and Joint Surgery*, **78A**(12), 1808–16.

Weinstein, D. M. *et al.* (1995) Surgical treatment of complete acromioclavicular dislocations. *American Journal of Sports Medicine*, **23**, 3.

Winters, J. C. *et al.* (1997) Comparison of physiotherapy, manipulation and corticosteroid injection for treating shoulder complaints in general practice: randomized single blind study. *BMJ*, **314**, 1320–5.

3.4.4 Glenohumeral instability

Roger Hackney

The shoulder has the greatest range of motion of any joint in the human body. This function allows use of the hand across a wide area, perhaps as essential in human development as any other advance. One consequence of the great mobility of the shoulder is the effect upon the stability of the joint. Medicine has classically focused upon the traumatic anterior dislocation of the shoulder. Over the last two decades it has increasingly been realized that there is a spectrum of instability.

The earliest report of anterior dislocation of the shoulder in found in the Edwin Smith Papyrus, dated 3000–2500 BCE. Hippocrates studied the shoulder and described the anatomy, the dislocations which may occur, a method of reduction, and a method of preventing recurrence of dislocation. The introduction of a red-hot poker into the anterior shoulder to induce scarring, thereby preventing recurrence, has not stood the test of time. The use of heat in management of instability has, however, had a rather poetic resurgence.

The incidence of anterior dislocation of the shoulder is roughly 1%, rising in certain sports, for example ice hockey, to 7%. In a unique study from Sweden, Hovelius (1987) followed every shoulder dislocation in patients between 18 and 70. He found general results of a 1.7% prevalence and recurrence rates of 20% overall; 60% of 20-year-olds had more than one subsequent dislocation. Other authors have found much higher rates of recurrence in a young active population, approaching 100% in teenagers.

Biomechanics of stability

An understanding of shoulder instability depends upon an understanding of the structures responsible for glenohumeral joint stability. The features responsible for stability can be conveniently divided into static and dynamic stabilizers.

Static stabilizers

Bony anatomy

The bony anatomy of the glenohumeral joint does not contribute greatly to stability. The acromion, together with the coracoacromial ligament, forms the roof of the shoulder preventing superior translation of the humerus. Movement in other directions is not restricted by bony anatomy. The glenoid is positioned in a variable amount of anteversion, and the humerus correspondingly retroverted.

Glenoid labrum

The glenoid is a shallow concavity. A rim of fibrocartilage called the glenoid labrum increases its depth. The articular surfaces of the glenoid and humerus are not fully congruent. When the humerus is pressed into the glenoid, there is a strong concavity compression effect, aided by the adhesion–cohesion mechanism of wet surfaces. This can be compared to the grip that the 'sucker' head of a child's arrow has when stuck on to a window. The negative pressure inside the glenohumeral joint has been measured at –31 mmHg. This provides a significant contribution to joint stability.

The superior portion of the labrum has the attachment of the long head of biceps.

Shoulder capsule

The shoulder capsule arises from, or just behind, the glenoid labrum. Ligaments are thickenings of the capsule. There are three named condensations whose function varies with different positions of the arm. With the arm hanging by the side, the superior glenohumeral ligament prevents inferior subluxation of the shoulder. The middle glenohumeral ligament is less consistently present, but tends to function with the arm partially abducted. The inferior glenohumeral ligament is said to act a sling or hammock, allowing for reciprocal tightening of the anterior and posterior elements in various positions of rotation. This ligament holds the arm in place with the shoulder in abduction. The posterior capsule is a relatively weak structure.

The inferior glenohumeral ligament has been extensively investigated because of its importance first in maintaining joint stability and second in sports involving overhead activity. The ligament has the property of becoming stronger and stiffer at high strain rates, resisting injury with fast, athletic activity. The ligament usually fails at the insertion onto the glenoid when loaded in tension, although tears in mid-substance also occur prior to avulsion.

The coracohumeral ligament has been described, running from the base of the coracoid to the lesser tuberosity where it combines with the superior glenohumeral ligament. It occupies the space between the subscapularis and supraspinatus muscles. The ligament is not thought to have a suspensory function, but has been implicated in the pathology of frozen shoulder.

Rotator interval

The rotator interval is a triangular area of capsule bordered superiorly by the edge of supraspinatus and inferiorly by subscapularis. Dividing the tissue occupying the rotator interval markedly increases translation in all directions.

Dynamic stabilizers

Rotator cuff

The rotator cuff is a group of four muscles arising from the scapula. They merge to form a cuff of tendon that envelops the humeral head. The primary function of the rotator cuff is to pull the humeral head into the glenoid, contributing to the concavity compression phenomenon. The compression effect is maintained throughout the range of motion by synchronous coordinated contraction of the rotator cuff group. An essential part of this is the position of the scapula. Although the rotator cuff does function to assist activities such as throwing, the primary task is to centre the humeral head within the glenoid. The glenohumeral joint does not act strictly as a ball and socket joint. There is approximately 4 mm of sliding movement of the humeral head across the glenoid in the vertical and horizontal planes during normal movement, which amounts to up to 50% of the width of the glenoid.

Scapula

Movement of the scapula on the chest wall allows the position of the glenoid to be varied. This ability allows much greater range of movement of the shoulder joint, and hence the position of the hand in space, whilst maintaining stability. The importance of the movement of the scapula in the maintenance of stability can be illustrated by considering the effect of scapula positioning with the arm abducted to 90° and in the sagittal plane, pointing forwards. With the scapula protracted, the humerus is aligned with the glenoid centre line, and the rotator cuff is nicely positioned to provide compression. When the scapula is fully retracted, the humerus is nearly at a right angle to the glenoid. The balance of the rotator cuff is awry and stability is jeopardized.

Long head of biceps

The long head of biceps is an intra-articular structure. When the biceps contracts, there is a downward force exerted on the humeral head. This adds to the superior stability of the shoulder, adding to the combined effects of the shape of the acromial arch and the rotator cuff.

Types of instability

The classification of instability must include the mechanism by which the instability occurs, the frequency, and the direction.

- **Laxity** is the asymptomatic translation of the head of the humerus over the glenoid. This varies greatly between individuals. Laxity may

be congenital or acquired, the latter especially in participants in throwing, swimming and gymnastic sports. Laxity in a given individual can be determined by noting the following signs:
   - the degree of external rotation of the shoulder with the elbow tucked into the side
   - the presence of a sulcus sign with gentle downwards traction on the shoulder
   - the anterior and posterior draw signs.

- **Instability** occurs when the laxity becomes symptomatic, causing pain or apprehension of movement of the shoulder.

- **Subluxation** is a symptomatic degree of instability. Dislocation is the complete separation of the articular surfaces. There is a spectrum of instability with a variety of causes. The idea of a shoulder either being unstable, dislocating or not has been superseded by a greater understanding of the subtlety of the concept of instability.

- Instability may be **anterior, posterior, or inferior**. A combination of more than one of these is defined to be multidirectional. Ninety-five per cent of all instability is anterior, though a degree of a secondary component is commonplace. Increased laxity of the shoulder predisposes to multidirectional instability, through the load-sharing concept of shoulder instability.

- <u>T</u>raumatic <u>u</u>nilateral with <u>B</u>ankart lesion treated by <u>s</u>urgery (TUBS) describes the dislocation of the glenohumeral joint where the forces acting at the joint are sufficiently severe to cause a capsular and bony injury sufficient to render the joint unstable.

- <u>A</u>traumatic <u>m</u>ultidirectional instability, <u>b</u>ilateral treated by <u>reha</u>bilitation and if surgery is necessary, with <u>i</u>nferior capsular shift (AMBRI) is the other extreme of a spectrum along which shoulder instability exists.

- **Habitual dislocation** describes the unstable shoulder where the individual is unable to maintain the stability of the joint during normal movement, or in extremes, at rest.

- **Voluntary dislocation** (Figure 3.4.12) exists when an individual is able to sublux, or rarely dislocate the shoulder at will. The direction of instability is almost invariably posterior.

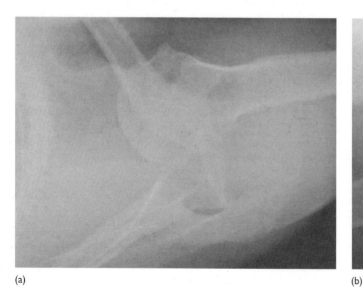

(a)

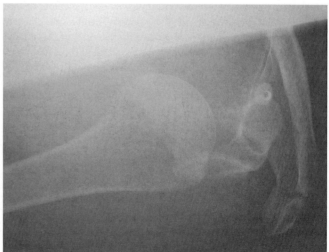

(b)

Figure 3.4.12 (a), (b) Voluntary dislocation.

● **Locked dislocations** occur both anteriorly and posteriorly. **Chronic anterior dislocation** occurs in elderly people, where a surprisingly full range of motion can be observed, or in the situation of major trauma when the shoulder injury has been missed. Chronic posterior dislocation is more common, as a result of trauma or epileptic seizure.

Pathophysiology of the unstable shoulder

Anterior

The damage caused by a traumatic shoulder dislocation depends to a significant degree upon the age of the individual. Below the age of 40 years, the major damage is to the capsulolabral attachment to the rim of the glenoid. The classic **Bankart tear** of the anterior labrum occurs in nearly 90% of traumatic dislocations. Although the labrum is an important structure in the stability of the shoulder, what seems to predispose the shoulder to further episodes of instability is the ripping of the attachment of the glenohumeral ligaments from the glenoid. The capsule remains attached to the glenoid, but much more medial and inferior to the original position. The lack of any anterior restraint allows subluxation and dislocation to occur at the same site with increasing ease. Occasionally the rotator interval may split rather than the capsule avulse. This tends to occur more in overhead athletes, or those with a lax joint.

A small but significant number also avulse the superior attachment of the labrum with the insertion of the long head of biceps, the so-called **SLAP lesion** (Figure 3.4.13). Steve Snyder first coined this term in 1990, though Andrews *et al.* described the lesion in 1985.

With increasing age, a tearing of the substance of the capsule is more likely. In elderly people, a Bankart lesion *per se* may be quite uncommon. The rotator cuff is far less pliable and will tear readily, not infrequently giving rise to a flail arm.

With anterior dislocation, the humeral head impacts upon the sharp anterior rim of the glenoid. The indentation of the soft bone of the humeral head is termed a **Hill–Sachs lesion** in the Anglo-American literature. This lesion can be large enough to destroy a large area of the articular surface, and predispose to easy recurrent dislocation. The engaging Hill–Sachs lesion in abduction and external rotation requires a separate management programme.

The rim of the glenoid along with the capsulolabral complex may be avulsed during dislocation, the so-called **bony Bankart**. This may reduce the width of the glenoid significantly, again predisposing to recurrent dislocation.

Posterior

The posterior capsule is less strong than the anterior capsule; nonetheless, it may be avulsed along with the posterior labrum and render the shoulder more liable to recurrence. The posterior dislocation seems more likely to lead to a significant indentation of the humeral head, the 'reverse' Hill–Sachs lesion.

Clinical assessment of the unstable shoulder

History

The purpose of taking a history in an individual with an unstable shoulder is to enable one to appreciate the aetiology of the instability and how it affects the patient.

The mechanism of the primary dislocation episode is important to understand. The story of the first instability episode is an essential part of the history. The age at the time of first dislocation or subluxation, the mechanism of injury, the method of reduction, and the treatment should all be documented. Anterior shoulder dislocation usually occurs in a position of abduction, extension, and external rotation. A fall on to an outstretched arm most frequently leads to an anterior dislocation. The age of first dislocation is important, because the risk of recurrence is highly dependent upon age of first dislocation. A teenager has an extremely high risk (90–100%) of further problems of the shoulder. In addition, one has to question the reason for such early dislocation. Unless there is a strong history of severe trauma, searching for a predisposing factor is indicated. A prior history of subluxation episodes or spontaneous reduction is commonplace. The ease of reduction does not necessarily reflect the severity of injury, but a history of frequent easy self-reduction indicates a significantly unstable joint.

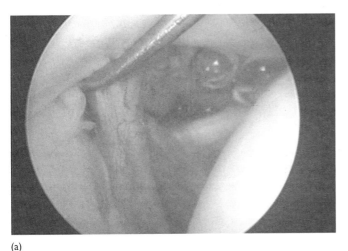

(a)

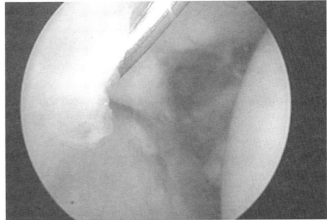

(b)

Figure 3.4.13a, b SLAP lesion.

The position of the shoulder in subsequent recurrent dislocations gives an indication of the direction of the dislocation. The instability may develop into the situation where the shoulder dislocates in certain positions, habitual dislocation. Reaching up to a high shelf may be enough to provoke a shoulder dislocation, which is obviously quite disabling. Subluxation or even dislocation may occur in sleep.

A history of joint laxity, subluxation or dislocation of the patella should prompt a search for laxity, even congenital hyperlaxity.

The more subtle instability patterns can be as disabling as frank dislocations. Appropriate treatment should not be withheld on the basis of the lack of radiographic evidence.

Acute posterior dislocations can be caused by direct or indirect force, for example, a direct blow to the anterior joint or a fall on to an adducted arm. A posterior dislocation may also occur as a result of a fit. The history is important and should arouse a degree of suspicion; nearly 50% of posterior dislocations are missed at first presentation. An inability to externally rotate the arm confirms the diagnosis.

A sporting history should detail overhead sporting activity. Swimming, throwing, and gymnastics all lead to secondary stretching of glenohumeral ligaments and an odd combination of instability and impingement.

Examination

The results of the history and examination should provide enough information to classify the dislocation.

Acute dislocation

The acute shoulder dislocation is usually painful, with obvious deformity. The patient is frequently aware of the nature of the injury. There are exceptions to this rule: recurrent dislocators, those with congenital laxity, and voluntary dislocators. With posterior dislocation, the deformity is less obvious and not infrequently missed.

The patient should be examined for neurovascular injury, and the findings documented. The common neurological injury is to the axillary nerve. The signs are of a numb area on the point of the shoulder and over the proximal deltoid, and weakness of deltoid. Up to 45% of acute anterior shoulder dislocations have electromyographic evidence of neurological damage. The peripheral pulses should also be checked prior to reduction. The possibility of an associated fracture should be considered, and a radiograph obtained before reduction. On the sports field, a gentle attempt at reduction may be made.

Observation

The shoulder should be examined for abnormal posture. The contours of the shoulder can look surprisingly normal in the presence of a chronically unreduced shoulder. Occasionally a patient with congenital hyperlaxity may present with the shoulder that subluxes with such ease that the patient is unable to control the position of the humeral head.

Movement

The shoulder should be assessed in flexion, abduction, and external and internal rotation.

The normal rhythm of shoulder movement may be compromised, as the subject struggles to maintain the head of the humerus in joint. The habitual dislocator will be aware that the shoulder subluxes during abduction in particular. External rotation greater than 45° in either shoulder must alert the examiner to the possibility of hypermobility of the shoulder.

The shoulder should be examined from the front and back. The rhythm of movement of the scapulothoracic and glenohumeral joints can be observed. The apposition of the scapula against the chest should be carefully scrutinized. Any degree of lifting away of the scapula from the chest should be compared with the other side. Full scapular winging is obvious and is associated with loss of function of the long thoracic nerve and paresis of serratus anterior. More subtle signs of winging are associated with glenohumeral instability, especially in those with ligamentous laxity.

Strength

The power of supraspinatus should be tested in the 'upturned beer glass' position. Infraspinatus is tested in resisted external rotation, and subscapularis with the lift-off test. In elderly people, the rotator cuff is liable to injury and power of the cuff must be formally examined. Weakness of deltoid may indicate an axillary nerve lesion. Subscapularis is tested by the lift-off test. The back of the hand is placed against the small of the back, and then pushed away from the body. The ability to perform this indicates an intact subscapularis; strength is tested by pushing the hand back towards the body.

Palpation

Little additional information can be gained from palpation of the unstable shoulder. There may be anterior joint line tenderness, but this is very non-specific. The tendon of biceps may be tender if it subluxes, when a palpable clunk may be detected. Crepitus may arise from a variety of sources, some distant from the shoulder, so is not a reliable localizing sign.

Instability tests

The sulcus sign indicates inferior laxity. This test is performed by applying gentle traction along the length of the arm, with the patient relaxed. The sign may be increased in the presence of hyperlaxity, a superior labral tear, or a very unstable shoulder.

The anterior and posterior draw signs require a relaxed patient. The humeral head is pushed anteriorly and posteriorly in turn, gauging the distance traversed across the glenoid:

- grade 0: normal, up to 50% of the diameter of the glenoid.
- grade 1: above 50% translation
- grade 2: the humeral head rides out to the rim of the glenoid
- grade 3: the humeral head sits over the edge of the glenoid.

These tests are most reliably performed under general anaesthetic, but if positive will indicate the amount of joint laxity. The quality of endstop is important to gauge the relative resistance of the patient's rotator cuff.

Posterior subluxation is tested by laying the patient supine, with the shoulder flexed to 90°. Direct pressure is applied along the humerus, intending to sublux the humeral head posteriorly. The arm is then brought around into abduction, maintaining the pressure. As the arm reaches 90°, a positive sign is produced if a palpable clunk is obtained as the shoulder relocates.

The classic apprehension test is performed with the shoulder in 90° of abduction and external rotation. The patient will feel a sense of impending instability. Pain is a less reliable guide to instability and may be due to a variety of causes, including subacromial and internal impingement as well as instability.

More subtle forms of instability are detected with the Jobe relocation test. This test was developed to try to determine the causation of the shoulder pain felt by throwing athletes. The original concept was that the position of abduction and external rotation produced an anterior subluxation, leading to a sensation of instability. By pressing down upon the humeral head it was thought that the humeral head could be relocated in the glenoid. Further external rotation is applied to the point of further discomfort. A positive test results when the pressure on the humeral head is removed and significant pain is produced.

Investigations

Plain radiography of an injured shoulder should always include two planes of view. The standard anteroposterior and axillary views allow easy diagnosis of the anterior dislocation. Difficulties arise in the diagnosis of posterior dislocation where only the anteroposterior view is obtained. The humeral head has the appearance of a light bulb, without an obvious joint space between the humeral head and glenoid. The diagnosis is easy with the axillary view, but nearly 50% of posterior dislocations are missed at initial presentation.

In the investigation of recurrent dislocation, the use of MRI has been widely proposed. CT with or without arthrography may also reveal the pathology. The use of MRI and CT is extremely common, but I question the necessity. In most cases, management is not affected by the results of such scans, which are expensive and, in the case of arthrography, invasive. There are a number of indications where the diagnosis is in doubt, but the use of examination under anaesthetic and arthroscopic examination by an experienced shoulder arthroscopist is undoubtedly superior. An ideal indication for MRI is where there is evidence of some weakness and wasting of the supra- and infraspinatus muscles. A cyst of the posterior glenoid leading to entrapment of the suprascapular nerve must not be missed.

A fracture of the glenoid rim, the bony Bankart lesion, may occur in 10% of cases of traumatic dislocation coming to surgery (W. A. Wallace, personal communication, 1995). In a few cases, the size of the bony avulsion is sufficient to reduce the diameter of the glenoid to the extent that recurrent dislocation occurs with extreme ease. Where a significant bony avulsion is seen on plain film, CT will reveal the true size of the lesion. Rowe and Sakellarides (1961) stated that up to one third of the width of the glenoid could be lost without compromising stability.

Complications of acute glenohumeral dislocation

Bony

Fractures of the glenoid may permit recurrent dislocation, and should be investigated with a plain radiograph followed by CT if surgical treatment is proposed.

Fractures of greater tuberosity are easily viewed on a plain anteroposterior radiograph, but the position can be misleading, and the tuberosity is dragged posteriorly as well and superiorly. Occasionally the posterior displacement is significant, and may displace further with time. An axillary view reveals the amount of displacement. A repeat radiograph should be taken at 3 weeks. If the displacement is greater than 1 cm, then surgical repair is recommended. Complications of an unreduced greater tuberosity are subacromial impingement and reduced external rotation. These injuries are more common with increasing age.

Humeral head fracture

When the humeral head impacts onto the glenoid rim, a dent in the soft cancellous bone of the head occurs. This is termed a **Hill–Sachs lesion**. The **reverse Hill–Sachs**, which occurs in posterior dislocation, tends to be larger. A significant Hill–Sachs lesion will predispose to recurrent instability. Surgical management is required for this complication

Neurological

The incidence of neurological injury in acute dislocation is up to 45% with EMG investigation. A number of nerves or plexus injuries have been described, but the axillary nerve is the most commonly injured (de Laat et al. 1994).

Axillary nerve injury

The axillary nerve is at risk of a traction injury with anterior dislocation. The clinical signs are of a numb patch over the lateral edge of the shoulder and weakness or paralysis of the deltoid. The paralysis may be present without the numb patch. The injury is usually a neuropraxia and recovers within 6 weeks. If recovery is delayed, then EMG studies should be undertaken. If there are no signs of electrical recovery then referral to an appropriate surgical specialist should be made.

Rotator cuff tears

Rotator cuff tears occur with increasing frequency with age. Above 40 years of age the incidence exceeds 30%; above 60 years the incidence is 80% (Itoi and Tabata 1992).

The presentation is of pain and weakness, which persists after the initial trauma has subsided, at about 3 weeks after injury. The primary deficit is in abduction and external rotation. Investigation in the form of an ultrasound scan will reveal the extent of the tear. The lesion may be an extension of a pre-existing tear or a new injury. Prompt surgical repair has been recommended, though the risk of adhesive capsulitis is increased with early surgery. Physiotherapy to gain as much benefit as possible with conservative management should be pursued for 6 weeks after diagnosis. A persisting flail shoulder should initiate further investigation for neurological injury and to ascertain the size and age of the tear. CT may determine whether there is any fatty atrophy and hence the suitability for repair.

Recurrent dislocation

The most significant factor when determining the risk of recurrent dislocation is the age of the patient. Several authors have demonstrated that the risk is 90% for those aged under 20, 60% for those aged 20–40, and 10–15% for those over 40. Hovelius (1987) reported figures much lower than other authors in a careful prospective study in Sweden: 33% for under 20 and 25% for those between 20 and 30 years. Most authors do not agree with these figures, but the study is important because of its prospective nature.

Sport is a further factor that influences recurrence. The recurrence rate is highest amongst sportsmen. The severity of the initial trauma also appears to be relevant.

Locked anterior dislocation and locked posterior dislocation

Locked dislocations occur in both directions. A locked posterior dislocation is associated with loss of external rotation and a large defect in the humeral head. Reduction may require surgical intervention, but the shoulder is often unstable after this. Transfer of the greater tuberosity into the defect of the reverse Hill–Sachs is frequently curative. Locked anterior dislocation is often found in elderly people. A surprisingly full range of motion can remain, and with reasonable comfort. Gentle rehabilitation may be all that is required.

Treatment of the unstable shoulder

Reduction of the acute anterior dislocation

A number of techniques have been described. The easiest is also the simplest. Lay the patient prone with the affected shoulder over the edge of a couch or suitable flat raised surface. Gentle encouragement to relax the arm, possibly supplemented by a mild intravenous sedative and analgesic, with the shoulder in an abducted position, will almost invariably result in an easy, atraumatic reduction. Using this technique, I have only failed to achieve reduction in two weightlifters whose upper arms were the same diameter as my thigh.

Immobilization

The traditional method of managing an acute traumatic dislocation has been a period of immobilization in a sling. The concept of holding the arm in internal rotation is to allow any avulsed ligaments to heal back to the rim of the glenoid. However, it is apparent from the incidence of recurrent dislocation in young people that this is not often the case. An interesting observation when viewing the position of the acutely avulsed labrum via the arthroscope is that the capsule is pulled away from the glenoid in the position of internal rotation, but pulled against the glenoid when the shoulder is externally rotated. It is therefore possible that immobilization may succeed, but only if the shoulder is placed in external rotation.

A number of authors have concluded that the incidence of recurrence is not related to either the type of immobilization used or the duration (McLaughlin and Cavallaro 1950, Rowe and Sakellarides 1961, Ehgartner 1977, Hovelius 1987). Fewer authors have shown that more than 3 weeks' immobilization may produce a reduced incidence of recurrence (Kazar and Relovsky 1969). The 10-year study by Hovelius (1987) failed to show any effect of immobilization.

I currently advise a week in a sling for older non-athletic individuals while the pain from the trauma of the dislocation settles.

Physiotherapy

There is little evidence to support the use of physiotherapy as a means of reducing the risk of recurrence. One study of US navy midshipmen supported the use of a 3-week period of immobilization followed by a progressive regimen of exercises (Aronen and Regan 1984). The subjects were only allowed to return to activities when there was no evidence of atrophy or apprehension. It should be noted that a military environment is the most suitable for such a regimen. From the perspective of patient compliance or resources, it may not be a practical solution for National Health Service patients.

Rehabilitation should take the form of scapular exercises for positional control, together with rotator cuff strengthening exercises

Surgery

Indications for surgery for the acute dislocation include a displaced greater tuberosity fracture and a large glenoid rim fracture of more than 30% of the width of the glenoid.

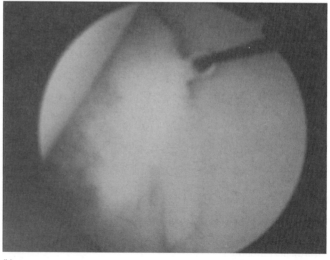

(a)

(b)

Figure 3.4.14 (a), (b) Arthroscopic labral repair.

The recommended procedure for recurrent instability is the reattachment of the avulsed labrum and capsule to the rim of the glenoid, the **Bankart repair** (Figure 3.4.14a,b). This can now be accomplished with suture anchors, which remain buried in subchondral bone and permit an anatomical repair. Range of motion remains within a few degrees of the uninjured side. The results of open surgery for stabilization of the shoulder are excellent with recurrence rates of 5% at 5 years reported for the Bankart repair. The early techniques for arthroscopic repair were not comparable. However, with the advancement of techniques, and more importantly the understanding of the pathology, recent publications cite recurrence rates as good as open surgery.

The high incidence of recurrent dislocation in young athletes, together with the advances in arthroscopic techniques, has led to the question of whether early arthroscopic surgery may be of benefit to that subgroup. A carefully selected group of cadets from West Point were selected for early arthroscopic surgery using the early techniques that proved so unreliable for recurrent dislocation. A recurrent dislocation rate of 82% in the control group was turned around to 14% in the surgical group. It is my belief that early arthroscopic surgery should be offered to young athletes, provided the surgeon has the appropriate experience and training in arthroscopic shoulder stabilization.

Scapula

Snapping scapula

Snapping scapula was first described by Boinet in 1867, according to Milch (1950). The syndrome consists of a painful rubbing sensation that may be audible, usually over the superomedial scapula. Overhead activity tends to be provocative, with pain and snapping.

A snapping or washer board scapula is not always symptomatic. Not infrequently there is a degree of snapping from the contralateral

---

Thermal capsular shrinkage

Collagen heated to around 62°C denatures and shrinks. Applying heat energy to the shoulder capsule arthroscopically in the form of diathermy or laser is currently under study for the management of instability in the group of multidirectional instability patients who fail to respond to rehabilitation techniques. Although this technique is still under study, it is unfortunately in widespread use. Published results do not go beyond 2 years, but it would appear to be of benefit, possibly allowing sufficient mechanical stability to be gained to allow the physiotherapists to be more effective with more conventional techniques.

Synovial ganglion cyst of the glenoid

This unusual finding presents with pain, atrophy, and weakness of the spinati. The cyst is usually caused by a leakage of synovial fluid from a tear of the posterior labrum, in much the same way as a meniscal cyst develops from a tear of a lateral meniscus. The nerve contains both sensory and motor components, so a mixture of clinical signs may develop. Surgical drainage can be accomplished quite easily by arthroscopic means.

Causes of snapping scapula

Bony

- Luschka's tubercle (a fibrocartilaginous nodule of the supero-medial angle of the scapula)
- Increase in curvature of the superior angle
- Exostosis
- Tumours
- Tuberculosis
- Spengel's deformity

Changes in the muscle

- Tendinitis of the scapular stabilizers
- Anatomical variations
- Muscle insertion avulsions and traction spurs

Bursal

- Scapulothoracic bursa
- Inflammation and adhesion formation

---

side, indeed the incidence has been described as high as 80%! Winging has an unclear association found in some series and not other (Percy *et al.* 1989).

Investigation includes a tangential radiograph of the scapula. A number of aetiologies have been described (see box).

Snapping scapula is thought to be a condition that usually resolves with time and physiotherapy. In some cases this does not occur. When the superomedial corner is clinically localized as the problematic area, conventional surgery involves an open incision. Reported results are good, but cosmetic appearance and postoperative recovery can be a problem. Arthroscopic surgery to the bursa is via a portal below the spine of the scapula to avoid the neurovascular structures and three finger breadths from the vertebral border of the scapula. The cosmesis is much improved over open techniques (Harper *et al.* 1999).

Winging of the scapula

Scapular winging occurs with paralysis of serratus anterior. The long thoracic nerve of Bell supplies serratus anterior via a long path along the midaxillary line. Serratus anterior arises from the first to ninth ribs and inserts onto the medial border of the scapula in three functional parts. The superior digitations insert onto the upper border and control the scapula during abduction, the middle fibres insert along the middle of the medial border and aid scapular protraction. The lower fibres rotate the scapula upwards during abduction.

The nerve can be injured by direct pressure: one particular individual suffered winging of the scapula after falling asleep on the hard edge of a seat. The nerve is also susceptible to traction injury in overhead sporting activity. A stretch beyond 10° will lead to a neuropraxia. Neuralgic amyotrophy is a commonly ascribed cause, a paralytic brachial neuritis.

Patients present with an obvious cosmetic deformity, a sensation of weakness and loss of control of the shoulder, and a generalized aching from the shoulder girdle. They are generally aware of the winging, which may not develop immediately. Scapular winging is obvious when the shoulder girdle is viewed from behind with forward flexion. Investigation may include EMG study, but the diagnosis is clinical.

Conventional management involves reassurance that many cases resolve spontaneously, and shoulder girdle rehabilitation. More recently, where EMG studies fail to show recovery, surgical neurolysis has given dramatic results. There is generally a leash of vessels running over the nerve in its mid course in the lower axilla. Release has led to recovery in a small series performed by Professor Wallace's team in Nottingham, UK.

Pseudo-winging

This phenomenon is found in individuals with an unstable glenohumeral joint (Figure 3.4.15a, b). The subjects either have a form of hyperlaxity or more usually associated with overhead sports such as swimming, throwing and racquet sports. The scapula lifts away from the chest wall, but to a minor degree compared with true winging. Pseudo-winging will resolve once glenohumeral stability is restored.

Calcific tendinitis

Deposition of calcium in the tendon of the rotator cuff, usually supraspinatus, is a common disorder. While the calcium is deposited the patient may complain of mild discomfort or be entirely pain free. Severe pain, in the so-called acute calcific tendonitis, occurs when the calcium undergoes resorption.

Incidence

The reported incidence varies according to the methods used and age of the subject. Figures vary from 2.7 to 20% (Bosworth 1941, Wefling *et al.* 1965). The vast majority of calcium deposits lie in the supraspinatus tendon. Women are affected more than men. The highest occurrence is in the age range 31–50, the right shoulder more than the left (Wefling *et al.* 1965). There appears to be no connection with trauma.

Pathophysiology

The aetiology of calcific tendinitis is unknown. There is some genetic predisposition, with an increase in HLA A1, but little else is known about the triggers for formation or resolution. What is known is that the calcific deposits are multifocal and that the deposits are surrounded by avascular areas of fibrocartilage containing chondrocytes. Ageing, degeneration, and necrosis probably precede calcification. The precalcific stage involves fibrocartilaginous transformation of degenerate tendon.

The deposition of calcium, the calcific stage, is not symptomatic. Surgery performed in this period will reveal chalky material, although not quite the solid lump that radiographic appearances would suggest. The resting period of the process ends with a resorptive phase that involves granulation tissue and scar formation with removal of the calcium deposits. By this time the calcium has the consistency of toothpaste.

There is no strong evidence of any correlation between frozen shoulder and calcific tendinitis or other diseases. A variety of classifications have been proposed, using size, chronicity or nature of deposition, localized or diffuse. Most surgeons managing this condition do not use any of these systems as they do not have a bearing on management or prognosis.

The natural progression of the condition is for spontaneous resolution, with 85% of fluffy deposits and 33% of dense deposits disappearing in 3 years (Gartner 1993).

History and examination

The stage of formation of the calcium deposits is probably asymptomatic, any discomfort being due to tendon degeneration or impingement which can occur with larger deposits. When the calcium resorbs, swelling occurs as a result of revascularization and accompanying oedema. This causes pain. The acute onset of severe pain is associated with shorter duration of symptoms, slower resorption gives rise to longer duration of pain. Severe pain tends to last about 2 weeks; less aggressive symptoms may persist for up to 3 months. Pain radiates to the insertion of deltoid and down the arm.

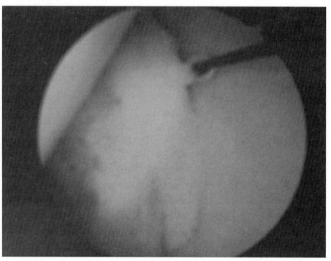

(a)   (b)

Figure 3.4.15 (a), (b) Pseudo-winging

The pain can be excruciating in its severity, with pain at rest and with activity. Patients hold their arm against the chest wall and resist any attempt at active or passive movement. As the pain subsides, a painful arc may become apparent. The acute onset has been thought to be due to rupture of the deposit into the bursa, though the bursa usually has little reaction. Pain may appear and disappear quite abruptly.

Investigation

Calcium deposits are found on plain radiograph in neutral rotation. They are usually located in the substance of the tendon of supraspinatus. The resorptive phase where the pain is most severe is characterized by removal of the calcium which appears to be diffuse, fluffy, and much less dense. Chronic cases without much discomfort tend to be much denser and with well-demarcated edges.

Calcific deposits which extend onto the tuberosity should be differentiated from other, more stippled deposits associated with other arthropathies. Rotator cuff tears with osteoarthritic changes will provide similar appearances.

Ultrasound will readily demonstrate calcification within the tendon, detecting very small quantities in expert hands. Dynamic ultrasound scanning will also demonstrate any subacromial impingement.

Using T2 weighted images, MRI will demonstrate increased signal intensity around the deposits the indicating oedema. The internal degeneration of the tendon will show easily on MRI.

Management

Conservative management

The initial management is along standard lines of shoulder physiotherapy. Initial pendular movements with passive then active range of motion exercises progress to muscle strengthening exercises focusing on the scapular and specific rotator cuff muscles. There is little if any evidence of efficacy of ultrasound or other electrotherapies, though heat may provide some pain relief.

Lithotripsy: extracorporeal shock wave therapy

This technique is well established in continental Europe, but less so in the UK. The aim is to focus acoustic energy to induce fragmentation of the calcific deposit and induce resorption. The short-term results are said to be excellent. There is considerable placebo effect, and in a carefully controlled trial Speed et al. (2002) failed to show any difference between extracorporeal shock wave therapy and sham treatment for non-calcific tendonitis. Only one study has assessed the long-term results (Deacke et al. 2002).

The outcome at 3 months is in line with other studies with improvement in pain and Constant scores. Longer term, however, only 23% of those receiving one dose and 37% of those receiving two doses had not received further treatment to the shoulder. The rate of surgical intervention was 20% for the 59% followed up, implying the rate is potentially much higher. Studies tend to concentrate on the disappearance of calcific deposits despite the evidence being that the deposits *per se* are asymptomatic.

Needling and injection

Release of a deposit under tension allows the material, which is the consistency of cream cheese, to spurt out under tension in acute cases. Needling the deposit can give short- and long-term relief (Pfister and Gerber 1994). These authors found that 60% of patients followed after 5 years were free of pain, though the follow-up rate was 70%.

The needle is inserted at the site of most tenderness, though optimum accuracy is obtained using ultrasound or radiological guidance. Lavage with local anaesthetic is recommended. The addition of corticosteroid is commonplace, but without much evidence to support its use. Some authors, e.g. Lippman (1961), warn that corticosteroids abort the cellular activity that leads to resorption.

Surgery

The extremely painful acute stages of resorption should be managed conservatively, with physiotherapy and ultrasound-guided needling and lavage with local anaesthetic. Surgery has been used to treat this problem, but the results, although good, take longer to achieve than with conservative measures.

Chronic pain in the presence of calcific deposits that has failed to respond to conservative measures may be treated surgically. The majority of surgeons focus on the calcific deposit, which can be identified at arthroscopy. Using a needle or arthroscopic shaver, the deposit can be decompressed and to a variable extent removed. Surgeons vary in their enthusiasm for the addition of a subacromial decompression; my personal practice is to do so, on the grounds that the evidence suggests that most patients with chronic calcific tendinitis in the resting phase are asymptomatic (Bosworth 1941). My investigation of choice is dynamic ultrasound scanning, which assesses the degree of subacromial impingement, more likely to be the cause of symptoms. Success rates for surgical decompression are in the region of 95%.

Coracoid impingement

Coracoid impingement was described in the 1930s by Meyer (1938). The subacromial arch extends as far anteriorly as the tip of the coracoid process, and the height and length of the coracoid helps to determine the size and shape of the subacromial outlet space. The coracoacromial ligament is variable in shape and not infrequently joins the tendon of coracobrachialis at the tip of the coracoid creating a sharp angle of firm fibrous tissue.

Pain is usually localized more anteriorly and inferiorly than the usual impingement pain. Pain may radiate down the forearm. The pain is aggravated by adduction combined with flexion and internal rotation.

Imaging techniques such as MRI have not been found to be helpful. There seem to be a variety of contributing anatomical variations. These include abnormal tendons including insertion of pectoralis minor, cysts of subscapularis, and iatrogenic causes following osteotomy. There may be an association with a weak or wide rotator interval (Dumontier et al. 1999).

The diagnosis is confirmed by injection of local anaesthetic under the coracoid. Where a diagnosis of bicipital tendinitis is made, there should be high index of suspicion for coracoid impingement.

Treatment consists of excision of the tip of the coracoid. This can be achieved through open or arthroscopic surgery.

Subacromial impingement

Subacromial impingement occurs when the rotator cuff is encroached by the surrounding bony and soft tissue structures. This may occur through interference with normal rotator cuff function that produces an abnormality of normal humeral head/glenoid mechanics, or a compromise of the subacromial outlet space through which the rotator cuff passes. The result is symptoms of shoulder pain associated with mechanical wear and tear. The syndrome is more common with increasing age, but there appears to be a separate problem in the young athletic population.

Aetiology

In the 1930s, Meyer identified the undersurface of the acromion as the source of friction on the rotator cuff and Codman identified a critical zone in the rotator cuff as the site of degeneration. This area is 1 cm lateral to the insertion of the supraspinatus tendon on the greater tuberosity. The classic paper in the history of understanding of sub-acromial impingement is that by Neer (1972). His theory was that the rotator cuff was damaged by the phenomenon of impingement by either outlet or non-outlet causes.

Outlet impingement is caused by mechanical damage to the superior surface of the rotator cuff by wear against the coracoacromial arch. Narrowing of the supraspinatus outlet is the most common cause. Abnormalities of the acromion have been described. Nicholson *et al.* (1996) used radiographic techniques to report three different shapes of the acromion: type 1 is flat, but types 2 and 3 are acquired. Type 2 is curved and type 3 hooked. The hooks are within the coraco-acromial ligament and are effectively traction spurs. Although there has been an increased association of rotator cuff tears with type 3 acromia, both are age related and a causal relationship is not certain.

The acromioclavicular joint can contribute to and be a direct cause of subacromial pain. Degenerative changes with in the joint may produce downwards-pointing osteophytes, which directly impinge upon the rotator cuff causing direct mechanical damage.

Non-outlet impingement is caused by a functional abnormality leading to friction and wear against the subacromial arch. A wide variety of causes are known (see box).

The rotator cuff degenerates with age. Several studies, both in the community and cadaver, have demonstrated the increasing incidence of rotator cuff tears with age, independent of symptoms. The natural history of the rotator cuff appears to be typical of tendon degeneration seen elsewhere in the body, but with a remarkably high incidence in elderly people, over 80% aged over 80 years (Milgrom *et al.* 1995). Chard and Hazleman (1991) used ultrasound to examine 644 subjects aged 70 or more: 21% complained of shoulder symptoms and 40% of these sought help. The tendinopathy appears as changes in cell arrangement with calcium deposition, fibrinoid thickening, fatty degeneration leading to necrosis and rents and eventually rotator cuff tears. Ageing appears to be the single most important contributing factor in the pathogenesis of tears of the cuff tendons.

Rathbun and MacNab (1970) demonstrated a critical zone of rela-tive avascularity near the insertion of the supraspinatus tendon, which

Neer's classification of subacromial impingement

1 Reversible cuff oedema
2 Fibrosis and tendinitis
3 Partial or full-thickness tears

Non-outlet impingement of the rotator cuff

- Abnormal mechanics
- Neurological injury, scapular rotators
- Mechanical traumatic injury, prominence of greater tuberosity from trauma
- Loss of humeral head depressor (cuff or long head of biceps)
- Acute injury to the rotator cuff losing normal force couple
- Loss of normal fulcrum, from glenohumeral instability or laxity
- Loss of normal suspensory mechanism from chronic grade 3 acromioclavicular joint injury
- Acromial defects, fracture, os acromiale
- Thickened bursa or cuff from calcium deposits, bursitis
- Increased workload from loss of lower limb with a weight bearing upper limb
- Rotator cuff tears as a cause of impingement

was thought to contribute to rotator cuff degeneration. Subsequent work has shown this to be an artefact, due to the position of the shoul-der during the injection process (Gerber *et al.* 1990), and no such arte-rial watershed area exists. There is probably an area of reduced vascularity at the site of the insertion of the tendon, which may be relevant in the aetiology of chronic tears.

Impingement can be thought of as a syndrome with a variety of causes and contributions leading to pain and reduced function of the rotator cuff.

A number of terms are associated with subacromial pain, which, although descriptive, do not constitute a diagnosis and are not necess-arily the true source of pain. These include **subacromial bursitis**. The subacromial bursa provides a frictionless interface for the rotator cuff and long head of biceps against the coracoacromial arch. The arch consists of the acromion, acromioclavicular joint, and undersurface of the coracoclavicular ligament. The bursa may become thickened and inflamed, but surgical removal of the bursa alone rarely gives relief of symptoms and the bursa is therefore probably not an important source of pain. **Rotator cuff tendinitis** occurs in stage 1 of Neer's classification, but the majority of patients present with degenerate rather than inflamed tendons.

History

The patient typically presents with a vague pain in the shoulder and difficulty with using the shoulder in an overhead position. There may be an element of night pain.

The pain is frequently poorly localized, but may present with pain in the region of the insertion of deltoid, anterolateral shoulder pain, or pain radiating either proximally or distally. Pain is relieved with rest. Weakness is not a common feature unless pain is severe.

Examination

Inspection is unlikely to reveal wasting of the rotator cuff muscles in the absence of a tear. Swelling may be observed over the acromioclav-icular joint. The rhythm of movement is usually abnormal, with a painful arc of movement. The patient may 'hitch' the shoulder in elevation to avoid the moment that reproduces the impingement, elevating the scapula with abduction. The classic painful arc of supra-spinatus tendinitis is 60–120° of abduction, but this is highly variable. The patient is usually able to get above the painful arc. Failure to achieve this indicates either severe pain or a crescendo arc from the acromioclavicular joint that occurs above 160°. Restriction of range of motion is uncommon unless the pain is severe. Painful limitation of flexion with the scapula stabilized by the examiner is Neer's test for impingement. Hawkin's test is more sensitive in detecting subacromial impingement. In this test, the examiner brings the shoulder passively to abduction of 90° and flexion of 30°. The examiner then moves the shoulder actively into internal rotation, directly compressing the cuff under the subacromial arch.

There may be pain on stressing supraspinatus and infraspinatus, but classically no weakness. Experience suggests that weakness can be present with an intact rotator cuff, whilst other individuals seem to be able to produce significant strength on formal testing despite the presence of a full thickness rotator cuff tear.

Investigation

Radiographs

A plain radiograph may reveal subacromial sclerosis and a correspond-ing greater tuberosity sclerosis/cyst. Specific subacromial outlet views may demonstrate an acromial spur and/or acromioclavicular joint osteo-phytes. The subacromial space is preserved in the absence of a cuff tear.

Ultrasound

Ultrasonography requires a degree of experience from the operator to provide reliable and repeatable reports, but has the major advantage over other modalities of being a dynamic examination. This technique can detect abnormalities of the structure of the tendon and direct evi-dence of impingement when bunching of supraspinatus in abduction is visible.

MRI

MRI has the advantage of demonstrating the amount of water or fat in a tissue and hence abnormalities of the internal structure. It is expen-sive, and not easily available for all practitioners. This is a very sensi-tive method of investigation, but it must be emphasized that the changes seen must be related to the clinical situation. This is particu-larly apposite with the rotator cuff, where changes in the rotator cuff tendon are more related to the age of the subject than the presence or absence of symptoms.

Subacromial local anaesthetic

The use of diagnostic local anaesthetic injection is an excellent method of differentiating subacromial sources of pain from other causes of shoulder pain, that is, in the absence of a rotator cuff tear. My practice is to inject 10 ml of bupivacaine into the subacromial space and re-examine the patient for signs of impingement after 20–30 minutes. Abolition of a painful arc and restoration of glenohumeral rhythm are positive findings to indicate that the source of pain is subacromial.

Technique

The anatomical landmarks are the anterolateral corner of the acromion and the humeral head. The skin is cleaned aseptically. The injection is given in the gap between the acromion 1–2 cm posterior to the anterolateral edge of the acromion. The needle points slightly superiorly. The bursal space will fill without backpressure, and the rotator cuff is not penetrated. The patient should be warned about rebound pain once the anaesthetic has worn off.

Accuracy of injection has been studied, and found to be wanting. Training and practice using ultrasound guidance is to be commended.

Management

Conservative

General principles of non-surgical management of shoulder pain and injury

- Reduce pain and inflammation
- Restore normal range of motion
- Regain rotator cuff and scapular strength
- Restore control movement patterns and rhythm
- Improve muscle strength
- Graduated return to activity

When managing impingement syndrome, it is vital to confirm the primary pathology. A young athlete with impingement pain secondary to instability will not return to full competitive activity until the primary instability has been addressed. Similarly, acromioclavicular joint osteophytes will prevent recovery unless they are removed.

The first principle is relative rest, avoiding any aggravating activity. Non-steroidal anti-inflammatory drugs (NSAIDS) for 3 weeks provide pain relief in addition to any anti-inflammatory effect. Local modali-ties such as cold and heat may help in pain relief. Stretching of poste-rior capsular tightness needs to be addressed early. Range of motion work with physiotherapy supervision will also address abnormalities of rhythm of movement. Physiotherapy should be pursued for up to 3 months before other treatments are considered. It is important to assess the quantity and quality of the physiotherapy before consider-ing the treatment has failed. The individual who does not continue the prescribed exercises away from the treatment room, or who has been offered mainly electrotherapy, has not received adequate treatment.

Local anaesthetic injection alone has benefits over placebo. The common management is to offer corticosteroid injection with the local anaesthetic. There is widespread use of these agents, but little more than anecdotal evidence for any benefit. A number of studies have tried to assess the results of various conservative modalities. Berry (1980) compared acupuncture, physiotherapy, steroid injec-tions, and anti-inflammatory medication, but found no difference in the results. Withrington (1985) found no evidence of efficacy for the use of corticosteroid injection with a double-blind trial.

One of the problems with such studies is the use of shoulder pain as a diagnosis and justification for a form of treatment. This is inade-quate, particularly given the wide variety of causes of shoulder pain and even impingement-type pain itself. Studies using shoulder pain as a patient source cannot be considered with any degree of reliability. Kirkley (1999) followed patients with a confirmed diagnosis of impingement for a year following an injection of local anaesthetic alone or with steroid. She found no statistical difference through the year, with just a trend for steroid to be better at 3 months.

Many papers have been published on the subject of the use of corti-costeroid in the treatment of subacromial pain. Some demonstrate a positive effect, and certainly the practice is well established. One has to question whether the effect is a local one, or whether the systemic effect of steroids is the factor that produces the anecdotal effect. Valtonen (1978) found no difference between subacromial and gluteal injections of steroids in the management of supraspinatus tendinitis.

Corticosteroids are not benign substances that may be given freely without fear of damage to the rotator cuff. The effect of steroids on tendon *in vitro* is harmful, and the risk of re-rupture of a rotator cuff tear is higher if steroids have been used (Kennedy and Willis 1976, Watson 1985). There is a need for well-structured research in this area. Currently, subacromial injection of corticosteroids, a standard method of treatment, has not been proven to be effective, but has been shown to be potentially harmful, both *in vitro* and *in vivo*.

Surgical

Surgical management is indicated where conservative treatment has been tried and failed. Surgery includes both open and arthroscopic options. Arthroscopic surgery is the preferred technique. The results are equally good when compared with open surgery and there are advantages of less pain and smaller scars. In addition the gleno-humeral joint can be inspected and other pathology identified and treated, if appropriate. The accuracy of the diagnosis of impingement can be confirmed as the lesion where the rotator cuff impacts can be seen at bursoscopy. The acromioclavicular joint can be assessed and treated by excision of the lateral end and debridement of any inferior osteophytes.

Satisfaction levels are in excess of 90% (Ryu 1992). The procedure has been accepted as the surgical treatment of choice.

References

Andrews, J. R. Carson, W. G., Mcleod, W. D. (1985) Glenoid labrum tears related to the long head of biceps. *Am J Sports Med*, 13, 337–341.

Aronen, J. G., Regan, K. (1984) Decreasing the incidence of recurrence of first anterior shoulder dislocations with rehabilitation. *Am J Sports Med*, 12, 283–291.

Berry, H. (1980) Clinical study comparing acupuncture physiotherapy injection and oral anti-inflammatory therapy in shoulder-cuff lesions. *Curr Med Res Opin*, 7, 121–126.

Bosworth, B. M. (1941) Calcium deposits in the shoulder and subacromial bursitis. A survey of 12,122 shoulders. *JAMA*, 116, 2477–2482.

Chard, M. D., Hazelman, R, Hazelman, B. L. (1991) Shoulder disorders in the elderly, a community survey. *Arthritis Rheum*, 34, 766–769.

de Laat, E. A. Visser, C. P. Coene, L. N. (1994) Nerve injuries in primary shoulder dislocations and humeral head fractures: A prospective clinical and EMG study. *J Bone Joint Surg*, 76, 381–383.

Deacke, W., Kusnierczak, D., Loew, M. (2002) Long term effects of extracorporeal shock wave therapy in chronic calcific tendinitis of the shoulder. *J Shoulder Elbow Surg*, 11, 476–480.

Dumontier, C., Sautet, A., Gagey, O., Apoil, A. (1999) Rotator interval lesions and their relation to coracoid impingement syndrome. *J Shoulder Elbow Surg*, 8, 130–135.

Ehgartner, K. (1977) Has the duration of cast fixation after shoulder dislocations had an influence on the frequency of recurrent dislocation? *Arch Orthop Unfallchir*, 80, 187–190.

Gartner, J. (1993) Tendinnosis Calcarea Behandlungsergebnisse mit dem Needling. *Z Orthop Ihre Grenzgeb*, 313, 461–469.

Gerber, C., Schneeberger, A. G., Vinh, T. S. (1990) The arterial vascularisation of the humeral head an anatomical study. *J Bone Joint Surg*, 72A, 1486–1494.

Harper, G. D., McIlroy, S., Bayley, J. I. L., Calvert, P. T. (1999) Arthroscopic partial resection of the scapula for snapping scapula. A new technique. *J Shoulder Elbow Surg*, 8, 53–57.

Hovelius, L (1987) Anterior dislocations of the shoulder in teenagers and young adults. Five years prognosis. *J Bone Joint Surg*, 69A, 393–399.

Itoi, E. A., Tabata, S. (1992) Rotator cuff tears in anterior dislocation of the shoulder. *Int Orthop*, 16, 240–244.

Kazar, B., Relovsky, E. (1969) Prognosis of primary dislocation of the shoulder. *Acta Orthop Scand*, 40, 216.

Kennedy, J. C., Willis, R. B. (1976) The effects of local steroid injections on tendons: a biomechanical and microscopic correlative study. *Am J Sports Med*, 4, 11–21.

Kirkley, S. (1999) *World Orthopaedic Congress of English Speaking Nations*, Auckland, New Zealand.

Lippman, R. K. (1961) Observations concerning the calcific cuff deposit. *Clin Orthop*, 20, 49–60.

McLaughlin Cavallaro, W. U. (1950) Primary anterior dislocation of the shoulder. *Am J Surg*, 80, 615–621.

Meyer, A. W. (1938) Chronic functional lesions of the shoulder. *Arch Surg*, 35, 646–674.

Milch, H. (1950) Partial scapulectomy for snapping. *J Bone Joint Surg*, 32A, 561–566.

Milgrom, C., Schaffer, M., Gilbert, S., van Holsbbeeck, M. (1995) Rotator cuff changes in asymptomatic adults. *J Bone Joint Surg*, 77B, 296–298.

Neer, C. S. (1972) Anterior acromioplasty for the chronic impingement syndrome in the shoulder. A preliminary report. *J Bone Joint Surg*, 79A, 41–50.

Nicholson, G. P., Goodman, D. A., Flatow, E. L., *et al.* (1996) The acromion: morphologic condition and age-related changes. A study of 420 scapulas. *J Shoulder Elbow Surg*, 5, 1–11.

Percy, E. C., Birbrager, D., Pitt, M. (1989) Snapping scapula, a review of the literature and presentation of 14 patients. *Can J Surg*, 247, 111–116.

Pfister, J., Gerber, H. (1994) Behandlung der Periarthropathia humeroscapularis calcarea mittels Schulterkalkspulung retrospektive Fragebogen analyse. *Z Orthop ihre Grenzgeb*, 132, 300–305.

Rathbun, J. B., MacNab, I. (1970) The microvascular pattern of the rotator cuff. *J Bone Joint Surg*, 52B, 540.

Rowe, C. R., Sakellarides, H. T. (1961) Factors related to recurrences of anterior dislocations of the shoulder. *Clin Orthop*, 20, 40–48.

Ryu, R. K. (1992) Arthroscopic subacromial decompression: a clinical review. *Arthroscopy*, 8, 141–147.

Snyder, S. J. (1990) SLAP lesions of the shoulder. *Arthroscopy*, 6, 274–279.

Speed, C., Richards, C., Nichols, D., Burnet, S., Wies, J. T., Humphreys, H., Hazleman, B. L. (2002) Extracorporeal shock wave therapy for tendonitis of the rotator cuff a double blind randonised trial. *J Bone Joint Surg*, 84B, 509–513.

Valtonen, E. J. (1978) Double acting betamethasone in the treatment of supraspinatus tendinitis: A comparison of subacromial and gluteal single injections with placebo. *J Int Med Res*, 6, 463–467.

Watson, M. (1985) Major ruptures of the rotator cuff: the results of surgical repair in 89 patients. *J Bone Joint Surg*, 67B, 618–624.

Wefling, J., Kahn, M. F., Desroy, M. (1965) Les calcifications de l'epaule. La maladie des calcifications multiples. *Rev Rheum*, 32, 325–334.

Withrington, R. H., Girgis, F. L., Seifert, M. H. (1985) A placebo controlled trial of steroid injections in the treatment of supraspinatus tendonitis. *Scand J Rheumotol*, 14, 76–78.

3.5 Upper limb disorders

Michael Hutson

The upper limb is a veritable treasure trove for neuromusculoskeletal pathology. Additionally, in terms of body posture and 'posturing', the upper limb acts as a barometer for the stresses and strains that are endemic in a 'civilized' environment.

The recognition that the hand acts as a diagnostic window for many systemic medical conditions and illnesses is an essential component of medical school training. The nails in particular are a flag for many types of pathology. Rheumatological and neurovascular conditions may be detected by inspection of the hand. Swellings, deformities, and contractures are often obvious to casual inspection. Both distress and impairment of function may be manifest and recorded by observing resting posture and the expressive use (or otherwise) of the hand and upper limb at interview, when undressing and dressing, and during formal examination of the patient.

Neuromusculoskeletal disorders in the upper limb are a frequent cause of discomfort and disability, reflecting our use of the hand and upper limb for virtually all domestic, recreational, and workplace tasks. They may be viewed according to a number of models: for instance, pathomorphological ('structural'), biomechanical, pathoneurophysiological ('dysfunctional'), and biopsychosocial. Dysfunction, the common theme throughout this book, is sometimes associated with pathomorphology, but not inevitably so. In the upper limb, dysfunction may have devastating consequences.

The disease–illness model, a central pillar of modernist medical thinking over several decades, is as inappropriate in many upper limb disorders as it is in the generality of neuromusculoskeletal disorders. The **biopsychosocial model**, on the other hand, takes account of the behavioural response to illness, injury, and dysfunction. It has a core holistic component and is the preferred model for clinical assessment of neck, shoulder, and arm symptoms, and the construction of appropriate management strategies.

The pathogenesis of neuromuscular disorders in the upper limb is often multifactorial. The time-honoured subdivision of structural pathology into degenerative, traumatic, neoplastic, infective, inflammatory – as taught in medical school – may be standard practice for the orthopaedic surgeon, but this categorization does not adapt easily to the study of neuromusculoskeletal dysfunction. Several of the following aetiological factors may coexist:

- **Overuse:** Repetitive microtrauma, whether associated with domestic activities, sport, leisure, or work, is the principal cause of tendinitis. Tendinopathies are frequently encountered at the shoulder, elbow, and wrist. Muscle hypertrophy is a consequence of repetitive forceful activities, and may give rise to nerve entrapment (Kopell and Thompson 1963).

- **Degeneration:** Tendinopathies and enthesopathies usually have a degenerative component. Fibroproliferative diseases (found predominantly in the hand) are also basically degenerative in type. Arthropathies may of course be degenerative.

- **Posture:** Adverse body posture at work, rest, or play, particularly at the proximal thoracic spine and shoulder girdle, should always be considered as a possible aetiological factor, hence the need for a thorough examination of the cervicodorsal spine and shoulder region in patients presenting with upper limb symptoms. The close anatomical relationship between neurovascular, myofascial, and osseous structures at the thoracic inlet, proximal thoracic cage, and pectoral girdle should raise clinical awareness at initial assessment of the potential for neuromuscular and/or vascular dysfunction. Postural vigilance by patient and medical attendant is required during rehabilitation from many upper limb problems to prevent recurrence of dysfunction.

- **Biomechanics/ergonomics:** A study of the technical aspects of gripping, lifting, and the use of the hand and arm during all manual activities is often revealing. A basic knowledge of ergonomics in the factory and at the keyboard is essential. Ergonomists may be recruited to assist in evaluation and management of upper limb disorders that are associated with work.

- **Comorbidity – systemic and psychiatric illness:** Systemic conditions that include diabetes, nutritional deficiencies, hormonal disturbances, alcohol abuse, and inflammatory joint disease contribute to increased vulnerability to neuromusculoskeletal dysfunction. Diabetes in particular, affecting a significant proportion of the population, is associated with an increased incidence of fibroproliferative conditions (such as trigger finger and Dupuytren's contracture), and also with carpal tunnel syndrome. Psychosocial factors are the principal cause of chronicity in many somatic syndromes, particularly back pain, whiplash, and upper limb disorders. Prognosis is substantively adversely affected by the coexistence of frank psychiatric illness.

- **Neural dysfunction:** Neural disturbances, whether playing a primary, secondary, or contributory role, are particularly common in the upper limb: hence the need to evaluate function at the cervical and proximal thoracic spines when presented with a symptomatic upper limb. The so-called **double crush phenomenon** (Upton and McComas 1973), although a somewhat crude label with regard to increased neural tension and neural plasticity, is a helpful concept to some clinicians. The possibility of the additive effect of nerve compression at diverse sites such as the intervertebral foramen, the brachial plexus, and the periphery needs to be considered in the aetiology of many conditions, particularly work-related. It is a reminder of the continuum of this delicate but vital structure throughout the upper limb. To others, the pathogenesis of non-specific upper limb pain is more easily understood when predicated on the hypothesis of abnormal sensory neural processing – in other words, a reduced threshold for pain perception (Mitchell *et al.* 2000) – a feature of central neurosensitization. The cause of central sensitization in patients with 'non-specific' arm pain is disputed. Indeed, it may vary from one patient to another. Cervical spinal nerve entrapment has to be considered (Smythe, see Chapter 2.2.3). Reduced median nerve mobility in the carpal tunnel is mooted as another possibility in some patients (Greening *et al.* 1999). In yet another vulnerable group, neural compression between neck and shoulder, often associated with poor upper body posture and adverse biomechanics, is a possibility.

- **Iatrogenesis:** Iatrogenesis is common and may be a major factor in the development, severity, and chronicity of upper limb disorders. The devastating potential of iatrogenesis may only be reduced by improved postgraduate tuition, leading to a better understanding by clinicians of the principles of neuromusculoskeletal medicine.

- **Beware: Neuropathic pain is common; iatrogenesis is common.**

The emphasis in this chapter is on those soft tissue and neural conditions of the upper limb that occur relatively frequently in family medical practice and also in secondary medical care. Conditions that primarily affect the joints of the elbow, wrist, and hand are excluded. (In general, these are associated with pathomorphology such as inflammatory joint disease, degenerative joint disease, and post-traumatic capsulitis, and are dealt with adequately elsewhere). Shoulder joint dysfunction is discussed in Chapter 3.4.

Examination of the elbow, wrist, and hand

The examiner observes demeanour, posture, and the use of the hand and arm at interview and during examination. In general, behaviour at interview and during examination is often as important as more formal functional assessment. By way of illustration: a weak, limp handshake is typical of neuropathic pain syndromes. The use of a wrist support could have similar connotations, or could indicate soft tissue pathology. The systemic manifestations of diseases such as rheumatoid arthritis, nodal osteoarthritis (of the hands), and endocrine disorders may be detected.

Elbow and forearm

Soft tissue swellings include olecranon bursitis, sometimes referred to as 'beat elbow'. A more modest degree of soft tissue swelling may be present over the common extensor origin in lateral epicondylitis. The range of active/passive movements at the elbow is −10/150°. More than 10° of extension is referred to as **hyperextension**. Sometimes this is a component of the hypermobility syndrome. The end-feel in flexion is soft, whereas the end-feel to extension should be hard. A springy block to extension is indicative of synovitis/capsulitis or an intraarticular loose body. The capsular pattern of joint dysfunction is a greater loss of flexion compared to extension.

Resisted elbow flexion and extension (testing biceps and triceps primarily) are undertaken routinely. Weakness may be caused by biceps/triceps muscle lesions or by nerve dysfunction (for a variety of reasons). Resisted supination and pronation are undertaken primarily to assist with the diagnosis of muscle lesions in the proximal forearm. Palpation of the lateral epicondyle, medial epicondyle and distal biceps tendon should be routine. Biceps tendonitis and distal biceps rupture are relatively uncommon but may cause long-term loss of function if not diagnosed. 'Tennis elbow' may give rise to tenderness of the extensor muscle mass as well as the lateral epicondyle. Tenderness at the head of the radius may be present in an atypical tennis elbow. Tenderness in golfer's elbow is usually maximal 0.5–1 cm distal to the point of the medial epicondyle. The presence of more widespread tenderness should alert the examiner to the possibility of neurogenic conditions. Palpation at the medial epicondyle may reveal a hypermobile ulnar nerve in the cubital tunnel.

Resisted dorsiflexion of the wrist and extension of the fingers is undertaken routinely in lateral epicondylitis. The examination should always include resisted forearm rotation (supination and pronation), resisted palmarflexion of the wrist, and resisted flexion of the fingers as the examiner may occasionally be caught out by neuropathic arm pain (in which all these manoeuvres are painful because there is regional mechanical hyperalgesia) manifesting as 'apparent' epicondylitis. In medial epicondylitis resisted pronation is very commonly more painful than resisted palmarflexion of the wrist or resisted flexion of the fingers, reflecting its causation in many cases originating in the pronator teres part of the common flexor origin.

Joint play (accessory) movements may (and should) be undertaken at the inferior radioulnar joint. The techniques described by John Mennell are to be commended (Mennell and Zohn 1976).

Wrist

Bony deformities may be the result of a previous fracture. Soft tissue swellings over the dorsum of the wrist are more common than swellings over the volar aspect. Diffuse synovial proliferation suggests an inflammatory disorder. The dorsum of the wrist is the most common site for a ganglion. The active movements of dorsiflexion, palmarflexion, radial deviation, and ulnar deviation are tested sequentially. Passive movements provide the examiner with a test of end-feel. Radial and ulnar deviation should be assessed with the wrist held in zero flexion. Comparison with the other side is recorded, as there is a considerable variation in the normal ranges of movement. Phalen's test demands full palmarflexion of the wrist for 1 minute. This should be undertaken with the arms held in a dependent position. The **reversed Phalen's test** is undertaken by combining wrist dorsiflexion with extension of the fingers and forearm, commonly uncomfortable with finger flexor tendonitis. **Finkelstein's test** is undertaken with the wrist passively ulnar deviated and the thumb passively opposed across the palm (held in position by active flexion of the fingers): discomfort (a positive test) is experienced in de Quervain's syndrome.

The joint play movements described by Mennell are again commended. Loss of anteroposterior glide is a useful indicator of dysfunction at the wrist. Palpation at the wrist should be undertaken gently but methodically. A heavy-handed approach will reveal spurious tenderness (for instance in the anatomical snuff box) (Hutson 1997). A careful progression by palpation along the bony and tendon landmarks is essential for confirmation of the provisional diagnoses that may have been made by history, movement assessment, and resisted muscle contraction. Careful palpation is required to detect localized tenderness and thickening of tendons, particularly when tendinopathy is at a subacute or chronic stage. A comparison should always be made with the asymptomatic contralateral wrist.

Hand

Neurological contractures are not described here. Thenar or hypothenar wasting are commonly observed, and should stimulate a search for the primary cause in the neurological system or an adjacent joint. Swellings of the finger joints are examined for the bony hardness of osteoarthritis, including Heberden's nodes, or the soft synovial swelling of inflammatory arthritis. The squaring at the base of the thumb indicative of osteoarthritis of the first carpometacarpal joint is noted. Vasomotor changes and palmar fascia thickening should also be recorded. Asking the patient to 'make a fist' is useful for demonstration of the movements at the carpometacarpal, metacarpophalangeal and interphalangeal joints of the thumb and fingers, but flexion can also be limited by the swelling of tenosynovitis in the palm and fingers. At the carpometacarpal joint of the thumb, the capsular pattern is more loss of abduction than extension. As at the hip joint, axial compression combined with rotation is often uncomfortable in osteoarthritis. Ulnar laxity at the first metacarpophalangeal joint may result from 'skier's thumb' when traumatic or from 'gamekeeper's thumb' as a consequence of repetitive stress.

Joint play movements at all the interphalangeal and metacarpal joints may be undertaken. Although such techniques are useful during workshop-type training, in practice they are often discarded because of their failure to contribute much to diagnosis.

Conventionally, neurological examination includes assessment of motor and sensory function. Motor function is routinely tested by resisted contraction during the examination of the joints and soft tissues. Whether formal sensory examination, for instance by the two-point discrimination test, yields much information is somewhat contentious. It is my opinion that the symptoms of sensory blunting reported by a patient are probably the most reliable guide to reduced sensation. Tinel's test for the median or ulnar nerves is notoriously unreliable. The concept of neural 'tension' in the upper limb is also a contentious issue; neural 'sensitivity' is a more appropriate concept. The test commonly referred to as **adverse neural tension** should be considered to reflect such upper limb neural sensitivity; when positive, it should stimulate the examiner to search for the cause of the sensitivity. For further information on neural tension tests and neural sensitivity, the reader is referred to Butler (Chapter 2.2.4).

Tendinopathies

At the hand, wrist, and forearm a frequently applied diagnostic label in family practice is tenosynovitis, tendinitis or 'teno'. Indeed, many patients suffering from unexplained wrist and forearm pain, particularly when they are engaged in repetitive stereotyped activities (most frequently in the workplace), are prescribed non-steroidal anti-inflammatory medication (NSAIDs) and frequently wrist supports on the basis of a presumed inflammatory tendinopathy.

There is in fact little evidence of an inflammatory reaction in tendinopathies in the upper limb other than for the inflammatory disorders such as rheumatoid arthritis. Should florid signs of inflammation be present, rheumatoid arthritis or an associated inflammatory condition is the most likely cause.

This book concentrates on non-inflammatory disorders, but it is always necessary for the musculoskeletal physician to exclude inflammatory arthritis, particularly with any degree of soft tissue swelling. The conventional view of tendinitis (more appropriately labelled tendinosis) is that cumulative stress or overload, often in the form of repetitive vigorous manual activities, gives rise to viscoelastic deformation of collagen. Compensatory mechanisms may be overwhelmed, causing collagen fibril microfailure. Light microscopy in surgical cases reveals frayed fibrils with disrupted architecture (Khan et al. 2002). Should a tendon be covered by a paratendon, a secondary inflammatory reaction may then occur, giving rise to paratendonitis as in Achilles paratendonitis in the lower limb.

When tendons run through fibro-osseous channels, they have a lining synovium in addition to a fibrous sheath. Although 'tenosynovitis' is an appropriate term for tendon pathology associated with inflammatory disorders such as rheumatoid arthritis, tendon degeneration (with no significant inflammation) is more accurately labelled 'tendinosis'. Conditions such as de Quervain's disease in which there is thickening of the tendon sheath should be labelled 'tenovaginitis'.

In the hand, thickening of the fibrous sheath may give rise to tenovaginitis stenosans, for instance trigger thumb or trigger finger. The association between repetitive manual activities and tenovaginitis is unclear. Many conditions that give rise to thickened collagenized fibrous structures, such as trigger finger and Dupuytren's contracture, are more common in diabetics.

Pathophysiologically, tendinosis may be seen to reflect functional failure as a consequence of uncompensatable viscoelastic deformation – in other words, when microstructural catabolism overcomes anabolic reconstitution. Biopsy findings in de Quervain's tenovaginitis reveal increased fibroblastic activity and vascular proliferation, but the more obvious features are an increase in glycosaminoglycan content (hyaluronic acid, condroitin sulfate and dermatin sulfate), synovial thickening, and fibrocartilaginous transformation.

Overuse leads to degradative changes (tendinosis). These should be interpreted as the response to stress and not merely the inevitable age-related changes of degeneration (Hutson 1997). In view of the morphology, it should come as no surprise to find that NSAIDs have little effect on symptoms or on chronicity. They are, however, associated with a significant morbidity.

De Quervain's disease

Fritz de Quervain described this condition in 1895. He called it 'fibrose, stenosierende tenovaginitis'. It is likely, however, that Tillaux (1892) described the same condition a few years previously.

De Quervain's disease is relatively common. Although it is seen most frequently in middle age, mothers of young children are at risk (Harvey et al. 1990). Symptomatic de Quervain's disease is seen in workers whose tasks include repetitive use of the thumb and hand, particularly repetitive use of the pinch grip and radioulnar deviations at the wrist. Although Leao (1958) stated that de Quervain's disease could be considered an occupational condition in many cases, it is unclear whether repetitive manual activities cause the condition or simply cause a (previously asymptomatic) condition to become symptomatic.

Discomfort at the radial wrist is predominantly activity related. Although crepitus is sometimes associated with the acute phase of the condition (and indeed Tillaux in his initial description of the condition labelled it as '*tenosynovitis crépitante*') the more commonly encountered chronic condition rarely exhibits crepitation on examination. Patients are nearly always aware of, and certainly complain of, 'swelling' of the distal forearm. Because the condition is work related, discomfort is maximal at work, lessening with rest. Manual activities in the kitchen are particularly stressful. Although pain may radiate proximally and distally, it is experienced maximally over the radial styloid and slightly distal to this.

The most reliable clinical features are thickening ('swelling') of the combined tendons of extensor pollicis brevis and abductor pollicis longus at the level of the radial styloid, and a positive Finkelstein's test. To experienced examiners, the thickened tendinous structures are not often a diagnostic challenge. Finkelstein's test, however, should always be undertaken with considerable care. A false positive test (when the patient complains of pain due to other conditions) may be the result

of a poor examination technique. A comparison should always be made with the other (presumably painless) side. The examiner should be careful to apply pressure to the radial margin of the second metacarpal to create ulnar deviation at the wrist once the thumb has been passively flexed across the palm and held there by the patient's fingers. My advice is to apply passive radial deviation in the first instance, and then ulnar deviation to distinguish between those conditions at the wrist that have an articular component and de Quervain's tenovaginitis.

The most common differential diagnosis is degenerative change (osteoarthritis) at the first carpometacarpal joint. Other degenerative changes within the carpus, such as scaphotrapezoid osteoarthritis, may also cause radial wrist pain. In these conditions tenderness is expected over the affected joint. However, in patients who are difficult to assess because of abnormal hyperalgesia, for instance when neurosensitized, tenderness may be somewhat diffuse. Under these circumstances, the clinical features of neurosensitization may be augmented by articular hyperalgesia (in which all passive movements and indeed virtually all examination procedures at the wrist, however gentle, evoke discomfort).

Management strategies include the use of NSAIDs, physiotherapy (usually disappointing), wrist support, steroid injections, and surgery. A trained musculoskeletal physician would usually treat by localized

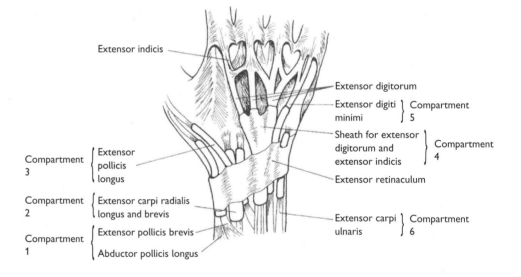

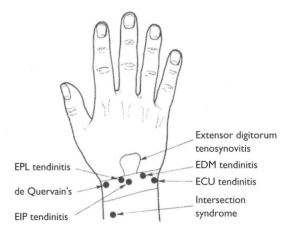

Figure 3.5.1 De Quervain's disease.

low-dose steroid (combined with local anaesthetic) infiltration around and along the line of the affected tendons, as most patients benefit from this. The injection may be given proximal-to-distal, or the other way around, at the level of the radial styloid or just proximal to the base of the first metacarpal. No more than 5–10 mg of triamcinolone is necessary. An 80% success rate for resolution of de Quervain's disease with steroid injections is quoted by Harvey *et al.* (1990). More than one injection may be necessary. A reasonable treatment protocol is to review the patient 1 month after the initial injection, and to repeat if symptoms persist. Should symptoms recur, surgical decompression is nearly always effective if the correct diagnosis is made.

A common clinical error is to confuse de Quervain's disease with intersection syndrome (see below). The conditions are at different anatomical sites, and it is in intersection syndrome that crepitus is a marked diagnostic feature. De Quervain's disease affects extensor pollicis brevis and abductor pollicis longus in the first dorsal compartment of the wrist (see Figure 3.5.1). An understanding of the dorsal compartments facilitates the assessment of wrist pain.

Intersection syndrome

This condition affects the tendons of the second dorsal compartment at the wrist, more accurately described as the distal forearm as this condition is situated more proximally than other tendinopathies at the wrist. The condition arises at the intersection between the extensor carpi radialis longus and brevis tendons, (by definition the tendons of the second dorsal compartment), and the tendons of extensor pollicis brevis and abductor pollicis longus. It is a crossover point, thus explaining the histopathological features of a sticky fibrinous deposit between these tendons. In a seminal article, Thompson *et al.* (1951) considered that unaccustomed work, or a return to work after a period of absence, was the stressor in a significant proportion of cases.

Intersection syndrome is otherwise known as peritendinitis crepitans, reflecting the clinical feature of crepitus secondary to an inflammatory reaction at the site of the musculotendinous junction of the affected tendons. Although first described by Velpeau (1841), it was probably Troell (1918) who used the term peritendinitis crepitans. Troell compared the condition to similar tendinopathies of the lower leg, including the Achilles tendon.

Intersection syndrome is an overuse condition. Patients complain of pain, swelling, tenderness, and 'creaking'(crepitus). As is common to other tendinopathies, not only in the upper limb but also throughout the body, patients usually complain of 'weakness', probably because of pain inhibition.

Manual workers constitute a high-risk group, though rowers and canoeists are frequently affected, as are weightlifters and dog handlers (Hutson 2001). In Thompson's series (Thompson *et al.* 1951), most of the 544 patients with forearm tendinitis (of which 419 cases were due to peritendinitis crepitans) worked in the Vauxhall motor factory.

Intersection syndrome is found approximately 6 cm proximal to Lister's tubercle at the wrist. Crepitus is a constant feature in the acute state. Tenderness and swelling are present, and Finkelstein's test may be positive.

Very slow progress is to be expected with splinting or physiotherapy. This is one of the few crepitating inflammatory conditions found in clinical practice that resolves within a few days of administering a steroid injection. Nevertheless, a full assessment of the aetiological factors is necessary to prevent recurrence. As with all

tendinopathies, an appropriate period of rest or at least reduction of biomechanical stresses is necessary to prevent recurrence. It is my experience that increased vulnerability to recurrence persists for months, possibly years.

Extensor pollicis longus tendinitis

The extensor pollicis longus lies in the third dorsal compartment. It was described by Dums (1896) in Prussian drummer boys in whom rupture occurred as a result of attrition at Lister's tubercle. Extensor pollicis longus rupture may also be a consequence of a fracture of the radial styloid, more commonly a minimally displaced Colles' fracture than a fracture requiring manipulative reduction. Gross weakness of active extension at the interphalangeal joint of the thumb is found in extensor pollicis longus rupture. The more classical findings (of tendinitis) are present with tendinosis: pain on passive flexion of the thumb and pain on resisted thumb extension.

Extensor digitorum tenosynovitis

The labelling of this fourth dorsal compartment tendinopathy reflects its aetiology. It is appropriately labelled tenosynovitis, as it is most commonly due to rheumatoid arthritis. The presentation, in the form of swelling, tenderness, and deformity, is often relatively florid. The swelling distal to the extensor retinaculum is often in the form of a goose foot when marked.

It may be an isolated lesion in the hand, but a high index of suspicion with respect to an inflammatory disorder should be present when there is swelling. Impairment of function is often severe in well-established rheumatoid arthritis.

Extensor digiti minimi tendinitis

This condition is rare, although it has been reported as a consequence of trauma or overuse (Hooper and McMaster (1979). Attempts to flex the wrist after making a fist are described as painful.

Extensor carpi ulnaris tendinitis

After de Quervain's tenovaginitis and intersection syndrome, extensor carpi ulnaris tendinitis is the next most common tendinopathy that is not due to inflammatory disease. It occurs in the sixth dorsal compartment of the wrist, giving rise to ulnar wrist pain. It is an overuse condition, occurring in work or recreational activity in which there are repetitive radioulnar wrist deviations, particularly when combined with rotation. It occurs in professional golfers who may need to revise grip and swing to offload the extensor carpi ulnaris as part of the management of this condition.

A reliable clinical finding is discomfort on passive radial deviation of the wrist with a fully pronated forearm/wrist. Full passive supination may also be painful. As with many tendinopathies at the wrist, resisted contraction of the affected tendon is not painful other than in the acute phase. Care needs to be taken to localize tenderness over the ulnar styloid. Clicking raises the possibility of recurrent subluxation of the extensor carpi ulnaris.

The most common differential diagnosis is a lesion of the inferior radioulnar joint. This condition also gives rise to discomfort on passive rotations of the forearm and to localized tenderness. Occasionally, a sprain of the ulnar collateral ligament at the wrist is found, although a ligamentous injury tends to be overdiagnosed by the inexperienced physician.

Flexor carpi ulnaris tendinitis

This condition may result from repetitive flexion movements of the wrist (as an overload phenomenon) or from repetitive direct trauma to the volar–ulnar aspect of the wrist (as in racquet players, golfers, or cricketers). In practice the at-risk group appears to be industrial workers, particularly those involved in the building and demolition industries. The use of a heavy hammer combines a high degree of force with repetition.

The flexor carpi ulnaris tendon is tender, maximally just proximal to the pisiform bone. In those activities in which compression of a tool or sporting implement is an aetiological factor, compression of the pisiform against the underlying triquetral may evoke discomfort. Stretching of the flexor carpi ulnaris tendon by combined extension and radial deviation of the wrist usually evokes discomfort.

As a consequence of the topographical relationship between the flexor carpi ulnaris tendon (and pisiform) and the ulnar nerve at the wrist, entrapment neuropathy of the deep branch of the ulnar nerve in Guyon's canal, during its course around the pisiform, is an occasional associated finding. A change in working or sporting technique is often necessary to reduce overload. Localized steroid/local anaesthetic injections are effective.

Flexor carpi radialis tendinitis

This is relatively uncommon. Figure 3.5.2 demonstrates a case of calcific flexor carpi radialis tendinitis at the volar aspect of the wrist that gave rise to acute pain and loss of function of the hand. This example reveals the usefulness of plain radiology in acute pain and swelling of the hand.

Flexor digitorum tendinitis

Although not often described as a discrete tendinopathy, flexor digitorum tendinitis is commonly found as a mild chronic condition in workers whose job tasks include repetitive grasping. Chronic tendinitis gives rise to a minor flexion contracture and a positive prayer sign. This stenosing form of tendinitis is found in a subgroup of patients with carpal tunnel syndrome. In the acute form, swelling may be observed proximal to the wrist creases (Kiefhaber and Stern 1992).

Power of finger flexion is retained. Attempts by the examiner to passively extend the fingers evoke discomfort. If detected early, a programme of graded stretching exercises is a logical management strategy, but it is apparent that patients appear to accept symptoms at a relatively minimal or nuisance level and rarely seek advice.

Stenosing tenovaginitis of the digital flexors (trigger finger; trigger thumb)

This condition is characterized by thickening of the first annular (A1) pulley of the fibrous flexor tendon sheath at the level of the metacarpophalangeal joint. Patients complain of triggering and clicking. The thumb, middle, or ring fingers are most commonly affected.

Repetitive compression during strong grasping is a logical, but unproven, aetiological factor. Bonnici and Spencer (1988) established an increased incidence in women and an association with occupations that require repetitive hand movements. There appears to be a subgroup of the population, particularly but not exclusively people with diabetes, who are vulnerable to fibroproliferative conditions of the hand such as trigger finger and Dupuytren's contracture. Low-dose steroid injections are effective. Early relief of discomfort and triggering is the expected outcome (Marks and Gunther 1989) although, as with de Quervain's tenovaginitis, cases that are refractory or recurrent may be treated by surgical decompression.

The most effective injection technique, using a 23-gauge needle, is to advance the tip of the needle at a more or less 90° angle to the palm, through the tendon, withdraw slightly from the bone and then inject 10 mg triamcinolone (or equivalent). Some practitioners prefer an angled technique, or an approach through the web between the digits.

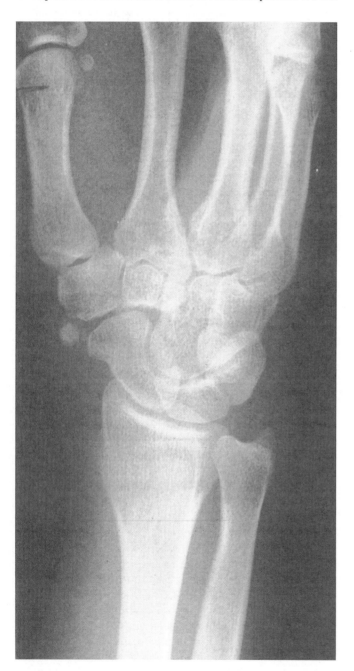

Figure 3.5.2 Calcific flexor carpi radialis tendinitis at the volar aspect of the wrist.

Dupuytren's contracture

Repetitive manual activities were considered by Baron Dupuytren (1834) to be the cause of this condition, which he described in a coachman and in a wine merchant. This association is now much more uncertain, although alcohol may be a causative factor (Noble *et al.* 1992). It is rarely seen in non-white people, and often has a familial distribution. The palmar condition is usually described, although the plantar fascia is also affected in many patients.

It is more common in men than women, and is usually found to be bilateral over time. The earliest feature, usually unnoticed initially by the patient, is thickening of the palmar fascia, often with a nodular component. Puckering soon becomes evident, and subsequently the characteristic flexion deformity of the right and little fingers.

Massage and stretching in the early stages may prevent or delay flexion contracture. There appears to be no inflammatory element, and steroid injections are ineffective. Pronounced contractures can only be effectively treated by surgery.

Ganglion (synovial cyst)

A ganglion is a tense cystic swelling, containing thick viscous fluid, associated with a joint or tendon sheath. Probably the most common site, certainly the most frequently described, is the dorsum of the wrist. Often there is tethering to the carpal joints. However, ganglia are also seen elsewhere, and are more common in women than men (Nelson *et al.* 1972).

Ganglia are not manifestations of rheumatoid arthritis or associated conditions. Distinguishing between a ganglion and a rheumatoid swelling is usually not difficult as the former is tense, and yields a sticky fluid when aspirated; rheumatoid swelling is typically soft, warm, and more diffuse. Ganglia are often painless, but their presence is often disturbing and cosmetically unsightly. They are also unpredictable with respect to their natural history. For the majority, spontaneous resolution is to be expected. However, many recur, and treatment is often sought.

Discomfort, particularly on manual activities, may develop and be associated with impairment of function at the wrist. In a subgroup of patients, dorsal wrist discomfort may precede the development of swelling. Localized tenderness may be present, also discomfort on dorsiflexion and palmarflexion at the wrist but there are no features of tendinitis or of synovitis. Aspiration with a 20-gauge needle, with or without a steroid injection, is often effective (Varley *et al.* 1997). The more traditional management strategy of 'bashing' with a heavy object (commonly a family bible in Victorian times) is outdated.

Although the majority of patients recover satisfactorily after surgical excision, dissection may be tedious, and recurrence is not unusual. In Nelson's series of 222 patients (in whom 50% of ganglia occurred over the dorsal aspect of the wrist) the cure rate of 94% with surgery under general anaesthesia was significantly better than other groups treated by digital pressure or by aspiration.

Peripheral nerve entrapment

The neural system in the upper limb should be viewed as a continuum, both anatomical and physiological, extending from the cervical spine to the fingertips. Nerve compression occurs at well-recognized sites at which constrictions and compressions result from a variety of osseous, muscle and fascial structures. Increased susceptibility to abnormal neural dynamics may be caused by the double crush phenomenon (in which there are multiple sites of neural compression or irritation). The following entrapment neuropathies are the most common, and will be dealt with in some detail, either in this chapter or elsewhere:

- **Intervertebral foramina of the cervical spine:** Nerve root compression is most commonly caused by degenerate bulging discs combined with fibro-osseous hypertrophy of the apophyseal joints. Cervical spinal extension and ipsilateral rotation reduce the dimensions of the foramina. Thus compressive (axial) injuries, particularly when associated with extension of the neck, often cause nerve root compression. Activities that are associated with prolonged flexion of the neck often provoke radicular symptoms, probably because of increased tautness of the spinal cord and the emerging roots. Unpleasant symptoms that radiate to the upper limb from the neck, whether radicular (dermatomal) or pseudoradicular ('sclerotomal') in type, do not always conform to recognized pathways (Slipman *et al.* 1998). It is often difficult on clinical grounds to state categorically whether such symptoms are arising in the neck, as it has been established that many tissues other than nerve roots may refer pain (Kellgren 1939, Feinstein *et al.* 1954), giving the clinician good cause to rely on an appropriate neuromusculoskeletal examination and not just on the presence of neurological signs. Symptoms in the arm that seem to be consistent with a radicular or pseudoradicular syndrome based on the clinical features of somatic dysfunction at the cervicodorsal spine, may have their origins elsewhere in the upper limb; a local cause of neural irritation in the arm must be excluded – an important theme of this text.

- **Brachial plexus/thoracic outlet syndrome:** The components of the brachial plexus may be compressed between the anterior and middle scalene muscles (the 'scalenous gap'), or under the pectoralis minor muscle, or between the clavicle and the first rib, or by compression from a cervical rib or fibrous band.

- **Median nerve entrapment:** The median nerve may be compressed just above the elbow by an accessory ligament from the tip of a supracondylar bony spur (the ligament of Struthers). At the elbow, compression may occur as the median nerve passes between the two heads of the pronator teres muscle, by a sharp lacertus fibrosus (the broad aponeurotic expansion of the distal biceps brachii), or under the edge of the flexor digitorum superficialis (Howard 1986). Occasionally, the anterior interosseous nerve – a branch of the median nerve, arising in the proximal forearm – is traumatized, giving rise to weakness of pinch grip. The most common site of median nerve compression is at the wrist, beneath the flexor retinaculum (transverse carpal ligament) where it is universally referred to as **carpal tunnel syndrome (CTS)**.

- **Ulnar nerve entrapment:** Because of its relatively exposed position the ulnar nerve is vulnerable to compression or trauma at the elbow: either in the condylar groove (cubital tunnel) behind the medial epicondyle, or as it pierces the flexor carpi ulnaris muscle. Another relatively common site is at the canal of Guyon at the wrist.

- **Radial nerve entrapment:** Most commonly, radial nerve compression occurs following injury, such as humeral fracture, in the upper arm. Compression injuries to the radial nerve as it winds around the humerus are sometimes referred to as 'Saturday night palsy'. At the elbow, compression occurs in the radial tunnel (giving rise to both motor and sensory components) at the arcade of Fröhse (the thickened superior edge of the supinator muscle) or by tightening of the fibrous edge of extensor carpi radialis brevis (Kopell and Thompson 1963), when a motor deficit only is the consequence. Occasionally compression of the superficial radial nerve occurs in the distal forearm, giving rise to paraesthesiae over the dorsal aspect of the base of the thumb.

As a general comment, frequent, repetitive and forceful movements of the hand, wrist, forearm, and elbow may give rise to muscle hypertrophy that has the capacity for constricting an adjacent nerve. This is the more likely with co-existent constitutional anatomical variants such as tight tunnels or fascial envelopes, resulting in a vulnerability to dynamic (in the first instance) and subsequently chronic (or fixed) nerve entrapment. These conditions are seen most frequently in sportsmen, and in assembly workers, construction engineers and the like.

Carpal tunnel syndrome

CTS is the most common peripheral nerve entrapment in the upper limb, affecting the middle-aged predominantly (but with a large overlap from the 30s to over 60). It affects women more commonly than men. It is not uncommonly bilateral. The essential characteristic is compression of the median nerve at the wrist in the carpal tunnel. At one end of the spectrum of severity, in the younger age groups, it may be dynamic (and reversible). At the other end it is refractory to management other than surgical decompression. Most cases of somewhat moderate severity are often helped by non-surgical management strategies.

The carpal tunnel is bounded to the radial side by the tuberosity of the navicular (scaphoid) bone and the trapezoid, and to the ulnar side by the pisiform bone and the hook of hamate. All but the trapezium are palpable. The musculoskeletal physician is recommended to become familiar with the surface anatomy. This is helpful when undertaking steroid injections.

At the wrist the median nerve has both sensory and motor components, supplying the muscles of thumb opposition. The manifestations of median nerve compression in the carpal tunnel include:

- Paraesthesiae and numbness in the distribution of the median nerve in the hand (usually the thumb and adjacent 2½ fingers, although it is well recognized that this is variable, and should not be relied upon for diagnosis).

- Discomfort in the wrist and hand, often with radiation proximally to the forearm, and sometimes to the shoulder and the neck.

- More intense nocturnal symptoms. Patients commonly wake and hang their hand out of bed for relief.

- Worsening of symptoms on elevation of the hand for everyday tasks.

- Clumsiness (as a consequence of altered superficial sensation distally) for intricate finger/manual activities.

- The onset is usually insidious, although it may sometimes follow trauma.

Although CTS is commonly labelled as idiopathic, there are a number of clinical conditions that reduce the space for the median nerve in the carpal tunnel and with which CTS is associated:

- rheumatoid arthritis
- non-specific tenosynovitis of the finger flexors
- pregnancy
- acromegaly
- hypothyroidism
- diabetes
- amyloidosis
- occasionally other space-occupying lesions within the carpal tunnel, such as a ganglion.

Of these conditions, the most contentious, principally because of the connotation of work relatedness, even a causal relationship with work, is 'non-specific' flexor tendonitis. I have no doubt that this is responsible for reversible CTS, usually seen in relatively young factory workers (referred to by Braun et al. 1989 as 'dynamic' CTS). These cases, incidentally, are not necessarily seen or recognized in hand clinics that are associated with long waiting lists. It also occurs in a subgroup of the more typical middle-aged CTS sufferers in whom chronic flexor tenosynovitis gives rise to fixed flexion contractures of the fingers (as demonstrated on examination by the 'prayer' sign).

Additionally, the so-called double crush syndrome (Upton and McComas 1973) may also play a role. This is not difficult to understand once the basic concepts of abnormal neurodynamics are understood. CTS is one cause of neural irritation in the upper limb. However, it does not take much imagination to appreciate that neural irritation in the upper limb may develop from compression at more than one site such as at the neck or the thoracic outlet. It follows that in some patients with demonstrable CTS, symptoms are also experienced in the neck and in the upper limb. A full evaluation of the possible additional sites for neural compression in the upper limb to identify a double crush phenomenon should be undertaken before patients are subjected to carpal tunnel decompression.

In view of the possible dual pathology the clinician should examine the cervicodorsal spine as well as the upper limb in patients with symptoms, however vague or diffuse, in the arm and hand. The 'specific' tests for CTS are:

- **Reproduction of symptoms** (burning, paraesthesiae, numbness in the thumb and fingers) by pressure over the volar aspect of the wrist. This is based on the same principle as the Tinel test (or sign), but I recommend that firm pressure over the volar aspect of the wrist for 30 seconds is preferable to tapping.

- **Positive Phalen's test** (Phalen 1966): This may be undertaken bilaterally and simultaneously by holding the dorsum of the palmarflexed wrists against each other during forward flexion at the shoulders and elbow flexion. However, this test may also be positive in the presence of neural compression proximally, and it is advisable to undertake the modified Phalen's test one arm at a time by active or passive palmarflexion of the wrist with the arm in the dependent position.

- Wasting of the thenar eminence.

- Weakness of opposition of the thumb and/or abduction of the thumb.

- Blunted sensation in the distribution of the median nerve.

None of these tests offers a better than 75% sensitivity or specificity (Katz et al. 1990). Muscle wasting and muscle weakness are late signs, and it is poor medical practice to await positive clinical findings in the form of sensory blunting or muscle weakness for the diagnosis of CTS.

The 'gold standard' is often considered to be positive neurophysiological studies. Beware, however, the possibility of minor neurophysiological abnormalities without symptoms (false positive test), and negative neurophysiological findings with characteristic symptoms (particularly in the younger dynamic reversible case). Be aware, too, of the not uncommon association with other conditions in the upper limb, particularly at the cervical and proximal dorsal spines, that contribute to neural tension (see relevant sections). Patients who unexpectedly do not improve following carpal tunnel decompression are often considered by their medical attendants to have alternative agendas (for instance compensation), but in fact the issue of adverse neural tension in the upper limb, and the possible contributory sites, may not have been explored.

Traditionally, allopathic medical management has been predicated on the use of night splints and decompression surgery. Patients often find that the maintenance of a flexed position of the wrist, or repetitive wrist flexion, is provocative (by further compression of the median nerve in the carpal tunnel), hence the usefulness of cock-up splints (to provide slight dorsiflexion at the wrist) at night.

I recommend the use of low-dose steroid injections (for instance 5 mg triamcinolone) to the carpal tunnel. When combined with a small amount of local anaesthetic, this management strategy has both diagnostic and therapeutic usefulness in the majority of patients. With practice, correct needle placement is not difficult. Imagine a vertical line dividing the carpal tunnel midway between the pisiform bone and the tuberosity of the navicular (more or less in the position of the palmaris longus tendon if present); then place the needle just to the ulnar side of this line between the proximal and distal wrist creases, angulating distally and dorsally at approximately 45°. The preferred technique of injecting the ulnar aspect of this vertical dividing line avoids impinging the needle on the median nerve.

Improvement or abolition of symptoms (even if only for a few days or a few weeks) is confirmatory diagnosis of CTS. In a significant proportion of patients, approximately 50% overall, one injection successfully abolishes symptoms or reduces them to a level that is compatible with normal day-to-day activities (Dammers *et al.* 1999). A minority of patients in whom the symptoms recur within a few months are helped on a long-term basis by further injections, but the law of diminishing returns usually applies, in which case surgical decompression is a reliable fallback procedure.

The disadvantages and/or side effects of the described management strategies are few, but they are more frequent after surgery than after non-surgical techniques. Median nerve damage has been reported after impingement by a needle, but the precaution of 'backing off' if electric shock feelings are experienced at the time of needle penetration should prevent this. Reflex sympathetic dystrophy may follow carpal tunnel decompression, and it is not unusual for patients to express dissatisfaction, either because of persistence or recurrence of symptoms, tenderness of the scar, or an unsatisfactory cosmetic result. Surgery is never without the occasional hazard. Traditional osteopathic approaches include neural mobilization of the median nerve in the carpal tunnel.

Upper limb symptoms due to neural irritation are often associated with cervical spinal dysfunction and/or proximal thoracic spinal dysfunction (but without substantive loss of spinal mobility, which is sometimes referred to as a 'hard' clinical sign by many orthopaedists).

Successful treatment often requires the combination of cervical spinal mobilization, thoracic spinal mobilization, paravertebral block injections in both the neck and upper thoracic spine, advice regarding postural awareness and ergonomic improvements, neural release and stretching, and carpal tunnel injections. The clinician should not be afraid to address a complex case in this manner. A satisfactory conclusion may be obtained by spinal mobilization alone, but it is my experience that in the entrenched case, usually in factory workers, a battery of treatments is necessary, combined with ergonomic advice and (often) liaison with employers or supervisors regarding work practices.

When assessing the relationship of CTS to work, both intrinsic factors ('constitutional' narrowing of the carpal tunnel or swelling of its contents) and external factors (repetitive flexion and extension of the wrist, long periods of wrist flexion, or repetitive grasping/finger flexion as in the pinch grip) should be considered. The studies by Silverstein *et al.* (1987) and Wieslander *et al.* (1989) are often cited. Silverstein identified a significant association between forceful use of the hand and repetitive wrist motion and symptoms in the wrist and hand, but a specific diagnosis of CTS was not made in the study population. Wieslander noted that CTS is most common in workers using hand-held vibrating tools, those undertaking repetitive and/or forceful hand/wrist movements such as assembly workers, grinders, keypunch operators, musicians, and bricklayers. Feldman *et al.* (1987) noted an increased incidence of symptoms and signs suggestive of CTS in workers with high-risk jobs.

The increased association with exposure to vibration is generally accepted (Koskimies *et al.* 1990, Rosenbaum and Ochoa 1993). There are numerous (anecdotal) accounts of a sudden painful flush of paraesthesiae in the hand from the unaccustomed use of vibrating equipment such as electric shears with the wrist flexed. For those exposed to the use of vibrating tools on a regular basis as part of their work, CTS is accepted as an industrial injury (PD A12) in the UK. Nevertheless, it has to be distinguished from the condition of hand/arm vibration syndrome that may also give rise to discomfort and paraesthesiae in the hand but, critically, also has a substantive component of circulatory disruption.

Pronator syndrome

Hypertrophy of the pronator teres muscle arises from repeated forceful pronation of the forearm, often accompanied by prolonged firm finger flexion, as in assembly workers, sports such as tennis, and also in musicians (Bejjani *et al.* 1996). Direct trauma or compression by fibrous bands is occasionally found. Both motor and sensory deficits may result, as in CTS, but in addition painful weakness of pronation is usually present. Most cases respond to local infiltration of steroid and local anaesthetic, failing which surgical exploration may be necessary.

Ulnar nerve entrapment

Ulnar nerve entrapment at the elbow is the second most common peripheral nerve entrapment in the upper limb. However, at least two other possibilities should always be considered for neuritic symptoms along the ulnar border of the hand: thoracic outlet syndrome and ulnar nerve entrapment in the canal of Guyon at the wrist.

The ulnar nerve enters the forearm via the fibro-osseous cubital tunnel in the groove behind the medial epicondyle. The boundaries are the elbow joint, a fascial arcade intimately associated with the heads of flexor carpi ulnaris, and the flexor carpi ulnaris muscles themselves. Compression by the fascial band, by muscle hypertrophy, and by osteophytic spurs in osteoarthritis are possibilities. Additionally, in evaluating the possible cause of ulnar nerve compression at the elbow, direct compression (usually repetitive in nature and work related) should be distinguished from the more occasional and unpredictable trauma to a hypermobile ulnar nerve. (Treatment of the two conditions may be radically different.)

Paraesthesiae and numbness of the little finger and the ulnar margin of the ring finger are virtually always present. An early presentation may be a manual worker's inability to undertake intricate or repetitive tasks as competently as previously. Symptoms from ulnar nerve compression at the elbow are always experienced distally, but also sometimes proximally (when additional or alternative causes of neural dysfunction have to be considered). Progressively, hypothenar wasting becomes apparent, and in the late stages clawing of the fingers due to weakness of the intrinsic hand muscles. Symptoms are often worse at night as the elbow is often held in the flexed position, in which the ulnar nerve at the elbow is relatively taut.

Workers at risk are those who rest their elbows on a work surface to stabilize their arms for manual activities. Baseball pitchers, tennis players, and field athletes are susceptible as a consequence of valgus forces at the elbow, causing fibrosis and in some cases osteophytosis. Symptoms may be aggravated (and, arguably, sometimes caused) by resting the medial aspect of the elbow on some part of the adjacent door when driving a car. Repetitive flexion and extension of the elbow are cited as provocative activities. This is based on the fact that the ulnar nerve moves in the cubital tunnel during sagittal plane movements, becoming relatively taut in flexion.

A standard neurological examination is necessary. An early feature is weakness of abductor digiti minimi. Sensory assessment usually reveals sensory blunting (although this part of the examination is often forgotten or deliberately ignored by many clinicians who feel that the subjective awareness of altered sensation is evidence enough of a sensory component to a neural problem). At the elbow, the ulnar nerve should be palpated for hypermobility, first in elbow flexion and then in extension, and also during the movement from flexion to extension. Tapping the ulnar nerve or compressing it digitally at the elbow may give rise to discomfort and/or paraesthesiae distally as a normal finding but patients with ulnar nerve entrapment experience increased discomfort when compared with the normal side. Nerve conduction studies are commonly undertaken but in many cases this confirmatory examination is unnecessary.

A conservative approach is reasonable in early cases, particularly when there is no (or no substantive) sensorimotor deficit. This is particularly important in those patients in whom compression of the nerve during daily activities, usually working at a bench, is considered to be an aetiological factor. Liaison with employers or with an ergonomist may need to be considered in order to reduce the stresses at the elbow.

The ulnar nerve may be compressed at the wrist as it passes through the canal of Guyon, possibly by the pisohamate ligament. Trauma, as a single event or repetitively, to the region of the hamate (for instance in golfers or cricketers) or repetitive compression at work, for instance when using a hammer or similar tool, may be the cause. In cyclists, 'handlebar palsy' may result from prolonged compression against dropped handlebars. The deep branch of the ulnar nerve as it traverses the palm may be compressed in those workers who hold an implement or tool in or across the palm; pizza-cutter's palsy has been described by Jones (1988).

Entrapment of the radial nerve and posterior interosseous nerve

The radial nerve curves round the humerus in the spiral groove, piercing the lateral intermuscular septum to lie in front of the elbow. It then enters the radial tunnel, bounded medially by the brachialis muscle and anterolaterally by the brachioradialis muscle and extensor carpi radialis longus. At the distal aspect of the tunnel it divides into a superficial branch and the deep branch – the posterior interosseous nerve.

In the radial tunnel, first described by Roles and Maudsley (1972), subsequently by Lister *et al.* (1979), compression may occur as a consequence of fibrous bands or arches including the arcade of Fröhse and by a sharp margin to the extensor carpi radialis. Compression of the radial nerve may give rise to mixed sensory and motor manifestations. However, when the posterior interosseous nerve is compressed (giving rise to the 'posterior interosseous nerve syndrome') the consequences are motor only. The posterior interosseous nerve is vulnerable to compression between the two heads of the supinator muscle in those athletes and workers whose supinator is hypertrophied. In my experience, this problem occurs most commonly in workers who use relatively heavy tools such as industrial hammers and who supinate their forearms repetitively (for instance in the tightening movement with a screwdriver), and occasionally in athletes. Roles and Maudsley reported cases of resistant tennis elbow that were helped by surgical decompression of the radial nerve. The diagnosis of tennis elbow is far more complex than might appear to the novice clinician; the possibility of nerve compression masquerading as tennis elbow should always be considered. In my experience, when muscle hyperalgesia is found around the elbow (particularly when accompanied by more extensive regional muscle hyperalgesia) this is most likely to be the consequence of proximal nerve compression or irritation; however, an index of suspicion with respect to the radial nerve and posterior interosseous nerve at and just below the elbow should always be maintained.

Neurological examination of the upper limb, particularly a search for motor defects, is paramount. Assessment of supination and dorsiflexion of the wrist is particularly important. Lesions of the radial nerve or posterior interosseous nerve commonly give rise to weakness of supination (often a reflection of pain inhibition, when it is accompanied by discomfort on resisted contraction), weakness of dorsiflexion of the wrist and sometimes of the finger extensors. The presence of paraesthesiae in the forearm or back of the hand suggests that the compression is occurring relatively proximally in the radial tunnel, affecting the radial nerve rather than the posterior interosseous nerve.

In the established case, ergonomic adjustments at work, or technical adjustments during sporting activity, for instance the backhand at tennis, are of prime importance. Partial relief of symptoms may be gained by intramuscular stimulation or injections (for instance of local anaesthetic) as the extensor muscle mass in the proximal forearm, including both the extensor carpi radialis muscles and the supinator muscle, are commonly hyperalgesic and hypertonic. Nerve conduction studies may be helpful. Surgical decompression should be considered in the established case that is refractory to conservative management.

The superficial radial nerve may be traumatized or compressed distally in the forearm. The condition is sometimes referred to as Wartenberg's syndrome. Paraesthesiae are experienced over the dorsi-radial aspect of the hand, frequently in occupations that require repetitive supination and pronation and/or hyperpronation (Dellon and Mackinnon 1986), and occasionally as a consequence of over-tight splints or even handcuffs.

Neuropathic arm pain

The regional pain syndrome, commonly referred to as neuropathic arm pain (NAP), 'RSI', or type II work-related upper limb disorder (WRULD) (Hutson 1997) to distinguish it from those upper limb disorders in which there is demonstrable pathomorphology (type I WRULD), is characterized by persistent pain and dysaesthesies. Initially experienced peripherally, often in the hand(s) or forearm(s), discomfort often extends diffusely to the shoulder, neck and upper back. In a minority of patients it is experienced in the contralateral upper limb. Usually the pain has a deep, burning, 'toothache' quality, sometimes accompanied by a subjective sensation of swelling and by a variable degree of numbness and tingling in the hand and/or fingers. It is commonly associated with repetitive stereotyped activities of the hands and digits, but perhaps more relevant in causation is the upper body posture that is maintained for long periods in office workers. The symptoms are often related to a particular task, for instance the use of a keyboard or mouse or (commonly) to an intensive spell of keyboard activities.

Initially the symptoms resolve with rest. Gradually, the symptoms become more persistent, intense, and refractory to either rest or conventional treatment. Sleep pattern is often disturbed. The discomfort becomes increasingly intrusive with respect to work and home activities. Psychological symptoms are commonly found at this stage – for instance, depression, headaches, chronic fatigue, and frustration. Not infrequently there is a history of unsuccessful surgery for suspected tennis elbow or CTS.

The pathogenesis is evident from the acronym NAP. It has long been established that pain and altered sensation following peripheral nerve damage results from pathophysiological changes within the nervous system. The hypothesis with respect to the pathogenesis of NAP is that these pathophysiological changes within the central nervous system, and possibly in the peripheral nervous system too, are precipitated by repetitive or prolonged stresses applied to the soft tissues of the upper limb. Afferent stimulation at a consistently intense level may arise in the hands and fingers, but may also arise proximally at the shoulder girdle or at the cervicodorsal spine. The overloaded sensorineural mechanisms for pain production and perception are augmented by sensitization of the wide dynamic range (WDR) neurones situated in the dorsal horns of the spinal cord. Pain amplification develops, resulting in allodynia (reduced threshold to painful stimuli) hyperalgesia (increased response to stimuli), wind-up (increased response to repeated stimulation), hyperpathia (prolonged response to stimuli), and the expansion of receptive fields (giving rise to relatively widespread symptoms).

It may be noted from the seminal work of Cohen and associates (1992) that the clinical features are remarkably consistent. Secondary hyperalgesia, manifesting as 'regional' muscle tenderness and sometimes terminal discomfort on joint movements, are present in the majority of patients. The proximal forearm muscles, extensor and flexor, are usually tender. The proximal scapular fixator muscles are also hyperalgesic. There are usually signs of segmental dysfunction in the cervical spine or proximal thoracic spine or both. Adverse neural tension is commonly present. It is noteworthy that although it is generally recognized that adverse neural tension may be associated with cervical spinal dysfunction, it is extremely common in this group of patients for proximal thoracic spinal dysfunction (between D3 and D5) to be present. It is hypothesized that in many patients poor work postures, associated with a proximal thoracic kyphosis and protracted shoulders, cause proximal thoracic spinal and cervical spinal dysfunction, and altered neurodynamics. The addition of repetitive stereotyped activity of the hands and fingers to the long periods of static muscle activity at the shoulder girdle overwhelm the already compromised peripheral nervous system, giving rise in vulnerable patients to neurosensitization.

Conventional investigations such as cervicodorsal spinal radiographs, nerve conduction studies, and MRI are negative. Occasionally nerve conduction studies may be equivocal for CTS, leading the unsuspecting orthopaedic surgeon to undertake carpal tunnel release. The condition, however, remains refractory to such operative intervention.

Other aetiological factors often play a role. These include psychosocial factors (such as premorbid psychological profile, environmental stresses, misattributions and beliefs, adverse posture and ergonomics, iatrogenesis, and litigation). Of these factors, iatrogenesis is often a powerful aggravating factor. Just when a patient sorely needs a knowledgeable medical practitioner in the early stages to deal with the described factors appropriately, help is not always to hand. Regrettably, the failure of the medical profession in general to recognize the early presence of neuropathic pain leads to misdiagnosis, inappropriate management, and an increasingly frustrated and despondent patient. It is not surprising that reactive depression often develops, sometimes compounded by the prescription for amitriptyline, useful in low dosages for pain relief, without an appropriate explanation of the use of a tricyclic antidepressant, thereby inculcating in the patient's mind the impression that the medical attendant believes 'it's all in the mind'.

The most appropriate management strategy is an explanation to the patient of the nature of the complaint. Attention to ergonomics and work environment in general is required if this has not already been undertaken. My preferred tricyclic is amitriptyline, commencing at 10–20 mg at night, gradually increasing in dose by titrating against tolerance and efficacy. Manual treatment includes neural stretching and treatment for spinal dysfunction. In my experience, spinal mobilization alone is insufficient. Localized paravertebral block injections of low-dose steroid and local anaesthetic to the appropriate cervical spinal or proximal thoracic spinal segments are often helpful. A pragmatic approach incorporating most if not all of these modalities combined with reduction of provocative physical stresses yields the best results. For patients with neuropathic arm pain I have found that the most effective physical therapy is the combination of neural blocks and neural mobilization (Hutson 1997).

Lateral epicondylitis

Lateral epicondylitis ('tennis elbow') is an enthesitis (otherwise referred to as an enthesopathy) at the common extensor origin from the lateral epicondyle of the humerus. It is sometimes associated with inflammatory disorders although, as its colloquial name suggests, it is usually the consequence of repetitive manual activities that cause overload of the collagenized tissues that form the teno-osseous unit at the lateral epicondyle. The extensor carpi radialis brevis (extensor carpi radialis brevis) tendon attachment at the lateral epicondyle appears to be affected more commonly than the extensor carpi radialis longus (extensor carpi radialis longus) attachment at the supracondylar ridge. Entheses are relatively avascular structures, and the pathomorphological changes include microtears of the tendon and disruption of the zone of calcification at the teno-osseous junction. Mesenchymal transformation, calcification, and new bone formation are described (Chard and Hazleman 1989). 'Angiofibroblastic hyperplasia' is the description used by Nirschl (1986). Occasionally, direct trauma is stated to be a precipitating event, though this is unlikely without underlying and pre-existing degenerative changes (albeit microscopic in the majority of cases).

As is well recognized, lateral epicondylitis is a very common condition, affecting at least 1% of manual workers (Kivi 1982). It occurs primarily in the dominant arm. Its maximal incidence is in the age group 40–55. It does of course occur in racquet sportsmen and was first described in the late 19th century in tennis players. However, sport is not the cause in the majority of sufferers. Women in their 40s are a significant subgroup, presumably the consequence of multitask manual activities, not least the modern trend for financially remunerative work by both partners. Lateral epicondylitis is primarily associated with repetitive firm grasping: both the power grip and the pinch grip are implicated. The condition is clearly work related in the majority of cases and caused by work in some, though given the current medicolegal culture it is worth stating that the development of lateral epicondylitis in an employee does not automatically imply culpability on the part of the employer.

Lateral epicondylitis is characterized by lateral elbow and adjacent proximal forearm pain, worse on gripping and sometimes sufficiently sharp to cause patients to release their grip and drop things. Discomfort commonly radiates distally, rarely proximally. A common complaint is that the use of a pinch grip, as in holding a cup, evokes pain. Patients also describe localized tenderness and swelling. More widespread symptoms, for instance discomfort in the neck and shoulder, or discomfort, paraesthesiae and numbness in the hand and fingers should alert the clinician to alternative causes for lateral elbow pain. The presence of concurrent ipsilateral medial elbow pain, or bilaterality also suggests that enthesitis is probably not the correct diagnosis. The natural history for true lateral epicondylitis is for gradual spontaneous resolution within 12–18 months but recurrence is common. Naturally, patients are often intolerant of an expectant approach, the majority seeking and receiving treatment whether it be by NSAIDs, steroid injections, physiotherapy, or osteopathy.

In the typical case the examination findings leave little room for doubt about the diagnosis. Patients accurately localize their symptoms to the lateral epicondyle, sometimes to the proximal common extensor muscle mass. In a subset of patients, passive extension at the elbow meets with terminal resistance. However, passive elbow flexion is normal. Resisted dorsiflexion of the wrist is painful; resisted finger extension is also painful, often less than resisted dorsiflexion of the wrist. Passive stretching of the common extensor origin (by pronation of the forearm, palmarflexion of the wrist and extension of the elbow) is uncomfortable. There is often slight soft tissue swelling overlying the

lateral epicondyle, and exquisite tenderness. In a subgroup of patients tenderness is also present (or even maximal) in the common extensor muscles 4–6 cm distant, but the finding of muscle hyperalgesia should alert the clinician to the possibility of a neurogenic aetiology. In the straightforward case of lateral epicondylitis, the upper limb neurodynamics are normal and there are no relevant or associated features in the cervicodorsal spine. Resisted supination of the forearm is painless. (Should this not be the case, posterior interosseous nerve entrapment in the proximal forearm is a likely cause.) Tenderness at the head of the radius is not present other than in a subgroup of atypical cases (considered by Roles and Maudsley 1972 to be due to radial tunnel syndrome).

The management of lateral epicondylitis is somewhat controversial, insofar as the standard management strategy of steroid injection has been questioned in recent years (Smidt et al. 2002). Cyriax (1969) advised treatment by low-dose steroid injections, although he noted that if left untreated the natural outcome is for gradual and spontaneous resolution over the course of approximately 1 year. Smidt identified a high recurrence rate following steroid injections, and a better outcome for a 'wait-and-see' policy or physiotherapy than with injections. To a large degree this is consistent with much anecdotal evidence that in those patients whose symptoms recur relatively early following a steroid injection, not only does the law of diminishing returns apply (with respect to effectiveness of further injections) there is also significant risk of delayed full recovery. In a small minority of patients symptoms persist for several years. Sclerotherapy or tendon-slide surgery may then be helpful.

My own preference is for a pragmatic management strategy. Decision-making is dependent upon individual circumstances rather than dogma. Some patients would prefer, quite understandably, to await natural spontaneous resolution rather than have steroid injections. Most practitioners find that physiotherapy is not effective but it does suit some. Intramuscular stimulation may be helpful, particularly if there is significant hyperalgesia of the common extensors. Should steroid injections be undertaken, low dosages (no more than 10 mg triamcinolone) should be used, using the Cyriax technique of droplet infiltration at the teno-osseous junction. Perhaps the most important advice is for a period of relative rest from forceful and repetitive manual activities of at least 3 weeks after injections, to maximize the effectiveness of treatment. There is a strong suspicion amongst many experienced musculoskeletal physicians that the recurrence rate is significantly raised by failure to implement appropriate ergonomic evaluation and common sense (with respect to a period of 'rest') following treatment. As is common with other upper limb disorders, the need for clinical re-evaluation is paramount.

Confounding factors with respect to diagnosis include widespread upper limb symptoms, cervicodorsal spinal discomfort, shoulder girdle discomfort, and bilaterality. Should any of these symptoms coexist, the clinician should have a high index of suspicion of referred (pseudoradicular or sclerotomal) symptoms in the upper limb that are secondary to cervicodorsal spinal dysfunction and/or abnormal neurodynamics. A common scenario is the combination of proximal dorsal spinal dysfunction, protracted shoulders, altered neurodynamics (detected clinically by the identification of adverse neural tension) and muscle hyperalgesia that commonly includes the proximal scapular fixator muscles and common extensor muscles in the forearm, not infrequently the common flexor origin at the elbow and other muscle groups. Lateral elbow discomfort under these circumstances is a manifestation of secondary hyperalgesia. The lateral epicondyle may be tender but the resisted muscle contraction tests are not specifically uncomfortable. Unsuspecting clinicians, who are not familiar with the possibility of a neurogenic model for elbow and forearm symptoms, commonly misattribute such symptoms to an enthesitis (tennis elbow) or 'tenosynovitis', thereby evoking uncertainties in some patients regarding causation (and frustration and despondency when their symptoms do not respond to localized steroid injections).

Medial epicondylitis

Medial epicondylitis ('golfer's elbow') is an enthesitis that affects the common flexor origin at the medial epicondyle of the humerus. It gives rise to medial elbow discomfort, sometimes radiating to the volar and ulnar aspects of the forearm. It is less common than lateral epicondylitis. It affects primarily the middle aged, and in particular those engaged in work or sport that involves repetitive forceful grasping and pronation of the forearm. Hence, it occurs in right-handed golfers with a 'strong' right hand: uncocking the wrist before ball contact is associated with greater pronation than is the case with a 'weak' grip on the club. (Right-handed golfers tend to experience medial epicondylitis of the right elbow or lateral epicondylitis of the left elbow.) As the name of the condition (medial epicondylitis) suggests, pathological changes may occur at the tendons attached to the medial epicondyle. These changes have been confirmed by the work of Nirschl (1986). The pronator teres muscle and the flexor carpi radialis are the principal muscles involved. Of these, it would appear to be the pronator teres that is the more important aetiologically. This is borne out by the clinical observation that resisted pronation is painful and weak, more so than resisted wrist or finger flexion, in these patients. Patients usually complain of medial elbow tenderness in addition to discomfort on manual activities.

Examination reveals a full range of movements at the elbow. There is rarely any significant swelling. Tenderness is localized to the tenoosseous junction, maximal 1 cm distal to the tip of the medial epicondyle. Resisted pronation is painful and associated with variable degrees of weakness on resisted contraction. There is rarely weakness of other muscle groups. Should weakness be apparent of the muscles used in the pinch grip (the muscles of flexion and opposition of the thumb, and flexion of the index finger) the **pronator syndrome** should be suspected. In this condition the median nerve is compressed during its passage through the pronator teres muscle. (According to Bejjani et al. 1996, musicians are a particularly vulnerable group as a consequence of frequent repetitive pronation of the forearm.) In a relatively straightforward case of medial epicondylitis there are no neuritic symptoms. Movements at the elbow and wrist are normal, although stretching the common flexor/pronator origin by the combination of passive extension of the elbow, supination of the forearm, and dorsiflexion of the wrist evokes medial elbow discomfort.

Management is much the same as for lateral epicondylitis. Although a low-dose steroid injection is expected to be symptomatically beneficial, a relapse of the condition is frequently found unless appropriate advice is given with respect to reduction of biomechanical loading of the common flexor origin. Tennis players with a wristy (heavily topspin) forehand usually benefit from an adjustment to their technique. Similarly, golfers often need to weaken their grip on the club. Factory workers, for instance those on assembly lines, often benefit from an ergonomic assessment, particularly with respect to the use of tools. Physiotherapy gives modest returns. Medial elbow pain

that is refractory to conventional treatment may be a manifestation of secondary hyperalgesia. A neurogenic aetiology is always a possibility in patients with elbow and forearm pain, hence the need for a comprehensive cervicodorsal spinal evaluation and an assessment of upper limb neurodynamics in all patients. Indications that abnormal neurodynamics are playing a significant role are:

- the coexistence of medial and lateral elbow pain
- bilaterality of symptoms
- relatively widespread upper limb symptoms and hyperalgesia, particularly the presence of hyperalgesia of the proximal scapular fixator muscles, and adverse neural tension
- an adverse upper body posture, particularly protracted shoulders.

References

Bejjani, F. J., Kaye, G. M., Benham, M. (1996) Musculoskeletal and neuromuscular conditions of instrumental musicians. *Arch. Phys. Med. Rehabil.*, 77, 406–13.

Bonnici, A. V., Spencer, J. D. (1988) A survey of trigger finger in adults. *J. Hand Surg.*, 13B, 202–3.

Braun, R. M., Davidson, K., Doehr, S. (1989) Provocative testing in the diagnosis of dynamic carpal tunnel syndrome. *J. Hand Surg.*, 14A, 195–7.

Chard, M. D., Hazleman, B. L. (1989) Tennis elbow – a reappraisal. *Br. J. Rheumatol.*, 28(3), 186–8.

Cohen, M. L., Arroyo, J. F., Champion, G. D., Browne, C. D. (1992) In search of the pathogenesis of refractory cervicobrachial pain syndrome. *Med. J. Aust.*, 156, 432–6.

Cyriax, J. H. (1969) *Textbook of Orthopaedic Medicine: diagnosis of soft-tissue lesions*, 5th edn. Baillière, Tindall, Cassell, London, p. 337.

Dammers, J. W. H. H., Veering, M. (1999) Injection with methylprednisolone proximal to the carpal tunnel tunnel. *BMJ*, 319, 884–6.

Dellon, A. L., Mackinnon, S. E. (1986) Radial sensory nerve entrapment in the forearm. *J. Hand Surg.*, 11A, 199–205.

Dums, F. (1896) Uber trommlerlahmungen. *Deutsch. Militarztliche Zeitschr.*, 25, 144–55.

Dupuytren, Baron G. (1834) Permanent retraction of the fingers, produced by an affection of the palmar fascia. *Lancet*, ii, 222–5.

Feinstein, B., Langton, J. N. K., Jameson, R. M. *et al.* (1954) Experiments on pain referred from deep somatic tissues. *J. Bone Joint Surg.*, 36A, 981–97.

Feldman, R. G., Travers, P. H., Chirico-Post, J., *et al.* (1987) Risk assessment in electronic assembly workers: carpal tunnel syndrome. *J. Hand Surg.*, 12A, 849–55.

Greening, J., Smart, S., Leary, R., Hall-Craggs, M., O'Higgins, P., Lynn, B. (1999) Reduced movement of median nerve in carpal tunnel during wrist flexion in patients with non-specific arm pain. *Lancet*, 354, 217–218.

Harvey, F. J., Harvey, P. M., Horsley, M. W. (1990) de Quervain's disease: surgical or non-surgical treatment. *J. Hand Surg.*, 15A, 83–7.

Hooper, G., McMaster, M. J. (1979) Stenosing tenovaginitis affecting the tendon of extensor digiti minimi at the wrist. *Hand*, 11, 29–301.

Howard, F. M. (1986) Controversies in nerve entrapment syndromes in the forearm and wrist. *Orthop. Clin. North Am.*, 17(3), 375–81.

Hutson, M. A. (1997) *Work-related upper limb disorders: recognition and management*. Butterworth Heinemann, Oxford.

Hutson, M. A. (2001) *Sports Injuries: recognition and management*, 3rd edn. Oxford University Press, Oxford.

Jones, H. R. (1988) Letter: Pizza-cutters's palsy. *N. Engl. J. Med.*, 319, 410.

Katz, J. N., Larson, M. G., Sabra, A. *et al.* (1990) The carpal tunnel syndrome: diagnostic utility of the history and physical examination findings. *Ann. Intern. Med.*, 112, 321–7.

Kellgren, J. H. (1939) On the description of pain arising from deep somatic structures with charts of segmental pain areas. *Clin. Sci.*, **4**, 35–46.

Khan, K. M. *et al.* (2002). Time to abandon the 'tendinitis' myth. *BMJ*, **324**, 627–8.

Kiefhaber, T. R., Stern, P. J. (1992) Upper extremity tendinitis and overuse syndromes in the athlete. *Clin. Sports Med.*, **11**(1), 39–55.

Kivi, P. (1982) The aetiology and conservative treatment of humeral epicondylitis. *Scand. J. Rehabil. Med.*, **15**, 37–41.

Kopell, H. P., Thompson, W. A.L. (1963) *Peripheral entrapment neuropathies.* Williams & Wilkins, Baltimore, MD.

Koskimies, K., Farkkila, M., Pyykko, J., Jantti, V. *et al.* (1990) Carpal tunnel syndrome in vibration disease. *Br. J. Industr. Med.*, **47**, 411–16.

Leao, L. (1958) de Quervain's disease: a clinical and anatomical study. *J. Bone Joint Surg.*, **40A**(5), 1063–70.

Lister, G. D., Belsole, R. B., Kleinert, H. E. (1979) The radial tunnel syndrome. *J. Hand, J.*, **4A.**, 52–9.

Marks, M. R., Gunther, S. F. (1989) Efficacy of cortisone treatment in treatment of trigger fingers and thumbs. *J. Hand Surg.*, **14A**, 722–7.

Mennell, J.McM., Zohn, D. A. (1976) *Diagnosis and physical treatment: musculoskeletal pain.* Little, Brown, Boston, MA.

Mitchell, S., Cooper, C., Martyn, C., Coggon, D. (2000) Sensory neural processing in work-related upper limb disorders. *Occup. Med.*, **50**(1), 30–32.

Nelson, C. L., Sawmiller, S., Phalen, G. S. (1972) Ganglions of the wrist and hand. *J. Bone Joint Surg.*, **54A**, 1459–64.

Nirschl, R. P. (1986) Soft-tissue injuries about the elbow. *Clin. Sports Med.*, **5**(4), 637–52.

Noble, J., Arafa, M., Royle, S. G., McGeorge, G., Crank, S. (1992) The association between alcohol, hepatic pathology and Dupuytren's disease. *J. Hand Surg.*, **17B**, 71–4.

Phalen, G. S. (1966) The carpal-tunnel syndrome – seventeen years' experience in diagnosis and treatment of six hundred and fifty-four hands. *J. Bone Joint Surg.*, **48A**, 211–28.

Roles, N. C., Maudsley, R. H. (1972) Radial tunnel syndrome: resistant tennis elbow as a nerve entrapment. *J. Bone Joint Surg.*, **54B**(3), 499–508.

Rosenbaum, R. B., Ochoa, J. L. (1993) *Carpal tunnel syndrome and other disorders of the median nerve.* Butterworth-Heinemann, Stoneham, MA, pp. 233–49.

Silverstein, B. A., Fine, L. J., Armstrong, T. J. (1987) Occupational factors and carpal tunnel syndrome. *Am. J. Ind. Med.*, **11**, 343–58.

Slipman, C. W., Plastaras, C. T., Palmitier, R. A., Huston, C. W., Sterenfeld, E. B. (1998) Symptom provocation of fluoroscopically guided cervical nerve root stimulation: are dynatomal maps identical to dermatomal maps? *Spine*, **23**(20), 2235–42.

Smidt, N., van der Windt, D. A.W. M., Assendaft, W. J. J., Deville, W. L. J. M. *et al.* (2002) Corticosteroid injections, physiotherapy, or a wait-and-see policy for lateral epicondylitis: a randomised controlled trial. *Lancet*, **359**, 657–62.

Thompson, A. R., Plewes, L. W., Shaw, E. G. (1951) Peritendinitis crepitans and simple tenosynovitis: a clinical study of 544 cases in industry. *Br. J. Ind. Med.*, **8**, 150–8.

Tillaux, P. (1892) *Traité d'anatomie topographique. Avec applications à la chirugie* (ed.), 7. Asselin et Houzeau, Paris.

Troell, A. (1918) Uber die sogenannte tendovaginitis crepitans. *Dtsch. Z. Chir.*, **143**, 125–62.

Upton, A. R. M., McComas, A. J. (1973) The double crush in nerve-entrapment syndromes. *Lancet*, **ii**, 359–62.

Varley, G. W., Needoff, M., Davis, T. R. C., Clay, N. R. (1997) Conservative management of wrist ganglia. *J. Hand Surg.*, **22B**(5), 636–7.

Velpeau, A. (1841) Crepitation douloureuse des tendons. Article 2, *Leçons orales de clinique chirurgicale a l'Hôpital de la Charité*, vol. 3, 94, Gernser-Baillière, Paris.

Wieslander, G., Norback, D., Gothe, C-J., Juhlin, L. (1989) Carpal tunnel syndrome and exposure to vibration, repetitive wrist movements, and heavy manual work: a case referent study. *Br. J. Ind. Med.*, **46**, 43–7.

3.6 The pelvis

Malcolm Read

The pelvis is formed from the sacrum and two innominate bones, the innominate being a composite of the ilium, ischium, and pubis, which fuse in the region of the acetabulum. Apart from protecting the viscera and providing attachment for muscles, the pelvis transmits the weight of the body from the vertebrae through the sacrum and onto the femora when standing, or the ischia when sitting. The sacrum forms an auricular L-shaped joint with the two iliac bones (Figure 3.6.1). This sacroiliac joint is a diarthrodial joint because it contains synovial fluid, and has matching articular surfaces. However, it is different from all other joints in the body because the ilial surface has fibrocartilage that articulates with the hyaline cartilage of the sacrum. The joint is synovial on its anterior aspect and fibrous on its posterior aspect.

The sacroiliac joints (SIJs) are capable of a nutational or nodding movement in the anteroposterior plane, but this movement is small, and is limited by the ridges and depressions which produce a rough surface that locks the joint into a stable position that will allow the transmission of impact forces from the leg to the body, and support the body weight. The anterior, posterior, and interosseous ligaments are associated functionally with the sacrotuberous and sacrospinous ligaments (Figure 3.6.2), and the fascia of the gluteals and hamstrings

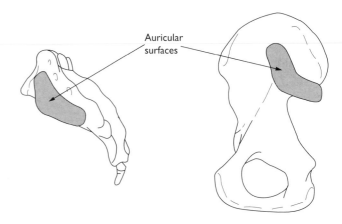

Figure 3.6.1   The auricular L shape sacroiliac joint.

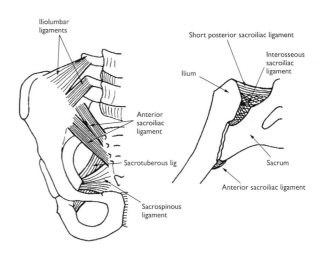

Figure 3.6.2   Ligaments of the sacroiliac joint.

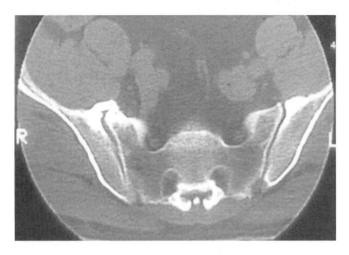

Figure 3.6.3   CT scan with large right and developing left osteophytes.

producing a linked stabilizing system. The anterior aspect of the pelvic ring is formed from the pubic bones on both sides meeting at the pubic symphysis. This joint is an ovoid synovial joint with strong ligaments forming the arcuate ligament inferiorly. The fascia over the adductors is contiguous with the abdominal fascia and it is this anatomical continuity, and the continuity of the gluteals and hamstrings with the sacrotuberous and sacrospinous ligaments and gluteal fascia, that produce diagnostically challenging disorders from the spine and hamstrings, and anteriorly the groin strain and adductor tear. This diagnostic conundrum is further complicated by referred pain from the discs, facet joints, and sacroiliac joints. The whole pelvis may be looked on as a ring, one feature of which is that it cannot be disturbed in only one place at a time, so that a disturbance in one area produces an associated disturbance in another part of the ring. These features of the ring mechanism, the fascial connections, and referred pain from disc, facet, and dura makes the management of pelvic injuries a problem, for it sometimes appears as though one injury improves only for another injury to appear in its stead. The apparent stability of the SIJ belies the fact that it can move and the stresses across the joint are manifest by osteophytes on its anterior surface (Figure 3.6.3). The joint can ankylose from ageing or from the effect of inflammatory arthropathies.

Pain may be referred from proximal structures to the pelvis. Accordingly, any examination of the pelvis must include an examination of the spine and particularly the thoracolumbar junction where the ilioinguinal nerve (T12) originates to supply the groin. Pain may be referred to the buttock and the groin from lumbar segmental disturbances such as discal pathology and facetal dysfunction as well as the connecting ligaments. Sometimes invasive diagnostic interventions, for instance infiltrating the facet joints under direct vision or even a provocative probe when the disc, facet joint and sacroiliac joint are stimulated under narcoleptic anaesthesia, may be required to establish the cause of pelvic pain. Those practitioners whose training conditions them to search for referred pain must be aware of local conditions that can also be a cause of pelvic pain.

Sacroiliac joint

Vleeming *et al.* (1997) and Bowen and Cassidy (1981) have demonstrated, by injecting the SIJ with contrast and steroid, that the SIJ is a source of pain. However, it is not quite so easy clinically to differentiate a sacroiliac lesion from facetal or discal pathology.

History

The patient's history can range from a diffuse sacroiliac or buttock pain, to pain referred down the leg as far as the ankle. However, the referred sacroiliac pain is not accompanied by pins and needles or numbness. The young age of a patient (especially if he is a man in his 20s), will raise the suspicion of ankylosing spondylitis, which has a male/female ratio of 8 : 1, but this condition can present in the 30s and 40s as undiagnosed back pain. Ankylosing spondylitis may be so severe that the patient is carried into the consulting room on a stretcher, exhibiting all the signs of an acute prolapsed disc with severe limitation of straight leg raise. Specifically, a young patient or a patient with undiagnosed back pain should be asked about any family history of ankylosis and whether there has been any history of iritis, urethritis, or bowel disease. Recurrent enthesitis affecting multiple sites and/or a groin strain also may be presenting features of ankylosing spondylitis. Schober's test and a reduced chest expansion (below 4 cm) are indicative.

Investigations include blood tests (for ESR, CRP, HLA B27), radiographs, and possibly CT scanning of the SIJ. The radiographs will show sclerosis on the ilial side of the SIJ and may also show irregularity and lytic areas within the joint (Figure 3.6.4). CT scanning may display these areas of erosion and sclerosis even in the presence of normal radiographs (Figure 3.6.5). MRI may not be quite so effective for displaying problems with cortical bone, but the inflammatory

> ### Schober's test
>
> Schober's test for the lumbar spine may be carried out by taking a lower mark in the standing position at the level of the posterior inferior iliac spines, measuring 15 cm up from this mark, and making another mark on the skin in the midline. The patient is then asked to flex their spine forwards towards their toes while the tape measure is held on the upper mark. The distance between the two marks should lengthen by at least 5 cm. Failure to do so suggests some degree of spinal ankylosis.

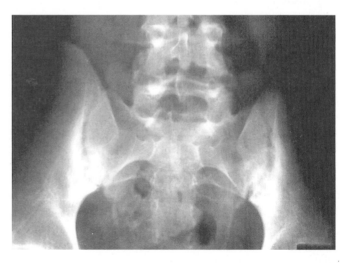

Figure 3.6.4   X ray of the SIJ's showing ileal sclerosis typical of ankylosing spondylitis.

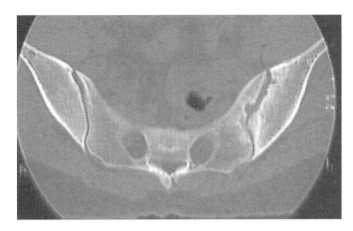

Figure 3.6.5 A CT scan showing ankylosing spondylitis. This 30 yr old female had normal X rays and MRI scan.

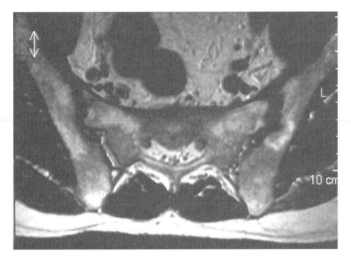

Figure 3.6.6 Increased signal can be seen in the left ileum in this seronegative sacroiliitis.

nature of ankylosing spondylitis can be seen on T2 weighted or STIR related sequences of the SIJ (Figure 3.6.6).

A history of direct trauma to the SIJ may indicate an apparent springing or crushing of the pelvis. On the other hand, falling off a horse but catching the foot in the stirrup, so that the limb is pulled out from the pelvis, will produce a distraction or shearing of the SIJ. Running downhill or driving the foot into the ground with the back in extension, as in the polevault take-off, produces a compressive shearing force. Compression and some shearing force to the right SIJ is probably applied by the right-handed golfer who is concentrating on coiling the pelvis at the top of the backswing. Here the hip is prevented from full internal rotation by the muscle tension, and the twisting force is transferred to the SIJ.

The hormone relaxin, which is secreted perimenstrually and in the latter stages of pregnancy, produces some relaxation of the pelvic ligaments. This may be reflected by perimenstrual backache and the backache of pregnancy experienced by some women. Though the lithotomy position may be used during delivery, especially with for-

ceps, there is an increased incidence of SIJ pain following this procedure. Care should be taken not to force the hips too far into abduction, so that the loads are transferred to the SIJ where they cause problems. This is particularly important when the patient is under general anaesthetic and has no ability to resist the abduction forces on the hips and subsequently the SIJ.

Examination

Assessment should always include examination of the spine to exclude segmental instability. However, weightbearing extension of the spine can produce pain from the SIJs and therefore the **one-legged extension test** and the **Fitch catch**, which require increased extension and rotation and are a test for a pars interarticularis defect, may also prove positive in SIJ problems. Both of these manoeuvres increase the extension of the spine with weightbearing; the Fitch catch adds rotation.

The **Piedallu sign** is perhaps more difficult to interpret. It is thought to be a consequence of SIJ fixation, but lumbar segmental disorders can produce the same response. Equally, a stance with one hemipelvis held forward of the other or one anterior superior iliac spine being rotated anteriorly or posteriorly, may be produced by SIJ dysfunction, a genuine short leg, segmental dysfunction, or muscular imbalance. Unfortunately this finding is often described osteopathically as a short leg, which leads to confusion. A true short leg can only be accurately assessed on a standing radiograph or light ray grid screen. Without a true short leg this sign only represents a **functional short leg**, which is what it should be called.

None of these tests for a short leg is accurate, and before the results are given credence at least three of the tests should indicate the same leg is short. Indeed, as many individuals have a leg length discrepancy that causes them no functional disability, leg length correction, as a therapeutic measure, should be approached with caution. Perhaps the quickest way to make a clinical assessment is to stand the patient, who should supinate their feet, in case any tendency to pronation has dropped one side lower than the other, and check iliac crest levels either by palpation or with a spirit level. Face them 180° in case the floor is not level, and repeat. Only if this gives a significant difference is it worth following through to further tests of true leg length difference.

The **Downing sign** is used by some to indicate SIJ fixation, but the accuracy of this sign has been called into question, suggesting that it is more related to the thoracolumbar junction (Sweetman 1998).

Pelvic spring is indicative of quite severe SIJ dysfunction, but the fifth lumbar segment disc or facet joint will also produce a positive pain response if inflamed. Pain that disappears on supporting the fifth segment is suggestive of segmental dysfunction.

Sacroiliac stress tests also load the sacrotuberous, sacroiliac, and iliolumbar ligaments. These may be a cause of pain when stressed. **Ongley's test** is performed with the patient supine. Direct pressure over the posterior aspect of the SIJ with the patient lying prone may also be painful, as may be compression of the ilial wing with the patient side lying.

Dural stress tests such as straight leg raising, Lasegue, and slump test are negative, but facet rocking tests can be equivocal. The dura is capable of sliding within the spinal canal, lateral canal, and fascia to accommodate movement, but if it is tethered then a pull is exerted on the nerve linings producing pain. Stretching of the dura and neural complex is the rationale behind dural stress tests. In the lower limb this can be performed by raising the straight leg of the supine lying

Tests for SIJ dysfunction

- The **one-legged hyperextension test** (Figure 3.6.7) is performed with the patient standing on one leg whilst the other leg is raised with the knee flexed to about 90°, and at this stage the patient extends the back.
- The **Fitch catch** (Figure 3.6.8) is performed with the patient standing with legs apart and leaning the back into extension, but at the same time the hand stretches backwards to reach for the contralateral Achilles. This is then repeated on the other side.
- The **Piedallu sign** test is performed with the patient standing, and the thumb of one hand is placed over the spinous process of the fifth, fourth, and third segment consecutively, while the thumb of the other hand is placed over the posterior inferior iliac spine (PIIS). The patient is asked to raise the ipsilateral knee towards the chest. The ischium will move outwards and the PIIS should swing downwards, but will rise cranially in the presence of a dysfunctional SIJ.
- For the **Downing sign** test, the patient is laid supine with ankles together, then the hip is flexed, externally rotated, and then abducted before the hip is returned to its position on the couch. A lengthening of the apparent leg length, as noted from the position of the medial malleoli as they lie together, is said to indicate a mobile joint whereas a fixed SIJ will produce shortening of the affected leg. With a reversal of this movement the apparent lengthening should return to its pre-test state.
- **Pelvic spring** is a provocative stress test that produces SIJ pain when the iliac crests are compressed or distracted in the supine patient. The patient should then be asked to lie on their hand, which supports the fifth segment, and the compression or distraction force reapplied. Pain that disappears on supporting the fifth segment is suggestive of segmental dysfunction.
- For **Ongley's test**, the hip on the side to be tested is flexed to 90° and then axial compression with some adduction is applied through the femur. At 90° of hip flexion this is thought to stress the sacroiliac ligaments, greater than 90° the sacrotuberous ligament, and less than 90° the iliolumbar ligaments.

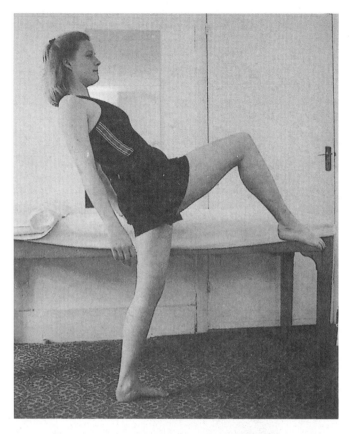

Figure 3.6.7 The one legged hyperextension test.

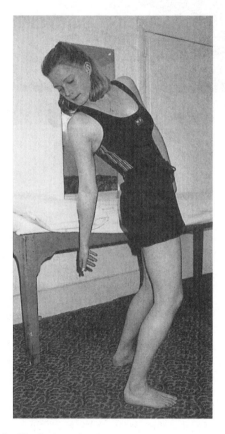

Figure 3.6.8 The Fitch catch.

Assessment of a short leg

Clinically, a **short leg** may be assessed somewhat inaccurately by comparing the measurements on each side from the umbilicus to the tip of each medial malleolus; from the anterior superior iliac spines to the tip of the medial malleolus; from the greater trochanter to the tip of the lateral malleolus and by placing the thumbs on the tips of the medial malleoli, while making certain they are level and then asking the patient to sit up. The malleoli should remain level and an alteration in their position with one rising cranially suggests a short leg on that side. Similarly, if the buttocks are actively raised off the couch and dropped back on the couch a malleolus may move cranially to indicate the short leg.

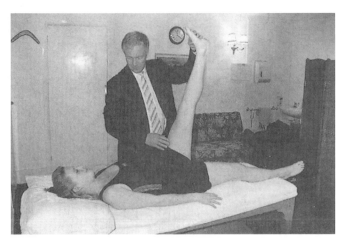

Figure 3.6.9 The Lasegue test. Straight leg raising tensions the sciatic nerve. This pull is increased by adding ankle dorsiflexion.

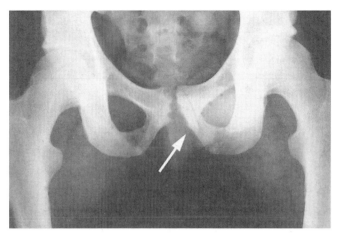

Figure 3.6.11 X rays show cysts and sclerosis with erosion of the gracilis margin (arrow) in a 19 yr old footballer with ankylosing spondylitis.

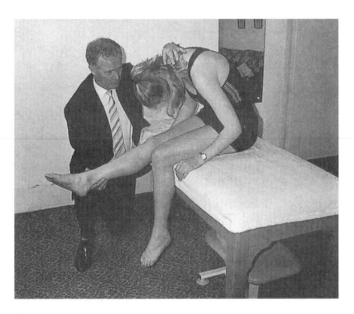

Figure 3.6.10 Slump test. A positive test eases the pain with neck extension and increases pain with neck flexion.

patient to stretch the sciatic nerve. The patient's pain is felt in the back and/or leg. Dorsiflexing the foot at the same time will stretch the sciatic nerve further, which is the **Lasegue test** (Figure 3.6.9). The dura may then be added to this test by sitting the patient on the couch with their back straight or in slight extension, and then raising the straight leg. This manoeuvre is then repeated with the patient's back curled into flexion and their chin on their chest (Figure 3.6.10). This position will be more painful if the dura is involved and will be relieved to some degree by raising the chin from the chest, whilst returning the chin to the chest reproduces the increased pain. This is the **slump test**.

Investigations

Plain radiographs may display the sclerosis on the ilial aspect of the SIJ that is associated with ankylosing spondylitis (Figure 3.6.4) and in severe cases irregular lytic areas may be visualized, until the joint reaches a state of ankylosis visible by radiography. Look also for verte-

bral signs of ankylosis plus any erosion of the gracilis margin of the pubic symphysis (Figure 3.6.11). Degenerative or adaptive changes may be demonstrated as inferior osteophytes which are virtually never reported upon by the radiologist as they are interpreted as normal changes, but presumably are representative of stress forces across the joint (Macdonald and Hunt 1951, Solonen 1957).

Bone scanning excludes any bone injury or disease such as Paget's disease, tumours, or stress fractures. The SIJ normally manifests an increased radiation count, or hot scan, on technetium-99 bone scanning, but local areas of increased signal may still be visualized within the SIJ and can then be further investigated with CT or MRI.

CT and MRI through the SIJ can display areas of sclerosis, lysis (Figure 3.6.5), and sacroiliitis (Figure 3.6.6) that may be missed on standard radiographs and MR scans of the spine. These areas of altered bone architecture presumably reflect the stresses transferred from the legs through the pelvis and on to the spine. CT examination of an area that has a 'hot' bone scan can differentiate the lesion further, such as an underlying stress fracture of the SIJ or ilial wing. MRI must be directed specifically at the SIJ as the standard lumbar views do not display this area well (Read 1998). They can demonstrate an increased T2 weighted signal with an inflammatory iliitis (Figure 3.6.6), but MRI is not as effective for cortical bone and may miss the areas of sclerosis and anterior osteophytosis.

Bone densitometry will be required when pelvic or SIJ stress fractures have been diagnosed and this must be accompanied by a dietary and hormonal profile and advice, as oligo- and amenorrhoeic athletes are susceptible to unusual stress fractures. Blood tests may reveal a raised ESR or CRP, RBC and WBC in leukaemia which may present as bone pain, and markers of bone activity such as alkaline phosphatase, myeloma fractions, and prostate specific antigen (PSA).

Treatment

Inflammatory sacroiliitis should be treated as appropriate for the underlying systemic disease, with non-steroidal anti-inflammatories (NSAIDs) as required for pain control. Exercise should in preference be non-impact and swimmers should avoid the breast stroke, though the reduced abduction and external rotation of the wedge kick, as opposed to the frog kick, may be tolerated. Spinal mobilization and muscle stretching exercises should be undertaken and maintained.

Dysfunctional SIJ pain may respond to manipulation both of the ileum and the sacrum itself, but excessive manipulation may well maintain an unstable and inflamed joint.

An acute flare of the joint can be treated with steroids injected into the posterior sacroiliac ligaments and the joint from the posterior superior aspect. These ligaments can be strengthened by sclerosant injections to the sacroiliac and iliolumbar ligaments. They are particularly useful for women who have perimenstrual or postpartum ligamentous insufficiency and SIJ instability (Cyriax and Cyriax 1983).

Posterior lumbar ligament strain

Posterior lumbosacral ligament strain occurs in the inter- and supraspinous ligaments, but particularly in the iliolumbar, lumbosacral, and sacroiliac ligaments (Figure 3.6.2). The diagnosis may be one of exclusion, as these ligaments can produce radiation of pain to the buttock, leg, or groin, and the nature of the pain may mimic other mechanical disorders; indeed, strain of these ligaments can accompany and be part of the pain complex from the intervertebral disc or facet joint.

History

Primarily, the history may be the persistence of symptoms following the resolution of a disc, facet joint or SIJ lesion. In its pure form, if that exists, it is rest pain relieved by movement. So the history of morning pain, and sitting pain that are relieved by movement, can be considered typical. Indeed, this ligamentous pain is sometimes referred to as the 'cocktail party' or 'theatregoer's' back, as the individual is not able to sit or stand for long without having to alter position. A less frequent presentation is a history of pain in the popliteal fossa that appears after a back lesion has settled, and this seems to respond to appropriate treatment to the posterior lumbar ligaments.

Examination

A principal requirement is the exclusion of disc, facet, or SIJ disorders, bony disease or neural referrals of pain, or their detection alongside features that could be associated with ligamentous dysfunction. The absence of mechanical signs apart from outer range discomfort on spinal flexion and extension in the presence of pain that has no other cause is suggestive of ligamentous strain.

Treatment

Correction of the primary underlying cause such as a disc lesion will enable the ligamentous pain to settle over time, but this may be aided by NSAIDs or a local intraligamentous cortisone injection. Electrotherapeutic physiotherapy modalities to reduce inflammation can be effective. Persistence of the pain suggests stress of the posterior lumbar ligaments, and these may be strengthened by sclerosant or proliferant injections (sclerotherapy, or prolotherapy). Following this the patient should be advised how to adopt their spinal neutral position whenever possible, and institute muscle balance work/core stability to stabilize the pelvic posture.

Side-lying external hip rotation

The patient lies on their side with the knees slightly bent, and the back is taken into lumbar neutral, and splinted into this position by tightening

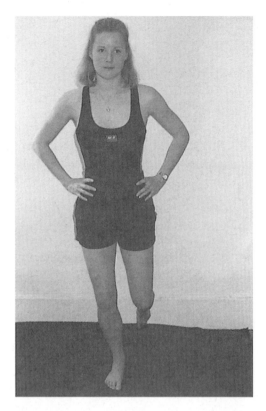

Figure 3.6.12   The half squat. The pelvis is straight and the knee in line with the foot. This works the hip stabilizers.

the abdominal muscles. The upper knee is then raised but the ankles are kept in contact, so that the external rotators of the hip work, but the lumbar spine is fixed in neutral. This should be repeated 30–40 times on each side.

One leg half-squat balancing

The patient stands evenly balanced on both legs and then tightens the gluteals, at which stage they balance on one leg and lower themselves into a half squat (Figure 3.6.12). This exercise is to strengthen the external rotators of the hips, so the pelvis must not be allowed to slide out sideways nor the ipsilateral anterior superior iliac spine to rotate forwards and medially. This should be held for 20 seconds. Repeat on the other side.

Super (wo)man

Kneel on all fours and hold the lumbar spine in neutral. Splint this position by tightening the abdominal muscles, and then raise one leg backwards followed by the contralateral arm forwards. (Figure 3.6.13) Care must be taken not to lose the horizontal plane of the pelvis or to lose spinal neutral. This balance should be held for 30–40 seconds.

Entrapment of the long cutaneous nerve of the thigh

The long cutaneous nerve to the thigh supplies an area over the posterolateral pelvis and the thigh. The area of pain referral overlies the tensor fascia lata and the iliotibial band.

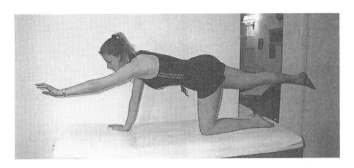

Figure 3.6.13 Super (wo)man. Exercises the pelvic and back stabilizer muscles.

History

The pain can radiate to the lateral aspect of the knee and is difficult to distinguish from the tensor fascia lata and the iliotibial tract syndrome. There may be some subjective awareness of numbness in this area. It is possible that continual pressure from clothing and local trauma may be causative.

Examination

The diagnosis is made by the absence of resisted abduction pain from the tensor fascia lata and absence of resisted hip external rotator pain. On palpation, it shows a non-tender trochanteric bursa and piriformis insertion. Hip pathology and referred pain from other sources such as the spine must be excluded. Palpation over the crest of the ileum shows a local tender area that may also refer pain down the outside of the thigh.

Treatment

A local cortisone injection may be effective. Sometimes a neuroma exists, or the nerve must be decompressed in its fascia.

Meralgia paraesthetica (compression of lateral cutaneous nerve of thigh)

The presenting symptoms are usually altered sensation and pain over the anterior thigh. The lateral cutaneous nerve to the thigh is commonly compressed as it emerges through the superficial fascia, but it may emerge near the anterior superior iliac spine or close to the groin crease. In sportspeople the tight elastic from clothing around the top of the leg can cause compression of the nerve, in which case it is cured by releasing the elastic tension in the clothing. It has also been noted in female gymnasts who compress the front of their thighs on the asymmetric bars during many of their gymnastic routines.

Examination

There is a delineated area of altered sensation over the anterior aspect of the thigh, commensurate with the lateral cutaneous nerve distribution. A small area of increased discomfort may be palpated somewhere from the anterior superior spine to the upper mid thigh, and this area of nerve entrapment can be further delineated by pressure from a blunt probe such as a retracted ballpoint pen.

Investigations

EMG is of little value.

Treatment

Simple alteration of clothing will suffice if the cause is pressure from the clothing. Local infiltration with corticosteroid around the fascial entrapment can help, but surgery to release the fascia may be required.

Gluteal bursitis

History

Occasionally after a lot of running or leg extension exercises the gluteal bursa may become inflamed, producing pain over the upper buttock that is worse on these movements and on local pressure.

Examination

Care must be taken to exclude spinal and SIJ pathology, but the diagnostic features are pain on active movement and resisted testing of the supine straight leg raising, with localized palpable tenderness over the upper outer quadrant of the buttock. [*Editor's note:* With respect to differential diagnosis, it is worthy of note that myofascial pain from the glutei is common in the population at large, often associated with low lumbar or sacroiliac dysfunction.]

Treatment

A reduction in gluteal exercises is required, especially in martial arts and circuit training exponents, who specifically exercise the gluteals. Electrotherapeutic modalities to settle inflammation and a cortisone injection into the upper, outer quadrant with the needle reaching the bone when allied to a diminution of gluteal specific exercises can be curative. Care must be taken to avoid the sciatic nerve during any massage or injection techniques.

Tensor fascia lata dysfunction

An uncommon source of lateral pelvic, hip, and lateral thigh pain.

History

Specifically occurring with gymnasium activities when abduction of the leg is overworked, it is often accompanied by trochanteric bursitis, and sometimes iliotibial band syndrome. It occurs in running when the tensor fascia lata is overworking to stabilize the pelvis. Camber running with the painful side lower than the pain-free side is contributory. Theoretically, a grossly supinated foot with weak external rotators may also overload the tensor fascia lata.

Examination

Both active movement of, and resisted abduction of the hip are painful. Maximum tenderness is under the lip of the ileum, though a more general tenderness may be present over the whole muscle. The **modified Thomas test** may reveal abnormal abduction of the thigh (Figure 3.6.20).

Treatment

The most effective treatment is massage and stretching by a physiotherapist of the straight leg into adduction behind the other leg, also by the patient standing with the affected leg crossed behind the other. The body is swung out and over the affected hip but the actual weight is still supported by the normal leg. Electrotherapeutic modalities to settle inflammation help. NSAIDs and a locally placed cortisone under the ilial rim ease the discomfort. Rehabilitation will include relaxing the hip during running and reducing exercises that abduct the leg.

Trochanteric bursitis

The trochanteric bursa lies over the greater trochanter and under the iliotibial band which originates from the tensor fascia lata and inserts at Gurney's tubercle at the knee. It is a strong ligamentous band that provides attachment to the lateral quadriceps and hamstrings, and its function is to stabilize the hip and leg against abduction forces. During hip movement, particularly walking and running, the iliotibial band moves across the greater trochanter from which it is separated by the trochanteric bursa. This bursa may become inflamed from increased friction or direct trauma when it may produce a haembursitis.

History

The history may include trauma from a fall, or hitting a wall or an individual with the hip. However, the bursitis comes on insidiously, though sometimes after increased uncommon activity. It is worse on walking and running, but is also painful to lie on or to cross the painful leg over the non-painful leg.

Examination

Examination should exclude referral of pain from the back and the hip joint, though the hip is less easy to exclude because internal rotation and flexion may produce pain from the bursa. Local tenderness to palpation directly over the greater trochanter is very suggestive. Sometimes resisted abduction of the hip may be painful.

Tests for trochanteric bursitis

- **Ober's test** is performed with the patient lying on their side. The lower leg is flexed at the knee and then at the hip. The upper femur is then taken into abduction and extended, and following this is then adducted behind the lower leg. A normal band should allow adduction beyond the upper aspect of the other leg. The tight iliotibial band either produces pain or does not adduct beyond the upper aspect of the other leg.
- The **modified Thomas test** can demonstrate a tight iliotibial band (Figure 3.6.14). The patient lies supine with their buttocks on the end of the couch but one leg bent at the hip and held into full flexion. The other hip is extended. The normal iliotibial band allows the extended leg to lie straight in line whereas the tight iliotibial band pulls the thigh into abduction.

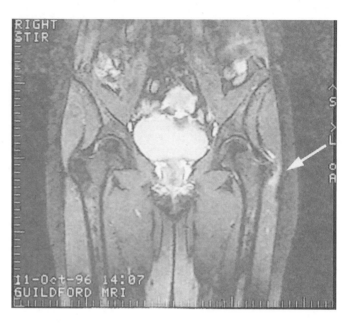

Figure 3.6.14   Stir sequence MRI displays left trochanteric bursitis (arrow).

Investigations

Investigations are undertaken to exclude underlying bony or hip pathology, but specific views of the bursa are best obtained with diagnostic ultrasound, especially with a haembursitis which may be aspirated at the same time. Like all haembursae they tend to recur and require further draining on a few occasions. Steroids into the haembursa may reduce the recurrence. Complications such as accompanying bony trauma or even an enthesitis from the external rotators of the hip may lead to a bone scan or MRI investigation being required, the inflamed bursa being best seen on T2 or STIR related sequences (Figure 3.6.14).

Treatment

Treatment of the bursitis may be with electrotherapeutic modalities to reduce inflammation, NSAIDs, or intrabursal cortisone. However, the iliotibial band may be tight and Ober's test positive, in which case stretching of the iliotibial band as described for tensor fascia lata is required. Frequently the external rotators of the hip and in particular the piriformis are weak, allowing the pelvis to slide outwards over an adducted and internally rotated hip. Thus, strengthening exercises to the hip stabilizers are essential. Having said this, race walkers, who particularly slide past their hip in this fashion, do not seem to produce this injury even in their early days of training. Surgical Z-plasty may be effective in recalcitrant cases.

Dysfunction of the external rotators of the hip

This group of deep pelvic muscles is probably as important as the rotator cuff is at the shoulder, and probably functions in a similar way to fix and stabilize the hip.

History

Patients may present with pain over the buttock, trochanter, and the line of the gluteal insertion along the lateral aspect of the femur, and may radiate down towards the ankle and foot. Painful external rotators are often seen in golfers who hit into a 'closed' left side, and this problem can be relieved by opening out the left foot at the stance, allowing the left side to swing through and out of the way. Unfortunately, established pain in the external rotators is difficult to handle and indeed to establish as a correct diagnosis. The patient may have pain at rest, lying in bed, and on walking. This pain is flared on climbing stairs when the painful hip leads on to the next stair and begins to raise the weight of the body.

Examination

External hip rotator dysfunction is a common finding that accompanies tracking problems at the knee. The weakness of the external rotators of the hip, rather than pain, may be the prime cause of the malfunction at the knee. During foot strike the external rotators should hold the hip firmly, but if they are weak the hip will be allowed to roll into internal rotation and the pelvis on that side moves anteriorly. This movement increases the functional anteversion of the femur which becomes translated into a valgus movement at the knee with increased Q angle (see p. 302, and Figure 3.7.10). Examination of the hip, produces an unclear pattern of painful movement that is suggestive of hip pathology but is not quite a capsular pattern, and hip flexion is often sore, producing Cyriax's sign of the buttock (Cyriax and Cyriax 1983).

Palpation demonstrates tenderness over the insertion of the piriformis at the posterolateral aspect of the greater trochanter, but there may also be tenderness over the gluteal insertions. Variably there is tenderness over the origin of the piriformis at the inferior medial margin of the ileum and SIJ, and often there is tenderness over the ischial aspect of the sacrotuberous ligament. *Per rectum* the obturator internus may be tender. Resisted external rotation of the hip is usually painful. The whole complex may be complicated by a trochanteric bursitis, and a tight iliotibial tract with a positive Obers' sign. Finally, as if there was not enough to confuse the diagnosis, the rare piriformis, and hamstring syndromes must be excluded (see below). Here straight leg raise and Lasegue tests should be positive but the slump test negative. Pelvic instability at the SIJ and pubic symphysis will often cause dysfunction in the external rotators.

Investigations

MRI is the investigation of choice in musculotendinous lesions, but usually shows no clinical evidence of inflammation or dysfunction in this condition (though abnormalities have been demonstrated in the quadratus femoris tendon) (Klinkert *et al.* 1997).

Hip pointer

According to American literature, baseball players who are likely to slide into the bases on their sides will often produce a haematoma over the iliac crest. Though this may be aspirated, surgical release of the haematoma may be required.

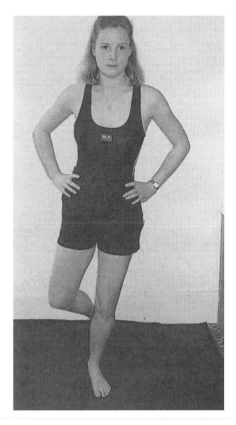

Figure 3.6.15 The left pelvis has swung forwards. Figure 3.6.12 shows the right external rotators stabilizing the hip.

Treatment

Correction of the hip weakness is required rather than exercises for the knee. Orthotics that prevent or limit this valgus movement at the knee will therefore be of value in the short term to the hip as well, but rehabilitation must be directed to retraining the strength of the external rotators of the hip. Techniques of side lying, maintaining pelvic stability, and then externally rotating the hip, or of balancing on one leg in a half squat, can aid strengthening of these hip rotators, as may step-ups on the affected side while taking care to maintain hip and pelvic stability (see posterior ligament strain, above). During the half squat, the ipsilateral anterior superior iliac spine must not be allowed to rotate forwards, the hip must not slide outwards, and the contralateral leg must not be permitted to swing behind the balancing leg, as all of these manoeuvres prevent the external rotators from working properly (Figures 3.6.12 and 3.6.15). Sitting with the affected leg crossed over the other leg, and the foot placed on the couch alongside the knee, permits an increased internal rotation to stretch the muscles, and the muscle may be strengthened by external rotation isometrics. The history of buttock pain and sometimes referral down the leg is similar to that produced by dural or SIJ irritation, and an injection of the piriformis insertion at the posterior lateral aspect of the greater trochanter can refer pain to the foot. Discomfort from these muscles can produce a painful straight leg raise, but Lasegue and slump tests are negative.

Treatment is difficult and lengthy for the painful syndromes, and involves stretching of the external rotators and iliotibial tract. The

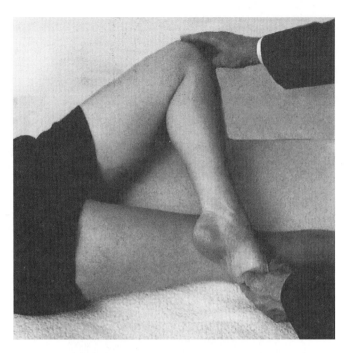

Figure 3.6.16   Figure of 4 test.

external rotators are stretched by sitting with the affected leg crossed over the straight extended contralateral leg. The ipsilateral foot is placed as proximal as possible on the couch alongside the lateral aspect of the contralateral leg. The knee is then pulled by the hands towards the midline to achieve a passive stretch. In the figure-of-four stretch, the patient lies supine with the foot of the hip to be stretched crossed over and resting just above the contralateral knee (Figure 3.6.16). The affected hip is externally rotated as far as possible and then the contralateral knee is pulled by the hands towards the chest, thus flexing the spine . As the pelvis becomes lifted off the couch by this manoeuvre, so the external rotators come under a stretch. This must be accompanied by isometric exercises to the piriformis and isotonic exercises with external rotation in side lying to the piriformis and obturator (posterior ligament strains). However, pelvic stability is a functional problem and the balancing exercises with a half squat as described above, and 'running tall', are essential. Running tall concentrates the running style on maintaining pelvic stability and moving over the hips, rather than sliding the hips outwards and rolling through the gait.

Like all inflammatory lesions, rehabilitation sometimes cannot continue until the inflammation has resolved, and massage, electrotherapeutic modalities, and cortisone to the piriformis origin and insertion or the sacrotuberous ligament and trochanteric bursa may be of value.

Sacrotuberous ligament sprain

The sacrotuberous ligament is a strong ligament running from the sacrum to the ischial tuberosity and is not frequently disturbed.

History

When this ligament is injured there is usually a history of an external rotation strain of the pelvis on a fixed, flexed, weightbearing hip. An example is digging out a trench with a spade, and throwing the soil out sideways and backwards towards the affected side, without fully straightening up.

Examination

Referred pain from the back must be excluded and any accompanying external hip rotator dysfunction must be dealt with, but the sacrotuberous ligament is locally tender to palpation over the superior surface of the ischial tuberosity. This can sometimes be palpated more easily with the patient kneeling on all fours, but lying the patient prone on the couch with the knee on the affected side dropped on to a chair placed alongside the couch will flex the hip to allow easy palpation of the sacrotuberous ligament and prove less threatening to the patient.

Treatment

The inflammation settles over time with physiotherapy to calm inflammation, but if resistant it can respond to a carefully placed steroid injection into the sacrotuberous insertion on the ischial tuberosity, being aware of the sciatic nerve approaching the lateral aspect of the tuberosity. Stretching as for external rotators of the hip is of benefit.

Piriformis and hamstring syndromes

The sciatic nerve may be trapped by the piriformis or gemelli as it passes between these muscles, this being an anatomical variant. It may also be bowed or tethered by the biceps femoris insertion on to the lateral aspect of the ischial tuberosity in athletes who have trained the hamstring.

History

The history is of sciatica with pain and perhaps pins and needles and numbness in the sciatic distribution, but there is no history of back pain. The piriformis syndrome may have some greater trochanteric element to the pain distribution.

Examination

Initially this is a diagnosis of exclusion, when the common causes of sciatic nerve entrapment are ruled out by normal back movements. The indicative findings are of a straight leg test and positive Lasegue test because the sciatic nerve is tethered, but the slump test is negative because there is no dural tethering. It is unusual to have signs of motor nerve involvement, but altered sensation may be detected. Sometimes resisted piriformis contraction tested with the ipsilateral hip flexed and the foot crossed beyond the contralateral thigh may reproduce the referred pain.

Investigation

Investigations are undertaken to exclude other causes of sciatica. EMG may be able to differentiate between an intraspinal lesion and this extraspinal cause.

Treatment

Stretching of the type used for adverse neural tension may benefit both conditions, but takes time. An injection close to the biceps femoris insertion can be curative, but the sciatic nerve must be avoided. Surgery may be required to release the nerve entrapment.

Stress fractures

History

Stress fractures of the pelvis seem to be confined to runners. They may occur in either sex but are predominant in oligo- or amenorrhoeic women, in whom atypical pelvic pain should immediately raise the possibility of a stress fracture. The pain is located over the site of the lesion and is worse with foot impact to the ground. Look particularly for sacral (Figure 3.6.17) and ileal stress fractures (Bottomley 1990), but more commonly inferior pubic ramus (Figure 3.6.18). Stress fractures of the superior pubic ramus are reported less commonly.

Examination

Examination may be confusing, with hip and lumbar spinal movements producing pain, as may pelvic compression tests. The lack of a clear diagnosis in the presence of pain on weightbearing or foot impaction in a runner should lead to a bone scan to exclude any underlying bony problems. Indeed, the lack of a clear diagnosis in a sports person should generally lead to a bone scan.

Investigation

The watershed diagnostic aid is a bone scan when the increased radiation from the active bone technetium-99 appears more intense (hot) on the scan. It may be necessary to scan the lesion further with CT or MRI to attempt to differentiate it from a tumour, bone cyst, or osteoid osteoma. Particular scrutiny should be made of the sacrum, the ilial wing, and the inferior pubic ramus, though stress fractures of the superior pubic rami do occasionally occur. Investigation of bone density and a dietary profile should be undertaken, especially looking at the calcium intake. Many runners are confused about power/weight ratio, as they believe that by losing weight they will have less bulk to carry around. Unfortunately for proponents of this theory, all racers have to be able to generate speed up to a sprint level to win high-class races, and the type 2 white fibres, which are required for sprinting, have bulk. Muscle weighs more than fat, but the athlete confuses the benefits of the muscle bulk with the weight of fat. Skin thickness monitoring rather than weight should be advocated for these individuals. Among this group there will also be some people with genuine anorexia nervosa, whose body image is acceptable to society as long as they run. These individuals respond quite well to a therapeutic approach orientated around their athletic performance, such as 'muscle needs to be provided with energy and this is carbohydrate', and discussions centred upon their running performance with positive support, as opposed to a dietary approach. However, there are hormonal problems within this group, and gynaecological and endocrinological opinions are of value.

Treatment

Impact training such as running should be suspended and the athlete cross-trained on non-impact modalities such as the bike, rowing machine, and swimming or pool running. Running is introduced and

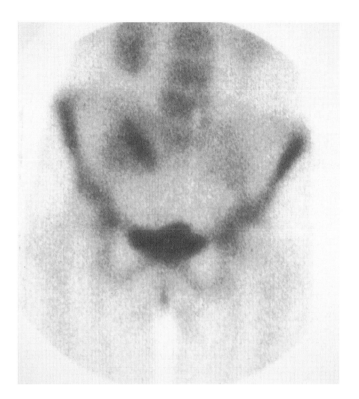

Figure 3.6.17 Bone scan shows the stress lesion across the right sacroiliac joint.

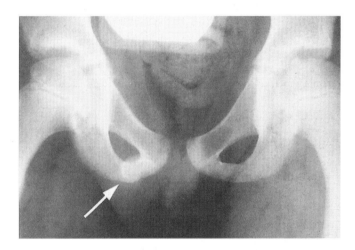

Figure 3.6.18 Callus in the inferior pubic ramus from a healing stress fracture (arrow).

increased incrementally against pain, and at this stage a biomechanical assessment of running style, muscle balance, and leg length should be undertaken.

Enthesopathies and avulsion apophysitides

During the growth phase children become less supple as the muscle–tendon complex grows more slowly than the bony length, but the muscle–tendon complex is stronger than the epiphysis so that the adolescent injury is usually entheseal. Particular problems occur around the pelvis in adolescence, which therefore require a radiograph to exclude an avulsion apophysitis. These same problems occur in adults, but they are more likely to be tendinous or muscle lesions rather than an apophysitis.

Therapy, in the adult or child without an avulsion, is directed towards stretching the muscle complex just to pain, and by strengthening the muscle group. The child with an avulsion must be rehabilitated carefully, with due attention to pain, and in the early stages TENS or interferential set to twitch the muscle may be sufficient to maintain muscle loading. As the injury improves, so isometrics within the restraints of pain and then isotonic exercises against resistance may be added. Later, controlled running ladders through to sprinting, and kicking ladders for those who require them, should be introduced (Read 2000).

Lesions of the rectus femoris origin

History

The acute injury presents as a sudden pain while sprinting or kicking, whereas the chronic onset often presents as weakness or fatigue when running accompanied by groin pain of a more diffuse nature.

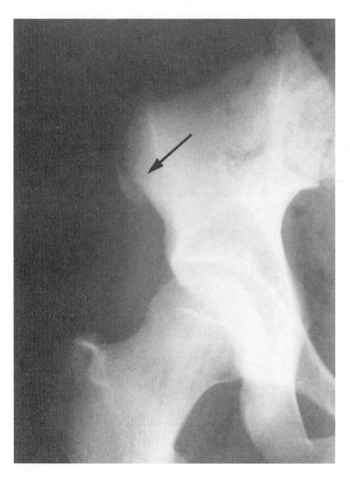

Figure 3.6.19   Anterior superior iliac spine avulsion in an adolescent following a sprint race.

Modified Thomas test

The patient sits on the end of the couch with the opposite knee pulled up to the chest. The patient is then laid down and the opposite leg stretched out with the knee straight. The amount of hip extension is a reflection of psoas tightness. The knee may then be flexed from this position and the degree of knee flexion is a function of quadriceps tightness. The good side should be compared to the bad side (Figure 3.6.20).

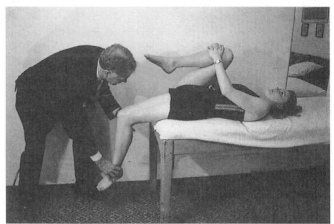

Figure 3.6.20   Modified Thomas test for quadriceps tightness.

Examination

The pain is centred over the anterior aspect of the hip, where it is tender to palpation over the anterior superior iliac spine or the reflected head of the rectus femoris from the acetabular lip (Figure 3.6.19). Active or resisted supine straight leg raising is painful, whereas a psoas lesion causes pain on resisted testing of the flexed hip as well as or instead of an extended hip. The **modified Thomas test** is painful and limited for quadriceps stretching.

Investigations

The more persistent chronic presentation with an acute initial onset, especially if getting worse over 5 days or so, should be radiographed, as myositis ossificans is a fairly common complication of this injury and will delay healing (Figure 3.6.21). Children must be radiographed for a possible avulsion lesion (Figure 3.6.19).

Treatment

The injury is treated as for any enthesopathy (see above) but particular attention should be paid to grade rehabilitation back into sprinting and kicking. Any myositis has the added requirement of rest in the initial stages, though indomethacin is reputed to be of benefit; if rehabilitation fails, surgical excision should be considered. The complication of surgery is that the lesion reforms if the surgery is performed too soon.

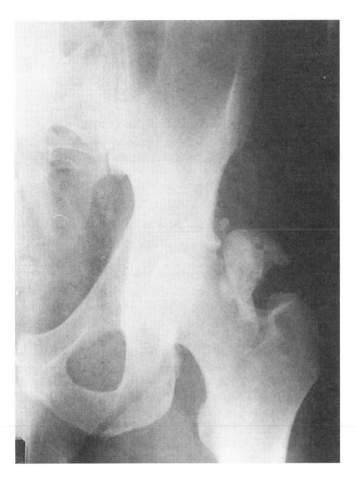

Figure 3.6.21 Myositis ossificans in the rectus femoris.

Psoas muscle lesions

History

The psoas is a flexor and external rotator of the hip, and it is injured during sprinting and kicking, but particularly in high knee lift exercises and running in mud, when the foot has to be pulled out of the clinging mud. Lesions arise after hill running and sometimes in half-bent running sports such as field hockey. Because the psoas, working on a fixed leg, aids abdominal curls, most sit-up exercises are done with the hips flexed, but sit-up exercises done with straight legs or leg raises may overload the psoas and may encourage extension of the spine, which is a problem for those suffering from extension-orientated spinal dysfunction.

Examination

The pain is located anteriorly and just lateral to the femoral canal in the groin. Passive hip flexion may be painful, which suggests the psoas bursa is inflamed. Resisted testing of the hip flexors at 90° of hip flexion indicates a muscle lesion or an enthesopathy at the psoas attachment at the lesser trochanter. However, this is a strong muscle and sometimes manual testing just does not produce sufficient tension across the enthesis to produce pain. The modified Thomas test for psoas tightness (see above) is restricted and painful.

Investigation

Radiography may show an avulsion at the lesser trochanter and bone scan may display a hot lesion in this area. MRI may reveal a psoas bursa on T2 weighted STIR sequences, but often no abnormality is detected.

Treatment

Management is to reduce the inflammation by electrotherapeutic modalities and then to gradually reintroduce resisted hip flexion as an isometric exercise followed by repetition of active high knee raises. Rehabilitation should then be graded into running drills that include high knee exercises, and finally incremental load increases up to sprinting and hill running. Stretching of the psoas and rectus femoris is required to lengthen the musculotendinous junction and to prevent scar tissue contraction. Localized tenderness over the psoas bursa, which lies below Poupart's (inguinal) ligament and approximately two fingerbreadths lateral to the femoral canal, may respond well to a cortisone injection placed on the surface of the muscle, and then followed by appropriate rehabilitation.

Adductor tendinitis

It is difficult to be accurate as to which adductor is involved in individual cases, as the muscles vary in their activity depending upon the degree of hip flexion at the time of testing, but the majority of localized palpable pain will centre over the adductor longus at the pubic symphyseal area and less frequently the adductor magnus insertion, with tenderness running along the inferior pubic ramus to the ischial tuberosity.

History

Adductor longus tendinitis, or tendinopathy, is situated at the enthesis, but there is frequently a musculotendinous variant that is locally tender about 6 cm distal to the origin. This can produce a partial rupture with bruising and a palpable gap. The cause may be acute, either from a blocked side foot tackle or a sudden sideways abduction stretch of the hip during a slip, or it may be caused by chronic overload from repetitive abduction stretches or adduction forces such as side-footing a ball. The fascia encasing the adductors is contiguous with the abdominal fascia, and the patient may also present with suprapubic abdominal pain. This pain can be difficult to distinguish from symphyseal pain and the pain from the conjoined tendon at the inguinal ring and pubic tubercle.

The adductor magnus injury does not seem to refer pain suprapubically; by contrast, it mimics a hamstring lesion. It is seen more frequently during fast acceleration where the adductors often contribute as much power as the hamstrings.

Examination

Adductor tendonitis is invariably tender to local palpation over the origin, whereas, the absence of localized tenderness but the presence of a history of groin pain suggests the adductors are not primarily involved. Examination may reveal hip discomfort, but not in a capsular pattern. Resisted adduction is painful when the supine lying patient squeezes a fist held between their knees, adducts the neutral hip from about 45° against resistance, and the 90° flexed hip is adducted against resistance. The pain produced by this resisted muscle testing is localized to the adductor areas. Tenderness is found over the adductor origin or about 6 cm from the origin in the case of a musculotendinous lesion. The adductor magnus lesion may also give rise to pain on resisted hamstring contraction as well as adduction, and tenderness is palpated along the inferior pubic ramus.

Treatment

Treatment is by electrotherapeutic modalities to settle inflammation, frictions to organize scar tissue, and stretching exercises of the adductors to prevent scar tissue contraction. An injection of cortisone at the adductor origin settles inflammation in the acute and chronic case and may be required in spite of extensive physiotherapy to this area. Resisted isometric adduction is then initiated at both inner and outer range to start therapy for any concomitant tendinopathy. This is followed by cross leg swinging in front and behind the uninvolved leg, crossover steps in front and behind the other leg, and sideways steps leading to sideways bounds. Running starts with the use of a rehabilitation ladder. When straight line sprints can be tolerated, side steps, figure-of-eight runs, and cutting runs should be added, as may a kicking ladder (Read 2000). The partial rupture will heal by itself and often leaves a palpable gap. Surgery is rarely required to close the defect. Rarely, surgical debridement of the adductor origin may be required.

Ischial tuberosity lesions

The hamstring origin may suffer from a traction apophysitis. In a child the apophyseal avulsion may remain unattached (Figure 3.6.22). The avulsion may be of sufficient force to separate the apophysis at such a distance that surgery to screw the apophysis back is required (Kurosawa *et al.* 1996). A localized tendinous tear adjacent to the origin occurs in the adult, and a bursitis between the hamstring tendon and the ischium can form (Figure 3.6.23).

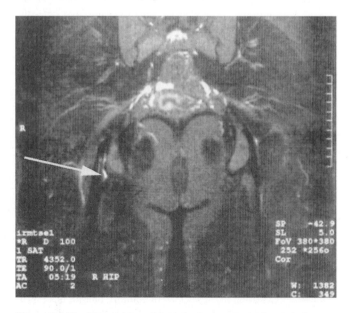

Figure 3.6.22 This avulsion of the ischeal tuberosity is chronic having remained detached during growth.

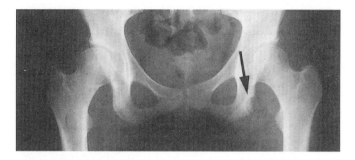

Figure 3.6.23 MRI shows a degenerative tear in the hamstring tendon and an ischeal bursa.

History

Great forces are applied to the hamstring origin by a fall that whips the hip into full flexion with extended knees, such as a fall on to the back. However, stretching exercises can also avulse the origin in moves such as the front/back splits of dancers (Figure 3.6.24), and the hurdle stretch, where the leg is raised on to an object and the body is flexed over the straight leg. Osternig *et al.* (1986) demonstrated coactivation between the ipsilateral hamstrings and quadriceps. Basically the hamstrings start contracting in the last third of knee extension to decelerate the swing phase and prepare to stabilize the leg for foot impact. Unfortunately the hurdles stretch, which requires knee extension and hip flexion can, if forced, provoke a coactivation contraction from the hamstring, the very muscle one is trying to stretch and thus a powerful eccentric force on the ischeal origin. **Lombard's paradox**, in which one end of a muscle is contracting whilst the other is relaxing, is exhibited by any muscle that crosses two joints. The hamstring contraction should produce extension of the hip and flexion of the knee, but some movement patterns, such as dipping for the line at the end of a race, or bending to pick up a ball at speed, require flexion of the knee and flexion of the hip. Mistiming of this muscle movement makes for a torn hamstring, and is the reason that rehabilitation drills must build up this paradoxical skill to higher speeds. The aetiology of an ischial lesion includes an acute episode of stretching or exercising the hamstring, though some martial art kicking drills may gradually overload the enthesis.

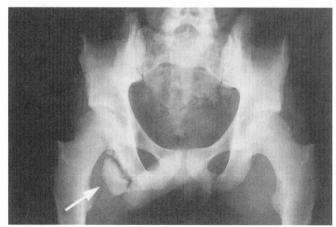

Figure 3.6.24 X ray shows a discrete avulsion of the ischeal tuberosity following 'front and back' splits.

Bowstring sign

Examination

Resisted testing of hamstrings in prone lying evokes pain at the tuberosity. Passive supine straight leg raising is painful, but the Lasegue and slump tests do not increase the pain. The primary posterolateral disc prolase, renowned for producing sciatica without lumbar pain, is often mistakenly diagnosed as a hamstring tear, and must be excluded. The use of the **bowstring sign** at this stage is perhaps most helpful.

Local palpation of the tuberosity or the tendinous junction is painful. The hamstring can maintain high loads and manual testing may be insufficient to produce pain.

Lie the patient on the floor with heels resting on a chair. The patient then raise the hips off the ground as high as possible. This test may be performed with one leg taking the load and the other raised clear of the chair. The extra power required for this manoeuvre may evoke the pain. It is also an excellent rehabilitation exercise.

Investigation

Radiography may demonstrate the avulsion, bone scan a hot tuberosity, and MRI the tendon tear and a bursitis. Real-time ultrasound in skilled hands may also be diagnostic. When healing has progressed to a sufficient level isokinetic dynamometry, tested sitting and prone, registers the muscle balance (or imbalance), both between the ipsilateral and contralateral hamstrings and quadriceps. It is important to assess muscle balance so that proper strategies for rehabilitation may be effected. It may be preferable for the muscle to be exercised with the hip flexed or extended, and either at slow or fast speeds. Some of our unpublished work with hamstring dynamometry indicates that the damaged leg may be weak or strong, so that a damaged hamstring in the strong leg will require strengthening of the non-damaged weak leg during rehabilitation.

Treatment

Treatment is directed to reducing inflammation with electrotherapy or cortisone injection, organizing scar tissue with isometrics and massage, and preventing scar contraction with stretching exercises. However, **ballistic stretching** is required for the hamstring so that both the range and control of hamstring coactivation is improved. A hamstring rehabilitation ladder through running drills is required to return the patient to full activities.

Ballistic stretching

Hip joint

The hip is a major load-bearing joint within the body, with ligamentous and bony configurations so strong that instability within the joint is almost unknown, except as a result of major trauma. It is, however, prone to its own peculiar pathologies.

The neonate

The standard assessments of the newborn baby include testing the hip for any clicking or limitation of abduction, in which case the baby is treated by frog splinting, and is under the care of the orthopaedic or paediatric department.

The toddler

The young child, up to about 6–8 years old, may present with a painful hip on load-bearing and on passive testing when a capsular pattern of pain is found. This requires radiography to exclude other pathology such as a tumour or infection. If a bone scan and blood test are normal, treatment for the symptomatic hip is non-weightbearing until the joint has settled, at which stage all may have returned to normal without future recurrence of the problem. As the mechanism is not well understood, this is referred to as an **irritable hip**.

From about 5–10 years children may have hip pain which in its early stage is associated with a normal radiograph, but bone scan may show a diminished uptake in the femoral head. This may be associated with an irritable hip. Alternatively, there may be no history of malfunction until examined as an adult who presents with an early degenerate hip with a flattened femoral head. This is the Legg–Calvé–Perthe malformed hip, where the normal rounded contour of the femoral head is replaced by a flattened elongated femoral head caused either by some degree of avascularization or even a mild slipped capital femoral epiphysis that was unrecognized and untreated. The Legg–Perthe hip, in the adult, is in itself not painful, but the joint is prone to early degenerative changes, which are painful.

Growth spurt

The growth spurt is generally thought to occur between the ages of 12 and 16, but as children develop at different rates, so the range of the age spectrum must always be considered. Knee pain in an adolescent that occurs during their growth spurt must always raise an index of suspicion about the hip. Clinical examination of all knee and thigh pain should begin by excluding hip pathology, and this is vital in an adolescent, who may sustain a slipped capital femoral epiphysis. Here, movement of the hip is immediately referred to the knee as pain. Internal rotation of the hip may be impossible, and there may be a fixed external rotation of the hip with shortening. Radiography may show a slipped capital femoral epiphysis. If there is any doubt about the diagnosis, it should be treated as a slipped capital epiphysis and a paediatric orthopaedic opinion sought for possible femoral capital epiphyseal pinning.

Avascular necrosis of the hip

Pain in the hip that presents soon after scuba diving should raise the possibility of avascular necrosis from the 'bends', a nitrogen gas infarct from depressurizing too rapidly. Avascular necrosis may be a long-term consequence of the use of alcohol, steroids, or barbiturates.

Osteoarthritis of the hip

The most common problem is the degenerate osteoarthritic hip. There appears to be a familial element to degenerative joint disease, but some research suggests that impact exercise may increase the likelihood of degenerative disease.

History

The pain usually starts with activity and presents as groin pain, but posterior hip pain is not uncommon. This pain may then become almost continuous, disturbing sleep. There are probably two elements to the pain source; osteochondral damage and the capsular soft tissue inflammation. The capsulitis causes the more continuous pain, and is present without loadbearing. It occurs when getting in or out of a car or crossing the legs one over the other, whereas the osteochondral damage gives rise to loadbearing pain and is often pain free at rest. This history can govern treatment, in that the capsular pain does respond to anti-inflammatories such as NSAIDs and intra-articular injection of cortisone, or electrotherapy, whereas the osteochondral joint damage may respond to electrotherapeutic measures such as interferential and short-wave diathermy, but does not respond so well to NSAIDs and cortisone.

Examination

Examination is always thought to be easy, but this is often not the case. The patient may enter the consulting room with pain or a limp, or with a Trendelenburg gait. Here the gluteal muscles are weak on the side of the lesion so that the patient cannot fix the pelvis to raise the leg, and thus leans towards the non-affected side to assist the raising of the painful side. The Trendelenburg gait is probably diagnostic, and the Trendelenburg sign is confirmatory, but the external rotators of the hip can mimic this sign when weak or painful, as can nerve damage to the gluteals. Hip flexion and rotation at its extreme end of range will be enhanced by flexion of the spine, and thus restriction of hip range can load the SIJ and vertebral column. Equally, testing the vertebral column with the patient standing may also place stresses throughout the hip, so the lumbar spine should be tested with the patient sitting, at which stage the pain from lumbar movements will not be influenced by hip movement. If the hip shows a capsular pattern, then the capsule is inflamed, but a degenerative osteochondral joint may not have a true capsular pattern. The finding of a capsular pattern is diagnostic of hip disease. Pain on flexion of the hip alone is difficult to interpret, as this may be relieved by adding slight external rotation suggesting some local impingement or labrial tear. MRI can display these possible lesions. Flexion pain of the hip that is felt in the buttock was described by Cyriax and Cyriax (1983) as 'the sign of the buttock': not diagnostic of a lesion in the buttock, but indicative that the lesion is not in the hip. Look elsewhere, such as the facet joints, external rotators of the hip, sacrotuberous ligament, or possibly a capsular impingement of the hip. Facet joint pain may be felt directly in the groin on hip flexion. The capsular pattern at the hip, with pain in all planes of movement, should be detected with the patient sitting on the edge of the couch, and while lying supine and lying prone. The passive movements include flexion and extension, internal and external rotation, plus abduction and adduction. When the examiner is unable to distinguish between the hip and the back as the cause of symptoms, then as a general rule of thumb the back should be treated first.

Investigation

Investigations of the hip are primarily by radiography, which will reveal narrowing of the joint space and osteophytic lipping in early degenerative disease. Cystic and sclerotic changes in the head of the femur and the acetabulum develop at a later state. Radiography may demonstrate the flattened femoral head of a Perthe's hip which is prone to early degenerative changes. Occasionally an os acetabulare is seen at the acetabular rim and though this is recognized as a normal variant it can limit abduction of the hip, with some discomfort, which in high-kicking sports such as martial arts, presents a long-term problem. The os acetabulare develops as an apophysis, and in some sports that require a large range of hip movements may produce pain on passive movement and on resisted muscle testing of the rectus femoris which attaches in this area. The apophysis fuses up to the age of 25, which can produce problems of management in the young professional sportsperson.

Treatment

It must be remembered that degeneration of a joint is a continuum that gets worse with time. Radiography may be normal, but capsular signs are present, in which case, the pain is predominantly from the soft tissues which will respond to conservative therapeutic measures. It is when bony changes occur that conservative measures are less effective, as they only treat the soft tissue elements. The extent of disability and amount of pain caused by osteochondral degeneration will govern the criteria for a possible surgical replacement of the hip. Activities should be encouraged but should be non-weightbearing and involve high repetitions and low-resistance work. This is best done on a cycle, or rowing ergometer, though swimming is of value as long as the outer ranges of the hip movement are not stressed. Because movements at the outer range of the joint range are painful, smaller walking paces are advised, as is getting out of the car with both legs together. A bicycle seat may have to be raised to accommodate limited hip flexion and the left foot turned further out at the golf address to permit a follow-through after ball-strike.

Stress fracture

Stress fractures of the hip occur through the femoral neck. They are divided into compression and tension fractures. The compression fracture lies on the inferior surface of the femoral neck (Figure 3.6.25) and the tension fracture on the superior surface (Figure 3.6.26). The tension stress fracture is more likely to convert to a complete fracture (Figure 3.6.27) with serious consequences, such as avascular necrosis of the femoral head.

History

A history of groin pain in an active 18–40-year old individual, especially a runner or military recruit (Stoneham and Morgan 1991), should raise the possibility of a stress fracture. The pain is relieved at rest and is worse on activities though, when severe, the pain may be present when moving the non-weightbearing hip. Sometimes this pain presents in the buttock as well.

Examination

Clinical findings will differ, depending on the extent of the lesion, but will be provoked by passive hip movements and weightbearing, but resisted hip muscle testing may flare the pain as it is impossible to prevent some movement at the hip. Most important of all is an aware-

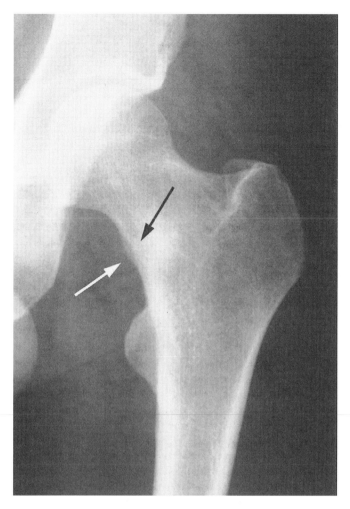

Figure 3.6.25 X ray showing a compression stress fracture with callus (arrow).

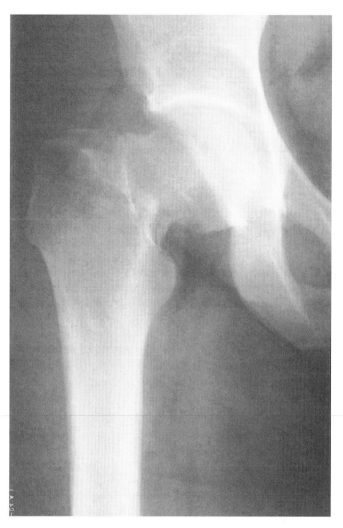

Figure 3.6.27 A disaster in a young athlete, this tension stress fracture has completed and needs surgery. Avascular necrosis may still occur.

ness of this lesion, and that the possibility of a stress fracture must be excluded from a presentation of hip pain because the missed diagnosis can lead to bony collapse of the femoral neck, avascular necrosis, and a replacement hip in a 20-year old. A disaster!

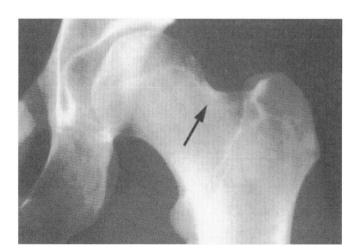

Figure 3.6.26 The sclerosis of this tension stress fracture suggests healing. A CT scan would exclude or display non-union (arrow).

Investigations

Investigations will be initially by radiography. In the subacute lesion callus or sclerosis at the superior or inferior femoral neck is revealed. However, during the early stages of this lesion radiographs may be negative, and the clinician should investigate further with a bone scan. This will demonstrate increased uptake of technetium-99 in the presence of a stress lesion. A tension stress fracture should then be CT scanned to assess whether a fracture line is apparent; if it is, then surgical pinning is probably required for this is a potentially unstable lesion. Though MRI may show the early stress lesion as medullary oedema, it may not display the extent of the fracture to a degree that a surgical opinion can be given with confidence.

Once the presence of a stress fracture has been established, a full menstrual history and hormonal balance, dietary regime, and possible bone density should be instigated. However, this lesion does appear in men and a training history of too rapid incrementation of loads should be sought, and biomechanical faults should also be corrected, together with biochemical bone markers.

Treatment

If there is no requirement for surgical pinning; the management is rest from all impact training. However, cross-training on a bicycle or rowing ergometer, or in water, is maintained. When impact pain from walking has settled, then gradual incrementation of impact loads may be considered.

Obturator neuropathy

The obturator nerve arises from the nerve roots L2–4 and exits the pelvis as an anterior and posterior branch, through the obturator foramen. It is thought that the anterior branch may become trapped at the level of the obturator foramen (Brukner *et al.* 1999).

History

The history is of exercise-related groin pain in a sportsperson, often of some months duration, centred on the adductor origin at the pubic bone. This may radiate down the medial aspect of the thigh to the knee.

Adductor spasm and weakness is more likely after exercise, and in long-standing cases there may be some paraesthesia over the medial thigh.

Examination

Obturator neuropathy is suspected when the patient stands in a partial lunge position with the affected leg backward, externally rotated and abducted and this position then produces the groin pain.

Investigations are undertaken to exclude other causes of groin pain. EMG may be diagnostic of denervation in the adductor longus and brevis muscles in long-standing cases. A nerve block injection under radiographic control into the roof of the obturator foramen, confirmed with radio-opaque dye, may block the post-exercise pain and reproduce the weakness.

Treatment

Conservative measures may fail, and surgical release of the nerve is then the treatment of choice, followed by early rehabilitation to jogging and running.

Pubic symphyseal lesions

Traumatic osteitis pubis symphysis (TOPS) and conjoined tendon disruption

Traumatic osteitis pubis symphysis consists of damage to the ligaments and or joint of the pubic symphysis, whereas damage to the conjoined tendon of the external inguinal ring, formed from the abdominal muscular and fascial insertions into the pubic tubercle, displays microtears and disruption to the enthesis and the tendon itself. Early papers that describe TOPS probably include cases of conjoined tendon disruption as well, and indeed there may well be a continuum of injury from the conjoined tendon disruption through to the unstable pubic symphysis. Certainly there seems now to be a plethora of conjoined tendon disruptions that either reflect altered training

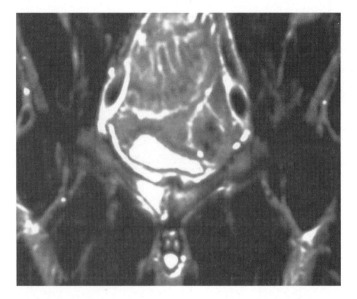

Figure 3.6.28   Oedema in the pubic bone with underlying adductor entheseal inflammation.

(perhaps too many sit-ups and crunches) or a failure to diagnose these in the past, when all groin strains were classified as TOPS. However, it must be remembered that many of these lesions get better with rest for 12–18 months. Harris and Murray (1953) described TOPS in footballers who had associated sacroiliac problems, which would support the hypothesis of a pelvic ring injury. This does appear to be a sporting problem, possibly from one-legged overload as in kicking a ball, but perhaps more pertinent is twisting over a fixed foot such as tackling an opponent in soccer. Here the support leg is moved into external rotation and abduction as the tackle leg is stretched out into abduction, and when the outer limits of the range of the hip movements are reached the load is transferred to the pelvic ring, producing a distraction force across the pubic symphysis. Indeed, MRI scanning has revealed several cases with oedema in the adjacent pubic bone (Figure 3.6.28).

History

The history of both lesions is of groin pain, and adductor muscle enthesitis may also be present, but the indicator of pelvic ring dysfunction is the accompanying low suprapubic abdominal pain. The apparent connection to the adductors may well come from the fact that the adductors are involved not only in stabilizing the pelvic ring, but also because the adductor fascia passes deep to the symphysis pubis and becomes contiguous with the abdominal fascia. In its mildest form, pain is produced by twisting and turning and by sprinting rather than just running, but as the lesion becomes more severe so there may be a constant suprapubic ache that is worse turning over in bed, sitting up, and walking. Some will complain of perineal or rectal pain, and I feel that this history is more indicative of TOPS rather than a conjoined tendon lesion. Coughing and especially sneezing are painful.

Examination

Clinically the patient indicates the site of pain as over the adductor origin and the pubic tubercle, and this pain is worse on resisted adduction and sitting up. However, with TOPS or a conjoined tendon lesion, the adductor origin is classically not tender to palpation whereas it is when the adductor origin lesion is present. The external inguinal ring palpated through the invaginated scrotum is tender. This sign may not be present if the patient has been resting, and a therapeutic trial of cortisone to the adductor origin followed by 10–14 days of incremental activities building up to sprints is a reasonable procedure at this stage. If there is a flare of symptoms, the diagnostic signs of a conjoined tendon lesion may then be found. TOPS is tender to palpation over the pubic symphysis, and the conjoined tendon lesion is tender over the pubic tubercle. There is usually no pathological cough impulse to be palpated through the inguinal canal in either case. The diagnosis is not easy and investigations may not be helpful.

Investigations

Investigations should include the one-legged standing radiograph (the **stork or flamingo test**). If there is symphyseal instability, there is a shift in the level of the contralateral two pubic bones by over 2 mm (Figure 3.6.29). The radiograph may reveal sclerosis and lysis through the symphysis indicative of TOPS, rheumatoid arthritis, or ankylos-

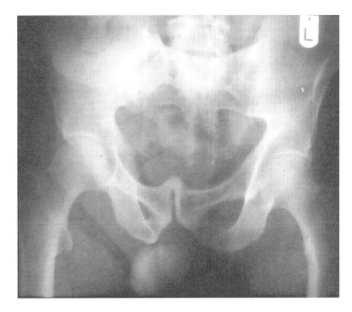

Figure 3.6.30   Ankylosis of the pubic symphysis.

ing spondylitis (Figure 3.6.11). Ankylosis of the pubic symphysis (Figure 3.6.30) and erosion of the gracilis margin are indicators of ankylosing spondylitis.

A bone scan excludes any other bony injury, in particular stress fractures of the femur and pelvis. The standard anteroposterior view of the bone scan does not separate the bladder from the symphysis and therefore a rather arbitrary assessment is made of a 'hot lesion'. The squat view separates the bladder signal from the pubic symphysis, and is therefore more reliable, but there are still problems of interpretation. I looked at a comparison of the radiation count between a select number of pixels of the pubic bone, left and right, and the humerus as an indicator of background radiation. Controls were those having bone scans for other reasons. Though there were differences in the ratios, with TOPS having higher counts, there was too much overlap to make this a useful investigation for diagnostic certainty. MRI can demonstrate pubic symphyseal shift, particularly in the horizontal plane, and can display bone marrow oedema. Careful assessment of the MRI can confirm disruption of the surrounding soft tissues.

Treatment

Sometimes circumstances require short-term treatment of the inflamed lesion. Cortisone and local anaesthetic may be injected into the pubic symphysis with or without ultrasound control for TOPS, or into the pubic tubercle for the conjoined tendon lesion (Holt *et al.* 1995). The vogue is for a surgical repair to the conjoined tendon, which returns players rapidly to their sport. However, it should be remembered that this lesion does get better with rest, albeit 12–18 months of controlled non-impact rest. Many sportsmen experience a contralateral injury, or a recurrence, presumably because the causative factors have not been identified and treated, or the sportsmen have been returned too soon to their causative sport. As yet, this is a very uncommon injury in women.

Some surgeons will not repair the conjoined tendon if the pubic symphysis shifts by more than 2 cm on the stork test, and then the treatment of the unstable pelvis becomes a problem. Rest from impact

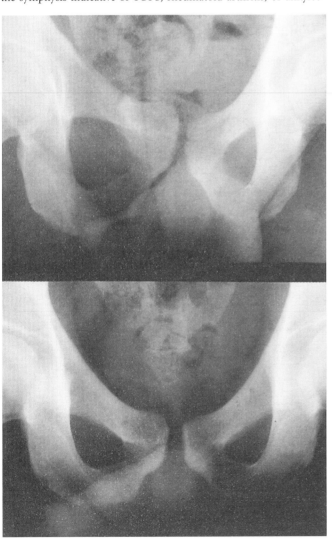

Figure 3.6.29   Flamingo or Stork views. Standing on one leg and then the other shows movement of the pubic symphysis greater than 2 mms.

is essential and any training should be by non-impact cross-training methods, although in the severe stages of TOPS swimming is also painful. It may be possible to stabilize the pelvis by sclerosing the SIJs with dextrose selerosant solution, on the principle that a ring cannot be disturbed in only one place, and that if the SIJ ligaments are strengthened then there is a stabilizing effect on the symphysis. Time and reduction in twisting and impaction exercises are essential, as is proper rehabilitation and a graded return to sporting activities. Rarely, the symphysis is surgically fused.

References

Bottomley, M. B. (1990) Sacral stress fracture in a runner. *Br. J. Sports Med.*, **24**(4), 243–244.

Bowen, V., Cassidy, J. D. (1981) Macroscopic and microscopic anatomy of the SIJ from embryonic life until the eighth decade. *Spine*, **6**(6), 620–628.

Brukner, P., Bradshaw, C., McCrory, P. (1999) Obturator neuropathy: a cause of exercise related groin pain. *Physician and Sportsmedicine*, **27**(5), 62–73.

Cyriax, J. H., Cyriax, P .J. (1983) *Illustrated manual of orthopaedic medicine*, 2nd edition, Butterworth Heinemann, Oxford.

Harris, N. H., Murray, R. O. (1953) Osteitis pubis of traumatic etiology. *J. Bone Joint Surg.*, **35A**, 685.

Holt, M. A., Keen, S. J., *et al.* (1995) Treatment of osteitis pubis in athletes. Results of corticosteroid injections. *Am.J. Sports Med.*, **23**(5), 601–606.

Klinkert, P., Porte, R., de Rooje T. P., deVries, A. G. (1997) Quadratus tendinitis as a cause of groin pain. *Br. J. Sports Med.*, **31**(4), 348–350.

Kurosawa, H., Nakasita, K., Saski, S., Takeda, S. (1996) Complete avulsion of the hamstring tendons from the ischial tuberosity. A report of two cases sustained in judo. *Br. J. Sports Med.*, **30**(1), 72–74.

Macdonald, G. R.. Hunt, T. E. (1951) Sacroiliac observations on the gross and histological changes in the various age groups. *Can. Med. Assoc. J.*, **66**, 157.

Osternig, L. R., Hamill, J., Lander, J. E., Robertson, R. (1986) Co-activation of sprinter and distance runner muscles in isokinetic exercise. *Med. Sci. Sport Exercise*, **18**(4), 431–435.

Read, M. T. F. (1998) Specific computerised tomographic views of the SIJ shows lesions that are undiagnosed with standard investigations of the lumbar spine. *J. Orthop. Med.*, **20**(1), 22–24.

Read, M. T. F. (2000) *A practical guide to sports injuries.* Butterworth Heinemann, Oxford.

Solonen, K. A. (1957) The SIJ in the light of anatomical roentgenological and clinical studies. *Acta Orthop. Scand*, **27** (suppl. 27), 1–127.

Stoneham, M. D.. Morgan, N. V. (1991). Stress fractures of the hip in Royal Marine recruits under training, a retrospective analysis. *Br. J. Sports Med.*, **25**(3), 145–148.

Sweetman, B. J. (1998) Low back pain and the leg twist test. *J. Orthop. Med.*, **20**(2), 3–9.

Vleeming, A., Mooney, V., Snijders, C., Dorman, T., Stoeckart, R. (eds) (1997). *Movement, stability and low back pain. The essential role of the pelvis.* Churchill Livingstone, Edinburgh.

Further reading

Brukner, P., Khan, K. (1993) *Clinical sports medicine.* McGraw-Hill, New York.

Reid, D. C. (1992) *Sports injury assessment and rehabilitation.* Churchill Livingstone, Edinburgh.

History

General questions

All histories begin with the presenting complaint and, in the case of a joint, the site and side affected. This is then followed by the patient's age, occupation and, specifically in knee-related problems, sporting participation (including type and intensity). The latter three are important in ascertaining the patient's degree of functional disability, which clearly has a bearing on the range of treatments offered. For instance, a 20-year old professional footballer with a tear of the anterior cruciate ligament (ACL) may be offered different advice from a 40-year old office worker who presents with the same injury but has no active sporting participation.

It is then important to ascertain the duration of symptoms, exact details of the precipitating injury, and then the general course of events including response to any treatment already received. It is through this aspect of the history that one obtains a clear picture of the degree of disability suffered by the patient.

Usually, patients present with a combination of symptoms relating to pain, swelling, locking, and giving way. The diagnostic specificity of each of these symptoms in isolation is poor; rather, they are used in combination to guide the examiner to a differential diagnosis. In addition, the presence and degree of each of these symptoms at presentation and then how they changed with the passage of time is important.

Specific questions

Pain

The site of pain within the knee is an indication as to the structure damaged but by no means diagnostic, particularly with traumatic disorders such as meniscal tears. As an example, lateral joint pain from a patellofemoral disorder is frequently mistaken for a lateral meniscal tear and, before the use of MRI and arthroscopy, resulted in unnecessary lateral meniscectomies. The site of pain following an episode of injury, such as a medial collateral ligament strain, is, however, a clear indication of the possible structures involved. It is useful to obtain a description of the pain at the time of injury or presentation and then how the pain has progressed. Of particular importance is whether the pain is constant and whether it occurs at night. For instance, these symptoms are an indication to recommend arthroplasty in assessing a patient with severe degenerative changes. Constant pain may indicate more sinister pathology, such as tumour or infection.

It is then important to relate the pain to the level and type of activity, such as whether the symptom appears after a few steps walking or only after running. In addition, questions about the pain related to specific actions such as twisting and turning may indicate a problem with the main weightbearing areas of the knee such as a meniscal tear or chondral defect. Bent-knee activities such as kneeling, crouching, or squatting may indicate a patellofemoral problem, though posterior horn tears of the medial meniscus are aggravated by loaded bent-knee activities such as coming up from a squatting position.

The examiner should always be aware of the possibility of referred pain from the hip or lumbar spine, particularly when assessing a patient with degenerative symptoms.

Swelling

Swelling can be localized, such as a lateral meniscal cyst, or generalized, such as a haemarthrosis. With regard to local swellings, it is important to ascertain the length of time the swelling has been present and whether it is increasing in size and painful. Localized swellings such as bursae, meniscal cysts, and ganglia may vary in size, sometimes associated with activity levels, and are common findings. Swellings which are constant and increasing in size should be investigated as a matter or urgency; soft tissue or bony tumours around the knee are rare but well reported. Some swellings, such as popliteal cysts, are associated with a generalized effusion and respond to treatment for the generalized inflammation.

Generalized swellings are effusions secondary to an inflammatory process. The commonest effusion is related to some mechanical derangement within the knee such as a meniscal tear or chondral damage. There is usually a history of injury with the effusion appearing within 24 hours. Effusions also occur secondary to inflammatory arthropathies and can be massive if chronic. There is usually no record of injury but a careful history should be taken to identify other features of rheumatoid arthritis or seronegative arthropathies. These generalized swellings are not necessarily pure effusions; at least part of the swelling may be synovial hypertrophy, which will become apparent on examination if suspected from the history.

Generalized swelling may be secondary to a haemarthrosis, which is generally defined as swelling appearing within 4 hours of an injury. The main differential diagnosis of a haemarthrosis is an ACL rupture, an osteochondral fracture (often associated with a patella dislocation), or a peripheral meniscal tear. Indeed, if an athlete gives a history of a twisting injury on the sports field followed by swelling within 4 hours, they have a 70–80% chance of having sustained an ACL rupture (Maffuli *et al.* 1993). The commonest misdiagnosis in this setting is to confuse an ACL rupture with a lateral patella dislocation; indeed, rarely both can occur together (Simonian *et al.* 1998). Both occur on the slightly flexed weightbearing knee forced into external rotation. This reinforces the need for a skyline radiograph in the acutely injured knee to identify a possible osteochondral fragment from the patellofemoral joint that occurs in patellar dislocation. This injury is best treated by early re-attachment.

Not surprisingly, haemarthroses are painful due to the degree of tension within the knee. A relatively painless diffuse swelling as opposed to a true haemarthrosis should alert the examiner to the possibility of a more extensive ligamentous injury with disruption of the capsule. The examiner can be lulled into thinking the injury is less severe than it really is.

Locking

Locking can be subdivided into true locking and pseudo-locking. True locking is relatively rare. It occurs when an intra-articular structure, loose body or meniscal tear interposes between the femoral condyle and tibial surface. Classically the patient loses terminal extension but is able to flex the knee (though usually also losing some terminal flexion, which is less noticeable). They may present with the knee locked, but more commonly are able to unlock the knee with a trick manoeuvre involving rotation of the tibia. When the knee unlocks it usually occurs with a clunk, and full movement is immediately restored. Loose bodies may also be felt by the patient in the suprapatellar pouch but more commonly in either the medial or lateral gutter. They are classically elusive and once found immediately move to another area, hence their eponym of 'joint mouse'.

Pseudo-locking is a far more common presentation, and usually occurs in patients with anterior knee pain secondary to some form of patella maltracking. Classically it is associated with marked pain and the knee is solidly locked. Over a period of time, often hours, the knee movement gradually returns. The patient usually rests the knee and may use massage and analgesia until the pain subsides. Often this type of locking occurs during some form of bent-knee activity, frequently when coming downstairs.

Giving way

There are two types of giving way: true giving way, which is usually associated with some form of ligamentous instability, and a buckling-type sensation, which is usually associated with anterior knee pain and the symptom of pseudo-locking previously described.

An example of true giving way is seen in ACL instability. The patient has no problem running in a straight line, but on planting the foot and twisting with the upper body internally rotating, the knee suddenly collapses, quickly followed by pain and later swelling. With the initial rupture there may be contact, but in the chronic cases this is often not the case. Indeed, in chronic cases, the knee may collapse in actions of everyday living. Once the swelling settles the knee apparently returns to normal until it gives way again. Again, it is worth bearing in mind the similarity between the symptoms of giving way in chronic ACL rupture and chronic patellar dislocation or subluxation (Simonian *et al.* 1998). If the patella spontaneously reduces and the patient cannot recall the position of the patella, the diagnosis can only be made by careful examination for stability.

Chronic medial instability usually presents with difficulty performing cutting movements rather than rotation. Isolated posterior cruciate ligament (PCL) rupture does not usually present with instability unless there is associated posterolateral or posteromedial instability. In these situations the knee again feels unstable with rotatory movements but also on walking downstairs, because of the unimpeded anterior displacement of the femur on the tibia. Often, patients with these complex problems present with marked instability with active daily living and may constantly need the use of a knee brace.

Buckling of the knee is seen in patients with anterior knee pain and is associated with pain. These patients often report their knee buckling without any rotary movement, usually occurring when walking in a straight line or downstairs. The knee buckling is rarely associated with an effusion.

Examination

Orthopaedic examination of the knee follows the usual routine of inspection, palpation, movement, and measurement. (*Editor's note:* The musculoskeletal physician may well be trained in the Cyriax routine of inspection, active movements, passive movements, stress tests, muscle contraction tests and palpation.) Specific tests for patellofemoral pathology and stability will also be addressed. One must always remember to use the opposite limb for comparison and (to gain the patient's trust) leave any possibly painful tests to the end. A tense patient will make any assessment of subtle instabilities impossible.

General examination

The examination should start immediately the patient enters the clinic to assess their gait, walking aids, and general mobility. Full assessment requires the patient to be undressed from mid-thigh; shorts are ideal.

Inspection

Initial inspection should begin with the patient standing to assess overall limb alignment and any shortening which can be assessed at this stage. Limb alignment includes any femoral or tibial rotational malalignments, which have a bearing particularly on patellofemoral function. In addition, the foot position should be assessed for evidence of any abnormalities such as hyperpronation which again can affect patellofemoral function. It is easier at this stage to assess the posterior aspect of the knee for scars, swellings, or bruising. The anterior aspect can be assessed now or later when the patient is supine. Gait pattern is observed when the patient walks both towards and away from the examiner.

The patient is now laid supine on the examination couch with their head relaxed on a pillow and their hands placed on their chest. A patient straining to watch an examination may increase muscle tone, affecting observations such as knee laxity. As well as inspecting the anterior aspect of the knee for scars, swellings or bruising, any quadriceps or calf wasting can be observed and measured if thought appropriate. Sometimes swellings, such as a lateral meniscal cyst, are best seen with the knee bent to 90° and in comparison with the opposite knee. With the knees flexed in this position they should be observed from the side to identify any posterior sag indicative of a posterior cruciate ligament rupture. A prominent tibial tubercle as seen in late Osgood–Schlatter's disease may make this assessment difficult.

Palpation

Palpation of the patella and associated structures will be dealt with later. There are two basic tests for the presence of an effusion. The first is balloting the patella on the femoral trochlea, having first emptied the medial and lateral gutters of synovial fluid. The second is stroking the lateral gutter to empty the fluid and watching for a fluid wave in the medial gutter. If there is the appearance of swelling in the knee and yet no effusion one must consider synovial hypertrophy, as seen in conditions such as pigmented villonodular synovitis (Flandrey *et al.* 1994).

The knee is largely subcutaneous apart from posteriorly, and many structures can therefore be palpated directly. This is best done with the knee flexed to 90° with the foot firmly planted on the examination couch in a neutral position. The fingers can then be used to palpate along the joint lines starting with the painless side. Tenderness along the joint line, particular posteromedially, may indicate a meniscal tear. The borders of the femoral and tibial condyles, the patellar tendon, and medial (MCL) and lateral (LCL) collateral ligaments can also be palpated for tenderness.

The site of tenderness is important in an MCL strain. Most commonly there is tenderness on the medial epicondyle at the site of the femoral attachment of the MCL. This can be confused with disruption of the medial patellofemoral ligament seen in lateral patellar dislocation. Tenderness along the medial joint line in an MCL strain is indicative of disruption of the deeper fibres and suggests a potentially more complicated injury. Disruption of the tibial insertion of the MCL and hence tenderness in this area is usually only seen in a major knee injury such as dislocation. The best way to isolate the lateral collateral ligament is to put the patient's leg in a figure-of-four position. This puts the ligament under tension, making it more pronounced and easier to palpate. The patellar tendon should be palpated in full extension and when tensed at 90° of flexion. In chronic patella tendinosis, tenderness at the proximal tendon is more noticeable in extension; in flexion the normal superficial fibres cover the damaged deep fibres, resulting in less pain on palpation.

The posterior aspect of the knee should also be palpated to identify soft tissue masses in the popliteal fossa, which may not have been evident on inspection.

Movement

The normal range of passive movement in the sagittal plane is assessed comparing both sides and including hyperextension. When performing this movement the hand should be placed over the patella to assess the presence and type of patellofemoral crepitus. The range can be noted as degrees of movement (e.g. −10° −0° −140°). Alternatively, hyperextension can be measured as the distance the heel can be lifted off the examination couch and flexion by the heel to buttock distance. A more precise technique is laying the patient prone with their knees level with the end of the examination couch and, as gravity extends the lower leg, observing the difference. The patient should be asked to actively perform a straight leg raise to assess the integrity of the extensor mechanism and flex the knee as far as possible.

Specific examination

Meniscal pathology

McMurray's test was intended to recreate displacement of a painful meniscal tear, and is probably not in the patient's best interests. A modification of this is a compression test to produce discomfort along the joint line, which may indicate pathology in the medial or lateral compartment. The patient is supine with the knee flexed. The examiner places one hand on the top of the knee with the fingers and thumbs positioned to palpate the joint line and the other under the heel. The examiner can then compress the joint by pushing down on the top hand while the lower hand controls flexion and can also provide a varus or valgus strain, thereby compressing each compartment in turn in varying degrees of flexion. This test is most specific for a tear of the posterior horn of the medial meniscus. The patient reports discomfort on the posteromedial joint line with the knee compressed in full flexion and external rotation. Similar compression of the joint can be achieved using **Apley's compression test** (Apley and Solomon 1982) with the patient prone. Compression, flexion, and rotation of the knee are controlled by the examiner's hand on the patient's heel.

Another less specific test is to ask the patient to fully squat, and if possible duck walk. This action compresses the posterior horns of the menisci but can also cause patellofemoral pain. No one test for meniscal pathology is absolutely diagnostic (Evans *et al.* 1993, Stratford and Binkley 1995). One usually makes a diagnosis from the history and looks for confirmatory tests on examination. The absence of positive signs does not definitely exclude a meniscal tear, but other investigations such as MRI should be undertaken.

Patellofemoral pathology

With the patient supine an assessment of the patella size, position (laterally displaced), and height is made in both extension and flexion, though this is done more accurately with radiographs. The patella is then observed with the patient flexing and extending the knee to observe patellar tracking. This is often easier done with the patient's knee flexed over the end of the couch. Rarely one can identify a sudden jerk of the patella as it moves from its laterally placed position into the trochlea at the onset of flexion. Medial displacement of the patella is extremely uncommon and usually iatrogenic. With the leg in this position the patient can then be asked to extend against resistance to induce pain with concentric loading and also slowly allow the leg to flex with the examiner forcibly flexing the knee against a quadriceps contracture to assess eccentric loading.

With the patient supine, the borders of the patella and the retinaculae are carefully palpated for tenderness. In acute patellar dislocation, there is a boggy feel to the medial retinaculum with tenderness along the medial border of the patella or over the medial epicondyle at the site of insertion of the medial patellofemoral ligament. With chronic anterior knee pain from maltracking there may be tenderness over the superolateral border of the patella.

An assessment should then be made of lateral retinacular tightness, which one finds with patellar tilting such as seen in excessive lateral pressure syndrome. To do this the patella should be just engaged in the femoral trochlea. The knee is flexed slightly by placing one hand balled into a fist under the knee while the other moves the patella maximally medially and laterally. If one imagines the patella split into quadrants, it should be able to move at least one quadrant medially; any less indicates lateral retinacular tightness. The medial retinaculum is naturally more lax, but movement of greater than two quadrants laterally indicates laxity in the medial retinaculum that one may see in recurrent patella dislocation. With the patella held in this lateral position, the knee is now flexed and the patient's reaction observed. A positive **patella apprehension test** is seen when the patient resists further flexion for fear of the patella dislocating.

Ligament instability

This is subdivided into ACL instability, MCL instability, and PCL instability, including posterolateral rotatory instability (PLRI).

ACL instability

Before assessing ACL or PCL instability, both knees are viewed from the side when flexed to 90° to identify any posterior sag indicating PCL instability. If this is not recognized, anterior movement from an abnormally posterior placed tibia may be misinterpreted as anterior instability.

The classic test for ACL instability is the **Lachman test** (Torg *et al.* 1976). With a normal-sized knee the best technique is to grasp the distal femur with one hand, holding the femur while flexing the knee to 20°; and then the other hand grasps the proximal tibia and displaces the tibia anteriorly. The amount of anterior displacement is then estimated and can be graded. One method of grading is: grade 0, 0–3 mm (normal); grade I, 3–5 mm; grade II, 5–10 mm; grade III, >10 mm, with no endpoint. These measurements are estimated on comparison with the uninjured knee. The amount of displacement is subjective and, although useful to the same examiner with subsequent examinations, is of little use to another examiner. True measurement of displacement is better undertaken with some form of laxity measurement device, though even these are subject to interobserver error. Of more importance on examination is whether there is definite anterior displacement and whether there is a soft or hard endpoint. A soft endpoint is indicative of a complete rupture. For patients with large thighs or examiners with small hands it is better to fix the femur over the examiner's flexed knee while displacing the tibia with the other hand (Draper and Schulthies 1995).

The other classic test for ACL instability is the **pivot shift test** (Galway and MacIntosh 1980), which can be performed in a number of different ways though the basic principle is the same. The pivot shift test recreates the anterolateral subluxation of the tibia on the femur which results in the giving way sensation experienced by the patient when twisting on a planted foot. The patient's leg is held in full extension, with the hands around the knee and the foot tucked under the arm. The lower leg is then internally rotated by twisting the examiner's body and a valgus strain applied to the knee via the laterally placed hand and the elbow and body. In this position, the tibia is anterolaterally subluxed. The knee is then flexed gently and at about 20° the tibia suddenly reduces, which can be seen in obvious cases (usually under anaesthetic), and palpated by the hands around the knee in more

subtle cases. The degree of instability is increased if the hip is abducted, as this decreases tension in the iliotibial band (Bach *et al.* 1988). It is not possible to perform this test with medial instability, as the medial pivot is lost. The key to this test is obtaining the patient's confidence, as if it is performed too forcibly can be distressing for the patient. With the leg securely held and the hands around the knee the patient feels more confident, allowing this test to be performed gently and quickly.

Some examiners prefer to undertake the **jerk test**, in which the knee is subluxed momentarily by the examiner when extending from a flexed position, but this can be more distressing to the patient.

MCL instability

This is the commonest form of knee instability. In the acute situation the patient guards the knee and although an impression of medial instability may be gained, the extent of the instability is difficult to assess. In the chronic setting the examination is much easier. The knee is held in the same manner as for performing the pivot shift test. Indeed it is my usual practice to assess collateral stability after the Lachman test and immediately before the pivot shift test, leaving the latter potentially more distressing examination until the end.

With the leg held as described, the knee is placed in full extension including hyperextension. A valgus force is then applied to the knee by pushing the lower leg held by the elbow and body against the laterally placed hand. The degree of opening can be assessed as described in the Lachman test, but the most important point is whether there is a soft or hard endpoint. If there is no endpoint with the leg in full extension, this signifies a major disruption of the knee with damage to the cruciate ligaments, which act as secondary stabilizers to valgus strain. Some opening with an endpoint may represent disruption of the deep fibres of the MCL. The test is then performed in 20° of flexion, which relaxes the secondary restraints and allows an assessment of the superficial fibres of the MCL. Again an assessment is made as to the degree of movement and the presence of an endpoint.

Posteromedial rotatory instability is a major instability in which there is damage to the posteromedial structures of the knee (Nielsen *et al.* 1984), principally the posterior oblique ligament, and occurs with severe ligament disruptions, usually affecting the PCL. As well as medial opening in extension and flexion, the posterior subluxation of the medial tibial plateau off the femur can be demonstrated using a **dial test**, which is described in the section on posterolateral instability.

Lateral collateral instability in isolation is unusual and associated with posterolateral instability, which is described in the next section. Essentially however, the test is the same as for the MCL. There is

Table 3.7.1. Clinical tests in posterior cruciate ligament (PCL)/posterolateral corner (PLC) instability

	PLC	PLC + PCL	PCL
Posterior sag at 90°	N	SP	SP
Posterior draw at 90°	N	SP	SP
Posterior draw at 20°	P	SP	N
Quadriceps active test	N	SP	SP
Valgus stress test	P	P	N
Passive external rotation at 30°	P	SP	N
Passive external rotation at 90°	P	SP	N

N, normal; P, positive; SP, strongly positive.

greater normal laxity in the lateral structures and care should be taken to compare movement with the uninjured knee.

PCL instability and PLRI

These two instabilities are described together as they frequently co-exist, but also because there are subtle differences in differentiating the two on examination. The examination for these instabilities should take place concurrently (Miller *et al.* 1999) (Table 3.7.1).

As described earlier, before cruciate ligament examination, both knees are flexed to 90° with the patient supine and both feet planted on the examination couch. In this **posterior sag test**, gravity displaces the tibia relative to the femur, indicating a PCL disruption.

One then proceeds with the **posterior drawer test** with the knees in this position and the feet planted in neutral rotation. The examiner sits on the feet with hands around the knee; the fingers can ensure the hamstrings are relaxed and the thumbs can palpate the joint line. At this angle of flexion the anterior tibial condyles should be anterior to the corresponding femoral condyles. The injured knee is compared with the normal knee and the posterior translation is measured, as described earlier for the Lachman test. Another method of grading is grade I if it is 0–5 mm (tibia still anterior to the femur), grade II if 5–10 mm (tibia flush with femur) and grade III if over 10 mm with no endpoint (tibial condyles sagging behind femoral condyles). In the PCL-deficient knee, the posterior drawer test at 20°, or **posterior Lachman test**, is also mildly positive, but it is more strongly positive in the presence of posterolateral rotatory instability.

In the **quadriceps active test**, the patient is positioned as previously. Anterior translation of the proximal tibia with quadriceps contraction indicates a PCL injury.

Although there are many tests described to diagnose posterolateral instability, I rely on three basic tests. The first, the posterior Lachman test, has already been described. This is most positive in combined PCL and PLRI, slightly less in isolated PLRI, and least in PCL instability.

The **varus stress test** is performed by positioning the patient in exactly the same way as for the valgus test described in the MCL section but with a varus force applied to the knee in full extension and 20° of flexion. Increased opening in flexion indicates injury to the LCL, which is usually associated with damage to the posterolateral

corner. Increased opening in extension may still be present in an isolated injury to these structures, but is more obvious when combined with anterior or posterior cruciate instability. Comparison with the normal side is important.

The **dial test** is passive external rotation of the tibia (relative to the femur), with the knee at 30° and 90° of flexion. This is best performed with the patient prone, when the feet indicate the degrees of rotation from neutral. In the rare case of isolated PLRI, increased external rotation is noted at 30° but less so at 90°. When combined PCL and PLRI are present, increased external rotation is noted in both positions (Staubli 1994, Veltri and Warren 1994).

Tests such as the **external rotation recurvatum test**, **reversed pivot shift test**, and a posterior drawer test performed with the foot in external rotation may also be performed for additional confirmation.

Limb alignment and gait pattern must be observed, to ensure there is no lateral thrust on walking which is seen in chronic PLRI, usually associated with PCL injury but also seen in ACL injury. If this is not recognized, the ligament reconstructions may fail in the absence of a corrective osteotomy.

PCL and posterolateral corner injuries are major events and in the acute setting particular care must be taken to ensure there is no neurovascular injury, in particular to the common peroneal nerve.

Meniscal lesions

Structure

The medial and lateral menisci lie interposed between the femur and tibia in their respective compartments of the knee. As with articular cartilage, they are specialized connective tissue structures, principally formed by type 1 collagen. They are crescent-shaped structures designed to resist compression forces and, by effectively increasing the surface area of the joint, avoid high-point contact and therefore spread the load applied across the joint. The majority of collagen fibres are orientated circumferentially around the meniscus in the shape of a hoop (Figure 3.7.1). These fibres are anchored to bone at the anterior and posterior horns of the meniscus and therefore, when a compres-

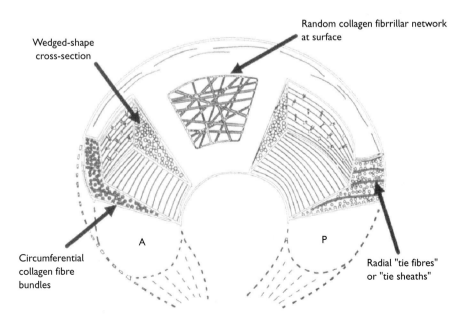

Figure 3.7.1 Ultrastructure of the meniscus.

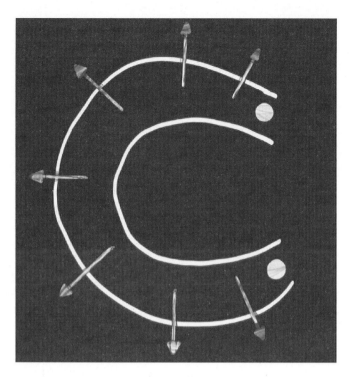

Figure 3.7.2 The meniscus resists radially orientated stresses by the attachment of the circumferentially orientated fibres to the anterior and posterior horns.

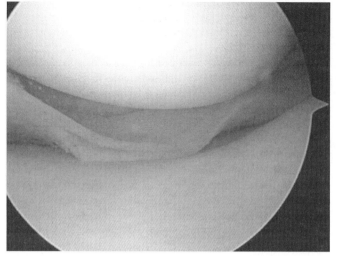

Figure 3.7.3 A longitudinal split towards the periphery of the meniscus associated with a horizontal cleavage tear.

sive load is applied, the hoop fibres effectively resist extrusion of the meniscus effectively sharing load across the joint (Figure 3.7.2). There are also radial tie fibres which tether the meniscus to the peripheral capsule, and a mesh of obliquely orientated fibres on the surface of the meniscus that resist shear forces.

The medial and lateral menisci are shaped differently, conforming to the respective joint surfaces. The lateral meniscus is generally more mobile than the medial, which reflects the increased laxity in the lateral compartment when compared to the medial. The peripheral attachments of the medial meniscus are therefore more secure, particularly in the posterior aspect, which may explain the higher incidence of meniscal tears in the posterior horn of the medial meniscus caused by a compressive and rotary force on a fixed structure.

Menisci are largely avascular except for the peripheral third (Arnoczky and Warren 1982), so it is only in this area that the normal reparative process occurs. More central tears, which include the vast majority, do not heal.

Pathology and presentation

Meniscal tears are common events and most commonly produced by rotation on the flexed loaded knee. Medial meniscal tears are 5–7 times more common than lateral tears, and the vast majority occur in the posterior third of the meniscus. The patterns of tear differ from side to side. There have been numerous classifications of tear, but most relate to the type of tear rather than aetiology. The basic types are longitudinal split, flap, radial, oblique, and horizontal cleavage (Figure 3.7.3; Dandy 1990). Degenerate tears can be a combination of tears occurring with chondral changes of early osteoarthritis. Cystic degeneration is a common finding on MRI scan and is believed to predispose a meniscus to tearing if sufficient load is applied. Cystic

degeneration is associated with a meniscal cyst that occurs more commonly in the lateral meniscus in its anterior third and when symptomatic is almost always associated with a tear, usually a horizontal tear. Discoid menisci occur in 5% of the population (rising to 20% in Japan), and 10 times more common in the lateral meniscus. They are usually only symptomatic when torn or, far more rarely, if the posterior horn attachments are deficient (Wrisberg type), with instability and locking.

Meniscal tears are commonly associated with injuries to other structures, notably the chondral surface or ACL, so evidence of injury must always be sought. This is particularly true of the ACL rupture, as this may be associated with a peripheral tear of the meniscus which may be reparable. The mechanism of injury has been described previously, but the degree of force required to tear a meniscus varies with age. In a younger athlete, there will be more record of a specific injury as a greater force is required to tear an otherwise normal meniscus. In an older person, there is often some cystic necrosis in the body of the meniscus that renders it softer and more liable to injury. As an example, simply squatting and twisting may supply sufficient force to tear the meniscus. Thereafter a torn meniscus may present in one of two ways: either as intermittent locking (see earlier) or simply pain with weightbearing activity, made worse by rotary movements and particularly bent-knee activities. This becomes a recurrent problem as if the patient rests the symptoms often resolve, only returning once activity is resumed. There may be an effusion in these acute episodes but this is usually mild unless associated with chondral damage. There is often a 'buckling' sensation, a sensation that the knee may collapse but in the absence of any ligamentous instability. The clinical signs of a meniscal tear have been dealt with earlier, but often the diagnosis is made from the history, as there may be few clinical signs at presentation. This is particularly true of the lateral meniscal tear where there is more recourse to additional investigations such as MRI. With regards to the medial meniscal tear, if there is tenderness in the posteromedial joint line with a positive compression rotation test as described earlier, then one can be confident of a tear of the posterior horn of the medial meniscus and the use of MRI is less evident.

MRI has been of great benefit in the diagnosis of knee pathology and has reduced the need for unnecessary arthroscopy. The sensitivity of the clinical diagnosis of meniscal tears is in the order of 75–80% compared with 88–90% for MRI. This does not mean that all knees need MRI. If there is a clear clinical need for an arthroscopy, then MRI will not alter the management and will only increase cost. If there is doubt, which is usually with lateral meniscal tears, then MRI is justified. It has been well demonstrated that a knee specialist has fewer negative arthroscopies and a greater number of positive MRI scans, indicating better clinical skills and a more economical use of resources (Dandy 1997).

Management

The initial management of a meniscal tear is conservative, with the usual regime of <u>r</u>est, <u>i</u>ce, <u>c</u>ompression, and <u>e</u>levation (RICE). The only exception to this is if the patient presents with a locked knee or with a peripheral tear of the meniscus. Attempts to try to manipulate the knee should be avoided, as this could potentially cause further damage. The patient should undergo surgery at the earliest opportunity, to unlock the knee and treat the tear with excision of the torn segment or suture. With the uncomplicated tear, the initial symptoms often resolve but may recur with increased activity. As meniscal tears do not heal, the patient often returns with further recurrent problems, or the tear may extend with an episode of further trauma. If a patient has such recurrent problems, the next stage in management is arthroscopic removal of the torn fragment.

Meniscal tears were originally thought to be of little function and were removed through an open arthrotomy. As the chondral surface became overloaded degenerative changes appeared within the knee which often, some 15–20 years later, became symptomatic. Over the past 30 years, with the advent of arthroscopic surgery, meniscal preservation has become the norm with removal of only the torn fragment or suturing of the meniscus if the tear was in the peripheral zone. Theoretically this should reduce the incidence of late degenerative changes, though, in view of the long time frame, few data are so far available to support this claim. It is a general clinical impression that even partial tears of the lateral meniscus in the adolescent athlete are not as benign as was hoped, even with the advent of partial meniscectomy.

Meniscal suturing is popular, and there should be no excuse for sacrificing the meniscus, particularly in the young athlete, if there is any chance of repairing it. However, the patient should be warned of the poor healing capacity of the meniscus. The chance of healing for a tear associated with an ACL rupture is in the order of 80%, but this drops to 50% for an isolated tear. In addition, the rehabilitation is far slower, with a return to contact sport at 6 months rather than 6 weeks if the tear is removed. This, and the consequences of a major meniscectomy, should be carefully explained to the patient but there is often pressure, particularly in the professional athlete, to return to sport quicker thus compromising the meniscal treatment. This should be resisted, in particular when treating an adolescent athlete.

If a meniscus is unavoidably lost, there is a place, particularly in the younger patient before degenerative changes ensue, to consider replacing the meniscus with an allograft. This is specialized surgery requiring a long rehabilitative programme and should be performed in recognized centres. The results are variable and there are few long-term data on the prevention of degenerative changes. Future research in this field is leading towards the development of a collagen-engineered meniscus.

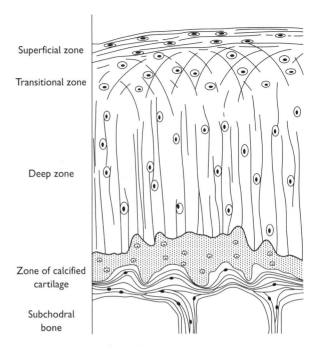

Figure 3.7.4 Diagrammatic representation of the articular cartilage.

Chondral lesions

Structure

Articular cartilage is a specialized connective tissue, the matrix of which consists of a gel of proteoglycan and water, reinforced by collagen fibres (Fig 3.7.4). These fibres are firmly anchored to the subchondral bone, giving stability to the cartilage. Chondrocytes synthesize and maintain the matrix of collagen and proteoglycan within which they lie. The collagen is predominantly of type II. The collagen fibres are arranged in the form of arcades that arise from subchondral bone. The proteoglycans and cells are embedded within the collagen fibres. The proteoglycans are long-chain polysaccharides linked to hyaluronate that are negatively charged and hold water within the cartilage. This proteoglycan–water gel gives the cartilage matrix a high osmotic pressure. The tendency of the proteoglycan to swell is balanced by the elastic resistance of the collagen network. The collagen arcades thus aid in absorption of compressive forces.

Pathology and presentation

Articular cartilage is avascular, aneural, and alymphatic, and nutrition must therefore be derived either deeply from blood vessels in the subchondral bone or from the synovial fluid bathing the cartilage surface. The chondroblasts in the cartilage tissue are relatively few and their metabolic rate is low. The capacity of chondrocytes to divide and migrate in the articular cartilage is restricted by the matrix fibres. As a consequence, the articular cartilage does not repair significantly after injury.

The proteoglycan structure can be damaged by trauma, or by enzymes from inflammatory disease and infection. If this happens, the proteoglycan structure disintegrates and the water-holding capacity is lost. Progressive breakdown of the collagen meshwork occurs, leading to exposure of bone, which is responsible for the symptoms of severe pain and disability. A number of classification systems are in use, but no single system seems to be universally applicable. The spectrum of grades is from softening and fissuring to fragmentation and erosion.

Partial-thickness injuries of the articular cartilage do not heal. They stimulate only a minimal and short-lived reaction in the adjacent chondrocytes in the form of increased cell replication and matrix turnover. Full-thickness injuries penetrating the subchondral bone produce the normal response associated with wound healing, including vascular invasion, cell migration, and inflammatory reaction, filling the defect with fibrocartilage. Fibrocartilage primarily functions as a resistor to tension, in contrast to hyaline cartilage which mainly resists compressive forces. The end product of fibrocartilage is thus inadequate biomechanically, and is bound to fail in the long term. Articular defects increase surface stresses in the remaining cartilage, increasing wear in the affected compartment.

Damage to articular cartilage is a common problem. In a review of 31 516 knee arthroscopies by Curl et al. (1997), 53 569 hyaline cartilage lesions were documented in 19 827 patients. Grade III lesions of the patella were the most common. Grade IV lesions were predominantly located on the medial femoral condyle. Patients under 40 years of age with grade IV lesions accounted for 5% of all arthroscopies, and 74% of these patients had a single chondral lesion (4% of the arthroscopies). No associated ligamentous or meniscal pathology was found in 36.6% of these patients. In another study (Hardaker et al. 1990), it was associated with 16% (21) of 132 injuries of the knee that were sufficient to cause intra-articular bleeding.

Levy et al. (1996) examined 23 isolated chondral defects in 15 soccer players. All players had knee pain, although 33% of the lesions were less than 10 mm in diameter. This study indicated that even small lesions are significant in producing symptoms. It appears that pain is caused by the stimulation of nerve endings in the subchondral bone as a result of compromised capabilities for transmitting loads and absorbing energy.

There is increasing clinical evidence that full thickness articular cartilage defects advance slowly and progressively, leading to premature arthritis. Twyman et al. (1991) prospectively followed 22 knees in which osteochondritis dissecans had been diagnosed before skeletal maturity; at an average of 34 years, 32% had radiographic evidence of moderate or severe osteoarthritis.

These lesions may be encountered incidentally during ligament or meniscal surgery, having been silent or asymptomatic for an unknown period of time, or they may mimic a meniscal tear in their presentation. The usual symptoms and signs include pain with weightbearing, mechanical catching, clicking or locking, and effusion. MRI using cartilage sequencing can provide reliable information on the state of articular cartilage (Potter et al. 1998). Direct arthroscopic visualization is confirmatory.

Management

To date, no peer reviewed, prospective, randomized, controlled studies of operative versus non-operative treatment for full-thickness articular cartilage lesions have been published. Even though the long-term results of surgical treatment for full-thickness articular surface lesions remain unknown, the early results are encouraging. Although most treatment options will produce fibrocartilage or hyaline-like cartilage, the elimination of pain, swelling, stiffness, grinding, and locking may enable people to return to work and sports, the resultant repairs

Treatment for full-thickness articular cartilage lesions

- Mechanical techniques
  - washout and debridement (trimming the loose tissue flaps)
  - refixation or removal of chondral fragments
- Marrow stimulation techniques (palliative, not curative)
  - subchondral drilling
  - abrasion arthroplasty
  - microfracture
- Resurfacing techniques
  - osteochondral autograft transplantation
  - autologous cultured chondrocyte implantation
  - perichondral / periosteal transplantation
  - allograft osteochondral transplantation
  - resurfacing with carbon fibre
- Late procedures
  - altering joint loading by osteotomies or joint distraction
  - joint replacement
  - arthrodesis
- Non-surgical methods to enhance healing
  - continuous passive motion
  - hyaluronate
  - implantation of growth factors
  - miscellaneous: steroids, electrical stimulation, lasers

remaining quite functional for varying periods of time. Most techniques (see box) report approximately 70% satisfactory results.

The outcome of articular cartilage repair depends on understanding the following complex issues: the size and thickness, the location and the degree of containment of the lesion, chronic versus acute condition, previous repair, ligament and meniscal integrity, and alignment. Femoral condylar defects of less than 2 cm² ('smaller lesions') have the best prognosis. If the lesion is stable and contained, simple debridement for low-demand patients and a bone marrow stimulating technique (e.g. microfracture) for higher-demand patients is appropriate. If these simpler procedures fail, the surgeon can offer osteochondral autograft transplantation (OAT, mosaicplasty) or autologous chondrocyte implantation (ACI). If there is no major associated ligament, meniscal, or alignment pathology, results should be reasonably successful in the short term (3–5 years), probably without progression to arthritis.

For lesions more than 2 cm² in size, the results of simpler procedures are less predictable. The probability of progressing to arthritis is higher, because repair tissue is unable to contain the defect. The surgeon can try debridement with or without subchondral perforation in low-demand patients. In the higher-demand group it may be appropriate to proceed to OAT, ACI, or another alternative as initial treatment if deemed cost-effective. In case of failure, it may be appropriate to attempt ACI or OAT again. Alternatively, one might proceed to osteochondral allograft transplantation. Tertiary failure of OAT or ACI transplantation may require realignment and block allograft or arthroplasty. For femoral osteochondritis dissecans lesions the initial approach should include refixation with bioabsorbable pins. This probably works only on relatively fresh osteochondral rather than chondral fragments. If this fails, OAT and ACI should be considered, especially in large and deep osteochondral lesions. It the lesion is particularly deep it may require a large cylindrical osteochondral allograft or staged procedure with an initial bone graft followed by ACI. There is still no satisfactory treatment for patellar chondral defects, and results are usually poor in the long run. The main problem is its thickness and shape, as well as the enormous compression and shearing forces inherent in the joint. Correcting patellofemoral malalignment is essential.

Areas of current research in cartilage repair include the use of cultured cells supported in engineered tissue. One approach is to massively increase the numbers of cells produced in culture by using bioreactors, mechanical devices that cause controlled movement of cells during culture, thereby improving their nutrition and allowing more rapid proliferation (Freed *et al.* 1993). Another source being explored is stem cells (Wakitani *et al.* 1994) taken from the bone marrow of the patient. These could be modified by culture conditions to produce cartilage cells and matrix. This method has the theoretical advantage of providing unlimited numbers of cells, avoiding the need to harvest them from the patient's joint.

Conclusion

At the current state of knowledge, it is probably not possible to recreate the anatomical structure of the articular cartilage with its collagen arcades, etc., even though it is possible to generate individual chondrocytes. At a recent conference of the International Cartilage Repair Society, all participants were in agreement that we are, as yet, unable to regenerate hyaline articular cartilage. This has been aptly summed up by Buckwalter (1999): 'the cells appear to produce the correct components, but they can't seem to put them together correctly to produce hyaline cartilage'. The outlook for the future is encouraging. However, as we understand this complex process, more questions will be raised than answered. Yet, efforts must go on to attempt answering these difficult questions if advances are to be made that could ultimately lead to replacement of damaged articular cartilage, restoration of joint function, and prevention of the development of arthritis. These developments in treating knee joints will in time have applications in other joints.

Knee instability

The normal stability and kinematics of the knee joint are maintained by the shape of the femoral and tibial condyles and the menisci in combination with the passive supporting structures consisting of the four major ligaments: ACL, PCL, MCL, and LCL. Significant contributions are also made by the posteromedial and posterolateral capsular components and the iliotibial tract. All of these structures provide primary static stability. The muscles acting over the joint provide secondary dynamic stability. Instability resulting from ligament injury results from both direct and indirect trauma. The non-contact mechanism is the most frequent, occurring with activities that involve cutting, twisting, jumping, and sudden deceleration.

In acute injuries, early swelling (indicative of a haemarthrosis) and hearing or feeling a 'pop' (highly suggestive of an ACL injury) are significant events. Chronic instabilities present with mechanical symptoms such as locking, catching, clicking, or giving way, particularly with twisting movements. Age, occupation, lifestyle, level of sporting activity, and past medical and surgical history should all be

noted, as all these factors are considered in the subsequent management. Investigations must include plain radiographs of the knee. Anteroposterior, lateral and skyline views are the minimum. These may show fractures, avulsions, osteochondral fragments, or a fluid level of a haemarthrosis. If these allow a clear diagnosis, a specific treatment can be started. If an adequate examination is possible, but diagnosis is inconclusive, an expectant policy of mobilization, physiotherapy, and re-evaluation in approximately 2 weeks may be adopted. If adequate examination is not possible due to pain, spasm, etc. in the acute case, the options available are: re-evaluation, MRI, or examination under anaesthetic and arthroscopy. MRI is particularly useful because of its non-invasive nature, but it is not universally available in the UK as an emergency investigation. MRI is valuable in making an early diagnosis in multiple ligament injuries and peripheral tears of the meniscus, thereby influencing management.

Medial collateral ligament

The MCL is attached proximally to the medial femoral condyle and distally to the tibial metaphysis, 4–5 cm distal to the medial joint line beneath the pes anserinus insertion. Posterior to the MCL is the posterior oblique ligament (POL), which is a thickening of the capsule. Immediately deep to the MCL is the medial capsular ligament. These constitute the medial ligament complex. The MCL has a superficial portion, (the primary static stabilizer to valgus stress) and the deeper meniscotibial and meniscofemoral portion. In full extension, the POL and the posteromedial capsule resist valgus stresses. These relax at 20–30° of flexion, when the MCL becomes the primary restraint. The MCL together with the POL resists abnormal internal tibial rotation. Isolated injuries occur usually as a result of a direct blow to the lateral aspect of the knee in a slightly flexed position. When the deforming force includes a rotational component, associated injuries to the cruciate ligaments can occur.

Assessment of the acute injury includes looking for a localized bruise or swelling, localized tenderness, and application of a gentle valgus force with the patient's knee in 15–20° of flexion (flexion beyond this tends to produce internal rotation of the limb at the hip). The degree of medial joint opening compared to the normal knee is a measure of damage to the MCL. A difference of only 5–8 mm is indicative of significant structural damage to the MCL because of its parallel collagen arrangement (Indelicato 1995). This is now repeated with the knee in full extension, to evaluate the extent of the medial soft tissue damage. Excessive opening in full extension is indicative of combined MCL and posterior oblique ligament damage, and should alert the examiner to the strong possibility of an associated ACL or PCL injury. If the knee is stable in full extension, one can safely assume that there is no significant damage to the posterior oblique ligament.

Treatment of acute, isolated MCL injury is conservative (Indelicato 1995). Incomplete tears (sprains) of the MCL without significant instability are treated with RICE during the first 48 hours. This is followed by temporary immobilization and the use of crutches for pain control. Weightbearing as tolerated is encouraged as soon as pain allows, followed by early functional rehabilitation.

Chronic MCL insufficiency is rare in isolation and is usually associated with ACL or PCL injury. Careful examination must differentiate between MCL with or without posteromedial rotary instability. Symptomatic medial instability not improved with conservative treatment usually requires surgery in the form of proximal advancement of the MCL (Shahane and Bickerstaff 1998). Posteromedial rotary instability may require reconstruction of posterior oblique ligament with free hamstring graft.

The anterior cruciate ligament

The ACL is intracapsular but extrasynovial. Its femoral attachment is on the lateral wall of the intercondylar notch at its posterior aspect. The tibial attachment is on the anterior aspect of the tibial plateau near the tibial spines. The ACL has been described as having an anteromedial band which is tighter in flexion and a posterolateral band which is tighter in extension (Amis *et al.* 1991). This arrangement of the fascicles allows different portions to be taut throughout the range of motion, allowing the ligament to be functional in all degrees of flexion and extension. Its main source of blood supply is the middle genicular artery, a branch of the popliteal artery that approaches by piercing the posterior capsule. It has also been shown to contain proprioceptive nerve endings (Biedert *et al.* 1992). The ACL is the primary restraint to anterior translation of the tibia on the femur and to hyperextension (Fu *et al.* 1993). It functions as a secondary restraint to varus or valgus angulation at full extension. It also resists internal and external rotation mostly near full extension than in early flexion.

Diagnosis is made by a positive **Lachman's test** and a positive **pivot shift (or jerk) test**. Plain radiographs may show an avulsion of the insertion of the ACL or a Segond fracture which is a lateral capsular avulsion fracture from the margin of the lateral tibial plateau that is often associated with an ACL injury. MRI has an overall accuracy of approximately 90% in assessing the ACL (Glashow *et al.* 1989) although this need not be used routinely. MRI also shows bone abnormalities not seen on conventional radiographs. These include 'bone bruises', seen in approximately 60% of ACL injuries (Graf *et al.* 1993), the significance and long-term sequelae of which have yet to be determined. Examination under anaesthetic and arthroscopy is only required if there is still doubt after clinical examination and/or MRI scan.

It is widely accepted that an acute repair is associated with poor results, including a higher re-rupture rate and arthrofibrosis (Harner *et al.* 1992). Hence the initial treatment is based on the reduction of pain and swelling and early restoration of normal joint movement. The goal of treatment for ACL deficiency is to prevent re-injury which otherwise may lead to chondral injuries, meniscal injuries, or laxity of secondary restraints. These secondary injuries are thought to lead to arthritis although progression to radiologically detectable osteoarthritis appears to be variable (Frank and Jackson 1997). I am aware of no study in the literature that suggests that ACL reconstruction to stabilize the knee prevents the development of arthritis. Once ACL deficiency is diagnosed, the decision between operative and non-operative treatment is based on variables that are unique to each individual. Among the factors considered are the patient's age, activity level (recreational/occupational), the degree of laxity, associated meniscal or ligamentous pathology, ability and willingness to participate in a physiotherapy programme, and future expectations including the type of sporting activity in which the patient wishes to participate.

One of the studies most useful in discussing the management of ACL deficiency with a patient is that by Daniel *et al.* (1994) which has shown that the ability of a patient to cope with ACL insufficiency is related to both the amount of instability present and to the type and

Sporting activities: high, medium, and low risk

Activities can be graded as low risk (level 3) to high risk (level 1) depending on the risk to the ACL-deficient knee.
- **Low-risk** activities such as cycling, swimming, stair-climbing and rowing are level 3 sports.
- **Medium-risk** activities such as skiing, tennis, and golf constitute level 2. Although level 2 sports involve pivoting this is predictable and a patient can usually prepare for it.
- Level 1 (**high-risk**) sports include high-level skiing, basketball, football, soccer, and volleyball where there is considerable risk that the patient can be caught off-guard and suffer a twisting injury without time to prepare for it. Patients with ACL insufficiency are best advised to avoid participation in level 1 sports unless the ACL is surgically reconstructed.

intensity of sports participation. This prospective outcome study followed up 292 patients for an average of 5 years. Those patients who had less than 5 mm anteroposterior movement and who participated for 50 hours or less in level 1 or 2 sports had a low risk of needing further surgery. Those patients with a 7 mm or greater anteroposterior movement with more than 50 hours of level 1 or 2 sporting activity were in the high risk group.

Older people are often more willing to modify their activities but surgery may be required even in these individuals, if the laxity level is so great that their activities of daily living are impaired or, as is increasingly seen, they are unwilling to stop pivoting sports. As patients do not tolerate instability in two major ligaments well, the presence of associated injuries also influences decision-making in the direction of surgery. Also in cases in which meniscal repair is undertaken, ACL reconstruction is advisable because the failure rate of meniscal repair is too large in the presence of ACL instability (Hanks *et al.* 1990).

Non-operative management of acute ACL tears is likely to be successful in those patients who have no associated injuries, and are willing to give up high-demand sports. The rehabilitation programme emphasizes proprioceptive muscle training to maximize the dynamic stability. Non-operative management also includes counselling concerning high-risk activities and measures to prevent recurrent injuries. The role of functional knee bracing remains controversial (Wojtys and Huston 1998). Braces were thought to provide protection by improving joint position sense and by providing mechanical constraint of joint motion. Some patients report they have less instability in a brace, allowing them to participate in an increased level of sporting activity. However, the use of a brace cannot substitute for lack of quadriceps or hamstring training and it certainly cannot assure protection from further injury.

Surgical techniques have been described for intra-articular and extra-articular reconstructions of the ACL using iliotibial band, the semitendinosus and gracilis tendons, the patellar tendon, allograft tissue, and various synthetic materials. Currently intra-articular techniques are most commonly used. The surgical technique requires proper placement and tensioning of the graft, avoidance of impingement, and stress risers on the implanted tissue and adequate fixation. The available graft materials are broadly divided into autografts, allografts, and synthetic grafts.

Autogenous grafts are most commonly employed in ACL reconstruction. They provide a framework for revascularization and regeneration of the ligament and with modern fixation techniques allow rapid rehabilitation. Allografts heal in a similar fashion but at a slower rate. There is also a risk of disease transmission. They are therefore more widely used when there are no autograft alternatives. Synthetic grafts, although the most attractive, have not proved successful in the long term. Surgeons differ in their preference of autogenous tissue. The patellar tendon graft (B-PT-B) has greater initial tensile strength and allows more secure bone-to-bone fixation. Most surgeons report 80–90% good or excellent results using autogenous B-PT-B. Patellar fracture, tendinitis, anterior knee pain, and increased incidence of infrapatellar contracture syndrome have been described with their use. Patellar fracture can usually be avoided by improved technique. Patellar tendinitis is usually short-lived and after 1 year is generally not a problem; however, anterior knee pain appears to be more significant with this graft source than with hamstring reconstruction.

Use of semitendinosus and gracilis tendon grafts for reconstruction of the ACL has now been well established as they have been postulated to offer certain advantages. They provide a stronger ACL substitute when both are used together. Their stiffness characteristics mimic the normal ACL more closely than does the stiffer patellar tendon graft. Multiple strands of the hamstring grafts also allow a better opportunity for revascularization. These offer an ideal alternative in skeletally immature patients (where harvesting patellar graft can jeopardize the tibial apophysis), in women for cosmetic reasons, or when there is extensor mechanism pathology. Hamstring harvest is associated with minimal graft site morbidity (Yasuda et al. 1995). Both direct and indirect clinical comparisons have shown that B-PT-B grafts and hamstring grafts have similar rates of effectiveness in adults, with only minimal variations in knee stability and muscle strength at an average of 3 years after implantation (Otero and Hutcheson 1993).

Postoperative rehabilitation is an important aspect of care of ACL-deficient patients. Previously, rehabilitation focused on protection of the new ligament with block to full extension and avoidance of active quadriceps contraction to prevent anterior tibial translation stressing the graft. This led to stiffness of the knees and patellofemoral problems. Shelbourne and Nitz (1990) advocated an accelerated rehabilitation protocol, the objective being early and long-term maintenance of full knee extension, improving results. This protocol was based on the use of patellar tendon graft, although the principles are similar with other types of grafts.

The lateral collateral ligament and the posterolateral corner

The LCL originates on the lateral epicondyle of the femur and is attached distally on the fibular head. The LCL is relatively rarely injured in isolation and is usually injured as part of a complex involving the posterolateral corner, the PCL, or the ACL. The posterolateral corner is a complex anatomical region of the knee consisting of the popliteus tendon, the popliteofibular ligament, the arcuate ligament, and the posterolateral joint capsule. The lateral and the posterolateral corner complex can be considered as consisting of three layers – the iliotibial tract and the superficial portion of the biceps femoris forming the first layer; the LCL as the second layer; and the joint capsule, the arcuate ligament, the popliteofibular ligament and the popliteal tendon as constituting the third layer. The LCL is the primary static stabilizer to the lateral opening of the joint supplemented by the popliteofibular ligament and the cruciates. The popliteofibular ligament is the primary restraint to posterolateral rotation, supplemented by the LCL and the popliteus tendon (Shahane et al. 1999).

The most useful tests in differentiating between isolated LCL, PCL, and PLC or combined PCL–PLC injuries are the varus stress test, passive external rotation of the tibia (relative to the femur) with the knee at 30° and 90° of flexion, and the reverse Lachman test (see earlier). Tests such as the **external rotation recurvatum test**, reversed pivot shift test, and a posterior drawer test performed with the foot in external rotation, i.e. the **posterolateral drawer test**, may also be performed for additional confirmation but are not particularly specific. The patient's limb alignment and gait pattern must be observed to ensure there is no lateral thrust on walking. If this is not recognized, the ligament reconstruction may fail in the absence of a corrective osteotomy. MRI is useful in the acute setting to identify associated cruciate injury, the site of injury to the structures in the posterolateral corner, which will help plan surgery.

The data available on surgical outcomes for posterolateral reconstruction is limited. The wide variety of procedures used to treat patients with posterolateral instability makes it difficult to derive a consensus on the most effective and appropriate approach to this clinical entity. With acute injuries of the posterolateral corner, surgical intervention within 2 weeks of the initial injuries is optimal (Jakob and Middleton 1998) with the direct repair of all injured structures where possible. If the LCL or the popliteofibular ligament is ruptured mid substance, then consideration should be given to reconstruction of these structures as direct repair in isolation may be insufficient. In the chronic setting direct repair is often not possible and a variety of techniques can be used, including tissue advancement and augmentation with autograft or allograft tissues. I use hamstring autografts to reconstruct the lateral collateral and the popliteofibular ligaments similar to the technique described by Larson (Kumar et al. 1999). If there is a varus thrust, I prefer to perform an opening medial wedge osteotomy to avoid any further slackening of the lateral structures one may see with a lateral closing wedge osteotomy.

Posterior cruciate ligament

PCL injuries account for 15–20% of knee ligament injuries (Cooper et al. 1991). They are increasingly recognized as occurring in sporting injuries. It is likely that the apparent increase in incidence is due to more frequent recognition. The PCL takes origin from the medial femoral condyle with its attachment in the shape of a semicircle. It inserts in a depression between the posterior aspect of the two tibial plateaus, approximately 1 cm below the articular surface. Functionally it is composed of two bundles, anterolateral and posteromedial. In mid range of flexion (40–120°) the anterolateral bundle is the primary restraint to posterior drawer. The posteromedial bundle increases its contribution towards full flexion (Race and Amis 1996). Earlier studies have shown that the anterolateral bundle to be structurally and biomechanically more significant (Harner and Xerogeanes 1995). Recent studies (Race et al. 1998) recommend reconstruction of both the bundles to restore the normal function of the PCL throughout the range of motion.

The PCL is the primary static restraint to posterior translation of the tibia. It is a secondary stabilizer to varus angulation and external tibial rotary displacement at 90° of knee flexion. The mechanism of most sporting PCL injuries is a fall on the flexed knee with the foot in plantar flexion. This imparts the force to the tibial tubercle, pushing the tibia posteriorly and usually resulting in an isolated PCL rupture. Hyperflexion of the knee without a direct blow to the tibia can also cause isolated PCL injury. Forced hyperextension can injure the PCL, but this usually is combined with injury to the ACL. Posteriorly directed force to the anteromedial tibia with the knee in hyperextension may also cause a posterolateral corner injury; this results in varus in external rotation knee instability. Significant varus or valgus stress will injure the PCL only after rupture of the appropriate collateral ligament. In isolation there is often little instability, whereas when associated with posterolateral or posteromedial injuries, stability of the knee is dramatically reduced.

Plain radiographs may show a PCL avulsion fracture. MRI has proved to be sensitive and specific for diagnosis of acute PCL injury. It can be used to confirm meniscal and chondral damage. Instrumented knee testing can also be used to confirm the diagnosis of PCL injury in combination with the quadriceps active test.

Management of **acute** isolated PCL injuries is conservative. Reconstruction is usually not required (Veltri and Warren 1993). If the degree of posterior translation is less than 10 mm, as in the majority of isolated injuries or even in those with small tibial PCL avulsion fractures, a non-operative aggressive rehabilitation programme is arranged. Following an initial period of RICE, an extension splint is worn for 3–4 weeks. Physiotherapy is focused especially on quadriceps strengthening. Close follow-up is necessary so that combined instability is not missed. If the avulsed fragment is large, it can be reduced and fixed through a posterior approach. If the posterior translation is greater than 10 mm without a firm endpoint, reconstruction is advised since it is likely that additional secondary restraints have been compromised. If significant chondral or meniscal injuries are suspected based on MRI, an arthroscopy is performed to deal with them. Acute surgical treatment of complete PCL tears can include primary repair or reconstruction depending on the location of injury. PCL reconstruction can be performed with a patellar tendon autograft, semitendinosus and gracilis autograft or a patella or achilles tendon allograft. The reconstruction of the PCL can be performed with open or arthroscopically assisted techniques. Arthroscopic procedure is performed under radiographic control using an additional posteromedial portal to assist in tibial tunnel preparation. This procedure is technically demanding. When an acute injury has posterolateral, ACL or grade III MCL components (that usually occurs in a spontaneously reduced dislocation of the knee), it appears best to operate early between 2–3 weeks to maximize healing potential and minimize stiffness (Good and Johnson 1995). One must particularly watch for any neurovascular injury.

For **chronic isolated PCL instability**, Parolie and Bergfeld (1986) reported good long-term results of non-operative treatment. At an average follow-up of 6.2 years, 80% of the patients were satisfied with their results and 84% had returned to their previous sport. Rehabilitation of the quadriceps to achieve the same strength as on the non-injured side correlated with successful results. Whether the PCL-deficient knee is at risk of the development of degenerative changes is currently not clear. Despite the lack of prospective studies it appears that progressive degenerative changes may occur in some PCL-deficient knees. Long-term results of surgical reconstructions for PCL instability remain unclear. I recommend non-operative treatment with quadriceps rehabilitation for the majority of patients initially. Recon-

struction is considered if the laxity is more than 10 mm at 90° of knee flexion or in the presence of symptoms that have not responded to rehabilitation treatment. Reconstruction is not performed if there is evidence of marked degenerative changes. No data are available to support reconstruction for pain, though corrective osteotomies are increasingly being performed. Hamstring autograft may be used for the reconstruction, reconstituting both the bundles of PCL with a suspensory form of fixation on the tibial side and interference fixation with bioabsorbable screws on the femoral side. Chronic combined injuries constitute a difficult problem. The principles of management include proper evaluation of the associated structures involved, and correction of limb alignment for reasons alluded to earlier.

Postoperative rehabilitation following PCL reconstruction is designed to restore range of motion without stressing the graft. Exercises that produce posterior tibial translation are avoided. Limited weightbearing using crutches is allowed with a PCL knee brace allowing full range of movements for 6 weeks. Following the early rehabilitation programme, running begins at about 5 months and sports and physical activity commences at 6–7 months. Full range of sports is allowed when adequate quadriceps and hamstrings strength is demonstrated after about 9 months.

Conclusion

It is hoped that future basic science and clinical studies and further technical experience with various reconstructive procedures will continue to improve both our understanding and surgical outcomes for the instabilities of the knee. Collagen engineering and developments in prosthetic ligaments are likely to play an increasing role, avoiding graft harvest. Long-term studies on the outcomes of PCL reconstruction may clarify whether early reconstruction of the PCL prevents late degenerative changes. Long-term studies to evaluate the role of factors other than mechanical, such as local intra-articular cytokines released at the time of injury, in the development of degenerative changes in chronic ligament injury are being explored. (Price *et al.* 1999) This could lead to prevention of early degenerative changes of articular cartilage following ligament injuries.

References

Amis, A. A. *et al.* (1991) Functional anatomy of ACL: fibre bundle action related to ligament replacement and injuries. *J. Bone Joint Surg.*, **73B**(2), 260–7.

Apley, A. G., Solomon, L. (1982) *Apley's system of orthopaedics and fractures*, 6th edn. Butterworths, London.

Arnoczky, S. P., Warren, R. F. (1982) Microvasculature of the human meniscus. *Am J. Sports Med.*, **10**, 90.

Bach, B. R. Jr, Warren, R. F., Wickiewicz, T. L. (1988) The pivot shift phenomenon: results and a description of a modified clinical test for anterior cruciate ligament instability. *Am. J. Sports Med.*, **16**(6), 571–6.

Biedert, R. M., Stauffer, E., Friederich, N. F. (1992) Occurrence of free nerve endings in the soft tissues of the knee joint – a histologic investigation. *Am. J. Sports Med.*, **20**, 430–3.

Buckwalter, J. A. (1999) Evaluating methods of restoring cartilaginous articular surfaces. *Clin. Orthop.*, **244**, 238.

Cooper, D. E., Warren, R. F. *et al.* (1991) The PCL and the posterolateral structures of the knee: anatomy, function and patterns of injury. *Instr. Course Lectures*, **40**, 249–70.

Curl, W. W., Krome, J., Gordon, S., Rushing, J., Smith, B. P., Poehling, G. G. (1997) Cartilage injuries: a review of 31, 516 knee arthroscopies. *Arthroscopy*, **13**, 456–60.

Dandy, D. J. (1990) The arthroscopic anatomy of the symptomatic meniscal lesion .J. Bone Joint Surg., **72B**(4), 628.

Dandy, D. J. (1997) Arthroscopy and MRI of the knee. *J. Bone Joint Surg.*, **79B**, 520.

Daniel, D. M., Stone, M. L. *et al.* (1994) Fate of the ACL injured patient – a prospective outcome study. *Am. J. Sports Med.*, **22**(5), 632–44.

Draper, D. O., Schulthies, S. S. (1995) Examiner proficiency in performing the anterior draw and Lachman tests. *J. Orthop. Sports Phys. Ther.*, **22**(6), 263–6.

Evans, P. J., Bell, G. D., Frank, C. (1993) Prospective evaluation of the McMurray test. *Am. J. Sports Med.*, **21**(4), 604–8.

Flandrey, F., Hughston, J. C., McCann, S. B., Kurtz, D. M. (1994) Diagnostic features of diffuse pigmented villonodular synovitis of the knee. *Clin. Orthop.*, **298**, 212–20.

Frank, C. B., Jackson, D. W. (1997) The science of reconstruction of ACL. *J. Bone Joint Surg.*, **79A**(10), 1556–76.

Freed, L. E., Vunjak-Novakovic, G., Langer, R. (1993) Cultivation of cell-polymer cartilage implants in bioreactors. *J. Cell. Biochem.*, **51**, 257–64.

Fu, F. H., Harner, C. D. *et al.* (1993) Biomechanics of knee ligaments – basic concepts and clinical applications, ICL. *J. Bone Joint Surg.*, **75A**(11), 1716–27.

Galway, H. R., MacIntosh, .D. L. (1980) The lateral pivot shift a symptom and sign of anterior cruciate ligament instability. *Clin. Orthop.*, **147**, 45–50.

Glashow, J. L. *et al.* (1989) Double blind assessment of the value of MRI in the diagnosis of ACL meniscal lesions. *J. Bone Joint Surg.*, **71A**, 113–19.

Good, L., Johnson, R. J. (1995) The dislocated knee. *J. Am. Acad. Orthop. Surg.*, **3**, 284–92.

Graf, B. K., Cook, D. A., De Smet, A. A. *et al.* (1993) Bone bruises on MRI evaluation of ACL injuries. *Am. J. Sports Med.*, **22**, 220–3.

Hanks, G. A., Gause, T. M., Handal, J. A. *et al.* (1990) Meniscus repair in the ACL deficient knee. *Am. J. Sports Med.*, **18**, 606–13.

Hardaker, W. T. Jr., Garrett, W. E. Jr., Bassett, F. H. (1990) I. I.I: Evaluation of acute traumatic haemarthrosis of the knee joint. *Southern Med. J.*, **83**, 640–4.

Harner, C. D., Irrgang, J. J., Paul, J. *et al.* (1992) Loss of motion after ACL reconstruction. *Am. J. Sports Med.*, **20**(5), 499–506.

Harner, C. D., Xerogeanes, J. W. (1995) The human PCL complex: an interdisciplinary study – ligament morphology and biomechanical events. *Am. J. Sports Med.*, **23**, 736–45.

Indelicato, P. A. (1995) Isolated MCL injuries in the knee. *J. Am. Acad. Orthop. Surg.*, **3**, 1.

Jakob, R. P., Middleton, R. G. (1998) Posterolateral instability. In: *Controversies in orthopaedic sports medicine.* Williams & Wilkins, Baltimore, MD, pp. 158–67.

Kumar, A., Jones, S., Bickerstaff, D. R. (1999) Posterolateral reconstruction of the knee: a tunnel technique for proximal fixation. The Knee, .

Levy, A. S., Lohnes, J., Sculley, S. *et al.* (1996) Chondral delamination of the knee in soccer players. *Am. J. Sports Med.*, **24**(5), 634–9.

Maffuli, N., Binfield, P. M., King, J. B., Good, C. J. (1993) Acute haemarthrosis of the knee in athletes. A prospective study of 106 cases. *J. Bone Joint Surg.*, **75B**(6), 945–9.

Miller, M. D., Bergfeld, J. A., Fowler, P. J., Harner, C. D., Noyes, F. R. (1999) The posterior cruciate ligament injured knee: principles of evaluation and treatment. *Instr. Course Lect.*, **48**, 199–207.

Nielsen, S., Rasmusson, O., Oveson, J., Andersen, K. (1984) Rotatory instability of cadaver knees after transection of collateral ligaments and capsule. *Arch. Orthop. Trauma Surg.*, **103**(3), 165–9.

Otero, A. L., Hutcheson, L. (1993) A comparison of the doubled semitendinosus/ gracilis and central third of the patellar tendon autografts in arthroscopic ACL reconstruction. *Arthroscopy*, **9**, 143–8.

Parolie, J. M., Bergfeld, J. A. (1986) Long term results of non-operative treatment of isolated PCL injuries in the athlete. *Am. J. Sports Med.*, **14**, 35–8.

Potter, H. G., Linklater, J. M., Allen, A. A. *et al.* (1998) Magnetic resonance imaging of articular cartilage in the knee. *J. Bone J. Surg.*, **80A**, 1276–84.

Price, J. S., Till, S. H., Bickerstaff, D. R. *et al.* (1999) Degradation of cartilage type II collagen precedes the onset of OA following ACL rupture. *Arthritis Rheum.*, **42**(11), 2390–8.

Race, A., Amis, A. A. (1996) Loading of the two bundles of the PCL – an analysis of bundle function in a posterior drawer. *J. Biomech.*, **29**(7), 873–9.

Race, A., Amis, A. A. *et al.* (1998) P. C.L reconstruction: In vitro biomechanical comparison of 'isometric' versus single and double bundle anatomic grafts. *J. Bone Joint Surg.*, **80B**(1), 173–9.

Shahane, S. A., Bickerstaff, D. R. (1998) Proximal advancement of the medial collateral ligament for chronic medial instability of the knee joint. *The Knee*, **5**, 191–7.

Shahane, S. A., Bickerstaff, D. R. *et al.* (1999) The popliteo-fibular ligament – an anatomic study of the posterolateral corner of the knee. *J. Bone Joint Surg.*, **81B**(4), 636–42.

Shelbourne, K. D., Nitz, P. (1990) Accelerated rehab after ACL reconstruction. *Am. J. Sports Medicine*, **18**, 292–9.

Simonian, P. T., Fealy, S., Hidaka, C., O'Brien, S. J.,Warren, R. F. (1998) Anterior cruciate ligament injury and patella dislocation: a report of nine cases. *Arthroscopy*, **14**(1), 80–4.

Staubli, H. U. (1994) Posteromedial and posterolateral capsular injuries associated with posterior cruciate ligament insufficiencies. *Sports Med. Arth. Rev.*, **2**, 146–64.

Stratford, P. W., Binkley, J. (1995) A review of the McMurray test definition, interpretation and clinical usefulness. *J. Orthop. Sports Phys. Ther.*, **22**(3), 116–20.

Torg, J. S., Conrad, W., Kalen, V. (1976) Clinical diagnosis of anterior cruciate ligament instability in athletes. *Am. J. Sports Med.*, **4**(2). 84–93.

Twyman, R. S., Desai, K., Aichroth, P. M. (1991) Osteochondritis dissecans of the knee. A long term study. *J.Bone J. Surg.*, **73B**(3), 461–4.

Veltri, D. M.,Warren, R. F. (1993) Isolated and combined PCL injuries. *J. Am. Acad. Orthop. Surg.*, **1**, 2.

Veltri, D. M., Warren, R. F. (1994) Posterolateral instability of the knee. *J. Bone Joint Surg.*, **76A**, 460–74.

Wakitani, S., Goto, T., Pineda, S., Young, R., Mansour, J., Caplan, A. *et al.* (1994) Mesenchymal cell-based repair of large, full thickness defects of articular cartilage. *J. Bone J. Surg.*, **76A**, 579–92.

Wojtys, E. M.. Huston, L. J. (1998) Functional knee braces – the 25 year controversy. In: *Controversies in orthopaedic sports medicine*, pp. 106–115, Williams & Wilkins, Baltimore, MD.

Yasuda, K., Tsujimo, J., *et al.* (1995) Graft site morbidity with autogenous semitendinosus/gracilis tendons. *Am. J. Sports Med.*, **23**(6), 206–14.

3.7.2 Patellofemoral disorders; chondromalacia dysfunction, maltracking and plica syndrome

Nicholas Peirce

It is clear that the patellofemoral joint is a complex articulation, depending on both dynamic and static restraints for stability. Consequently, classifications of patellofemoral disorders have been numerous and somewhat confusing. Several attempts to classify patellofemoral disorders have been made, including those by Fulkerson and Shea (1990). In order to facilitate appropriate treatment, patellofemoral problems in the skeletally mature patient can be divided into three broad categories, as shown in Figure 3.7.5, which can usually be ascertained from the history and examination:

- patellofemoral pain with instability, i.e. subluxation or dislocation
- patellofemoral pain with malalignment but no episodes of instability
- patellofemoral pain without malalignment.

Patellofemoral disorders

Anterior knee pain has received extensive attention over the years, both in the clinical and the academic setting. It represents up to 50% of all knee injuries, and is the most common presentation to sports injuries clinics, accounting for 25–33% of all visits.(Kannus *et al.* 1987, Hahn and Foldspang 1998, Mummery *et al.* 1998) Anterior knee pain customarily follows chronic overload of the extensor mechanism, including the patellofemoral joint, the patellar tendon, and its bony attachments, but can be associated with traumatic episodes. As the name implies, it is very much an umbrella term encompassing a huge variety of disorders of the extensor mechanism, patellofemoral joint, and associated structures outlined in Table 3.7.2. In this chapter an attempt will be made to distinguish between the different conditions that predispose to anterior knee pain including patellofemoral pain, patella dislocations, synovial plica, extensor mechanism pains including patella tendonitis, and some of the uncommon but important differential diagnoses to consider. After an injury has been defined as traumatic or non-traumatic, the anterior knee pain can be classified using the algorithm in Figure 3.7.5.

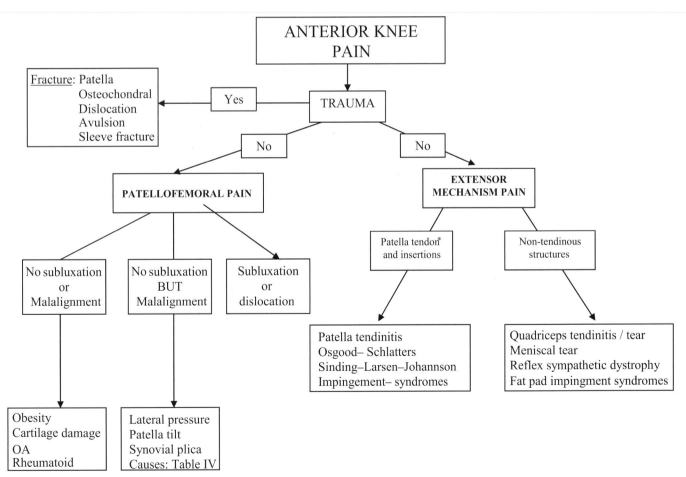

Figure 3.7.5 Anterior knee pain algorithm.

Table 3.7.2. Causes of anterior knee pain

Common cause	Moderately common	Rare
Patellofemoral pain syndrome	Bursae: prepatellar superior/deep infrapatellar	Reflex sympathetic dystrophy
Patella tendonosis (jumper's knee)	Lateral retinacular / medial plicae	Referred pain
Osgood–Schlatters disease	Sinding-Larsen–Johansson syndrome	Malignancy
Patellar subluxation/dislocation	Fat pad syndrome Quadriceps tendinitis/rupture	Anterior impingement Nerve injuries

Patellofemoral pain

Aetiology

Patellofemoral pain syndrome (PFPS) has become increasingly accepted as a unifying description of any condition that produces retropatellar pain and possible cartilage changes, excluding acute episodes of dislocation of the patella. Despite the prevalence of PFPS, there is still some controversy over its aetiology and diagnosis. This is highlighted by the huge variety of titles that have been used to describe the spectrum of retropatellar discomfort: chondromalacia patellae, patellar chondropathy, patellofemoral arthralgia, patellalgia, lateral pressure syndrome, runner's knee, retropatellar knee pain. What is certain is that PFPS causes significant morbidity, threatening both routine activities and sporting ambitions typically in adolescents of both sexes, although with greater severity in young women.

The cause of pain is unknown, although until recently it was thought to relate to the softening of the patella cartilage, chondromalacia patella, originally described by Koenig in 1924 (Owre 1934). Although this clinical condition does exist, cadaveric, imaging, and arthroscopic studies have clearly demonstrated it to be an incidental finding in asymptomatic individuals and have conversely demonstrated normal cartilage in patients with longstanding anterior knee pain (Casscells 1975, McGinty and McCarthy 1981, Bentley and Dowd 1984). Early changes in cartilage (softening, fissuring, and blister-like formations) have sometimes been shown to progress to underlying bone changes, appearing frequently over the areas of increased lateral pressure. Consequently, numerous studies have attempted both to map these changes and correlate them with patient symptoms and sites of established loading, with only partial success. Furthermore, as the cartilage itself has no neural innervation, mechanisms for retropatellar pain are only speculation and may be multifactorial, such as trauma-induced irritation of the retinacular nerves (Fulkerson *et al.* 1985), osteochondral microfractures, marginal synovitis, (Radin *et al.* 1984), and painful retinacular structures. What is strikingly apparent, however, is the correlation of anterior knee pain with increased activity and hours of participation in sport (Milgrom *et al.* 1996, Mummery *et al.* 1998).

Anatomy

The patellofemoral joint represents a functionally distinct articulation separate from the tibiofemoral joint, and some authors have considered it to be insufficiently advanced for the loads delivered by erect activity in humans (Dye 1987). The anterior distal femur forms a saddle-shaped trochlear groove in which the patella glides, with the lateral femoral condyle slightly more prominent to ensure midline

patella tracking and prevent lateral subluxation (Figure 3.7.6 opposite). (Tria *et al.* 1992) As the femoral sulcus increases beyond 150°, the patella is increasingly likely to subluxate or dislocate laterally (Figure 3.7.7), referred to as the **glide** of the patella (Figure 3.7.8). The patella

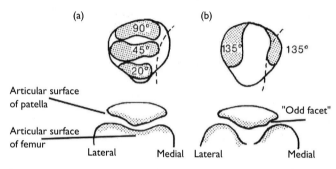

Figure 3.7.7 Articular surfaces of the patella during flexion: (at 80° flexion, (b) at 135° flexion. Contact remains minimal, until 10–20° of flexion, when the inferior pole of the patella and the femoral condyle meet. As flexion continues, contact is made between the middle and finally superior facets, only making contact with the odd facet after 120°. Modified from Ficat and Hungerford (1977).

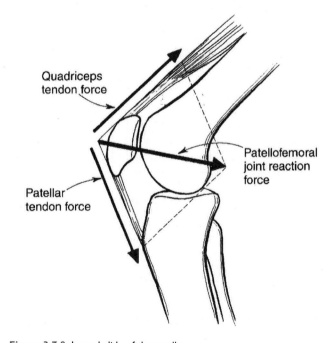

Figure 3.7.8 Lateral glide of the patella.

View	Knee flexion	Technique and position	Measurement	Implications
AP	0°	Standing feel straight ahead	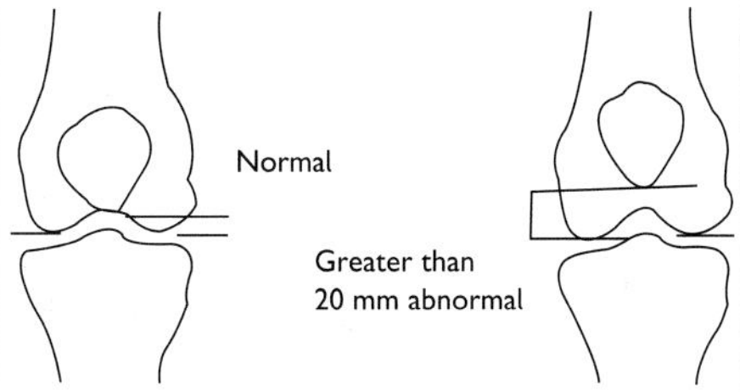 Normal — Greater than 20 mm abnormal	– Hypoplastic patella – Lateral subluxation patella – Biparlite patella – Asymmetry of femoral condylar (abnormal femoral anteversion or femoral rotation)
	90°	Supine	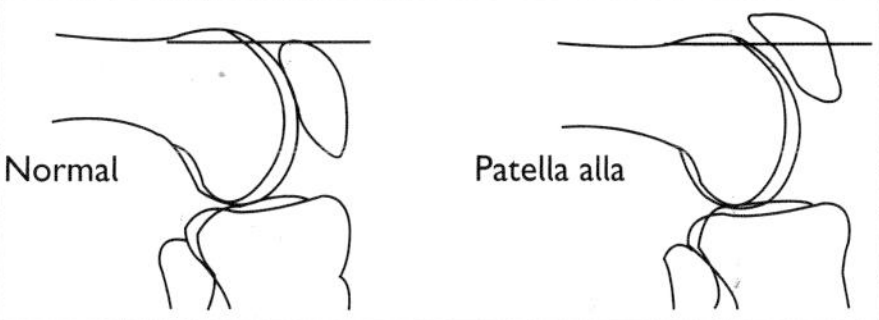 Normal — Patella alla	– Patella intera – Patellar tracture
Lateral	Approx 30°	Supine (Insali-Salvati)	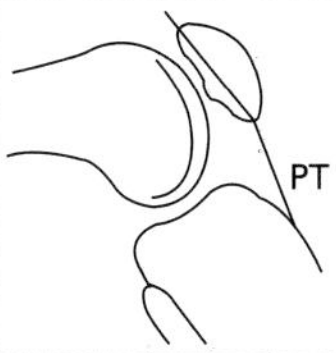 Ratio of P PT = 10 More than 20% vanation is abnormal	
	30°	Supine	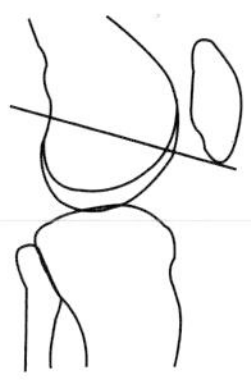 Blumensaat's line (see text)	
(Hughston) Tangenfial	55°	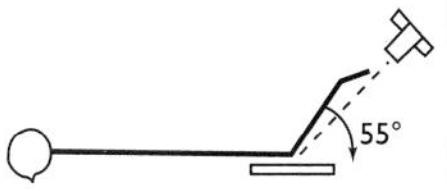 Prone position Beam duecled cephalad and intenor. 45 degrees from vertical	1) Sulcus angle: 118° 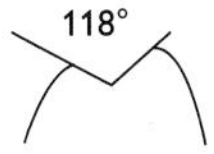 2) Patella index: 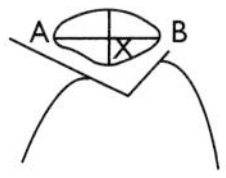 $$\frac{AB}{XB - XA}$$ NL Male 15 Female 17	– Patellar dislocation – Osteochondral tracture – Soft tissue calciticalion (old dislocated patella or tracture) – Patellar subluxation Patellar lilt Increased medial joint space Apex of patella lateral to apex of femoral sulcus Lateral patella edge lateral to femoral condyle Hypoptastic lateral lemoral condyle (usually proximal) – Patellofemoral osleophyles – Subchondral trabeculae onentation (increase or decrease) – Patellar configuration (Wiberg-Baugarll) 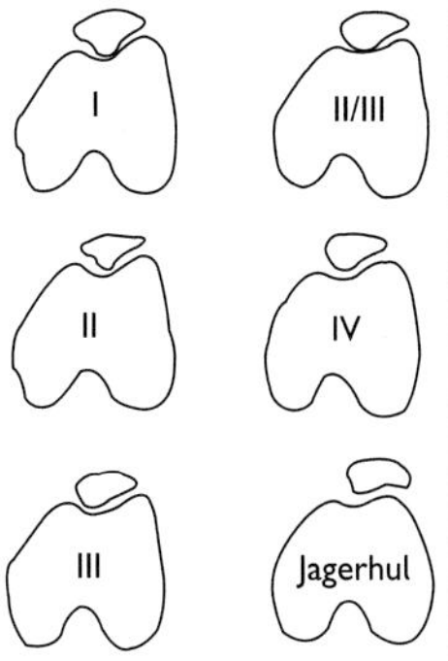
(Merchant) Tangenfial	45°	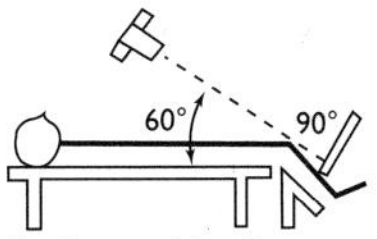 Supine position Beam duecled caudal and intenor. 30 degrees from vertical	1) Sulcus angle: 138° 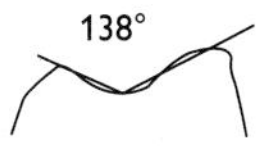 2) Congruence angle: 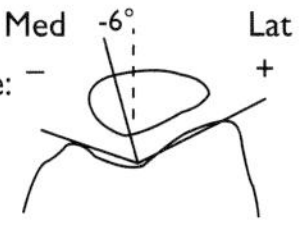 Med –6° Lat	
(Laurin) Tangenfial	20°	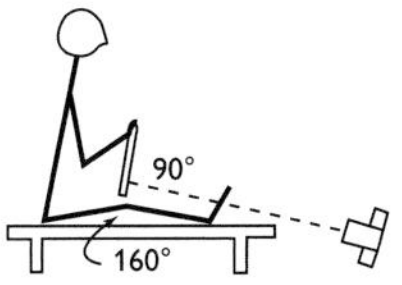 Sitting posilion Beam duecled cephaled and supenor. 160 degrees from vertical	1) Lateral patellofemoral angle: LAT 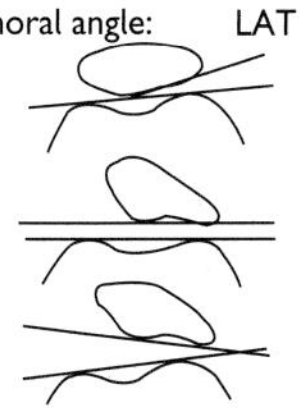 NL ABNL ABNL 2) Patellofemoral index: 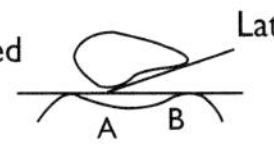 Ratro A/B Med Lat Normal = 16 or less	

Figure 3.7.6 Summary of radiological views and patellofemoral indices predisposing to patellofemoral disorders. (Adapted from Carson et al, with permission.)

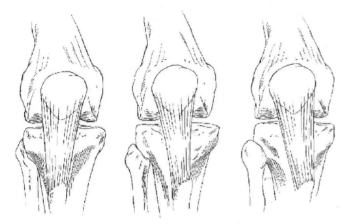

Figure 3.7.9 Patellofemoral joint reaction force. (Reprinted with permission from Chan *et al.*)

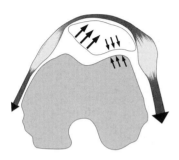

Figure 3.7.10 Normal alignment. Patellofemoral alignment is maintained by the Q angle, the angle formed between the line of the quadriceps (superior anterior iliac spine to the mid-patella) and the patellar tendon (mid-patella to tibial tuberosity) produces a resultant lateral force. Angles greater than 10° in men and 15° in women are considered abnormal and predispose to malalignment and an increasing displacement of the patella laterally (reprinted from Chan et al with permission).

tubercle), the **Q angle** (Figure 3.7.10) (Kaufner and Arbor 1971, Grabiner *et al.* 1994) . An excessive angle (more than 10° in men and 15° in women) encourages the patella to subluxate laterally, normally abolished after 30° flexion.

Patella maltracking

There now seems to be a general acceptance of the relationship between maltracking and PFPS, although there is a variety of possible causes for pain (Fulkerson and Shea 1990, Kannus and Nittymaki 1994). Increased patella height has been also shown to correlate with unilateral PFPS as determined by lateral radiographs. Patella height, defined as the ratio of the patellar ligament to the length of the patella, is measured by the Insall–Salvatti index. A value of greater than 1.2 is referred to as **patella alta**. This condition may predispose to subluxation, with a mean index of 1.17 for normal subjects and 1.30 for those with anterior knee pain (Kannus and Nittymaki 1994). The relationship between the patella configuration and the sulcus angle is also referred to as the **patella congruence** and can be represented by a variety of measurements outlined in Figure 3.7.10. These have been extensively described by Laurin *et al.* (1979) and Merchant (1988) and also include additional radiographic measures such as the lateral patellofemoral angle and patellofemoral index (Laurin *et al.* 1979) (Figure 3.7.6). Together these may be used to try and predict a tendency to subluxate, as well as the degree of patella tilt and glide. Maltracking and PFPS are also thought to arise from an imbalance of the medial restraints of the patella (53% of the total soft tissue restraining force derived from the medial patellofemoral ligament, with a small contribution from the medial patellomeniscal ligament and retinaculum; Conlan *et al.* 1993). Additionally, maltracking clearly appears to arise from inaction of the VMO (Lieb and Perry 1968), and it is widely recognized that weakness of the VMO and imbalance of the quadriceps musculature predisposes to maltracking

itself is in essence a large sesamoid bone within the extensor mechanism that articulates through the medial (convex) and lateral (concave) facets (Figure 3.7.6). Only distinct parts of these surfaces are in contact with the trochlea during flexion, further increasing the loading across the joint. This can reach up to 7–8 times body weight during jumping and squatting (reflected in the thickness of the articulator cartilage) and is often referred to as the patellofemoral joint reaction force (Figure 3.7.9). Thus the joint is exposed to significant stresses that may be exacerbated by uneven load distribution, produced by abnormalities in patella shape, malalignment, obesity, overuse, and subluxation or dislocation of the patella. An enormous continuum of patella shapes has been classified, e.g. by Wiberg (1941). Those that are most likely to produce problems are the dysplastic shapes such as patella magna and parva, and dysplasia of the femoral condyles (Figure 3.7.6) (Ficat and Hungerford 1977). Maintenance of normal patellar alignment and tracking within the trochlear groove is achieved by the V of the lateral and medial walls of the trochlear groove, the control of the quadriceps muscle groups, in particular the vastus medialis oblique (VMO), and the relative mobility of the medial and lateral retinaculum. Maltracking nevertheless appears to be common and is, in part, dependent on the resultant of the forces formed by the angle between the quadriceps insertion (anterior superior iliac spine and the mid-patella) and that of the patellar tendon (mid-patella to tibial

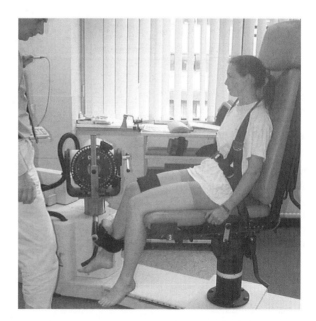

Figure 3.7.11 Lateral pressure syndrome and VMO dysplasia. Excessive lateral pressure can result from tight lateral retinacular structures, VMO dysplasia resulting in lateral glide, maltracking seen and lateral facet overload.

Table 3.7.3. Causes of patella malalignment

Structure	Condition
Pelvis/hip/lumbar spine	Gynecoid pelvis
Tibia	Genu varus/valgum/recurvatum
	Tibia vara/torsion
	Hyperpronation
Femur	Anteversion/retroversion
	Trochlear dysplasia
	Sulcus angle: widening
	Previous fractures/shortening
Quadriceps	VMO dysplasia/weakness/atrophy
	Vastus lateralis hypertrophy
	Rectus femoris tightness
Patella	Alta/baja/parva
	Dysplasia/odd facet
	Tilt
	Dysplasia/odd facet
Lateral structures	Tight ITB
	Tight lateral retinaculum

(Figure 3.7.11). VMO weakness can occur as a result of disuse atrophy, congenital dystrophy, or reflex pain inhibition and may not be detectable unless end-of-range and variable testing is undertaken with EMG and isokinetic measurements. Some of the many causes of malalignment are shown in Table 3.7.3.

Lateral patellar pressure syndrome

Also referred to as lateral compression syndrome, this condition describes PFPS that may arise from a tight lateral retinaculum, tight iliotibial band, and patella tilt (Figure 3.7.11). The distinguishing feature is no history of subluxation or variable maltracking, but instead constant loading of the lateral facets. This condition, characteristically, is no longer considered separately from PFPS and they will be considered together.

History

The patient with PFPS often has a variety of nondescript pains with an insidious onset and present since childhood. Crepitus, clicking, and pseudo-locking may all be associated with the dull aching, which is frequently bilateral. However, a history of trauma may be present, including a direct blow to the patella that may indicate localized articular cartilage changes. Otherwise patellofemoral pain is associated with eccentric activity, ascending and especially descending stairs, squatting, or prolonged flexion such as with sitting and driving. This has led to the term 'movie-goer's sign', when extension of the knee in an aisle seat may relieve patellofemoral pressure. Many of the symptoms are also found in inflamed plicae, which can also be associated with clicking and locking. Patella subluxation or dislocation is important to distinguish and is most commonly accompanied by subjective episode of 'giving way', often not associated with rotation. The patient may feel a popping sensation and often pain cause the knee to buckle,

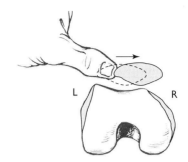

Figure 3.7.12 Glide/dislocation of the patella. Lateral displacement of the patella demonstrates the glide of the patella and may reproduce apprehension of an impending dislocation.

probably as a result of inhibition of the quadriceps mechanism. Swelling may also be seen occasionally in all forms of patellofemoral pain.

Examination

The assessment of patellofemoral pain is dependent on a careful analysis of the gait and alignment of the lower limb of the individual. As well as routine observation of effusions, deformity, and bruising, the tracking of the patella can be observed in standing, walking, and squatting. Sit the subject over the edge of a couch and palpate the femoral condyles. The lateral should be higher than the medial and in this position the knee can be taken through resisted extension with any lateral deviation or glide provoked. Palpate the medial edges for plica and retropatellar articular changes while assessing the glide and mobility of the patella and any apprehension indicative of subluxation (Figure 3.7.12). Inspection of the quadriceps musculature bulk, strength, flexibility and the activity during contractions is also important as well as assessing the tilt of the patella that may be associated with tight lateral retinaculum and iliotibial bands (Figure 3.7.13). The key examination points are outlined in Table 3.7.4.

Investigations

The radiographic imaging of patellofemoral disorders includes standard radiographs taken through the sulcus of the femoral condyle at varying degrees. These include skyline views at 30° and further views

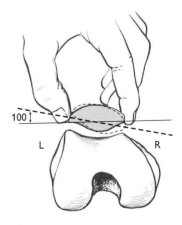

Figure 3.7.13 Tilt of the patella. Excessive tilt is demonstrated by deviation of more than 100° around the central axis. (Modified from Post *et al.*)

Table 3.7.4. Key examination points

Palpation	
Patella	Shape ?Hypotrophic ?Bipartite ?Dystrophic
	Bony tenderness ?apophysitis/stress fracture/ avulsion ?Trauma
	Inferior and superior poles ?apophysitis/ enthesopathy ?tendonopathy
Medial/Lateral Patella Joint Line	Plica, Retropatella Discomfort, ITB referred pain
Surrounding Structures	Tibio-femoral joint line, condylees, superior tibio-fibular joint, quadriceps muscle
Observation	
Alignment: (Static and Dynamic)	Medialisation/Lateralisation/Q-angle
	Alta/Baja/Tilt/Rotation
	Quadriceps tone and contractile activity
Inflammation	Bursa/Inflammation/Deformity/atrophy/Chronic Pain Syndrome
Gait	Hind-foot, forefoot pronation, hip ante-retroversion, leg length descrepancy, gluteal control, antalgia
Tibia/Ankle/Foot	Tibial torsion, cavoid foot, pes planus
Test	
Neural Tests	Femoral Nerve/Slump/SLR ?referred lumbar spine component
Active Test	Clarks Compression ?patello-femoral joint pain, crepitus
	Apprehension Test ?instability
	Plica fold test (lateral stretch of plica)
	Resisted Muscle tone
	Squatting/duck walk
Ultrasound	Routine observation of apophyseal/tendon pathology
Other Tests	Joint Hypermobility, local anaesthetic test, heel wedge/orthotic tests, taping, isokinetic, aspiration, activity provocation

at 40° and 60° that may show tilting or displacement of the patella. These are illustrated in Figure 3.7.6 (Insall and Salvati 1971, Hughston and Walsh 1979, Laurin *et al.* 1979, Merchant 1988). Recently ultrasound has been tried with varying success (Joshi and Heatley 1998) and most promising may be results from dynamic imaging using MRI (Miller *et al.* 1998).

Treatment

Non-surgical treatment

Non-surgical management of the PFPS centres on correcting any maltracking, improving tracking, and removing abnormal loads from the lateral facets and retinaculum. Provided gross traumatic changes of the cartilage and significant subluxating or dislocating individuals are identified, conservative measures for the treatment of patellofemoral pain are often successful and in up to 95% of cases produce resolution or significant improvement in symptoms (Natri *et al.* 1998, Post 1998). This

may also reflect the self-limiting nature of PFP. A wide variety of different management strategies is practised, reflecting the lack of consensus and evidence for consistent benefit from each technique. In a series of recent reviews, no one treatment strategy has been shown to be consistently effective when subject to randomized prospective study (Powers 1998). Treatment regimes include activity modification, exercises, stretches and regional soft tissue mobilization, orthotics, analgesia, and taping and bracing techniques, with only 2–3% requiring surgical intervention. A recent meta-analysis of clinical studies of many of these techniques found only five trials matched strict methodological criteria. Of these only strengthening exercises and injections with glycosaminoglycan polysulfate produced short-term benefits, with the remainder producing equivocal results (Arroll *et al.* 1997).

The mainstay of non-surgical treatment remains the correction of maltracking which can arise from VMO dysplasia or disuse atrophy. McConnell reported 96% success rate with an exercise and taping regime that is now extensively incorporated into many rehabilitation protocols. (McConnell 1986, Crichton 1989, Gerrard 1989) The purpose of the programme is to improve the timing, strength, and coordination of VMO/vastus lateralis contractions which have a reciprocal action in controlling patellar position. A normal ratio of contractile activity is reported as 1 : 1, which may be reduced in people with PFPS, although others have questioned this association with PFPS (Herrington 1998). Certainly the results of taping and VMO strengthening have not always been reproduced (Wood 1998, Hilyard *et al.* 1989) and taping has been shown to produce no change in EMG activity (Herrington and Payton 1997, Powers 1998). In addition, VMO strengthening is arguably difficult to achieve in isolation. Nevertheless there is no doubt that both passive stretching and active training, preferably in the last 30° of extension, can provide painless and impressive results in some individuals (Voigt and Wieder 1991, Morrish and Woledge 1997, Natri *et al.* 1998).

Closed chain programmes incorporating electrical stimulation may also be helpful, although biofeedback techniques have met with variable success, but the use of open chain techniques such as isokinetics remains controversial. Anti-inflammatory modalities such as ice, cryocuffs, interferential, and ultrasound have a limited role in immediate management. Braces are now widely used in the management of PFPS, acting as biomechanical restraints and corrective devices, and corrective orthotics have been reported to have positive benefits. A variety of sleeve devices are also used in an attempt to relocate and maintain the patella within the femoral sulcus. The Palumbo lateral buttress brace (Palumbo 1981) is well known, with one study suggesting that muscle activation of the VMO and vastus lateralis was reduced with the use of the brace (Gulling *et al.* 1996). There are now a variety of different devices including devices to correct tilt, glide, and even rotation. Stretching of the lateral structures, including the iliotibial band, is also part of most physiotherapy protocols. Stretching is centred on quadriceps, hamstrings, calf muscles, and lateral structures that may cause maltracking, rotation of the tibia or femur, and lateral deviation of the patella during contraction (Gose and Schweizer 1989). Hydrotherapy may have a strong place in rehabilitation, but access to it is limited.

Conservative measures appear to benefit many people. Those with negative findings in the clinical tests of patellar pain and crepitation, non-appearance of bilateral symptoms during the follow-up, low body height, and young age are associated with good long-term outcome (Natri *et al.* 1998).

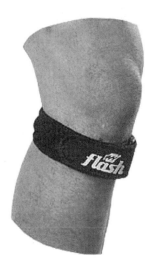

Figure 3.7.14 Patella control brace. Knee braces can help prevent lateral displacement. The above brace (Dynev Tilt and Glide Brace, Promedics Ltd) also helps prevent tilt as well as glide (reprinted with permission from Promedics Ltd).

In a recent study, at 7 years follow-up, Kannus and colleagues found that glycosaminoglycan polysulfate injection, combined with intensive quadriceps-muscle exercises, compared favourably to injections of a placebo combined with exercises, and to exercises alone. At 6 months, complete subjective, functional, and clinical recovery had occurred in almost three quarters of the patients and the 7-year overall outcome was good in approximately two thirds of the patients. Interestingly the remaining patients who still had symptoms or objective signs of a patellofemoral disorder had an increased appearance of overt signs of osteoarthritis (Kannus *et al.* 1999). One should also remember that many patients with patellofemoral pain might have a chronic maladaptive syndrome and an increased likelihood of a variety of underlying psychological problems (Witonski *et al.* 1999).

Surgical treatment

Surgical treatment may sometimes be necessary. In the chronic and extreme patella subluxer or dislocator, surgical procedures may be clearly indicated. However, surgical treatment for PFPS should be reserved for (1) failure of conservative management, (2) unremitting pain localized to patella, (3) pain with activities of daily living, (3) patellar subluxation/dislocation, or (4) associated trauma. Only 2–3% of patellofemoral pain normally requires surgery. For those patients with lateral patellar pressure, odd facet syndrome, and tight lateral retinaculum, a lateral retinacular release can reduce lateral tension and improve tracking. First advocated in 1970, this procedure has now been widely adopted as the technique of choice (Wilner 1970, Harwin and Stern 1981, Krompinger and Fulkerson 1983, Christensen *et al.* 1988, Hughston *et al.* 1996, Fu and Maday 1992). It can be performed openly, arthroscopically, or subcutaneously, and is a relatively safe procedure. Nevertheless it is sometimes used indiscrimately and can produce haemarthrosis, vastus lateralis disruption, medial instability, and postoperative stiffness (Post 1997). The exact mechanism for improvement is unknown, but destruction of pain fibres and restoration of normal alignment in lateral patellar tilt has been suggested.

A large number of other surgical procedures are used, including arthroscopic debridement, tibial transfer procedures such as a Maquet procedure (tibial advancement), Elmslie–Trillat procedure (medializa-

tion of the tibial tuberosity), lowering of the patella, vastus medialis plasty, and trochleoplasties. The huge variety of treatments again reflects the individual nature of each case and underlying malalignment as well as the variable success of each procedure.

Patellar subluxation/dislocation

This most commonly occurs in a lateral direction accompanying direct trauma to the knee, or with forced external rotation of the tibia. The subject normally experiences extreme pain, may cry out, and will often notice a spontaneous reduction. An immediate effusion usually develops and there may be considerable tenderness along the medial border after disruption of the meniscofemoral ligaments and medial retinaculum. Radiographs are important to exclude osteochondral lesions, and additional damage to ligaments including cruciates and collaterals should be considered.

If the patella remains dislocated, gentle medial pressure, with the knee in full extension, followed by a PRICE regime to help reduce haemarthrosis is valuable. Many dislocations can be managed conservatively with initial immobilization and casting or bracing followed by an intense mobilization and quadriceps strengthening programme. At long-term follow-up, good to excellent results have been seen in 75% of patients (Henry and Craven 1981, Hawkins *et al.* 1986). Nevertheless, in the presence of considerable soft tissue disruption, osteochondral fractures, inadequate reduction, or recurrent dislocation, realignment of the extensor mechanism may be necessary and is often successful (Metcalf 1982). Interestingly, recurrent dislocations are not more likely to produce osteoarthritis changes but may require surgical intervention to correct underlying malalignment abnormalities (Maenpaa and Lehto 1997).

Plica (synovial)

During fetal development, three synovial compartments fuse within the knee. Remnants can be left overlying medial retinaculae. Plicae are some of the normal synovial structures of the knee joint cavity. They are remnants of the mesenchymal tissue that occupies the space between the distal femoral and proximal tibial epiphyses in the

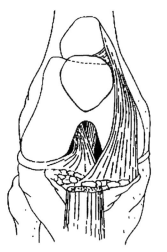
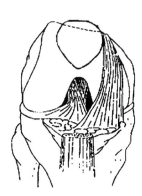

Figure 3.7.15 Medial plicae. Synovial plicae are vestigial remnants found superolaterally and medially. During flexion, loading of the plicae between the patella and femoral condyle increases and can produce pain, clicking, and even locking sensations.

8-week-old embryo. The incomplete resorption leaves synovial pleats in most of the knees (Figure 3.7.15). The superior and the inferior plicae are the most common (50–65%) but have little clinical relevance. There are many morphologic types. The lateral plica is rare (1–3%). The medial plica is present at autopsies in one of every three or four knees. It also is of various types, wide and thick in one of every fifteen knees. Arthrography, ultrasonography, CT scan with arthrography, and MR imaging can demonstrate their presence and measure their size with good accuracy. Arthroscopy allows a very precise assessment of the plica, including dynamic examination. It may detect medial impingement against the patellofemoral articular surfaces and secondary (localized chondromalacia) as well as other incidentally associated pathologic conditions of the knee. Medial plicae rarely become symptomatic, but can follow blunt trauma. Nevertheless, no predisposing factors are necessary. The plica causes symptoms such as pain, crepitus, snapping, or popping and may be seen with an effusion related to patellofemoral joint motion. The clinical picture mimics a torn medial meniscus or a maltracking patella. Clinical examination is extremely helpful if the snapping plica is palpated at the medial edge of the patella, reproducing the patient's symptoms. If chronic, these symptoms may be treated with NSAIDs, physiotherapy, electrophoresis, or local injection. Surgical treatment is indicated if conservative therapy fails. Arthroscopic complete resection of the plica cures the symptoms in a few days, thereby confirming the correct diagnosis and the effectiveness of the treatment. Histological examination often confirms chronic irritation between the plica and the femoral condyle. The syndrome probably only occurs in one in ten medial plicae, and less than 3% of arthroscopies for patellofemoral pain. In addition, associated lesions are very common, which makes it difficult to evaluate the role of the plica in the production of symptoms.

Patella hypertension

Patella hypertension was first voiced as a possible cause of anterior knee pain in humans when Lempberg and Arnoldi (1978) identified a rise in interosseous venous pressure in association with anterior knee pain, and in the absence of articular degeneration. Raised bone marrow pressure has also been identified with hip pathology and several studies have shown changes in interosseous pressure, possibly caused by delayed venous blood flow of the patella during flexion and kneeling. Several studies have demonstrated an association with anterior knee pain and articular changes, but at present clinical identification of the affected individual, measurements of interosseous pressure and treatment through drilling or osteotomy remains uncertain.

Bipartite patella

The patella initially ossifies at between 3 and 5 years of age, commencing as multiple foci that rapidly coalesce. As the patellar ossification centre enlarges, the expanding margins may be irregular and associated with accessory ossification centres. These are most common superolaterally and may lead to the development of a bipartite patella, which has cartilaginous continuity despite the appearance of osseous discontinuity. During development, cartilage may not be replaced in the superior two thirds of the articular surface (the lower one third is covered by the fat pad) (Ogden 1984). These are frequent

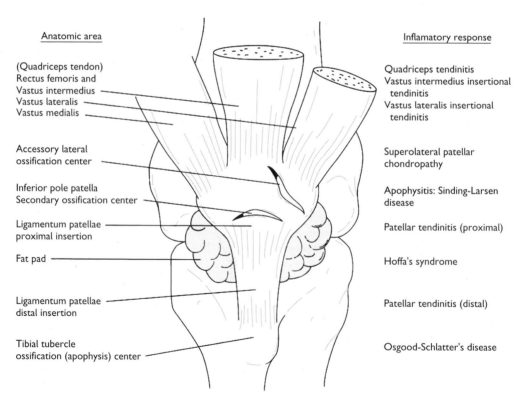

Figure 3.7.16 Extensor mechanism. Anterior knee pain includes inflammation and trauma to the extensor apparatus. A spectrum of conditions can disrupt the quadriceps musculature, patellar tendon and secondary ossification centres. The regional areas are highlighted on the left and the corresponding pathological entity on the right. (Modified from Reid 1992).

incidental findings on radiography and are unlikely to contribute to symptoms. Occasionally a fracture must be considered.

Extensor mechanism pain

The extensor mechanism of the knee comprises the quadriceps musculature, the patella, and the patellar tendon. Rectus femoris, VMO, vastus intermedius, and vastus lateralis unite to form a single tendon (the quadriceps tendon) that inserts into the superior pole of the patella with the superficial fibres forming a sheath over the patella and dispersing as the medial and lateral retinaculum (Figure 3.7.16). These fibres then align together, at the inferior pole, to become the patellar tendon (patellar ligament) that runs distally, 6–8 cm long and 2.5–3 cm wide, to insert into the tibial tuberosity. The forces transmitted through the patellar tendon can exceed eight times body weight during eccentric activities, such as jumping and landing. Inferior fibres of the patellar tendon insert into the posterior surface of the patella apex through a gradual transition from tendon to fibrocartilage and mineralized fibrocartilage to bone, dispersing stress evenly from tendon to bone (Roels *et al.* 1978). The conditions that affect the extensor mechanism are less common than those of the patellofemoral joint, producing significant morbidity and occasionally catastrophic failure. They are often predictable through chronology with the enthesopathies. Osgood–Schlatter's disease and Sinding–Larsen–Johannson syndrome present in the prepubertal child, quadriceps and patellar tendinitis in early adult life, and fractures or rupture usually in the middle decades.

Patellar tendinitis

Patellar tendinitis can often refer to a number of conditions affecting the patellar tendon, but specifically refers to an inflammation of the patellar tendon at its proximal insertion, of less than 1 year's duration. 'Jumper's knee' is often used as a synonym for patellar tendinitis but, originally described by Blazina in 1973, it is a non-specific name for inflammation of the extensor mechanism. Both are relatively uncommon in the general population but have an extremely high incidence in specific sports (including basketball, volleyball, football, and dancing) that provide repetitive and explosive eccentric quadriceps activity (Blazina *et al.* 1973, Stanish and Curwin 1984). Increasingly it is also seen in sports that have moved from grass to artificial surfaces, such as field hockey. Histological abnormalities are usually found at the bone–tendon junction and consist of an absence of the normal blue line between the zones, sometimes with the presence of cystic degeneration (Ferretti *et al.* 1983). MRI also demonstrates changes within the centre of the tendon. Stress fractures may also be noted at the distal patellar pole as well as tendon calcification and complete (sleeve) fractures of the distal pole. The initiation of tendinitis may result from microfractures and tears of the teno-osseous junction, with subsequent ingrowth of fibroblasts, mucoid degeneration, and cyst formation.

Patellar tendinitis frequently presents with aching during activity. Studies of volleyball and basketball players have described up to 40% with 'jumper's knee', 65% with pain over the inferior pole, 25% over the quadriceps tendon insertion, and 10% over the tibial tuberosity (Neri 1991). Conditions that appear to predispose to injury include four or more training sessions per week, deconditioning, concrete floors, and patellar abnormalities. In recent years Laduron and Johnson have both suggested that patellar tendinitis may in part relate to impingement between the inferior pole of the patella and the femoral trochlea. However, although MRI appearances confirm compatible lesions, this possibility has not been confirmed in anatomical studies (Johnson *et al.* 1996).

Classification

Attempts have been made to grade patellar tendinitis, in an attempt to help with the management. (Blazina *et al.* 1973, Roels *et al.* 1978) The likelihood of achieving full recovery diminishes from 83% for grade 1 and 78% for grade II to 58% for grade III.

- stage 1: pain after athletic activity
- stage 2: pain at the beginning of activity, disappears during and returns after activity
- stage 3: pain remains during and after activity and unable to compete
- stage 4: complete rupture of the patellar tendon.

Treatment

Non-surgical treatment

Investigations often do not change management, but can include plain radiographs to demonstrate an associated traction enthesopathy or calcification, ultrasound and MRI to demonstrate soft tissue changes including tendon thickness, cyst formation, mucoid degeneration, and possible tears. Conservative management is indicated for stages I–III and centres on initial restriction of provocative activities, anti-inflammatory modalities, and non-steroidal anti-inflammatories (NSAIDs). Addition of cushioning insoles and phonophoresis of NSAID or steroid aqueous solutions may be considered if symptoms persist. Traditionally low-dose steroid injections have been considered for stage III, but this is no longer common practice, with a possible link to tendon disruption and rupture. In one study 4 out of 5 patients with stage IV had previously received injections (Martens 1982). Instead, biomechanical assessments, cushioning insoles, and eccentric strengthening programmes through 'minidips' are now widely prescribed. The use of patellar tendon clasps is also extremely popular in certain sports such as basketball, although the clinical evidence of benefit has not been widely published. Acute inflammation of the paratenon is rare but is the one scenario where steroid injection may be appropriate.

Surgical treatment

Surgery is occasionally indicated for those who have failed conservative treatment or have ruptured the ligament. Most operative techniques focus on removal or debridement of abnormal tissue and re-stimulating healing, and indications for surgery vary. In one study in which 31 knees in 29 patients were treated with surgical resection of degenerate tissue for patellar tendonitis, the results were very good in 26 knees, good in 1, and poor in 4 (Roels *et al.* 1978). Persistent patellofemoral pain was considered the most important cause leading to a poor result (Roels *et al.* 1978, Verheyden *et al.* 1997). Other techniques include open resection of the inferior pole (Johnson) and arthroscopic resection of the inferior pole (Johnson) (Roels *et al.* 1978, Blazina *et al.* 1973).

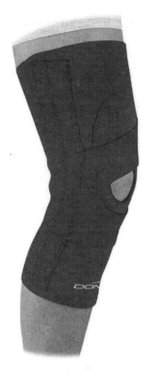

Figure 3.7.17 Patellar tendon clasp. A variety of patellar tendon clasps are used in jumping sports such as basketball and volleyball. They can provide considerable relief of discomfort during activity (reprinted with permission from Promedics Ltd).

Unexplained tendinitis must be always be considered as an indicator of underlying systemic disease such as rheumatoid or seronegative arthritis, systemic lupus, gout, diabetes mellitus, steroid abuse, or rare conditions such as alpha-1-antitrypsin deficiency. In addition iatrogenic causes, such as the side effects of ciprofloxacin, have been reported (Naessens *et al.* 1995).

Osgood–Schlatter's disease

This is one of the most common apophysitides. It is an exercise-induced growth disorder primarily affecting boys aged 10–15 years and girls aged 8–13, with pain and swelling of the tibial tubercle most commonly reported in the active individual (18%) (Kannus *et al.* 1988).

The tibial tuberosity begins ossification at 7–9 years of age as a distal focus. This progressively enlarges proximally and anteriorly, while the main tibial ossification centre concomitantly expands downward into the tuberosity (Figure 3.7.16). A section of epiphyseal cartilage (Henke's disk) usually remains between these two ossification centres until close to physeal maturity (as late as 19 years of age) and as such the anterior chondro-osseous region at the site of patellar tendon attachment is a susceptible region. This may be acutely or chronically traumatized to create an Osgood–Schlatter lesion, which can eventually elongate to form an enlarged ossicle. The closure of the tuberosity physis occurs at puberty and usually resolves the problem (Ogden 1984).

The most common presenting symptom is pain. In a survey of 412 young athletes, symptoms first occurred at 13.1 years on average. Several biomechanical associations have been made, including patella alta (Aparicio *et al.* 1997). Initially pain is managed by activity modification, NSAIDs, and icing as well as US and interferential treatment, while cross-training with avoidance of loading activities. Infrapatellar braces may be used (Levine and Kashyap 1981). Occasionally there may be severe night pain, and the differential diagnosis of malignancy must be considered. Bone scans are usually unhelpful because of the activity of the apophysis, and plain radiograph and MRI are more appropriate. Successful reduction in symptoms has been reported in one study with cessation of training for an average of 3.2 months, and interference with activity for an average of 7.3 months. Pain is typically found in 21% of those physically active and 4.5% in the inactive. Interestingly, the incidence appears higher in siblings (45%) and those who suffer from Sever's disease (calcaneal apophysitis) (68%) (Kujala *et al.* 1985) although is more common in soccer, volleyball, and basketball players. Occasionally surgical removal of painful ossicles is considered (Fisher 1980, King and Blundell-Jones 1981), although the treatment is usually delayed until after puberty. Initially drilling of the tuberosity was largely unsuccessful, but results from surgery are now encouragingly good (Fisher 1980, King and Blundell-Jones 1981, Glynn and Regan 1983).

Sinding–Larsen–Johannson syndrome

This condition, described by Sinding and Larsen in 1920 and Johannson in 1921, occurs as a result of traction enthesopathy of the inferior pole of the patella. The pathological process is similar to Osgood–Schlatter's disease, and is a result of overuse in the prepubertal child. It is similar in presentation to patellar tendinitis and management remains consistent with treatment protocols for patellar tendinitis and Osgood–Schlatter's disease (Araldi *et al.* 1989, Traverso *et al.* 1990). Occasionally sleeve fractures occur in conjunction with pre-existing Sinding–Larsen–Johannson syndrome (Gardiner *et al.* 1990).

Failure of the extensor mechanism; fractures

The patellar tendon, insertions, and quadriceps musculature can all rupture in extreme cases of sudden overload or trauma. Fortunately rare in athletes, these failures can occur in the presence of pre-existing disease states, with quadriceps ruptures most likely in the over-40s and patellar tendon ruptures in younger people. A variety of systemic disease conditions, as described above, may predispose to this condition and the implication that previous steroid injections can induce rupture still remains controversial. Occasionally the distal pole of the patella or the tibial tubercles can be avulsed, which is usually managed conservatively in the prepubertal child. One example is the sleeve fracture.

Fat pad syndrome (Hoffa's disease)

Hoffa's disease, an obscure cause of anterior knee pain, may result from impingement and inflammation of the infrapatellar fat pad (Figure 3.7.16). First reported by Albert Hoffa in 1904, the condition remains uncommon, is infrequently reported, and is sometimes seen in association with surgical procedures (Tsirbas *et al.* 1991, Jerosch and Schroder 1996, Faletti *et al.* 1998). The exact role of the fat pad is ill defined, although it may act in helping anterior stability of the soft tissue structures. Inflammation of this structure often follows direct trauma or surgery, producing ill-defined pain. This may be antero-lateral or anteromedial and can be accompanied by considerable stiffness. Occasionally a bulging fat pad can be identified but often the diagnosis is missed, leading to chronic changes and disability. Regional injections of anaesthetic may help establish the diagnosis, although concomitant pathology such as with patellar tendonitis and adjacent bursa are frequently well established (Duri *et al.* 1997). A possible relationship between impingement of the infrapatellar fat pad and the development of ossifying chondroma has also been reported (Krebs and Parker 1994). Treatment includes initial rest from provocative activities with quadriceps stretching, patella mobilization, regional anti-inflammatory modalities, steroid injection, and occasionally surgical resection. Fat pad entrapment may also mimic anterior meniscal pathology and can produce catching, jumping, and locking sensations as well as a positive McMurray's test.

Differential diagnosis

Anterior knee pain is commonly seen in the adolescent, and a variety of different underlying diagnoses must therefore always be borne in mind (see Table 3.7.2). Osteochondritis dissecans of the tibiofemoral and less commonly the patellofemoral joint (not dealt with in this book) are essential to identify early. Probably more important are tumours of the soft tissue and bone that, although infrequent, occur most commonly in the long bones of the femur and tibia. Thus night pain, pain unrelated to activity, and pain that is failing conservative treatment with no obvious malalignment should always flag up possible underlying pathology. Patella fractures, non-ossifying fibromas, necrosing lipomas, infection, and neuritis may all present with anterior knee pain. With surgery and arthroscopy frequently performed, the possible sequel must also be considered including infrapatellar contracture syndrome and infrapatellar neuritis, nerve root entrapment of lumbosacral nerve roots L2–4, and the poorly understood reflex sympathetic dystrophy, now classified as chronic pain syndrome (CPS) type 1 (Youmans 1989).

References

Abril, J. C., Calvo, E. and Alvarez, L. (1997) *Journal of Pediatric Orthopedics*, 17, 63–66.

Aparicio, G., Abril, J. C., Calvo, E., Alvarez, L. (1997) Radiologic study of patellar height in Osgood-Schlatter disease. *J. Pediatr. Orthop.*, 17, 63–6.

Araldi, R., Martoni, S., and Motta, E. (1989) *Ortopedia e Traumatologia Oggi*, 9, 29–32.

Arroll, B., Ellis-Pegler, E., Edwards, A., and Sutcliffe, G. (1997) *American Journal of Sports Medicine*, 25, 207–212.

Bentley, G. and Dowd, G. (1984) *Clinical Orthopaedics*, 189, 209–228.

Blazina, M. E., Kerlan, R. K., Jobe, F. W., Carter, V. S., and Carlson, G. J. (1973) *Orthopedic Clinics of North America*, 4, 665–678.

Casscells, W. (1975) *Journal of Bone and Joint Surgery*, 57, 1033.

Christensen, F., Soballe, K., and Snerum, L. (1988) *Clinical Orthopaedics and Related Research Issue* 234.

Conlan, T., Garth, W. P., and Lemons, J. E. (1993) *Journal of Bone and Joint Surgery*, 75A, 682–693.

Crichton, K. (1989) *Australian Journal of Physiotherapy*, 35.

Duri, Z. A.A., Aichroth, P. M., Dowd, G., and Ware, H. (1997) *Knee*, 4, 227–236.

Dye, S. F. (1987) *Journal of Bone and Joint Surgery*, 69A, 976–983.

Faletti, C., De Stefano, N., Giudice, G., and Larciprete, M. (1998) *European Journal of Radiology*, 27, S60–69.

Ferretti, A., Ippolito, E., Mariani, P., and Puddu, G. (1983) *American Journal of Sports Medicine*, 11, 58–62.

Ficat, R. P. and Hungerford, D. S. (1977) *Disorders of the Patellofemoral Joint.* Williams and Wilkins, Baltimore.

Fisher, R. L. (1980) *Orthopaedic Review*, 9, 93–96.

Fu, F. H. and Maday, M. G. (1992) *Orthopedic Clinics of North America*, 23, 601–612.

Fulkerson, J. P. and Shea, K. P. (1990) *Journal of Bone and Joint Surgery*, 72A, 1424–1429.

Fulkerson, J. P., Tennant, R., Jaivin, J. S., and Grunnet, M. (1985) *Clinical Orthopaedics and Related Research, N. O.,* .

Gardiner, J. S., McInerney, V. K., Avella, D. G., and Valdez, N. A. (1990) *Orthopaedic Review* 19.

Gerrard, B. (1989) *Australian Journal of Physiotherapy*, 35, 71–80.

Glynn, M. K. and Regan, B. F. (1983) *Journal of Pediatric Orthopedics*, 3, 216–219.

Gose, J. C. and Schweizer, P. (1989) *Journal of Orthopaedic and Sports Physical Therapy*, 10, 10.

Grabiner, M. D., Koh, T. J., and Draganich, L. F. (1994) *Medicine Science Sport and Exercise*, 26, 10–21.

Gulling, L. K., Lephart, S. M., Stone, D. A., Irrgang, J. J., and Pincivero, D. M. (1996) *Isokinetics and Exercise Science*, 6, 133–138.

Hahn, T. and Foldspang, A. (1998) *Scandinavian Journal of Social Medicine*, 26, 44–52.

Harwin, S. F. and Stern, R. E. (1981) *Clinical Orthopaedics and Related Research* No, .?????

Hawkins, R. J., Bell, R. H., and Anisette, G. (1986) *American Journal of Sports Medicine*, 14, 117.

Henry, J. H. and Craven, P. R. (1981) *American Journal of Sports Medicine*, 9, 82.

Herrington, L. (1998) *Critical Reviews in Physical and Rehabilitation Medicine*, 10, 257–263.

Herrington, L. and Payton, C. J. (1997) *Physiotherapy*, 83, 566–572.

Hilyard, A., Moore, C., and Pope, J. (1989) *Australian Journal of Physiotherapy*, 35.

Hughston, J. C., Flandry, F., Brinker, M. R., Terry, G. C., and Mills, I. J. (1996) *American Journal of Sports Medicine*, 24, 486–491.

Hughston, J. C. and Walsh, W. M. (1979) *Clinical Orthopaedics*, 144, 36.

Insall, J. and Salvati, E. (1971) *Radiology*, 101, 101.

Jerosch, J. and Schroder, M. (1996) *Archives of Orthopaedic and Traumatic Surgery*, 115 195–198.

Johnson, D. P., Wakeley, C. J., and Watt, I. (1996) *Journal of Bone and Joint Surgery*, 78B, 452–457.

Joshi, R. P. and Heatley, F. W. (1998) *Knee*, 5, 129–135.

Kannus, P., Aho, H., Jarvinen, M., *et al.* (1987) *American Journal of Sports Medicine*, 15, 79–85.

Kannus, P., Natri, A., Paakkala, T., and Jarvinen, M. (1999) *Journal of Bone and Joint Surgery*, 81A, 355–363.

Kannus, P., Niittymaki, S., and Jarvinen, M. (1988) *Clinical Pediatrics*, 27, 333–337.

Kannus, P. A. and Nittymaki, S. (1994) *Medicine Science Sport and Exercise*, 26, 289–296.

Kaufner, H. and Arbor, A. (1971) *Journal of Bone and Joint Surgery*, 63, 1551–1560.

King, A. G. and Blundell-Jones, G. (1981) *American Journal of Sports Medicine*, 9, 250–253.

Krebs, V. E. and Parker, R. D. (1994) *Arthroscopy*, 10, 301–304.

Krompinger, W. J. and Fulkerson, J. P. (1983) Lateral retinacular release for intractable lateral retinacular pain. *Clinical Orthopaedics and Related Research*, 179, 191–3.

Kujala, U. M., Kvist, M., and Heinonen, O. (1985) *American Journal of Sports Medicine*, 13, 236–241.

Laurin, C. A., Dussault, R., and Levesque, H. P. (1979) *Clinical Orthopaedics*, **144**, 16–26.

Lempberg, R. K. and Arnoldi, C. C. (1978) *Clinical Orthopaedics*, **136**, 143–156.

Levine, J. and Kashyap, S. (1981) A new conservative treatment of Osgood-Schlatter disease. *Clinical Orthopaedics and Related Research, N. O.*, **158**, 126–8.

Lieb, F. and Perry, J. (1968) *Journal of Bone and Joint Surgery*, **50A**, 1535.

Maenpaa, H. and Lehto, M. U. K. (1997) *Clinical Orthopaedics and Related Research Issue*, **339**.

Martens, M. (1982) *Acta Orthopaedica Belgica*, **48**, 453–454.

McConnell, J. (1986) *Australian Journal of Physiotherapy*, **32**, 215–223.

McGinty, J. B. and McCarthy, J. C. (1981) *Clinical Orthopaedics*, **167**, 9–18.

Merchant, A. C. (1988) *Arthroscopy*, **4**, 235.

Metcalf, R. (1982) *Clinical Orthopaedics*, **167**, 9.

Milgrom, C., Finestone, A., Shlamkovitch, N., Giladi, M., and Radin, E. (1996) *Clinical Orthopaedics and Related Research*, **331**, 256–260.

Miller, T. T., Shapiro, M. A., Schultz, E., Crider, R., and Paley, D. (1998) *American Journal of Roentgenology*, **171**, 739–742.

Morrish, G. M. and Woledge, R. C. (1997) *Scandinavian Journal of Rehabilitation Medicine*, **29**, 43–48.

Mummery, W. K., Spence, J. C., Vincenten, J. A. and Voaklander (1998) *Canadian Journal of Public Health*, **89**, 53–6.

Naessens, G., Hansen, L., De Bruyne, J., Deckers, K., and Driessens, M. (1995) *European Journal of Physical Medicine and Rehabilitation*, **5**, 200–202.

Natri, A., Kannus, P., and Jarvinen, M. (1998) *Medicine and Science in Sports and Exercise*, **30**, 1572–1577.

Neri, M. (1991) *Journal of Sports Traumatology and Related Research*, **13**, 95–101.

Ogden, J. A. (1984) *Skeletal Radiology*, **11**, 246–257.

Owre, A. (1934) *Acta Chiolurgica Scandinavica*, **77**.

Palumbo, P. M. (1981) *American Journal of Sports Medicine*, **9**, 1.

Post, W. R. (1997) *Techniques in Orthopaedics*, **12**, 145–150.

Post, W. R. (1998) *Physician and Sports Medicine*, **26**, 68–78.

Powers, C. M. (1998) *Journal of Orthopaedic and Sports Physical Therapy*, **28**, 345–354.

Radin, E. L., Pail, I. L., and Lowy, M. (1984) *Journal of Bone and Joint Surgery*, **B**, 660.

Reid, D. C. (1992) *Sport Injury Assessment and Rehabilitation*. Churchill Livingstone, New York.

Roels, J., Martens, M., Mulier, J. C., and Burssens, A. (1978) *American Journal of Sports Medicine*, **6**, 362–368.

Stanish, W. D. and Curwin, S. (1984) *Tendonitis: its etiology and treatment*. Collamore Press, Lexington, MA.

Traverso, A., Baldari, A., and Catalani, F. (1990) *Journal of Sports Medicine and Physical Fitness*, **30**, 331–333.

Tria, A. J., Palumbo, N. C. and Alicea, J. A. (1992) *Orthopedic Clinics of North America*, **24**, 545–553.

Tsirbas, A., Paterson, R. S., and Keene, G. C. R. (1991) *Australian Journal of Science and Medicine in Sport*, **23**, 24–26.

Verheyden, F., Geens, G., and Nelen, G. (1997) *Acta Orthopaedica Belgica*, **63**, 102–105.

Voigt, M. L. and Wieder, D. L. (1991) *American Journal of Sports Medicine*, **19**, 131–137.

Wilner, P. (1970) *Clinical Orthopaedics*, **669**, 213.

Witonski, D., Karlinska, I., and Musial, A. (1999) *Medicine and Science Monitor*, **4**, 1019–1023.

Wood, A. (1998) *Journal of Sports Chiropractic and Rehabilitation*, **12**, 1–14.

Wiberg, G. (1941) *Acta Orthopodica Scandinavica*, **XII**, 319.

Youmans, W. T. (1989) *Clinics in Sports Medicine*, **8**, 331–342.

3.7.3 Superior tibiofibular joint

Mark Batt

Anatomy

The superior tibiofibular joint is a diarthrodial plane joint between the medial facet of the head of the fibula and the tibial facet on the posterolateral tibial condyle. The joint has a synovial lining which is separate from the knee joint cavity. The joint is inherently stable, with a fibrous capsule reinforced by anterior and posterior superior tibiofibular ligaments and tendinous insertions. The stronger anterior superior tibiofibular ligaments are comprised of three bands, whereas the posterior superior tibiofibular ligament is a relatively weak single band, augmented by the popliteus tendon. Additional stability is provided superiorly by the lateral collateral ligament, medially by the interosseous membrane, and anterolaterally by the biceps femoris insertion. The joint size, shape, and orientation are variable, classified by Ogden (1974a) as either horizontal or oblique. The oblique orientation is characterized by relative immobility and a smaller joint surface, which diminishes in size as the angle of inclination increases.

Biomechanics

Ogden (1974a) described three key functions of the superior tibiofibular joint: (1) dissipation of torsional stresses at the ankle, (2) dissipation of lateral bending moments of the tibia, and (3) tensile, rather than compressive weightbearing. The fibula externally rotates

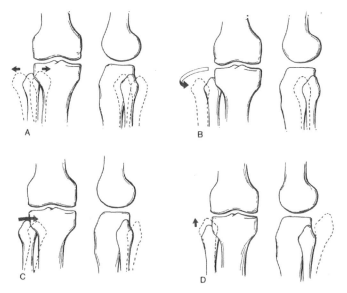

Figure 3.7.18 Injuries to the superior tibiofibular joint: subluxation and anterior, posterior, or superior dislocation.

and the joint glides laterally as the ankle dorsiflexes. Additionally, there is distal migration secondary to contraction of muscles attached to the fibula. The joint does not sit in the true sagittal plane, so the gliding motions are anterolateral and posteromedial, the latter occurring naturally as the knee extends in response to the pull of biceps femoris and the lateral collateral ligament.

Injuries

Injuries to the superior tibiofibular joint are relatively uncommon and are more typically acute than chronic. Their incidence as a cause of lateral knee pain may be under-reported, reflecting a lack of knowledge of this joint and associated injury. The principle pathology is laxity of the joint, which may arise from direct or indirect, acute, or chronic trauma producing subluxation or dislocation. Ogden described four types of injury: subluxation and anterior, posterior, or superior dislocation (Ogden 1974b) (Figure 3.7.18).

Acute injuries

The joint may be injured by direct or more commonly indirect trauma. Acute injuries tend to be clear-cut, although delayed presentation and complication can make assessment problematic.

Mechanism

Indirect injuries may occur in combination with fracture of the tibia, or fibula, or fracture-dislocation of the ankle (producing superior laxity), but more commonly in the sporting setting they occur when an athlete falls on a flexed, adducted leg with ankle inversion. This latter sliding mechanism is seen with the sliding tackle in soccer or base-slides in baseball or softball, or following awkward falls in water-skiing or parachuting. In this position the knee is flexed, relaxing the biceps femoris tendon and the lateral collateral ligament, and the ankle is inverted and plantarflexed, producing tension on the muscle origins of the anterolateral muscle compartments. When combined with an external rotation torque on the tibia, anterolateral instability ensues. Anterolateral subluxation or dislocation is much the more common type of instability, occurring in 90% of patients. Direct injury to the joint is less common than indirect injury and results from a direct blow to the flexed knee when in a sitting position, as in horse riding or jet-skiing. This produces posteromedial dislocation and carries higher morbidity due to associated peroneal nerve injury and persistent instability.

A self-limiting, typically bilateral, atraumatic subluxation is also described in adolescents with generalized ligamentous laxity. This tends to resolve with skeletal maturation. A further injury specific to this age group is an epiphyseal fracture of the proximal fibula.

Evaluation

An awareness of these injuries and their mechanism will facilitate their recognition. The description by the patient of symptoms referable to the 'knee' may lead to confusion as pain, giving way, and locking may occur at both the knee and the tibiofibular joint. However, the lack of knee joint effusion is a clue to superior tibiofibular joint injury. Additionally patients may complain of ankle problems in association with lateral knee pain. Physical examination is crucial, as patients' symptoms may be vague without recollection of a specific injury episode. Acutely, there may be a tender swelling over the proximal fibula with associated hypermobility and pain. Forced dorsiflexion of the ankle may cause pain, and care should be taken to exclude common peroneal nerve damage. Open-chain knee flexion may be reduced and painful with a 'pinch' at end of range. Closed-chain knee flexion as a single leg mini-dip may be impaired because of pain and instability. Comparison should be made with the normal limb, as these signs may be soft. Specific plain radiograph views for the superior tibiofibular joint have been described, but instability is commonly demonstrated on bilateral anteroposterior and lateral views without resort to internal rotation, oblique, or fluoroscopic views.

Treatment

Acute dislocations require closed reduction by manipulation, which produces pain relief and sometimes audible relocation. This is achieved by flexing the knee to 90° with the ankle dorsiflexed and everted. After reduction, the joint is generally stable, but casting in near full extension (non-weightbearing) for 3 weeks may aid healing and prevent recurrence. After the cast is removed, structured rehabilitation should be undertaken, avoiding early hamstring work in the case of posteromedial laxity. A counterforce brace may be used during rehabilitation to aid subsequent return to sport, which should be possible at 6–12 weeks.

Chronic injuries

Chronic injuries may arise as complications of acute injuries or *de novo* as overuse injuries. As there may be no clear history of trauma, the diagnosis of chronic superior tibiofibular joint injury may be challenging. The differential diagnosis is extensive, including lateral meniscus tear and cysts, popliteus tendonitis, iliotibial band syndrome, lateral collateral ligament sprain, posterolateral knee instability, arthritis, fabella syndrome, and ganglions. Chronic superior tibiofibular joint injuries described by Wong and Weiner (1978) include recurrent subluxation or dislocation, idiopathic subluxation, and proximal tibiofibular synostosis.

Mechanism

Idiopathic subluxation may occur as an overuse injury due to training errors in association with adverse lower limb biomechanics resulting in excessive fibular rotation. Posteromedial subluxation results from stretching of the anterior capsule and ligaments of the superior tibiofibular joint in conjunction with sustained posterior pull of biceps femoris and soleus muscles.

Evaluation

Assessment of chronic laxity of the superior tibiofibular joint requires the knee to be flexed to 90° with relaxation of the hamstrings. Comparing with the contralateral side, the examiner then attempts to translate the fibular head anterolaterally.

Treatment

Taping or use of a counterforce brace may help the unstable joint. Physiotherapy to strengthen biceps femoris and activity modification may also provide satisfactory results (Halbrecht and Jackson 1991). When this fails and chronic debilitating instability persists, a variety of surgical procedures to either excise or stabilize the fibular head have been advocated. No large series comparing different surgical procedures exists, making informed comparisons impossible (Weinert and Raczka 1986, Shapiro *et al.* 1993). Resection of the fibular head is avoided in athletes because of the requirement to reattach the lateral collateral ligament and biceps femoris tendon. Similarly, fusion of the joint is avoided to prevent subsequent ankle symptoms.

References

Halbrecht, J. and Jackson, D. (1991) Recurrent dislocation of the proximal tibiofibular joint. *Orthop. Rev.,* **20**(11), 957–960.

Ogden, J. (1974a) The anatomy and function of the proximal tibiofibular joint. *Clin. Orthop.,* **101**, 186–191.

Ogden, J. (1974b) Subluxation of the proximal tibiofibular joint. *Clin. Orthop.,* **101**, 192–197.

Shapiro, G., Fanton, G. *et al.* (1993) Reconstruction for recurrent dislocation of the proximal tibiofibular joint. *Orthop. Rev.,* **22**(11), 1229–1232.

Weinert, C. and Raczka, R. (1986) Recurrent dislocation of the superior tibiofibular joint. *J. Bone Joint Surg.,* **68A**(1), 126–128.

Wong, K. and Weiner, D. (1978) Proximal tibiofibular synostosis. *Clin. Orthop.,* **135**, 45–47.

3.7.4 Exertional lower leg pain

Mark Batt

Stress fractures

Tibial stress fracture

Stress fractures are common overuse injuries that may account for 5–10% of all sports injuries. The tibia is the most common site, accounting for 31–50% of diagnosed stress fractures (Hulkko and Orava 1987, Ha *et al.* 1991). Somewhat lower relative incidences of tibial stress fractures are reported in the military, where the incidence of foot stress fractures is higher (Wilson and Fn 1969). The cause of these injuries is repetitive loading, typically occurring in the athlete or military recruit who suddenly increases training load and volume. The role of adverse biomechanics as a precipitant has yet to be scientifically proven. The normal response of bone to repetitive loading is to undergo physiological remodelling; however, this may become pathological when resorption (osteoclastic activity) outstrips the laying down of new bone (osteoblastic activity). Physiological bone remod-

elling is an asymptomatic process. Accelerated bone remodelling becomes symptomatic with localized bone pain, the precise cause of which is unclear. Local discomfort may reflect a periosteal reaction, which occurs concomitantly with cortical bone remodelling and reflects the laying down of subperiosteal woven bone. This bone activity is part of a spectrum and it is incorrect to consider a stress fracture as an all-or-nothing event. It is better to consider the spectrum of bone stress from physiological remodelling through to frank cortical disruption (Figure 3.7.19). Tibial stress fractures have been described in athletes, military recruits, and performing artists. Most patients present with posteromedial tibial pain, although a small subgroup presents with anterior midtibial stress fractures; these are liable to progress to non-union with pain localized to the anterior crest of the tibia. They are often known as 'dreaded black line fractures', which in part reflects their poor prognosis.

Tibial stress fractures present with the progressive onset of tibial pain, associated with a history of increased physical activity. In about 15% of cases these injuries may occur bilaterally (Matheson *et al.* 1987). A typical history of 'crescendo pain' is described and this is associated with examination findings of localized tibial tenderness made worse by percussion or hopping. The patient history may reflect training errors in addition to unforgiving running surfaces, inappropriate shoes, dietary issues and, in women, poor bone health resulting from menstrual irregularity.

Investigations

The usefulness of various radiographic techniques in the diagnosis and confirmation of tibial stress fractures is dependent upon the time course of the injury (Figure 3.7.19). Accelerated physiological bone remodelling may be demonstrated on triple-phase bone scan (TPBS) and it is important to consider the likely presence of asymptomatic foci when interpreting these scans. Alternatively, MRI may be used and

Bone stress	Normal	Increased load/Repetitive loading		Failure
Bone remodelling	Physiological	Accelerated	Fatigue	Fracture
	RES=REP	RES>REP	RES>>REP	
Bone pain	**Asymptomatic**	**Pain relieved by rest**		**Constant pain**
Radiography		Cortical lucency	Periosteal reaction	Cortical disruption
TPBS		Increased diffuse uptake		Intense focal uptake
MRI	Marrow oedema	Subperiosteal signal		Cortical signal

Figure 3.7.19 Continuum of bone response to increased loading. Adapted from Daffner (1992) and Anderson and Greenspan (1996).

has been demonstrated to provide similar sensitivity and specificity to TPBS in the diagnosis of shin splints (Batt 1995). Caution should be exercised, however, as the extent of MRI findings in asymptomatic subjects is not known, leading to oversensitivity and a lack of specificity. Plain radiographs may be positive after as little as 4–6 weeks of pain, with a blurred periosteal margin representing the earliest change. At this stage one would anticipate a discrete hot spot on TPBS, and bone marrow oedema and subperiosteal changes on MRI. Subsequent plain radiograph findings may include cortical hypertrophy, medullary canal narrowing, and periosteal elevation. Typically anteroposterior and lateral projections will suffice, although on occasions oblique projections may provide additional periosteal information.

Management

Treatment should focus on two inter-related areas: first, management of the fracture (or bone stress injury); and second, investigation and correction of precipitants. Fracture management should include a period of non-weightbearing if walking produces significant pain. Healing is typically accelerated with the use of a pneumatic leg brace and this allows for an earlier return to pain-free activity (Swenson *et al.* 1997). During the period of fracture healing, fitness may be maintained with cross-training; the use of non-impact activities such as cycle and an upper body ergometer is encouraged. Similarly, swimming, and aquatherapy may be used. After a period of modified rest, a graduated return to physical activity should be made. During this time, both intrinsic and extrinsic precipitants of these overuse injuries should be sought. Typical intrinsic factors include adverse lower limb and foot biomechanics (cavoid or hyperpronating foot), hormonal disruption, and nutritional deficiencies. External factors include inappropriate shoe and orthotic use, running surface, and training error.

Fibula stress fracture

Fibula stress fractures are commonly reported, accounting for 12–20% of stress fractures in runners and 8% in the military. Once dubbed the 'runner's fracture', fibula stress fractures most commonly occur in the distal third of the fibula. They are also reported to occur in figure skating, aerobics, and ballet. These fractures present typically with a history of crescendo pain and localized tenderness. They most commonly occur in the distal third of the fibula, although they have been described in the proximal third. With modified rest and a graduated return to full activity once pain-free, the prognosis for these fractures is good.

Chronic compartment syndrome

The lower limb consists of four compartments, classically described as anterior, lateral, deep, and superficial posterior. The presence of separate posterior compartments is debated, and indeed some believe that tibialis posterior has its own fascial investment (Figure 3.7.20). The pattern of pain of chronic compartment syndrome (CCS) is different from that of a stress fracture. Whereas the discomfort experienced by the patient with a stress fracture typically continues after the physical activity, patients with CCS have severe crescendo pain that is ischaemic in nature, but which typically resolves rapidly on stopping activity, with only dull residual pain after activity. Associated with this activity-related discomfort, and particularly in the anterior compart-

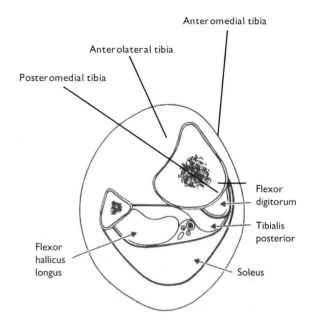

Figure 3.7.20 Diagrammatic representation of axial cut of left mid-tibia to demonstrate muscle compartments. Adapted from Detmer (1986).

ment syndrome, there may be a sensation of muscle rigidity. The recurrence of exertional pain when re-exercising is predictable.

CCS is defined as increased intramuscular pressure associated with pain, swelling, impaired muscle function, and frequently dysaesthesiae. These signs and symptoms occur due to excessive exercise-induced pressure increases in skeletal muscle fascial compartments. The cause of pain is unclear; although ischaemic pain is described, involvement of fascial and periosteal pain nociceptors may also occur. Predisposing factors include muscle hypertrophy, fascial or periosteal thickening, and a small compartment. Compromise of the arteriovenous pressure gradient results in elevated venous and intracompartmental pressure rises with a corresponding decrease in local blood flow.

There are reports in the literature of anterior, lateral, and deep posterior compartment syndrome. Chronic anterior compartment syndrome is most commonly reported and may be seen in running athletes as well as rowers. Lateral compartment syndrome is uncommon and the existence of deep posterior compartment syndrome is subject to considerable debate.

Investigation and management

Typically intracompartmental pressure measurements are undertaken to confirm the diagnosis of CCS. History and clinical findings are often insufficient to make a definitive diagnosis, with the exception of patients with anterior CCS who may provide a classical history and a set of physical examination findings. The physical examination findings should include exercise-induced muscle pain and swelling with muscle dysfunction resulting from ischaemia and pain. Measurement of intramuscular pressure may be achieved via a variety of techniques including injection, infusion, non-infusion, and pressure transducer (Styf 1989). Irrespective of technique used, each laboratory should develop a standard protocol: patients should be exercised into pain and measurements made when the patient is symptomatic. It is difficult to meta-analyse normal and abnormal pressure recordings in the

COMPARTMENT PRESSURE TEST

Name :   Date :

GP :   Hospital No. :

Symptoms : Side :   Duration :   (months)

Describe :

TEST : Compartment (specify) :

                              RIGHT (mm Hg)   LEFT (mm Hg)

At rest supine :

During exercise :

Post exercise immediate :

Post exercise 1min :

Post exercise 2 min :

Post exercise 3 min :

Post exercise 5 min :

Post exercise 10 min :

Exercise : Supine/Standing (Delete)   Type :

Medications used :

Test performed by :

Additional comments :

Figure 3.7.21 Protocol used for compartment pressure testing.

literature, as different equipment and techniques may give rise to different sets of baseline and exercise data. Furthermore, different lower leg compartments produce different results. I use a hand-held non-infusion technique that lends itself to measurements during exercise. Measurements are taken according to a standard protocol and these are compared to a matrix of values obtained from the literature. (Figure 3.7.21, Table 3.7.5) (Pedowitz *et al.* 1990, Reid 1992, Styf 1995). It is not my practice to measure the deep posterior compartment, as the validity of the measurement is uncertain (Styf 1988, Melberg and Styf 1989). If abnormal pressures are measured within one or more muscle compartment, the patients are referred for fasciotomy. This procedure, performed under general anaesthetic, involves fasciotomy of the affected compartment with or without periosteal stripping or cautery. Typically this provides good results with a lowering of intracompartment pressures in those instances where postoperative measurements have been obtained. Before surgery, patients should be warned that there will be scarring of the legs and in addition some bulging of the released muscle compartment. Conservative management of compartment syndrome may be tried before surgery and this should include soft tissue massage and the use of orthotics where biomechanical abnormalities exist.

Table 3.7.5. Comparison of compartment pressure values (mmHg)

| Values | Author | | |
	Reid	Pedowitz	Styf
Rest	>30	>15	Unreliable
1 min after exertion	>60	–	>30–35
2 min after exertion	>20	>30	–
5 min after exertion	–	>20	> Rest

Shin splints

This term is descriptive, not diagnostic and should be used to describe exertional lower leg pain not attributable to bone stress injury, compartment syndrome, or muscle hernia (Batt 1995). Despite a similar definition offered by the American Medical Association in 1966, the term has been subject to misuse and probably reflects the confusion surrounding the various conditions presenting with exertional lower limb pain. The term 'shin splints' is generic, representing a heterogeneous group of conditions, some of which may be inter-related with bone stress injury and compartment syndrome. Various authors in the past have used the term synonymously with medial tibial stress syndrome, medial tibial syndrome, periostitis, periostalgia, without specific evidence for the relationship. Furthermore, other authors have attributed shin splints to variable anatomy and have led to terms such as 'soleus syndrome' (Michael and Holder 1985). Typically, patients manifest chronic or acute-on-chronic symptoms of posteromedial tibial pain that is diffuse, linear, and sometimes bilateral. The diagnosis of shin splints is one of exclusion of bone stress injury and compartment syndrome; history and examination are helpful. The presentation of diffuse rather than localized pain leads one away from the diagnosis of bone stress injury or stress fracture. On examination there is diffuse linear posteromedial tibial tenderness that may be accompanied by periosteal irregularity. Resisted muscle testing is seldom rewarding, but lower limb malalignment may be seen. Patients affected are often runners and other athletes who are involved in stop/start activity such as hockey, basketball, and tennis. Radiographs are normal, and TPBS may demonstrate diffuse linear posteromedial uptake of tracer, which is usually bilateral, reflecting the patients' symptoms. Patients frequently complain of bilateral symptoms, although one leg may be disproportionately symptomatic. The absence of focal transcortical TPBS uptake should lead the clinician away from the diagnosis of a bone stress injury. Furthermore, the history is typically chronic with symptoms present over months or years. MRI studies have helped rationalize the management of patients presenting with shin splints. Batt et al. (1998) found that patients with short-lived symptoms had MRI findings compatible with a bone stress injury, whereas those with chronic symptoms had normal scans. Indeed, the MRI scan showed no evidence of periosteal thickening or subperiosteal fat deposition. Management of these difficult patients includes fascial stripping or cautery and may produce good results. It is unclear why these patients improve, and it is thought that denervation may be responsible.

Other considerations

Fascial hernias

Most fascial defects are asymptomatic. They are most commonly seen involving tibialis anterior, but may involve other compartments. Their occurrence is often in association with venous perforations of the fascia or at the site of the exit of the superficial peroneal nerve. Such fascial defects may give rise to symptoms, and indeed have been reported to be present in 20–60% of patients with chronic anterior compartment syndrome and 5% of patients with anterior lower leg pain from other causes (Styf 1989). Herniations may only become evident with physical activity and may result from muscle hypertrophy following intense training. They typically present as a painful tender mass after activity, which is reducible. If bothersome they are best treated by longitudinal fasciotomy of the compartment (Berlund and Stocks 1993). Closure of the fascial deficits causing local muscle hernia is not recommended as this may lead to decreased compartment size and subsequent compartment syndrome (Miniaci and Rorabeck 1986).

Popliteal artery entrapment

This unusual syndrome occurs when an abnormal anatomical relationship exists between the popliteal artery and surrounding musculature. Patients are usually young men involved in physical activity who complain of progressive posterior lower limb claudication when exercising. Depending on the anatomy, walking may produce more profound symptoms than running, reflecting a more sustained gastrocnemius contraction. There are approximately 300 reported cases in the literature and there is a diversity of symptoms, which probably reflects variable anatomy in addition to other variable causal factors. Screening may be undertaken by duplex ultrasound, which is non-invasive and increasingly reliable. Angiography (+/– MRI) typically provides a definitive diagnosis and should be considered before surgery. The treatment of this condition involves release of the entrapped vessels and repair of the arterial lumen where appropriate. The prognosis depends on the anatomy and degree of arterial damage.

Pseudoradicular syndromes/nerve entrapments

Peripheral nerve entrapments may give rise to leg pain and should be considered as part of the differential diagnosis of exertional lower leg pain. In a large series of patients with complaints of lower extremity pain with suspected lumbar radiculopathy, peripheral nerve entrapments were found as a sole cause of leg pain in over 1% of this group; 50% also had concomitant back pain. The peroneal nerve was most commonly involved, followed by femoral and tibial nerves (Saal et al. 1988). Compression of the superficial peroneal nerve may be associated with a fascial defect and muscle herniation, or an anomalous course of the nerve. It may also arise after ankle sprain, or as a complication following fasciotomy of the anterior compartment (Styf 1989). Superficial peroneal nerve entrapment is characterized by sensory disturbance over the dorsum of the foot during exercise and some positional dysaesthesiae at rest. The latter symptom is of particular diagnostic importance, as compartment syndrome never begins before exercise commences. There may be localized discomfort over the anterior intermuscular septum with an associated positive Tinel's sign. Pain may occur when the ankle joint is passively flexed and supinated. Evaluation of nerve conduction velocities may improve diagnostic specificity and are recommended prior to decompression. Surgical release of the lateral compartment may provide relief of symptoms in up to 50% of cases.

References

Anderson, M. and Greenspan, A. (1996) State of the art: stress fractures. *Radiology*, **199**, 1–12.

Batt M., Ugalde, V., Anderson, M. (1998) A prospective controlled study of diagnostic imaging for acute shin splint. *Med Sci Sports Exercise*, **30**(11), 1564–71.

Batt, M. (1995) Shin splints: a review of terminology. *Clin J Sport Med*, **5**(1), 53–7.

Berlund, H., Stocks, G. (1993) Muscle hernia in a recreational athlete. *Orthop Rev*, **11**, 1246–8.

Daffner, R. (1992) Stress Fractures: Current concepts. *AJR*, **159**, 245–52.

Detmer, D. (1986) Chronic shin splints – classification and management of medial tibial stress syndrome. *Sports Med*, **3**, 436–46.

Ha, K. I., *et al.* (1991) A clinical study of stress fractures in sports activities. *Orthopaedics*, **14**, 1089–95.

Hulkko, A., Orava, S. (1987) Stress fractures in athletes. *Int J Sports Med*, **8**, 221–6.

Matheson, G., Clement, D., McKenzie, D. (1987) Stress fractures in athletes: a study of 320 cases. *Am J Sports Med*, **15**, 46–58.

Melberg, P.E., Styf, J. (1989) Posteromedial pain in the lower leg. *Am J Sports Med*, **17**(6), 747–750.

Michael, R., Holder, L. (1985) The soleus syndrome – a cause of medial tibial stress (shin splints). *Am J Sports Med*, **13**(2), 87–94.

Miniaci, A., Rorabeck, C. (1986) Compartment syndrome as a complication of repair of hernia of the tibialis anterior. *J Bone Joint Surg*, **68A**(9), 1444–1445.

Pedowitz, S. R., *et al.* (1990) Modified criteria for the objective diagnosis of chronic compartment syndrome of the leg. *Am J Sports Med*, **18**(1), 35–40.

Reid, D. (1992) *Sports injury assessment and rehabilitation.* Churchill Livingstone, New York.

Saal, J. A., Dillingham, M. F., Gamburd, R. S., Fanton, G. S. (1988) The pseudo-radicular syndromes. *Spine*, **13**(8), 926–930.

Styf, J. (1989) Chronic exercise-induced pain in the anterior aspect of the lower leg. *Sports Med*, **7**, 331–339.

Styf, J. (1995) Intramuscular pressure measurements during exercise. *Operat Technique Sports Med*, **3**(4), 243–249.

Styf, J. (1988) Diagnosis of exercise-induced pain in the anterior aspect of the lower leg. *Am J Sports Med*, **16**(2), 165–169.

Swenson, E., *et al.* (1997) The effect of a pneumatic leg brace on return to play in athletes with tibial stress fractures. *Am J Sports Med*, **25**(3), 322–328.

U.S. Department of Health and Human Services. *International classification of diseases (9th rev). Clinical modification, 4th ed.* Washington, DC: DHHS Publication No. (PHS)91–1260.

Wilson, E.S., Katz, F. N. (1969) Stress fractures – an analysis of 250 consecutive cases. *Radiology*, **92**, 481–486.

3.8 Foot and ankle

3.8.1 Biomechanics of the foot and ankle

Bryan English

Understanding the biomechanics of the foot and ankle is of great importance when considering musculoskeletal complaints of the lower limb in particular. The search for structural pathology may be a fruitless exercise if the underlying aetiology is a functional problem. Because of the complexity of the structure, the biomechanics are different from individual to individual. In effect, the biomechanics of the foot are as unique as a fingerprint.

The foot and ankle consists of 26 bones, 57 joints, 32 muscles, and a network of ligaments. This complex has to work harmoniously to create bipedal ambulation. Any alteration in the biomechanics will result in an alteration of forces throughout the lower kinetic chain (the lower limb) that predominantly functions as a closed kinetic chain (i.e. the foot is in contact with the floor), and not as an open chain like the upper limb (the hand being free and not 'fixed' on a surface). This alteration of forces will therefore affect and possibly disrupt the biomechanics of the rest of the body. If the body is unable to adapt to an alteration or disturbance in biomechanics, then a normal or an abnormal compensation will take place somewhere in the chain. An abnormal compensation will lead to injury.

The foot/ankle complex provides:

- support and adaptation to terrain/surface
- balance
- shock absorbency, with differing landfall patterns depending on the activity
- force production/propulsion in a multitude of directions.

The forces that have to be absorbed in this area consist of:

- the body weight and the effects due to gravity
- the ground reaction force, i.e. the force that is generated by the ground against the body (Newton's third law: 'To each action there is an equal and opposite reaction.')
- compressive forces applied across the complex due to muscle contraction producing a co-contraction of forces assisting in stability.

These forces are amplified up to five times during running. In a pes cavus foot type, which is a rigid structure and therefore a poor shock absorber, the ankle (which is the size of a postage stamp) has to absorb the force. This illustrates one of the functions of articular cartilage.

Before discussing the biomechanics, some terminology must be introduced:

- **rear foot**: loose term usually meaning the hind and midfoot, or purely as the calcaneus when viewed from behind
- **hindfoot**: the talus and the calcaneus
- **midfoot**: the navicular, cuboid, and cuneiforms
- **forefoot**: the metatarsal 'rays' and the phalanges.

Positions of the foot

Figure 3.8.1 and 3.8.2 shows various rear and forefoot positions. Note that the terminology is used as though the foot is a vertical continuum of the lower leg (and not at right angles to the coronal/frontal plane;

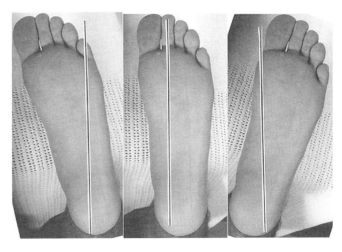

Figure 3.8.1 Positions of the left foot in the transverse plane: (a) adducted, (b) midline, (c) abducted.. The normal axis of the foot passes through the second ray. The diagrams should be visualized as though looking at the right lower limb from behind.

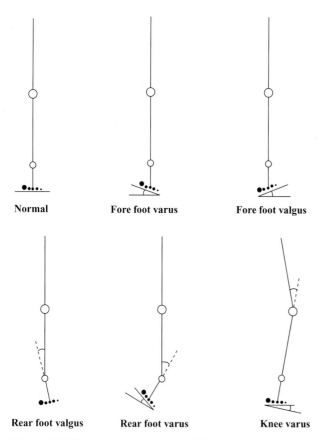

Figure 3.8.2 Varus and valgus positions of the foot.

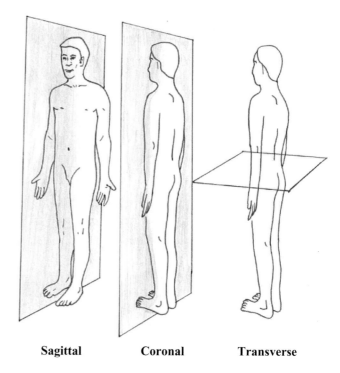

Figure 3.8.3 Anatomical positions.

Figure 3.8.3). Therefore abduction of the foot occurs in the transverse plane and not in the coronal plane, as is the case with abduction of the lower leg.

- Varus and valgus positions of the foot occur in the coronal plane.
- Inversion and eversion are the terms of movement that create a rear foot varus and valgus respectively, and therefore they occur in the coronal plane.
- Plantarflexion and dorsiflexion of the foot occur in the sagittal plane.
- Abduction and adduction of the foot occur in the transverse plane.

Pronation and supination

- A **supinated foot** is a rigid lever. This form is useful for stability and 'push off' and consists of plantar flexion combined with inversion and adduction of the foot. The appearance is of a high arched foot.
- Pronation consists of dorsiflexion, eversion, and abduction of the foot. The **pronated foot** is a loose 'bag of bones', acting as an effective shock absorber. The appearance is of a flat foot.

Joint axes within the foot and ankle

This section provides a guide to the complexities involved within the moving foot. The reader should also appreciate how orthotic or sur-

gical interference of the structure and mechanics of the foot will lead to an alteration of this refined system. A normal or abnormal adaptation may then take place. (Note that figures quoted for the angle of the axis of a joint are generalized, because of the variability of human structure.)

- The complexity of lower limb biomechanics is partly predetermined by the axis of each joint as well as the levers that act across the joint.
- The closer a joint is to a body plane, the less movement will take place in that plane.
- The axis of the ankle joint descends at a 20° angle in the frontal plane, from the medial malleolus, through the talus to the tip of the lateral malleolus. Therefore, dorsiflexion (20°) of the ankle joint is accompanied by abduction of the foot. Plantarflexion (45°) is accompanied by adduction of the foot.

Subtalar joint

The subtalar joint has a triplanar axis (as it does not run in any of the cardinal axes of the body). This runs from the posterolateral-plantar aspect to the anteromedial-dorsal aspect. It is angled at 16° medially from the sagittal plane, 42° upwards from the transverse plane and therefore 48° and 74° from the frontal plane (Figure 3.8.4).

The only movement that is measurable, from a clinical point of view, is the degree of inversion and eversion (functionally this is a rear foot varus and valgus respectively) that occurs (in the coronal plane)

Talo-calcaneo-navicular complex

This has a similar axis to the subtalar joint. The inclination and anterior angle is 40°, with a medial deviation of 30° from the sagittal plane. This axis allows pronation and supination to occur.

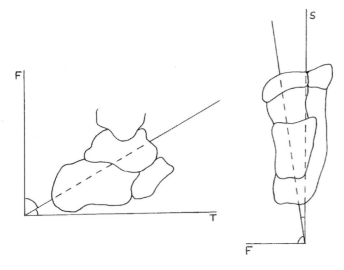

Figure 3.8.4 The triplanar axis of the subtalar joint.

Transverse tarsal complex

This is an S-shaped structure created by the talonavicular joint and the calcaneocuboid joint. There are two axes about which the foot pronates and supinates: the longitudinal axis, which inclines upwards and medially in the anteroposterior direction, and the oblique axis, which is at a similar angle to that of the talo-calcaneo-navicular joint.

When weightbearing the cuboid does not move, but the calcaneus and talus move on the navicular and cuboid. Movement at the transverse tarsal complex, which can contribute up to one third of the pronation and supination of the talo-calcaneo-navicular complex, is dependent on subtalar position.

Tarsometatarsal joints and metatarsals (rays)

- The first three rays involve the first three metatarsals and the medial, intermediate, and lateral cuneiforms respectively. The fourth and fifth metatarsals form joints with the cuboid.

- The axis of the first ray is oblique and allows dorsiflexion with inversion and adduction, plantarflexion with eversion and abduction. The fifth ray has an oblique axis nearly perpendicular to that of the first, hence the movements are opposite in that dorsiflexion will be accompanied by eversion and abduction, plantarflexion with inversion and adduction.

- The second and the fourth metatarsals have axes that are less oblique in that they are more perpendicular to the longditudunal axis of the foot. The axis of the thirrd ray is perpendicular, so the movement is predominantly into plantar and dorsiflexion.

- The second tarsometatarsal joint is wedged in between the three cuneiforms and the first and third metatarsal. This is useful for stability, but may result in increased stress going through the second metatarsal (especially if it is longer than the first metatarsal, as in a Morton's foot) and the resulting susceptibility to a stress fracture (March fracture).

Metatarsophalangeal joints

These allow abduction and adduction. However, plantar and dorsiflexion are the main movements creating the hinge type of move-ment during ambulation. The windlass mechanism involving these joints and the plantar fascia are discussed in the section on heel pain.

Arches of the foot

- The medial longitudinal arch is higher 'off the ground' and more flexible than the lateral arch. This flexibility allows pronation. The arch is supported by the bony configuration as well as the soft tissues, thereby creating a degree of elastic recoil as the foot returns to supination.

- The transverse arch is perpendicular to the longitudinal arch, and is most obvious in the mid- and forefoot. The bony configuration of the cuneiforms and the cuboid creates a concavity of the rays on the plantar aspect of the foot. This allows a fan-like spread of the forefoot during weightbearing, which contributes towards shock absorbency.

Muscles of the foot

- There are 13 extrinsic muscles and 19 intrinsic muscles of the foot. The details of their relative actions on the foot are discussed in greater detail elsewhere in this chapter.

- The extrinsic muscles of the posterior compartment act as plantar-flexors (mainly via gastrocnemius, soleus) and toe flexors (flexor digitorum longus and flexor hallucis longus), and provide stability to the ankle and the longitudinal arch (tibialis posterior).

- The lateral compartment muscles act as evertors of the foot and ankle; peroneus longus also acts as a plantarflexor at the midtarsal joint.

- The anterior compartment muscles act as dorsiflexors of the foot (tibialis anterior) and extensors of the toes (extensor hallucis longus and extensor digitorum longus). Tibialis anterior contributes to inversion of the foot, extensor hallucis longus to eversion.

- The intrinsic muscles provide specific movements. For example, the flexor hallucis brevis flexes the proximal phalanx of the great toe, and its tendons house the sesamoid bones. The extensor digitorum brevis extends the medial four toes at the proximal phalanx.

Biomechanical analysis

The neuromuscular structures control foot and ankle movement about a predetermined axis. This can be assessed kinematically and kinetically, and has been extensively investigated and analysed in humans. The following paragraphs provide a brief generalization of the biomechanics that may be observed.

People vary a great deal in relation to how their foot comes into contact with the ground. For example, most runners will strike the ground with the heel followed by distribution of force throughout the foot prior to toe off. This is called a **heel–toe technique** and will be used as the example in the following paragraphs. Other patterns include a **forefoot technique** (where the heel does not actually strike the floor, but descends sufficiently to allow eccentric stretch of the ankle dorsiflexors) and a **toe–heel–toe technique** (with the initial strike taking place at the midfoot or forefoot).

A functional model

The heel strikes the ground on the lateral border of the heel. The supinated foot, with an inverted rear foot, starts to pronate. The degree of pronation will be dictated by the subtalar joint. If no movement occurs here, then the only way the foot can pronate is by internal rotation of the lower leg. The subtalar joint is a **torque convertor** (see section on the subtalar joint). Movement here will unlock the foot for pronation and lock the foot for supination.

- As foot pronation occurs, there is internal rotation of the lower leg. This rotation increases if there is limited subtalar joint movement. This internal rotation results in a functional knee valgus and an increase in the Q angle of the knee(see Chapter 3.7).

> Most causes of bilateral anterior knee pain are due to a high Q angle that is increased by excessive pronation

- Excessive subtalar movement will put increased stress on the medial aspect of the ankle and/or lower leg.

> Insertional tendonitis of tibialis posterior and/or medial shin pain, may be due to excessive pronation with the action of tibialis posterior being overcome by the body weight and the ground reaction force.

- Excessive pronation will also put increased stress on the medial aspect of the Achilles tendon.

> Palpate the sore tendon of a distance runner. If the tendon is just tender medially, then excessive pronation is probably the cause of the excess strain.

- As the excessively pronated foot with limited subtalar movement and functional knee valgus now attempts to supinate, the lower leg will start to externally rotate whilst the femur wants to stay internally rotating to create knee extension.

> Could there be a mistiming of thigh on lower leg movements here? Is the knee being forced to perform a pivot shift manoeuvre? Is this a possible reason why 80% of anterior cruciate ligaments tear as a result of non-contact injuries?

- With the foot excessively pronated with a functional knee valgus, the abductor muscles of the buttock are attempting to abduct the adducted thigh.

> Is pronation, aided by excessive weight, the reason why the sedentary population suffer from lateral buttock pain?

- Due to the above effects of pronation, functional shortening of the lower leg can occur causing a strain to the pelvis, lumbar spine and beyond.

> If people get pain in the lower back and lower limb that is aggravated by exercise, have a look at the lower limb biomechanics, i.e. examine them whilst they are experiencing their pain and not just standing or lying on a couch when they have told you that these positions do not cause pain.

All these components will be magnified with increased activity such as running. So often, we are dealing with functional problems caused by a functional and/or structural problem within the foot.

Kinematics

> Kinematics can be defined as the branch of mechanics concerned with the motion of objects without reference to the forces which cause the motion.

Gait can be broken down to a stance phase and a swing phase (Figure 3.8.5). The stance phase lasts for approximately 65% of the gait cycle in walking. This percentage decreases with running. The phase con-

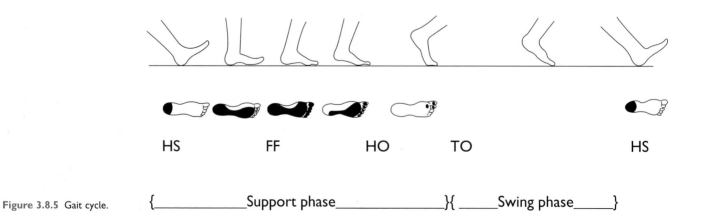

HS   FF   HO   TO   HS

Figure 3.8.5 Gait cycle.   {_____Support phase_____}{ _____Swing phase_____}

sists of heel strike, flat foot, mid stance, heel off, and toe off. Each section of the phase is dependent on many factors such as foot anatomy, type of footwear, and type of surface.

Heel strike

Most muscular activity as the foot adapts to the surface occurs in the first 15% of the cycle that follows heel strike (Figure 3.8.6). The graphs

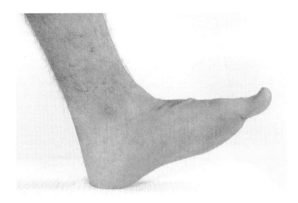

Figure 3.8.6 Heel strike.

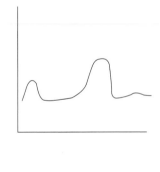

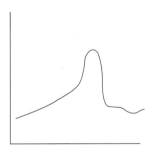

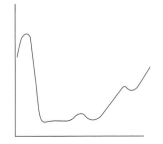

Figure 3.8.7 (a) The activity of peroneus longus, which is active at heel strike and toe off, acting as a stabilizer to the ankle joint. (b) Gastrocnemius acting eccentrically during weightbearing before maximal activity at toe off. (c) Initial high eccentric activity of tibialis anterior to prevent foot slap and activity during the swing phase to keep the foot off the ground.

in Figure 3.8.7 are a simple representation of the activity within the peroneus longus, gastrocnemius and tibialis anterior muscles during the cycle. The heel strikes the ground in a more or less vertical plane. The vectors of the ground force reaction are mentioned later in this chapter in the discussion of force plate studies.

The heel strikes on the lateral border of the rear foot as the leg is swinging towards the line of progression (external rotation of the thigh to counteract the transverse plane rotation of the pelvis, and also the foot is supinated at this point). Wearing out of the lateral border of a shoe is therefore a normal phenomenon. Soon after heel strike the rear foot starts to move from an inverted towards an everted position, thus producing fairly rapid pronation (a useful way to absorb shock).

Flat foot

As pronation is starting to occur when approaching flat foot (Figure 3.8.8a), the lower leg is starting to internally rotate (due to the torque convertor effect of the subtalar joint). The timing of the joint movements during this phase is important as the foot adapts to the surface. Internal rotation of both the femur and tibia on a partly flexed knee incorporates more force down on to the talus, encouraging more pronation and an 'unlocking' of the foot.

After **mid stance** (where the lower leg is perpendicular to the ground), ankle dorsiflexion produces a degree of locking of its mortise. The lower leg starts to externally rotate on the ankle, resulting in a return towards supination (Figure 3.8.8b).

Heel off

Plantarflexion is initiated along with dorsiflexion of the metatarso-phalangeal joints which stretches the plantar fascia encouraging

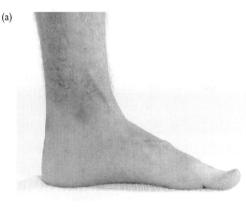

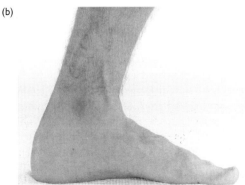

Figure 3.8.8 (a) Flat foot. (b) Ankle dorsiflexion in flat foot.

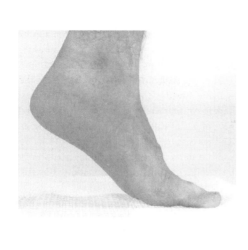

Figure 3.8.9 Heel off.

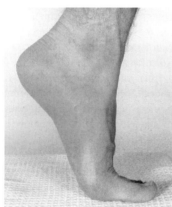

Figure 3.8.10 Toe off.

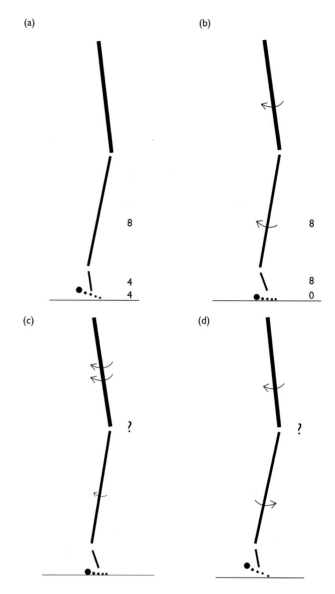

Figure 3.8.11 The biomechanics of a left lower limb (see text for details).

increased supination. This more rigid foot is ideal for the propulsive action that is about to take place. Ideally the heel is in the neutral position at this stage to prevent excessive forces occurring on either the medial aspect (if the foot remains in pronation) or the lateral aspect (rapid movement over to supination with an inverted rear foot). **Toe off** is the end of the stance phase, and usually occurs at the great toe.

Swing phase

The main concern during this phase is to prevent the foot from catching the floor, so the ankle returns from a highly plantarflexed position at toe off, to a dorsiflexed position in the middle of the swing phase.

Normally the ankle is in a more stable dorsiflexed position before heel strike. However, when landing from a jump 80% of individuals have the foot plantarflexed. This position allows the foot and ankle to absorb the increased force of landing from a height.[1]

Figure 3.8.11 shows stick diagrams representing the biomechanics of a left lower limb viewed from the front (running towards the reader): (a) a 4° forefoot varus, 4° rear foot valgus, and 8° tibial varus at heel strike; (b) for the foot to reach the floor, 8° of rear foot valgus will be required, resulting in increased internal tibial rotation; (c) the foot may start to supinate with tibial external rotation, while the femur is still internally rotating to create knee extension; (d) the foot may remain pronated, so knee extension is possible only with increased

internal rotation of the femur (i.e. self-inflicted pivot shift manoeuvre). Is this a possible reason for the 'mistiming' of joints, considering that many ligamentous injuries to the knee are non-contact injuries? Using the above model, would an orthotic controlling rear and forefoot movement have a beneficial effect on abnormal knee rotation?

Methods for measuring kinematics

- **Observation**: Inexpensive, but very subjective.

- **Multiple exposure**: Inexpensive basic camera required with reflective markers on the patient. Gait cannot be observed.

- **Cinematography/television**: Relatively inexpensive cine camera with video playback analysis. The most commonly employed system for the clinician. Body markers may be placed on bony anatomical landmarks (to minimize the movement of the soft tissues), or the body can be marked with ink. This analysis in its basic form is sub-jective to an extent, useful for high-speed sporting activities, but tedious frame by frame visualization of playback is required if statistical analysis is to take place (in which case body markers need to be used). However, computer software systems are now available that will digitize from a video with markers.

- **Television/computer:** Expensive. Cameras emit infrared light on to reflective body markers, and the reflection is received by the same camera. Six cameras appears to be the minimum required for sophisticated analysis of all the body planes and ensuring that the body markers are always visible.

- **Active marker systems:** These markers emit their own characteristic signal so the cameras can easily tag each marker separately. A power source has to be carried by the patient.

Kinetics

> Kinetics can be defined as the branch of mechanics concerned with the motion of bodies under the action of forces.

Lower limb kinetics can be complex. It is still very much in the realms of research, and could form the subject of an entire textbook. The following few paragraphs are aimed at the clinician, as an introduction to the possibilities of scientific assessment and how these are best applied in the clinical setting.

When requesting dynamic computer-assisted analysis, it is best for the clinician to request that specific clinical questions be answered if at all possible. Scientific analysis will produce vast reams of data that may overcomplicate the situation if it is not communicated well for the benefit of the patient.[2]

Ground reaction force

This force can be measured with a rectangular force plate/platform which is embedded into the floor, so the patient is unaware that they are walking upon the 'chosen' surface. The plate has pressure transducers at each corner. Data collected will be the magnitude, direction, line of action, and point of application of the ground reaction force.

Newton's third law (quoted at the beginning of this section) states that to each action there is an equal and opposite reaction. The force of the body hitting the floor is met by an equal and opposite ground reaction force.

force = mass × acceleration

The ground force measured is therefore a measure of the acceleration of the centre of mass of the body (the mass being easily determined by body weight).

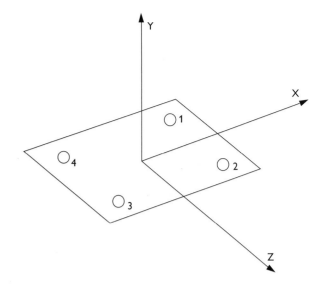

Figure 3.8.12 Measuring forces in three dimensions.

Vertical, horizontal, and translational forces can be measured (Figure 3.8.12). The vertical force (F_Y) is usually the greatest force and includes the effects due to gravity. The horizontal force (F_X) includes forces in the direction of movement plus frictional forces. The translational force (F_Z) is the sideways movement that occurs on contact with the ground, and obviously this also consists of a frictional force (enabling the body to change directions quickly without the foot slipping).

The resulting graphs of the ground reaction force (Figure 3.8.13) are characteristic for human gait and certain forms of foot strike. With a heel strike, for example, there is an initial spike as the foot 'strikes' the plate (this is termed a passive peak) followed by a curve as the whole foot contacts the ground (this active peak being under muscular control). In Figure 3.8.13 the active peak occurs twice. This occurs when walking as there is a double support phase (i.e. weightbearing on the other leg). It does not occur with a stance phase during running.

Graphs such as these are useful for assessing the effectiveness of an amputee gait, for example (affected or unaffected limb). The prosthesis can be altered to recreate a relatively normal ground reaction force.

Types of force

Internal forces: muscle action; friction between soft tissues; elastic/stored energy

External forces: gravity; ground reaction force; external friction

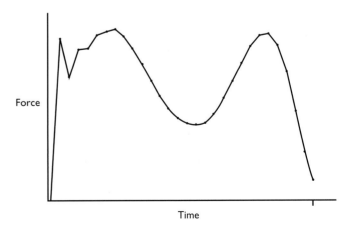

Figure 3.8.13 Ground reaction force.

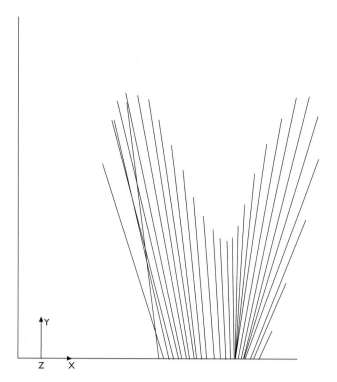

Figure 3.8.14 Butterfly diagram.

These diagrams are not useful in determining what part of the foot is undergoing pressure, after the initial contact.

Excessive force on heel strike may also be a reason for athletic-induced injuries. For example, basketball players who land with a flat foot after a jump have been observed to produce a ground reaction force up to 30% greater than those who land toe to heel. Admittedly one cannot rule out the effects of inertia (the effect that gravity has on the limb), but there may be a problem of technique. Runners can have problems with this, especially after an injury.

Vector forces

Knowing the direction of the forces that have to be absorbed is of particular value, especially when considering gait analysis of athletes as well as amputees and patients with cerebral palsy. Vector diagrams can be extrapolated to form 'butterfly diagrams' (directions of force throughout the stance phase) (Figure 3.8.14). They are useful to determine when the body's centre of gravity comes across the midline.

A vector is a force with a direction. In vector diagrams such as Figure 3.8.15 the length of the line is proportionate to the degree of force, relative to the other lines of the diagram (hence the line R is longer than v and h). For example, according to the equation of a right-angled triangle, the resultant force vector R in the figure can be derived using the following simple equation:

$$F_R = \surd(\Sigma F_h^2 + \Sigma F_v^2)$$

where F_R is the resultant and ground reaction force and F_h and F_v are the horizontal and vertical forces that are detected by the force plate. Further algebraic manipulation will also reveal the angle of F_R.

The examples given above are for movements in the sagittal plane. Medial and lateral movement in the coronal plane can also be assessed. Details have been published elsewhere.[1,3–5]

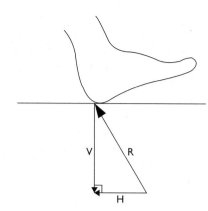

Figure 3.8.15 Vector of forces diagram.

Free-body diagrams

After the vector forces have been obtained, the effect of these forces on one body segment can be determined (Figure 3.8.16). In the figure, R is the ground reaction force/vector, A is the muscle force required to resist plantarflexion (eccentric tibialis anterior work), and C is the weightbearing load. It can be seen from the diagram that R acts behind the centre of the ankle joint. This will result in a moment of force in the clockwise direction to produce plantarflexion.

If the compressive force C acts through the centre of the joint, then force A has to equal R in order to prevent a rapid plantarflexion manoeuvre.

Pressure measurement at the foot

So far we have only discussed the forces that are distributed to the ankle and leg.

Pressure-sensitive materials

Measurement of the pressure distribution at the foot can be performed with pressure-sensitive materials that, for example, will release a certain amount of ink on to the mat placed above them (the greater the pressure, the more ink is released).

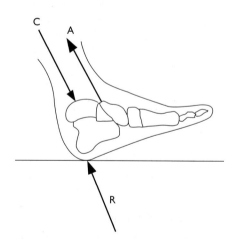

Figure 3.8.16
Free-body diagram.

Moment = force × distance (measured in newton metres)

Dynamic pressure measurement

A more sophisticated, dynamic method of measuring pressure distribution is to use a pedobarograph. This device consists of a layer of plastic placed above a sheet of glass. The plastic distorts under pressure, distorting the light passing through. The results are digitized and presented as a colour print-out. This is useful to determine time under pressure at a particular site, for example when assessing the cause of undue pressure due to a 'dropped' metatarsal head.

Other devices for dynamic testing consist of materials made up of a few hundred isolated cells (each acting as its own pressure transducer), which react when weight is placed upon them. Shear forces make actual pressure transducer insoles difficult to employ. They also require the patient to be electrically linked to the recording device. Any device that the patient is aware of may alter the gait.

Treatment for abnormalities of lower limb biomechanics

History

There may be several pointers in the history that should lead the clinician to suspect the possibility of a biomechanical problem.

Bilateral pain

It would be unusual for a structural disorder to occur on both sides unless it is congenital or developmental in the growing years. Bilateral anterior knee pain, for example, is a biomechanical disorder until proved otherwise, in my opinion. Other examples would be bilateral tibialis posterior tendonitis and bilateral lateral buttock pain. Spinal pathologies may present with bilateral pain, but other aspects of the history will differentiate them.

Pain with exercise

With biomechanical problems, exercise is often the aggravating factor, but non-weightbearing exercise will be painless. Problems simply with going up and down stairs are suggestive of such problems. The clinician should therefore examine the patient when they are ambulant. Too often the patient is examined standing and lying down only, i.e. when they do not have pain. Examination while the pain is being produced can produce a totally different set of observations.

Exercise-related pain may also be associated with other diagnoses, such as compartment syndrome or a stress fracture, that have been dealt with in Chapter 3.7.

No trauma

Often the history is of an insidious onset when the musculoskeletal system has been subjected to increased demand. The body may adapt to biomechanical abnormalities until the stage is reached when an increased load will result in breakdown. This may be due to increased demand, increased weight, or a change in surface (such as a mountain runner starting to train on concrete).

Previous multiple assessments and investigations

The following clinical case represents such a scenario.

A 22-year-old woman presented to the orthopaedic department with bilateral anterior knee pain of 4 years' duration. The pain was exacerbated by exercise. She had been given various forms of self-management exercises and several courses of manual and electrical physiotherapy. Following the lack of response to this treatment, she underwent the following investigations:

- skyline X-rays followed by serial skyline radiographs (20°, 40°, 60°)
- CT scan of the patellofemoral joint followed by serial CT (0–20°)

As these investigations were normal, a decision was made to perform bilateral arthroscopies that demonstrated a normal knee and patellofemoral joint. Subsequently surgical lateral release was undertaken bilaterally. This had no effect on the patient's pain. Before examination, the patient was asked if anyone had ever looked at her feet, or watched her walking or running. She answered that this had not been the case. Standing examination demonstrated a mild degree of overpronation that was notably exaggerated on walking, producing functional maltracking of the patella. The patient was provided with foot orthotics for walking and for exercise and became symptom-free within 2 months.

Not all cases will be as straightforward. However, a simple history and examination can avoid unnecessary investigations, unnecessary radiation, and unnecessary surgery.

Examination

Standing

Asymmetry is very common in the musculoskeletal system (Figure 3.8.17). Moderate asymmetry is obvious to the naked eye and can detect scoliosis, spinal movement asymmetry, pelvic level, internal femoral torsion, tibial varus, pronated or supinated feet, and a relaxed calcaneal stance position (when viewed from behind, as demonstrated in the middle photograph of Figure 3.8.18). A useful tip is to talk to the patient, allowing them to relax into a position that is normal for them. Pronation will occur as the patient relaxes and becomes used to being observed.

When the patient is standing, the movements of the foot and especially the ankle can be observed by:

- **Standing on tiptoes:** This demonstrates plantarflexion of the ankle and hyperextension of the great toe (Figure 3.8.19). In this relatively supinated position the arches of the foot and the soft tissues of the fascial layers may be observed for their integrity.

- **Flexing the knee and moving the knee joint as far over the front of the foot as possible:** This is useful to detect the degree of dorsiflexion of the ankle and the degree of pronation that may occur (Figure 3.8.20). To prevent the patient from avoiding painful anterior impingement of the ankle, the instruction should be to produce this movement in the sagittal plane initially and then to allow pronation with subtalar joint movement.

Sitting

A functional scoliosis will become straight if the pelvis becomes level as in sitting.

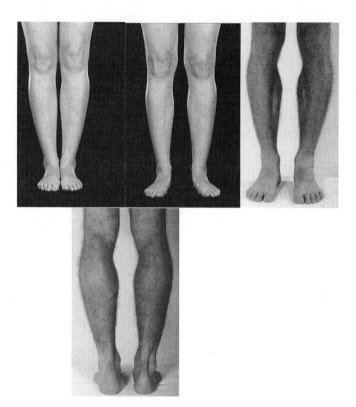

Figure 3.8.17 Asymmetry in the musculoskeletal system.

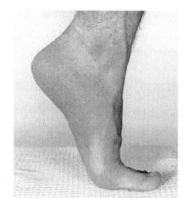

Figure 3.8.19 Standing on tiptoe.

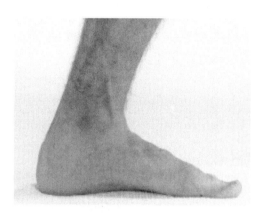

Figure 3.8.20 Ankle dorsiflexion

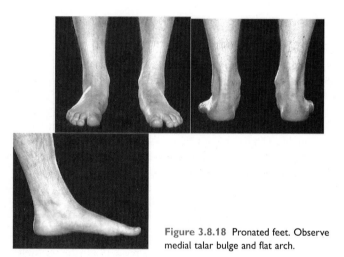

Figure 3.8.18 Pronated feet. Observe medial talar bulge and flat arch.

- **Midfoot movement** is difficult to detect, but testing one side compared to the other is useful. Shearing (translatory) movements of the navicular, cuboid, and cuneiforms on their neighbouring bones may produce pain in a symptomatic patient.

- **Forefoot movement** consists of shearing movements of the metatarsals on one another. The first tarsometatarsal joint is the only one that has substantial movement (10–25°). There is relatively no movement of the second tarsometatarsal joint as it is fixed in position by the neighbouring bones. The movements of the metatarsophalangeal joints are of importance especially that involving dorsiflexion of the first metatarsophalangeal joint.

Supine

Pelvic level, hips, knees, and limb length deformity can be examined with the patient supine. The ankle and foot can be examined passively:

- **Malleolar position** should be approximately 13–18° but will be decreased for example by internal tibial torsion. This is an angle of inclination going from the lateral malleolus to the medial malleolus.

- **Ankle dorsiflexion** with the knee flexed (otherwise a tight gastrocnemius/soleus complex may limit the movement). This movement may be easier in the prone position.

- **Plantarflexion** of the ankle ensuring that the movement comes from the talocrural area and not the midfoot/forefoot.

Prone

Sacroiliac joints and pelvic level can be examined. This position is particularly useful for examining the relationship between the lower leg, rear foot, and forefoot (Figure 3.8.21). Lines bisecting the lower leg and rear foot may be drawn on the skin to assist with the visual inspection. Tibia varus of up to 8° is normal, and the range of subtalar joint movement can be detected using a protractor. The range of subtalar joint movement is divided into two thirds inversion and one third eversion The rear foot to forefoot relationship is observed with the subtalar joint in the neutral position and the talus fixed into the mortise of the ankle joint. A typical forefoot varus is demonstrated in Figure 3.8.22.

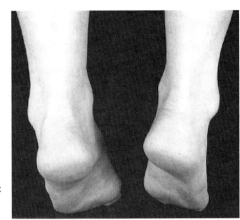

Figure 3.8.21 Lower leg, rear foot and forefoot relationship.

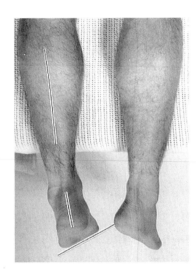

Figure 3.8.22 Lower leg, rear foot and forefoot relationship.

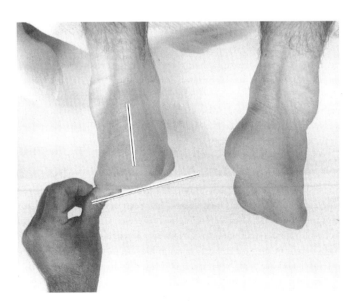

Figure 3.8.23 Typical forefoot varus.

Walking

Functional abnormalities may be highlighted by ambulation, which can take place in a consulting room with or without a treadmill. The numerous possible observations include increased pronation, abduction of the feet on ambulation, early heel rise (due to tight gastrocnemius), functional knee valgus/squinting of the patella, and excessive strain/bowing of the Achilles tendon due to rearfoot valgus (Figure 3.8.23).

Running

Abnormalities on running may have to be detected by video analysis, as the more subtle problems cannot be detected by the naked eye at the speeds that may be involved. All the above factors may be further pronounced because of the higher impact forces (up to five times body weight).

Assessment

The various forms of functional assessment have been discussed elsewhere in this section.

Radiographs of the foot and ankle with the patient weightbearing may be useful. The talar declination angle and the calcaneal inclination angle (Figure 3.8.24) will confirm the degree of supination/pronation that is present. Radiography may also detect congenital abnormalities such as tarsal coalition.

Treatment

Self-management

With any biomechanical disorder, the neuromuscular system is a determinant of movement of the structure. An individual may look after their own system by complying with flexibility work and general body conditioning. A muscle will never produce 100% power without 100% flexibility. Neuromuscular stretches should be part of a daily routine for anyone who presents with biomechanical problems.

Physician advice: type of exercise, footwear, terrain, sport

Some individuals are not designed to run marathons. The morphology of an individual, plus various anthropometric measurements, may suggest that certain activities may lead to problems whether there is a biomechanical problem or not. The symptoms from a lower limb disorder may be aggravated by running on concrete, and the athlete would be advised to cross-train (i.e. spend some time doing other sports or competing on a different, more forgiving, surface).

Footwear is also a crucial factor. A patient walking in a pair of worn-out shoes (specifically if they are worn out on the lateral aspect of the heel where heel strike occurs) will be liable to problems. Modern footwear can consist of sophisticated shock-absorbing material as well as providing 'support' for those with biomechanical problems.

Physiotherapy muscle work, etc.

Self-management may not be sufficient. Manual work on areas of specifically tight musculature will be of benefit in releasing tension. Detection of muscle tightness and dysfunction will lead to a more prescriptive phase of post-injury rehabilitation.

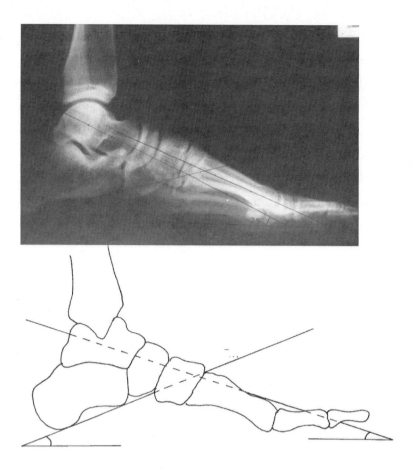

Figure 3.8.24 Calcaneal inclination angle and talar declination angle

Talar declination angle

Calcaneal inclination angle

Podiatry, orthotics

This area of treatment and the speciality of podiatry can be the key to most of the clinical dilemmas presenting as biomechanical disorders. The basis behind corrective orthotics is to bring the floor up to the foot and prevent the foot from having to drop to the floor. The orthotic is a sophisticated device that will control and guide movement throughout the foot. Hence the effects of the orthotic will be 'felt' in the whole of the lower limb and beyond.[6,7]

Orthoses consist of shock absorbing materials that also provide stability for support. Carbon fibre is used for those orthotics requiring a firmer degree of control.

There is a great deal of anecdotal evidence of benefit from the use of orthoses, but there is still a great deal of work to be done to prove their value scientifically.[8,9] Precision making of the device is ruled out by the interobserver error in measuring range of movement of the subtalar joint, for example. For this reason, off-the-shelf orthotics for the most common abnormality (a forefoot varus) will often suffice, providing the gross adjustment and allowing the body to make the finer adjustments. For more unusual abnormalities, casting of

devices by a practitioner experienced with the technique is recommended.

When orthoses have been prescribed, the patient should gradually be introduced to wearing them (i.e. 15 minutes on the first day, increasing by a further 15 minutes on subsequent days). The patient should be wearing walking orthotics for several weeks before running orthotics are prescribed. Wearing orthotics too much too soon may cause discomfort, blistering, and biomechanical problems elsewhere in the body if there has been insufficient time to adjust.

Surgical treatment

Structural adjustment of a biomechanical abnormality is required when all else has failed. Once surgery has been performed, the rehabilitation phase has to be carefully monitored as the body adjusts and hopefully adapts to the new forces to which it will be subject. The technical details of surgical correction for ankle and foot abnormalities are extensive and are dealt with in many other reference books.[3,10,11]

Surgery may sort out one problem only to cause another. The patient should be advised carefully before any form of surgery.

References

1. Valiant, G. A., Cavanagh, P. R. A study of landing from a jump: implications for design of a basketball shoe. In: Winter D. A. *et al.* (eds) *Biomechanics IX-B*, Human Kinetics, Champaign, IL, 1985.

2. Hamill, J., Knutzen, K. M. *Biomechanical basis of human movement.* Williams and Wilkins, Baltimore, MD, 1995.

3. Subotnik, S. (ed.) *Sports medicine of the lower extremity.* Churchill Livingstone, Edinburgh, 1989.

4. Palastagna, N., Field, D., Soames, R. *Anatomy and human movement*, 2nd edn. Butterworth-Heinemann, Oxford, 1994.

5. Sammarco, G. J. *Rehabilitation of the foot and ankle.* Mosby, St Louis, 1995.

6. McPhoil, T. G., Cornwall, M. W. The effect of foot orthoses on transverse tibial rotation during walking. *Journal of the American Podiatry Association*, 2000, **90**, 2–11.

7. Rodger, M. M., Leveau, B. F. Effectiveness of foot orthotic devices used to modify pronation in runners. *Journal of Orthopaedic and Sports Physical Therapy*, 1982, **4**, 86–90.

8. Nawoczenski, D. A., Cook, T. M., Slatzman C. L. The effect of foot orthotics on three-dimensional kinematics of the leg and rear foot during running. *Journal of Orthopaedic and Sports Physical Therapy*, 1995, **21**, 317–327.

9. Stacoff, A., Reinschmidt, C., Nigg B. M. Effects of foot orthoses on skeletal motion during running. *Clinical Biomechanics*, 2000, **15**, 54–64.

10. Baxter, D. E. *The foot and ankle in sport.* Mosby, St Louis, 1995.

11. McGlamry, E. D., Banks, A. S., Downey M. S. *Comprehensive textbook in foot surgery*, 2nd edn. Williams and Wilkins, Baltimore, MD, 1992.

3.8.2 **The ankle joint**

Richard Higgins

Anatomy

The ankle joint, or talocrural joint, is a hinged synovial joint consisting of a complex combination of articular surfaces. The stability of the joint is reliant on its position. In dorsiflexion the talus is squeezed by the malleoli, as because of its shape it spreads the mortice, tightening the interosseous and anterior and posterior tibiofibular ligaments, securely locking the joint. This contrasts with the relative instability experienced in plantarflexion. Contributing to the adjustment to uneven surfaces and assisting in shock absorption are additional important functions of the ankle joint.

During sporting activity, the lateral ankle complex is more frequently injured than any other major structure.[1] Forces generated when landing from a jump are absorbed through the kinetic chain via the foot and ankle complex, as it progresses from plantarflexion through to dorsiflexion and pronation. Landing flatfooted would therefore transmit most of these forces proximally to other structures. Situations in which this occurs are common in many sports, and with up to 80% of players landing in a significantly plantarflexed position,[2] any additional factors such as the player attempting a sudden turn, or landing being affected by contact with another player, can increase lateral movement and further increase the chances of sustaining an inversion injury.

The talus, wider anteriorly than posteriorly, slots into the ankle mortice, formed by the distal tibial and fibular surfaces, articulating superiorly via its trochlear surface. Its medial and lateral surfaces bear facets that articulate with their respective malleoli.

Joint movements available are those of dorsiflexion, primarily produced by tibialis anterior, during which the malleoli are forced slightly apart, and plantarflexion, with gastrocnemius and soleus acting as the prime movers. In addition, rotation in the transverse plain, abduction, and adduction also occur in plantarflexion, with most inversion and eversion occurring at the subtalar joint.

The capsule derives its strength from local ligamentous structures. Medially the deltoid ligament consists of three superficial and two deep components, fanning out in a triangular fashion from the medial malleolus, inserting into the navicular, calcaneum, and talus respectively, with each reflection being named accordingly. In addition to conferring significant stability to the medial side of the joint, the deltoid ligament provides support to the medial longitudinal arch while securing the calcaneum and navicular to the talus.

The lateral or tripartite ligament (Figure 3.8.25) is a less substantial structure. It comprises the relatively weak anterior talofibular liga-

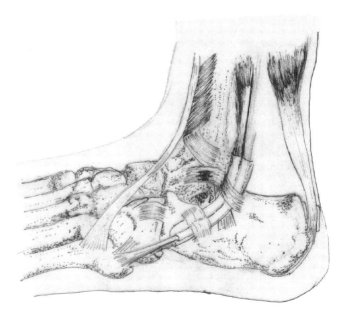

Figure 3.8.25 Anatomy of the lateral ligament.

ment, a capsular thickening passing anteromedially to the talus, the stronger posterior talofibular ligament passing almost horizontally, and the cord-like calcaneofibular ligament, which passes postero-inferiorly, being crossed superficially by the tendons of peroneous longus and brevis and blending with the medial wall of their tendon sheath.

The anterior and posterior portions of the capsule remain relatively thin and the synovial capsule is somewhat superficial in these areas, so if there is any swelling it is often evident here.

Inversion injuries

Aetiology

Inversion injuries, or acute lateral ligament sprains, are the commonest form of sporting injury,[3] accounting for on average 40% of all injuries and up to 85% of ankle sprains,[4] which in themselves are responsible for over 15% of all time lost from sport.[1] The injury occurs when the athlete lands with the foot plantarflexed and slightly inverted, a position that unlocks the joint. Of factors thought to confer increased risk of sustaining an inversion injury, muscle imbalance relating eversion to inversion strength appears to be particularly significant.

Disruption of the anterior talofibular ligament is most frequently encountered and will involve capsular damage. A more severe injury includes damage to the calcaneofibular ligament, which is rarely injured on its own, and involving the peroneal tendon sheath because of its confluence. This is easily demonstrated on arthrography. Additional injury to the posterior talofibular ligament is the least common finding, occurring relatively infrequently.

Classification of lateral ligamentous injuries is variable. Injuries are described as primary, secondary, or tertiary or grade 1, 2, or 3, in order of increasing severity. Grading also reflects the combination of ligaments involved, progressing from a single-ligament injury to complete disruption.

Diagnosis

This is based on the clinical history, with the patient's description of mechanism of injury directing the clinician towards the possibility of associated damage, such as syndesmotic rupture. Examination findings then help to confirm suspicions, as described below. Rushed history-taking, and subsequent failure to accurately elucidate the mechanism of injury, often leads to the assumption that this is just another 'simple ankle sprain'. Associated injuries may be missed, at best leading to confusion and embarrassment when symptoms are slow to resolve, at worse leading to possible legal implications.

> Most sports physicians enjoy having some involvement as a team physician to complete their professional development, and realize its necessity. However, it is in this environment that mistakes most often occur. Lunchtime visits, dealing with multiple complaints, tempt one to cut corners. Adequate time and private consultation facilities, away from interfering enthusiasts, are essential.

Examination findings

Associated swelling around the lateral malleolus is usually present even in grade 1 injuries, often extending proximally. Palpation will reveal tenderness over the respective ligaments, pain over the anterior joint line possibly suggesting a talar dome injury. Inversion will often be painful when tested both actively and passively.

When an anterior drawer is undertaken (Figure 3.8.26), it should always be compared with the other side, as normal variations in ligamentous laxity may produce false positives. A movement of 5–10 mm is considered abnormal, most of the research findings falling within this range, though as with many tests there is an element of subjectivity. Equipment cannot replace experience. A positive test undertaken in slight plantarflexion indicates a complete tear of the anterior talofibular ligament. Further investigations such as talar tilt are sometimes used in helping to confirm the diagnosis.

The distal tibiofibular syndesmosis should be palpated. Specific tenderness in association with either a positive squeeze test (which compresses the fibula to the tibia above the midpoint of the calf,

causing pain distally) or external rotation of the foot in dorsiflexion (the external rotation stress test), similarly causing local discomfort, are indicative of disruption. Always palpate the base of the fifth metatarsal to exclude an associated fracture.

Investigations

Plain radiographs should be undertaken if there is suspicion of a fracture. An inability to weightbear continuing on arrival in the emergency department, alongside bony tenderness on either malleolus, form the basis of the Ottawa rules, a scoring system which gives a good indication as to whether there may be an underlying fracture and has been shown to decrease requests for unnecessary investigations. At least two views should be requested, fields extending to include the base of the fifth metatarsal, with stress radiographs being undertaken if significant instability is suspected.

Talar dome injuries are best imaged using MRI. Widening of the ankle mortice indicates a rupture of the syndesmosis, complete disruption indicating surgical intervention.

Treatment

Initial treatment of an acute inversion injury or simple ankle sprain follows the usual regime of rest, ice, compression, elevation (RICE). This regime is often not undertaken aggressively enough. Ice is beneficial immediately after injury, decreasing swelling and helping with pain relief.[5] However, blood flow does not decrease significantly for about 10 minutes after the application of ice, by which time considerable bleeding may already have occurred, so the compressive element becomes equally important as an aid to restricting haemorrhage.[6] If sports related, the athlete should be removed from the field of play without placing weight on the joint, the limb being elevated as soon as possible and compression applied. Cryocuffs (Figure 3.8.27) are often used in this situation and although some of the research is conflicting, experience shows that they are a useful adjunct in the initial 24–48-hour period. Non-steroidal anti-inflammatories are also of benefit at this time.

During the acute phase compression is achieved by taping, with the addition of a U-shaped stirrup (Figure 3.8.28) to produce a more local application of pressure around the lateral malleolus; this has been shown to be more beneficial than non-specific compression.[7]

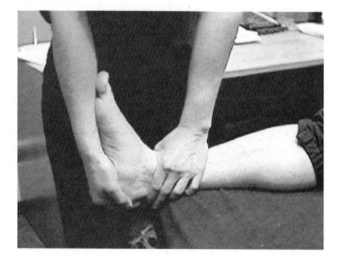

Figure 3.8.26 Anterior drawer sign.

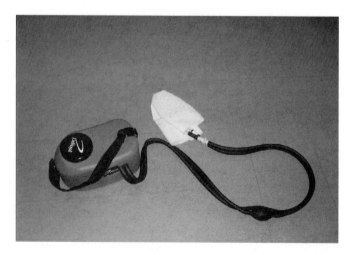

Figure 3.8.27 Cryocuff.

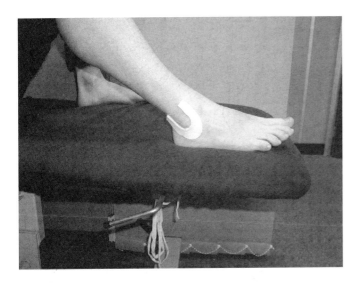

Figure 3.8.28 U-shaped stirrup.

peutic benefit experienced.[10] Its non-thermal effects are still not clearly understood and, although some research has been published to the contrary, it most probably provides little or no benefit.

The athlete should also be taken through passive and active assisted exercises, to improve range of motion. All these steps must be followed aggressively, each being of vital importance in the acute-phase of the rehabilitation programme.

Unfortunately it is still not uncommon to see an athlete hobbling into the clinic on crutches a week after an inversion injury; the local emergency department is often the culprit, with recovery already having been compromised. Management regimes such as this, comprising prolonged non-weightbearing or cast immobilization, are still advised, but are unacceptable. Observation and review of these cases, backed by research,[11] show that this approach leads only to ongoing pain and dysfunction.

The recovery phase then begins, introducing multidirectional activities. Weightbearing exercise is undertaken using an airbrace or taping as support, early mobilization being essential as it decreases

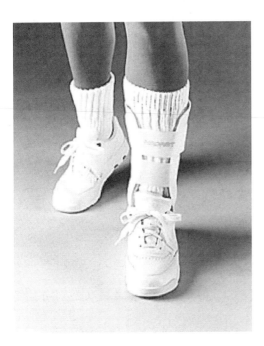

Figure 3.8.29 Aircast brace.

Air splints (Figure 3.8.29) are often used as rehabilitation progresses and have been shown to be protective against re-injury in many studies. The suggestion is that they should be worn for at least 6 months after moderate to severe injuries, although in many sports this is not practical.[8]

Contrast baths are sometimes suggested as treatment after the acute phase, but research does not support this, in some cases indicating an increase in swelling after use,[9] confirming the thinking that ice and compression are the most appropriate modalities during this phase.

Heat produces analgesia and decreases muscle spasm, but should not be used while swelling is still present. Electrical treatments such as ultrasound are often used in the post-acute stage. Ultrasound has thermal effects which are probably responsible for most of the thera-

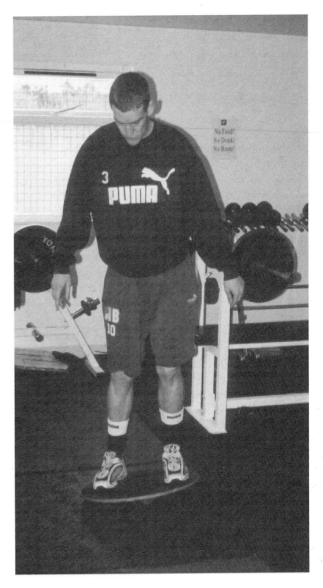

Figure 3.8.30 Wobble board.

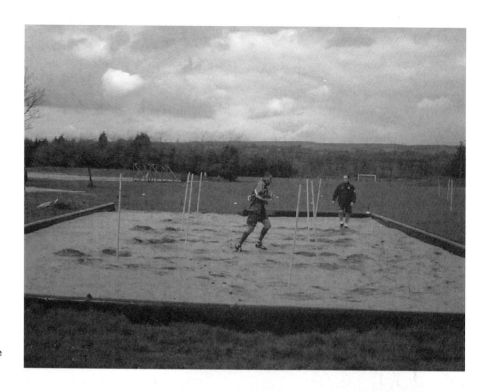

Figure 3.8.31 Training in sand. (Courtesy Dave Ferre, Blackburn Rovers F. C.)

recovery time. Proprioceptive exercises are added, which may begin as alphabet writing (balancing on the affected side whilst spelling out letters with the other foot) or heel walking, progressing to various wobble boards (Figure 3.8.30) with differing degrees of difficulty.

Muscle strengthening is imperative at this stage, starting with isometric-type exercises, then gradually progressing to both closed and open kinetic chain exercises, strengthening of the peroneals proving very important in future ankle stability.

Finally, the athlete progresses through to the functional phase, which aims at restoring a full range of motion in all positions. Proprioceptive exercises are essential, with various techniques being used to increase load and difficulty by adding external forces. The activities undertaken aim to improve agility, with the intensity of exercise being increased. Eccentric loads are applied at this stage. The result is an increase in contractile strength of the peroneals and improved neuromuscular function, similar effects also having been demonstrated contralaterally, with speed of contraction increasing significantly after such a regime.[12]

Once activities using equipment such as a wobble board or a Pilates board or fitter (a curved board with foot plates on runners) have been completed, a progression is followed through to trampete exercises, then increasing eccentric loading and difficulty through various functional activities. Sandpit exercises (Figure 3.2.31) have been used successfully by an inventive physiotherapist involved with professional soccer.

After an initial injury the risk of recurrence doubles,[13] so only when all stages have been satisfactorily completed may the athlete return to competition. At this time a full range of motion should be accompanied by adequate joint stability, proprioception, and muscle strength. Failure to achieve this can lead to recurrent injury with the possible sequelae being ankle instability due to ligamentous laxity and a 'chronic ankle sprain', a scenario that should never occur.

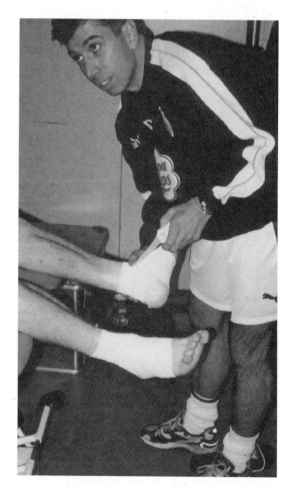

Figure 3.8.32 Ankle strapping.

Many sportsmen tape their ankles prophylactically after an inversion injury (Figure 3.8.32). The usefulness of this practice is much debated. Although some research has shown taping to improve stability, it has also demonstrated that the supportive effect becomes negligible after approximately 20 minutes.[14] The presumption therefore is that it works by improving proprioception, in much the same way that patella taping appears to produce a cure in anterior knee pain. The frantic demand for strapping in the treatment room before a professional soccer game lends weight to this theory. Although support is anecdotal in the main, it would not be wise to refute the practice; experience shows that the professional sportsman's intuition sometimes proves to be more informed than a plethora of conflicting and inconclusive research.

Should it be advised that a career-long preventive programme should be the aim? Anecdotal evidence suggests that players seen in the gym after training seem to suffer fewer recurrences after their return to play than their less conscientious colleagues, who, though keen to return to competition, tend also to return to the physio's table at an earlier date. Supporting this observation, 'focused conditioning', involving specific exercises aimed at prevention alongside education, has been shown to produce a decrease in injury rate.[15]

Surgery

Osteochondral fractures of the talar dome can be a consequence of a severe inversion injury and are classified according to their severity and displacement, with lateral lesions proving more unstable and requiring surgical intervention at an earlier stage than medial lesions. Symptoms suggesting referral for arthroscopic examination are recurrent swelling, stiffness, instability, clicking or locking, and ongoing pain. Chondroplasty is undertaken for chondral lesions, with a number of procedures being available to correct ligamentous instability, an unnecessary sequela of inadequate rehabilitation.

Anterolateral impingement syndrome, described below, is sometimes associated and may require arthroscopic debridement.

Other associated injuries

Syndesmotic injury

This is most commonly caused during a collision in which the ankle is forcefully externally rotated or dorsiflexed, either individually or in combination. These injuries are thought to comprise up to 10% of 'ankle sprains'. Inversion injury can also cause disruption of the syndesmosis, with the anterior inferior tibiofibular ligament sometimes being torn.[16]

The syndesmosis consists of the anterior inferior tibiofibular ligament, posterior inferior tibiofibular ligament, transverse ligament, and interosseous ligament and membrane. Disruption follows a characteristic pattern, in a similar manner to lateral ligament tears, with damage occurring initially to the anterior inferior tibiofibular ligament followed by the interosseous ligament. Diagnosis is confirmed as described above.

A Maisonneuve fracture, which is a fracture of the proximal fibula, is sometimes present in association with complete syndesmotic rupture.

Peroneal subluxation

This is a possible complication following an inversion injury. If recurrent, it may require surgery, both to prevent further episodes of sub-

luxation and to repair any tear within the tendon or sheath that may have accompanied the injury, with the same occasionally happening to the tibialis posterior tendon after a significant eversion stress.

Sinus tarsi syndrome may also occur as a consequence of an inversion injury, sometimes complicating the picture (see Chapter 3.8.3).

Impingement syndromes

Anterior and posterior

Aetiology

Anterior and posterior impingement syndromes, particularly common in soccer and ballet and often called 'footballer's ankle', may occur in any sport that entails forceful plantarflexion and dorsiflexion of the foot at the ankle joint. Initial impingement of the soft tissues progresses, with the development of osteophytes anteriorly and posteriorly at the articular margins, as a result of the bony impact in these regions. A sequela of this can be the production of associated loose bodies. Additional complications in relation to posterior impingement may be the presence of an os trigonum (Figure 3.8.33), an unfused ossification centre, posterior to the talus, present in 7–10% of the population. This may be the cause of the symptoms, or an addition to them. Recent studies have shown an ostrigonum to be present

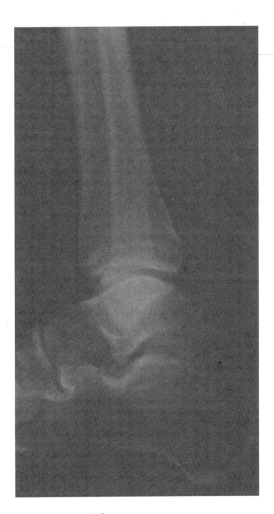

Figure 3.8.33 Radiograph of os trigonum.

more frequently in soccer players, suggesting that the nature of the sport may be causal.

Examination

Clinical presentation is that of localized joint line tenderness, with passive plantarflexion reproducing the pain in posterior impingement, and dorsiflexion the pain in anterior impingement.

Investigation

Plain radiographs demonstrate the abnormality quite clearly, with further investigation often being unnecessary, as damage to the articular cartilage is not a part of the pathology, the osteophytes being unrelated to an osteoarthritic process. Isotope bone scan is sometimes useful in helping to decide the contribution of an os trigonum to the athlete's posterior ankle pain.

Treatment

Initial management is conservative, with restriction of aggravating factors, non-steroidal anti-inflammatory medication, and localized physiotherapeutic modalities. If symptoms fail to resolve, a well-directed injection of a long-acting corticosteroid is often beneficial. In the more chronic cases, usually demonstrating radiographic changes, treatment tends to be surgical once symptoms become persistent and the osteophytes restrict movement. Arthroscopic removal of any loose bodies with removal of the osteophytes is undertaken. Persistent posterior impingement in the presence of an os trigonum may require its removal. Surprisingly, although gross radiographic

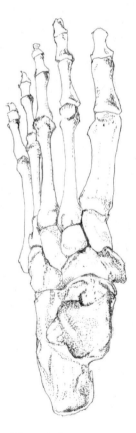

Figure 3.8.34 Anatomy of the navicular.

changes are often noted incidentally in players in their early twenties, the majority remain asymptomatic, with surgery being less prevalent than one would expect. Although it is common practice to order plain radiographs of the ankles in pre-signing medicals for professional soccer clubs, this practice therefore appears to be unfounded.

Anterolateral

Anterolateral impingement syndrome occurs after injury to the lateral ligamentous structures.[17] Inadequate rehabilitation after an inversion injury may potentiate recurrent injury to the region, with the subsequent development of chronic inflammatory changes within the tissues, leading to the production of scar tissue, which is repeatedly trapped in the lateral gutter. The result is persistent lateral ankle pain. Again the initial approach is physiotherapeutic, with the correction of any biomechanical abnormalities being important. Localized steroidal injection into the area, also injecting into the sinus tarsi in case of associated pathology, may achieve a cure. However, persistence of symptoms suggests that surgical intervention may be necessary. Arthroscopic debridement has a high success rate; most patients become symptom free.[17]

Midfoot pain

Stress fractures occur as overuse injuries, with different sports producing this effect in different regions. One of the most important midfoot stress fractures is that of the navicular (Figure 3.8.34), because of its tendency to progress to fracture with non-union, with avascular necrosis being an unfortunate sequela. The navicular is easily located, with its prominent tuberosity medially, surrounded by the talus, cuboid, and three cuneiforms, and articulating with all.

Aetiology

Navicular stress fractures are found in a variety of sports, commonly those entailing forceful dorsiflexion of the foot as the athlete pushes off. They predominate in track and field athletes, but are not particularly common in soccer. In my experience, however, they are becoming increasingly common in rugby league as the pace and intensity of the game increase.

History and examination

Diagnosis is mainly a clinical one, with a history of pain on exercise, crescendoing if the athlete attempts to persist with their training regime, culminating in pain both at rest and at night. Any degree of discomfort on palpation in this region warrants caution and further investigation. Classically tenderness is felt over the proximal portion of the navicular, in the midline, the region in which the stress fracture most commonly occurs, often described as the N spot.

Investigation

Isotope bone scan will confirm the suspicion, though it often remains 'hot' long after healing has occurred. MRI is becoming the investigation of choice, revealing early stress reactions that may suggest caution, though plain radiographs and CT should be used to image the bony disruption accurately in definite cases.

Treatment

An aggressive approach must be undertaken to prevent the debilitating sequelae mentioned above. A non-weightbearing cast is applied for 6–8 weeks. Occasionally even prolonged immobilization is unsuccessful and surgical intervention with bone grafting becomes necessary.

Cuboid syndrome

Ongoing discomfort in the lateral midfoot may indicate subluxation of the cuboid, the normal articulations of which are the navicular and lateral cuneiform medially, the calcaneum posteriorly, and the fourth and fifth metatarsals anteriorly. Often following an inversion injury and frequently presenting in ballet dancers, the cuboid is subluxed in a plantarwards direction, the medial portion occasionally being rotated dorsally. Using direct pressure over the bone and directing it upward in the reverse direction to the subluxation, manipulation often produces a successful reduction, the foot being simultaneously plantarflexed during the manoeuvre, with an associated clunk and an immediate relief of symptoms being the result. Taping techniques may help to help prevent recurrence.

A differential diagnosis of cuboid stress fracture is rare but has been reported and so should be born in mind, with cases sometimes mimicking peroneal tendinitis. Both CT and isotope bone scan have proved useful in helping achieve a diagnosis.[18,19]

Occasional occurrences

- **Talar stress fractures** occasionally occur, presenting with ankle pain more severe when hopping.

- **Midtarsal sprains** quite commonly prove to be the cause of midfoot pain, either in association with an acute injury or due to more chronic biomechanical deficiencies.

- **Tarsal coalition** must be considered as a possible cause of midfoot or ankle pain, and although the cuneiforms are not often included in this, rarely they may be implicated. I have experienced one case producing symptoms and findings on isotope bone scan that were markedly similar to those of a metatarsal stress fracture.

References

1. Liu, S. H., Jason, W. J. Lateral ankle sprains and instability problems. *Clinics in Sports Medicine*, 1994, **13**(4), 793–809.

2. Valiant, G. A., Cavanagh, P. R. A study of landing from a jump. In: *Biomechanics IX-B*. Human Kinetics, Champaign, IL, 1985.

3. Barker, H. B. *et al.* Ankle injury risk factors in sports. *Sports Medicine*, 1997, **23**, 69–74.

4. Garrick, J. G. The frequency of injury, mechanism of injury and epidemiology of ankle sprains. *American Journal of Sports Medicine*, 1977, **5**, 241–2.

5. Hocutt, J. E. *et al.* Cryotherapy in ankle sprains. *American Journal of Sports Medicine*, 1982, **10**, 316.

6. Lehmann, J. F. *et al.*, Cryotherapy. In: *Therapeutic heat and cold*, 4th edn, Williams and Wilkins, Baltimore, 1990.

7. Wilkerson, G. B., Horn- Kingery, H. M. Treatment of the inversion ankle sprain: comparison of different modes of compression and cryotherapy. *Journal of Orthopaedic and Sports Physical Therapy*, 1993, **17**(5), 240–6.

8. Bahr, R. *et al.* A two fold reduction in the incidence of acute ankle sprains in volleyball after the introduction of an injury prevention programme: A prospective cohort study. *Scandinavian Journal of Medicine and Science in Sports*, 1997, **7**, 172–177.

9. Cote, D. J. *et al.* Comparison of three treatment procedures for minimizing ankle sprain swelling. *Physical Therapy*, 1988, **68**, 1072.

10. Coakley, W. T. Biophysical effects of ultrasound at therapeutic intensities. *Physiotherapy*, 1978, **64**, 166.

11. Kannus, P., Renstrom, P. Treatment for acute tears of the lateral ligaments of the ankle. Operation, cast, or early controlled mobilisation. *Journal of Bone and Joint Surgery*, 1991, **73A**, 305–12.

12. Benjamin, S. *et al.* The benefit of a single-leg strength training programme for the muscles around the untrained ankle. *American Journal of Sports Medicine*, 2000, **28**(4), 568–73.

13. Milgrom, C., *et al.* Risk factors for lateral ankle sprain: a prospective study among military recruits. *Foot and Ankle*, 1991, **12**, 26–30.

14. Greene, T. A., Hillman, S. K. Comparison of support provided by a semi-rigid orthosis and adhesive ankle taping before, during and after exercise. *American Journal of Sports Medicine*, 1990, **18**(5), 498–506.

15. Bahr, R. *et al.* Incidence of acute volleyball injuries. *Scandinavian Journal of Medicine and Science in Sports*, 1997, **7**, 166–171; Ekstrand, J. *et al.*, Prevention of soccer injuries. *American Journal of Sports Medicine*, 1983, **11**, 116–20.

16. Cox, J. S. Surgical and nonsurgical treatment of acute ankle sprains. *Clinical Orthopaedics*, 1985, **188**, 88–96.

17. Jacobson, K. E., Lui, S. H. Anterolateral impingement of the ankle. *Journal of the Medical Association of Georgia*, 1992, **81**(6), 297–9.

18. Beaman, D. N., Roeser, W. M., Holmes, J. R., Saltzman, C. L. Cuboid stress fractures: a report of two cases. *Foot and Ankle*, 1993, **14**(9), 525–8.

19. Mahler, P., Fricker, P. Case report: cuboid stress fracture. *Excel*, 1993, **8**(3), 147–8.

3.8.3 The subtalar joint

Bryan English

Anatomy

The inferior aspect of the talus and the superior aspect of the calcaneum form this joint. Normally the surface consists of three facets and an accessory joint along the mid sulcus of the calcaneum:

- **posterior facet**: biconvex calcaneum opposing biconcave talus
- **anteromedial facet**: biconcave calcaneum opposing biconvex talus
- **anterolateral facet**: concave calcaneum opposing convex talus.

Arthroscopy has demonstrated that although most people have three facets to this joint, a small proportion have only two (the anterior facets being combined). The three-facet joint in supination forms an osseous block. An interesting hypothesis is that the two-facet joint has a greater surface area and will allow more movement as the axis of the joint will move towards the transverse plane and away from the coronal plane (see section on joint axis in Chapter 3.8.1). It follows that people who pronate excessively may have a higher incidence of only one anterior facet.

Anterior to the posterior facet is the sinus tarsi (which acts like an accessory joint). Two thickenings of the capsule of the joint at this site form the anterior and posterior interosseous ligaments, which provide the majority of support for the subtalar joint.[1] They protect the joint during inversion and restrain possible joint separation. Other ligament supports to the joint are listed in Table 3.8.1.

Movements

No muscle inserts onto the talus, so any ankle movement has to be mediated via the subtalar joint. Closed kinetic chain movement occurs with heel strike. The movement at the subtalar joint will determine the action of the foot and the lower leg. It therefore acts as a torque con-

vertor. If there is very little subtalar movement, the foot and lower leg will move early to compensate. If there is excessive subtalar movement, the movement of the lower leg and foot will be dragged along with the subtalar joint and lower limb joint movements may be mistimed.

As mentioned in Chapter 3.8.1, the subtalar joint has a triplanar axis, but the only axis of movement that can be detected on examination is that in the coronal plane, involving eversion and inversion. The range varies from 6° to 25°, with two thirds of the movement being into inversion and one third into eversion.

Injuries

Inversion injury

Considering the importance of its role, the subtalar joint is remarkably 'uncomplaining'. It is most commonly injured as a result of an inversion injury to the ankle. If the lateral collateral ligament of the ankle is ruptured, the subtalar joint may undergo ligament damage. Subsequent hypermobility of this joint will lead to ongoing symptoms and instability of the ankle during the rehabilitation process.[2] Strapping, temporary or permanent, may be required to 'ease' the joint. As with all joints, good proprioceptive function is important to assist in recovery.

Ligament damage may be difficult to detect clinically without the assistance of further imaging such as MRI.

Stress fracture

The subtalar joint is a good shock absorber, but regular excessive loading may lead to stress fracture, presenting with diffuse heel pain that is worse at night.[3] MRI is diagnostic, although CT and isotope bone scans are still commonly used. If there is no obvious cause for the fracture, such as excessive loading, then further investigations of bone density and hormonal status should be considered.

Conservative treatment would be to avoid activity that causes pain, and the wearing of shock-absorbing insoles. Immobilization in a plaster of Paris slipper or non-weightbearing foot brace for up to 12 weeks is the treatment of choice, but may be viewed by some as too aggressive. Others would allow weightbearing if this was asymptomatic.

Sinus tarsi syndrome

This often follows trauma and occasionally presents as an overuse injury.[4] The pathology of the condition is open to debate. Inflammation of the synovium, the interosseous ligaments, and the chondral

Table 3.8.1. Ligament supports of the subtalar joint

Ligament	Protects joint from
Lateral talocalcaneal	Inversion and dorsiflexion
Anterior talocalcaneal	Inversion
Medial talocalcaneal	Eversion
Posterior talocalcaneal	Inversion and dorsiflexion
Calcaneofibular ligament (lateral collateral of the ankle)	Inversion and dorsiflexion
Deltoid/tibiocalcaneal ligament (medial collateral of the ankle)	Eversion and abduction

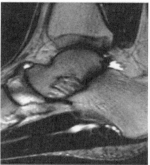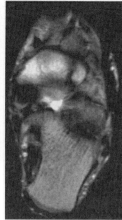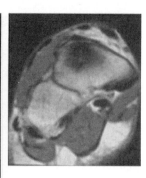

Figure 3.8.35 Chondral bruising of the subtalar joint.

surface of the joint have all been suggested, along with a further postulation of entrapment of a branch of the peroneal nerve.[2] My opinion is that chondral inflammation/bony bruising is the most common cause detected on MRI (Figure 3.8.35), further aggravated by hypermobility of the joint due to ligamentous damage.

The symptoms are diverse, but often consist of pain on weightbearing with lateral and/or medial heel pain. There may be tenderness over the sinus tarsi, indicating inflammation of this accessory joint. The location is most easily palpated just above the sustentaculum talus (a projection of the calcaneum) and some way below the medial malleolus. Detection of the swelling and bony oedema within the area is best detected by MRI.

Forced eversion of the ankle can cause pain, and hypermobility of the joint can be detected by passive movements comparing subtalar movements of both limbs.[4]

The treatment is conservative before considering immobilization. The use of an orthotic device may be of use if the rear foot demonstrates a chronic valgus deformity, for example.[5] Other anti-inflammatory modalities and medication should be considered along with appropriate footwear.

A cortisone injection under radiographic screening can be diagnostic as well as therapeutic. One technique for injecting the joint is via the posterolateral approach. The point of entry is approximately 2.5 cm above the tip of the lateral malleolus and 1 cm medial to the posterior border of the fibula. The needle is introduced at a 55° angle until the resistance of the chondral surface is felt.

Other approaches to the joint can be directly from the medial and lateral aspect of the subtalar joint, detecting the route via surface anatomy and checking the progress of the needle with imaging. These approaches are difficult because the bony contours vary from patient to patient.[6]

References

1. Sarrafian, S. S. *Anatomy of the foot and ankle*, 2nd edn. Lippincott, Philadelphia, 1983.

2. Heilman, A. E., Braly, W. G., Bishop, J. O., Noble, P. C., Tullos, H. S. An anatomic study of subtalar instability. *Foot and Ankle*, 1990, **10**(4), 224–8.

3. Eisle, S. A., Sammarco, G. J. Fatigue fractures of the foot and ankle in the athlete. *Journal of Bone and Joint Surgery*, 1993, **75A**, 290–98.

4. Shear, M. S., Baitch, S. P., Shear, D. B. Sinus tarsi syndrome. The importance of biomechanically based evaluation and treatment. *Archives of Physical Medicine and Rehabilitation*, 1993, **74**, 777–81.

5. Wooten, B., Uhl, T., Chandler, J. Use of an orthotic device in treatment of posterior heel pain. *Journal of Orthopaedic and Sports Physical Therapy*, 1990, **11**, 410–13.

6. Cyriax, J. H., Cyriax, P. J. *Cyriax's illustrated manual of orthopaedic medicine*, 2nd edn. Butterworth-Heinemann, Oxford, 1993.

3.8.4 Plantar fasciitis and heel pain

Bryan English

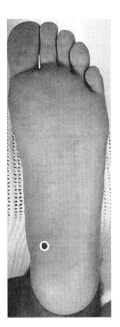

Figure 3.8.36 The classic site for plantar fasciitis is the anteromedial border of the calcaneum.

Plantar fasciitis

The fascial layers within the foot have several functions:

- shock absorbency by limiting displacement of the fat pads under the calcaneum and metatarsal heads

- site for muscle attachments

- protection of the plantar vessels, nerves and muscles from excessive compressive forces

- facilitation of tendon movement and 'holding down' of muscles and tendons in the sole of the foot

- creation of optimal transmission of biomechanical forces.

The fascial layers consist of interdigitating fibrous tissue. The main fascial layer is the plantar aponeurosis, which consists of medial, lateral, and central portions. Only the central section is truly aponeurotic. The origin of this tissue, at the medial process of the medial calcaneal tuberosity, is the site of the most common type of plantar fasciitis (Figure 3.8.36). The fascia may also be inflamed elsewhere along its length, when it is painful on stretching with dorsiflexion of the toes. The insertion of the fascia is partly via the superficial stratum that inserts into the dermis (under and distal to the metatarsophalangeal joints) and partly via the deep stratum that inserts into the plantar ligaments of the metatarsophalangeal joints, the flexor tendon sheaths and the periosteal layer of the proximal phalanges.

Aetiology

Table 3.8.2 lists causes of plantar fasciitis. The condition can be very resistant to treatment. It may occur in the flat (pronated) foot as well as the high-arched (supinated) foot. However, a common fault is a failure to address the biomechanical abnormalities or variants that may be present.

As stated in Chapter 3.8.1, excessive strain can be put on the fascia by alteration of rear foot and/or forefoot mechanics. Excessive or repetitive stretch on the fascia will lead to microtrauma and inflammation.

The windlass mechanism (Figure 3.8.37) is widely mentioned in literature on the foot and ankle. The mechanical dynamics of this system are worth mentioning in this chapter in relation to heel pain. As a consequence of the sites of origin and insertion of the plantar fascia, there is supination of the foot during toe off in the gait cycle. At toe off there is dorsiflexion of the metatarsophalangeal joints, thereby tensioning the plantar fascia, which in turn decreases the distance of the fascial length between the calcaneum and the metatarsophalangeal joints. The result is a supinated foot, which is a rigid lever and therefore the most appropriate structure to transmit forces during the propulsive phase of gait. Excessive dorsiflexion of the metatarsophalangeal joints may occur in an effort to maintain the duration of the weightbearing phase and to transmit the maximum forces possible. For example, decreased ankle dorsiflexion due to a tight gastrocnemius–soleus complex will result in an increased dorsiflexion of the metatarsophalangeal joints during gait. This excessive movement in turn results in extra stretch on the plantar fascia due to the windlass mechanism. The resulting microtrauma leads to inflammation at the calcaneal insertion of the fascia.

Table 3.8.2. Causes of plantar fasciitis

Structural	Supinated foot with poor flexibility of fascia
	Excess weight
Structure leading to a functional disorder	Pronated foot due to rear/forefoot abnormality
	Tight plantar fascia
	Decreased dorsiflexion at the ankle
Functional disorder	Overuse injury due to excessive training/poor footwear/hard surface
	Hypertonic gastrocnemius/soleus complex
	Hypertonic deep flexors of the lower leg
Systemic	Enthesopathy due to rheumatological disorder

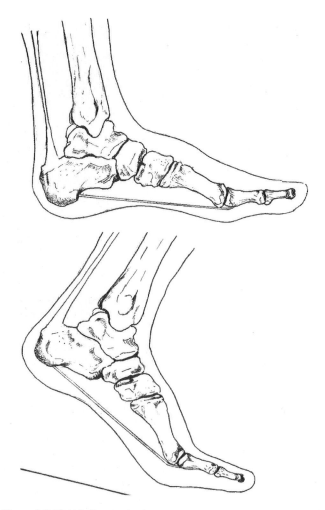

Figure 3.8.37 Windlass mechanism.

The valgus heel or excessive functional pronation of the foot can result in excess strain of the plantar fascia because of the increased distance between the origin and insertion. However, when the foot remains in pronation excessive work is performed by the muscles to transmit the necessary forces. The pronated foot is a non-rigid lever. The mechanical inefficiency that is therefore present may also lead to microtrauma within the foot or lower leg.

Increased tension with great toe hyperextension encourages a supinated foot.

Diagnosis

This is confirmed by history and examination. The patient will describe pain and an inability to walk normally for several minutes on rising in the morning and after several minutes' sitting during waking hours. The pain will ease to an extent after walking for several minutes.

Examination demonstrates an area of specific tenderness at the insertion of the aponeurosis at the heel. It is common for stretching of the fascia to be painless, whereas palpation of the plantar fascia itself may detect other areas of tenderness due to microtrauma, and also tightness that can be visible (especially with passive dorsiflexion of the toes) and palpable comparing one side to the other (compared to a

boggy sensation if there has been a medial band rupture). Interestingly, passive dorsiflexion of the toes does not cause pain at the insertion of the calcaneum; however, there is pain if there is a plantar fasciitis in the midfoot.

Investigations

These are of limited value for this condition. The presence of a calcaneal spur on a lateral radiograph is normally irrelevant, although a tumour or stress fracture of the calcaneum would be excluded as part of the differential diagnosis. The resistant fasciitis, however, may be due to the presence of a rheumatological disorder. An enthesopathy may be present in conditions such as the seropositive and seronegative arthritides. A plain radiograph will show furring at the site of inflammation and this pathology may be confirmed with appropriate serological investigations and an isotope bone scan, although this latter investigation may be positive with a purely trauma-induced periostitis.

Treatment

This is related to the aetiology.[1] It is important to establish realistic goal-setting; the individual may find it hard to accept that this 'injury' may take 6 months to heal. The basic principle here is to decrease the forces that go through the plantar fascia. Correction of biomechanical abnormalities has been discussed earlier. If the condition occurs as a result of overuse, then once again temporary or permanent orthoses may be used to take the strain off the fascia. As this condition often proves resistant to treatment, a multidisciplinary approach is indicated, as is the case with most enthesopathies (e.g. compare with lateral epicondylitis).

Self-management

This may be the key. It consists of self-massage to the length of the fascia (with fingers or rolling the foot over a golf ball), self-articulation to the joints of the ankle and foot (to result in a more compliant and shock absorbing-structure), stretching of the calf muscles and deep flexors, decreasing excess body weight, and wearing shoes with good shock absorbency (such as marathon running shoes or devices with viscoelastic insoles). Avoiding aggravating factors (such as running on roads) must also be considered. Anti-inflammatory drugs may be prescribed for a 4 week period at a maximum dose.

If there is a degree of success with self-management, then the patient should be introduced to a rehabilitation programme that will gradually increase the stress on the fascia, so that it may remodel and begin to cope with increased force. Progress may seem painfully slow, especially for the impatient athlete. Long-distance walking should be employed well before running. Adequate explanation to the patient will often result in increased compliance. Use of a night splint or strapping techniques will maintain fascial stretch when at rest.

Orthotics

These may then present a second line of treatment, used in conjunction with self-management. It must be pointed out that although examination of the foot may demonstrate no biomechanical abnormalities, visualization of the foot when walking or running may demonstrate notable overpronation that may be the cause of the plantar fasciitis.

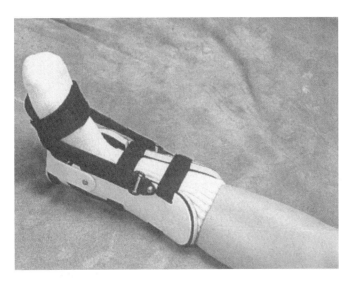

Figure 3.8.38 Night splint.

Other methods of treatments

If there is no success with these treatments, then the use of a **cortisone injection** may have greater success than if it were used as a first line of treatment. The injection should be directed to the site of tenderness preferably from the medial aspect of the calcaneum, with an administration of 1.5 ml of local anaesthetic plus 10 mg of triamcinolone, for example. Injections directly into the inferior aspect of the foot can be very painful and cause degeneration of the shock-absorbing fat pads within the area.

Immobilization of the foot in a slipper cast is a method of alleviating forces through the fascia if the pathology appears to be purely chronic inflammation. A more popular method of 'scientific' immobilization is with the use of a night splint (Figure 3.8.38) that creates a stretch on the fascia when at rest.

Surgery to the plantar fascia must be avoided if at all possible. The alteration of the foot biomechanics in the absence of an effective aponeurosis will result in increased compressive forces in the midfoot, plus a decreased arch height and an increased susceptibility to metatarsalgia. Incision of the plantar fascia using a medial approach can be used, taking care to avoid damage to the medial calcaneal branch of the posterior tibial nerve (damage to the nerve may result in a painful neuroma) and the first branch of the lateral plantar nerve.

Other causes of heel pain[2,3]

Entrapment of the first branch of the lateral plantar nerve

This nerve innervates the medial aspect of the calcaneum, the long plantar ligament, and the muscles of flexor brevis and abductor digiti quinti.[4] The nerve may become trapped between the muscles of quadratus plantaris, superiorly, and the muscles of abductor hallucis and flexor brevis inferiorly (Figure 3.8.39). These muscles may become particularly hypertonic in athletes such as sprinters. A calcaneal spur may also add a compression element in this narrow space, and the local inflammatory changes of a plantar fasciitis may also be a causative factor.

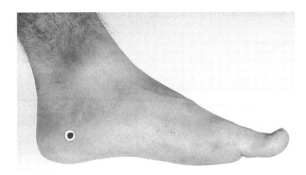

Figure 3.8.39 Site of tenderness and of entrapment.

This pathology is differentiated from a plantar fasciitis on clinical grounds. The site of tenderness is medial and superior to the origin of the plantar fascia. Pressure at this site may also produce referred pain to the heel. Paraesthesia is rare, and not a reliable diagnostic feature. Correspondingly, nerve conduction studies are not sufficiently sophisticated to isolate this branch.

Treatment of this lesion is very similar to that of plantar fasciitis. Physical therapy to the relevant musculature can also be of great benefit. If self-management, manual treatment, orthotics, and injections have not succeeded, then surgical release of the nerve is indicated. This consists of release of the fascial layers of the muscles compressing the nerve, along with removal of a heel spur if present.

Tarsal tunnel syndrome

The posterior tibial nerve may be trapped as it passes beneath the flexor retinaculum due to the anatomical restrictions within the tarsal tunnel (Figure 3.8.40). The compression of the nerve is commonly due to increased pressure within the tunnel, this in turn being due to swelling or inflammation as a result of acute or chronic trauma. The symptoms are of a diffuse heel pain/burning plus paraesthesia or numbness of the lateral and plantar aspect of the foot and toes. The symptoms may be reproduced by percussion over the nerve (Tinel's sign). Tenderness over the heel is rare.

Other than pure compression, causes of tarsal tunnel syndrome comprise varicose vein, bony fracture/osseous encroachment, ganglion (or other space-occupying lesion), and systemic pathologies such as myxoedema.

The diagnosis tends to be made from the history and examination findings. Nerve conduction tests are unreliable and if anything are used to confirm a diagnosis, not to make one (as for carpal tunnel

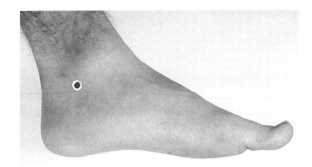

Figure 3.8.40 Tarsal tunnel syndrome.

syndrome). An injection of local anaesthetic into the tarsal tunnel may alleviate the distal symptoms and further substantiate the diagnosis.

Treatment is initially by relieving the pressure on the nerve. In a patient who overpronates, the use of a corrective orthotic can solve the problem. Cortisone may be only a temporary measure. Surgical release of the retinaculum is the treatment of choice if other measures have failed. Once again the benefit of a good history and precise examination, including a functional analysis, will assist the practitioner in differentiating one of the less common pathologies associated with heel pain.

Fat pad atrophy

The fat pad is a 'cushion' consisting of a series of spirals of vertically orientated elastic adipose tissue, connecting the calcaneum to the skin. The pad is an effective shock absorber that deteriorates with increasing age. The pain and tenderness are situated directly under the body of the calcaneum (Figure 3.8.41), but in some patients the pain and tenderness can be diffuse. Patients with atrophy or degeneration of the fat pad can be diagnosed by palpation. Rather than a density of 'rubbery' soft tissue under the heel, there is a sensation of a thin dermal layer overlying the bone. Indeed, the calcaneal tuberosities are easily palpable through this tissue.

Treatment for this condition is limited. Shock-absorbing heel cups are of benefit, with footwear that is made with highly attenuating material (that is, with viscoelastic properties).

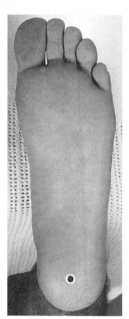

Figure 3.8.41 Central site for heel tenderness with fat pad atrophy.

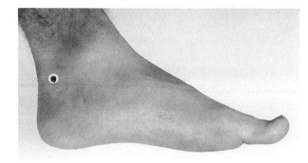

Figure 3.8.42 Retrocalcaneal bursitis.

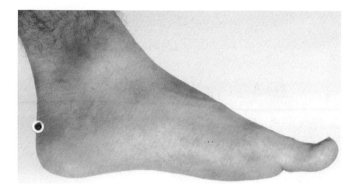

Figure 3.8.43 Achilles bursitis.

Immobilization in a plaster of Paris slipper relieves the area of weightbearing for a period of 4–6 weeks. The concern over injecting cortisone into this area is the direct association with fat degeneration. Such a treatment can give marked relief, but there is a lack of controlled studies and long-term follow-up with this treatment. Injectable anti-inflammatory homeopathic remedies, such as Traumeel, have been advocated by those who fear the adverse side effects of cortisone.

Retrocalcaneal bursitis

This occurs due to repetitive motion of the Achilles tendon over the back of the calcaneum. Patients may have a prominence of the superior angle of the calcaneum (Figure 3.8.42).

Adequate stretching of the calf muscles is advised. A temporary heel raise may prevent excessive dorsiflexion. Injection therapy may be of benefit; otherwise, the superior angle of the calcaneum may be surgically removed.

Achilles (postcalcaneal) bursitis

Direct pressure of footwear over the back of the tendon, with the prominent bone beneath, may result in this condition (Figure 3.8.43). Avoiding pressure to the area is an obvious treatment, so removal of a heel tab on running shoes can provide a 'useful cure'. Injection therapy may alleviate the acute symptoms if more invasive treatment is sought. The lesion may become chronic and lead to the development of granulation/fibrous tissue and bone bossing resulting in a lesion called a 'pump bump'. This disorder is common in sports such as ice hockey, and with people who wear footwear that is too tight. Surgical excision of the excess soft tissue, along with excision of the bony prominences, is sometimes the only way to restore comfort.

References

1. Batt, M. E., Tanji, J. L. Management options for plantar fasciitis. *The Physician and Sports Medicine*, 1995, **23**, 77–86

2. Doxey, G. E. Calcaneal pain: a review of various disorders. *Journal of Orthopaedic and Sports Physical Therapy*, 1987, **9**, 25–32

3. Leach, R. E., Delorio, E., Harney, R. A. Pathologic hindfoot conditions in the athlete. *Clinical Orthopaedics*, 1983, **177**, 116

4. Henricson, A. S., Westlin, N. E. Chronic calcaneal pain in athletes. Entrapment of the calcaneal nerve? *American Journal of Sports Medicine*, 1984, **12**, 152–4

3.8.5 **Tendonopathies**

Bryan English

Pathology within the tendons of the foot and ankle is often a consequence of excess strain on the musculotendinous unit. This may be due to increased duration and intensity of athletic training. Excessive body weight and biomechanical abnormalities of the foot may also be predisposing factors. As with most tendon pathologies there are also systemic causes of a tendonopathy, such as rheumatoid arthritis and systemic lupus erythematosus.[1]

Tendinitis can be treated by addressing the aggravating factors. If the patient is poorly conditioned, there should be a period of flexibility work followed by gradual return to weightbearing activities. The use of anti-inflammatory measures (ice packs, oral and topical anti-inflammatory medication) will help to decrease the swelling and pain in the area. Strapping and braces can take the strain off the tendon temporarily or permanently. Cortisone injections should be used with great care. Attention must be given to the inherent risks of injecting around tendons that have intrasubstance tears or substantive degeneration.

Tears of the tendon can be treated in a similar way. Complete tears have to be assessed as to whether the function of the foot is sufficiently impaired to require surgical correction. Obviously lesions of the Achilles tendon will require surgical repair, but other tendons such as extensor hallucis longus may not interfere with the functional demands of an individual.

Self-management strategies, including the use of appropriate footwear, are crucial in avoiding and treating disorders of the tendons.

Achilles tendon

The Achilles tendon or tendocalcaneus is the strongest tendon in humans. The origin of the tendon is the musculotendinous junction of the gastrocnemius, approximately 15 cm proximal to the calcaneum. Muscle fibres from soleus join the anterior aspect of the tendon along its upper aspect. Towards the lower end the tendon becomes more oval before its attachment to the posterior aspect of the calcaneum. The insertion is slightly to one side of midline, resulting in both inversion and plantarflexion of the ankle when the muscles of the gastrocnemius/soleus complex are contracted.

The blood supply to the tendon is from both superior and inferior aspects. Approximately 4 cm above the insertion of the tendon, there is a site of possibly limited blood supply where the bidirectional supply anastomoses. This is one reason why the tendon is susceptible to chronic inflammation.

Adolescents appear to be susceptible to inflammation at the insertion of the tendon. Adults suffer more from a classic tendinitis 2–3 cm proximal to the insertion, and elderly people more commonly present with a tear to the musculotendinous junction of the gastrocnemius.

Mechanics

The tendon is important in reducing the energy costs during locomotion. It acts like a spring and will only stretch to about 8% of its length. Before this elastic limit, the tendon will store energy and release it at a specific stage during the gait cycle. Fortunately, thanks to the properties of mammalian tendon,[2] this mechanism produces very little heat and up to 93% of stored energy is returned to assist locomotion.[3]

Good flexibility of the tendon and its associated musculature, plus maximum range of movement of the ankle and subtalar joints, will potentiate the viscoelastic mechanism.[4] Increased flexibility will result in the potential for increased power and increased stamina. As a consequence, this should reduce the possibility of acute or chronic pathology within the tendon.

Achilles tendinitis

Aetiology

Stress applied to the structure of a tendon will lead to microtrauma. Excessive and repetitive force may lead to a failure of the healing process, thereby causing acute, acute on chronic, and chronic inflammation of this tendon. Excessive load may be due to an increased level of weightbearing exercise (increased speed, increased power, or increased duration). Alteration of the training surface or a change of footwear can also be aggravating factors. Inherent problems such as excess bodyweight, poor lower limb flexibility, and/or abnormal lower limb biomechanics are factors that must also be addressed. This condition can prove resistant to treatment unless a multifactorial approach is adopted.

With regards to the biomechanics, there are various foot patterns that may aggravate an Achilles tendinitis. A supinated foot, for example, is a poor shock absorber. The 'shock' on walking and running has to be absorbed somewhere, and the tendon (tendinitis) or bone (stress fracture) may be unable to cope with poor foot compliance. A pronated foot due to a rear foot valgus, or a combined rear and forefoot varus, may put excessive strain on the medial aspect of the Achilles tendon.

Diagnosis

The history should reveal the classic story of pain being worse 'first thing in the morning' and after a period of 'rest'. The pain is often easier after several minutes of walking and is not aggravated during sport. However, stiffness after exercise is another common feature.

It is important to consider details of footwear, training patterns, and any possible trauma to the area. Previous injury to either lower limb will also indicate whether a problem proximal or distal to the tendon may be the primary cause of excessive loading of the Achilles tendon.

Examination will demonstrate thickening of the tendon, most commonly a fusiform swelling 2–3 cm proximal to its insertion. The non-diseased tendon may often be tender, but the inflamed tendon is acutely tender. The examiner should detect whether this tenderness is medial and/or lateral, as this may be a pointer to the biomechanical origin.

Investigation

An ultrasound scan is a dynamic investigation that is useful to detect whether the tendon is thickened and inflamed or whether there is any true degeneration of the tendon itself. This is an important distinction when considering treatment options.

MRI has the benefit of demonstrating the whole tendon complex and can therefore demonstrate intraluminal tears within the tendon with less dependence on operator reliability than is required with the ultrasound scan. I believe that the ultrasound is the first-line investigation, especially as the dynamic image may pick up an impingement that can occur at the superior angle of the calcaneum. Individual tendon fibres are also more easily detected with ultrasound because of the high resolution that is available.

With a more acute history, such as 'a sensation of something tearing' or a direct kick on to the tendon, then MRI will be of additional use to assess intrasubstance pathology.

Treatment

It is imperative to find the cause of the inflammation. If it is due to inappropriate exercise, then the individual has to address this issue and take responsibility for self-management. This would consist of decreasing the intensity and duration of exercise levels and complying with flexibility work.

Appliances that may be used are shock-absorbing insoles, a temporary heel raise, and a suitable orthosis if a biomechanical disorder, such as overpronation, is to be corrected. The use of a night splint (see Figure 3.8.38, p. 345) will keep the tendon on a light stretch, and avoid the foot adopting the plantarflexed position that is the norm when asleep.

The response to anti-inflammatory agents, such as ice and topical and oral non-steroidal anti-inflammatories, is varied, but these therapeutic modalities should be included as part of the treatment.

Injection of cortisone to the medial or lateral aspect of the tendon may be considered, but with caution. Rupture of the tendon is a genuine concern if the tendon itself degenerates. If the ultrasound scan confirms thickening of the tendon only, then cortisone injected alongside the inflamed tendon sheath can offer great relief and a cure for this resistant problem. The non-diseased tendon cannot be injected, as the collagen structure is too thick to inject fluid into. Mucinoid degeneration of the tendon will allow an ill-advised injection to enter the tendon, this may then lead to rupture of a structure that is already susceptible to such a traumatic event. An extensive review of literature reveals no evidence that 'healthy' human tendons will rupture following a cortisone injection.[5–9]

Ohberg and Alfredson found that injection of sclerosant material alleviates the symptoms in those tendons that have developed a neovascularization.[10] They describe how the sclerosant produces a neurolysis and devascularization of the area (which is the outcome of any surgical procedure). This theory flies in the face of previous theories of treating tendonopathies, and further studies into this technique are awaited with interest.

Immobilization of the tendon in a plaster of Paris cast is out of favour because of the known local and regional side effects of such a treatment. Rehabilitation after immobilization can cause more problems than an isolated Achilles tendinitis.

Surgery, consisting of removal or splitting of the thickened paratenon, may be considered for the most resistant of chronic problems. The main problems with the procedure is the risk of necrosis at the site of the wound or development of a painful scar. Rehabilitation after Achilles surgery is far more complex, and therefore difficult to implement, than the surgery itself. The success of operative procedures should be measured on return to the type of function that is satisfactory to the patient.

Degeneration

Mucinoid degeneration will occur after repeated intrasubstance tear. If the condition is painful and causes restriction of daily activities, then surgical removal of the degenerative tissue is indicated and often very successful. Tender nodules on the tendon may be visible as well as palpable. Confirmation of diagnosis is available with an ultrasound scan or MRI. A protracted recovery with conservative management may indicate that a surgical option is more realistic. After surgery, rehabilitation is active with early stretching and mobilization.

Rupture

Ambroise Paré in 1579 gave one of the first descriptions of rupture of the tendon.[11] Causes included 'slipping when mounting a horse', 'too quick mounting', and 'false steps'. Treatment was by bed rest, which resulted in a permanent limp as the tendon failed to unite. His description of the event remains classic: the noise of the rupture compared to a whiplash, the local pain, and the depression over the heel.

The injury appears to be caused by mechanical overload, poor blood supply, degenerative change within the tendon, or a mixture of all these factors. It often occurs in a previously fit individual who has gone through an injury phase resulting in decreased conditioning of the tendon. Resumption of demanding exercise then causes a rupture.

Surgical repair of the tendon was developed in the late nineteenth century. Throughout the twentieth century there was continuing controversy over conservative versus surgical treatment. In the late 1950s and through the 1960s there were numerous scientific articles demonstrating the benefits of surgical repair.[12,13] The reasons for a nonsurgical approach were the 'side effects' of any surgical procedure such as tissue necrosis, recurrent ruptures, and nerve injuries. Immobilization in a plaster of Paris cast with the ankle initially in plantarflexion, followed by a series of further plasters with the ankle in decreasing degrees of plantarflexion, followed by increasing degrees of dorsiflexion, was advocated by some authorities. However, as surgical techniques have improved, it is now generally held that surgery is the treatment of choice, especially for athletes.[14–20]

Postoperatively the area can be mobilized relatively quickly, with the use of various appliances (Figure 3.8.44) that will allow partial weightbearing with controlled ankle dorsiflexion and plantarflexion.

Degenerative tissue within the tendon will also be excised at operation. Surgical removal of an inflamed retrocalcaneal bursa and the posterior angle of the os calcis (which may be acting like a fulcrum, causing trauma to the Achilles tendon during dorsiflexion) are other procedures that may be performed, depending on the pathology and pathomechanics.

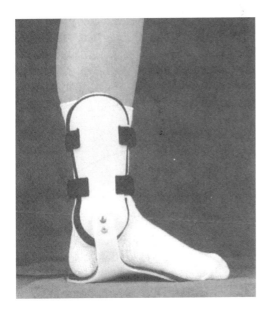

Figure 3.8.44 Fixed-position Sure Step.

Tibialis posterior tendon

Tibialis posterior dysfunction begins with an insidious course of inflammation, followed by degeneration and eventual tendon rupture which is mechanically a disaster for foot function (Table 3.8.3). The resulting and progressive planovalgus deformity (and later forefoot abduction) is an avoidable problem if early diagnosis of dysfunction is made. All too often, however, this is not the case because an accurate diagnosis is not made.

Tibialis posterior produces plantarflexion and inversion of the ankle and rear foot. It performs this manoeuvre by locking the midtarsal joints and causing a transfer of plantarflexion forces to the metatarsals.[21] Failure to perform this function results in rear foot eversion, the midtarsal area does not lock, and therefore the plantarflexion forces act on the talonavicular joint and the medial ligamentous structures thus producing a flat foot deformity.[22] Tibialis posterior also acts with other muscles to produce a co-contraction of forces about the ankle to add to the stability of the ankle joint.

The tibialis posterior tendon may become symptomatic towards its insertion at the navicular. The tendon also inserts onto the three cuneiforms, the base of the second, third, and fourth metatarsals, and has a further attachment to the inferior calcaneonavicular ligament.

The tendon has an area of hypovascularity proximal to the sustantaculum talus.[23] There is a bowstring effect due to the tethering action of the flexor retinaculum. The above two factors are further reasons for excessive loading and chronic inflammatory change occurring in this tendon in a biomechanically inefficient foot and ankle.

The tendon may become symptomatic as a consequence of direct trauma or an overuse injury. As for the Achilles tendon, the pathology may be one of inflammation or degeneration.

The history is of medial foot pain exacerbated by exercise. There is tenderness and swelling along the path of the tendon. The lower limb biomechanics must be assessed on standing and with the patient walking, as notable overpronation may be the cause of the problem.

Early diagnosis of the condition and its aetiology is the key to success. Active resisted movements may demonstrate weakness, and the tendon may not be palpable in the case of a rupture. Forefoot abduction may be observed by the 'too many toes' sign when the patient is observed from behind. Another useful test for this condition is the one foot raise test. The patient stands on the affected leg only and then attempts to heel raise (Figure 3.8.45). This will demonstrate a degree of weakness and pain along the medial border of the foot. In severe tibialis posterior tendinitis/rupture, this manoeuvre may not be possible. This would normally be associated with longstanding rear foot abnormalities such as a rear foot valgus, which produces a diseased and elongated tendon.

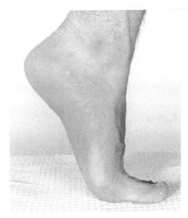

Figure 3.8.45 One foot raise test.

Table 3.8.3. Stages of tibialis posterior tendon degeneration[24]

	Stage 1	Stage 2	Stage 3	Stage 4
Condition of tendon	Tendinitis and/or degeneration	Elongation	Elongation	Rupture
Rearfoot	Mobile. Normal alignment	Mobile valgus position	Fixed valgus position	Fixed valgus position
Pain	Medial, focal and mild	Medial along the tendon and moderate	Medial sometimes lateral and moderate	Medial sometimes lateral and moderate
Heel raise test	Mild weakness	Moderate weakness	Marked weakness	Inability to perform
'Too many toes' sign	Normal	Positive	Positive	Positive
Pathology	Synovial proliferation, degeneration	Moderate degeneration	Marked degeneration	Rupture and marked degeneration

Investigation

Weightbearing radiographs may demonstrate collapse of the medial foot joints. Ultrasound scan may demonstrate intra- or extrasubstance tear of the tendon. The dynamic aspect of this investigation is useful to assess areas of tethering. MRI provides information on the contour of the tendon and is also more precise with regard to the extent of intrasubstance pathology. Correlation of MRI findings and the staging of the disease process have been documented.[25]

Treatment

This may take the form of an orthosis to correct any abnormal biomechanics (particularly to correct the rear foot valgus), local modalities to alleviate the inflammation, and a cessation or reduction of the aggravating activities. After a period of relative rest, a rehabilitation regime of lower limb flexibility and a graded return to weightbearing exercise should be recommended.

In severe disorders, immobilization for up to 4 weeks with a lower leg brace or plaster of Paris can be considered, creating a degree of rearfoot inversion and foot plantarflexion.

Chronic inflammation will cause further degeneration, which is when surgery should be considered before the deformity becomes too severe.

Surgery

Rupture of the tendon itself may be repaired. Transferring the tendons of flexor digitorum or tibialis anterior to assist in plantarflexion plus inversion of the rearfoot may be incorporated, should the tibialis posterior be irreparable. Reconstructive osteotomies can be used alongside soft tissue repair. Arthrodesis may consist of isolated arthrodesis of the talonavicular or the subtalar joint, double arthrodesis, or triple arthrodesis.

As with all surgical procedures, the patient must be evaluated as an individual. The patient's age, occupation, activity level, and expectations should be considered.

Tibialis anterior tendon

This tendon takes origin from the anterior aspect of the tibia, interosseous membrane, and crural fascia (Figure 3.8.46). The insertion is on the medial cuneiform and proximal first metatarsal. The tendon and its muscle act as an eccentric decelerator at heel strike, as a stabilizer during stance, and as an invertor and dorsiflexor (supinator) before and during the swing phase.

The tendon is susceptible to trauma in its exposed position over the anteromedial aspect of the ankle. It may be traumatized by kicking, or the front of the ankle may be struck by another player. Laceration occasionally occurs, and will result in retraction of the tendon several centimetres up the lower leg (Figure 3.8.47). The other foot extensors may compensate to a degree; however, on examination the definition/surface anatomy of the tendon is absent.

Surgical repair of rupture is reserved for young people and athletes. Early diagnosis is essential, otherwise a tendon graft will be required to approximate the ends of the damaged tendon. Conservative therapy is indicated for lesions in the older and more sedentary population, where functional disturbance is barely noticeable.

Avulsion of the tendon from its insertion presents with pain and decreased function in young people. In older patients, the presenta-

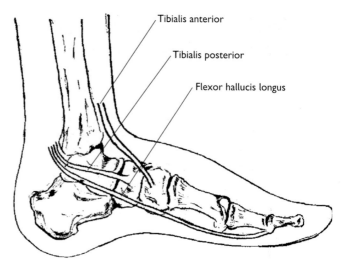

Figure 3.8.46 Anatomy of the tibialis anterior, tibialis posterior, and flexor hallucis longus tendons.

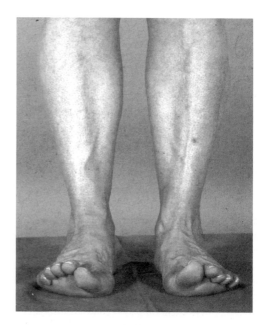

Figure 3.8.47 Rupture of tibialis anterior on right leg.

tion may be that of a mass that has developed over the anterior aspect of the ankle. This mass is the retracted tendon underlying the extensor retinaculum. A useful test for an avulsed tibialis anterior is that dorsiflexion of the foot cannot be performed without extension of the toes. Treatment is again conservative, except in young people and athletes. Other causes of a soft tissue mass around the ankle, related to a tendon, are a ganglion, mucinoid degeneration, and rarely a giant cell tumour of the tendon sheath.

Tendinitis occurs in the acute and chronic forms. Pain with active resisted movements may be evident. Crepitus may also be present, but swelling may be absent as the tendon is covered by the extensor retinaculum. As with most tendinitis, the cause is usually due to overuse or poor conditioning. Symptomatic treatment and a few days of decreased activity followed by functional rehabilitation including flexibility and strength training should suffice.

Extensor digitorum longus and extensor hallucis longus tendons

Lesions at these tendons are rare and usually result from direct trauma similar to that found with tibialis anterior. Tendinitis may result from overtight shoelaces. Loss of extension of the toes associated with substantive disturbance of function of the tendon(s) may cause problems, especially at the hallux where tripping may occur along with difficulty putting the foot into the shoe. However, if performance is not hindered, management is conservative.

Peroneus brevis tendon

The muscle arises from the lower two thirds of the fibula and intermuscular septae of the lateral compartment. The tendon lies next to the lateral malleolus in the peroneal groove and then passes over the calcaneofibular ligament and the trochlea lateralis of the calcaneum before inserting onto the styloid of the fifth metatarsal. Peroneus brevis is the most powerful abductor of the foot and also acts as a secondary flexor and evertor.

Tendinitis occurs after unaccustomed activity in the unconditioned individual. Swelling and tenderness can be located over the tendon which is superficial and wrapped in its own tendon sheath over the lateral aspect of the calcaneum and cuboid. As with most tendons the underlying pathology may be due to one of the arthritides, in which case ultrasound or MRI diagnosis may be required. However, if the history is classically that of an overuse injury, of which peroneus brevis tendinitis in ballet dancers is a classic example, then the usual anti-inflammatory modalities should be employed. plus the use of foot taping to prevent excessive stretch on the tendon. Tenosynovectomy may be considered in resistant cases.

The peroneus brevis is susceptible to trauma around the ankle as it is compressed in the fibular groove by the peroneus longus (Figure 3.8.48). Trauma will result in longitudinal tearing of the tendon. Recurrent inversion injuries in an ageing tendon with a decreased blood supply are all factors that can lead to a chronic tear within the tendon and resulting degenerative change. Thickening, tenderness, and pain with active resisted movements will occur, along with lateral

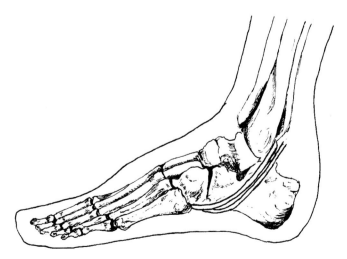

Figure 3.8.48 Peroneus brevis is compressed into the fibular groove by peroneus longus.

ankle pain that may radiate a few centimetres up the back of the fibula. Radiographs will reveal any bony prominences that may have caused the chronic tear. MRI or an ultrasound scan will assist the diagnosis. Conservative treatment consists of anti-inflammatory modalities plus the use of an ankle brace and/or basketball-type boots that will restrict ankle inversion and eversion. Manual treatment to the area will be beneficial, as these muscles are not easy to stretch without assistance. Surgery is considered only if the pain persists or when function is substantively impaired.

Because there is posterolateral lower leg pain, pain with active resisted movement, and tenderness over the back of the fibula, the differential diagnosis includes a stress facture of the fibula.

A complete rupture of the tendon is treated surgically by attachment to the calcaneum of those tendons that become retracted, or by the use of a tendon graft. Avulsion of the insertion of the tendon on the styloid process of the fifth metatarsal can occur with sudden inversion of an ankle against contraction of the peroneus brevis. Tenderness over the styloid should lead to a diagnostic radiograph. The fracture may be treated with an elasticated support if the patient is non-weightbearing, or a cast boot if the patient is to weightbear. Remember, however that an accessory sesamoid (os vesalianum) and an apophysis in a young patient may result in a 'false positive' radiograph.

Subluxation of the peroneal tendons may occur when there is a shallow fibular groove and inefficient superior peroneal retinaculum. The dislocating tendons can be observed especially during dorsiflexion and eversion. In an asymptomatic individual there is no need for treatment. If there is pain or recurrent instability, surgery may deepen the groove and tighten the retinaculum. Once again the rehabilitation phase is important, and will involve flexibility work and graded power training.

Peroneus longus tendon

The origin of the muscle is from the lateral head and proximal two thirds of the fibula. The tendon lies behind the lateral malleolus and over the tendon of peroneus brevis. It then runs below the trochlea lateralis of the calcaneum, under the inferior peroneal retinaculum and brevis tendon, before turning underneath the foot through a groove in the cuboid. The tendon passes under the long plantar ligament to be inserted on the first metatarsal and medial cuneiform. This complex, tortuous path enables the muscle and tendon to act as an abductor and pronator of the foot and a plantarflexor of the ankle.

Tendinitis often occurs in the patient who lacks conditioning and then overloads the musculotendinous unit. Pain is experienced over the lateral aspect of the foot and ankle, especially when the foot is pushing off. Tenderness is present along the tendon. Cessation of aggravating activities, anti-inflammatory modalities, and the provision of an orthosis correcting excessive pronation will alleviate the strain on the tendon. This is to maintain a neutral position and thus partially deactivate the peroneus longus eccentric activity (the orthotic therefore assisting in ankle stabilization). The eccentric function of peroneus longus can easily be observed when the patient balances on one leg.

As peroneus longus also plantarflexes the first metatarsal, an overpronated foot results in forced dorsiflexion of the first ray, thus overriding the action of the muscle. This another reason why the orthotic should be helpful.

A tear or rupture of the tendon is usually preceded by several days of pain within the area. The site of the tear is often at the os perineum, a sesamoid bone that commonly lies within the tendon under the cuboid. With a rupture, the site of the os peroneum will migrate towards the trochlea lateralis and then further up towards the ankle. This can be detected on serial radiographs. Ultrasound and MRI will also aid diagnosis. Anti-inflammatory agents, relative immobilization in a brace or cast, and an orthosis to prevent excess pronation will be beneficial. Surgical repair is considered if pain and impaired function are severe and persistent. Surgery for a tear may consist of debridement and tenosynovectomy. A rupture will result in impaired function and stabilization of the ankle. Reattaching the torn tendon may require a tendon graft if retraction has occurred. Rarely there may be retraction and fixation of the tendon, in which case reattachment to the lateral aspect of the calcaneum will at least restore plantarflexion and lateral stabilization.

Flexor hallucis longus tendon

From its origin in the deep posterior compartment of the lower leg (lower two thirds of the fibula and intermuscular septae) the tendon of the muscle passes behind the talus, beneath the sustentaculum tali of the calcaneum, and then deep to the flexor digitorum longus before passing between the sesamoids of the hallux to insert into the distal phalanx (Figure 3.8.46). This pathway results in flexion of the joints of the great toe as well as supination of the foot (flexion of the midtarsal joints) plus plantarflexion of the ankle.

Tendinitis of this tendon causes posterior ankle pain. Active plantarflexion of the ankle and flexion of the foot causes pain. There will be tenderness anterior to the Achilles tendon, with crepitus on occasions. The differential diagnosis of posterior ankle pain requires careful attention. Tendinitis is one of the less common causes of impingement. A radiograph would rule out the possibility of an os trigonum and arthritis of the subtalar joint.

The musculotendonous junction is relatively low at this site, so as they pass through the narrow groove the hypertrophied muscle fibres may impinge on the posterior aspect of the talus. Other areas of tendinitis can occur where the tendon is surrounded by a fibrous pulley, namely in the midfoot and metatarsophalangeal joint. Before considering surgery, for instance tenosynovectomy, the tendon should be subjected to stretching, flexibility work, and the usual anti-inflammatory measures plus avoidance of the aggravating factors.

Trigger toe occurs when there is thickening of the tendon following a partial tear. The thickening causes friction as it passes back and forth under the sustentaculum tali. Pain is experienced when weightbearing; the classic example is a dancer attempting to go from half pointe to full pointe. There will be posterior ankle pain and the sensation of a snap as the tendon passes through the area of stenosis. The diagnosis of this lesion can be aided by palpation of the tendon at the sustentaculum tali during active and passive great toe flexion and extension. Flexion of the toe may not be possible, or a pop will be felt over the tendon during toe flexion.

Rupture of the tendon is rare and may be an incidental finding in sedentary individuals. If there is impairment of function then surgical correction may be undertaken.

Flexor digitorum longus tendon

The muscle originates from the posterior aspect of the tibia and fibula in the deep posterior compartment. The tendon runs medially to the tendon of flexor hallucis longus and close to tibialis posterior at the sustentaculum tali level. The tendon splits into four and provides the origin for the lumbrical muscles that attach to the extensor hoods of the four lesser toes. The four tendons terminate at the distal phalanx of the four lesser toes after passing through the tendon slips of flexor digitorum brevis. The tendons act as flexors of the toes and foot as well as a stabilizer for the ankle during the stance phase.

Lesions of this tendon are rare. Tendinitis and tears are often associated with pathology within other tendons.

References

1. Meyerson, M., Solomon, G., Shereff, M. Posterior tibial tendon dysfunction: its association with sero-negative inflammatory disease. *Foot and Ankle*, 1989, **9**, 219–225.

2. Bennett, M. B., Ker, R. F., Dimery, N. J., Alexander R. McN. Mechanical properties of various mammalian tendons. *Journal of Zoology, London A*, 1986, **209**, 537–48.

3. Cavanagh, P. R., Lafortune, M.A. Ground reaction forces in long distance running. *Journal of Biomechanics*, 1980, **13**, 397–406.

4. Alexander, R. McN. The spring in your step. *New Scientist*, 1989, **114**(1558), 45–6.

5. Shrier, I., Matheson, G. O., Kohl, H. W. 3rd. Achilles tendonitis: are corticosteroid injections useful or harmful? *Clinical Journal of Sports Medicine*, 1996, **6**(4), 254–50.

6. Fredburg, U. Local corticosteroid injection in sport: review of literature and guidelines for treatment. *Scandinavian Journal of Medicine and Science in Sports* 1997, 7(3), 131–9.

7. McWhorter, J. W., Francis, R. S., Heckman, R. A. Influence of local steroid injections on traumatised tendon properties. A biomechanical and histological study. *American Journal of Sports Medicine*, 1991, **19**(5), 435–9.

8. Read, M. T. Safe relief of rest pain that eases with activity in achillodynia by intrabursal or peritendinous steroid injection: the rupture rate was not increased by these steroid injections. *British Journal of Sports Medicine*, 1999, **33**(2), 134–5.

9. Assendelft, W. J., Hay, E. M., Adshear, R., Bouter, L. M. Corticosteroid injections for lateral epicondylitis: a systematic overview. *British Journal of General Practice*, 1996, **46**(405), 209–16.

10. Ohberg, L., Alfredson, H. Ultrasound guided sclerosis of neovessels in painful chronic Achilles tendinosis: pilot study of a new treatment. *British Journal of Sports Medicine*, 2000, **36**(3), 173–7.

11. Paré, A. *Oeuvres completes*, ed. 8ème livre, chapitre XXXVII. J. F. Malgaigne, Paris, 1840–41, pp.110–11.

12. Lea, R. B., Smith, L. Rupture of the Achilles tendon. Non surgical treatment. *Clinical Orthopaedics*, 1968, **60**, 115–18.

13. Gillies, H., Chalmers, J. The management of fresh ruptures of the tendon Achilles. *Journal of Bone and Joint Surgery*, 1970, **52A**, 227–43.

14. Nellen, G., Martens, M., Bursens, A. Surgical treatment of chronic achilles tendinitis. *American Journal of Sports Medicine*, 1989, **17**, 754–9.

15. Cetti, R. Ruptured Achilles tendon. Preliminary results of a new treatment. *British Journal of Sports Medicine*, 1988, **22**, 6–9.

16. Schram, A. *et al.* Complete rupture of the Achilles tendon. A new modification for primary surgical repair. *Journal of Foot Surgery*, 1988, **27**(5), 453–7.

17. Bradley, J., Tibone, J. Percutaneous and open surgical repairs of Achilles tendon ruptures. A comparative study. *American Journal of Sports Medicine*, 1984, **18**(2), 188–95.

18. Hattrup, S., Johnson, K. A. Review of ruptures of the Achilles tendon. *Journal of Foot and Ankle*, 1985, **6**(1), 34–8.

19. Kellam, J. F., Hunter, G. A., McElwain, J. P. Review of the operative treatment of Achilles tendon rupture. *Clinical Orthopaedics*, 1985, **201**, 80–3.

20. Schepsis, A., Leach, R. E. Surgical management of Achilles tendinitis. *American Journal of Sports Medicine*, 1987, **15**, 308–15.

21. Kaye, R. A., Jahss, M. H. Tibialis posterior: a review of anatomy and biomechanics in relation to the support of the medial longitudinal arch. *Foot and Ankle*, 1991, **11**(4), 244–7.

22. Funk, D. A., Cass, J. R., Johnson K. A. Acquired adult flatfoot secondary to posterior tibial tendon pathology. *Journal of Bone and Joint Surgery*, 1986, **68A**, 95–102.

23. Frey, C., Shereff, M., Greenridge, N. Vascularity of the posterior tibial tendon. *Journal of Bone and Joint Surgery*, 1990, **72A**, 884–8.

24. Johnson, K. A. Tibialis posterior tendon rupture. *Clinical Orthopaedics*, 1983, **177**, 140.

25. Rosenberg, Z. S., Cheung, Y., Jahss, M. H. *et al.* Rupture of the posterior tibial tendon: CT and MR imaging with surgical correlation. *Radiology*, 1988, **169**, 229–35.

3.8.6 Metatarsalgia

Bryan English

The true definition of metatarsalgia is 'pain in the forefoot in the region of the heads of the metatarsals'. The term is subject to abuse, and patients may present with a diagnosis of metatarsalgia with any forefoot pain.

Metatarsophalangeal joint capsulitis

This condition is often due to trauma, but inflammation and a capsulitis at this site can be due to an underlying inflammatory arthropathy. A non-traumatic onset of problems at this site should alert the diagnostician to consider rheumatological investigations including radiographs and possibly an isotope bone scan.

Traumatic capsulitis of the joints is due to excessive forces being applied to this area. Sports people may develop this condition if their footwear lacks adequate shock absorbency. A sudden increase in mileage, a change of footwear, an alteration of terrain, and a recent increase in body weight are all factors that must be taken into account with sports-related overuse trauma. In the sedentary population, excessive body weight and unsuitable footwear (Figure 3.8.49) are the main causative factors.

As this type of capsulitis is due to excessive loading, any device that will decrease the shock that has to be absorbed will be of great assistance.

The assessment of metatarsal position is important, along with assessment of metatarsal length. A typical presentation of length (numbering the metatarsals from great toe to little toe) is 2 > 1 = 3 > 4 > 5.[1]

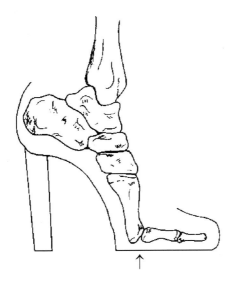

Figure 3.8.49
Footwear can have a profound affect on the pressure placed on the metatarsophalangeal joints.

Interdigital neuroma

Neuritic pain in the region of the metatarsal heads will suggest the presence of a neuroma between two of the metatarsal heads (usually 2/3 or 3/4). The neuroma occurs at the anastomoses of the medial and lateral plantar nerves. Other symptoms are paraesthesiae spreading along the two toes that are supplied by the interdigital nerve. The symptoms are aggravated by walking with shoes on.

To confirm this diagnosis, a squeeze test may be performed by clasping the forefoot in one hand and applying pressure to compress the enlarged nerve between the metatarsal heads. Palpation may reveal tenderness over the nerve. This may recreate the pain and/or produce a click (Mulder's sign). The neuroma is a space-occupying lesion and may therefore separate the toes. This is called Winston Churchill sign, for obvious reasons.

One must also take care to elicit any signs of peripheral neuropathy or vascular insufficiency with neuritic pain. Instability of the metatarsal head may also present in a similar way. Finally, the diagnosis of neuroma may be confirmed by injecting local anaesthetic into the metatarsal space. Ultrasound and MRI investigation will demonstrate the pathology.

Treatment of an interdigital neuroma should initially be conservative. The patient must address the issue of footwear. Shoes that are ill-fitting, especially if they are too tight, may be the cause of the problem. A reduction in those activities that bring on the pain will help, along with a temporary orthotic placed just proximal to the affected interspace. If the pain is due to inflammation, then local infiltration of cortisone can be beneficial. Infiltration would be indicated on up to three occasions at 4-weekly intervals, with the access to the interdigital space being from the dorsal aspect of the foot.

If conservative therapy fails, surgical excision of the neuroma should be considered. The dorsal approach is preferable to the plantar approach. Although the former is technically a more difficult procedure, the latter may produce a painful scar on the weightbearing surface.

Metatarsophalangeal joint instability

This is not an easy diagnosis to make, especially in the early stages. The most common site for the lesion is the second metatarsophalangeal joint. The reason for this that in many people the second metatarsal is longer than the first. This fact, plus excessive loading (for example, in long-distance runners with pronated feet) may lead to joint instability due to collateral ligamentous insufficiency and laxity/disruption of the volar plate.[2] The presentation is of a vague forefoot pain often exacerbated by weightbearing.

There will be tenderness over the joint involved, but no referred neuritic pain (differentiating this disorder from a neuroma) and no tenderness over other metatarsophalangeal joints (as would normally be the case with an inflammatory arthropathy). On examination, the drawer sign will stress the joint in the dorsiplantar direction. Not only will there be excessive movement, but also pain may be intense at the end of range when stretching the joint capsule and/or collateral ligaments. At a later stage there will be deviation of the second toe due to medial malalignment. The exact site of the pain can be determined by infiltrating local anaesthetic. Radiological investigation would consist of an arthrogram.

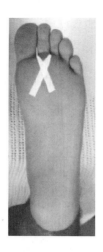

Figure 3.8.50 Sling taping device.

Treatment for this disorder is conservative if the condition is diagnosed in the early stages. A decrease in activity (if exercise has been an aggravating factor) will be part of the self-management for such a condition. Taping the toe to a neighbouring toe, or using a sling taping device which wraps around the base of the toe (Figure 3.8.50) may be helpful.

A metatarsal pad placed proximal to the metatarsophalangeal joint, or a more formal orthotic, will limit the degree of dorsal and plantarflexion thereby providing a degree of stability. These devices may be used for several months. However, if the symptoms do not resolve, and if the patient requires a high level of activity, then surgery may have to be considered.[3] This would take the form of capsular reefing (with a flexor tendon transfer if hyperextension/dorsiplantar instability persists) which tightens the part of the capsule of the joint that has been overstretched. This procedure may not be advisable for a serious athlete, as a return to previous function and the demands of weight-bearing sport may not be possible. Surgery would normally be withheld until the end of the athlete's career.

Disorders of the great toe

Hallux rigidus

Degenerative change of the first metatarsophalangeal joint occurs insidiously in some individuals. Various predisposing factors have been suggested, such as osteochondritis of the metatarsal head, a flattened metatarsal head, an overpronated foot, and metatarsus primus elevatus.

The more dramatic presentation follows trauma. An acute synovitis occurs with tenderness specifically over the dorsal and lateral aspect of the joint. Later there is bony overgrowth that causes painful impingement, again specifically at the dorsal and lateral aspect of the joint where an exostosis will be visible and palpable. The exostosis may cause discomfort because it forms a pressure point against footwear. Hyperextension of the interphalangeal joint is present.

Decreased dorsiflexion of the first metatarsophalangeal joint can be due to bony proliferation at the superior aspect of the joint, as well as due to arthritic degeneration.

The decreased range of movement is very restricting to ambulation and effective use of the foot as an energy return system. This condition is disastrous for athletes, because of the functional restrictions it imposes on jumping, turning, accelerating, etc. Other problems may

occur as the individual attempts to compensate for the restriction by walking on the outside of the foot, or by externally rotating the lower limb, i.e. walking with the foot in an abducted position thereby avoiding a dorsiflexion strain on the first metatarsophalangeal joint.

Diagnosis may be confirmed by radiography. However, in the early stages of the condition one must rely more on clinical evaluation as the chondral changes will not be evident. Bony spurs or exostoses will appear later, along with a decreased joint space of a degenerate joint. Care is necessary in making the diagnosis, in order to take into account other pathologies that occur in this area, such as gout, sesamoiditis, or a fracture within the joint.

Treatment may be conservative. Orthoses may be used to aid dorsiflexion, but firm insoles will decrease the function of the foot as a loading structure. Mobilization by a manual therapist will help in the mild forms before a cortisone injection into the joint is considered. The footwear must be addressed: shoes that are too small compress the first metatarsalphalangeal joint, further aggravating the symptoms.

Surgical intervention is often successful if the restriction to movement is bony. There are joint-preserving or joint-destroying surgical techniques. The latter, typically consisting of an arthrodesis, have been extensively studied.[3] However, the joint-preserving procedures such as cheilectomy[4] and/or osteotomy, should not be overlooked.[5] A cheilectomy removes the bony growth that is causing the impingement, and this is the operation of choice as a percentage of joint range of movement will be restored . The individual may return to full function, although the degenerative change will continue. Joint replacement, such as a Keller's excisional arthroplasty, is considered in more elderly patients.[6]

Turf toe

This term was introduced by Bowers and Martin in their 1976 study into shoe-related injuries in American football.[7] They found that up to 45% of players had sustained an injury to the great toe at some stage of their career. The term 'turf toe' is open to excessive use, as with other non-specific terms such as shin splints and frozen shoulder. I prefer to use this term to apply to inflammation of the capsule of the first metatarsophalangeal joint, with damage to the capsulo-ligamentous structures more commonly on the plantar aspect.[8] I would also prefer to rename it 'Astroturf toe' as the greatest incidence appears to occur in sports that are played on this surface.[9] An important consideration is that arthritis of this joint (and restricted range of movement) is not necessarily a painful condition. However, a painful capsulitis can be an extremely disabling condition and will cause greater morbidity than many other injuries around the foot and ankle complex.

The cause of turf toe is trauma. Hyperextension, forced abduction, forced adduction (and occasionally hyperflexion[10]) can result in excess strain to the strong supportive capsuloligamentous complex that supports this joint.[11] The sesamoid ligaments are part of this complex and will be addressed later in this section. Compression injury (stubbing of the toe) and a direct blow (kicking the side of the joint against a post, for example) are other mechanisms of injury.

The effects of trauma may also be exacerbated by certain types of footwear that apply excessive pressure to the joint (footwear that is too small) or lack adequate support (flimsy lightweight shoes such as running spikes). Football boots may aggravate the condition because of the location of the screw-in stud.

The training surface is also important. Astroturf is an unforgiving surface that allows little or no foot movement once the foot is planted on the ground. The compressive forces and effects of body loading therefore have to be absorbed throughout the musculoskeletal system. As the first metatarsophalangeal joint is the first and last point of contact in speed sports, and most pivotal manoeuvres emanate from this area when the joint is in hyperextension, it is not surprising that turf toe can be a career-threatening injury. Anything that can dissipate these forces, such as playing sport on a grass surface with adequate shock absorbers within the shoe, will be of use in preventing injury.

Diagnosis begins with a concise history. The biomechanics of the injury should be ascertained, if possible. The more chronic presentations are characterized by pain and stiffness of the joint after rest. Pain after exercise may be profound, and the athlete will point to the site of the pain. There may be a degree of swelling around the joint. The end of range of movement in all directions may be painful, especially if there has been a capsuloligamentous injury. Valgus and varus testing will detect collateral instabiltity. Crepitus on movement will raise the question of a possible bony injury. Palpation will reveal if the area affected is localized (such as a collateral ligament injury) or whether another pathology of close proximity is suspected (such as a sesamoiditis). The differential diagnosis of pain in this area includes sesamoiditis/fracture and osteochondritis/fracture.

If a bony pathology is suspected, then radiographs of the area (anteroposterior, lateral, oblique, and sesamoid views) should be requested. Fracture, degenerative change, or bony avulsion (due to ligamentous injury) may be present. The sesamoid views will be addressed in the next section. The lateral view in neutral and hyperextension of the joint may indicate if there has been ligamentous avulsion of the sesamoid ligamentous complex (Figure 3.8.51).

Initial treatment is aimed at decreasing the inflammation and stress placed on the joint, such as the NICER regime (non-steroidals, ice, compression, elevation, and relative rest). A rigid full-length orthotic will be of great benefit to prevent the joint being forced into hyperextension on general ambulation. Immobilization should be considered if significant ligamentous damage has occurred (3–6 weeks) or if a chondral pathology or sesamoid fracture has been detected (6 weeks). Gradual return to exercise is then advised with a graded, carefully planned rehabilitation package. At all stages, if the area is not being totally immobilized, the joint should be gently mobilized by the therapist and the athlete. This involves passive movements towards the end of range, employed with and without a gentle traction force applied across the joint (some practitioners will call this a distraction technique). Biomechanical evaluation may suggest the use of tempo-

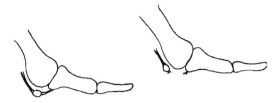

Figure 3.8.51 Lateral radiograph of the great toe can demonstrate avulsion of the sesamoid ligament complex.

rary or permanent orthotics. Finally, the prescription of 'sensible' footwear is essential along with advice on how to avoid further stress and injury.

Sesamoiditis

This condition can be confused with turf toe. Indeed, the symptoms may be similar, although examination findings should easily differentiate one condition from another. The end of range of movement of the first metatarsophalangeal joint does not cause pain with a sesamoiditis, except possibly at the end of range of hyperextension. With sesamoiditis, the tenderness is specifically on the plantar aspect of the joint, and indeed the sesamoid itself may be palpable. Inflammation of this area results from excessive loading. Therefore, as with turf toe, orthotics, local therapy, and corrective footwear may be helpful. A local cortisone injection may resolve particularly resistant cases.

The sesamoid radiographic views on are useful, especially if fracture is suspected (Figure 3.8.52). Bipartite sesamoids are not unusual, and may occur on both sides of the great toe.[12] The smooth appearance of the bones will suggest that the structure is bipartite and not fractured. If the clinical suspicion is of a fracture or stress fracture, an isotope bone scan is diagnostic.[13] The treatment of a fracture is a minimum of 6 weeks' immobilization or surgical removal of the bone.

Hallux valgus

The normal range of valgus for this joint is up to 12°. In hallus valgus the great toe is displaced laterally and rotated medially in a valgus position. The first metatarsal is displaced medially in a varus position. In this position the abductor hallucis longus is displaced inferiorly, resulting in its action becoming that of a flexor rather than as an abductor. The flexor and extensor hallucis longus and the flexor hallucis brevis muscles are displaced laterally increasing abduction.

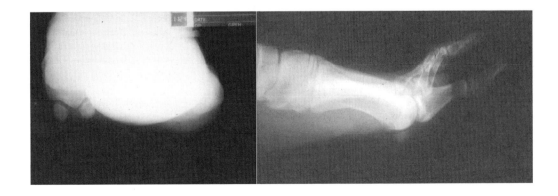

Figure 3.8.52 Sesamoiditis.

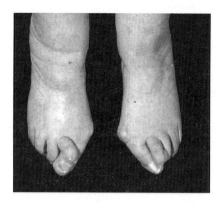

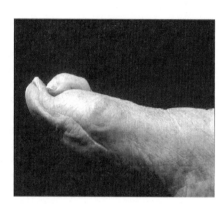

Figure 3.8.53 Hallux valgus.

Treatment

Preventing this condition is the ideal, hence the benefit of good footwear advice from a young age. An excessively pronating foot may result in hallux valgus, and the use of foot orthotics may prevent this. Orthoses may also be used to prevent the worsening of an established case of this condition. However, should the deformity accelerate, then surgical intervention should be considered to prevent disorders spreading to other toes within the foot. Various osteotomy procedures are available such as Reverdin and Austin.[15,16] A concise text on forefoot surgery is the book by Dalton McGlamry, Banks, and Downey.[17] Hetherington[18] is also recommended.

References

1. Bjosen-Moller, F. Calcaneocuboid joint and stability of the longditudinal arch of the foot at high and low gear push off. *Journal of Anatomy*, 1979, **129**(1), 165–76.

2. Coughlin, M. J. Metatarsophalangeal joint instability in the athlete. *Foot and Ankle*, 1993, **14**, 309.

3. Shereff, M. J., Baumhauer, J. F. Hallux rigidus and osteoarthrosis of the first metatarsophalangeal joint. *Journal of Bone and Joint Surgery*, 1998, **80A**, 898–908.

4. Hattrup, S. J., Johnson, K. A. Subjective results of hallux rigidus following treatment with cheilectomy. *Clinical Orthopaedics*, 1988, **226**, 182–5.

5. Thomas, P. J., Smith, R. W. Proximal phalanx osteotomy for the surgical treatment of hallux rigidus. *Foot and Ankle International*, 1999, **20**, 3–12.

6. Kilmartin, T. Metatarsal osteotomy for hallux rigidus. An outcome study of three different osteotomy techniques compared with Keller's excisional arthroplasty. *British Journal of Podiatry*, 2000, 3(4), 95–101.

7. Bowers, K. D., Martin, R. B. Turf toe: a shoe related football injury. *Medicine Science Sports and Exercise*, 1976, **6**, 81–3.

8. Haverstock, B. D. Turf toe-injury of the first metatarsophalangeal joint. *British Journal of Podiatry*, 1998, 2(1), 46–9.

9. Ekstrand, J., Nigg, B. M. Surface related injuries in soccer. *Sports Medicine*, 1989, **8**, 56–62.

10. Frey, C., Anderson, G. D., Feder, K. S. Plantarflexion injury to the first metatarsophalangeal joint (sand toe). *Foot and Ankle International*, 1996, **17**, 576–81.

11. Coker, T. P., Arnold, J. A., Weber, D. L. Traumatic lesions of the metatarsophalangeal joints in athletes. *American Journal of Sports Medicine*, 1978, **6**, 326–34.

12. Frankel, J. P., Harrington, J. Symptomatic bipartite sesamoids. *Journal of Foot Surgery*, 1990, **29**, 318–23.

13. Van Hal, M. E., Keene, J. S., Lange, T. A., Clancy, W. G. Stress fractures of the great toe sesamoids. *American Journal of Sports Medicine*, 1982, **10**, 122–8.

14. Shaw, A. H. The biomechanics of hallux valgus in pronated feet. *Journal of the American Podiatry Association*, 1974, **64**, 193–201.

15. Beck, E. L. Modified Riverdin technique for hallux abducto-valgus (with increased proximal articular set angle of the first metatarsophalangeal joint). *Journal of the American Podiatry Association*, 1974, **64**, 657–66.

16. Austin, D. W., Leventen, E. O. A new osteotomy for hallux valgus. *Clinical Orthopaedics*, 1981, **157**, 25–30.

17. Dalton McGlamry, E., Banks, L., Downey, M. *Comprehensive textbook of foot surgery*. 3rd edn, Vol. 1. Williams & Wilkins, Baltimore, 2001.

18. Hetherington, V. J. (ed.). *Hallux valgus and forefoot surgery*. Churchill Livingstone, Edinburgh. 1994.

Collectively the alteration in forces causes increased valgus strain on the great toe.[14] Encroachment on the second toe may then occur as the hallux causes dorsal subluxation of the second metatarsophalangeal joint. The base of the second proximal phalanx is then displaced superiorly and lies over the metatarsal head, and the pull of the lumbricals and dorsal interossei then causes hyperextension of the metatarsophalangeal joint and flexion of the proximal and distal interphalangeal joint (i.e. 'a claw toe'). Incidentally, if flexion does not occur at the distal interphalangeal joint, the deformity is termed a 'hammer toe'.

Associated with a valgus deformity is the development of inflammation of the medial collateral ligament of the metatarsophalangeal joint, the joint capsule, and the medial soft tissues. The swelling is called a bunion. The partly exposed medial metatarsal head and a resulting exostosis are also aggravating factors leading to a bunion.

Hallux valgus is all too often an acquired condition that will lead to increased stress on the joint and the progression of degenerative change (Figure 3.8.53). Inappropriate, tight-fitting footwear can cause this deformity. Court shoes were designed with fashion in mind, with no consideration for the anatomy of the foot. If a patient stands barefoot next to their shoes, and the feet are wider than the shoe, then obviously there will be compressive forces applied throughout the forefoot. Therefore, useful advise to the patient is that there should be space (approximately the width of the thumb) at the end of the shoe to allow movement, backed up by appropriate width.

Part 4

Management strategies

4.1 Triage

Richard M. Ellis

Musculoskeletal complaints are so prevalent in the 'normal' community, (a Swedish study showing that the 45–64 age group had a 50% incidence in the period of their study[1]), that it is easy for the medical services to become overwhelmed, from constraints of either personnel or finance. In order to give the best care within the resources available, a robust system of triage at the person's first point of professional contact is valuable. Care pathways, where investigations, treatments, or return to work are instigated according to agreed guidelines, have been shown to improve rates of return to work substantially. A 54% reduction in days lost from work was reported in one study.[2]

Between the professionals most widely used in our system, there is potential flexibility in roles, which can be used to advantage according to the setting. In the industrial environment, a back pain case may often have a nurse or physiotherapist as first point of contact. In the UK, a family doctor is the usual first contact, but in other countries a specialist may be the first, at least for some segments of the population. Each professional group has unique advantages for certain roles.

The role of the family doctor

The primary care doctor is variously seen as the provider of almost all medical services, or as the sorter for referral to the specialist in the appropriate body system. Even if the latter is the case, or is perceived to be the case, the success or failure of the management of that case is still in the doctor's hands. For back pain at least, and quite possibly for other musculoskeletal complaints (at least in Western society), the prognosis depends on psychosocial variables and perceptions of general health.[3] The family doctor, who sees the person for many health conditions, and over a long period of time, is most likely to know about these factors, even if they are not measured. For back pain accompanied by the 'yellow flags' for poor prognosis, active early management will provide the return to work; if this is delayed, the prognosis greatly worsens. Ill health in the family may be an important factor for a worker who perceives that there is an option whether or not to continue at work with a chronic condition. Once again, the doctor who has treated or is currently treating other members of the family will have a more informed view on these aspects.

Treatment for most musculoskeletal conditions usually requires no special equipment, and since speed of starting treatment is a factor in its success,[4] the family doctor is also best placed to undertake management for most of these conditions: thus the delays which are inherent in a referral to a specialist are avoided.

It is a mistake to see certain procedures as 'specialist', as the essential criterion of safety depends on training. By attending appropriate training, a family doctor can become competent in the various manipulative and injection techniques.

The more that professionals see themselves as a team treating musculoskeletal problems, the better: thus the family doctor should promote the accessibility of physical treatments for patients. The family doctor should liaise with specialist and physiotherapist personnel to work out the most cost-effective plan for musculoskeletal cases.

The role of the specialist

The authors of this book contend that a doctor specializing in musculoskeletal medicine can provide better care for the abundant causes of locomotor pain, as shown by controlled trials and audit.[5,6]

A specialist in any area of medicine:

- spends most of their professional time with that type of case
- has an expert knowledge of the conditions of that type
- is an expert in the specifics of diagnosis and special investigations
- is expert in technical procedures for that area of medicine
- undertakes research in the subject, where possible
- undertakes continuing medical education in the subject.

In terms of the team treating musculoskeletal cases, the specialist may have fewer conflicting demands on their professional time, and may be best placed to coordinate activity between the primary and secondary care systems. Constant updating of new research will put the specialist in the most informed position to develop care pathways for maximum cost-effectiveness.

The role of the therapist

Much of the improved care of musculoskeletal conditions in recent years is due to improved research and education in physiotherapy, which has enabled us to discard ineffective treatments and introduce new, effective ones.

- **Manual skills:** As an expert in manual skills, the therapist is in an advantageous position to play an important part in management of cases.

- **The psychosocial advantage:** During manual treatment, the therapist's fingers can pick up valuable indications of the patient's psychological state; the patient probably spends more time with this health professional than any other. Thus the therapist can incorporate what is learnt about that person's home life and hopes and fears into the educational process of managing the musculoskeletal problem.

- **Education:** Handouts and leaflets can certainly help in training a person to learn exercises and postural control, but supervision produces better results.[7]

- **Professionalism:** Just as the doctor must realize that unsupervised exercise may not be adequate, the therapist will know the limitations of each type of treatment, and refer back: this teamwork is most advantageous to the patient. Also from the knowledge-base of efficacy of treatments, the therapist is in the right position to counsel the patient when it is clear that active treatment no longer has anything to offer.

References

1. Brattberg, G., Thorslund, M., Wikman, A. The prevalence of pain in a general population. *Pain*, 1989, **37**, 215–22.

2. Weisel, S., Feffer, H., Rothman, R. Low back pain: development and five year prospective application of a computerized quality based diagnostic and treatment protocol. *J Spinal Dis*, 1988, **1**, 50–8.

3. Thomas, E., Silman, A., Croft, P. R., *et al.* Predicting who develops chronic low back pain in primary care: follow-up. *BMJ*, 1999, **318**, 1662–7.

4. Linton, S. J., Hellsing A-L., Andersson, D. A controlled study of the effects of an early intervention on acute musculoskeletal pain problems. *Pain*, 1993, **54**, 353–9.

5. Blomberg, S., Hallin, G., Grann, K., *et al.* Manual therapy with steroid injections: a new approach to treatment of low back pain. *Spine*, 1994, **19**, 569–77.

6. Chakraverty, R., Parsons, C. J. An acute spinal pain service set up in accordance with the CSAG guidelines. *J Orthop Med*, 1999, **21**, 7–12.

7. Frost, H., Klaber Moffett, J., Moser, J., Fairbank, J. Evaluation of a fitness programme for patients with chronic low back pain. *BMJ*, 1995, **310**, 151–4.

4.2 Patient education and self care

Jennifer Klaber Moffett

Appropriate patient education is an essential part of managing musculoskeletal conditions effectively. If someone has insight into their problem and how to deal with it, the disorder is likely to improve more quickly. Effective patient education is likely to depend as much on the method of delivery as the content (Klaber Moffett 1989, Nordin 1995, di Blasi and Kleinen 2000). The first part of this chapter deals with the problem of successfully delivering the message. In the remainder of the chapter the content of the message is then addressed, using research-based evidence and personal clinical experience. Many of the examples are directly related to back pain, which often forms at least 50% of a musculoskeletal workload. Another reason for this emphasis is that much more research has been done on back pain than on other musculoskeletal conditions. It seems that much of the research and resulting principles could often safely be applied to other conditions.

Unfortunately, patient education, care, and self-care is not always optimal because individuals may:

- have **inappropriate beliefs and misconceptions** about their condition

- not have **understood** exactly what the clinician wanted them to do

- believe the advice was not **relevant** for them, and anyway would not help

- not feel able to carry out the advice because it seemed **impractical**, i.e. there are physical barriers

- find it would be too much effort.

If people are not doing as much as they might to help themselves, then the efforts of clinicians, regardless of expertise and skill, will be largely wasted.

The patient's perspective

Inappropriate beliefs and misconceptions

One of the first aims of patient education is to dispel misconceptions that may act as a barrier to recovery. Frequently this may relate to the attribution or cause of the condition with which the individual is consulting. Misconceptions need to be replaced with an explanation that is credible and will provide the individual with confidence to carry out an active rehabilitation programme and encourage them to return to normal activities as soon as possible.

The cause of pain, and pain mechanisms

Misconceptions about the cause of pain need to be addressed. Some insight into how pain is perceived and sustained can be helpful, especially in chronic pain. The individual needs to understand that pain is not processed through a simple mechanical pathway, but is a complex process that can be modified at many different levels of the nervous system. The pain experienced is modulated in the higher centres of the brain by such factors as distraction and suggestion. A large series of fascinating experiments have confirmed the powerful effect of such psychological variables on the reporting of physical symptoms (Pennebaker 1982, 1984). Patient education could include a simple description of the pain gate theory (Melzack and Wall 1982), which provides an explanation of how the mind influences the pain experience.

Most people have a working hypothesis, and if they don't they will be searching for an explanation for their condition. If the clinician's explanation is in conflict with the individual's expectations, it will be seen as irrelevant and any advice will probably be rejected. A very useful question to ask is, 'What is it that concerns you about the pain?' This is not a loaded question, and could be asked of anyone. It is a useful way of eliciting beliefs that might otherwise remain hidden.

Fear of movement and re-injury

If the indivdual believes that their back pain is due to an injury received at work, they may well believe that continuing with this work would be damaging. Similarly, if someone has apparently damaged their back while rowing they may be afraid of returning to this activity. Back pain is now considered more often than not to be accumulative strain, influenced by psychosocial factors, rather than a simple one-off biomechanical problem (Burton 1987, Waddell 1998). It has therefore been suggested that it is better not to use the term 'back injury', as this is inaccurate and encourages the fear and avoidance of movement (Hadler 1987, Hadler 1997). The individual may be afraid of movement that appears to reproduce the pain, associating it with further damage and preventing healing. Compare this to the sportsman's attitude when recovering from an injury: he will expect movements to be sore until the full range of movement is gained. He will not be surprised to find that unaccustomed exercise is usually slightly painful. With his coach, he will work through a carefully prepared training package. Such sportsmen – who of course have the advantage also of being highly motivated – generally recover even from quite major trauma much faster than other people. It is necessary for individuals to understand and believe that any advice to exercise will actually assist the healing process. Research is emerging which shows that people who can overcome a fear of movement and physical activity have better outcomes (Indahl, Haldorsen *et al.* 1998, Burton, Waddell *et al.* 1999, Vlaeyen and Linton 2000).

Fear of wear and tear

People who have been told they have arthritis or 'wear and tear' may believe that they should reduce their levels of physical activity in order to save the joints. Most people appreciate that exercise can strengthen muscles, but they do not realize that exercise and movement also play a very important role in the healing of other structures such as ligaments and even bone. People with arthritis need to be told that the right sort of exercise increases the lubrication in the joint space rather than wearing down the joint surfaces. For each condition, an explanation to suit that individual needs to be offered in the context of the person's own belief patterns.

Fear of a progressive condition

Another fear and misconception that may hinder recovery, especially if the person does not relate the pain to a physical incident or injury, is the unspoken possibility of the presence of some dreaded progressive disease. An individual may fear ending up in a wheelchair, or suspect that their pain must be due to cancer. Since these fears may not be voiced, it is incumbent on the clinician to elicit any such beliefs so that they can be dispelled. After a brief but appropriate history-taking and examination, the clinician is then in a good position to offer a credible and non-threatening explanation of the condition to reassure the person. In some cases no further treatment will then be required. However, for most people the rehabilitation process then can begin. For someone who is suitably motivated, much of this can be carried out at home with suitable guidance. This will be considered further under 'home exercise programmes'.

Understanding the message

The commonest reason for not 'complying with advice' may be to do with how the message is received and interpreted. The clinician may believe that they have clearly asked the person to carry out a few simple exercises and given specific advice about activities or positions to avoid. However, if the receiver is on a different waveband from the one the message was sent out on, the advice will not be received. Generally patients want to please and certainly do not want to look foolish, so they will usually appear to cooperate and maybe only when they get home realize how blurred the message was. An anxious person who feels insecure in the presence of the 'expert' may be unable to take in any details at all. The more relaxed and at ease an individual feels with the clinician, the more likely they are to be receptive to the message.

Language or jargon may be a problem. Words that are familiar to a clinician may be meaningless to a lay person, or be interpreted in quite a different way from how they were meant. A different problem arises when the clinician provides a message that conflicts with the patient's beliefs. In this case the individual may find it difficult to make sense of information because of their prior mindset and beliefs.

Advice perceived not to be relevant

If the advice given does not fit with the individual's understanding of their problem, commitment to it will be lacking. The individual will perceive that the advice is irrelevant and will not believe that the effort involved will be worthwhile. The advice must be credible in the patient's eyes. This can be achieved after assessment of the condition, which includes asking appropriate questions and a physical examination, followed by a brief non-threatening explanation of the problem.

Impractical advice: physical and perceived barriers

Practical reasons for not following the advice given could include:

Forgetting to do it

This could be because the person leads a busy life with many work and/or domestic commitments. The suggested programme may have a low priority on their schedule and thus may be overlooked. For others, including older people, memory may be a problem and methods of reminding themselves to do things may be necessary. The home programme needs to be written down and appropriate times negotiated and set by the patient. The time for doing the exercises then becomes part of a daily routine, with specific cues to aid memory. For example, 'I do this postural correction while the kettle boils'; 'I stand up and do my stretches every time someone leaves my office.' The chances of continuing with a programme of exercises long term increases if they are always done at the same time of the day and therefore linked with another activity. The habit or behaviour is reinforced if it is followed by an activity that the person enjoys or finds rewarding, such as having a cup of tea.

Exercise or advice is difficult to follow for a physical reason, e.g. obesity, ill-health

It is important that the clinician does not ask someone to carry out an activity without checking that it is within their perceived capability.

Time not available

The clinician should be realistic in prescribing how much exercise to expect someone to carry out. If an individual is asked to carry out an exercise programme every hour while they are at work, not only may this be unrealistic but also it could be disadvantageous because the person has to focus on their disorder rather than on their work. Another major disadvantage in making excessive demands is that the therapist may lose credibility in the patient's eyes.

Too expensive

Using a special facility such as a gym may be expensive. If an individual does not rate the activity as being very important or desirable, they will not think it is worth the money.

Lack of transport

For someone without a car, the additional effort of walking and using public transport may be perceived as an impossible barrier.

Lack of suitable space

It may difficult for someone to find space and privacy to carry out a routine conveniently. A mother with young children and little support at home may not have the necessary space and time to carry out the programme. People at work may have similar difficulties.

Lack of social support

In addition to any or all the previously discussed reasons for not complying with an exercise programme, social support is an important factor. If family, friends, and work colleagues understand the importance of carrying out the routine, they are more likely to be encouraging. In contrast, if they do not perceive the exercise programme to be important they may very easily act as a major antagonist.

In order to encourage family and friends to be supportive, it can be very helpful to involve them in the rehabilitation process. Commonly, the individual's family and work colleagues may be overprotective and may provide more sympathy than is helpful. They may encourage the individual in an invalid role by regularly offering to do tasks for them. This does not aid the rehabilitation process, and can also be quite demoralizing for the individual. If they understand the issues better, family, friends, and colleagues may be able to support and help the person in a much more appropriate way. They should at least have access to written information, which the individual should be encouraged to show them. A useful example of this is *The Back Book* (see subsection below on encouraging early return to activity). This provides evidence based information and positive messages to encourage recovery.

Effort and motivation

The aim of patient education aim is to provide people with information and increase their knowledge and understanding of their condition. It can influence their attitude to their disorder. However, although knowledge and attitudes are important, they do not necessarily predict behaviour. An individual may have been told that they should do exercises and know that this could be helpful, but for a number of different reasons there may be barriers, both mental and physical, that prevent them from doing the prescribed exercises. This is a key issue that health professionals need to address more closely. It is essential that the individual believes that it is worth putting the effort into doing the exercises. The chances of carrying out a new programme and maintaining it can be predicted using the Health Beliefs model (Janz and Becker 1984, Becker 1985). The key variables included in this model are:

- the perceived costs and effort required, balanced by

- the perceived benefit likely to be achieved, and

- the seriousness of the condition as perceived by the individual, and

- perceived barriers.

Techniques such as motivational interviewing can be used to improve the chances of a person taking on a new programme (Rollnick, Heather *et al.* 1992, Smith, Heckemeyer *et al.* 1997) and will be discussed under the heading of 'compliance or concordance?'

Clinician's perspective and approach

Effective communication

Effective patient education depends on effective communication. Most of us like to believe that we are good communicators, even though we may have had little or no training in this skill. A skilfully conducted interview is an essential starting point for optimal management of a musculoskeletal condition. If this is not done well, subsequent advice and management may well be inappropriate.

Time may be a real barrier for clinicians, but if patient education is considered to be an essential part of treatment intervention rather than a nice extra (Lorig 1995), it might be given greater priority. In the longer term it has been shown that effective communication can cut down on the use of health care resources, improving both patient satisfaction and treatment outcomes. In a study by Daltroy, Katz *et al.* (1992) it was found that if a rheumatologist made a clear statement about the purpose of a non-specific anti-inflammatory (NSAID) 79% of patients were compliant, compared with 33% where no clear statement was made. Also it has been shown that after a consultation the **doctor's perception** of what they told the patient may vary significantly from the **patient's perception** of what they have been told. The way in which information is provided is at least as important as the content of the information. Some clinicians may believe they should give each patient as much information as possible, whereas others commonly underestimate the amount of information that patients want. In either case the best approach is to find out what the individual's current understanding is and what other information they require. Open-ended questions such as 'what do you know about your condition?' may be a useful starting point.

A number of benefits may result from improved communication (Ley 1988), including:

- increased patient understanding and recall

- increased patient satisfaction

- less ill-informed consent

- increased patient compliance

- quicker and less stressful recovery from illness and surgery.

Patient–practitioner interaction

The health professional can influence the outcome of treatment by shaping beliefs, and providing support alongside physical care. These concepts have been highlighted in a recent systematic review (di Blasi and Kleinen 2000) and linked into Leventhal's self-regulatory model (Leventhal 1985, Leventhal and Cameron 1987). A combination of cognitive care, emotional care, and physical care has been reported to improve recovery in surgical cases and cardiac patients and probably applies also to people with musculoskeletal disorders. It seems likely that how the practitioner provides the information is as important as what material is provided. Di Blasi and Kleinen (2000) postulate that accompanying supportive care is an important aspect that is under-researched and could have an impact on successful outcome of treatment.

The most important goal in arthritis patient education, according to Daltroy (1993), is to develop a cooperative relationship between the physician and patient so that the patient will adhere to a mutually agreed regimen, and the regimen is guided by accurate feedback from the patient. In this way the symptoms can be monitored and managed most effectively. The patient needs to be asked what they see as their goal of treatment. The clinician needs to explain what is possible, including implications and limitations. The patient's preferences need to be taken into account, so alternative possibilities need to be discussed. In this way an adult–adult relationship is encouraged rather than a child–adult relationship implying undue dependency on the clinician (Klaber Moffett and Richardson 1997).

Providing the information

When providing patient education and advice, it is very tempting to think that the 'best' education is providing the individual with all the information that is available. However, this is a mistake, albeit one that some of us have taken many years of practice to appreciate. We have tended to spend time imparting a great deal of information and may have at times been surprised and disappointed at the result. The information is generally designed to provide a background and explanation to the person's disorder, in order to encourage them to carry out an exercise programme or modify their lifestyle or posture in some way. However, the key is not to give too much information. The person is likely to remember the first or the last piece of information they are given. Most of the rest will be forgotten, or may never even have been processed.

It is essential to find out what the person would like to know. They should be given only strictly relevant information, and it should not be thrust on them. It is likely to be much more useful to provide people with a small piece of information at each visit rather than a large amount of information at one visit. People learn better if they take an active role in seeking information. For this reason techniques such as motivational interviewing may be useful, where a change in behaviour would be desirable but may be difficult to achieve.

Labels, explanations, and the meaning of words

Both in an individual situation and in a group situation such as a Back School, explanations about the anatomy, biomechanics, and pathology can be provided in a simplified form. Great care and consideration needs to go into this process. Words may often be interpreted in a way that was not intended. People are very concerned to have a label to attach to their condition, so they can tell their neighbour what is wrong with them. They will then behave in a way that seems to fit the label, and the recovery rate may therefore hinge on the patient's understanding of their problem.

Radiographs

These are very frequently taken unnecessarily, but people who believe that a radiograph would show exactly what is wrong with them will be very keen to have one. It is therefore important for the practitioner to explain the limited usefulness of radiography. The clinical guidelines produced by the Royal College of General Practitioners on the management of low back pain recommend that radiographs should not be routinely taken unless there is a specific indication (Waddell, Feder *et al.* 1996), and this is consistent with the recommendations of the Royal College of Radiologists (Chisholm 1991). In fact it has been

estimated that 19 lives per year are sacrificed to the effects of unnecessary radiation. Many people are unaware that lumbar spine radiographs involve 120 times more radiation than chest radiographs. Less dramatically, radiography may have negative effects because the individual may understand that the radiograph shows they have a 'degenerative spine' and infer from this that their spine is nearly 'worn out'. The message can be a powerful and very negative one, if the corollary is understood as 'I had better save my back and not do too much physical activity or exercise in case I damage it further'.

Compliance or concordance?

The term 'compliance' is an unfortunate one, implying that the health professional is in a superior position, the expert, and the patient is the recipient. It implies an unfortunate adult–child relationship rather the adult–adult one which is desirable if the person is to not to become dependent on the health professional. The word 'patient' itself implies helplessness and long-suffering and is therefore a very unfortunate term, for which a more positive one should be substituted wherever possible.

The interaction of the relationship between the health professional and the individual is very important in successful treatment outcomes (Klaber Moffett and Richardson 1997). The term 'adherence' or 'concordance' is more consistent with a relationship based on an equal partnership. It is then acknowledged that the health professional is an expert in one respect but the patient is the expert relating to their own particular condition, and is the only person who knows what it feels like. Someone with a failed knee replacement that needs to be revised and is currently causing excessive swelling, loss of range of movement, and pain may not welcome the well-meaning physiotherapist saying, 'I know just how it feels'. In one particular case the response to this was direct and educational: 'You do *not* know how it feels'. A more appropriate way of expressing empathy might have been to say, 'It must be really very unpleasant/difficult for you'.

Having decided what to tell the patient, the problem in the clinician's mind remains 'how am I going to get them to do it?' It is known from the literature on compliance with taking drugs, that often less than 50% of the tablets prescribed are taken. This could be partly because many people don't like taking drugs. On the other hand, it is often much easier to swallow a pill than to follow an exercise programme. In a study of exercise compliance it was found that providing written information as well as oral information increased compliance from 33% to 77%. Many other studies have shown the importance of providing written material (Ley 1988).

A number of other factors are likely to influence whether a person carries out an exercise programme and maintains it over a longer period of time. The latter is much less likely. 'Concordance' implies that a programme has been discussed and negotiated with the full involvement of the individual, so its likelihood of successful uptake and maintenance is much greater. As far as longer-term maintenance is concerned, ownership of the programme is important. It is also more likely to be tailored to the needs of the individual as it has been agreed through discussion and is therefore more likely to be acceptable and realistic for that person.

Motivational interviewing

The basis of this counselling technique, which has been developed for use by busy doctors to use in short (5–15-minute) consultations is that the interview is not dominated by the clinician but rather appears to be led by the patient. Motivational interviewing was originally developed in the

Motivational interviewing

You ask: 'On a scale of 0–10, How ready would you say you are to change?'

If the person says 3, then you ask, 'Why 3 and not 0?'

He may say, 'Because I know that going for a swim three times a week, like I used to, would help my shoulder problem.'

'So why 3 and not 10?'

He then replies, 'Well, its 3 and not 10 because I couldn't have the car when I would like to go swimming immediately after work.'

Then you would explore what other options there might be.

field of addiction for helping people deal with ambivalence about behaviour change (Rollnick, Heather et al. 1992). It is based on the premise that many people are not ready to change when they consult a health care professional. It can be applied to education messages such as physical activity and exercise. The technique is to ask the individual about their readiness to change (or carry out a particular change in lifestyle).

If the individual is not ready to change at present, it may be most sensible for the clinician and patient to openly accept this. Through this non-judgmental discussion, the door is left open for the person to return when they feel ready to change. **Confidence of success**, which is another key concept to successful adherence in making lifestyle changes, is also explored in a similar way, asking them how confident they are that they could succeed in bringing that change about, or taking up a new activity and sticking with it.

Information-giving is a central part of the motivational interviewing technique, but is patient-centred and maximizes the freedom of choice for the individual. It avoids a judgmental or authoritarian approach. It can also be more satisfying for the practitioner who does not need to feel he has failed if the person is not able to take on the suggested advice at present. It is often argued that the technique is too time consuming, but in fact time can be saved as soon as the practitioner accepts that not all patients will be receptive to advice all the time.

Home exercise programmes

Home programmes form an essential part of most patient education and often include exercises. These need to be carefully taught: each exercise should be demonstrated, and then tried out with guidance from the practitioner. The purpose of each exercise should be clearly explained, and the programme should be written down and illustrated.

A home programme should be developed by the practitioner together with the patient and will be based on certain guiding principles such as: (1) setting specific and realistic goals, (2) working in a disciplined way gradually increasing the amount of exercise or activity and its grade of difficulty, and (3) using positive support systems to provide encouragement and feedback.

Setting realistic goals

The first task is to find out what it is that the individual would like to achieve. Specific and realistic goals need to be set. These should also be fulfilling, and if possible enjoyable, for the person who needs to carry them out. Once the goals (not more than three) have been arrived at, they need to be written down. It is important also to write down **when**,

i.e. how many times a week or times a day and for **how long, how far**, etc., the activity will be carried out. The task – say, doing the shopping – may need to be broken down into components, looking at what is required in order to carry out that activity. This includes walking to the bus stop, waiting at the bus stop, getting on to the bus, walking to the shops and round the shops, carrying shopping, and so on. Similarly, other activities such as playing a round of golf can be broken down into smaller components that the person can be guided to achieve gradually over a period of several weeks or months. With any exercise or activity it is essential to start at a very low base line that is certain to be manageable in order to avoid failure, which can be detrimental. Clear quotas of gradually increasing activity levels are then set. The person should keep careful records, noting exactly what they have achieved each day and each week. It is helpful if the activity can be easily measured in distance and or time, so that even small improvements can be recognized. Immediate feedback is a very important factor in encouraging and motivating an individual to continue with an activity.

Graded activity

Any new exercise or activity needs to be introduced in a graded fashion.

Advice needs to be quite carefully thought through, and details need to be carefully explained in order to avoid such a situation. The same principles of graded activity can be applied to gardening, tennis, walking, running, and even housework. All these activities need to be built up in a stepwise fashion, while successively spreading the load and effort to different parts of the body and different areas of soft tissue (muscle and its associated tissue as well as ligaments) and bone and cartilage. Walking on hard regular surfaces such as city pavements repetitively loads the same part of the joint, and can be uncomfortable. Experience shows that joints may more happily tolerate walking longer distances in the countryside than on pavements.

Use of positive support systems to provide rewards

Long-term adherence with exercise is dependent on perceived benefits and rewards. Positive feedback and a sense of self-efficacy are predictors of outcome (Bandura 1982, O'Leary 1985, Dolce, Crocker et al. 1986, Dolce 1987, Kores, Murphy et al. 1990, Jensen, Turner et al.

Introducing exercise gradually

A woman tells her physiotherapist that she was advised to go swimming but found it made her neck and back pain worse. On closer questioning it turns out that she had attempted to do 15 lengths of the pool although she had not done any swimming for several years. When asked what stroke she swam, she explained that she could only do breast stroke and didn't like to get her hair wet, so swam with her head and trunk held in extreme extension. Advice to alternate different strokes, or to devise a simple programme that includes different positions, is important. This woman can be advised to intersperse her breast stroke with walking in chest-deep water and floating on her back. She may be encouraged to join classes, which are now widely available for adults of all levels of ability, to improve her swimming technique.

1991). Social support from family or friends can help a great deal. Without the possibility of encouragement and rewards for the effort, as we have already seen, success with a home programme is less likely. Even worse than lack of support is a situation that actually discourages the individual from carrying out their home programme. For example, if the person perceives that the family is laughing at their efforts, the chances of adherence are very slim. This is a reason why it may be helpful to involve the partner in the self-management programme to get their support in encouraging the patient. This is especially important in long-term adherence.

Patient education for an acute problem

Rest

Rest may be necessary because of pain or a very extensive injury or surgical wound, but very rarely for more than 24 hours. For upper and lower limb extremities, the advice to apply ice, compression and elevation is still sensible. For the back, in very severe cases as much as 3 days' bed rest may be needed but generally it is better to allow as much movement as the individual can tolerate. For the neck, a collar may be worn to provide the person with a feeling of protection but not for more that a day or two and only if the pain is very acute.

Ice

In the presence of heated or inflamed tissue, ice may be more useful than heat. The individual may wish to purchase an ice pack from a local sports shop or pharmacy, which can be kept in the freezer between uses. Instructions for its safe use need to be given: applying an ice pack directly to the skin can easily cause a burn, but this can be avoided by placing the ice pack in a wet towel. As many experienced clinicians, sportsmen, and others will know, the application of ice can have quite a dramatic effect, for example in reducing an Achilles tendon swelling. It is more likely to be effective if the painful and inflamed tissue is fairly superficial.

In some instances ice may be a good substitute for anti-inflammatories, particularly for people who tend to suffer from the common side effects of these drugs. It is worth discussing this point with the patient, in order to check that they have not developed gastrointestinal symptoms. They may not be aware why they had developed pains in this region, possibly together with loss of appetite. It is does not appear to be common knowledge that NSAIDs, if taken over a long period of time, can cause bleeding and gastrointestinal ulcers in more vulnerable people (Rodriguez and Jick 1994). It should never be taken for granted that the general practitioner has found the time to discuss these side effects.

Heat

Applying heat in the form of a hot shower has some advantages over soaking in a bath, since the heat can be directed on to the painful area while the person can move, rather than being restrained to a fixed and possibly awkward position in the bath tub. Another method is to apply heat via a small towel placed in hand-hot water, wrung out and placed over the painful area. It should be placed directly in contact with the skin with another dry towel over it, to prevent the loss of heat being too rapid. Some people prefer to use a hot-water bottle, although this is not so malleable. Heat may often be used as a substitute for painkillers. It should be used before doing stretching exercises.

Stretching exercises

Stretching exercises are an important part of the rapid recovery process and need to be taught very carefully. Most people carry out their stretches too quickly, as most of us are far too impatient! Each stretch should be held for at least 15 seconds and repeated three times. A cold muscle should not be stretched; warm tissue has more elastic properties and is less likely to be injured. There are several different methods of stretching each muscle group in the body, but whichever method is chosen it is important to do it correctly. The patient needs to shown exactly how to do it, pointing out common errors such as turning the foot out when carrying out a calf muscle stretch instead of pointing the toes straight ahead. They should also be provided with diagrams and detailed instructions of when and how often to carry out the exercises. A well-illustrated book on the subject can be very useful (Anderson 1981).

Posture and ergonomic advice

Posture

A great deal of emphasis is often put on this aspects of patient education, without considering how effective it is likely to be. Ergonomic advice on its own may not be sufficient, as psychosocial aspects may be more important (Burton, Symonds et al. 1997).

It is difficult to change an individual's habitual posture, and attempts to do so may even be counterproductive. Successful techniques use training methods which involve repeating movements and positions over and over again, over a long period of time, with guidance and encouragement. Fast results are not expected but high levels of motivation, patience, and persistence are necessary. One such technique is the Alexander technique, which can be used to improve the posture and use of the spine and rest of the body. Oriental teachings such as yoga and tai chi can also train better posture. A clinician attempting to correct a poor posture in the course of a conventional consultation is less likely to succeed in making changes to the habitual stance of the individual.

It is often forgotten that posture is likely to be influenced by other factors:

- **Emotional status:** If a person is unhappy or insecure they may tend to fold their arms and stoop, whereas a happy confident person is more likely to be upright and maintain a more relaxed posture. The clinician treating a person with a musculoskeletal disorder should take this into account. It is important to be sensitive to body language. It may be counterproductive to tell a person who is depressed that their posture is bad and that they should stand up straighter. At the least it may just be a waste of time.

- **Genetics:** Observation shows us that members of some families tend to have a very hollow lumbar spine, with a marked forward incline of the pelvis. Others have a much flatter lumbar spine. This is at least in part due to tight hamstrings. Teaching the person to do effective hamstring stretching exercises may be the key to helping them.

Habits: Posture is habitual, and training plays an important role if maintained over a long enough period of time. Ballet dancers, army personnel, and Alexander teachers are examples of people who can be recognized by their 'good' posture, which is learnt over many years.

Strengthening and training specific muscle groups

Theoretically it should be possible to improve posture by strengthening particular muscles that help to maintain the body in a state of equilibrium. Some specific techniques put a great deal of emphasis on training individual muscles, such as the transversus abdominus and the multifidus muscles, which are deep segmental muscles of the trunk and are considered to act as trunk stabilizers (Jull and Richardson 1994, Hides, Richardson et al. 1995, Hides, Richardson et al. 1996). Pilates technique, which is currently very popular, aims to teach control of pelvic, abdominal, and trunk muscles by 'zipping and tucking' the pelvic area in order to learn to maintain a neutral position of the pelvis.

The workplace

It is important that the practitioner should explore the patient's work circumstances, both physical and psychosocial. For those in paid employment, recent guidance produced by the Faculty of Occupational Medicine could be useful (Carter and Birrell 2000, Waddell and Burton 2000). Liaison with the workplace (the occupational health department or the supervisor) can make a huge difference in helping the person to get back to work.

Office environment

It may be possible through simple advice to improve, for example, the working position of an individual who spends their whole day at a desk. A few very basic rules are worth considering. Ideally it is helpful to observe the individual in their working situation, in order to be able to make specific recommendations. One visit to the workplace may be worth half a dozen sessions in a clinic. If a visit is not possible, a detailed discussion is necessary to find out whether there could be some simple adaptation of the working environment. Unless the changes are very small it will be necessary to involve the supervisor or human resources department. The UK Health and Safety at Work legislation makes it the duty of the employer to respond to reasonable requests for new equipment to make the employee more comfortable. It is now accepted by most employers that this is actually to their advantage, as it may avoid the person going off sick. They should appreciate that buying a new chair for a sedentary worker could represent a cost saving if the alternative is for that employee to be off work for 6 months.

Seating at work

Making sure that the chair is suitable in height relative to the desk and the computer is a basic necessity that is sometimes overlooked. Someone who is shorter or larger than average is more likely to have problems achieving a good position. A taller person may require the desk to be raised.

Mandal (1985), in an interesting little book on seating, analyses different postures in children and adults seated in a variety of different chairs. He argues that the traditional furniture found in schools and offices does not meet the requirements of most people. Rather, he has found most people would benefit from higher chairs that tilt forward. He emphasizes that lumbar supports, when provided, are rarely used and are not a realistic requirement. Furthermore, he recommends the use of a tilting chair that moves with the person. My personal experience has been that the use of such an office chair (which tilts forward and backwards through about 15°) immediately reduced longstanding backache and referred pain in the hip area. It has continued to be comfortable over a period of 5 years, a fact emphasized by the discomfort I feel when sitting in long meetings in ordinary chairs. There has been considerable interest in 'alternative seating' such as kneeling chairs which originated from Scandinavia. Some people find these useful, but few people are comfortable on them for long periods. The design was thought to reduce stress on the spine because the angle between the thighs and the trunk is greater than 90°, making it easier to maintain a lordosis. More recent research (Althoff et al. 1992) does not support this theory.

Physiotherapists and doctors have used findings based on the work of Nachemson (1960) to advise patients that standing puts less strain on the spine than sitting. They also have advised people to sit up straight. However, recent research challenges these principles (Althoff, Brinckmann et al. 1992, Wilke, Neef et al. 1999). Althoff and colleagues used a stadiometer to measure stature for assessing spinal loading. These researchers validated a technique previously developed by Eklund and Corlett (1984). The research by Althoff is very interesting, as the findings appear to contradict some of the widely accepted findings published by Nachemson (1960) four decades ago. Nachemson inserted a needle in the L3/4 disc space and measured intradiscal pressure in different postures. Classically he reported that the intradiscal pressure was 30% greater in unsupported sitting than in standing. Althoff's more recent work refutes this, and furthermore two other recent studies support these findings (Rohlmann, Bergmann et al. 1995, Wilke, Neef et al. 1999). Wilke and colleagues used a more refined method of measuring intradiscal pressure by surgical implantation (see Fig. 4.2.1). The latest research continues to support the idea that pressure on the spine is reduced by keeping the load closer to the body and bending the knees rather than the back.

It is commonly recommended by physiotherapists and other practitioners that a good posture of the spine requires a lordosis to be maintained all the time (McKenzie 1981). This is not easy to do when sitting. However, a relaxed sitting posture has been shown to put less pressure on the disc than sitting upright (Wilke, Neef et al. 1999). This is probably related to muscle tension. The most important advice is probably to avoid maintaining any fixed posture for longer than necessary. The body, and especially the spine, likes movement, and this needs to be encouraged. For many people, physical activity is becoming less and less a part of their lives. Particularly in later life, people who are total couch potatoes may have to pay the price of being much less able-bodied, overweight, and generally more at risk of most life-threatening conditions.

Manual handling

There is evidence that heavy and frequent lifting of loads in excess of 50 kg can lead to a reduction in overall disc height in the entire lumbar

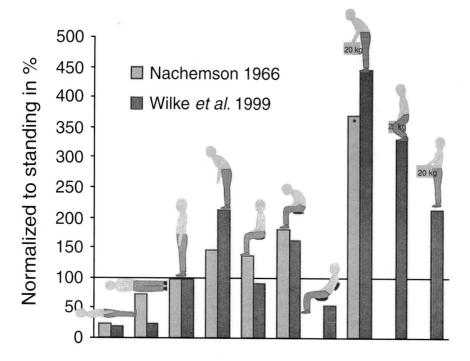

Figure 4.2.1 A comparison between Nachemson (1966) and Wilke *et al.* (1999) (both for 70 kg individuals) regarding intradiscal pressure in common postures and activities, normalized to standing.

spine (Brinckmann, Frobin *et al.* 1998). Workers lifting in cramped conditions or on uneven ground are also at risk. Further, research on miners has shown that whole-body vibration can result in damage to the discs.

The UK Health and Safety Executive guidance on regulations for manual handling does not set specific requirements such as weight limits (HSE 1992). They simply recommend that hazardous manual handling should be avoided where possible. They recommend the threshold limits of weights and related manoeuvres which if exceeded require individual assessments. These depend not only on the weight of the object but also the height and distance from the body. Physiotherapists and doctors have traditionally recommended people always to lift with a straight back and bent knees, and theoretically this can reduce pressure on the discs. However, workers often find this technique is not feasible. Indeed, for many women and older people of both genders the 'squat' technique is impossible, as it requires considerable strength in the quadriceps muscle to raise the weight of the body as well as the external load. It requires good flexibility of the ankles, knees, and hips. Finally, it requires skill, together with good balance and coordination. A recent review of the literature has examined the data on spinal compression, bending moments, net moments, and shear forces during 'stoop' lifting and 'squat' lifting (van Dieen, Hoozemans *et al.* 1999). These authors confirm that the biomechanical literature does not support recommending the use of the squat lift. It did not reduce the net moments and compression forces, the main problem being that the load is usually some distance from the body. The actual energy expenditure and the perceived exertion is greater for the squat lift (Welbergen, Kemper *et al.* 1991). In any case, this technique is unlikely to be complied with.

Group education programmes

Back schools

A back school is a popular method of providing group education for people with back pain. It was first described by a physiotherapist in Sweden (Zachrisson-Forsell 1980) and is popular with physiotherapists throughout the Western world. Some back schools, particularly in the US and Scandinavia, are multidisciplinary in their approach; the programme is delivered by a physiotherapist, an occupational therapist, a psychologist, a nurse, and a doctor. In the UK, back schools are usually run by physiotherapists. They were originally set up and evaluated in a Volvo factory, and found to be effective (Berquist-Ullman and Larsson 1977). Since then a number of other trials have been conducted, with varied findings, and these have been evaluated in several systematic reviews of the literature on back schools (Linton and Kamwendo 1987, Keijsers, Bouter *et al.* 1991, Cohen, Goel *et al.* 1994, Koes, van Tulder *et al.* 1994)). The evidence for their effectiveness is unclear. This is not too surprising, as back schools vary considerably; their success will depend on both the contents and the method of delivery (Klaber Moffett 1989, Nordin, Cedraschi *et al.* 1992, Nordin 1995). Back schools which are based in the occupational setting are more likely to be effective. This could be because the advice is likely to be seen to be more relevant to the individual's needs in the workplace, and also because the employers are seen to be interested and involved in the workers' problem. Having a supervisor and employee who care, appears to be an important variable in the equation. A back school is more likely to be successful if it includes an exercise programme encouraging normal activity and fitness (Frost, Klaber Moffett *et al.* 1995, Frost, Lamb *et al.* 1998, Lonn 1999). Just telling people to become more active and exercise more may not be sufficient. Trying to change people's attitudes and behaviour is difficult, especially in the longer term. Knowledge on its own does not necessarily bring about a change in attitudes or behaviour (Mazzuca 1982). Young people often know about the serious health risks associated with smoking, but this does not stop them doing it. Similarly, people with back pain may know that sitting in front of a computer all day and then slumping on to a sofa to watch television may not help their back problem, but they often continue to do so. Conversely, a new behaviour can influence attitudes. Experience shows that if people carry out exercises at a class and find – to their surprise – that the exercises, although they may hurt a bit at the time, do not make the back pain worse, their attitude and beliefs may be radically altered. They may re-evaluate their problem and realize that they can function normally again, and no longer think of themselves as a person with a serious problem.

Long-term adherence in particular needs to be addressed when setting up a programme.

Back to Fitness programmes

Over the past 10 years exercise programmes for people with back pain have been developed which are an important substitute or adjunct to back schools. They aim to help participants overcome the fear of damaging their spine by using cognitive-behavioural principles to restore confidence in using the back normally. Research on these programmes, which are now referred to as Back to Fitness programmes, is promising. Maintenance of beneficial effects of the exercise classes has been demonstrated at 1 year and even 2 years later (Frost, Klaber Moffett et al. 1995, Frost, Lamb et al. 1998, Klaber Moffett, Torgerson et al. 1999). The programme is led by physiotherapists and the manual for setting it up has been published (Klaber Moffett and Frost, 2000).

Other forms of group education

Considerable clinical experience has now been documented showing the value of self-management programmes for back pain, chronic arthritis, and other chronic diseases. The development of these programmes and their evaluation is described in a 12-year case study (Lorig and Gonzalez 1992). The key to the success of the programmes seems to be that they are patient centred. Indeed, all patient education needs to be patient centred so that individuals can receive the advice and information that they require rather than the information the health professional perceives they require.

This appears to be a very promising area for further research and development, particularly as demands for health care continue to increase. It could also be a way of reducing the gap between the public's expectations of health and health care and what is actually possible in reality (Coulter, 2000, Klaber Moffett and Frost, 2000).

Pain and discomfort at night or on rising: positioning at night

Personal experience over many years has shown that providing relevant advice about placing pillows to provide suitable support during the night can make a big difference to a person's comfort and dramatically reduce pain. The individual may be suffering disturbed and uncomfortable nights with a lot of stiffness or pain on awakening. This can often be reduced if the following tips are carefully conveyed and the principle of keeping the joints in neutral positions is understood.

Neck pain

Many acute neck problems result from sleeping in an awkward position such as (1) sleeping with the head in extreme flexion (too many pillows), or (2) sleeping on the side with too few pillows to support the head, or (3) worst of all, sleeping face down with a pillow which puts the head in an extreme position of extension and rotation.

Different possibilities will suit different people, and the following may be suggested:

- If using a feather pillow, tie it in the middle to make a 'butterfly' pillow. Use the 'wings' of the pillow to support the head and prevent it rolling into an awkward position.

- Explain the principle that pillows can be used to maintain a comfortable position and avoid putting structures into a stretched or stressed position. If this happens, the person will either be woken up by discomfort or find that the pain may be bad in the morning.

Sleeping prone – face down

Some people say they cannot get to sleep unless they sleep face down. This seems to be one of commonest causes of neck pain, as the head is forced into rotation. Using pillows under the head makes it worse, as the head is then also forced into extension. These are positions that most people's cervical spines cannot tolerate, especially in middle age.

Careful placing of two pillows can reduce the ill-effects of sleeping prone. One is placed lengthways under the person's torso. The other is under the head but mostly under the ear, allowing the nose to point down into the mattress. This provides two important advantages: the neck is only slightly rotated, and the person can breathe easily.

Foam pillows

These are better for anyone who suspects they may be allergic to feathers. It is important that they are put in the correct place, and are of the right proportion to suit the individual. Once the principle of support is understood, the person should be able to find out what suits them best.

Pillows are available in various shapes, but the principle is always the same. The purpose of the pillow is to support the neck and head in a neutral position while maintaining a cervical lordosis. They can be purchased as a large foam roll which is placed under the neck. A thin pillow may be used to support the head.

Shoulder disorders, e.g. 'frozen shoulder' or rotator cuff syndrome

These conditions can be very painful, especially at night time, causing distress and all the problems associated with a sleep deficit. Advice about placing pillows can be very useful. The aim is mainly to avoid the arm falling backwards into extension in the night and to maintain it in a neutral position.

The individual can be advised to use a substantial pillow under the arm, with the arm flexed at the elbow to 90°, and slightly flexed at the shoulder. It can be helpful to put the arm inside the pillowcase so that a restless sleeper will still maintain the support of the pillow even when moving around in the night.

Lower limb disorders

Painful hips or knees similarly can be supported on a pillow to maintain the joints in a neutral position. A pillow between the legs can usefully support the upper leg when the individual mostly sleeps on their side. The thickness of the pillow is important, and the individual should be encouraged to experiment with different-sized pillows.

A painful foot may not be able to tolerate any weight of bedclothes. A cradle can be improvised at home using a cardboard box with two sides cut out and placed over the feet under the bedclothes. Personal experience of working on orthopaedic wards has shown that nurses are often unhappy for a patient to use pillows under the leg, possibly because of a fear of putting extra pressure on the leg and especially the calf. This does not seem relevant for anyone who is moving around during the day.

Back pain

If sleep is disturbed by back pain, positioning needs to be considered. The mattress might need changing to provide suitable support to the spine. A heavier person needs a firmer mattress; couples may each require mattresses of different densities. If one mattress is shared in a double bed, an adaptation can be made by removing some of the slats under the mattress of the lighter partner. This will have a similar effect to lying on a softer mattress.

It is not essential to spend large sums of money on new mattresses or beds. An orthopaedic bed is certain to be very expensive, but is not certain to bring relief of pain and a good night's sleep. Better shops will encourage beds and mattresses to be tried out in the shop. They will also allow them to be loaned out for a couple of nights for a trial.

Some people with back pain find that a roll or thin pillow under the waist is useful, especially for side-lying positions. A larger pillow will be needed for women if the hips are much wider than the waist, in order to maintain the spine in a neutral position. A large pillow may also be needed under the upper leg, to avoid it dragging on the lumbar spine and causing discomfort.

Encouraging an early return to activity for people with back pain

Aiming to help patients take responsibility and cope with acute back pain, the Royal College of General Practitioners in the UK in conjunction with the Department of Health have produced a booklet called *The Back Book* (Roland, Waddell *et al.* 1996, updated 1999). It is written by a multidisciplinary group of back pain researchers and contains very simple messages. Based on the research evidence for the management of back pain and linked with the UK clinical guidelines (Royal College of General Practitioners 1996) it is designed to be given to patients by general proactitioners and therapists. It has been carefully designed to be easily read and accessible to most of the population. It encourages positive attitudes, and emphasizes the benefits of an early

return to activity. Preliminary surveys of users of this booklet show that they understand the messages and that it can result in a positive shift in attitudes towards back pain (Burton, Waddell *et al.* 1996). Also it has been shown in a randomized controlled trial that it can alter patients' knowledge and beliefs about back pain (Burton, Waddell *et al.* 1999). It is likely to be most effective if it is used as a back-up to oral advice on back care encouraging a return to physical activity. The book also provides advice on how to cope with an acute attack of back pain.

The advice to return to normal activities is probably relevant for conditions other than back pain, including, for example, ankle sprains, knee problems, and shoulder problems. However, of course the clinician will need to provide individual advice depending on the particular condition and the patient's situation. It is important for the clinician to bear in mind that the reported pain is only one factor in the equation predicting outcome. Many other factors are more influential, including psychosocial factors such as attitudes and beliefs, and patient's circumstances, and their environment (Waddell 1987, Burton, Tillotson *et al.* 1994).

Aiming to prevent recurrences – learning to cope

It may be difficult to prevent recurrences. However, disciplined approaches to exercise, physical activity, and sport can help to cut down on recurrences. Learning to cope with recurrences is of fundamental importance. Much of this is about building self-confidence. Longer-term maintenance is very often forgotten, but is important if one aim is to avoid repeated referrals and visits.

Conclusions

Patient education is a key part of the management of musculoskeletal conditions. Its success will depend on how it is delivered, and this requires some thought.

Simple advice that is appropriate to the needs of the individual can make the difference between long-drawn-out periods of treatment with slow recovery, and a quick return to optimal function. One of the main advantages of effective patient education is that a sense of self-efficacy and coping will be achieved. Passive dependency can then be translated into a sense of control and acceptance of responsibility for dealing with the problem.

Acknowledgement

Thanks are due to Kim Burton, Director of the Spinal Research Unit, Huddersfield, for his helpful comment and for providing additional evidence on biomechanical issues.

References

Althoff, I., Brinckmann, P., Frobin, W., Sandover, J., Burton, K. (1992) An improved method of stature measurement for quantitative determination of spinal loading. Application to sitting postures. *Spine*, 17, 682–93.

Anderson, J. (1981). "Low back pain - cause and prevention of long-term handicap (a critical review)." *Int. Rehab. Med.* **3**: 89-93.

Bandura, A. (1982) Self-efficacy mechanism in human agency. *American Psychologist*, 37(2), 122–47.

Becker, M. (1985) Patient adherence to prescribed therapies. *Medical Care*, **23**, 539–55.

Berquist-Ullman, M., Larsson, U. (1977) Acute low back pain in industry. *Acta Orthopaedica Scandinavica (Suppl)*, 170, 1-117.

Brinckmann, P., Frobin, W., Biggemann, M., Tillotson, M., Burton, K. (1998) Quantification of overload injuries to thoracolumbar vertebrae and discs in persons exposed to heavy physical exertions or vibration at the workplace: Part II. Occurrence and magnitude of overload injury in exposed cohorts. *Clinical Biomechanics*, 13(Suppl 2), 1–36.

Burton, K. (1997) Spine update. Back injury and work loss. Biomechanical and psychosocial influences. *Spine*, 22(21), 2575–580.

Burton, A., Tillotson, K., Main, C., Hollis, S. (1994) Psychosocial predictors of outcome in acute and sub-chronic low-back trouble. *Spine*, 20, 722–8.

Burton, A., Waddell, G., Burtt, R., Blair, M. (1996) Patient education material in the management of low back pain in primary care. *Bulletin of Hospitals for Joint Diseases*, 55(3), 138-41.

Burton, K., Symonds, T., Zinzen, E., *et al.* (1997) Is ergonomic intervention alone sufficient to limit musculoskeletal problems in nurses? *Occupational Medicine*, 47, 25–32.

Burton, A. K., Waddell, G., Tillotson, K. M., Summerton, N. (1999) Information and advice to patients with back pain can have a positive effect. A randomized controlled trial of a novel educational booklet in primary care. *Spine*, 24(23), 2484–91.

Carter, J., Birrell, L. (2000) *Occupational health guidelines for the management of low back pain at work – principal recommendations.* Faculty of Occupational Medicine, London.

Chisholm, R. (1991) Guidelines for radiological investigations. *BMJ*, 303, 797–8.

Cohen, J., Goel, V., Frank, J., Bombardier, C., Peloso, Guillemin, F. (1994) Group education interventions for people with low back pain. An overview of the literature. *Spine*, 19, 1214–22.

Coulter, A. (2000) Editorial: Promoting realistic expectations. *Health Expectations*, 3, 159–60.

Daltroy, L. (1993) Doctor–patient communication in rheumatological disorders. *Bailliere's Clinical Rheumatology*, 7(2), 221–39.

Daltroy, L., Katz, J., Liang, M. (1992) Doctor–patient communication and adherence to arthritis treatments. *Arthritis Care and Research*, 5(S19).

diBlasi, Z. and J. Kleinen (2000). Patient-practitioner interactions: A Systematic Review. York, University of York.

Dolce, J. (1987) Self-efficacy and disability beliefs in behavioral treatment of pain. *Behavioural Research and Therapy*, 25, 289–99.

Dolce, J., Crocker, M., Moletierre, C., Doleys, D. (1986) Exercise quotas, anticipatory concern and self-efficacy expectations in chronic pain: a preliminary report. *Pain*, 24, 365–72.

Eklund, J., Corlett, E. (1984) Shrinkage as a measure of load on the spine. *Spine*, 9, 184–94.

Frost, H., Klaber Moffett, J., Moser, J., Fairbank, J. (1995b) Randomised controlled trial for evaluation of fitness programme for patients with chronic low back pain. *BMJ*, 310, 151–4.

Frost, H., Lamb, S., Klaber Moffett, J., Fairbank, J., Moser, J. (1998) A fitness programme for patients with chronic low back pain: 2 year follow-up of a randomised controlled trial. *Pain*, 75, 273–279.

Hadler, N. (1987) Regional musculoskeletal diseases of the low back. Cumulative trauma versus single incident. *Clinics in Orthopaedics and Related Research*, 221, 33–41.

Hadler, N. (1997) Workers with disabling back pain. *New England Journal of Medicine*, 337(5), 341–3.

Hides, J., C. Richardson, et al. (1996). "Multifidus muscle recovery is not automatic after resolution of acute, first episode low back pain." *Spine* **21**: 2763-69.

Hides, J., C. A. Richardson, et al. (1995). *Multifidus inhibition in acute low back pain: recovery is not spontaneous.* MPAA Ninth Biennial Conference Proceedings, Gold Coast Queensland.

HSE (1992) *Manual handling operations regulations. Guidance on regulations.* Health and Safety Executive, Sheffield.

Indahl, A., Halderson, E. H., Holm, S., et al. (1988) Five-year follow-up study of a controlled trial using light mobilisation and an informative approach to low back pain. Spine, 23, 2625–30.

Janz, N., Becker, M. (1984) The health belief model: a decade later. *Health Education Quarterly*, 11, 1–47.

Jensen, M., Turner, J., Romano, J. (1991) Self-efficacy and outcome expectancies: relationship to chronic pain coping strategies and adjustment. *Pain*, 44, 263–9.

Jull, G. and C. Richardson (1994). Rehabilitation of active stabilization of the lumbar spine. *Physical therapy of the low back.* L. Twomey and J. Taylor: 251-273.

Keijsers, J., Bouter, L., Meertens, R. (1991) Validity and comparability of studies on the effects of back schools. *Physiotherapy Theory and Practice*, 7, 177–84.

Klaber Moffett, J. (1989) Backschools. In: Roland, M., Morris, J., editors. *Back Pain. New approaches to rehabilitation and education*: University of Manchester Press, Manchester.

Klaber Moffett, J., Frost, H. (2000) Back to Fitness Programme. The manual for physiotherapists to set up the classes. *Physiotherapy*, 86, 295-305.

Klaber Moffett, J., Richardson, P. (1997) The influence of the physiotherapist–patient relationship on pain and disability. *Physiotherapy Theory and Practice*, 13, 89–96.

Klaber Moffett, J., Torgerson, D., Bell-Syer, S., *et al.* (1999) A randomised trial of exercise for primary care back pain patients: Clinical outcomes, costs and preferences. *BMJ*, **319**, 279–83.

Koes, B., Bouter, L., Van, M. H., Essers, A., *et al.* (1992) Randomised clinical trial of manipulative therapy and physiotherapy for persistent back and neck complaints: Results of one year follow up. *BMJ*, 304, 601–5.

Koes, B., M. van Tulder, et al. (1994). "The efficacy of back schools: a review of randomised clinical trials." *Journal of Clinical Epidemiology* 47: 851-862.

Kores, R., Murphy, W., Rosenthal, T., *et al.* (1990) Predicting outcome of chronic pain treatment via a modified self-efficacy scale. *Behavior Research and Therapy*, 28(2), 165–9.

Leventhal, H., Cameron, L. (1987) Behavioral theories and the problem of compliance. *Patient Education and Counseling*, 10, 117–38.

Leventhal, H. (1985) The role of theory in the study of adherence to treatment and doctor-patient interactions. *Medical Care*, 23, 556–63.

Ley, P. (1988) *Communicating with patients. Improving communication, satisfaction and compliance.* Croom Helm, London.

Linton, S., Kamwendo, K. (1987) Low back schools. A critical review. *Physical Therapy*, 67(9), 1375–383.

Lonn J.H., Glomsrod B., Soukup M.G., Bo K., Larsen S. (1999) Active back school: prophylactic management for low back pain. A randomized, controlled, 1-year follow-up study. *Spine* 24(9):865-71

Lorig, K. (1995) Patient education: treatment or nice extra. *British Journal of Rheumatology*, 34, 703–6.

Lorig, K., Gonzalez, V. (1992) The integration of theory with practice: a 12-year case study. *Health Education Quarterly*, 19(3), 355–68.

Mandal, A. (1985) *The seated man.* Dafnia Publications, Klampenborg.

Mazzuca, S. (1982) Does patient education in chronic disease have therapeutic value? *Journal of Chronic Disability*, 35, 521–9.

McKenzie, R. (1981) *The lumbar spine.* Spinal Publications New Zealand.

Melzack, R., Wall, P. (1982) *The challenge of pain.* Penguin, Harmondsworth.

Nachemson, A. (1960) Lumbar intradiscal pressure. *Acta Orthopaedica Scandinavica Suppl*, 43, 1–93.

Nordin, M. (1995) Back pain: lessons from patient education. *Patient Education and Counseling*, 27, 67–70.

Nordin, M., C. Cedraschi, et al. (1992). "Back schools in prevention of chronicity." *Clinical Rheumatology* 6: 685-703.

O'Leary, A. (1985) Self-efficacy and health. *Behavior Research and Therapy*, **23**(4), 437–51.

Pennebaker, J. (1982) *The psychology of physical symptoms.* Springer-Verlag, New York.

Pennebaker, J. (1984) Accuracy of symptom perception. In: Baum, A., Tayler, S., Singer, J., editors. *Handbook of psychology and health.* Lawrence Erlbaum Associates, New Jersey.

Rodriguez, L., Jick, H. (1994) Risk of upper gastrointestinal bleeding and perforation associated with individual non-steroidal anti-inflammatory drugs. *Lancet*, **343**, 769–72.

Rohlmann, A., Bergmann, G., Graichen, F., Weber, U. (1995) In vivo measurement of implant loads in a patient with a fractured vertebral body. *European Spine Journal*, **4**, 347–53.

Roland, M., Waddell, G., Klaber Moffett, J., Burton, K., Main, C., Cantrell E. (1996) *The back book.* The Stationery Office, London.

Rollnick, S., Heather, N., Bell, A. (1992) Negotiating behaviour change in medical settings: The development of brief motivational interviewing. *Journal of Mental Health*, **1**, 25–37.

Royal College of General Practitioners (1996) *Clinical guidelines for the management of low back pain.* London: Royal College of General Practitioners, London.

Smith, D., Heckemeyer, C., Kratt, P., Mason, D. (1997) Motivational interviewing to improve adherence to a behavioural weight-control program for older obese women with NIDDM. *Diabetes Care*, **20**(1), 52–4.

van Dieen, J., Hoozemans, M., Toussaint, H. (1999) Stoop or squat: a review of biomechanical studies on lifting technique. *Clinical Biomechanics*, **14**, 685–96.

Vlaeyen, J., Linton, S. (2000) Fear-avoidance and its consequences in chronic musculosketal pain: a state of the art. *Pain*, **85**, 317–332.

Waddell, G. (1987) A new clinical model for the treatment of low back pain. *Spine*, **12**(7), 632–44.

Waddell, G. (1998) *The back pain revolution.* Churchill Livingstone, Edinburgh.

Waddell, G., Burton, K. (2000) *Occupational health guidelines for the management of low back pain at work – leaflet for practitioners.* Faculty of Occupational Medicine, London.

Waddell, G., Feder, G., McIntosh, A., Lewis, M., Hutchinson, A. (1996) Low back pain evidence review. Royal College of General Practitioners, London.

Welbergen, E., Kemper, H., Knibbe, J., Toussaint, H., Clijssen, L. (1991) Efficiency and effectiveness of stoop and squat lifting at different techniques. *Ergonomics*, **34**, 613–24.

Wilke, H., Neef, P., Caimi, M., Hoogland, T., Claes, L. (1999) New in vivo measurement of pressures in the intervertebral disc in daily life. *Spine*, **24**, 755–62.

Zachrisson-Forsell, M. (1980) The Swedish back school. *Physiotherapy*, **66**, 112–14.

4.3 Management

4.3.1 Manual treatment of somatic dysfunction

Michael L. Kuchera

The role of manual techniques

The medical history of manipulation dates back to the ancients and is a part of every culture's healing tradition even today. Manipulation under anesthesia of the shoulders (as in adhesive capsulitis) and of the low back (as in specific disk disorders) are part of the current armamentarium of the modern orthopedic surgeon. Likewise, manual reduction of various anatomically displaced somatic structures – fractures, dislocations, and subluxations – are common conservative treatment modalities. The use of manual treatment techniques to improve muscle function and balance, reduce fibrous adhesions or contractures, and relieve pain and joint dysfunction figures strongly in today's physical medicine and rehabilitation strategies. As an internal medicine specialist, Janet Travell pioneered the use of manual and needling techniques to address myofascial pain and dysfunction – even to modify somatovisceral reflex phenomena. In their first 4 years of training, all American-trained osteopathic physicians are taught the diagnostic and manual treatment skills (osteopathic manipulative treatment) to identify and address primary or secondary somatic dysfunction in patients with somatic, somatovisceral, or viscerosomatic complaints.

Worldwide, physician practitioners of musculoskeletal medicine are exploring the optimum role for the use of manual techniques in the conservative management of somatic dysfunction and pain. In the right hands and used for the proper reasons, these techniques can increase patient satisfaction and lead to symptomatic relief. They can remove the underlying somatic component maintaining a significant patient problem with pain or dysfunction. And they can be a significant option in part of a total physician-directed treatment program to enhance health and well-being.

Manual technique alone does not constitute manual medicine. Manual techniques applied to the musculoskeletal system may be delivered by any number of lay people – by coaches or sports trainers, by a variety of therapists in a systematic manner, or even by well-meaning family members. Furthermore, a number of allied health therapists spend a significant portion of their training using their hands applying manual techniques. Manual techniques are applied by therapists as 'massage therapy', or 'physical therapy', or as a specific school of therapy (e.g. Rolfing). Conversely, manual techniques applied by physicians constitute 'manual medicine'. Physicians treat, therapists provide therapy. Physicians incorporate the choice of treatment – manual or otherwise – into a complex algorithm of diagnostic and treatment choices, incorporating differential diagnoses followed by assessment of indications and contraindications (see Chapter 4.4). Physicians employing manual medicine incorporate manual techniques into a larger field of medicine such as 'physical medicine and rehabilitation', 'neuromusculoskeletal medicine', or 'orthopaedic medicine', or, in the case of American osteopathic physicians, incorporate manual diagnostic and treatment techniques as an integral approach throughout primary patient care.

Unfortunately, the proliferation of various practitioners with varying educational backgrounds employing an expanding portfolio of hands-on techniques with variable therapeutic (and less-than-therapeutic) results has been the source of growing confusion. The public has difficulty in differentiating between 'manual medicine' and use of a manual technique by a non-physician. A further complication, beyond physician delivery of a given manual 'maneuver or technique', is the issue of whether the physicians themselves have the training or ability to apply manual techniques within the larger field of medicine, or even the background to recognize somatic dysfunction requiring such treatment. Other than members of the International Federation of Manual/Musculoskeletal Medicine (FIMM) and American-trained osteopathic physicians and surgeons, few fully licensed physicians have adequate training in the palpation of somatic dysfunction; even fewer have skills in effectively delivering manipulative techniques. (FIMM physicians generally receive their manual medicine training after receiving their professional degree; US-trained osteopathic physicians have integrated training throughout both their professional degree program and afterwards.)

In the wrong hands, manipulative techniques can be benignly ineffective; at worst, they could be dangerous, even lethal.[1] In the absence of a well-thought-out treatment plan, manipulative techniques alone are only maneuvers with little likelihood of prolonged benefit. The confusion raises serious implications ranging from standardization of nomenclature to issues dealing with training, licensing, certification, research, reimbursement, and allocation of resources.

Nomenclature issues

Confusion in nomenclature is the easiest area to address. Manipulation is a generic word that in medicine historically denoted the use of 'therapeutic application of manual force.'[2] Different connotations are now associated with this and other 'hands-on' terms. 'Manipulative **treatment**', in contradistinction to 'manual **therapy**', was one attempt to make a semantic distinction between physician-applied 'treatment' rather than a therapist applying a technique. In some circles, 'manipulation' is specifically reserved as a term for a high-velocity, low-amplitude (HVLA) thrust-type technique, but in other circles it remains a generic term for all forms of hands-on therapeutic technique. The chiropractic profession (from the Greek root *chiros*, meaning hand) refers to its manipulative techniques as 'chiropractic adjustments'; not to be confused with the manual medicine techniques performed by German physicians, known as 'chiropraktikers', who incorporate 'chiropraxis'.

Osteopathic physicians in the USA employing 'osteopathic manipulative treatment' (OMT) sought through that specific nomenclature to convey that guiding osteopathic principles and therapeutic goals were a component part of the manual techniques they deliver. The difference between a physical therapist applying a counterstrain technique and an osteopathic physician performing OMT using that same counterstrain technique lay in the physician-level differential diagnosis, weighing of treatment options, and integration of the technique and its outcome with the ongoing plan applied during a patient visit. It is this difference that practitioners of musculoskeletal medicine seek to convey in their management. Throughout this chapter, I will refer to MMMT (musculoskeletal medicine manipulative treatment) in recognition of the physician-level differential diagnosis and therapeutic choice that precedes each MMMT prescription for and delivery of manual techniques.

The musculoskeletal medicine manipulative treatment (MMMT) prescription

The MMMT prescription is best directed by a physician working toward definitive goals. In order to do this properly, a working diagnosis derived from historical, physical, and palpatory findings is essential (see Chapter 3.3). As with any prescription, the physician must select the best therapeutic agent for the situation, must calculate the appropriate dose and frequency for the agent, and must both educate the patient and be prepared to deal with any potential side effects or untoward results.

The MMMT prescription consists of:

- **Setting goals:** What area would benefit from MMMT? What general indications are being addressed and what contraindications need to be avoided? What physiologic or biomechanical end result is desired?

- **Choosing methods:** What form of MMMT is indicated? Is the tissue texture change associated with an underlying physiologic status that is acute, chronic, or mixed? What techniques are most likely to accomplish the goal(s) with the fewest side effects?

- **Determining dose:** How long should each MMMT session last? What is the homeostatic reserve of the patient available to respond to the choice of method?

- **Prognosticating frequency:** How frequently should the MMMT be repeated? When can and should the patient return? When should the patient be re-evaluated?

- **Recognizing potential side-effects or complications:** Are there potential risk factors posed by underlying host factors (age, health status, concomitant pathology, etc.)? Might the technique or its outcome lead or mislead the patient to ignore other important factors in their presenting or ongoing condition?

Common MMMT-related questions and clinical experiences are outlined in Table 4.3.1.

The most commonly used methods are either direct or indirect. In **direct method techniques**, the set-up engages the somatic dysfunction barrier and then the physician applies an activating force that moves through the barrier to re-establish motion. In **indirect method techniques**, the set-up requires the physician to move away from the barrier to a specific site ('balance point') where various physiologic or inherent mechanisms cause the somatic dysfunction barrier to dissipate.

The **exaggeration method** is essentially an exaggerated indirect method wherein the set-up moves in the direction of freedom, past the balance point, to the normal physiologic barrier opposite the motion loss barrier. At this point, an activating force is applied. The exaggeration method is rarely used in some systems of manual medicine while in others, activating forces (typically thrust) are provided only in the direction of pain-free motion.

Physiologic response method techniques depend upon careful patient positioning and movement to obtain a therapeutic result. The lumbosacral junction, for example, may be positioned to limit physiologic motion of the sacrum to a single desired response. Motion induced actively or passively would then cause the sacrum to move in the specific direction needed to restore its normal motion characteristics.

Sometimes a single technique incorporates more than one of the methods above. For example, the technique may start by loading the tissues with the restrictive barrier being engaged in the manner of a direct method technique but then the regional soft tissues are moved to maintain the indirect balance point. Thus the description of this form of myofascial release (MFR) technique, also called 'myofascial unwinding' because of its appearance, best fits a **combined method technique** classification. Combined methods techniques include integrated neuromusculoskeletal release and myofascial release techniques[5] as well as Still technique.[6]

Activating forces include:

- HVLA or thrust[7]

- low-velocity, moderate-amplitude (springing or articulation)[8]

- various applications of patient-assisted muscle energy (especially isometric resistance or rhythmic resistive duction)[9]

- respiratory cooperation or force (inhalation causing spinal curves to straighten and extremities to externally rotate; exhalation causing spinal curves to accentuate and extremities to internally rotate)

- inherent forces or the body's tendency toward balance and homeostasis (certain positioning seems to enhance inherent activities associated with normal breathing, vascular pulsations, proprioceptive resetting, central response to reduction of afferent load, enhancement of lymphatic return, and other homeostatic mechanisms to dissipate barriers to functional motion)

Table 4.3.1. Clinical experiences modifying musculoskeletal medicine manipulative treatment

Question or option	Clinical experience (generalities and guidelines only)
Selection of direct or indirect method	Indirect or direct techniques are of no value to a physician who lacks the skill to use that technique[3]
	Indirect techniques may be especially helpful in somatic dysfunction manifesting acute, edematous tissue texture changes
	Direct techniques may be especially helpful in somatic dysfunction with chronic changes such as fibrosis
How much force should be used in an HVLA thrust?	'. . . enough to affect a physiologic response (increased joint mobility, produce a vasomotor flush, produce palpable circulatory changes in periarticular tissues, and/or provide pain relief) but not enough to overwhelm the patient.'[4]
Parameters modifying dose or frequency in the MMMT?[3]	The sicker the patient the less the dose
	Pediatric patients can be treated more frequently
	Geriatric patients require a longer interval between treatments to respond
	Acute cases should have a shorter interval between treatments initially
General guidelines for treatment order based upon regional affects?	In the chest cage, generally treat somatic dysfunction in this order: thoracic vertebrae, ribs, sternum
	In the pelvis, generally treat 'nonphysiologic' somatic dysfunctions (shears) before other dysfunctions
	For **very** acute somatic dysfunction, it may be necessary to treat secondary or peripheral areas first to allow access to the acute site
	In lymphatic goals, open fascial drainage pathways before enhancing the effects of diaphragmatic or augmented lymphatic pumps; local effleurage or other local tissue drainage is best done after other lymphatic techniques designed to achieve tissue drainage
What side-effects alert the clinician to modify the MMMT?	If the patient reports a flare-up of discomfort for more than 24 hours, modify the dosage, choice of activating method, and/or duration of treatment as needed
	In set-up and activating phases, it is best to avoid certain positions that aggravate otherwise intermittent radiculopathic signs (cervical or lumbar spine) in patients with spinal DJD or herniated nucleus pulposus
	Care must be paramount if HVLA is selected in a patient suspected to harbor significant osteoporosis; often forward bending pressures should be avoided as well
Guidelines: how long to treat?	Caring, compassionate novices often err on the side of overdosage
	Chronic conditions usually require chronic treatment; one rule of thumb suggests that it may take as many treatment sessions as years of dysfunction
Risk-to-benefit issues	An appropriate assessment and diagnostic examination before, during, and after an MMMT permits accurate risk-to-benefit decision-making regarding indications, relative contraindications, and absolute contraindications
	Manipulative treatment is among the safest treatments that a physician can administer (serious adverse response report 1 : 400 000 to 1 : 1 000 000)[1]

DJD = degenerative joint disease, HVLA = high velocity, low amplitude (thrust) manipulation.

- patient cooperative reflex activities (including eye movements and activation of other specific muscles in specific directions and/or at a specific time).

As with methods, a combination of activating forces may be more effective than repeated use of a single activating force. For example, in a direct method upper cervical technique using combined activating forces, the somatic dysfunction restrictive barrier should be optimally engaged. The initial activating force may be a request for one to three 3-second isometric muscle energy activations in a direction away from the barrier, with the physician carefully re-engaging the 'new' barrier site after each muscle energy activation. Combining forces simultaneously by having the patient look in the same direction that they are pushing engages oculocervical reflex connections to the small suboccipital muscles. Immediately after the last relaxation of muscle energy, the physician may apply an HVLA through any remaining barrier. Approaching the same evolving barrier with a single technique employing this combination of activating forces may be more effective (and certainly more time efficient) than attempting three separate direct-method techniques with three separate activating forces.

Selection of methods and activating forces to accomplish specific physiologic goals often depends on whether the tissue texture changes reflect acute, chronic, or mixed pathophysiologic findings. Such tissue texture changes influence the underlying viscoelastic properties of tissues and seem to affect the postulated mechanisms of action in manual medicine approaches, including tissue decongestion, viscoelastic creep, muscle guarding, central neurologic gate phenomena, etc.

In addition to the choice of method and activating force, the dose and frequency used in an MMMT prescription are also often determined by the host and their underlying constellation of pathophysiologic changes. Key considerations include the age and health status of the patient, individual homeostatic reserve, accompanying systemic or regional rheumatologic or vascular pathophysiology, and prior response to particular MMMT methods or activating forces. The most common response to a less-than-optimal choice of method, activating force, or dose is a flare-up of muscle soreness or whatever symptoms brought the patient to the office. Although this is the most common side effect of an MMMT, it is usually a minor annoyance to the patient and, in capable hands, not a frequent occurrence. A flare-up is never desirable, and any flare-up lasting more than 24 hours probably warrants reconsideration of the MMMT prescription. Usually modifications of the activating force, method, and/or dose during the next visit eliminate the problem.

Finally, one other major variable plays into the ability to deliver an appropriate MMMT prescription – the physician. The ability of a physician to effectively and efficiently accomplish the treatment procedures includes:

- personal stature, strength, and sense of balance
- palpatory ability to sense subtle tissue texture, symmetry, and motion changes in tissues before, during, and after treatment
- training level and mastery of a variety of techniques, methods, and activating forces
- knowledge of functional anatomy, physiology, and pathophysiology
- level of experience in problem-solving situations involving patients with primary and compensatory somatic dysfunction.

Other issues

The discussion of other issues identified in the introduction to this chapter – training, licensing, certification, research, reimbursement, and allocation of resources – is beyond the scope of this chapter. Throughout this chapter, the use of MMMT and discussion of manipulative techniques are presented in the context of their use by fully trained, fully licensed physicians and/or surgeons. MMMT integration with musculoskeletal medicine management approaches will represent, whenever possible, peer consensus of specialists, research evidence, and/or cost-effective perspectives.

Musculoskeletal medicine manipulative treatment (MMMT) techniques

The bulk of this section consists of individual MMMT techniques which must be applied within the context of a larger physician-level field of knowledge such as musculoskeletal medicine, neuromusculoskeletal medicine, orthopedic medicine, osteopathic medicine, physical medicine, rehabilitation medicine, orthopedic surgery, family practice, etc. The techniques below are not meant to be all-inclusive; rather, each is illustrative of manual medicine applications employing various combinations of technique methods and activating forces in different regions with the patient in different positions. Unless otherwise noted, all illustrations used in this Chapter have been selected from the text by Kimberly and Funk[10] or by Nicholas.[11]

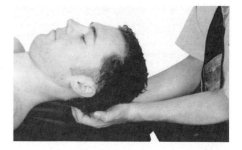

Figure 4.3.1 Basilar decompression technique (direct method).[11]

Head region

Basilar decompression technique (direct method)

Diagnosis: Occipitoatlantal backward bending somatic dysfunction with compression of the occipital condyles. Tension is palpated at the base of the skull. There is freedom of backward bending of the occiput upon the atlas with restriction to forward bending.
Patient position: Supine.
Operator position: Seated at head of table/bed.
Contact: Middle fingers placed at base of skull (occiput) pointed anteromedial in line with the occipital condyles (Figure 4.3.1).
Position to initiate technique: Patient is asked to draw chin toward chest as the operator's fingers are drawn posterolateral to hold the point of tissue tension.
Activation: Operator brings wrists together, pulling occipital condyles posterolateral in the direction of the facet motion allowed. As the tissues soften, slack is gradually taken up drawing the head further into forward bending on the neck.

Temporomandibular joint (TMJ) muscle energy technique

Diagnosis: Left TMJ restricted; jaw deviates to the left when opened.
Patient position: Supine.
Operator position: At head of table/bed.
Contact: Operator's right hand supports right side of patient's head. Left hand contacts left mandible (Figure 4.3.2).
Position to initiate technique: Patient instructed to open mouth until mandible first begins to deviate to the left. Operator's left hand applies pressure to the right until the dysfunctional barrier is reached.

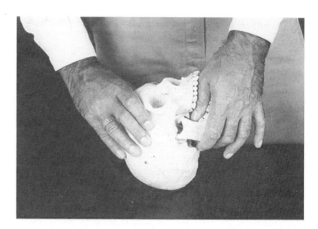

Figure 4.3.2 TMJ muscle energy technique.[11]

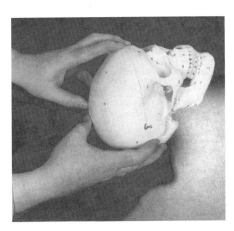

Figure 4.3.3 OM sutural V-spread technique.[11]

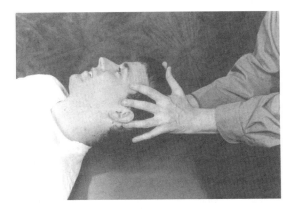

Figure 4.3.4 SBS indirect technique (e.g. right SBS torsion).[11]

Activation: Patient is instructed to gently push the chin for approximately 3 seconds to the left against isometric pressure from the operator's hand and then relax. During relaxation phase, a new barrier is engaged by removing slack by increasing pressure to the right. Repeat three times.

Follow-up: Re-evaluate S.T.A.R. characteristics (se Chapter 2.2.1). Instruct avoidance of repetitive asymmetrical chewing activities (gum).

Occipitomastoid (OM) sutural V-spread technique

Diagnosis: Tenderness and bogginess over OM suture on the right.
Patient position: Supine.
Operator position: At head of table/bed.
Contact: Operator's right index and middle finger pads on opposite sides of OM suture at site of maximum tenderness and tissue texture change. Left index and middle finger pads resting gently over left frontal eminence (Figure 4.3.3).
Activation: Right finger pads create tension across suture site by operator attempting to spread index and middle fingers apart into a 'V', left fingers place 5 g pressure in synchrony with extension phase of the cranial mechanism. Tension maintained on left and rhythmic pressure on left until right side releases.
Follow-up: Recheck S.T.A.R. characteristics.

Sphenobasilar synchondrosis (SBS) indirect technique (e.g. right SBS torsion)

Diagnosis: SBS prefers right torsion and is restricted in left torsion.
Patient position: Supine.
Operator position: Seated at head of table/bed.
Contact: Vault hold with index finger pads bilaterally over greater wings of sphenoid; middle and ring fingers straddling the ear with respective volar MCPs over the squamous portion of the temporal bones; pads of the fifth digit over the squamous occiput (Figure 4.3.4).
Position to initiate technique: Right index and left fifth digits drawn superiorly; left index and right fifth digits drawn inferiorly to point of balanced dural tension.
Activation: Patient instructed to hold respiration in inhalation or exhalation (whichever provides greatest tension release) as long as possible with continuous minor adjustment of hands to maintain balance point as release is accomplished.
Follow-up: Recheck asymmetry and motion characteristics.

Sphenopalatine ganglion (lateral pterygoid) pressure technique

Diagnosis: tension and tenderness over left lateral pterygoid muscle; excessive maxillary sinus secretion.
Patient position: Seated.
Operator position: Standing, facing patient.
Contact: Operator's gloved or sheathed right fifth digit is passed along the outside of the patient's gum line, beyond the last molar, and tipped superior, posterior, and medial to contact the left lateral pterygoid muscle (Figure 4.3.5).
Activation: Patient tips head to the left against the operator's fingertip for 2–3 seconds. This procedure is repeated three times.
Follow-up: Observe for unilateral lacrimation indicative of parasympathetic stimulation and then repeat on opposite side.

Frontal lift

Diagnosis: Restricted motion of the frontal bone; dural imbalance; ethmoidal–frontal restriction.
Patient position: Supine.
Operator position: Seated, at head of patient.
Contact: Operator's index fingers are placed at glabella with thumbs placed in the midline immediately anterior to the coronal suture; middle fingers hook around the orbital process of the frontal bone (at the edge of the brow) (Figure 4.3.6).
Position to initiate technique: Operator lightly compresses middle fingers medially to disengage the frontals from the parietals.
Activation: Lift the frontal bone anteriorly (toward the ceiling) and seek balanced membranous tension.
Follow-up: Recheck overall motion characteristics with frontal and vault holds.

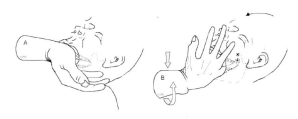

Figure 4.3.5 Sphenopalatine ganglion (lateral pterygoid) pressure technique.

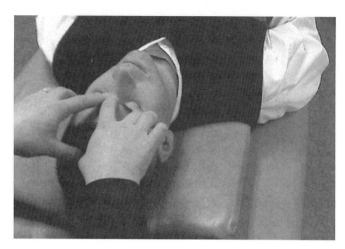

Figure 4.3.6 Frontal lift.[11]

'CV 4'

Diagnosis: Low amplitude or asymmetrical cranial rhythmic impulse (CRI). Used also for homeostatic enhancement.
Patient position: Supine.
Operator position: Seated at head of table/bed.
Contact: Operator's hands are gently overlapped to place thenar eminences over the squamous occiput bilaterally immediately medial to each mastoid process (Figure 4.3.7).
Position to initiate technique: Gentle pressure from each thenar eminence triangulating the anatomic location of the fourth ventricle.
Activation: Compression dampening cranial rhythmic impulse continues until a 'still point' is reached; increased warmth is often felt and the patient will often express a sigh at this point. Pressure is then released.
Follow-up: Reassess the CRI; specifically rule out iatrogenic introduction of cranial extension somatic dysfunction.

Craniocervical junction and cervical region

Superior cervical segment

OA muscle energy with oculocervical reflex muscle energy activation

Diagnosis: OA sidebending left, rotation right.
Patient position: Supine.
Operator position: Seated at head of table.
Contact: One hand forms a 'V' with the thumb and index finger of one hand and supports the posterior arch and lateral masses. Use other hand to control the head (Figure 4.3.8).
Position to initiate technique: Adjust flexion/extension to localize at the dysfunctional segment; induce right sidebending and left rotation of the occiput to engage the restrictive barrier and provide counterforce.
Activation: Activate the oculocervical reflex by instructing the patient to look to the right while the physician offers isometric counterforce for 3–5 seconds. The patient ceases the directed gaze force and the operator simultaneously ceases the counterforce.
Follow-up: Operator waits for tissue relaxation and then moves the head to the new restrictive barrier (all three planes) repeating activation and follow-up until normal motion is returned (average three times).

OA indirect method with respiratory cooperation

Diagnosis: OA sidebending left, rotation right.
Patient position: Supine.
Operator position: Seated at head of table.
Contact: Hand resting on the table forms a 'V' with the thumb and index finger supporting the posterior arch and lateral masses. Use other hand to control the head (Figure 4.3.9).
Position to initiate technique: Using the head, sidebend the OA joint to the left and rotate it to the right to the point of balanced ligamentous tension. Minor adjustments of flexion or extension may be needed.
Activation: Test respiratory phases and instruct patient to breath-hold as long as possible in the phase that provides the best ligamentous balance. Make minor adjustments in all three planes as needed to maintain ligamentous balance.
Follow-up: Repeat activating step as needed until the best motion is obtained.

OA HVLA

Diagnosis: OA sidebending left, rotation right.
Patient position: Supine.
Operator position: Standing at head of table.
Contact: Right hand contacts patient's right posterior occiput posterior to, but not on, the mastoid process. Physician's left hand cradles the head (Figure 4.3.10).
Position to initiate technique: Sidebend the occiput to the right on the atlas, adjust flexion or extension and rotate it to the left to localize at the restrictive barrier.
Activation: A HVLA left sidebending thrust is applied, directed medially, anteriorly and superiorly (towards opposite eye).
Follow-up: Recheck motion characteristics.

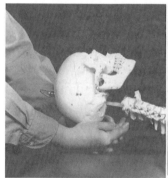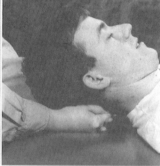

Figure 4.3.7 'CV 4'.[11]

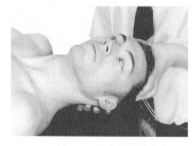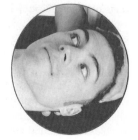

Figure 4.3.8 OA muscle energy with oculocervical reflex muscle energy activation ($S_L R_R$).[10]

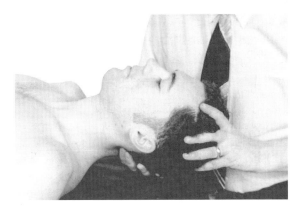

Figure 4.3.9 OA indirect method with respiratory cooperation (e.g. S$_L$R$_R$).[10]

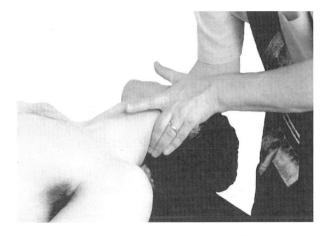

Figure 4.3.11 AA muscle energy (e.g. AA rotated left).[10]

Atlantoaxial muscle energy

Diagnosis: AA left rotation.

Patient position: Supine.

Operator position: Standing at head of table.

Contact: Place palms on each side of the patient's head and contact both lateral masses of the atlas with the lateral margin of the index or middle fingers (Figure 4.3.11).

Position to initiate technique: Extend head minimally over contact fingers and rotate the atlas to the restrictive barrier.

Activation: Patient is instructed to turn the head to the left while the physician offers isometric counterforce for 3–5 seconds sensing that the patient's contractile force is localized at the AA joint.

Follow-up: After the patient ceases the directive force and the operator simultaneously ceases the counterforce and moves the head and atlas to the new restrictive barrier, repeating until the best motion is obtained (average three times).

AA indirect method with respiratory cooperation

Diagnosis: AA left rotation.

Patient position: Supine.

Operator position: Seated at head of table.

Contact: Cradle the patient's head in both palms and contact both lateral masses of the atlas with the fingertips (Figure 4.3.12).

Position to initiate technique: Rotate the atlas to the left to the point of balanced ligamentous tension (slight adjustments of sidebending and flexion or extension may be needed).

Activation: Test respiratory phases and instruct to hold breath as long as possible in the phase that provides the best ligamentous balance (make minor adjustments in all three planes as needed to maintain ligamentous balance).

Follow-up: Recheck and repeat as needed to achieve optimal motion.

Lower cervical segment

Typical cervical HVLA (rotation activation)

Diagnosis: C2–3 extension rotation left, sidebending left.

Patient position: Supine.

Operator position: Standing at head of table.

Contact: Support head with wrists/forearms while contacting both articular pillars of the dysfunctional vertebra with the index fingers (Figure 4.3.13).

Position to initiate technique: Flex head/neck until motion is localized at the dysfunctional segment. Operator maintains flexion at the dysfunctional segment and extends the vertebral segments above. (This isolates the dysfunctional segment to enable rotation while the fingers act as fulcrums.) Sidebend the neck slightly to the left to lock the vertebrae above the dysfunction; then rotate the neck to the right to the restrictive barrier.

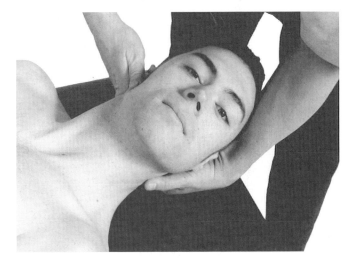

Figure 4.3.10 OA HVLA (e.g. S$_L$R$_R$).[10]

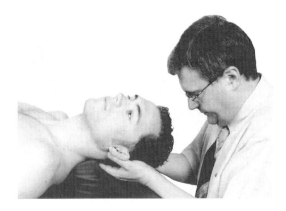

Figure 4.3.12 AA indirect method with respiratory cooperation.[10]

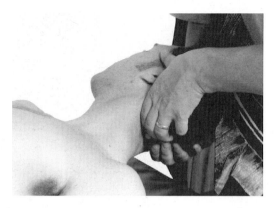

Figure 4.3.13 Typical cervical HVLA rotation activation (e.g. C2 ER$_L$S$_L$).[10]

Activation: HVLA rotational thrust is applied through both hands with the force directed along the plane of the facets. (Note: Rotation in the typical cervical spine is automatically accompanied by sidebending to the same side; therefore, correction of the sidebending component automatically occurs at the localized segment when the rotational thrust is applied.)

Follow-up: Recheck motion characteristics; if no improvement, then consider a sidebending activation alternative.

Typical cervical HVLA (sidebending activation)

Diagnosis: C4–5 neutral rotation left, sidebending left.
Patient position: Supine.
Operator position: Standing at head of table.
Contact: Support the head with wrist/forearm while contacting the articular pillars of the dysfunctional vertebra with the lateral margin of the index fingers (Figure 4.3.14).
Position to initiate technique: Lift the head to flex the neck and sidebend the neck to the right to the restrictive barrier. Then rotate the neck to the left to lock the vertebrae above the dysfunction. (Adjust flexion or extension within the neutral range as needed to localize all three planes at the dysfunctional segment.)
Activation: A HVLA sidebending thrust is applied to the articular pillar. (Note: Sidebending in the typical cervical spine is automatically accompanied by rotation to the same side; therefore, correction of the rotational component automatically occurs at the localized segment when the sidebending thrust is applied.)

Follow-up: Recheck motion characteristics; if no improvement consider rotational activation alternative.

Typical cervical muscle energy

Diagnosis: C3 neutral rotation left, sidebending left.
Patient position: Supine.
Operator position: Seated at head of table.
Contact: Sidebending is introduced at the dysfunctional segment using one of the following:

- Reach under the cervical spine to contact the right side of the articular column with the finger pads. Pull the cervical spine toward the left, inducing right sidebending to the restrictive barrier; **or**

- Place the pad of the thumb on the lateral margin of the right articular pillar of the dysfunctional vertebra. Push the articular column to the left, inducing right sidebending to the restrictive barrier.

Position to initiate technique: In addition to sidebending right, rotate right and flex or extend the neck as needed to localize to the dysfunctional segment; other hand grasps the head for counterforce (Figure 4.3.15).
Activation: Instruct to gently rotate left or sidebend left down to that vertebral unit for 3–5 seconds. Then cease the directive force and simultaneously cease counterforce.
Follow-up: Sidebend, rotate, and adjust the sagittal plane to the new barrier, repeating activating force until best motion is obtained (average three times).

Typical cervical counterstrain

Diagnosis: Tender right AC4 (anterior lateral mass of C4).
Patient position: Supine.
Operator position: Seated at head of table.
Contact: Right finger over tender AC4 site; left hand cupping and controlling the posterior aspect of the skull (Figure 4.3.16).
Position to initiate technique: Flex the patient's neck to the level of the tender point. Sidebend and rotate the patient's neck away (left, in this example) until the patient expresses at least 70% reduction of tenderness to pressure palpation.

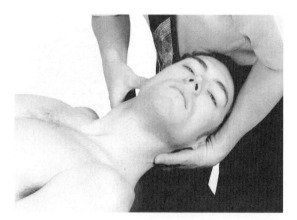

Figure 4.3.14 Typical cervical HVLA sidebending activation (e.g. C4 NR$_L$S$_L$).[10]

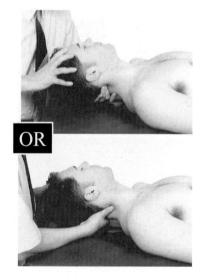

Figure 4.3.15 Typical cervical muscle energy (e.g. C3 NR$_L$S$_L$).[10]

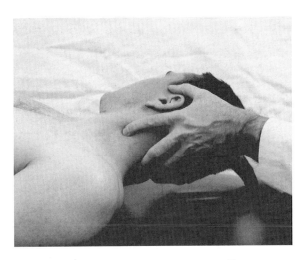

Figure 4.3.16 Typical cervical counterstrain (e.g. AC4).[11]

Activation: Hold position for 90 seconds and slowly return the head and neck to the neutral position.

Follow-up: Confirm at least 70% reduction to pressure palpation in the neutral position.

Typical cervical indirect method with respiratory cooperation

Diagnosis: C3 neutral rotation left, sidebending left.

Patient position: Supine.

Operator position: Seated at head of table.

Contact: Support the head with palms, wrists, or forearms; contact the articular pillars bilaterally with the index fingers (Figure 4.3.17).

Position to initiate technique: Sidebend neck left, rotate it left and flex/extend as needed to balance ligamentous tension in all three planes at the dysfunctional segment.

Activation: Test respiratory phases and instruct to hold breath as long as possible in the phase that provides the best ligamentous balance. (Make minor adjustments in all three planes as needed to maintain ligamentous balance.) Await tissue release.

Follow-up: Recheck motion for success.

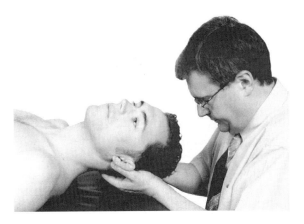

Figure 4.3.17 Typical cervical indirect method with respiratory cooperation (e.g. C3 NR$_L$S$_L$).[10]

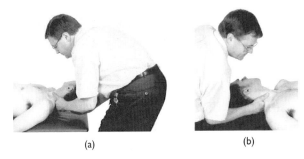

(a)   (b)

Figure 4.3.18 Superior thoracic inlet HVLA (two-step technique S$_R$R$_R$)[10]: (a) sidebending component; (b) rotation component.

Cervicothoracic junction and upper thoracic cage

Cervicothoracic junction, superior thoracic inlet

Superior thoracic inlet HVLA (two-step technique)

Diagnosis: Thoracic inlet sidebent and rotated right.

Patient position: Supine.

Operator position: Standing at head of table (Figure 4.3.18).

Step 1 Contact (sidebending component): Cradle patient's head with the right palm and place the web between the left thumb and index finger on the soft tissues at the cervical–thoracic junction (as a fulcrum).

Step 1 Position to initiate technique: Sidebend the neck and thoracic inlet over the fulcrum to the fascia's restrictive barrier while rotating the head and neck in the opposite direction to lock the cervical spine. Add flexion or extension to localize to the restrictive barrier.

Step 1 Activation: HVLA thrust is applied through the left hand inferiorly and slightly medial.

Step 2 Contact (rotation component): Transfer support of the patient's head to the left hand placing the web between the right thumb and index finger over the soft tissues at the cervical–thoracic junction.

Step 2 Positioning: Rotate the neck and thoracic inlet to the left to engage the fascial restrictive barrier; sidebend the head and neck to the right to lock the cervical spine adding flexion or extension to localize to the restrictive barrier.

Step 2 Activation: HVLA thrust is applied through the right hand carrying the thoracic inlet in a rotational direction anteriorly and medial (the left hand on the head maintains tissue tension only as the region is rotated).

Superior thoracic inlet indirect technique with respiratory cooperation.

Diagnosis: Thoracic inlet sidebent and rotated right.

Patient position: Supine.

Operator position: Seated at head of table.

Contact: Place hands over the thoracic inlet with fingers spread over the anterior thorax and thumbs over the posterior thorax (Figure 4.3.19).

Position to initiate technique: Carry the thoracic inlet region into right rotation and right sidebending (with left translation); add flexion or extension until all three planes are at ligamentous balance.

Activation: Test respiratory phases and instruct the patient to hold breath as long as possible in the phase that provides the best ligamentous balance until maximal tissue response has been obtained. Follow tissue release.

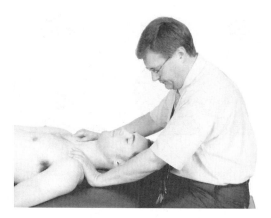

Figure 4.3.19 Superior thoracic inlet indirect technique with respiratory cooperation (e.g. inlet S_RR_R).[10]

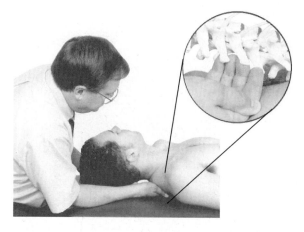

Figure 4.3.21 Upper thoracic muscle energy (e.g. T3 N S_LR_R).[10]

Thoracic spine T1–4

Upper thoracic HVLA

Diagnosis: T2 flexed, sidebent left, rotated right.

Patient position: Supine with elbows together.

Operator position: Standing on the patient's left side.

Contact: Contact the right transverse process of the dysfunctional segment with the left thenar prominence near the proximal phalanx of the thumb (Figure 4.3.20).

Position to initiate technique: Sidebend right down to the restrictive barrier and lift the head with the left hand (or ask patient to lift their own head) until pressure accumulates at the operator's left hand.

Activation: HVLA thrust is applied through the patient's elbows into the operator's hand to induce vertebral rotation to the left.

Upper thoracic muscle energy

Diagnosis: T3 neutral, sidebent left, rotated right.

Patient position: Supine.

Operator position: Seated at head of table.

Contact: Place the pad of a finger of the right hand on the left side of the spinous process of the dysfunctional segment to monitor and to induce left rotation and extension (Figure 4.3.21).

Position to initiate technique: Left hand is placed on patient's head and upper neck so that the neck can be moved into left rotation and right sidebending down to the dysfunctional segment.

Activation: Patient is instructed to push their head to the left against an isometric counterforce for 3–5 seconds.

Follow-up: After the patient and operator cease mutual isometric counterforces, the segment is sidebent right and rotated left to engage the new restrictive barrier. Slight flexion or extension adjustment may also be required. Repeat 2–3 times.

Upper thoracic indirect with respiratory cooperation

Diagnosis: T3 neutral, sidebent left, rotated right.

Patient position: Supine (Note: This technique is especially useful in acute traumatic situations and can also be performed in the seated position. The technique can also be used with the patient supine and the patient's head supported beyond the end of the table if additional extension is required.)

Operator position: Seated at head of table.

Contact: Support the head with left hand and reach under the neck to place the pad of the right index or middle finger on the left transverse process of the dysfunctional segment (Figure 4.3.22).

Position to initiate technique: Position in flexion or extension, as needed, as well as right rotation and left sidebending to the point of balanced ligamentous tension.

Activation: Test respiratory phases and instruct to hold breath as long as possible in the phase that provides the best ligamentous balance. Make minor adjustments in all three planes, as needed, to maintain ligamentous balance.

Upper thoracic counterstrain

Diagnosis: Right posterior third thoracic (PT3) – tenderness over T3 spinous process or right transverse process of T3.

Patient position: Prone.

Operator position: Standing on same side as tender point with knee on table to support the patient's right shoulder.

Contact: Right finger monitoring most tender point (Figure 4.3.23).

Position to initiate technique: Extend, rotate away, and sidebend slightly away from the tender point until patient expresses at least a 70% reduction of tenderness in pressure palpation.

Activation: Hold the position for 90 seconds and then slowly return the patient to the neutral position.

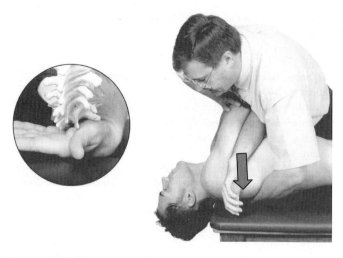

Figure 4.3.20 Upper thoracic HVLA (e.g. T2 $N_FS_LR_R$).[10]

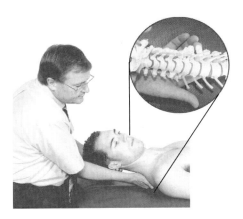

Figure 4.3.22 Upper thoracic indirect with respiratory cooperation (e.g. T3 N S$_L$R$_R$).[10]

Follow-up: Reconfirm at least a 70% reduction in tenderness to pressure palpation.

Rib cage R1–2

Rib 1: HVLA

Diagnosis: Right first rib elevated posteriorly.
Patient position: Seated (may be modified for supine).
Operator position: Standing behind patient.
Contact: Physician contacts the superior part of the posterior surface of the right first rib with the metacarpophalangeal joint of his/her index finger. The elbow is elevated and directed inferiorly toward the dysfunctional rib. The elbow of the other hand rests on the patient's shoulder and the hand controls head motion (Figure 4.3.24).
Position to initiate technique: Move neck into sidebending toward and rotation away from the dysfunctional rib. Tension is increased with both hands until the rib is carried to the restrictive barrier.
Activation: A HVLA thrust is applied to the rib inferiorly, anteriorly and medially to the rib (in a direction toward the opposite nipple).

Rib 1: Patient cooperation muscle energy with respiratory cooperation

Diagnosis: Bilaterally elevated first ribs (may be modified for unilateral elevation).
Patient position: Supine.
Operator position: Seated at head of table.
Contact: Operator contacts the posterior margins of both first ribs with thumbs in front of the trapezius and the pad of the index finger

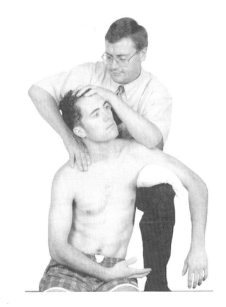

Figure 4.3.24 HVLA (elevated right first rib).[10]

over the anterior end of the first rib near the sternoclavicular joints (Figure 4.3.25).
Position to initiate technique: To modify for unilateral elevated first rib, sidebend patient's neck toward the involved rib (to remove scalene pull) and rotate head away from involved rib (to free costovertebral articulation).
Activation: Patient is instructed to shrug shoulder(s) towards ears while inhaling as operator maintains firm caudad pressure. The patient exhales and relaxes shoulders as the operator follows the ribs caudally. Repeat three times.

Thoracic cage

Thoracic spine T4–12

Mid–lower thoracic: HVLA

Diagnosis: T7 neutral, sidebending left, rotation right.
Patient position: Supine.
Operator position: Stand on the side opposite the rotation (for this diagnosis, on patient's left side).

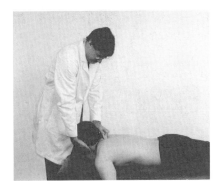

Figure 4.3.23 Upper thoracic counterstrain (e.g. PT3).[11]

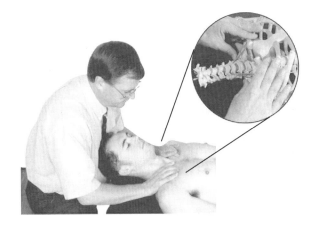

Figure 4.3.25 Rib 1: patient cooperation muscle energy with respiratory cooperation.[10]

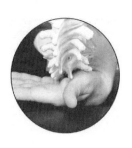
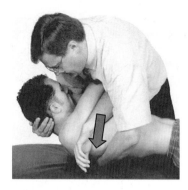

Figure 4.3.26 Mid–lower thoracic: HVLA (e.g. T7 N S$_L$R$_R$).[10]

Contact: Patient crosses arms across the chest with the opposite arm on top. (For this diagnosis the right arm is on top.) Operator's right hand lifts and rolls the patient forward placing the left thenar eminence (as a fulcrum) posterior to the right transverse process and articular facets of the dysfunctional segment. Fingers are extended over the left paraspinal region. Patient is rolled back on to the table, resting on the fulcrum (Figure 4.3.26).

Position to initiate technique: Patient's elbows are placed in the operator's epigastric region (or on the sternum or in the left axilla). The spine is extended at the level of the dysfunction while maintaining flexion above. Sidebend right to engage the restrictive barrier. Transfer tension through the patient's elbows into the fulcrum hand while maintaining localization of extension, right sidebending, and left rotation at the dysfunctional segment.

Activation: A HVLA thrust is applied through the patient's elbows into the fulcrum. This will result in left rotation, right sidebending, and extension of the dysfunctional unit.

Mid–lower thoracic: HVLA

Diagnosis: T7 extended (non-neutral), rotation and sidebending left.
Patient position: Supine.
Operator position: Stand on the side opposite the rotation (patient's right side, in this example).
Contact: Patient crosses arms across the chest with the opposite arm on top. (For this diagnosis the left arm is on top.) Operator's uses the left hand to grasp patient's left shoulder and rolls the patient into flexion to place the right thenar eminence posterior to the left transverse process and articular facets of the dysfunctional segment. Extended fingers are laid across the spine to the patient's right paraspinal region (Figure 4.3.27).

Position to initiate technique: Patient's elbows are placed in the operator's epigastric region (or on the sternum or in the left axilla). The patient is rolled back on to the table until flexion is localized at the dysfunctional unit. Flexion is maintained while the head and neck are used to introduce right sidebending down to the dysfunctional segment. The operator's body weight is applied through the epigastrium, sternum, or axilla to induce right rotation into the restrictive barrier.

Activation: A HVLA thrust is applied posterosuperiorly through the patient's elbows into the fulcrum at approximately a 45–60° angle to the table.

Mid–lower thoracic: muscle energy

Diagnosis: T11 neutral, sidebending left, rotation right.
Patient position: Seated on table.
Operator position: Standing behind patient.
Contact: Patient places right hand behind head or neck and grasps the elbow with the other hand. Operator reaches under patient's left arm across the chest grasping the right shoulder. The operator's right thumb is placed over the right transverse process of the dysfunctional segment (Figure 4.3.28).

Position to initiate technique: The thoracic spine is flexed or extended within the neutral range, as needed, to localize the sagittal plane. The patient is then sidebent right and rotated left until the restrictive barrier is engaged in all three planes.

Activation: Patient is instructed to turn to the right and/or sidebend to the left while the operator offers isometric resistance. The operator has the patient maintain the force long enough to sense that the patient's contractile force is localized at the dysfunctional segment (typically 3–5 seconds).

Follow-up: After simultaneously discontinuing isometric counter-forces, the operator waits for the tissues to relax completely (about 2 seconds) and then moves the dysfunctional segment to the new restrictive barrier. Activation and follow-up are repeated until best motion is obtained (average three times).

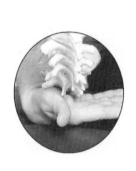
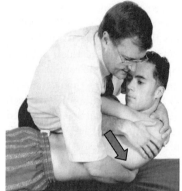

Figure 4.3.27 Mid–lower thoracic: HVLA (e.g. T7 E R$_L$S$_L$).[10]

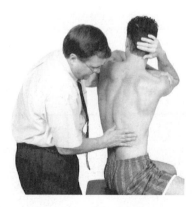

Figure 4.3.28 Mid–lower thoracic: muscle energy (e.g. T11 N S$_L$R$_R$).[10]

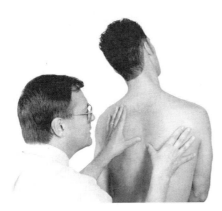

Figure 4.3.29 Mid–lower thoracic: indirect with respiratory cooperation (e.g. T6 N S$_L$R$_R$).[10]

Mid–lower thoracic: indirect with respiratory cooperation

Diagnosis: T6 neutral, sidebending left, rotation right.
Patient position: Seated.
Operator position: Seated or standing behind patient.
Contact: Right thumb contacts the right transverse process of the lower vertebra of the dysfunctional unit; left thumb contacts the left transverse process of the upper vertebra of the dysfunctional unit (Figure 4.3.29).
Position to initiate technique: Patient leans backward at the hips to establish firm contact, then sits up straighter or slouches forward slightly to localize the sagittal plane at the dysfunctional unit. The patient is instructed to lean left or right in small increments until all three planes are at the point of balanced ligamentous tension.
Activation: Test respiratory phases and instruct patient to hold breath (as long as possible) in the phase providing the best ligamentous balance. The physician makes continuous minor adjustments in the patient's position to maintain tissue balance.

Rib cage R3–12

Rib cage: HVLA

Diagnosis: Rib 4 exhalation somatic dysfunction on the right.
Patient position: Supine.
Operator position: Standing on opposite side.
Contact: Cross patient's arms in front of the chest, with the patient's forearm opposite the physician placed on top of the other forearm (Figure 4.3.30).

Position to initiate technique: Grasp patient's arms, roll patient to place thenar eminence, as a fulcrum, on the superior margin of the posterior angle of the rib involved, if single. In rib groups the thenar eminence is placed on the highest rib of the group. Roll patient back onto the fulcrum hand which should apply caudal traction on the rib. Compress through the patient's upper arm to the fulcrum.
Activation: A HVLA thrust is applied from above while a caudal force on angle of the rib is created by a quick wrist abduction or caudal motion.

Rib cage: muscle energy

Diagnosis: Rib 6 exhalation somatic dysfunction on the right.
Patient position: Supine.
Operator position: On same side as involved rib.
Contact: Hook fingers of caudad hand over the superior margin of the angle of the dysfunctional rib or the upper rib of a group and apply caudad tension (Figure 4.3.31).
Position to initiate technique: Patient's head is turned away from the dysfunctional rib; forearm is placed over forehead on the side of the dysfunction; Operator's cephalad hand holds patient's elbow and forearm.
Activation: Patient is instructed to press elbow into operator's hand (towards umbilicus for upper ribs and towards hip in lower ribs) at a vector that transfers the most muscle tension to the dysfunctional rib, while the physician offers isometric counterforce. Hold for 3–5 seconds, wait for tissues to relax completely, and then take up the slack with the caudad hand at the rib angle to the new restrictive barrier. Repeat 3–5 times.

Rib cage: muscle energy

Diagnosis: Rib 6 inhalation somatic dysfunction on the right.
Patient position: Supine.
Operator position: Near head of table on same side as involved rib.
Contact: hook fingers of cephalad hand over the inferior margin of the angle of the dysfunctional rib or the lower rib of a group and apply cephalad tension (Figure 4.3.32).
Position to initiate technique: Patient's head is turned away from the dysfunctional rib; forearm is placed along lateral or anterolateral thigh on the side of the dysfunction; operator's caudad hand contact the anterolateral rib involved.
Activation: The patient exhales and reaches with the left hand toward the foot of the table at a vector that puts the most muscle tension on

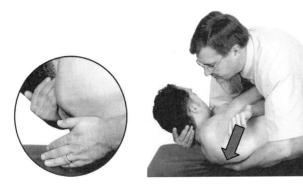

Figure 4.3.30 Rib cage: HVLA (e.g. right exhalation rib 4).[10]

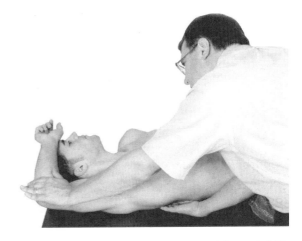

Figure 4.3.31 Rib cage: muscle energy (e.g. right exhalation rib 6).[10]

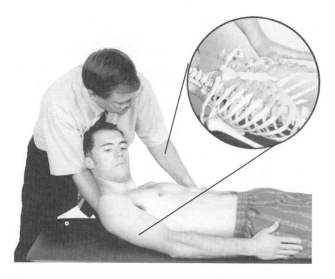

Figure 4.3.32 Rib cage: muscle energy (e.g. left inhalation rib 6).[10]

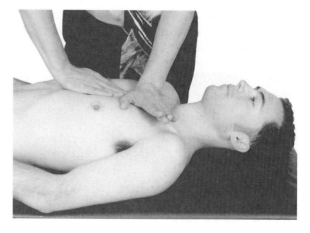

Figure 4.3.34 Sternum: indirect 'stacking' technique.[10]

the dysfunctional rib. The physician offers isometric counterforce. Hold for 3–5 seconds.

Follow-up: As patient relaxes, wait for tissues to relax completely, and then take up the slack with both rib contacts to the new restrictive barrier. Repeat 3–5 times.

Rib cage: indirect with respiratory cooperation

Diagnosis: Rib 4 dysfunction (inhalation or exhalation).
Patient position: Supine or seated.
Operator position: Seated beside patient on side of involved rib.
Contact: Passes posterior hand behind the patient and contact the inferior aspect of the angle of the involved rib with the lateral margin of the index finger; Place lateral margin of index finger of the anterior hand on the superior aspect of the dysfunctional rib at the mid-clavicular line. The thumbs are on the shaft at the midaxillary line (Figure 4.3.33).
Position to initiate technique: Use both hands to simultaneously move the rib angle medial and anterior to the point of balanced ligamentous tension. (Adjust towards inhalation in that dysfunction and towards exhalation in an exhalation dysfunction).
Activation: Patient is instructed to inhale for an inhalation dysfunction (or exhale for exhalation dysfunction) with operator continuously adjusting tension as needed to maintain ligamentous balance until tissues release and dysfunction resolves.
Follow-up: Repeat as needed.

Sternum

Sternum: indirect 'stacking' technique

Diagnosis: Somatic dysfunction in sagittal, coronal, and horizontal planes of the manubrium and of the sternal body; angle of Louis dysfunction; useful after motor vehicle accident with seat harness, after sternotomy patients, and after cardiopulmonary chest compressions).
Patient position: Supine.
Operator position: Standing beside patient.
Contact: Place the heel of one hand on the manubrium and the palm of the other hand on the sternal body with the fingers along its long axis (pointing toward the sternal angle) (Figure 4.3.34).
Position to initiate technique: Simultaneously carry both the sternal body and manubrium to the point of balanced ligamentous tension.
Activation: Test respiratory phases instructing patient to hold the breath as long as possible in the phase that provides the best ligamentous balance. Make continuous minor adjustments between hands as the tissues release to maintain ligamentous balance.

Sternum: 'plastic hand' indirect technique

Diagnosis: Restricted sternal motion within chest cage (this is also a treatment for the superior mediastinum).
Patient position: Supine.
Operator position: Seated at head of table.
Contact: Palm of one hand is placed over the sternum (heel of hand over the manubrium and the fingers on the sternal body along its long

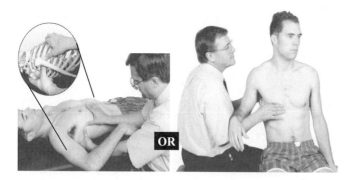

Figure 4.3.33 Rib cage: indirect with respiratory cooperation.[10]

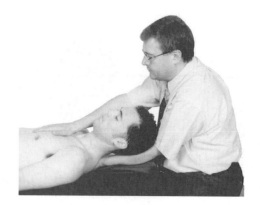

Figure 4.3.35 Sternum: 'plastic hand' indirect technique.[10]

axis). The other hand is placed on the back extending from T1 to T4. Patient's head is supported by operator's forearm (Figure 4.3.35).

Position to initiate technique: Sternal hand carries sternum and overlying soft tissues to the point of balanced ligamentous tension in three planes. The posterior hand provides counterforce and assists in positioning to ligamentous balance.

Activation: Test respiratory phases instructing patient to hold the breath as long as possible in the phase that provides the best ligamentous balance. Make continuous minor adjustments between hands as the tissues release to maintain ligamentous balance.

Thoracolumbar junction, inferior thoracic outlet, and lumbar spine

Thoracolumbar junction/inferior thoracic outlet

Thoracolumbar regional (indirect loading) myofascial release (including diaphragm redoming)

Diagnosis: Fascial dysfunction (left rotation and sidebending) of the inferior thoracic outlet region with or without diaphragm dysfunction.

Patient position: Supine.

Operator position: Standing on either side of patient (Figure 4.3.36).

Contact #1 (lateral): Grasp the lateral sides of the patient's rib cage with palms, fingers spread apart.

Alternate contact #2 (anteroposterior): Place one hand posteriorly to cup L1–3 vertebral column with fingers contacting paraspinal muscles on one side and the heel of the hand contacting the opposite muscles; Fingers of the anterior hand broadly contact the subxiphoid region.

Position to initiate technique:

- **#1 lateral hand-hold:** Carry the lower chest cage fasciae to the point of balanced ligamentous tension by rotating and sidebending further to the left. Translate tissues right to create left sidebending while simultaneously rotating the lower chest cage and fasciae to the left.

- **#2 anteroposterior hand-hold:** Rotate one hand clockwise and the opposite hand counterclockwise (whichever is indicated by testing fascial drag); also add any superior–inferior and left–right translation of the soft tissues needed to establish a sense of balance between anterior and posterior hands.

Activation: Closely monitor tissue balance with normal respiration and follow the tissues in their ease of motion as the patient exhales continuously adjusting minor motions as the tissues release.

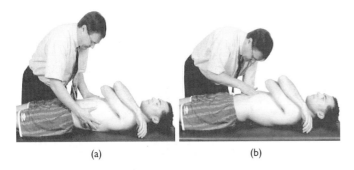

Figure 4.3.36 Thoracolumbar regional (indirect loading) myofascial release (including diaphragm redoming): (a) lateral hold; (b) anteroposterior hold.[10]

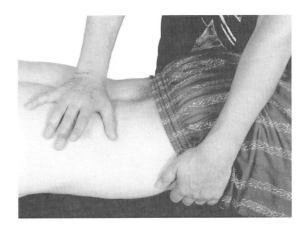

Figure 4.3.37 Quadratus lumborum soft tissue technique (e.g. hypertonic quadratus lumborum muscle or twelfth rib dysfunction in downward pincer position).[10] Contact entire twelfth rib.

Follow-up: Hold through several respiratory cycles until tissues under both hands release completely (both hand-holds) and there is a sense of equal motion during inhalation from both sides of the diaphragm (lateral hold).

Quadratus lumborum soft tissue/twelfth rib technique

Diagnosis: Left twelfth rib somatic dysfunction in downward pincer position **or** tight left quadratus lumborum muscle without rib dysfunction.

Patient position: Prone with the left arm extended and resting along side their head; lower extremities moved to the patient's right to induce lumbar sidebending and traction on the left quadratus lumborum muscle.

Operator position: On side opposite the involved rib (right side).

Contact: Contact the inferior margin of the shaft of the left twelfth rib with the full length of the right thumb to stabilize the entire rib. Grasp the anterior-superior iliac spine (ASIS) with the left hand (Figure 4.3.37).

Position to initiate technique: Lift the pelvis with the left hand while the right thumb maintains an anterior and superior pressure against the twelfth rib at the restrictive barrier.

Activation: Instruct the patient to breathe in deeply. The patient may also be instructed to pull their ASIS toward the table against isometric resistance.

Follow-up: After activation the patient relaxes and new barriers are engaged to repeat the procedure until the quadratus releases the rib (average 3 times).

Thoracolumbar region/twelfth rib: muscle energy technique

Diagnosis: Left twelfth rib in upward pincer position.

Patient position: Prone with lower extremities positioned to induce right lumbar sidebending and traction on the left quadratus lumborum muscle.

Operator position: Standing on side opposite involved rib (patient's right side in this example).

Contact: Place right thumb pad near the costotransverse joint of rib 12 to serve as a fulcrum; left hand grasps the left anterior superior iliac spine (Figure 4.3.38).

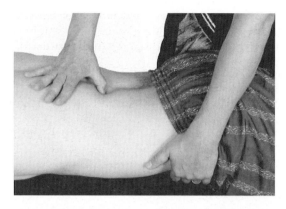

Figure 4.3.38 Thoracolumbar region/twelfth rib: muscle energy technique (left twelfth rib in upward pincer position[10]). Contact costotransverse junction with thumb tip.

Position to initiate technique: Lift pelvis until tension is palpated at fulcrum.

Activation: As patient exhales, operator further lifts the hip posteriorly (to new tissue tension). The quadratus lumborum will pull the rib shaft in a caudad direction rotating around the fulcrum into an exhalation position.

Follow-up: Repeat until the best motion is obtained (average three times).

Lumbar spine L1–5

Lumbar: HVLA

Diagnosis: L2 neutral, sidebending left, rotation right (L2 N_E $S_L R_R$).
Patient position: Left lateral recumbent.
Operator position: Standing in front of patient.
Contact: Fingers of right hand monitor motion contacting the interspinous ligament of the dysfunctional segment (Figure 4.3.39).

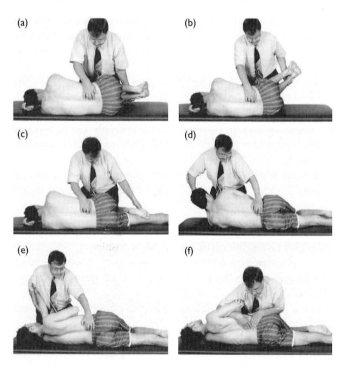

Figure 4.3.39 Lumbar: HVLA. See text for details.[10]

Position to initiate technique: Draw the patient's knees and hips into flexion until motion is palpated at the dysfunctional segment (Figure 4.3.39a). Grasp patient's ankles and lift them toward the ceiling to sidebend the lumbosacral region until localized at the dysfunctional segment (Figure 4.3.39b) This introduces right sidebending below the dysfunction. Ask the patient to straighten the left lower extremity (Figure 4.3.39c). Pull the patient's left shoulder superiorly (Figure 4.3.39d) to maintain right sidebending. Without increasing or decreasing the sagittal plane position, pull the shoulder anteriorly (Figure 4.3.39e) to rotate the thoracic and upper lumbar spine down to the dysfunctional site. As shown in Figure 4.3.39f, the physician's right forearm is placed in front of the patient's right shoulder with the patient's right forearm resting over the physician's. Tension is focused on the dysfunctional segment by rolling the patient slightly forward while maintaining posterior pressure against the patient's right shoulder and simultaneous anterosuperior pressure against the patient's pelvis behind the greater trochanter. Optimally this will be accomplished by the physician's upper torso turning as a unit in a counterclockwise direction around the fingers localized at the site of dysfunction.

Activation: A HVLA thrust is applied anterosuperiorly to the pelvis while providing counterforce through the patient's shoulder. Because the patient is rolled slightly forward to vertically align the plane of the facet joints, this allows the activating force to be directed toward the floor.

Lumbar: HVLA

Diagnosis: L2 nonneutral, flexion, rotation left, sidebending left (L2 NN_F $R_L S_L$).
Patient position: seated straddling table maintaining shoulders over hips as much as possible for balance throughout procedure.
Operator position: standing behind and to patient's right.
Contact: The physician's left hypothenar eminence is placed on the left transverse process of the dysfunctional segment bracing the left elbow on the left hip for support (Figure 4.3.40).
Position to initiate technique: The physician's right axilla or anterior shoulder is placed over the cap of the patient's right shoulder while reaching across the chest to grasp the patient's left shoulder. Pull the patient's left shoulder forward to induce varying increments of right rotation. Introduce right sidebending to the barrier by depressing the patient's right shoulder and by translating the lumbar region using

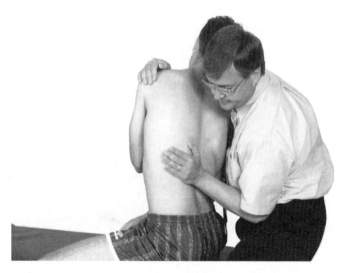

Figure 4.3.40 Lumbar: HVLA (e.g. L2 F $R_L S_L$).[10]

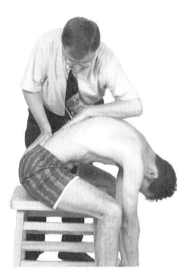

Figure 4.3.41 Lumbar: muscle energy (e.g. L3 E).[10]

the hypothenar eminence of the left braced arm. Add sagittal plane localization to fully engage the restrictive barrier.

Activation: HVLA thrust is directed anteriorly and superiorly by introducing a full body motion through the left braced hypothenar eminence.

Lumbar: muscle energy

Diagnosis: L3 extension (L3 E).
Patient position: Seated on stool with knees apart.
Operator position: Standing beside the patient.
Contact: Physician's caudad hand contacts the lumbar spine (or sacrum) one segment below the dysfunctional segment. Physician uses the other hand to apply superior traction in the midline and to tap the patient's back over the spine of the dysfunctional segment to inform the patient where to concentrate their attempts at motion (Figure 4.3.41).
Position to initiate technique: Patient bends forward allowing hands to fall toward the floor.
Activation: Patient is instructed to 'arch your back like a cat' to push the identified site posteriorly while the physician provides isometric counterforce (typically 3–5 seconds).

Follow-up: Upon simultaneous relaxation, wait for tissues to relax completely and then increase flexion to the new restrictive barrier. Repeat until the best motion is obtained (average three times).

Lumbar: muscle energy

Diagnosis: L2 neutral, sidebending left, rotation right (L2 N_E $S_L R_R$).
Patient position: Seated on stool or straddling table maintaining shoulders over hips as much as possible for balance throughout procedure.
Operator position: Standing behind and to patient's left.
Contact: Place right thumb pad on transverse process of the dysfunctional segment to monitor motion and provide a fulcrum; reach across the patient's chest with left hand to grasp the patient's right shoulder or arm (Figure 4.3.42).
Position to initiate technique: Use patient's left shoulder to induce varying increments of left rotation, right sidebending, and flexion or extension to fully engage the restrictive barrier.
Activation: Patient is instructed to bend to the left, **or** turn to the right localized against an isometric counterforce through the physician's thumb (typically 3–5 seconds).
Follow-up: Upon simultaneous relaxation wait for tissues to relax completely, reposition all planes to the new restrictive barrier, and repeat until the best motion is obtained (average three times).

Lumbar: muscle energy

Diagnosis: L2 non-neutral with flexion, rotation left, sidebending left (L2 NN_F $R_L S_L$).
Patient position: Seated straddling table maintaining shoulders over hips as much as possible for balance throughout procedure.
Operator position: Standing or seated behind.
Contact: Left thumb pad contacts the right side of the spinous process of the dysfunctional segment to induce right rotation (Figure 4.3.43).
Position to initiate technique: Physician's right hand grasps the patient's right shoulder and guides the patient's lumbar spine into right sidebending, right rotation, and extension, as needed, until all three planes are localized at the restrictive barrier.
Activation: Patient is instructed to bend to the left **or** turn to the left localized against an isometric counterforce through the physician's thumb (typically 3–5 seconds).
Follow-up: Upon simultaneous relaxation wait for tissues to relax completely, reposition all planes to the new restrictive barrier, and repeat until the best motion is obtained (average three times).

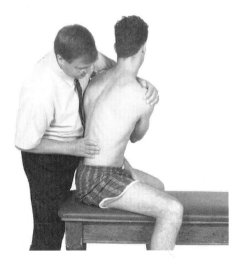

Figure 4.3.42 Lumbar: muscle energy (e.g. L2 N $S_L R_R$).[10]

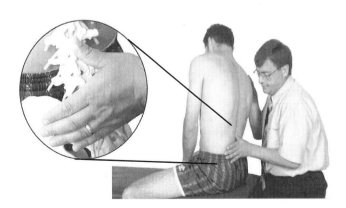

Figure 4.3.43 Lumbar: muscle energy (e.g. L2 NN_F $R_L S_L$).[10]

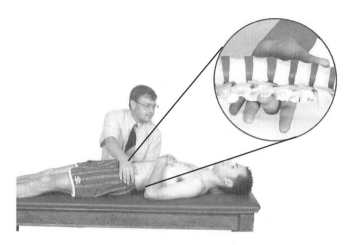

Figure 4.3.44 Lumbar: indirect with respiratory cooperation(e.g. L1 N_E $S_L R_R$).[10]

Lumbar: indirect with respiratory cooperation

Diagnosis: L1 neutral, sidebending left, rotation right (L1 N_E $S_L R_R$).
Patient position: Supine
Operator position: Seated to patient's right.
Contact: Reach under patient and places the pad of a finger on the left transverse process of the dysfunctional segment (Figure 4.3.44).
Position to initiate technique: Patient is instructed to arch or flatten back to balance ligamentous tension in the sagittal plane. Physician applies anterior pressure against the left transverse process (creating right rotation) and pulls the area gently toward him/her (creating left sidebending) to the point of balanced ligamentous tension.
Activation: The respiratory phases are tested and the breath is held as long as possible in the phase providing optimal ligamentous balance. The physician makes minor adjustments in all three planes as needed to maintain ligamentous balance as release is palpated.
Follow-up: Positioning and activation may be required through more than one respiratory session to reintroduce motion.

Lumbar: indirect with respiratory cooperation

Diagnosis: L2 non-neutral, rotation left, sidebending left (L2 NN_F $R_L S_L$).

Patient position: Seated
Operator position: Seated behind patient.
Contact: Physician's left thumb pad contacts the left transverse process of the lower segment of the dysfunctional unit; the right thumb pad contacts the right transverse process of the upper segment (Figure 4.3.45).
Position to initiate technique: Patient is instructed to lean backwards against both thumbs and then to slump slightly to localize the sagittal plane. Further patient instruction to slightly bend to the left and/or to turn to the left accompanies slight additional pressure through the right thumb (to create left rotation of the dysfunctional segment). Fine-tune these minor positional and pressure changes to achieve optimal balanced ligamentous tension.
Activation: The respiratory phases are tested and the breath is held as long as possible in the phase providing optimal ligamentous balance. The physician makes minor adjustments in all three planes as needed to maintain ligamentous balance as release is palpated.
Follow-up: Positioning and activation may be required through more than one respiratory session to reintroduce motion.

Lumbopelvic junction and pelvis

Lumbopelvic junction

Lumbopelvic region: muscle energy or springing (low velocity, moderate amplitude) physiologic method.

Diagnosis: Left on left lumbosacral 'torsion' (this is a combined diagnosis of L5 $NS_L R_R$ **and** the sacrum rotating left around a left oblique sacral axis).
Patient position: Prone
Operator position: Standing at patient's right side.
Preparation for technique: Patient flexes knees and raises the right hip (Figure 4.3.46a) as the physician flexes the hips to at least 90° and guides the knees to the right side of the table (Figure 4.3.46b).
Contact: Physician supports the patient's knees on his/her right thigh to provide a fulcrum for the activating force and to protect the patient's thigh from the edge of the table.

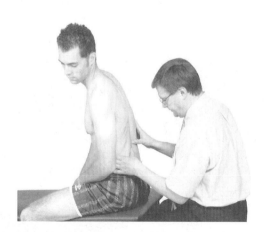

Figure 4.3.45 Lumbar: indirect with respiratory cooperation (e.g. L2 NN_F $R_L S_L$).[10]

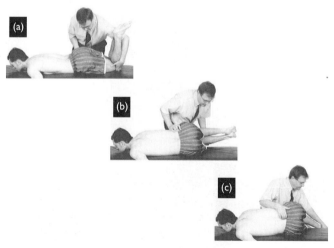

Figure 4.3.46 Lumbopelvic region: muscle energy or springing (low velocity, moderate amplitude) physiologic method (e.g. left sacral torsion).[10]

Position to initiate technique Physician monitors motion and flexes the hips until motion localizes at the lumbosacral junction. Physician grasps the spinous process of L5 with the fingers of the right hand to induce left rotation of vertebral bodies and lets the legs drop over the fulcrum inducing left sidebending.

Activation: Low velocity, moderate amplitude springing is applied toward the floor to the patient's feet or legs. Physician uses right hand to pull the spinous process of L5 into rotation left. (Alternatively, activation may benefit from respiratory activation in which the patient inhales and upon exhalation, reaches for the floor with the right hand; or the patient is instructed, 'Lift your feet toward the ceiling' while the physician offers isometric counterforce for 3–5 seconds.)

Follow-up: Repositioning to the new barrier in all three planes is usually required with 3–4 repeated activations. Physician carefully assists the patient to the prone position again with the legs extended on the table.

Lumbopelvic region: springing (low velocity, moderate amplitude) or muscle energy physiologic method.

Diagnosis Right on left lumbosacral torsion (this is a combined diagnosis of L5 NR$_L$S$_L$ and the sacrum rotating right around a left oblique sacral axis).

Patient position: Left lateral recumbent.

Operator position: Standing in front of the patient.

Position to initiate technique: Patient's left shoulder is drawn forward to induce right rotation down to the lumbosacral junction and the physician's right forearm stabilizes the patient's upper body. Patient's knees and hips are flexed just enough to allow the legs and feet to drop downward over the edge of the table. Flexion must be slight so that nonneutral sacral mechanics will not be induced.

Contact: Fingers of the right hand monitor the lumbosacral junction and sacral base (Figure 4.3.47).

Activation: Patient is instructed to breathe in. As they subsequently exhale, the physician pushes the patient's right shoulder further posterior and springs the feet toward the floor increasing the left sidebending. Alternatively, the physician may instruct the patient to lift their ankles towards the ceiling against isometric resistance (held 3–5 seconds) localized to the physician's monitoring hand.

Follow-up: repeat one or both activating forces until the best motion is obtained (average three times). Assist back to lateral recumbent position.

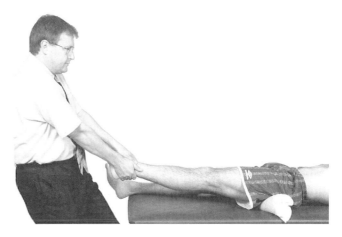

Figure 4.3.48 Sacrum: HVLA (e.g. left sacral shear or left superior innominate shear).[10]

Sacrum

Sacrum: HVLA

Note: This technique is contraindicated in a patient with primary or metastatic bone cancer, severe arthritis of the hip or knee, or an artificial knee or hip.

Diagnosis: Left unilateral sacral flexion **or** left superior (upslipped) innominate shear.

Patient position: Supine.

Operator position: Standing at foot of the table.

Contact: Physician places a pressure pad (such as a small rolled towel) under the left inferolateral angle (ILA) so the patient's body weight moves the left ILA anteriorly and stabilizes the sacrum. Physician grasps the left leg just above the ankle with both hands (Figure 4.3.48).

Position to initiate technique: Physician abducts (tight-packs) the leg slightly and internally rotates (loose-packs) the hip to gap the sacroiliac joint. With the patient relaxing, traction along the long axis of the lower extremity is applied to localize forces up to the pelvis. The patient is instructed to take a very deep and full breath but with pelvic and lower extremity muscles relaxed. (Sometimes mildly shaking the patient's leg along with the continued traction helps the physician to sense relaxation of the patient's muscles and localization to the restrictive barrier.)

Activation: An HVLA tug is applied through the lower extremity to gap the sacroiliac joint and glide the innominate inferior in relation to the sacrum.

Sacrum: HVLA

Diagnosis: Left sacral margin posterior.

Patient position: Supine with hands clasped behind neck.

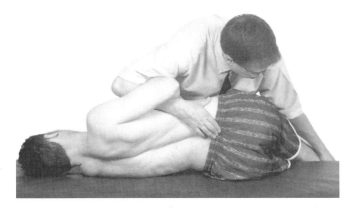

Figure 4.3.47 Lumbopelvic region: springing (low velocity, moderate amplitude) or muscle energy physiologic method (e.g. right rotation on left oblique axis or right backwards torsion).[10]

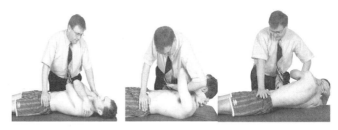

Figure 4.3.49 Sacrum: HVLA (e.g. left sacral margin posterior).[10]

Operator position: Standing on the side opposite the dysfunction (the right side, in this example).

Initial positioning: Pull the patient's hips toward and push the patient's legs and shoulders away to create left sidebending (concavity on the side of the posterior sacral margin).

Contact: Physician bends over the patient, reaches across to insert the cephalad (left, in this example) hand and forearm, from lateral to medial, into the space between the patient's arm and forearm, resting the dorsum of the left hand on the patient's chest. Physician's other hand cups the patient's anterior superior iliac spine on the side of the posterior margin (Figure 4.3.49).

Position to initiate technique: Physician rotates the patient's torso toward him/her to induce right rotation of the spine and sacrum sufficiently to just initiate a lift of the innominate off the table. The innominate is carried posteriorly by the physician's right hand to reach and maintain a restrictive barrier.

Activation: At the moment the innominate starts to lift, an HVLA thrust is applied posteriorly through the ASIS. (Note that the initial positioning assures that the thoracolumbar spine will be essentially vertical to the sacrum and pelvis at the time that the thrust is applied).

Sacrum: HVLA

Diagnosis: Bilateral sacral extension (sacral base posterior).

Patient position: Prone, supporting upper trunk on elbows (the patient's chin may be cradled in the palms of their hands to increase lumbar extension).

Operator position: Standing at the side of the table near the patient's knees.

Contact: Physician places the heel of the cephalad (left, in this example) hand on the sacral base; the other hand provides a counterforce with placement on the patient's ankle or leg (Figure 4.3.50).

Position to initiate technique: The sacral base is carried anteriorly to the restrictive barrier as the physician leans simultaneously onto the sacrum and lower extremity to apply a traction counterforce between both contact hands. The patient is instructed to take a very deep breath while the physician resists the posterior motion of the sacral base and then exhale while the physician follows the sacral base anteriorly.

Activation: At full exhalation, while maintaining traction between both contact hands, the physician applies a HVLA anterior thrust to the sacral base.

Sacrum: muscle energy

Diagnosis: Bilateral sacral extension (sacral base posterior)

Patient position: Seated with knees apart, the lumbosacral junction is flexed and the patient's arms are allowed to hang freely.

Operator position: Standing beside patient.

Contact: Physician places his/her caudad (left, in this example) hand on the patient's sacrum with the heel of that hand below the middle transverse axis of the sacrum. (It helps if this hand can grasp the edge of the stool with fingertips to allow better stabilization of the sacrum.) Physician places cephalad (right, in this example) forearm along the vertebral column.

Position to initiate technique: Traction is applied through the cephalad arm, and caudad hand stabilizes the sacrum.

Activation: Patient is instructed to push the lowest portion of their back backwards (localized at the lumbosacral junction) while the physician offers isometric counterforce (typically for 3–5 seconds).

Follow-up: Physician waits for the tissues to relax completely (about 2 seconds) and then flexes the lumbosacral joint to the new restrictive barrier. The technique is repeated until the best motion is obtained (average three times).

Sacrum: indirect with respiratory cooperation

Diagnosis: Sacrum left on a left oblique axis.

Patient position: Supine.

Operator position: Seated at the patient's left side (Figure 4.3.51b).

Initial positioning: Physician has the patient flex the right leg. Physician grasps the right knee, further flexes it and pulls it toward him/her, rolling the patient's hips toward the side of the table. This allows the physician to easily place a left hand under the sacrum. The patient is rolled back to a supine position with both legs extended.

Contact: The physician's fingers are specifically placed at the sacral base (typically with the index and ring fingers over the right and left aspects of S1 respectively) and the palm cupping the sacral apex. The physician's cephalad (right, in this example) hand may be used with the same forearm to bridge and compress the ASIS's towards one another attempting to gap both SI joints (Figure 4.3.51a) or may alternatively be placed under the sacrum to reinforce the left lifting fingers (Figure 4.3.51c).

Position to initiate technique: Physician lifts the index (and possibly the middle) finger of the left hand, applying anterior pressure to the right sacral base (at S1) to the point of balanced ligamentous tension. This rotates the sacrum to the left on the left oblique axis. Adjustments

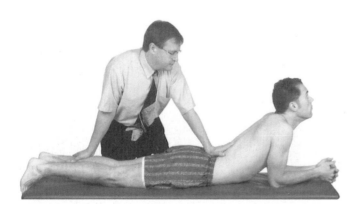

Figure 4.3.50 Sacrum: HVLA (e.g. sacral base posterior).[10]

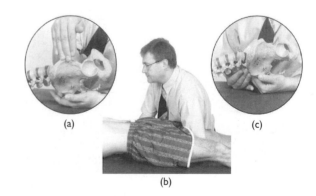

(a) (b) (c)

Figure 4.3.51 Sacrum: indirect with respiratory cooperation (e.g. left rotation on a left oblique axis).[10]

of flexion and extension may also be needed to obtain the best ligamentous balance.

Activation: The respiratory phases are tested and the patient is instructed to hold the phase that provides the best ligamentous balance for as long as possible. As tissues release, the physician continuously modifies finger/hand pressures to insure that the minor motions of the joint are maintained at the shifting point of balanced ligamentous tension.

Follow-up: The technique may be repeated until the best possible motion is obtained.

Sacrum: indirect with respiratory cooperation

Diagnosis: Sacrum right on a left oblique axis.
Patient position: Supine
Operator position: Seated at the patient's right side (Figure 4.3.52b).
Initial positioning: Physician has the patient flex the left leg. Physician grasps the left knee, further flexes it and pulls it toward him/her, rolling the patient's hips toward the side of the table. This allows the physician to easily place a right hand under the sacrum. The patient is rolled back to a supine position with both legs extended.
Contact: The physician's fingers are specifically placed at the sacral base (typically with the index and ring fingers over the left and right aspects of S1 respectively) and the palm cupping the sacral apex. The physician's cephalad (left, in this example) hand may be used with the same forearm to bridge and compress the ASIS's towards one another attempting to 'gap' both sacroiliac joints (Figure 4.3.52a) or may alternatively be placed to reduce lumbosacral pressure (Figure 4.3.52c).
Position to initiate technique: Physician lifts the thenar eminence of the right hand, applying anterior pressure to the left ILA, encouraging right rotation on the left oblique axis to the point of balanced ligamentous tension. Adjustments of flexion and extension may also be needed to obtain the best ligamentous balance.
Activation: The respiratory phases are tested and the patient is instructed to hold the phase that provides the best ligamentous balance for as long as possible. As tissues release, the physicians continuously modifies finger/hand pressures to insure that the minor motions of the joint are maintained at the shifting point of balanced ligamentous tension.
Follow-up: The technique may be repeated until the best possible motion is obtained.

Sacrum: counterstrain

Diagnosis: Tender point over one sacral pole.
Patient position: Supine.
Operator position: Standing at the patient's side.

Contact: While contacting the tender pole with one finger, place the heel of the opposite hand (pisiform or thenar) in point contact with the sacrum over the pole diagonal to the involved pole; for example, for left lower pole tenderness, contact the right upper pole.
Position to initiate technique: Pressure is applied through the heel of the hand until pressure with the monitoring single digit elicits tenderness at the original point that is reduced by 70% or more.
Activation: Maintain for a period of 90 seconds that amount of pressure through the heel of the hand needed to reduce the point tenderness by 70% with no pressure through the digit monitoring the tender point. After 90 seconds, gradually release the pressure.
Follow-up: Recheck to insure that there is only 30% or less tenderness at the original site. It is possible to repeat the technique or select another to affect arthrodial somatic dysfunction. Alternatively, the possibility of a posterior sacroiliac ligament strain might be considered.

Sacrum: direct method – respiratory force and low velocity, medium amplitude (springing)

Diagnosis: Left unilateral sacral flexion (left sacral shear).
Patient position: Prone.
Operator position: Standing on the side of the dysfunction (patient's left, in this example).
Contact: Physician places his/her thumb or fingers over the left sacroiliac joint to monitor motion. Physician positions self against the medial aspect of the patient's flexed leg to maintain internal rotation at the hip and left innominate. Physician places his/her right hypothenar eminence on the inferior aspect of the patient's left ILA and applies superior and anterior pressure (avoid pressure on the coccyx). The right hand may be reinforced with the left or, alternatively (as pictured), the left fingers may pull laterally on the PSIS to enhance gapping of the SI joint (Figure 4.3.53).
Position to initiate technique: Physician flexes the patient's knee, abducts and internally rotates the hip until gapping is palpated at the left sacroiliac joint. The knee is placed back onto the table at that point.
Activation: Patient is instructed to take a very deep breath. When they think they have taken a full breath, challenge them to add even further inhalation to encourage the sacral base to move posteriorly and engage the restrictive barrier. While relaxed but still holding the breath at full inhalation, the physician applies a superior and anterior low velocity, medium amplitude springing force through the left ILA.
Follow-up: The physician instructs the patient to exhale while maintaining a superior and anterior pressure on the left ILA. The activation procedure is repeated immediately another two times or until motion and better symmetry are reestablished.

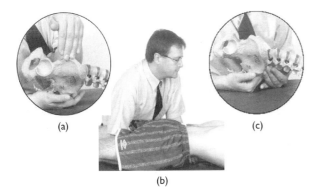

(a) (c)

(b)

Figure 4.3.52 Sacrum: indirect with respiratory cooperation (e.g. sacral rotation right on a left oblique axis).[10]

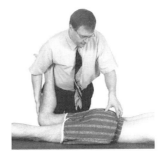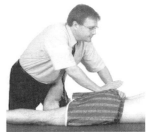

Figure 4.3.53 Sacrum: direct method – respiratory force and low velocity, medium amplitude (springing) (e.g. left unilateral sacral flexion).[10]

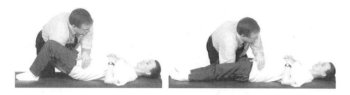

Figure 4.3.54 Sacrum: articulatory technique with respiratory cooperation (e.g. anterior sacral base).[10]

Sacrum: articulatory technique with respiratory cooperation

Note: This technique is especially useful in the severe sacral base anterior somatic dysfunction that may complicate late-term pregnancy or the postpartum period.

Diagnosis: Bilateral sacral flexion (anterior sacral base).

Patient position: supine with knees and hips flexed, feet flat on the table, and knees slightly apart.

Operator position: standing at the side of the patient.

Preparatory positioning:. Patient lifts the pelvis off the table to allow the physician to place a hand between the thighs and under the sacrum.

Contact: The physician's index, middle, and ring fingers of one hand contact on the sacral base above the middle transverse axis with the palm positioned at the sacral apex. The opposite forearm and fingertips bridge the ASIS applying compression to bring the ASIS together and to attempt to 'gap' the sacroiliac joints bilaterally (Figure 4.3.54).

Position to initiate technique: After physician hand and arm placements, the patient's pelvis is lowered to the table and the knees are allowed to fall laterally and the soles of the feet are brought together (sometimes called the 'frog' position).

Activation: Patient is instructed to take a deep breath and hold it as the physician applies long axis traction down the arm holding the sacrum. This directly rotates the sacrum posteriorly. While the physician maintains traction, the patient (with knees hanging laterally) is instructed to exhale while rapidly sliding both feet simultaneously toward the foot of the table. The final position will result in the physician still maintaining traction (to encourage a posterior position of the sacral base) and the patient will have an anatomical supine position with both lower extremities fully extended.

Follow-up: The patient can be instructed in a sacral gapping exercise in the supine position, hips and knees bent with feet on the floor spaced slightly more than shoulder width but knees together. Long deep breathes help to rock the sacrum around transverse axes.

Pubic symphysis

Pubic symphysis: muscle energy

Diagnosis: Left inferior pubic shear.

Patient position: Supine.

Operator position: Standing on side of dysfunction (patient's left).

Contact: Patient's left knee is placed against the physician's chest. Physician cups the right hand over the patient's left ASIS and grasps the left ischial tuberosity with the other hand (Figure 4.3.55).

Position to initiate technique: The left lower extremity is flexed at the knee and hip and the thigh is abducted to with just enough tension to gently 'gap' at the pubic symphysis. Rotate the innominate posteriorly (which carries the pubic ramus superiorly to the restrictive barrier) using the physician's hand contacts with the ASIS and ischial tuberosity and the chest contact with the patient's knee.

Activation: Patient is instructed to push with the knee toward the end of the table against an isometric counterforce provided by the physician's chest (typically for 3–5 seconds).

Follow-up: Physician waits for tissues to relax completely (about 2 seconds) and then rotates the innominate posteriorly to the new restrictive barrier using both contact hands and chest. This carries the pubic ramus superiorly. Repeat until the best motion is obtained (average three times).

Pubic symphysis: muscle energy

Diagnosis: Right superior pubic shear.

Patient position: Supine with the dysfunctional side near the edge of the table.

Operator position: Standing on the side of the dysfunction (patient's right).

Contact: Physician contacts the opposite (left) ASIS to stabilize the left hemipelvis and instructs the patient to move to the edge of the table until the right ischial tuberosity is over the edge. The patient may feel the need to 'hold on' to the table with one or both hands for stability. Physician's left hand is placed on the knee of the right (dysfunctional) extremity (Figure 4.3.56).

Position to initiate technique: Physician abducts the right lower extremity to localize 'gapping' at the pubic symphysis. The thigh is

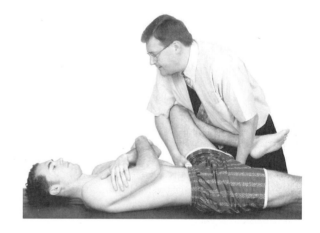

Figure 4.3.55 Pubic symphysis: muscle energy (e.g. left inferior pubic shear).[10]

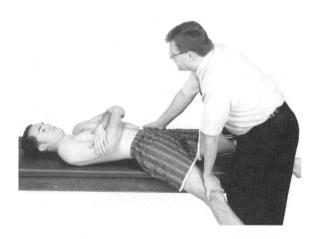

Figure 4.3.56 Pubic symphysis: muscle energy (e.g. right superior pubic shear).[10]

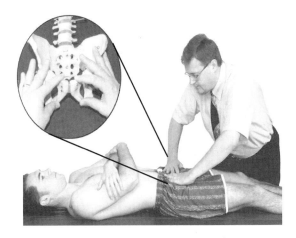

Figure 4.3.57 Pubic symphysis: indirect method, respiratory cooperation (e.g. inferior or superior pubic shear).[10]

extended off the table to tissue tension. (This rotates the innominate anteriorly and carries the pubic symphysis inferiorly to the restrictive barrier).

Activation: Patient is instructed to push with the knee toward the ceiling and medially against an isometric counterforce provided by the physician's left hand (typically for 3–5 seconds).

Follow-up: Physician waits for tissues to relax completely (about 2 seconds) and then rotates the innominate anteriorly to the new restrictive barrier using the contact hand above the knee. This carries the right pubic ramus inferiorly. Repeat until the best motion is obtained (average is 3 times). The patient's extremity is placed back on the table.

Pubic symphysis: indirect method, respiratory cooperation

Diagnosis: Inferior or superior pubic shear.

Patient position: Supine.

Operator position: Standing beside table.

Contact: Physician grasps each pubic bone with thumbs on the lower margins of each inferior ramus and index fingers on the superior margin of each superior ramus (Figure 4.3.57).

Position to initiate technique: Introduce appropriate superior and inferior glides by moving the pubic bones in opposite directions to the point of balanced ligamentous tension.

Activation: The respiratory phases are tested and the breath is held as long as possible in the phase that provides the best ligamentous balance. During this time the physician makes minor adjustments of the pubic bones to maintain ligamentous balance.

Follow-up: Repeat if needed to obtain the best motion.

Pubic symphysis: muscle energy, direct method

Diagnosis: Compression of the pubic symphysis.

Patient position: Supine with the hips and knees flexed 25–30 cm (10–12 inches) apart and the feet are flat on the table.

Operator position: Standing at the side of the table near the patient's hips.

Preparatory action: Physician grasps both knees, holds them together and instructs the patient to gently try to abduct both knees against an isometric counterforce (held approximately 3 seconds and repeated an average of three times). This prepares the adductor muscles and the pubic symphysis for the activating portion of the corrective technique.

Contact: The heel of the physician's cephalad hand is placed on the medial side of the knee opposite him/her. The palm of the other hand

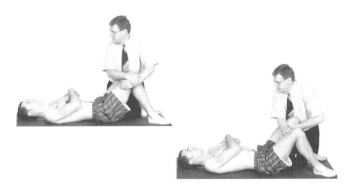

Figure 4.3.58 Pubic symphysis: muscle energy, direct method (e.g. pubic compression).[10]

is placed on the medial aspect of the other knee with the thumb abducted, grasping the other forearm (Figure 4.3.58).

Position to initiate technique: Physician spreads the knees 25–30 cm (10–12 inches) apart and adjusts the forearm grasp to brace the knees.

Activation: Patient is instructed to try to adduct both knees together against a simultaneous isometric counterforce. Physician has the patient maintain the force long enough to sense that the patient's contractile force is localized at the pubic symphysis (typically 3–5 seconds). An audible release may or may not occur during this procedure.

Follow-up: Physician waits for the tissues to relax completely (about 2 seconds) and then moves the feet and the knees a few inches farther apart. The technique may be repeated as needed to achieve return of motion and reduction of symphyseal tenderness.

Innominate

Innominate: HVLA

Note: This technique is contraindicated in a patient with primary or metastatic bone cancer, severe arthritis of the hip or knee, or an artificial knee or hip.

Diagnosis: Left superior (upslipped) innominate shear or left unilateral sacral flexion.

Patient position: Lateral recumbent.

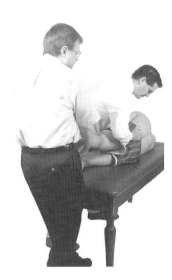

Figure 4.3.59 Innominate: HVLA (e.g. left upslipped innominate or left sacral shear.[10]

Operator and assistant positions: Physician stands at the foot of the table; an assistant stands in front or behind the patient (Figure 4.3.59).

Assistant contact: Places the hypothenar eminence of one hand on the inferior aspect of the inferolateral angle on the side of the dysfunction applying a firm cephalad pressure. The assistant's other hand contacts the superior margin of the iliac crest, pulling it inferiorly and compressing it against the cephalad sacral pressure to the restrictive barrier.

Physician contact: Grasps the patient's leg above the ankle on the dysfunctional side.

Position to initiate technique: Physician abducts and internally rotates the patient's leg slightly and applies steady traction along the long axis of the extremity to localize forces into the pelvis. The patient is instructed to take a very deep and full breath but with pelvic and lower extremity muscles relaxed. (Sometimes mildly shaking the patient's leg along with the continued traction helps the physician to sense relaxation of the patient's muscles and localization to the restrictive barrier.)

Activation: An HVLA tug is applied through the lower extremity to gap the sacroiliac joint and glide the innominate inferior in relation to the sacrum.

Innominate: muscle energy

Diagnosis: Anteriorly rotated right innominate.

Patient position: Supine, lower extremity on the side of the dysfunction is flexed at the knee and hip to bring the knee over the patient's abdomen.

Operator position: Standing on the side of the dysfunction (the right side, in this example).

Contact: Physician holds the patient's flexed knee in that position with his/her shoulder against the leg while cupping the anterior superior iliac spine (ASIS) with the cephalad hand (the left, in this example). The fingers of the other hand grasp the posterior aspect of the right ischial tuberosity (Figure 4.3.60).

Position to initiate technique: Tension is increased at all contact points and the innominate is rotated posteriorly to the restrictive barrier.

Activation: Patient is instructed to push the knee against the physician's chest that, along with hand contacts, offers isometric counterforce for 3–5 seconds.

Follow-up: The physician waits for the tissues to relax completely (about 2 seconds) and then slightly flexes the hip while concentrating on rotating the innominate posteriorly to the new restrictive barrier with both hand contacts. Activation and follow-up steps should be repeated until the best motion is obtained (average three times).

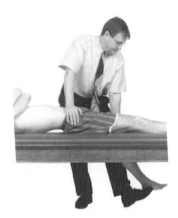

Figure 4.3.61 Innominate: muscle energy (e.g. posterior left innominate rotation).[10]

Innominate: muscle energy

Diagnosis: Posteriorly rotated left innominate.

Patient position: Supine. The patient is positioned at the edge of the table, close enough to permit the ischial tuberosity to be clear of the edge. (The patient may feel the need to grasp the table for stability.) The leg is allowed to hang freely.

Operator position: Standing on the side of the dysfunction (the left, in this example).

Contact: Physician reaches across the patient with one hand to cup the patient's opposite ASIS (for stability on the table) and places the other hand on the thigh of the dysfunctional extremity just above patient's knee. If necessary, the physician's foot is placed under the patient's foot to prevent it from touching the floor.

Position to initiate technique: Tension and a force directed toward the floor is applied to the thigh, rotating the innominate anteriorly to the restrictive barrier. The opposite hand maintains the pelvis from rolling up off the table.

Activation: Patient is instructed to pull the knee up toward the ceiling while the physician simultaneously offers isometric counterforce for 3–5 seconds through the thigh–hand contact (Figure 4.3.61).

Follow-up: The physician waits for the tissues to relax completely (about 2 seconds) and then slightly extends the hip while concentrating on rotating the innominate anteriorly to the new restrictive barrier. Activation and follow-up steps should be repeated until the best motion is obtained (average is three times).

Pelvic floor and coccyx

Ischiorectal fossa technique

Diagnosis: Tight pelvic floor with poor motion.

Patient position: Supine with knees and hips flexed and feet flat on table or bed.

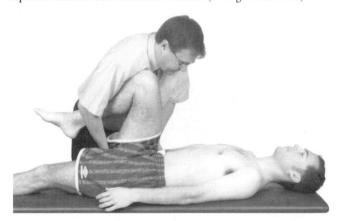

Figure 4.3.60 Innominate: muscle energy (e.g. anterior right innominate rotation).[10]

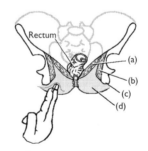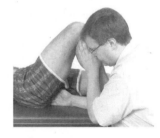

Figure 4.3.62 Ischiorectal fossa technique. (a = pelvic floor; b = obturator internus; c = ischial tuberosity; d = ischiorectal fat)

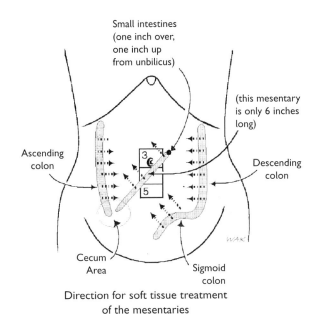

Figure 4.3.63 Mesenteric lift techniques: fascial release.

Operator position: Seated beside patient.

Contact: Physician's fingers are extended well into the ischiorectal fossa traveling along the inner aspect of the ischial tuberosity to avoid midline structures (Figure 4.3.62).

Position to initiate technique: The physician uses extended fingers to compress the ischiorectal fat against the pelvic floor muscles. Compression is increased until the muscular barrier is encountered.

Activation: The patient is instructed to take in a big breath while the physician's fingers resist the inferior excursion of the pelvic floor that this initiates. During exhalation, the extended fingers press superiorly to 'take up the slack' and to encounter the new barrier.

Follow-up: Repeat three or more times as needed to release the pelvic floor and then recheck the excursion allowed. (At the end of the last cycle of inhalation, the patient may be instructed to cough against a continuous finger pressure to stretch the pelvic floor more completely. This latter maneuver should not be attempted if there is a history or palpatory evidence of significant pelvic floor hyperreactivity.)

Coccyx: indirect

Diagnosis: Coccygeal somatic dysfunction (Diagnosis and treatment are done simultaneously in this technique. Please note that treatment of the coccyx is most effectively performed after treating all other pelvic dysfunction, including the pelvic floor, as described above. If this technique is used, treatment of the coccyx should follow completion of inhibition over areas of the pelvic floor palpated to have tension or pelvic floor myofascial trigger points.)

Patient position: Lateral recumbent position with knees and hips comfortably flexed.

Operator position: Seated behind patient.

Contact: Using caudal gloved hand, a lubricated finger (usually the index) is passed into the rectum to contact the anterior surface of the coccyx. The thumb of the cephalad hand is placed externally over the skin covering the posterior coccyx. (For some patients and physicians, respective sizes allow the physician to contact these two sites with the same caudad hand.)

Position to initiate technique: The physician gently checks flexion–extension, right and left sidebending, and right and left rotation of the coccyx on the sacrum. Somatic dysfunction permits motion in one direction of each paired motion and a restricted barrier in the other. Maintaining the finger–thumb contacts, each permitted motion is simultaneously stacked to the point of ligamentous balance.

Activation: The respiratory phases are tested and the breath is held as long as possible in the phase that provides the best ligamentous balance. During this time the physician makes minor adjustments of the coccyx to maintain balanced ligamentous tension.

Follow-up: Recheck motion and consider repeating until the best motion is obtained.

Abdominal region

Somatic

Mesenteric lift techniques: fascial release

Diagnosis: Poor lymphatic drainage within mesenteries containing the small and/or large intestines.

Patient position: Supine with knees bent and feet on table/bed.

Operator position: Standing on patient's right side.

Contact: Pads of operator's fingers (or edges of entire fifth digits) creating soft tissue slack in superficial abdominal tissues to allow deeper contact to viscera involved (small bowel; cecal area; ascending colon; or descending colon) (Figure 4.3.63).

Position to initiate technique: Draw viscera (contacted as described above) in the direction towards its mesenteric attachment to a point of balanced fascial tension; a small amount of torsion may need to be instituted for balance.

Activation: Hold tissues at balance point and follow any viscoelastic creep.

Follow-up: Check other areas; often follow-through with each mesentery throughout the gastrointestinal tract for a clinical effect in patients with constipation or with irritable bowel syndrome.

Visceral reflex

Collateral ganglion inhibition techniques

Note 1: This technique is contraindicated in the presence of an abdominal aneurysm, certain other visceral pathologies, or in the imme-

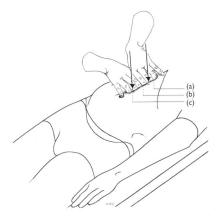

Figure 4.3.64 Collateral ganglion inhibition techniques. (from Kuchera M. L., Kuchera W. A. *Osteopathic considerations in systemic dysfunction*, 2nd edn. Greyden Press, Columbus, OH, 1994.)

diate postoperative healing stages; it is expected that a preliminary palpatory diagnosis of the abdomen shall have been made.

Diagnosis: Tension over one of three midline abdominal sites between the xiphoid process and umbilicus (a = celiac ganglion site; b = superior mesenteric ganglion site; c = inferior mesenteric ganglion site).

Note 2: In the viscerosomatic reflex model, these sites may correspond with vicerosomatic reflexes from T5–9 (a); T10–11 (b); or T1–L2 (c) other palpatory clues including somatic clues (Chapman's reflexes and/or related spinal somatic dysfunction) and visceral clues (organ palpation and other traditional physical examination) might be warranted or advisable before treating.

Patient position: Supine with knees bent and feet flat on table/bed.

Operator position: Standing at patient's side.

Contact: Maintaining all fingers the same length by gently bending several, compress gently in the midline over the involved ganglion/ganglia towards the abdominal aorta (Figure 4.3.64).

Position to initiate technique: Compress with enough pressure that the tissues gently resist, then ask the patient to take a half-breath to increase the tension to their tolerance.

Activation: Hold the inhibitory pressure as they hold their breath and when they exhale, follow the tissue tension in the direction of tissue release and then repeat the cycle a few more times or until the area over the site softens.

Follow-up: If the problem was truly viscerosomatic in nature (due to a primary visceral pathology), the reflex findings will typically recur. While treatment of the secondary recurrent somatic findings in a viscerosomatic reflex may play an adjunctive role in MMMT, the underlying primary cause of this type of reflex should be sought and treated appropriately according to the accepted standard of medical care.

Conclusion

The examples of manual medicine techniques in this chapter are illustrative of applying general principles as they might be used by manual medicine physicians to correct single somatic dysfunctions palpated and deemed clinically relevant. These and other manual medicine techniques can be integrated and used as valuable adjunctive tools in the complete management of patients with a wide variety of complaints. They have been shown to be capable of playing a role in reducing pain and improving function within the neuromusculoskeletal system as well as in supporting certain self-healing mechanisms.

An integrated musculoskeletal manipulative medicine treatment (MMMT) is most commonly prescribed within the context of its risk-to-benefit therapeutic ratio. It is deemed to be adjunctive or primary to the care of the patient (or even contra-indicated) by physicians who have undertaken at least several hundreds of additional hours learning palpatory diagnosis and can make this determination based upon the entirety of the clinical context, the host factors involved, and the range of approaches available. Such extensive training also extends to skills needed to safely and effectively administer manual technique and integrated regimens to remove somatic dysfunction. The form that the treatment protocol may take, the goals selected, and the choice of techniques used to accomplish those goals are part of the science, philosophy, and art of the attending physician and the clinical specialty context in which he or she is practicing.

Acknowledgements

The author extends his thanks to the Kirksville College of Osteopathic Medicine (KCOM) for their permission to use the many illustrations of the author applying technique.[10] The original color photographs and more detailed treatment directions for these and many more techniques can be found in the text for which they were originally taken: Kimberly P, Funk SF (eds). *Outline of Osteopathic Manipulative Procedures: The Kimberly Manual Millennium Edition* (2000), Walsworth Publishing Company, Marceline, MO.[10] This text is available from the Department of Osteopathic Manipulative Medicine of KCOM at 800 W. Jefferson, Kirksville, MO 63501, USA.

Gratitude is also extended by the author to the Philadelphia College of Osteopathic Medicine (PCOM) for the permission of departmental chairperson, Professor Alexander Nicholas, P.O., F.A.A.O. to release pictures for the upcoming Nicholas manual.

References

1. Kuchera, M. L., DiGiovanna, E. L., Greenman, P. E. Efficacy and complications. Chapter 72: in Ward, R. C. *Foundations for osteopathic medicine*, 2nd edn. Lippincott, Williams and Wilkins, Baltimore, MD, 2002, pp. 1143–52.

2. Education Council on Osteopathic Principles. Glossary of osteopathic terminology. In: Ward, R. C. (editor). *Foundations for osteopathic medicine*, 2nd edn. Lippincott, Williams and Wilkins, Baltimore, MD, 2002.

3. Kappler, R. E., Kuchera, W. A. Diagnosis and plan for manual treatment: a prescription. Chapter 40 in: Ward, R. C. *Foundations for osteopathic medicine*, 2nd edn. Lippincott, Williams and Wilkins, Baltimore, MD, 2002, pp. 574–9.

4. Kimberly, P. Forming a prescription for osteopathic manipulative treatment. *Journal of the American Osteopathic Association*, 1980, **79**, 512.

5. Ward R. C. integrated neuromusculoskeletal release and myofascial release. Chapter 60 in: Ward, R. C. *Foundations for osteopathic medicine*, 2nd edn. Lippincott, Williams and Wilkins, Baltimore, MD, 2002, pp. 931–68.

6. Van Buskirk, R. L. Treatment of somatic dysfunction with an osteopathic manipulative method of Dr. Andrew Taylor Still. Chapter 70 in: Ward, R. C. *Foundations for osteopathic medicine*, 2nd edn. Lippincott, Williams and Wilkins, Baltimore, MD, 2002, pp. 994–1114.

7. Kappler, R. E., Jones, J. M. Thrust (high-velocity/low-amplitude) techniques. Chapter 56 in: Ward, R. C. *Foundations for osteopathic medicine*, 2nd edn. Lippincott, Williams and Wilkins, Baltimore, MD, 2002, pp. 852–80.

8. Patriquin, D. A., Jones, J. M. Articulatory techniques. Chapter 55 in: Ward, R. C. *Foundations for osteopathic medicine*, 2nd edn. Lippincott, Williams and Wilkins, Baltimore, MD, 2002, pp. 834–51.

9. Ehrenfeuchter, W. C., Sandhouse M. Chapter 57 in: Ward, R. C. *Foundations for osteopathic medicine*, 2nd edn. Lippincott, Williams and Wilkins, Baltimore, MD, 2002, pp. 881–907.

10. Kimberly, P., Funk S. F. (eds). *Outline of osteopathic manipulative procedures: the Kimberly manual millennium edition* (2000). Walsworth Publishing Company, Marceline MO.

11. Nicholas, A., Nicholas, E. *The Nicholas atlas of osteopathic manipulative technique*, in press.

4.3.2 Injection of steroid and local anaesthetic

Richard M. Ellis

Joint injection for relief of pain has a satisfactory record of effectiveness: the most frequent injection used is one including corticosteroids, but other solutions, including saline, local anaesthetic, hyaluronate[1] and prolotherapy solutions[2] (see later) are used also. Patients are regularly grateful for this intervention, and so the aspiring musculoskeletal physician should not be put off by undue concern about expertise, desirable though that is: in a study of accuracy for true intraarticular placement, the most and least experienced members of a British medical team both achieved about 50% success.[3]

Efficacy

Local anaesthetic solutions are mainly used as a diagnostic test, confirming that the joint is a source of the person's symptoms. In the experimental situation, control injections with saline or an anaesthetic of different duration of action is used.[4] Although spinal diagnosis lends itself well to this approach, differential diagnosis between peripheral joints which are anatomically close, such as the trapeziometacarpal versus the trapezioscaphoid, or the ankle (tibiotalar) versus the subtalar, can also be made.

Saline injection

Isotonic saline injections have been noted to be beneficial in osteoarthritis, and the mechanism of action may be the removal of debris suspended in the joint fluid: the saline irrigation of a joint regularly carried out at arthroscopy is frequently followed by sustained relief. Dechow[5] found benefit to be maintained over 6 months in osteoarthritic knees irrigated with a litre of saline.

Corticosteroid injections

In inflammatory arthritis, efficacy of steroid injections is greatest if a depot preparation is used:[6] the larger molecular size maintains a greater concentration in the joint for longer. This benefit of duration of the drug intra-articularly can be enhanced further by bed rest, e.g. for 24 hours.[7]

In osteoarthritis, benefit occurs in a proportion of cases.[8] The benefit is more likely in cases without gross joint destruction, but other prognostic factors for a good response are not known.

Osteoarthritis can be complicated by pseudogout, where intra-articular steroid injection is the treatment of choice. In gout, injection is a useful option, if oral drugs are unsuitable, or an attack is slow to clear.

In self-limiting conditions, such as post-traumatic capsulitis, or idiopathic capsulitis of the shoulder (frozen shoulder), steroid injections can speed recovery and thereby maintain function of the other soft tissues.[9]

Hyaluronate injections

Hyaluronic acid is a component of normal synovial fluid and is depleted in osteoarthritic joints; it has been postulated that in osteoarthritis injection of hyaluronate of high molecular weight will be retained in the joint and will be beneficial. The turnover of hyaluronate in the joint is relatively rapid, but significant clinical benefit is obtained by a series of five, weekly intra-articular injections to a degree similar to oral anti-inflammatories[1] or a single corticosteroid injection. The mechanism of action remains unknown.

Complications

Infection

Intra-articular injection should always be carried out with an aseptic technique. Nevertheless, infection occasionally enters the joint. The frequency of infection is estimated to be only 1 in 17 000 to 77 000 cases, using normal precautions.[10,11] If there is diagnostic uncertainty, is it necessary for the aspirate to be cultured before steroid can be injected? In a study of 507 cases, all those aspirates which did give growth on culture were those clinically suspected.[12] If the aspirate is clear, and the cause of joint pain is thought not to be infective, it is reasonable to inject steroid at the first attendance.

Possible damage to articular cartilage

There has been considerable anxiety that steroid injection may accelerate loss of articular cartilage in a joint. Early reports detailed gross destruction of weightbearing joints with injections carried out frequently, such as weekly. This frequency of injection implied that the duration of relief was very short, and in retrospect it would seem that these were joints with advanced degenerative change, which were, by modern standards, unresponsive to the injection. Subsequent studies have refuted that premature destruction will take place. In one report of 30 osteoarthritic knees and 35 rheumatoid arthritic knees given up to 167 injections in 12 years, no evidence of accelerated deterioration was found.[13] Judicious use of steroids implies that repeat injections are not used unless substantial benefit resulted from the previous injection, and that there is an interval of over four weeks between injections. If adequate control of joint pain is not achieved, complicating factors must be considered, such as infection, hyperuricaemia or bone destruction: and other methods of relief must be considered, including physical relief by use of a walking stick, orthoses, or by other injection such as hyaluronate, or by surgery.

Haemarthrosis

Bleeding into the joint is a potential complication of any joint injection, but symptomatic reaction is rare. In cases with clotting abnormality or in those on anticoagulant therapy, the risk is much greater, so the doctor and patient must discuss the potential for painful haemarthrosis resulting. If one or two prior anticoagulant doses can be omitted, the risk will be much less.

Soft tissue or skin atrophy

Atrophy can occur with periarticular leakage of steroid preparations (or with soft tissue injection). This is more frequent and easily detected with superficially placed injections such as the wrist (or tennis elbow). The skin becomes thinner and depigmented, sometimes with telangiectasia. The patient should be warned about the possibility when the superficially-sited injections are to be repeated. Atrophy of muscle occurs rarely and unpredictably with some deeper injections.

Technique

Our preferred technique for intra-articular injection is:

1 Identify the joint line. The joint line, if not superficial and obvious, is best searched for by passive movement of the distal bone, while the examiner's thumbnail, of the hand stabilizing the proximal bone, is moved distally or proximally: when the thumbnail senses the distal bone abutting it (rather than lifting it), the line for injection is marked.

2 Avoid blood vessels and nerves. The extensor surface of the joint is normally clear of these vital structures, and is generally favoured, except for the hip joint.

3 Mark the skin point for injection, so that it is never touched after skin sterilization, before the injection. We favour using the point of a retracted ball-point pen, on the spot, using sustained gentle pressure for 10 seconds: the indentation is easily seen and remains for some minutes.

4 Sterilize the skin with an antiseptic solution, waiting a sufficient time for its action.

5 Use preliminary local anaesthetic if the joint is unduly sensitive, or the patient is apprehensive, or the doctor is relatively inexperienced.

6 Consider distraction of the joint by an assistant, to open up the joint space a little, if wished.

7 Insert the needle. Use the smallest needle that will reach the joint and allow the required volume of solution to pass quickly into the joint. For a small, superficial joint like the trapeziometacarpal, a 12-mm 25-gauge needle is easiest, but for the posterior approach to the shoulder, a 50-mm 21-gauge needle is usually needed.

8 If the needle does not immediately enter the joint (allowing fluid to be aspirated), first alter the angle of the needle without withdrawing it: this will often allow the needle to be advanced correctly.

9 After aspiration shows no blood (or only lightly blood-stained joint fluid), inject the solution.

10 Counsel the patient to avoid strain on the joint, especially for the first 24 hours, and to report any unusual reaction.

Although some texts advise the use of surgical gloves and a face mask, and for the injector not to talk during the procedure, I have found that the injection is safe and more relaxing for the patient without these extra precautions.

Radiographic or ultrasound guidance for injection

An injection may be ineffective because of a technical failure. Radiological or ultrasound screening is necessary for safety and/or accuracy of some spinal joint injections, but can be very useful for some peripheral joint injections: I use them most frequently for hip, shoulder, and subtalar injections.

References

1. Altman, R. D., Moskowitz, R. and the Hyalgan Study Group. Intra-articular sodium hyaluraonate in the treatment of osteoarthritis of the knee. *J Rheumatol*, 1998, **25**, 2203–12.

2. Stav, A., Sternberg, A., Landau, M., *et al.* Intra-articular injection of a proliferant for pain relief in patients with rheumatoid arthritis. Preliminary results. *The Pain Clinic*, 1992, **5**, 85–9.

3. Jones, A., Regan, M., Ledingham, J., *et al.* Importance of placement of intra-articular steroid injections. *BMJ*, 1993, **307**, 1329–30.

4. Lord, S. M., Barnsley, L., Bogduk, N. The utility of comparative local anesthetic blocks versus placebo-controlled blocks for the diagnosis of cervical zygapophysial joint pain. *Clin J Pain*, 1995, **11**, 208–13.

5. Ravaud, P., Moulinier, L., *et al.* Effects of joint lavage and steroid injection. *Arthritis Rheum*, 1999, **42**, 475–82.

6. Blyth, T., Hunter, J. A., Stirling, A. Pain relief in the rheumatoid knee after steroid injection. *Br J Rheumatol*, 1994, **33**, 461–3.

7. Chakravarty, K., Pharaoh, P. D. P., Scott, D. G. I. A randomized controlled trial of post-injection rest following intra-articular steroid therapy for knee synovitis. *Br J Rheumatol*, 1994, **33**, 464–8.

8. Freidman, D. M., Moore, M. E. The efficacy of intra-articular steroids in osteoarthritis. *J Rheumatol*, 1980, **7**, 850–6.

9. Jacobs, L. G. H., Barton, M. A. J., Wallace, W. A., *et al.* Intra-articular distension and steroids in the management of capsulitis of the shoulder. *BMJ*, 1991, **302**, 1498–501.

10. Haslock, I., MacFarlane, D., Speed, C. Intra-articular and soft tissue injections: a survey of current practice. *Br J Rheumatol*, 1995, **34**, 449–52.

11. Seror, P., Pluvinage, P., Lecoq d'Andre, F., *et al.* Frequency of sepsis after local corticosteroid injection. *Rheumatology*, 1999, **38**, 1272–4.

12. Pal, B., Nash, E. J., Oppenheim, S., *et al.* Routine synovial fluid culture: is it necessary? *Br J Rheumatol*, 1997, **36**, 1116–17.

13. Balch, H. W., Gibson J. M. C., El-Ghobarey, A. F., *et al.* Repeated corticosteroid injections into knee joints. *Rheum Rehab*, 1977, **16**, 137–40.

4.3.3 Soft tissue injections

John Tanner

Rationale

There is no doubt that the careful placement of a small dose of local anaesthetic with corticosteroid in a painful and inflamed soft tissue can provide early and effective symptomatic relief. Other soft tissue injection treatments are discussed later in this section, including trigger point injection and intramuscular needling. Steroid injections are the most commonly used, however, and are the best researched.

Mason *et al.* (1980), Nevelos (1980), and Staff and Nilsson (1980) report on the use of corticosteroids in the treatment of a variety of soft tissue inflammatory conditions with a high success rate. Staff reported the success of treating iliotibial band friction syndrome in long-distance runners with betamethasone. He emphasized, however, that the use of steroid medication is to give temporary relief of symptoms. It does not afford lasting relief unless the mechanical problem that is causing the symptoms is alleviated. Goupille and Sibilia (1996) reviewed all controlled studies between 1955 and 1993 on the efficacy of local corticosteroid injections in the treatment of rotator cuff tendinitis (excluding capsulitis and calcific tendinitis). They concluded that local corticosteroid injections were more effective than placebo and oral non-steroidal antiinflammatories (NSAIDs), especially for pain. However, they raised the question of whether local corticosteroid injections have a deleterious long-term effect on the rotator cuff, and it would seem logical to limit the number of local corticosteroid injections. Watson (1985) showed that poor surgical results were associated with a greater number of preoperative steroid injections, especially five or more. However it is likely that the worse results are more closely correlated with the intensity or severity of the rotator cuff lesions, justifying more frequent symptomatic relief. Chard *et al.* (1988) showed that the natural history of non-operated rotator cuff tendinitis revealed no worse clinical outcome in those patients who had received a greater number of local steroid injections.

Muscle injections

Infiltrations of local anaesthetic alone are more commonly used for trigger point deactivation in myofascial dysfunction. The alternative to the use of local anaesthetic is to dry-needle the muscle trigger point with an acupuncture needle; many authorities would regard this as at least as effective, if not more so (see Chapter 4.3.8). There is no known indication for the use of depot steroid or hydrocortisone directly into muscle tissue other than its use for systemic effects.

Ligaments, tendon sheaths, and bursae

These are the structures most commonly treated by direct corticosteroid infiltration. It has long been known that the direct intratendinous injection of corticosteroid can cause weakening and necrosis of collagen, significantly increasing the chance of tendon disruption, particularly in athletes. Perhaps one of the most commonly injected sites in entire musculoskeletal practice is the musculotendinous origin, the enthesis of the common extensor origin, at the lateral epicondyle for the treatment of 'tennis elbow'. Other entheses commonly treated are the common flexor origin at the medial elbow epicondyle ('golfer's elbow'), the plantar fascia origin on the calcaneal tubercle, or the insertion of the external hip rotators to the posterior greater trochanter.

However, in most instances the role of such infiltrations should be seen as ancillary to the overall therapeutic strategy. Better results will be achieved if account is taken of the functional and biomechanical factors involved in pathogenesis, which will indicate the underlying regimen for rehabilitation.

The rationale that lies behind the use of corticosteroids is based on the observation that many soft tissue lesions, which have traditionally been regarded as self-limiting, continue to cause symptoms long after normal healing should have occurred. As a result of the poor vascularity of dense collagenous tissue found in ligaments and entheses the healing process is delayed or inadequate, leading to a chronic low grade inflammatory response.

An anti-inflammatory agent such as corticosteroid blocks this response, reducing pain and allowing earlier motion. Earlier mobilization is believed to accelerate healing. This theory is both supported and contradicted by various authors who have looked at the effect of steroid on ligaments and tendons in the laboratory. Steroids are known to inhibit collagen synthesis (McCoy *et al.* 1980, Oikarinen *et al.* 1988) but we do not know whether the anti-inflammatory effect of corticosteroid can be separated from the collagen inhibition effect. Furthermore, we know that inflammation is the first phase of healing for collagenous tissues and if this is inhibited by steroids we do not know whether the repair process is simply delayed or permanently altered. The anti-inflammatory action is mediated by inhibition of phospholipase A2 which catalyses the breakdown of membrane phospholipid to arachidonic acid. In contrast, NSAIDs inhibit inflammation at the next step by blocking the enzyme cyclo-oxygenase. Hence corticosteroids inhibit both cyclo-oxygenase and lipo-oxygenase pathways and therefore inhibit the synthesis of leukotrienes in addition to prostaglandins and thromboxanes.

Corticosteroids: animal experiments

Wiggins *et al.* (1994) examined the healing characteristics of the New Zealand white rabbit medial collateral ligament after transection. One group was injected with saline, the second group with a dose of betamethasone, which from an earlier study had been shown to be sufficient to inhibit fibroblastic collagen synthesis, and the third group with a human-equivalent dose of betamethasone. The animals were killed at 10 days and 3 weeks postoperatively and were then subjected to biomechanical testing, collagen ratio analysis, and histological analysis. At 10 days all injected groups showed biomechanical properties significantly inferior to those of non-injected controls. At 3 weeks the human-equivalent steroid group continued to demonstrate significantly inferior properties. The histological appearance of the non-injected specimens at 10 days typically represented the late inflammatory healing phase: i.e. plump fibroblasts predominated, which under electron microscopy contained abundant rough endoplasmic reticulum indicating that they were synthesizing collagen actively. The higher-dose steroid group demonstrated minimal healing with fewer fibroblasts, more disorganization, and substantial oedema. In other words, the inflammatory phase appeared to be delayed or halted. At 3 weeks all the non-injected rabbits demonstrated the typical appearance of remodelling with alignment of collagen fibres and reduced vascularity. The lower-dose steroid group remained hypercellular with immature cells consistent with the proliferative phase of healing. The higher-dose steroid group were even more delayed and less mature than even the 10-day low-dose steroid specimens. Wiggins *et al.* concluded from this study that the anti-inflammatory and collagen- inhibiting properties of steroids cannot be separated and that loss of the inflammatory phase of healing occurs with corticosteroid treatment. This prob-ably represents only delay in healing and not true irreversible inhibition of healing, and what happens in the later phases of remodelling and maturation cannot be determined from this study. One might criticize this study on the basis that surgical transection of a ligament is not typical of the usual kinds of trauma treated in medical practice.

McWhorter *et al.* (1991) investigated the affect of hydrocortisone acetate injected around the Achilles tendon of the adult male rat after blunt trauma. He used 135 rats assigned to three groups. Groups 1 and 2 received a blunt trauma (a weight dropped on to the Achilles tendon). In Group I hydrocortisone in a dose of 12.5 mg was given either once or five times at weekly intervals adjacent to the tendon but not intrasubstance. Group 2 received trauma only. Group 3 received neither trauma or injections. The animals were killed at 3, 6, and 9 weeks, and histological and biomechanical analyses were performed. Hydrocortisone did not adversely affect the strength of the Achilles tendon of animals in this study except during week 6 when the control group demonstrated greater tendon strength than animals that had received trauma but not received injections. Histologically McWhorter *et al.* found that the use of steroids inhibited the presence of some cell types associated with healing. They concluded that if corticosteroid injections are used to treat acute tendinitis their study recommends temporary immobilization and protection of the tendon from stress allowing for natural healing to occur. However, the results of this study seriously question the claims of Wrenn *et al.* (1954), Sweetnam (1969), and Halpern *et al.* (1977), that corticosteroids inhibit the healing process of tendons.

In a follow-up study of the long-term effects of a single injection of corticosteroid on ligament healing in rabbits, Wiggins *et al.* (1995) examined the remodelling and maturation phases and found that the tensile strength of the specimens that had been injected with steroids returned to a value that was equal to that of the controls; however, the resistance to repeated deformation and load remained inferior to that of the controls. This was accompanied by a lag in histological maturation. These studies were performed 84 days after collateral ligament transection and injection with steroid. They concluded that acute corticosteroid treatment of an injured ligament is detrimental to the healing process in both the early and the later phase of healing.

Whether these animal experiments have direct relationship to clinical practice remains uncertain. In reviewing the literature on the use of steroids for Achilles tendon pain, Read and Motto (1992) concluded that steroids can be used safely.

Guidelines for soft-tissue injections

Any practitioner who is willing to perform local anaesthetic and/or corticosteroid infiltrations should be fully conversant with the physico-chemical properties such as time of onset, duration of action, degree of sensory and motor blockade, potency, and lipid solubility. They should be aware of the pros and cons of the use of a vasoconstrictor such as epinephrine (adrenaline), and the potency and potential to cause toxic reactions affecting the central nervous system and cardiovascular system, and to cause allergy. Any practitioner performing injections needs to observe strict aseptic technique and be fully prepared to deal with the possible and occasionally life-threatening complications which can occur such as anaphylaxis, cerebral convulsions, and hypotension. Oxygen, basic resuscitation equipment, airways, intravenous fluids and emergency drugs such as chlorpheniramine, epinephrine, hydrocortisone succinate, atropine, and diazepam should be available in the treatment room.

With our present state of knowledge it is possible to recommend the following basic guidelines when considering the appropriateness of local corticosteroid injection:

1 Perform a full functional assessment of the region concerned including the governing spinal segments. Search for evidence of proximal and distal dysfunctions. Identify biomechanical factors that may predispose to the condition or delay recovery.

2 Consider a trial of physical therapy including mobilizations and manipulation, local anaesthetic trigger point needling, and other approaches before resorting to a steroid injection. If active mobilization is not possible because of acute inflammation, judicious use of a small dose of corticosteroid to the affected site may allow earlier graduated progression of exercise.

3 Use the minimum dose necessary to achieve the therapeutic affect, i.e. no more than 10–20 mg of triamcinolone or 25–50 mg of hydrocortisone for ligament/bursa injection. Increase volume where necessary with local anaesthetic dilution.

4 Avoid intratendinous injection.

5 Recommend avoidance of vigorous exercise of the temporarily weakened tissue for at least 2–3 weeks following injection. However, functional movement of the area encourages new collagen formation with orientation in the lines of stress, to make a more effective repair.

6 As a rule, no more than a series of three injections is advised without a review of the diagnosis and treatment (Woo *et al.* 1975). If relief provided is no more than temporary and the condition continues to relapse, other forms of therapy should be sought, but if there has been good remission for some months or years then a further 1–2 injections could be considered.

Local corticosteroid therapy

Injectable corticosteroid preparations suitable for joint or soft tissue injection are listed in Table 4.3.2. It is generally recommended that the longest-acting preparations are not injected into tendon sheaths as they are less soluble and cause more soft tissue atrophy or chance of tendon rupture. The longest acting, least soluble preparations are typically used for intra-articular injections for a more powerful and long-lasting effect is sought.

Guidelines for the appropriate dose of corticosteroid to be injected as given in Table 4.3.3. Anaesthetic preparations can be safely combined or mixed with a corticosteroid preparation. However, if the corticosteroid preparation contains a paraben compound as a preservative, flocculation of the suspension is likely to occur. In practice

Table 4.3.2. Injectable corticosteroid preparations suitable for joint or soft tissue injection

Preparation	Strengths (mg/ml)	Prednisolone equivalent (mg)
Short acting, soluble		
Dexamethasone sodium phosphate	4	40
Hydrocortisone acetate	25	5
Long acting, less soluble		
Methylprednisolone acetate	20, 40, 80	25, 50, 100
Dexamethasone acetate	8	80
Longest acting, least soluble		
Triamcinolone acetonide	10, 40	12.5, 50
Triamcinolone hexacetonide	20	25
Betamethasone sodium phosphate	6	50

Table 4.3.3. Guidelines for the appropriate dose of corticosteroid to be injected

Site	Prednisolone equivalent dose (mg)
Bursa	10–20
Tendon sheath	10–20
Small joints of hands and feet	5–15
Medium-sized joints	15–25
Large joints	20–50

for the examples given in Table 4.3.3, it is recommended to use 1% lidocaine (lignocaine) either with hydrocortisone or triamcinolone since flocculation or precipitation of the particle does not occur with this combination.

Entheses

Injection of musculotendinous attachments, such as the common extensor origin at the lateral epicondyle, are a useful adjunctive therapy in the management of these common musculoskeletal conditions. A maximum of 10–20 mg of depot steroid such as triamcinolone acetonide, which may be mixed with 1–2 ml of 1% lidocaine (lignocaine), is delivered by meticulous infiltration in a 'peppering' fashion to the site of maximum tenderness. A small-gauge needle is used to deliver 0.1 ml at a time to the length, breadth, and depth of the involved tissue.

The patient should be advised that there may be a temporary exacerbation of pain lasting 12–24 hours; this occurs in a proportion of patients. If severe, this can be treated with application of ice and anti-inflammatories. Care must be taken to ensure that the dose is not delivered in the subcutaneous tissue to avoid the complications of fat atrophy. The patient should be advised to avoid heavy use of the structure for the following 2 weeks. When all or most of the pain has cleared, a programme of stretching and strengthening exercises should be instituted as well as attention to occupation or sports that may involve activities which could cause a recurrence.

Ligaments

Ligament sprains, whether acute or chronic, can be treated effectively with local corticosteroid infiltration. If clinical examination reveals signs of an unstable joint then it is wise to avoid the use of corticosteroids since further weakening of the soft tissue restraints may occur. Such injections are therefore best reserved for first-degree strains of ligaments of peripheral joints, such as the knee or ankle, which are not settling with physiotherapy. A similar dose and method of administration is used as described above with the needle directed towards the ligament attachment to the bone rather than mid substance. This is the area of the ligament that is most richly innervated with pain receptors. In the spine, interspinous ligaments, supraspinous ligaments, iliolumbar and sacroiliac ligaments all respond well to this form of therapy: at peripheral joints the commonest ligaments to be injected are those of the lateral ankle, the meniscotibial ligaments of the knee, the medial collateral ligaments, the ligaments of the wrist and of the acromioclavicular joint. An alternative approach is the use of prolotherapy (see Chapter 4.3.5).

After injection with corticosteroid, a period of up to 2 weeks relative rest of the affected part should be advised before progressing with stronger rehabilitation programmes.

Peritendinous injections

Perhaps the most commonly treated condition in this category is De Quervain's tenosynovitis of the wrist, but all the flexor and extensor tendons of the wrist and fingers can be successfully treated by corticosteroid injections when inflamed. The siting of the injection can be more contained in the portions surrounded by the synovial sheath, often affected where it is under a retinaculum, but small doses can be placed alongside the tendons in other areas. Around the ankle, the peroneal tendons, medial tibial tendons, and extensor tendons of the ankle slide within their sheath, showing swelling, heat and tenderness when inflamed. Using a 23-gauge needle is often ideal: it may be bent to a 25° angle in order to allow insertion into the skin and then to follow a direction parallel with the tendon, so that a bolus dose of 1–2 ml of corticosteroid with local anaesthetic can be given. Patients should be warned of a possible flare-up for 24 hours after the injection, followed by a gradual resolution of symptoms. During the first

2 weeks the affected region should be rested as far as possible in order to avoid undue physical stresses on the tendons.

Bursae

Many of the common sites of bursitis, both superficial and deep, can be identified through standard clinical examination and palpation techniques. In some cases, such as the prepatellar bursa or the olecranon bursa, aspiration of fluid should be attempted and if there is any suspicion of infection corticosteroids should be withheld and the fluid should be sent for microscopy and culture. Less superficial bursae rarely become infected and respond very promptly to appropriate corticosteroid treatment, since these conditions clearly demonstrate the classic signs of acute inflammation. In large bursae such as the subgluteal bursa, up to 20 ml of low-concentration local anaesthetic, such as 0.5% lidocaine (lignocaine), should be administered with 10–20 mg of depot steroid in order to ensure spread of the fluid throughout the bursa. In conditions such as trochanteric bursitis it is rarely possible to aspirate fluid since this is commonly recognized as a 'dry bursitis' except in the instance of rheumatoid or other inflammatory disease.

A stretching routine for the adjacent musculature appears to increase efficacy.

Complications

- **Infection** is rarely encountered with the use of sterile disposable syringes and needles and strict aseptic technique. The frequency of infection is probably the same as with joint injection (see Chapter 4.3.2).

- **Exacerbation of pain:** This is usually temporary, settling in 1–2 days: it occurs more frequently at entheses where ligaments or tendons insert.

- **Steroid flush** of the face may occur for 24–48 hours with higher doses, particularly in women of perimenopausal age.

- **Menstrual irregularities** may follow the use of higher-dose corticosteroid injections or where the series of injections is given over a relatively short period of time. It is important to be aware of this possibility particularly, when the patient is postmenopausal and complains of a bleed for the first time in some years, since it may precipitate gynaecological investigations.

- **Systemic effects of corticosteroids:** These are rarely seen with the low dosages used in this form of injection therapy.

- **Diabetics** should be warned that because of the small amount of steroid that can be absorbed, the blood glucose level will increase slightly for 2–3 days but it is not normally necessary to adjust the insulin regime.

- **Allergy:** This is a rare complication and may be due to the local anaesthetic (more commonly the esters such as procaine), or to the corticoids and any or all of the preservatives contained in the preparations

- **Haematoma:** Danger of haematoma formation is increased by anticoagulant therapy, which is a relative contra-indication to the treatment.

- **Lipoid atrophy:** This occurs particularly with the use of the less soluble steroids rather than hydrocortisone, and is most likely in superficial injections where some of the solution may track back under the skin. In a series of 53 tennis elbow injections Hay et al. (1999) reported that 2 cases showed evidence of skin atrophy at 6 months, and 1 case at 12 months. It is associated with hypopigmentation (more noticable if the adjacent skin is sun-tanned), thinning of the subdermal tissue and telangiectasiae.

References

Chard, M. D et al. (1988) The long term outcome of rotator cuff tendinitis. A review study. Br J Rheumatol, 27, 385–9.

Goupille, P. and Sibilia, J. (1996) Local corticosteroid injections in the treatment of rotator cuff tendinitis, except for frozen shoulder and calcific tendinitis. Clin Exp Rheum, 14, 561–6.

Hay, E. M., Paterson, S. M., Lewis, P., et al. (1999) Pragmatic randomised trial of local corticosteroid injection and naproxen for treatment of lateral epicondylitis of elbow in primary care. BMJ, 319, 964–8.

Halpern, A. A et al. (1977) Tendon ruptures associated with corticosteroid therapy. West J Med, 127, 378–82.

Mason, J. O. et al. (1980) The management of supraspinatus tendinitis in general practice. J Irish Med Assoc, 73(1), 23–4.

McCoy, B. J et al. (1980) In vitro inhibition of cell growth collagen synthesis and prolylhydroxylase activity by triamcinolone acetonide. Proc Soc Exp Biol Med, 163, 216–22.

McWhorter, J. W et al. (1991) Influence of local steroid injections on traumatized tendon properties: A biomechanical and histological study. Am J Sports Med, 19, 435–9.

Nevelos, A. B (1980) The treatment of tennis elbow with triamcinolone acetonide. Curr Med Res Opin, 6, 507–9.

Oikarinen, A. I. et al. (1988) Modulation of collagen metabolism by glucocorticoids. Receptor mediated effects of dexamethasone on collagen biosynthesis in chick embryo fibroblasts and chondrocytes. Biochem Pharmacol, 37, 1451–62.

Read M. T. F., Motto, S. G. (1992) Tendo achillis pain: steroids and outcome. Br J Sports Med, 26, 15–21.

Staff, P. H., Nilsson, S. (1980). Tendoperiostitis in the lateral femoral condyle in long distance runners. Br J Sports Medicine, 14, 38–40.

Sweetnam, R. (1969) Corticosteroid arthropathy and tendon rupture. J Bone Joint Surg, 51B, 397–8.

Watson, M. (1985) Major ruptures of the rotator cuff. J Bone Joint Surg, 67B, 618–24.

Wiggins, M. E. et al. (1994). Healing characteristics of a type 1 collagenous structure treated with corticosteroids. Am J Sports Med, 22, 279–88.

Wiggins, M. E. et al. (1995). Effects of local injection of corticosteroids on the healing of ligaments. J Bone and Joint Surg, 77A, 1682–90.

Woo, S. L.-Y., Matthews, J., Akeson, W., Amiel, D., Convery, R. (1975) Connective tissue response to immobility: correlative study of the biomechanical and biochemical measurements of normal and immobilised rabbit knees. Arthritis Rheum, 18, 257–64.

Wrenn, R. N et al. (1954). An experimental study of the effect of cortisone on the healing process and tensile strength of tendons. J Bone Joint Surg, 35A, 588–601.

4.3.4 **Epidural injections**
Keith Bush

The epidural space is the potential space surrounding the theca in the vertebral canal and runs from the foramen magnum to the sacral hiatus. It therefore forms a useful route whereby drugs that may influence the theca or surrounding tissues can be specifically delivered.

Traditionally, epidural injections have been associated with childbirth and surgical procedures, when local anaesthetic is injected to block the appropriate spinal nerve roots. However, the use of epidural injections in the management of spinal pain goes back to 1901 when Sicard described the introduction of cocaine through the caudal hiatus at the base of the spine.[1] There follows an extensive and enthusiastic literature primarily documenting the use of local anaesthetic and normal saline[2–4] until the addition of corticosteroids in the 1950s.[5–15] Some important clinical syndromes best managed by epidural injections are:

- sciatica
- cervical radiculopathy
- spinal claudication
- acute discogenic back pain
- acute discogenic neck or thoracic spinal pain.

Pathology

In broad terms, much spinal pain can be attributed to either mechanical or inflammatory pathology. Mixter and Barr[16] first drew attention to nerve root compression by a disc herniation as the cause for sciatica in 1934. Subsequently, Rydevick *et al.*[17] expanded upon the pathoanatomy and pathophysiology of nerve root compression. However, access to non-invasive imaging such as CT and MRI has demonstrated that many people with no symptoms may have apparent compressive pathology such as intervertebral disc herniations.[18,19] There are therefore alternative pathologies to pure compression. Recent research has demonstrated that inflammation can play a major role.[20] Olmarker *et al.*[21] have demonstrated that nuclear cell membranes from the nucleus pulposus are neurotoxic, both producing inflammatory and neurophysiological changes. Furthermore, these reactions are blocked by corticosteroids.[22]

Thus nuclear material which herniates into the vertebral canal through a crack in the annulus fibrosus may both compress and irritate the nerve roots and dura, resulting in back pain or sciatica and of course neck pain or brachialgia. Furthermore, repeat scanning has demonstrated that a high proportion of large disc herniations naturally regress with time.[6,23–28] Thus it is perfectly rational to place corticosteroids at the disc–nerve root interface to control inflammation and thus pain, while nature deals with the mechanical issues. However, surgical decompression is still required in some patients.

Indications

Most controlled studies addressing the efficacy of epidural injections for disc lesions have related to the management of sciatica.[5,8–14] Results remain conflicting, but meta-analysis supports the use of epidural corticosteroids in the management of sciatica.[15] Their positive effect is in the intermediate term; over weeks and months.[5,8]

There is therefore a place for repeating epidural injections over several months to control inflammation and thus pain. When this philosophy was applied to the management of 165 patients with sciatica, 86% made a satisfactory recovery without the need for surgical decompression with an average of 3 injections.[6] When managing 68 patients with cervical radiculopathy, the non-surgical outcome was satisfactory in all patients with an average of 2.5 injections.[7]

Thus, in broad terms, all patients with radicular syndromes or dural irritation manifesting as spinal pain are suitable candidates for a trial of epidural injections. Indeed, these injections are useful diagnostically as well as therapeutically in that during the procedure, if the diagnosis is correct, the patient's symptoms may be replicated and then immediately blocked by the anaesthetic.

Patients with cauda equina syndrome (with bowel or bladder dysfunction) or cervical/thoracic myelopathy (with long tract symptoms or signs) may require urgent decompression, but in the common types of sciatica, surgical intervention does not influence the ultimate neurological outcome.[29,30] Thus neurological signs in the form of reduced sensation, reduced power or reflexes are not a contraindication to conservative management: we obtain a surgical opinion in cases with acute and complete foot drop, as urgent decompression may offer the best chance of recovery.

Techniques

Asepsis

When performing epidural injections it is important to have a fastidious aseptic technique. Although infection is very rare, epidural abscess has been reported, leading to severe and permanent neurological deficit. A solution of 0.5% chlorhexidine in 70% alcohol has been shown to be effective against the usual flora to be found on the back. Both the vial tops and the skin should be swabbed with this and allowed to dry before the drugs are aspirated and then injected. A non-touch technique is perfectly adequate: however, sterile gloves should be worn for more intricate, protracted procedures such as selective epidurals/dorsal root ganglion blocks (DRGB). In addition to further protecting the patient from infection, the gloves protect the physician from the occasional flow-back of blood through the needle.

Caudal approach

For lumbar lesions, the caudal epidural injection technique has several advantages. Because the theca generally terminates several centimetres above the sacral hiatus, there is very little chance of intrathecal injection which is more of a hazard with the interlaminar approach. If 0.5%

procaine or lidocaine (lignocaine) without preservative is used, only the unmyelinated, nociceptive C fibres are blocked. There is therefore no loss of sensation or power and the blood pressure is not influenced.[3] The procedure can therefore safely be performed on an outpatient basis, with patients being able to get up and walk out shortly afterwards.

Nevertheless, it is useful to monitor the patients with pulse oximetry, which will draw early attention to a vasovagal attack or other complication. Furthermore, facilities to resuscitate the patient should be available in case of anaphylaxis or spinal block.

- 20 ml 0.5% procaine in normal saline with the addition of a corticosteroid such as 40 mg of triamcinolone is commonly used for the caudal route: this volume should spread to L1–2, covering the usual levels of pathology.[31]

- 10 ml will normally cover to L4–5, thus reaching 90% of discs responsible for sciatica.

Although epidural steroid injections have been performed as a standard procedure over the past four to five decades, no steroid preparation has actually been licensed for use in the epidural space. Methylprednisolone has been extensively used and triamcinolone to a lesser extent. Recently, some controversy has arisen as to whether epidural corticosteroids or the additional constituents of the preparations may be detrimental. However, an extensive report prepared on behalf of the Australian National Health and Medical Research Council has vindicated their use in the epidural space.[32] There is, however, some evidence to suggest that intrathecal corticosteroids may occasionally produce arachnoiditis.

Interlaminar approach

The interlaminar approach is the route preferred by many anaesthetists. However, there is certainly a higher incidence of inadvertent thecal puncture because the distance between the ligamentum flavum and the dura is only millimetres. This should of course be recognized by the experienced injector, but a small dural tear may not be, so that a 'spinal' headache will result. If the injection solution contains anaesthetic, this technique should therefore be only practised in a hospital setting, for fear of a spinal block.

Use of imaging

Accuracy of epidural needle placement can be tested by contrast media and imaging. Stitz and Sommer[33] reported a 74% success rate overall, but higher correct positioning in cases with easily identified bony landmarks. Intravenous injection occurred in 3.7% of their cases. Poor needle placement may be one of the explanations for the lack of efficacy reported by some researchers. There is therefore an argument for performing epidural injections under radiographic control (image intensifier C arm or CT) with the use of contrast media to confirm that the drug has reached the suspected pathology. Either the caudal (Figure 4.3.65) or interlaminar (Figure 4.3.66) route can be used. Furthermore, the intraforamenal route (selective epidural/DRGB) may also prove to be very useful, particularly in cases of lateral recess stenosis and far lateral disc herniation (Figure 4.3.67).

Choice of technique

Fluoroscopy and the specific techniques are obviously more time-consuming and expensive. For this reason it has been our practice first to perform a standard caudal epidural injection when managing appropriate lumbosacral pathology. However, if the response is unsatisfactory a more specific approach can be performed under radiographic control once MRI or CT has been performed to localize the pathology. This allows for a higher concentration of drug to be introduced: 1 ml of 1% lidocaine (lignocaine) without preservative with

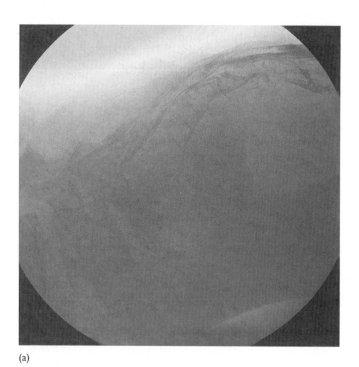

(a)

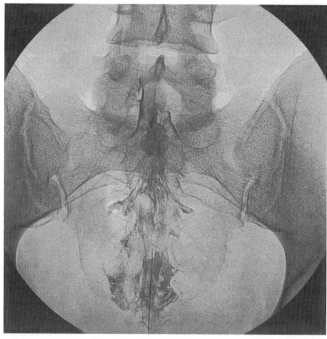

(b)

Figure 4.3.65 Caudal epidurogram demonstrating the satisfactory spread of 5 ml of contrast medium to L5. (a) lateral view; (b) anteroposterior view.

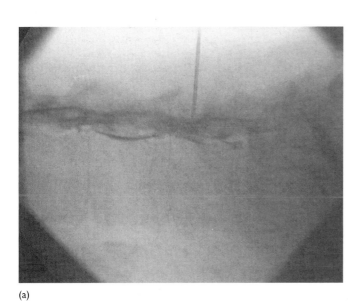

(a)

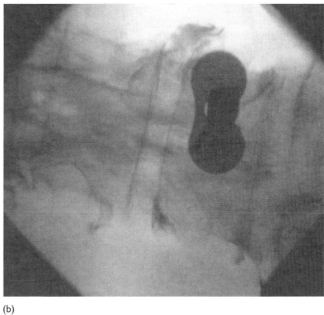

(b)

Figure 4.3.66 Lumbar L3/4 interlaminar epidurogram in a patient with a degree of spinal stenosis: (a) lateral view; (b) anteroposterior view.

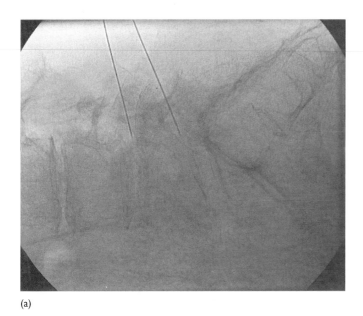

(a)

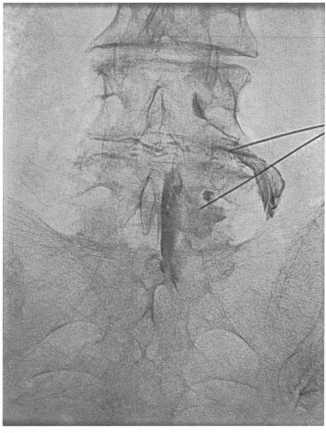

(b)

Figure 4.3.67 Lumbar selective epidurogram/DJRB: two-needle approach to introduce drugs to the L45 intervertebral disc/L5 nerve root interface. Note that the needle posterior to the L4/5 intervertebral disc has entered the herniation and initially, the introduction of contrast has resulted in a discogram until the needle was withdrawn. The lower needle is placed at the 6 o'clock position just below the L5 pedicle: (a) lateral view; (b) anteroposterior view.

40 mg triamcinolone being appropriate for a selective epidural/DRGB after confirming position with 0.5–1 ml of contrast medium (Figure 4.3.67).

In managing a series of 165 patients with sciatica, we found it necessary to resort to more specific injection techniques under radiographic control in 24% of cases.[6] However, of 68 cervical radiculopathies, less than 30% responded to the simple paravertebral block approach with over 70% responding to more specific injection techniques; either interlaminar[7] or intraforamenal (Figure 4.3.68).

The cervical radiculopathies seem to respond even better than the sciaticas, possibly because the cervical root canals are relatively larger than the lumbar root canals, the cervical nerve roots being surrounded by venous sinuses. Radiological contrast adds safety to selective epidurals/DRGB in the cervical spine, where inadvertent intravenous injection occurs more easily and frequently.

Besides steroid and local anaesthetics, other drugs such as morphine, clonidine, and hyaluronidase have been introduced into the epidural space. At present the literature does not present a convincing case for their use.

Caudal epidural injection technique

Caudal epidural injections are best performed with the patient lying prone. This allows for easy identification of the sacral hiatus in the midline. A pillow placed under the pelvis, or breaking the couch to raise the pelvis, is also helpful in bringing the sacral hiatus to prominence. This position is also more comfortable for the occasional patient whose pain is aggravated by spinal extension, but some will still have to lie in the lateral decubitus position to achieve reasonable comfort: in this position the soft tissues fall laterally, making identification of the sacral hiatus more difficult.

The sacral cornua can usually be palpated with the left thumb, bringing the thumb cephalad up the natal cleft. The skin is then marked with a thumbnail imprint which remains evident after the skin is swabbed with antiseptic. If the sacral hiatus is accurately identified, additional local anaesthetic is rarely required when using a 21-gauge 50-mm needle or a 22-gauge 90-mm spinal needle. The needle is introduced with the bevel facing down. This allows it to slide up the sacral canal without embedding into the periosteum. It is usually possible to feel the needle penetrating the membrane over the hiatus and it is then introduced a further 1 cm or so. In the more sensitive patient, 1–2 ml of 1% lidocaine (lignocaine) can be introduced superficially with a 23-gauge 25-mm needle.

Once the needle is in place, the syringe of local anaesthetic and steroid is connected. There is usually a moderate resistance to injection. However, resistance may be very high if the needle is subperiosteal and this can usually be relieved by turning the needle through 180°. It is not uncommon for the needle to be intravenous, and it is therefore most important to aspirate and disconnect the syringe to check for blood flow-back. This problem can usually be resolved by introducing the needle further or slightly retracting it. It is very rare for it to be intrathecal, because the theca usually terminates several centimetres above the sacral hiatus, but if there is any doubt, the procedure should be abandoned and repeated with care a few days later (with minimal distance insertion, possibly using imaging).

The drugs are introduced slowly, but can often exacerbate the patient's back pain or sciatica. This is a good sign, indicating that they have reached the appropriate disc–dural interface. The patient should be told that the faster the injection, the sooner it will be over but the

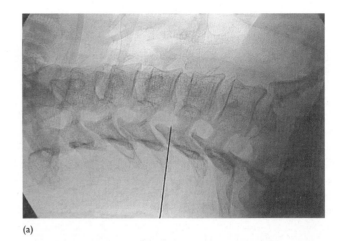

(a)

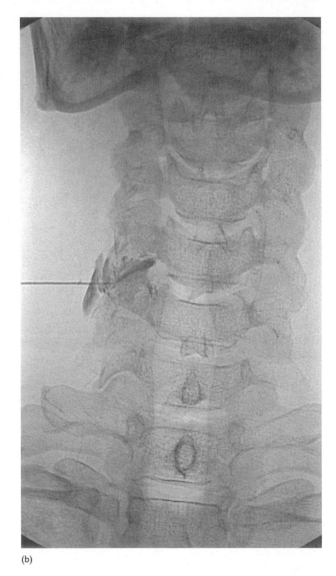

(b)

Figure 4.3.68 Cervical selective epidurogram/DRGB at the C6 level: (a) oblique view – note that the needle is along the posterior surface of the root canal. (b) anteroposterior view – note that contrast has initially spread into the paravertebral tissues until the needle was introduced further up the root canal ensuring placement of drugs at the intervertebral disc/nerve root interface.

more it may hurt and so a balance needs to be struck. Palpating over the sacrum with the left hand can detect an extrasacral injection. If there is any doubt, a woosh test should be performed: once it has been ascertained that the needle is not intravenous, a 10-ml syringe filled with air is connected and this is introduced while auscultating with a stethoscope over the midlumbar spine. A clear 'woosh' should be heard if the needle is correctly in the epidural space. Epidurography is the ultimate confirmation (Figure 4.3.65).

During the procedure, conversation with the patient and additional pulse oximetry leads to early detection of complications. The level of monitoring should reflect the potential for problems (for example in the dosage and siting of local anaesthetic used) with this generally benign procedure. Maximum safety will be achieved by pulse oximetry, blood pressure and cardiac monitor, intravenous line, and the availability of resuscitation equipment and drugs. If there is any concern about the patient's reaction, the procedure should be terminated. The inadvertent intravenous injection of procaine or lidocaine (lignocaine) leads to a feeling of panic with ringing in the ears which passes rapidly if identified early. We avoid the use of bupivacaine because it has cardiotoxic properties.

It usually takes no more than 5 minutes to introduce 20 ml of steroid and local anaesthetic except in patients with very severe sciatica. As stated above, a smaller volume such as 10 ml will give added safety and probably adequate effect. On completion the patient should remain lying down for 10–30 minutes. If straight leg raises were limited, these can then be re-tested to detect improvement due to the anaesthetic effect (and some authors believe this is therapeutic). Although the patient may feel some numbness of the buttocks for half an hour with 0.5% procaine or 0.5% lidocaine (lignocaine), it is very rare for there to be any weakness of the legs. If this does occur, the patient will have to rest until it resolves. The patient must not drive for a few hours.

Patients are instructed to proceed with care and lead a mobile but quiet lifestyle if the back condition allows. They are warned that when the anaesthetic wears off there may be an initial exacerbation of symptoms for up to a few days. There is potential for improvement over a few weeks when using a depot steroid such as triamcinolone. If some improvement is achieved, but not enough, the procedure can be repeated on several further occasions ranging from a few weeks to a few months.

Interlaminar epidural injection technique

Lumbar and thoracic interlaminar epidural injections are best performed with the patient lying in the lateral decubitus position with the symptomatic side lowermost. Cervical epidural injections are best performed with the patient lying prone and the neck in flexion, which is aided by a break in the table. Radiographic control can confirm the spinal level and contrast medium can illustrate correct position in the epidural space (Fig 4.3.66).

Using a non-touch technique, 5 ml of 1% lidocaine (lignocaine) is introduced into the soft tissues, confirming the level with lateral and anteroposterior screening. After the operator has scrubbed up and put on sterile gloves, a 16-gauge Tuohy needle (18-gauge with cervical epidurals) is then introduced using a loss of resistance technique with normal saline. Up to 5 ml of contrast medium is then introduced to absolutely confirm position before introducing 40–80 mg triamcinolone and 5 ml 1% lidocaine (lignocaine) isotonic (without preservative) – or normal saline if preferred. In the cervical spine a mixture of 1 ml 1% lidocaine (lignocaine) and 50 mg (5 ml) triamcinolone is used.

There is no need to introduce a catheter in the lumbar and thoracic spines, but in the cervical spine it is best because the needle is not so well supported and the epidural position may be lost when changing syringes. It is best for the patient to rest and be monitored for 2 hours after the procedure, but otherwise the same postinjection instructions apply as for caudal epidural injections.

Lumbar selective epidural injections

Lumbar selective epidural injections/DRGB are best performed with the patient lying in the prone position and screening in the anteroposterior and lateral planes. A butterfly needle serves as a marker to aim for the '6 o'clock' position just caudad of the appropriate pedicle, in the intervertebral foramen. The skin can then be marked a handsbreadth lateral to the spinous processes.

In selecting the level to be injected, we target the exiting nerve, e.g. L4 (at the L4–5 foramen) although the imaging usually shows that the nerve is embarrassed by the disc above (L3–4) – and the fluid tracks upward along the nerve.

Using an appropriate aseptic technique, a 22-gauge 90-mm spinal needle is introduced at about 45° with alternate screening in the anteroposterior and lateral planes. Occasionally a 125-mm needle is required. The needle can be steered away from the bevel to achieve correct position before introducing between 0.5–1 ml contrast medium which may exacerbate the patient's sciatica (Figure 4.3.67). If need be, additional 1% lidocaine (lignocaine) can be introduced into the paraspinal tissues but great care must be exercised not to injure the nerve root. It is therefore not appropriate to introduce local anaesthetic too close to the root canal until the needle is in place, and when close to the root canal the needle is introduced very slowly. For the S1 nerve root, commonly affected by L5–S1 disc prolapse, the approach is almost vertically into the first sacral foramen. Because the sacrum usually tilts forward, best visualization of the foramen may need up to 45° angle of the X-ray beam. A mixture of just 1 ml 1% lidocaine (lignocaine) isotonic (without preservative) with 40 mg (1 ml) triamcinolone is injected around the appropriate nerve root and a similar injection can be made at the next foramen up, e.g. L5, giving a double chance of reaching the disc–nerve root interface (Figure 4.3.67). Occasionally patients experience some leg numbness and weakness from the local anaesthetic.

Cervical selective epidural injection technique

Cervical selective epidural injections/DRGB are best performed with the patient lying supine with the head and neck on a completely radiolucent table to allow for oblique as well as anteroposterior and lateral screening. The cricoid is a guide to the C6 level and the C7 transverse process can usually be palpated in the interscalene space between scalenus anterior and scalenus medius.

Using an appropriate aseptic technique, a 22-gauge 90-mm needle is introduced laterally at the appropriate level into the interscalene space, avoiding the external jugular vein. It is directed slightly posteriorly and the level checked by screening in the lateral plane. The root canals are best viewed in the oblique plane: about 30° from the lateral plane (Figure 4.3.68).

The needle is introduced until it abuts the posterior canal wall. The bevel is then turned to face posteriorly and the needle is stepped over the edge and introduced very slowly along the posterior surface of the root canal so as to avoid piercing the nerve root. It is introduced about halfway down the canal as assessed in the anteroposterior plane. It is very common for the needle to be intravenous, and it needs to be adjusted in or out until contrast flows up the root canal (it may exacerbate the patient's arm symptoms) (Figure 4.3.68). Aspiration and observation is made for flow-back of venous or arterial blood and cerebrospinal fluid. Then 1 ml of 1% lidocaine (lignocaine) isotonic (without preservative) plus 40 mg (1 ml) of triamcinolone is introduced slowly. This may also exacerbate the patient's usual arm symptoms.

After the procedure the patient may experience some arm numbness and weakness for half an hour or so.

Side effects

In reviewing over 10 000 epidural procedures before 1982, Corrigan et al.[34] point out that reports of major complications are exceedingly rare. Abram et al.[35] also confirmed this in their 1996 review of the literature. This has certainly been my experience in performing some 14 000 procedures over the past two decades. However, technique should be fastidious. Anyone intending to perform these techniques should seek appropriate instruction and only attempt injections in the cervical spine under supervision.

There are a number of minor side effects, such as initial exacerbation of symptoms usually for a few hours to a few days, and menstrual irregularity. The incidence of side effects was calculated by Tanner[36] in a survey of almost 75 000 epidural procedures (see Table 4.3.4). Side effects can be broadly classified into those resulting from the corticosteroid, from the local anaesthetic, and from the physical effects of the procedure. Some physicians choose to avoid the potential for side effects of local anaesthetic by using normal saline for making up the solution to be injected epidurally.

Diabetes

People with diabetes should be warned that their blood sugar may increase for a few days or weeks, according to the corticosteroid dose and preparation. Insulin may need to be increased over this period. Some authorities have also suggested the use of prophylactic antibiotics in diabetics.

Anticoagulants

Patients on warfarin should stop this for 4 days before the injection, if their specialist agrees. This precaution reduces the chances of an epidural haematoma.

Table 4.3.4. Complications of epidural injections

Anaphylaxis	0.01%
Hypersensitivity	0.01%
Prolonged hypotension	0.02%
Epidural abscess	0.005%
Headaches	0.07%
Severe aggravation of pain	
for under 24 hours	1%
for over 72 hours	0.29%

Conclusions

Epidural steroid injection remains a most useful procedure when dealing with carefully selected spinal syndromes, but the benefit to the individual seems poorly conveyed by the controlled trials. A grateful ENT surgeon crystallized this sentiment: 'I am hard pushed to think of one procedure in my specialty which has such a dramatic and immediate benefit with so few possible side effects. I envy you.'

References

1. Sicard, A. Les injections medicamenteuses extra-durales par voie sacro-coccygienne. *Comptes Rendus Hebdomadaires des Séances et Mémoires de la Société de Biologie*, 1901, **53**, 396–8.

2. Bhatia, M. T, Parikh, L. C. J. Epidural saline therapy in lumbo-sciatic syndrome. *Journal of the Indian Medical Association*, 1966, **47**(11), 537–42.

3. Cyriax, J. *Textbook of orthopaedic medicine*, Vol 1, 8th edn. Baillière Tindall, London, 1984, pp. 319–26

4. Gupta, A. K. *et al.* Observations on the management of lumbosciatic syndromes (sciatica) by epidural saline. *Journal of the Indian Medical Association*, 1970, **54**, 194–6.

5. Bush, K., Hillier, S. A controlled study of caudal epidural injections of triamcinolone plus procaine in the management of intractable sciatica. *Spine*, 1991, **16**, 572–5.

6. Bush, K. *et al.* The natural history of sciatica associated with disc pathology. A prospective study with clinical and independent radiologic follow-up. *Spine*, 1992, **17**, 1205–12.

7. Bush, K., Hillier, S. Outcome of cervical radiculopathy treatd with peri-radicular/epidural corticosteroid injections: a prospective study with independent clinical review. *European Spine Journal*, 1996, **5**, 319–25.

8. Carette, S. *et al.* Epidural corticosteroid injections for sciatica due to herniated nucleus pulposus. *New England Journal of Medicine*, 1997, **336**(23), 1634–40.

9. Cuckler, J. M. The use of epidural steroids in the treatment of lumbar radicular pain. *Journal of Bone and Joint Surgery*, 1986, **67A**, 6306–12.

10. Dilke, T. FW. *et al.* Extradural corticosteroid injection management of lumbar nerve root compression. *British Medical Journal*, 1973, **2**, 635–7.

11. Klenerman, C. *et al.* Lumbar epidural injection in the treatment of sciatica. *British Journal of Rheumatology*, 1984, **23**, 35–8.

12. Koes, B. W. *et al.* Efficacy of epidural steroid injections for low back pain and sciatica: a systematic review of randomized clinical trials. *Pain*, 1995, **63**, 279–88.

13. Ridley, M. G. *et al.* Out-patient lumbar epidural corticosteroid injection in the management of sciatica. *British Journal of Rheumatology*, 1998, **27**, 295–301.

14. Snoek, W. *et al.* Double blind evaluation of extradural methylprednisolone for herniated lumbar discs. *Acta Orthopaedica Scandinavica*, 1977, **48**, 535–41.

15. Watts, R. W, Silagy, C. A. A meta-analysis on the efficacy of epidural corticosteroids in the treatment of sciatica. *Anaesthesia and Intensive Care*, 1995, **23**, 564–9.

16. Mixter, W. J., Barr, J. A. Rupture of the intervertebral disc with involvement of the spinal canal. *New England Journal of Medicine*, 1934, **211**, 210–15.

17. Rydevick, B. *et al.* Patho-anatomy and pathophysiology of nerve root compression. *Spine*, 1984, **9**, 7–17.

18. Jensen, M. C. Magnetic resonance imaging of the lumbar spine in people without back pain. *New England Journal of Medicine*, 1994, **331**, 69–73.

19. Wiesel, S. W *et al.* A study of computer assisted tomography. 1: The incidence of positive CAT scans in an asymptomatic group of patients. *Spine*, 1984, **9**, 549–51.

20. McCarron, R. F *et al.* The inflammatory effect of the nucleus pulposus. *Spine*, 1987, **12**, 758–64.

21. Olmarker, K. *et al.* Autologous nucleus pulposus induced neurophysiologic and histologic changes in porcine cauda equina nerve roots. *Spine*, 1993, **18**, 1425–9.

22. Olmarker, K. *et al.* Effects of methylprednisolone on nucleus pulposus-induced nerve root injury. *Spine*, 1994, **19**, 1803–8.

23. Bozzao, A *et al.* Lumbar disc herniation: MR imaging assessment of natural history in patients treated without surgery. *Radiology*, 1992, **185**, 135–41.

24. Bush, K. *et al.* The pathomorphologic changes that accompany the resolution of cervical radiculopathy. *Spine*, 1997, **22**, 183–6.

25. Delauche-Cavalier, M. C. *et al.* (1992). Lumbar disc herniation. Computed tomography scan changes after conservative treatment of nerve root compression. *Spine*, **17**, 927–32.

26. Maigne, J. V *et al.* Computed tomographic follow-up study of forty eight cases of non-operatively treated lumbar intervertebral disc herniation. *Spine*, 1992, **17**, 1071–8.

27. Maigne, J. V., Deligne, L. Computed tomographic follow-up study of 21 cases of non-operatively treated cervical intervertebral soft disc herniation. *Spine*, 1994. **19**, 189–91.

28. Saal, J. A. *et al.* The natural history of lumbar disc extrusions treated non-operatively. Spine, 1990, **15**, 683–6.

29. Hakelius, A. Prognosis in sciatica. *Acta Orthopaedica Scandinavica (Suppl)*, 1970, **129**, 1–76.

30. Weber, H. Lumbar disc herniation: A controlled prospective study with ten years of observation. *Spine*, 1983, **2**, 131–40.

31. Burn, J. M. *et al.* The spread of solutions injected into the epidural space. *British Journal of Anaesthesiology*, 1973, **45**, 338–45.

32. *Epidural use of steroids in the management of back pain.* National Health and Medical Research Council Australia, 1994, pp. 1–76.

33. Stitz, M. Y., Sommer, H. M. Accuracy of blind versus fluoroscopically guided caudal epidural injection. *Spine*, 1999, **24**, 1371–6.

34. Corrigan, B. *et al.* Intraspinal corticosteroid injections. *Medical Journal of Australia*, 1982, Mar 6, 224–5.

35. Abram, S. E., O'Connor, T. Complications associated with epidural steroid injections. *Regional Anaesthesia*, 1966, 21(2), 149–62.

36. Tanner, J. A. Epidural injections. A new survey of complications and analysis of the literature. *Journal of Orthopaedic Medicine*, 1996, **18**, 78–82.

4.3.5 Spinal injections

John Tanner

Anyone considering performing spinal injections needs proper training to achieve a defined level of competence. This is usually available within a specialty or may be provided by a multidisciplinary organization (such as BIMM in the UK).

Spinal injections usually involve the use of local anaesthetics within or close to the epidural space, and so entail potential risks. The operator therefore needs to have available a skilled nurse or assistant, intravenous fluids, oxygen, emergency drugs including adrenaline (epinephrine), hydrocortisone succinate, diazepam and others, as well as resuscitation equipment, and needs to regularly update on Advanced Life Support courses (run by the Resuscitation Council in the UK).

The descriptions of techniques outlined below, although detailed, are no substitute for proper training under supervision.

Cervical facet joint injection

These joints can be readily palpated between the muscles and the tender levels identified.

Indications

'Mechanical' pain, i.e. pain on active movement felt in the cervico-scapular/upper thoracic area that is resistant to manual therapy and postural re-training, in the absence of disc signs such as radiculopathy, with positive evidence of tenderness over specific levels in the articular column. (common in limited chronic whiplash-associated disorders). Extension, rotation, and sidebending may be painful and limited.

When performing cervical facet joint injections 'blind' (without fluoroscopic control), levels above C2/3 should not be attempted, for obvious reasons.

Materials

A 5-ml syringe, a 90-mm 22-gauge spinal needle (or 21-gauge hypodermic 40-mm needle for a thinner person), 10 mg depot steroid (per joint), 1% lignocaine (lidocaine).

Technique

Sit the patient leaning over the side of a raised treatment table so as to flex the neck, with the head supported on back of hands or a firm pillow. If the patient is liable to faint, lie them prone over a couch with a breathing hole and support the upper chest to achieve neck flexion.

Even with the neck flexed in this way, the cervical laminae overlap to such an extent that providing one approaches the lateral articular column from a perpendicular angle, there is no chance of passing between the articular processes and into the spinal canal.

A thorough working knowledge of anatomy is required, in particular identification of bony landmarks such as the C2 and C7 spinous processes. With the cervical lordosis flattened, the C2/3 facet joint lies on a line drawn between the C2 and C3 spinous processes. Because of the increasing length and slope of the distal spinous processes, the interarticular line tends to lie closer to the line drawn at the level of the lower end of the upper spinous process (see Figure 4.3.69).

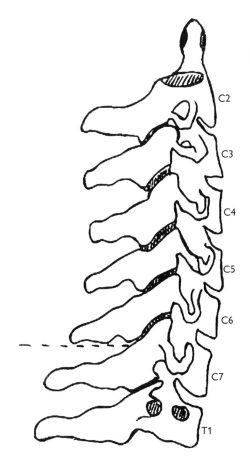

Figure 4.3.69

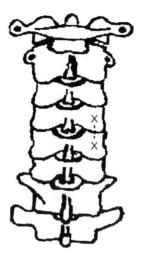

Figure 4.3.70 (R) C_{4-5} perifacetal injection.

Mark the tender levels, and prepare the skin with full aseptic technique.

Local anaesthetic can be infiltrated into skin and overlying muscle to raise a bleb at least one fingerbreadth (patient's finger size) from the midline.

The spinal needle is then directed through this wheal perpendicularly until it contacts bone. The stylet is withdrawn, the syringe with medication is fitted to the needle hub, and 0.3 ml of the mixture of steroid and local anaesthetic is injected after careful aspiration. The needle is walked up and down the articular column, staying parallel to the midline, depositing 0.2–0.3 ml at each point after careful aspiration. A total of 2 ml of local anaesthetic with steroid is deposited in this 'peri-facetal' intracapsular area. Care must be taken not to stray medially or laterally off the imaginary line parallel to the spinous processes, injecting only when in contact with bone (see Figure 4.3.70).

Complications

- **Intravascular injection:** The posterior route is unlikely to risk vertebral artery trespass unless the needle strays above C2.

- **Dural puncture:** A possible complication if needle strays towards the midline. Should be recognized early if slow and careful aspiration is performed regularly. No injection should be made unless the needle is in contact with bone.

- **Postoperative care:** Loss of balance and dizziness may occur if too many joints are injected in one session. This is due to local anaesthesia of joint proprioceptors. The patient should be escorted home and not permitted to drive.

Cervical facet joint injection under fluoroscopic control

These joints can be approached from a posterior or lateral approach. (Injection of the atlanto-occipital and atlantoaxial joints require special knowledge and skills which will not be covered in this section).

Indications

As for cervical facet joint injection (above).

Materials

Two 5 ml syringes, a 22-gauge or 25-gauge 90-mm spinal needle, 1% lignocaine (lidocaine), depot steroid, contrast medium.

Technique

Posterior approach

The patient lies prone with a pillow under the sternum to flex the neck.

Anteroposterior screening with intensifier directed craniad will identify the characteristic corrugated lateral edge of the articular columns. The joint margins lie at the convex points and the medial branches of the posterior primary ramus at the concave or waisted areas.

Raise a bleb over the midpoint of the designated facet joints viewed under this anteroposterior cranially oriented angle. Direct the needle to the posterior aspect of the joint. If these are not well visualized because of the mandible and metalware in the mouth, rotate the patient's head and jaw to the contralateral side. This also helps 'open' the lateral margin of the joints.

The needle tip should be insinuated carefully and slowly between the articular processes; a 25-gauge needle may be easier in very degenerated joints. The needle should not be passed too far into the joint, to avoid traversing it entirely and penetrating the root canal space or dura. A test dose of contrast (0.1–0.2 ml) should be used to obtain an arthrogram before injecting 1 ml or so of local anaesthetic and steroid (Figures 4.3.71 and 4.3.72).

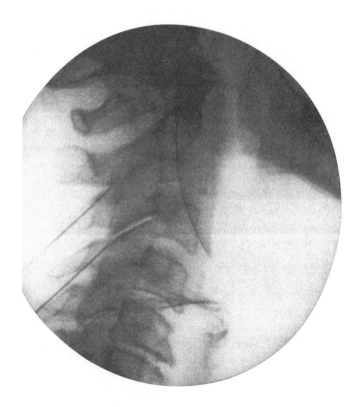

Figure 4.3.71 Posterior approach to C_{2-3} and C_{3-4}.

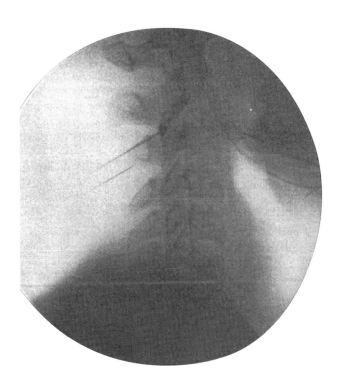

Figure 4.3.72 C$_{2-3}$ arthrogram — right.

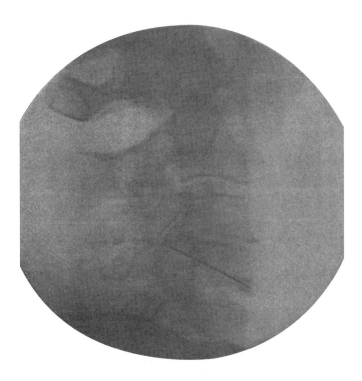

Figure 4.3.73

Lateral approach

This is more comfortable for the patient, and makes it easier to visualize the joints. If it s possible to get a view straight through both joints, then placement is easy. If not, rotate the C-arm of the image intensifier a few degrees, and the uppermost level will move towards the same side of the rotation, separating the two sets of joint margins. C2–3 is often approached more easily in this way (Figure 4.3.73).

Lumbar facet joints

Indications

'Mechanical' pain in the absence of signs of disc prolapse or radicular irritation, not responsive to manual therapy or therapeutic exercise. Pain usually refers only to the back or pelvic area, occasionally more distally into the limb. Features of the history include pain on upright activity, relief with recumbency, and older age group. Contrary to widely held belief, pain on active extension and/or rotation is no predictor of response to facet joint blocks.

Tenderness may be found directly on deep palpation of the affected levels or by performing the Mennell facet rock test. Radiological changes of degeneration are not helpful in determining the affected levels, but SPECT may be.

Meticulous intra-articular blocks using double-blinded, double-block design (one trial with short-acting, another with long-acting anaesthetic) suggests that facet joint pain is responsible for between 15% and 40% of a population with chronic 'non-specific' low back pain. However, perifacetal blocks, as outlined below, being less specific, may ameliorate a wider range of problems related to the posterior spinal column.

Materials

A 5-ml syringe, a 22-gauge 90-mm spinal needle, 1% lignocaine (lidocaine), 10–20 mg triamcinolone (per joint).

Technique

It is useful to have a plain anteroposterior radiograph to hand to check for any bony anomalies or significant rotational scoliosis (Do not attempt 'blind' perifacetal injection in the latter case).

The patient lies prone over a pillow or wedge to flatten out the lumbar region. The spinous processes are palpated and intersecting lines marked between them (see Figure 4.3.74). The facet joints lie approximately 2–2.5 cm from the midline at their intersections, slightly less at the upper lumbar levels and slightly more at the lumbosacral level, taking into account the size of the patient.

Raise a bleb with local anaesthetic overlying the target facet joints. Direct the 22-gauge 90-mm spinal needle perpendicularly on to the articular processes. In a thin person, you will contact bone at half penetration, i.e. 4–4.5 cm, but in a more obese or well-muscled person you may reach 8–9 cm before striking bone. Using the same technique of walking the needle up and down a line parallel to the midline, you can verify whether you are indeed on the articular processes which lie more superficial or on the lamina, which lies deeper ('up the mountain, down the valley'). In this way, you can infiltrate the pericarticular tissues with a total of 2-3 ml of a 50 : 50 mixture of local anaesthetic and triamcinolone, and reach the proximal or distal facet joint to cover two

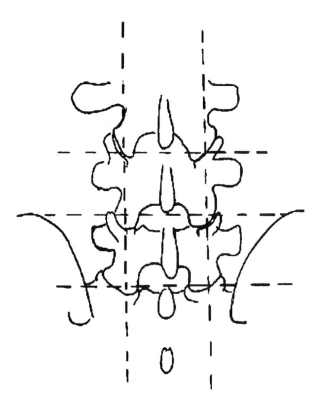

Figure 4.3.74 'Blind' lumbar facet joint approach, grid drawing.

Remember always to aspirate slowly before injecting and never to inject unless you are on bone.

levels. It is inadvisable to angle the needle too far cranially since it increases the risk of straying medially and through the ligamentum flavum.

If at first pass the needle does not contact bone, the chances are that you are too wide, in which case withdraw the needle almost to the skin and slide the skin with needle 0.5 cm medial so that you can make your second pass maintaining a perpendicular angle rather than simply angling the needle more medially.

Sometimes the needle tip can conveniently be 'snuck in' between the articular processes and come to rest after 2–3 mm against bone. Injecting the medication there will meet high resistance, indicating a true intra-articular facet injection. The joint normally admits no more than 1–1.5 ml, unless there is capsular rupture.

Try to ensure you are always directing the needle perpendicular to the plane of the lumbar spine, avoid directing the needle medially or too far cranially for obvious reasons.

Lumbar facet joints injection under fluoroscopic control

Indications

As for lumbar facet joints, above.

Materials

Two 5-ml syringes, 22-gauge 90-mm spinal needles, 1% lignocaine (lidocaine), depot steroid, water-soluble contrast medium.

Technique

The patient lies prone. Take an anteroposterior view initially and raise a bleb overlying the inferior aspect of the designated facet joints. The sagittal plane of the joint is easy to identify in the upper lumbar levels but is usually oblique and not readily visualized at L4–5 and L5–S1. Follow the line of the lamina down to the tip of the inferior articular process and mark the entry point there.

Direct the spinal needle perpendicularly down to bone and directly into the inferior recess of the capsule. The characteristic feel of the tip snicking into this cleft is reassuring, but not always reliable. Inject a test dose of contrast (0.2 ml) and screen. If a facet arthrogram is obtained, inject 1–1.5 ml of steroid and local anaesthetic against the usual high resistance. At the lower lumbar levels, once the needle tip is on bone but no arthrogram has been obtained, rotate the C-arm of the image intensifier obliquely to the respective side while screening until the plane of the joint is identified. Re-site the needle tip until it lies at the inferior recess of the joint and inject a test dose of contrast to obtain an arthrogram.

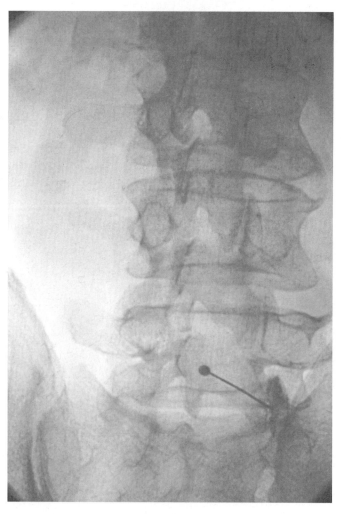

Figure 4.3.75 Right L5-S1 facet joint arthrogram.

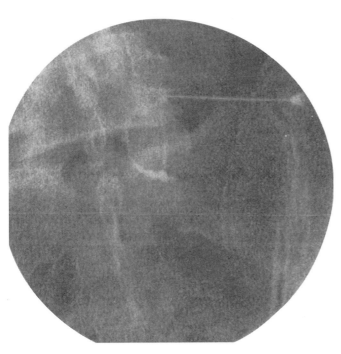

Figure 4.3.76 Facet arthrogram L₅–S₁ superior approach.

At L5–S1 you may need more than 45° rotation to see the parallel joint surfaces of the articular processes. Occasionally, even when in the joint, the contrast does not show. This indicates that the needle is intravascular. Reposition the needle towards the superior recess, taking care not to pass too far over the top and into the lateral root canal (Figures 4.3.75 and 4.3.76).

Paralaminar or paravertebral lumbar nerve block

Indications

Leg pain due to radicular irritation or compression that is not responsive to epidural steroid injection; lateral canal sterotic syndrome; far lateral disc hemiation.

It is useful to have CT or MRI confirmation of the nerve root involved, although imaging does not always provide conclusive information.

Materials

A 5 ml syringe, a 22-gauge 90-mm spinal needle, 1% lignocaine (lidocaine), 20 mg triamcinolone.

Technique

The patient lies prone over a pillow.

Mark out the intersecting horizontal lines between the spinous processes that you have identified (as for facet injections). Mark the spot 2–2.5 cm lateral to the midline that lies midway between these lines on the relevant side. This should overlie the edge of the lamina just below the origin of the transverse process. Raise a bleb at this

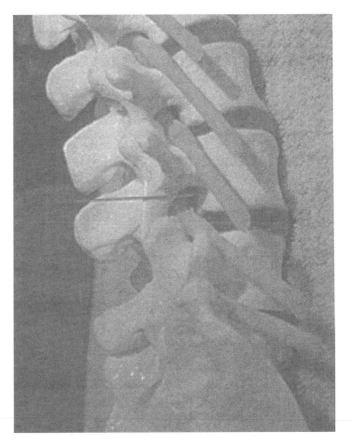

Figure 4.3.77

point and direct the needle perpendicularly downwards till it contacts bone. You should be on the lamina of the vertebra of the relevant emerging spinal nerve. Note depth of penetration. Withdraw almost to skin, perform the same skin-slide technique 0.5 cm laterally and direct perpendicularly to 1 cm deeper than your presumed lamina depth achieved at first pass. Advance very slowly for this last 1 cm in case you hit the nerve (Figure 4.3.77).

If you strike bone again at the same depth, repeat the skin-slide technique 0.5 cm laterally. If you hit bone again at the same depth and you are 3–3.5 cm lateral to the midline, you are on the transverse process. Therefore withdraw again almost to the skin, skin-slide caudally 0.5 cm and you should pass deeper. Aspirate slowly.

Injection in this extraforaminal plane meets little or no resistance and may stimulate paraesthesiae and eventually numbness or weakness in the relevant dermatome (if you have used local anaesthetic to confirm effect).

C7 paravertebral nerve block

Indications

C7 radiculopathy

Materials

A 5 ml syringe, a 23-gauge 2.5 cm hypodermic needle, 1% lignocaine (lidocaine), depot steroid.

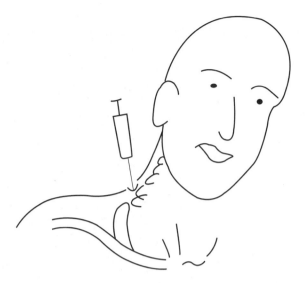

Figure 4.3.78 C₇ paravertebral block.

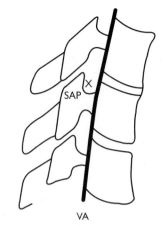

Figure 4.3.79 Oblique view mid cervical foramina. X – marks needle tip placement; SAP – superior articular process; VA – vertebral artery.

Technique

Sit the patient up with shoulder girdles relaxed. From behind, palpate the C7 transverse process in the supraclavicular fossa at the root of the neck. This is found by downward pressure midway between the clavicle and border of the descending trapezius. Mark the entry point. Raise a bleb with local anaesthetic. Direct the 23-gauge 2.5-cm needle attached to a syringe filled with 20 mg depot steroid and 1.5 ml 1% lignocaine (lidocaine) about 30° caudal and medially until you strike the tip of the articular process at C7. Aspirate slowly; if negative, inject slowly (Figure 4.3.78).

Complications

Too inferiorly directed a path may lead to pneumothorax. Starting too anterior to the transverse process line risks passing up the root canal or puncturing the vertebral artery. Both complications are avoidable by starting just posterior to the lateral prominence of the transverse process.

Cervical transforaminal (intraforaminal) nerve root blocks under fluoroscopic control

Indications

Cervical nerve root foraminal encroachment; compression or irritation due to disc protrusion.

Materials

Two 5-ml syringes, a 5-cm 25-gauge spinal needle, 1% lignocaine (lidocaine) or saline (preservative free), non-particulate steroid, contrast medium.

Technique

The patient lies supine on a radiolucent trolley, with the head and neck supported on an extended section.

Identify target level under lateral screening. Rotate the C-arm to an oblique position until the foramina are well visualized. This may require rotating the intensifier caudally 10° or so to 'look up' the foramina.

Mark the entry point directly over anterior margin of superior articular process. Slowly direct the spinal needle 'down the beam' to the articular process. Once you have contacted bone, rotate the C-arm to the anteroposterior position and redirect the needle slightly anteriorly to slip off the posterior column into the foramen. The ideal position is in the posterior part of the foraminal floor (see Figure 4.3.79).

Inject 0.5 ml contrast to display dorsal root ganglion and root. Ensure that the needle tip is not intravascular and has not strayed medially past the mid-zygoapophyseal 'line', as viewed under anteroposterior screening. This reduces the chance of intrathecal injection, although it does not eliminate it.

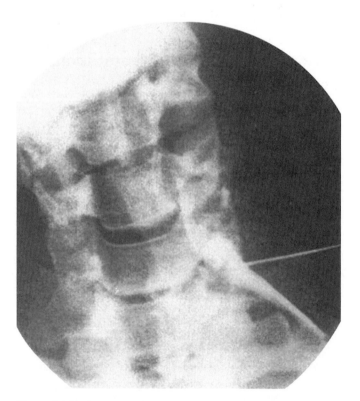

Figure 4.3.80 C₇ neurogram.

It is vitally important to ensure that the needle is not intradural or intravascular before injecting medication, particularly if local anaesthetics is being used. Contrast medium should always be used (Figure 4.3.80).

Complications

- Avoid lignocaine (lidocaine) with adrenaline and particulate steroids in all spinal nerve blocks because of the risk of radicular spinal artery injection causing ischaemia.

- Intradural injection, leading to spinal hypotension and cardiac arrest.

- Intravascular injection, leading to toxicity, or cord ischaemia.

- Haematoma of soft tissues, leading to airways obstruction.

Lumbar transforaminal (intraforaminal) nerve root block under fluoroscopic control

Indications

As for paravertebral nerve block. (NB: The use of the term 'selective nerve root block' should be reserved for small-volume extraforaminal injection.)

In the foramen the injected solution clearly spreads to more than one level, anaesthetizing the sinuvertebral nerve, and at L2 the afferents from most of the anterior spinal column in the lumbar region. A positive analgesic response does not necessarily inculpate that particular segment as the sole or main pain generator.

Materials

Two 5-ml syringes, a 22-gauge spinal needle, 1% lignocaine (lidocaine) or saline (preservative free), depot steroid, 90 mm contrast medium.

Technique

The patient lies prone with lumbar spine flattened. Use anteroposterior fluoroscopy to identify target level and rotate the C-arm obliquely to the required side to about 30–45°.

The superior articular process (SAP, Scottie dog's ear) points to the target of the emerging nerve root under the pedicle (see Figure 4.3.81). Mark the skin, and direct the 22-gauge spinal needle down the tunnel of the beam. Once you have passed the SAP, that is passed over the top of the zygoapophyseal joint, or when you have reached sufficient depth (in larger patients you may need a 120-mm or even a 150-mm needle), redirect the C-arm to anteroposterior viewing.

Guide the needle carefully to the 6 o'clock position just under the face of the pedicle. Ideally, 1 ml of contrast injection should flow centrally and peripherally to outline the nerve root (Figure 4.3.82).

Any pain or resistance to injection requires adjustment of the needle tip position. (In sterotic canals or where there is fibrosis, it may not be possible to eliminate these obstructions entirely).

Once you are satisfied with the neurogram obtained, inject 2–3 ml of local anaesthetic mixed with corticosteroid. Injection of larger

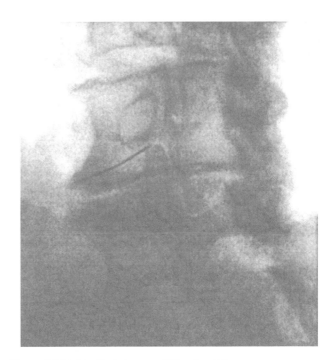

Figure 4.3.81 Needle tip between SAP and pedicle.

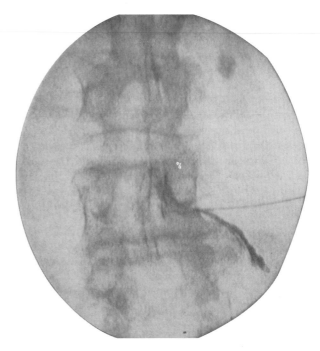

Figure 4.3.82 (R) L$_4$ foraminal injection. Note contrast flow centrally and peripherally with marked deviation around lateral osteophyte.

volumes or concentrations is not necessary, and increases the risk of complications.

Complications

- Intravascular injection: local anaesthetic toxicity (avoid by using contrast).

420

- Intraneural injection: nerve damage (avoid by adjusting needle position if painful).
- Intradural injection: can be avoided by checking contrast flow and not passing needle medial to the 6 o'clock position under pedicle.

First sacral root block (without fluoroscopic control)

Indications

As for paralaminar (paravertebral) lumbar nerve root block when the first sacral root is irritated or compressed.

Materials

As for lumbar nerve root.

Technique

Raise a wheal with local anaesthetic 1 fingerbreadth lateral to the S1 spinous process approximately midway between posterior superior iliac spine and mid-line of sacrum. This should overlie the S1 posterior foramen.

Direct the 22-gauge 90-mm spinal needle perpendicularly down until it contacts bone. The depth at which you contact the posterior surface of the sacrum should be noted. Withdraw almost to the skin and redirect slightly caudal, aiming to slip the needle off the sacrum 1–1.5 cm deeper into the foramen.

Aspirate slowly, ensuring the needle is not in a vessel (this is more likely here than at other segmental levels). Inject your mixture of steroid and local anaesthetic/saline slowly. There should be little or no resistance to flow. If the needle is close to the nerve root there may be some tingling or mild pain.

If you experience difficulty in locating the foramen, withdraw the needle to the skin and slide skin and needle laterally 1 cm, redirect the needle slightly medially and caudally to enter the foramen. Occasionally the posterior foramen is too small or even absent, making this route impossible (Figure 4.3.83).

Complications

- Intravascular, intrathecal, or intraneural injection can occur (see above).
- There is a theoretical complication of large-bowel perforation through passing the needle right through the sacrum into the pelvis. As far as I am aware, this has never actually happened.

First sacral root block (with fluoroscopic control)

Indications

As above.

Materials

As above.

Technique

The patient lies prone. Use anteroposterior screening, and screen caudally until the S1 translucent shadow is identified. It is significantly smaller than the S2 foramen which, in contrast, is easily identifiable. If the S1 foramen cannot be seen equidistant from the L5 pedicle and S2 foramen, rotate the C-arm 5–10° to the side being sought. This often identifies the foramen. Too oblique a view may result in the posterior superior iliac spine obscuring direct passage of the needle. Direct the spinal needle down the tunnel of the beam until you have contacted bone adjacent to the foramen. Note the depth. Withdraw slightly and bend the needle towards the foramen (using curved needle technique). Once the needle has entered by 1.5 cm, aspirate slowly and then inject contrast if placement

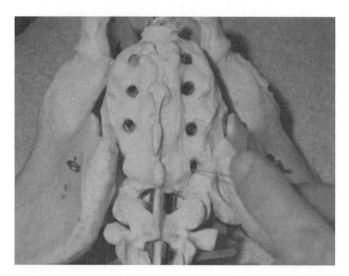

Figure 4.3.83

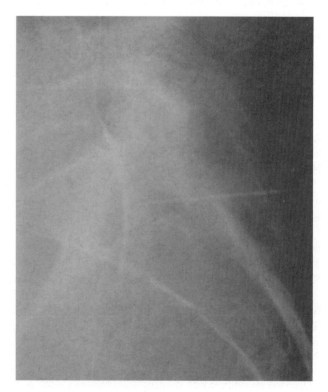

Figure 4.3.84

is not intravascular. Sometimes, despite negative aspiration, contrast does not appear on re-screening, indicating intravascular placement. Reposition the needle tip and try again. Success is marked by cranial flow of contrast outlining the nerve root. Inject medication slowly. No more than 20 mg depot steroid and 2 ml of local anaesthetic or normal saline is required (Figure 4.3.84).

Complications

As above.

Sacroiliac joint injection (without radiographic control)

Indications

Pain in the sacroiliac region or referred from that region which has not responded to manual/manipulative therapy or other treatment to the lumbar–pelvic region. Clinical diagnosis of mechanical dysfunction is not a certain diagnosis. Refractory pain may be abolished by prognostic blocks and may respond to intra-articular steroid. Prolotherapy or denervation, rarely fusion surgery, may be logical steps in treatment for difficult cases. Radiographic, CT or MRI evidence of inflammatory changes may lead to a trial of local treatment when systemic treatment is ineffective.

Materials

A 5 ml Luer-locking syringe, a 90-mm 21-gauge hypodermic or 22-gauge 90mm spinal needle, local anaesthetic, depot steroid.

Technique

The patient lies supine over a pillow to reduce lumbar lordosis. Mark the L5 spinous process and the PSIS. The needle is directed from the L5 spine laterally to the PSIS about 45° caudally, at an angle of 30–45° degrees to the skin, aiming to achieve the greatest depth through the posterior ligamentous tissue, into the cleft between ilium and sacrum.

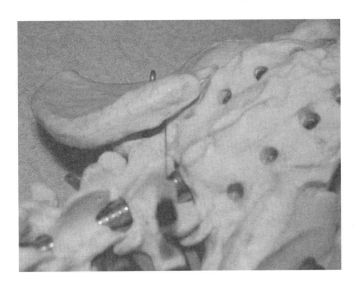

Figure 4.3.85

It is rarely possible to enter the joint proper in this way, but in cases of sacroiliitis a good therapeutic result is usually obtained.

Injection of 3–4 ml of a mixture of local anaesthetic and steroid (20 mg triamcinolone) is quite adequate (Figure 4.3.85).

Complications

- Minor: haematoma.

Sacroiliac joint (with fluoroscopic control)

Indications

As above.

Materials

As above, but 50-mm 25-gauge needle plus contrast medium.

Technique

Patient lies prone. Use anteroposterior screening. Identify inferior pole of joint and mark the skin directly over the lower end of the posterior joint line (this should lie slightly medial). Direct the 25-gauge needle directly to the lower end of this medial line and into the joint. Having entered the lower limb of the L-shaped joint, there is high resistance to contrast injection: 0.2– 0.5 ml should be enough to demonstrate an arthrogram (Figure 4.3.86).

Rotate the C-arm 30° to the same side to obtain an 'en face' view to visualize for contrast leakage indicating capsular rupture (Figure 4.3.87). This is relatively common. Injection of 2–2.4 ml medication is all an intact joint will allow.

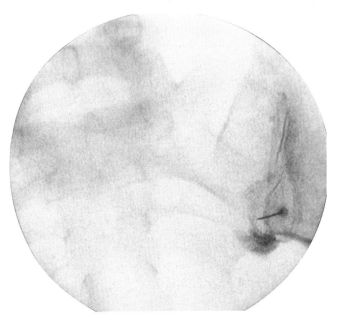

Figure 4.3.86

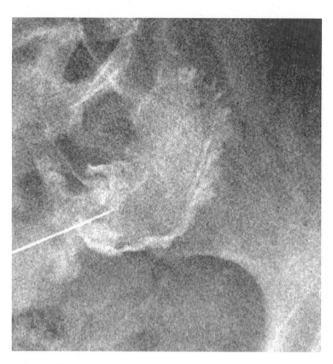

Figure 4.3.87 Right sacroiliac – en face view (note: anterior capsular leakage).

Complications

Minor: haematoma.

Other spinal injections

For techniques of injecting the thoracic spine, zygoapophyseal joints and spinal nerve roots, the reader is referred to other texts such as Lennard (2000). The principles, however, are the same.

Other diagnostic and therapeutic techniques rightfully constitute the domain of a musculoskeletal specialist's work – namely, the diagnosis and treatment of benign spinal pain whether acute or chronic. These include sympathetic blocks, medial branch blocks of the posterior primary ramus, thermal denervation of facet joints, provocative discography and therapeutic intradiscal procedures.

References

Lennard, T. A. (2000) *Pain procedures in clinical practice.* Hanley and Belfus.

For training, the British Institute of Musculoskeletal Medicine (BIMM) (UK) and the International Society for Spinal Injection (ISIS) (USA and Europe) are organizations that can provide a systematic approach under expert tutelage for the acquisition of these skills.

4.3.6 Prolotherapy

Thomas Dorman

Historical review

The first description of the intentional provocation of scar formation is found in the writings of Hippocrates two and a half millennia ago. Hippocrates describes the insertion of searing needles into the anterior capsule of the shoulder in order to stabilize shoulders in javelin throwers, the warriors of Sparta. The irritant can be introduced in a more sophisticated manner by injection through a hollow needle to the appropriate site. The modern use of **sclerotherapy** hails from the herniologists of the era that antedated antiseptic surgery. In 1837 Valpeau of Paris described the use of scar formation for their repair of hernias. The genealogy of herniology, and later the management of hydroceles and a variety of vein sclerosis techniques, was extensively reviewed by Yeomans (1939) and the tradition of vein sclerosis persists into contemporary medical times. Earl Gedney (1937), an osteopath from Philadelphia familiar with the sclerosing techniques of herniologists and venologists, was the first to introduce injection techniques for ligaments. Gedney injected a 'hypermobile sacroiliac joint (SIJ)' first, with salutary results. The term 'sclerotherapy' continued to be used until the mid-1950s when the great organizer of prolotherapy, George Hackett, acquired the skills of injection techniques from the osteopathic profession, evaluated its benefit in an initial series of studies, and published a number of articles about his experiences. This culminated in a short textbook, the third edition of which was published in 1958, and the tradition of his textbook has been maintained into modern times.

Optimal healing

Scar tissue has a number of mechanical properties which differ from those of normal connective tissue and are considered disadvantageous. Scars can be recognized histologically as different from normal connective tissue. It was Hackett who realized that in situations where ligaments are 'relaxed' (his term for ligament insufficiency), hypertrophy of the ligament represented an advantage, contrasting with scar formation which would be a disadvantage.

The therapeutic window

Following this 'road map,' there evolved quite rapidly in the 1940s and 1950s a series of informal empiric trials, first in animals and later in patients with injured ligaments, of the use of a number of sclerosing agents which were now renamed **proliferant agents** by Hackett. It transpired that a great deal of benefit could be achieved clinically by the use of a number of agents. These include extracts from several plants, the least unfamiliar being psyllium seed extract or Sylnasol, a product no longer available, and sodium morrhuate an extract from fish oil, still available in the pharmacopeia. As judged by the frequency of usage, the chief proliferant agents are (1) glucose, (2) glycerin, and (3) phenol. They are usually used in combination (1.25% phenol, 12.5% glucose, 12.5% glycerin) made up with 0.5% of lidocaine (lignocaine) for local analgesia in water. This preparation is also called P25G or P2G.

Klein (1995) and Banks (1991) have classified the injectable proliferating solutions that initiate the wound-healing cascade as follows:

- **Irritants**, which cause a direct chemical tissue injury that attracts granulocytes. Phenol, quinine, and tannic acid come into this category.

- **Osmotic shock agents**, which cause bursting of cell membranes leading to local tissue damage. Hyperosmolar dextrose (12.5–15% maximum) and glycerin are examples of the most commonly used agents in this category.

- **Chemotactic agents**, which activate the inflammatory cascade. Sodium morrhuate is a prototype of this group. These compounds are the direct biosynthetic precursors of the mediators of inflammation, i.e. prostaglandins, leukotrienes, and thromboxanes.

- **Particulates**, such as pumice flour: these are small particles of the order of 1 μm, which lead to longer-lasting irritation and the attraction of macrophages to the site.

Several other materials were previously used, including zinc, Sylnasol and sodium morrhuate. None of these offer any advantage and several have some distinct disadvantages, particularly the risk of allergic reactions.

Evidence of proliferant effect

George Hackett (1958) reported on the histological changes of the Achilles tendon of rats treated with proliferant therapy. These were uncontrolled studies. The next landmark in the study of prolotherapy was a blinded animal study combining histology, electron microscopy, and mechanical evaluation of rabbit ligaments. King Liu and his team (1983) used sodium morrhuate in the medial collateral ligaments of rabbit knees. The histological and mechanical beneficial effects of proliferant therapy in this experimental model were established categorically. The parallel effect on human tissues was established by taking biopsies of posterior SI ligaments which were performed before and after treatment in three patients with chronic low back pain (Oliver and Coughlin 1985). Treatment consisted of a series of six weekly injections into lumbar and SI ligaments, fascia, and facet capsular sites using a connective tissue proliferant (dextrose–glycerine–phenol) combined with mobilization and flexion/extension exercises. Biopsies carried out 3 months after completion of injections demonstrated fibroblastic hyperplasia on light microscopy and increases in average ligament diameter on electron microscopy from a pretreatment value of 0.055 ± 0.26 μm to 0.087 ± 0.041 μm after treatment ($P < 0.001$). Range of motion significantly improved after treatment in rotation ($P < 0.001$), flexion ($P < 0.015$) and side flexion ($P < 0.001$), as did visual analogue pain ($P < 0.001$) and disability ($P < 0.001$) scores.

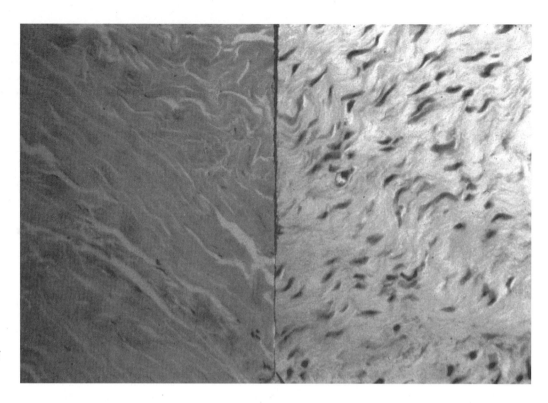

Figure 4.3.88 The histology of human ligaments (a) before and (b) after prolotherapy.

Figure 4.3.88 illustrates the histology of human ligaments before and after prolotherapy.

The use of the dextrose–glycerine–phenol proliferant, as practiced by a number of doctors in California, was found to have a salutary effect, and a double-blind clinical study was conducted. This study confirmed the initial clinical impression of the experimenters of its benefit (Ongley *et al.* 1987). A criticism (which in my view was inapplicable) leveled at the study was that it combined four components of treatment: manipulation, local anesthesia, select use of triamcinolone, and prolotherapy. I believe that the study evaluated a method, so a logical separation of the components is inappropriate. Nevertheless the criticism was accepted by two of the coauthors, and a second double-blind study was conducted to evaluate prolotherapy as a single variable. These results were also statistically meaningful, but the disparity between the groups was much less than in the first study (Klein *et al.* 1993).

Low back syndromes: treatment by prolotherapy

Orthopedic physicians recognize a large inventory of syndromes – clusters of symptoms and signs usually matching distinct pain diagrams which characterize specific mechanical dysfunctions. Some of these syndromes are dominated by symptoms which are secondary to the underlying mechanical cause. Many of these have been outlined by Cyriax (1983) or Dorman (1991) and are not considered in detail in this chapter.

Common to the sacroiliac dysfunction syndromes is one underlying phenomenon: that of ligament relaxation and **asymlocation** in the pelvis. This is the term used to convey the concept that in the **tensegrity model**, which we call the human pelvis, the sacrum is held

or trapped between the ilia. It is prone to being held in a somewhat asymmetric position between them. This tends to place an asymmetric strain on the soft tissues, the fasciae and ligaments. With a certain degree of relaxation of the ligaments, this asymmetry tends to advance to a point of exaggeration, akin to the phenomenon of fault propagation in mechanics. When this threshold is passed, recurrent entrapment of the sacrum asymmetrically amounts to a mechanical dysfunction, i.e. to **somatic dysfunction** in musculoskeletal terminology. This in turn is apt to provoke secondary phenomena which have been listed here as the 'mini'-syndromes characteristic of the human pelvis. Some of these show themselves with ligament symptoms alone, some by muscle dysfunction or spasm, and some, through the phenomenon of transfer of torque through the axial skeleton, are manifested in the neck or the thoracolumbar junction.

Patients with these dysfunctions frequently report that manipulation in the hands of a manual therapist allows them temporary, intermittent relief from pain. Not infrequently, the situation worsens gradually over the years, so that patients seen after one or two decades of recurrent episodes of pain report that the pain has become continuous. Nonetheless, the hallmark of this syndrome is that the pain was intermittently, temporarily relieved early in the history. The improvement from manual therapy is due to a realignment of the pelvic bones. The recurrences are due to ligament relaxation which allows recurrent dysfunctions. The specific characteristic of the dysfunction at one time might vary. It is proposed here, however, that the episodic improvement with manipulation is the hallmark of the ligament dysfunction in the axial skeleton, usually in the pelvic ring. A few examples of these syndromes are given below.

Recurrent sacroiliac strain

In this syndrome, patients report episodes where unexpectedly and suddenly following a slight movement – most characteristically rising

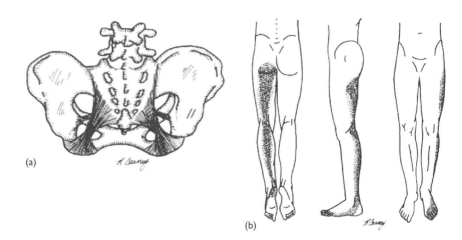

Figure 4.3.89 Sacrotuberous ligament strain in sacroliliac joint dysfunction.

(a)

(b)

from a stooped position with a slight degree of rotation in a casual manner and without a great weight – they feel severe, sudden-onset, asymmetric back pain, usually with radiating pain via one buttock down the leg. They are unable to stand straight. When examined acutely, these individuals are unable to form the normal lumbosacral lordosis, are able to flex forward, have marked asymmetry in sidebending and rotation at the lumbopelvic level, frequently suffer from marked limitation of straight leg raising on the painful side, may have secondary weakness due to pain, but do not suffer reflex suppression or sensory deficits. These individuals are frequently responsive to manipulative therapy. In its absence, the episodes typically recover in 2 weeks to 2 months, but are liable to recur. On detailed musculoskeletal examination, marked dysfunctions in the pelvis are always identifiable in the acute state. It is the thesis of this chapter that the phenomenon is one whereby the sacrum becomes entrapped asymmetrically. Forces acting in the soft tissues, particularly in the upright human, are adducting. (This becomes obvious in viewing the sacrum as suspended between the ilia.) The pelvis, being a tensegrity ring, functions as a whole. When pain occurs, secondary muscle spasm disallows relaxation and restoration of symmetry of the sacrum between the ilia. Such an episode typically resolves in about 2 weeks. It is proposed here that the mechanism(s) of this resolution include one or more of the following factors: (1) bone and ligament molding occurring within 2 weeks, (2) natural slippage of the displaced parts or (3) parts returning to normal through relaxation of the soft tissues or (4) through manipulation or (5) through a combination of all of these.

Sacrotuberous ligament

This ligament, or distal 'stay' of the pelvis, is often strained in SIJ dysfunction because it is further out in the radius of the pelvis (Figure 4.3.89). There is more than one pattern of pain, and individuals may vary as to how it affects them, although the repertoire of patterns is small. The diagnosis is made by the combination of local tenderness and the pain referral pattern.

Iliolumbar ligament sprain

This ligament, being the major stay of the relationship of the pelvis to the lower lumbar vertebrae, is frequently involved as a source of pain in pelvic dysfunctions. Marked local tenderness suggests the diagnosis. Of interest is that an asymmetry in physical findings is usual on exam-

ination when the subject is tested standing. It will be found that sidebending to one side provokes the pain, while rotation to the other side does so. (Note that I have not specified in which direction it is provoked. The ligament is a twisted three-dimensional structure, and the only consistent finding is that sidebending is painful in the direction opposite to which rotation is.)

Sciatica

This term implies pain in the low back with radiation down the lower limb posteriorly via the buttock. It is well recognized that **radiculopathy**, usually due to pressure on the dural sleeve of one of the lumbar nerve roots, can be responsible for this pain. On the other hand, 'sciatica' is more often due to referred pain from the sacrotuberous ligament. In this case, the pain may 'skip' the popliteal space, but often the patterns of pain are indistinguishable on pain diagrams. Straight leg raising is also not a useful discriminant, though stretching the sciatic nerve in the popliteal fossa or through dorsiflexing the foot at a strategic position of straight leg raising is a better differentiator. (Both maneuvers stretch the fascial sleeve of the leg and the branches of the sciatic nerve.) The absence or presence of neurological signs, the presence of tenderness at the attachment of the sacrotuberous ligament at the inferolateral angle of the sacrum, as well as clues from the medical history, are more useful.

Gluteus medius syndrome

As the gluteus medius has a specific role in locking the sacroiliac articulation on the stance side, it is subject to reflex inhibition when the ilium on the affected side is in a forward position (DonTigny 1993). This can be manifested clinically by an alteration in its contraction visible over the buttocks as an individual bends forward, but is also identifiable on examination in the side-lying position (Dorman 1994). Tenderness is found on deep palpation just under the rim of the upper portion of the iliac crest as well.

Piriformis syndrome

As the piriformis muscle plays a major role in stabilizing the pelvis and is an important muscle traversing the sacroiliac joint, it is not surprising that it is strained at times when the pelvis is dysfunctional. The patient reports pain in the middle of the buttock, down the middle aspect of the thigh to the level of the popliteal fossa, affected by certain movements. Testing the muscle when maximally stretched provokes severe pain and yields the diagnosis.

Slipping clutch syndrome

This newly recognized syndrome is characteristic of about 15% of subjects suffering from back pain due to sacroiliac ligamentous dysfunction (Dorman 1994). Patients report episodes of one leg giving way. This is painless, although occasionally patients are injured after a fall. They may not fall down, as they often catch themselves. The phenomenon of the limb giving way occurs invariably as the affected side enters into stance and is thought to represent slight slippage due to failure of the **force closure** of the joint which should occur normally at this moment. As force closure is dependent, amongst other things, on the normal elastic function of the posterior sacroiliac ligaments, it is not surprising that relaxation of these structures can be responsible for mechanical dysfunction, as well as a source of pain.

The response to manipulation

Most of the syndromes surrounding the pelvis, as well as those created remotely through the axial skeleton through the tensegrity and fault propagation phenomena discussed earlier, are due to a single cause: relaxation of the ligaments controlling the tensegrity unit we call the pelvis. This is the source of all mechanical dysfunctions. The dysfunctions themselves lead to, or aggravate strains of fasciae and ligaments. A vicious cycle develops. Muscle spasm is secondary. Its manifestations are well recognized in pain management circles.

Ongley's technique

From the discussion in this chapter so far, the reader will have drawn the logical conclusion that the optimal management should be restoration of symmetry followed by some measure to maintain the improved position. This, indeed, is exactly what is achieved with Ongley's technique. It goes without saying that the steps in this routine start with diagnosis. The diagnosis has to be based on a clinical assessment of the cause of the back pain, followed by a manipulation that should be so vigorous as to restore the pelvis to full symmetry and abolish any tendency for recurrence, which might be due to adhesions. Accordingly, it is an advantage if the patient can be maximally relaxed. A manipulation by the more popular and more gentle techniques of muscle energy, or even gentle thrust techniques, might be quite sufficient to restore a patient to temporary comfort but in my opinion might not restore the joint to optimal alignment nor completely release any adhesions which might be formed from prolonged malalignment. With this technique, therefore, the manipulation is vigorous. In order to facilitate this manipulation (and it is intended to be performed once only), there is an advantage if dilute lidocaine (lignocaine) is injected into the soft tissues guarding the pelvis, particularly the posterior sacroiliac articulation, but also the ligaments around the lumbosacral junction, the iliolumbar ligaments, and the capsules of the zygoapophyseal joints at the two lowest levels of the spine. The details of the injection routine are detailed elsewhere (Dorman 1991). At times, individuals suffer from marked pain from a peripheral fascial strain, such as the fascia overlying the gluteus medius muscle as along the iliac crest. This can be relieved with a local anesthetic injection, usually including small amounts of triamcinolone. It is important, however, not to place steroid injections into mechanically essential ligaments such as the posterior sacroiliac ligaments. A manipulation, which is a modification of an osteopathic technique, is used next, restoring the pelvis to as much symmetry as possible, and in turn this treatment is followed with proliferant therapy injections to the stabilizing ligaments of the pelvis, in particular the three layers of the posterior sacroiliac ligaments, with particular attention to the deepest and central part. Droplet infiltration of proliferant injections is also placed along the iliolumbar ligaments, the zygoapophyseal joint capsules of the two lowest levels of the lumbar spine, and the transverse processes to make contact with the intertransverse ligaments at their periosteal attachments, and into the supraspinous and interspinous ligaments of the lowest levels, and the fascia over the erector spinae at the upper level of the sacrum is also treated. This can be achieved through a single needle insertion point in the midline opposite L5.

A treatment session

Light conscious sedation is used. After a general review of the status of the patient's health and establishing normal vital signs, the patient is sedated with an intravenous injection of 3 mg of midazolam and 25 mg of ketamine. The patient is placed in the prone position and continuously monitored with oximetry for pulse rate and oxygen saturation.

A total of 50 ml of 0.5% lidocaine (lignocaine) is used by droplet infiltration. The operator utilizes a 10-ml Luer-Lock syringe with refills. The medication is distributed by droplet via one needle insertion point, at the spinous process of L5 in the midline with the patient lying prone. The needle is advanced first by stepwise movements with droplet infiltration down the lateral aspect of the spinous process on the left side, making contact with the lamina and with each needle contact a droplet of the anesthetic is dispensed (0.1–0.2 ml). Six such steps are made until the step-off at the zygoapophyseal joint. Here, a maneuver is performed to aim the needle into a somewhat more anterior direction as it is advanced. To achieve this, pressure is placed with the operator's left thumb over the skin at the estimated site of the tip of the needle. During this time the syringe and needle are curved by a flexing maneuver of the syringe-holding hand while advancing the syringe and needle. This causes the needle to curve forward, and contact can be made with the tip of the transverse process of L5 at an appropriate depth. Another droplet of anesthetic is deposited here. The needle is then withdrawn to the subcutaneous situation. The operator's hands are reversed and the maneuver repeated on the patient's right side. This being completed, the needle is again withdrawn to the subcutaneous level and the needle is now directed at an angle of about 45° caudad and laterally to the left and about 30° anteriorly, the palpating (left) thumb is held over the skin of the iliac crest as it curves from horizontal to vertical and anteriorly, aiming at the insertion of the iliolumbar ligament at the top of the iliac crest. Droplet infiltrations are deposited here. This having been completed, the needle tip is again withdrawn to a subcutaneous level and the procedure repeated (with reversed hands) to the right side. The needle is again withdrawn to the subcutaneous level and aimed at the posterior sacroiliac ligaments, first on the left side by a similar maneuver, again with a sentinel (left) thumb over the posterior-superior iliac spine. The needle is aimed in the crevasse (cave) consisting of the dorsal attachment of the superficial layer of the posterior sacroiliac ligament. Droplet infiltration of local anesthetic is deposited at this site, and by withdrawal and reinsertion the needle is maneuvered not only along the several points of insertion against the overhanging ilium, but also against the deeper recessed sacral attachment of the posterior sacroiliac ligaments in three layers. About 20 droplet infiltrations are deposited on this side by these maneuvers. Now the needle is again withdrawn to the subcutaneous level, still being inserted at the midline at the spinous process of L5, the hands are reversed and a similar maneuver is performed on the right. This routine takes about 40 ml of lidocaine (lignocaine). The needle is now withdrawn and a suitable dressing applied at the needle insertion site. In cases where an injection is required for a ligament causing pain, such as the sacrotuberous ligament, a separate injection is performed. In the case of the sacrotuberous ligament this is best done in the side lying position. The use of some triamcinolone at these sites is discretionary. After this is completed, the patient is returned into a supine position and a mobilization undertaken. On this occasion, the patient is rolled onto one side, say the right, with the shoulder remaining supine, so torque can be applied to the torso. An assistant standing on the patient's left applies a cushion across the patient's chest and places her body in such a position as to maintain firm contact between the patient's left shoulder and the couch. The physician places his right hand so the tip of the middle finger is at the lumbosacral junction. The patient's lower (left) thigh remains stretched out on the couch close to its margin on the side close to the physician. The operator's right hand flexes the thigh until tension is noted at the lumbosacral junction by the palpating hand. With the thigh in this position, adduction is now applied to it until the slack of the thoracic and lumbar spine is completely taken up, the forces concentrating at the lumbosacral junction and below them predominantly at the sacroiliac joint. The left hand is now placed over the patient's left greater trochanter and the right hand over the knee, the leg remaining flexed on the knee. At a moment of body relaxation at the end of expiration, force is applied firmly along the line of shear of the left sacroiliac joint, the assistant maintaining firm control of the patient's shoulder and upper torso. After this is done, the patient is placed in the supine position and if no substantial change in the alignment of the low back is achieved, as judged by apparent leg length discrepancy, the maneuver is repeated on the other side. This usually achieves satisfactory mobilization of the sacroiliac joints.

Flexion maneuver

The assistant places herself at the patient's feet. The patient's outstretched hands are grasped by the assistant's one hand and the knees firmly held flat on the couch with the other. The physician brings the patient to the sitting position and with the hands over the low lumbar spine induces gentle repeated flexion movements. This usually increases the range of flexion of the patient's lumbar spine. The patient is restored to the supine.

The routine prolotherapy follow-up described next is typically used on the first day after the local anesthesia and mobilization and weekly for a total of six sessions. It consists of 20 ml of P2G distributed by droplet infiltration through one needle insertion point at the spinous process of L5 in the midline with the patient lying prone. The needle is advanced first by stepwise movements with droplet infiltration down the lateral aspect of the spinous process on the left side, making contact with the lamina and with each needle contact a droplet (0.1–0.2 ml) of proliferant is dispensed. Six such steps are made until the step-off at the zygoapophyseal joint. Here, a maneuver is performed to aim the needle into a somewhat more anterior direction as it is advanced. To achieve this, pressure is placed with the operator's left thumb over the skin at the estimated site of the tip of the needle. During this time the syringe and needle are curved by a flexing maneuver of the syringe-holding hand while advancing the syringe and needle. This causes the needle to curve forward and contact is made with the transverse process of L5 at an appropriate depth by careful manipulation. Another droplet of proliferant is deposited here. The needle is then withdrawn to the subcutaneous situation. The operator's hands are reversed and the maneuver repeated on the patient's right side. It is usual at this time to repeat the maneuver at the L4 level. It is not always necessary to make another cutaneous needle insertion. There is usually enough laxity in the skin to slide it cephalad, while holding the tip just deep enough to pass through the upper dermis. The interspinous ligaments of the two to three lowest lumbar levels need to be infiltrated at this time. The operator will have gained a sense of the depth of the lamina. On no account should an injection stray into the lumbar theca. It is best to place the tip of the needle onto the inferior surface of the spinous process above and the superior surface of the spinous process below at each level. This can be facilitated by having the prone patient positioned passively for this portion of the injection into trunk flexion. Many suitable treatment couches are available for this; some practitioners use an inflatable pillow. Next, the iliolumbar ligament is injected as described in the section on the infiltration of the local anesthesia. The needle is again withdrawn to the subcutaneous level and aimed at the posterior sacroiliac ligaments. The routine here also follows that described above. This is the most important part of the proliferant injection. Particular care must be given to reach the deep innominate sacroiliac ligaments. It is important not to exceed about 20 ml of P2G in any one session to the back.

Finally, the patient is encouraged to perform full range of movement 'exercises' to encourage healing in the natural lines of strain.

The special case of the neck

Though prolotherapy has been used for cervical and referred upper thoracic pain since the 1950s, this difficult area of treatment has received even less attention than the low back. Nonetheless, a few practitioners, who have followed an analytic process outlined here for the identification of the ligamentous structures responsible for pain after whiplash and allied cervical injuries, have had excellent results (Kayfetz et al. 1963). In whiplash injuries, where the integrated function of the motion segments is disturbed by damage (e.g. to the capsules of the zygapophyseal joints and/or the attachments of the annulus of the disc to the vertebral endplate) there is likely to be associated ligament injury.

The asymmetry in range of movement at the segment can frequently be improved by manipulation with slight cervical extension under traction by the methods developed in the Cyriax school. However, when the correction is only temporary, consideration should be given to refurbishing the ligaments with prolotherapy. As in the case of the sacral dysfunction in the low back, Ongley has developed a routine for the neck.

Prolotherapy to the neck

The routine for light conscious sedation outlined under the section for the low back is followed.

For the initial treatment of the neck, the patient lies prone with the assistant sitting at the head of the treatment table which is elevated to the mid-waist level of the operator. It is best to use a treatment table with an appropriate opening for breathing. Local anesthesia is applied with the air gun to the midline opposite the spinous process of C2 and another bleb opposite the spinous process of C5. A total of about 50 ml of 0.5% lidocaine (lignocaine) can be used. The superior segment is treated first. A 19-gauge 75-mm needle attached to a 10-ml Luer-Lock syringe is charged with 0.5% lidocaine (lignocaine). Needle contact is first made with the spinous process of C2 opposite the anesthetic bleb. For accuracy of fine manual control, the neck is flexed, the assistant using her right hand on the back of the patient's head in the prone position. The assistant maintains pressure so that the neck remains flexed. Her left hand is placed flat in the midline, palm down, opposite T1 and T2, so that the operator can grasp the assistant's index finger for stability with the medial fingers of his left hand, the fifth finger serving as a sensory prod close to the site of the needle insertion. The operator's right hand is braced on the patient's right shoulder, or as appropriate the forearm is braced, and the right hand serves for needle placement. With this routine, the whole injection procedure is undertaken. At first, 20 ml of 0.5% lidocaine (lignocaine) are infiltrated into the upper cervical segment. The needle is first carefully passed through the skin at the C2 level and then directed to multiple sites of ligament attachment to bone in the neck. It is first directed anteriorly until contact is made at a depth of about 3 mm with the spinous process of C2. When the site has been defined, a droplet of local anesthetic is inserted here and a further droplet cephalad into the interspinous ligament at this depth. The needle is withdrawn marginally and directed laterally to the patient's left. After passing over the lateral component of the bifurcate spinous process, the needle is now curved by a combined maneuver of the right (syringe-holding) hand and the palpating tip of the operator's left fifth finger, pressing over the skin lateral to the site of the insertion. This directs the needle anteriorly so it makes contact with the lateral aspect of the spinous process of C2. Here another droplet of local anesthetic is deposited and the needle is advanced stepwise, contact with bone being made at each step, until a change of angle is encountered – the lamina. Further droplets of local anesthetic are deposited at these sites and the needle is advanced to the prominence of the zygoapophyseal joint of the C1–2 level. Here further droplets of local anesthetic are applied and the needle is then passed more laterally so it just passed over the bulge of the joint. The small transverse process of C2 is palpated with the needle tip and a final droplet of local anesthetic is applied here. This being established, the needle is withdrawn to the subcutaneous level and an equivalent maneuver is performed on the right side. The needle is then again withdrawn subcutaneously and directed cephalad, the palpating tip of the operator's left fifth finger being applied firmly to the posterior prominence of the atlas. By gentle encroachment at a superficial level, the needle is brought in contact with the arch of the atlas. A droplet of local anesthetic is applied here and the needle is 'walked' across the arch of the atlas carefully until the lateral side, or mass of the atlas, is reached. At this point advancement is stopped (because of the vertebral artery) and the needle is applied more superficially, advanced beyond the expected site of the vertebral artery, and then directed anteriorly to the tip or posterior surface of the lateral mass, curving over the

expected site of the vertebral artery. Another droplet of local anesthetic infiltration is applied here and the needle is withdrawn to the midline subcutaneous position. The equivalent maneuver is performed on the right-hand side. Throughout, the assistant is holding the neck in a firmly flexed position with her right hand, the left hand remaining on the dorsal aspect of the patient's upper thoracic spine as an anchor for the operator's directing left hand, the index finger being grasped between thumb and forefinger.

This maneuver having been completed, the needle (again withdrawn to the subcutaneous site) is directed caudad to the spinous process of C3. A similar maneuver of walking down the spinous process and lamina to the zygoapophyseal joint is performed first to the patient's left and finally to the patient's right. This having been accomplished, the needle is withdrawn entirely from the C2 insertion site. A cotton swab and dressing are applied. The patient's neck is maintained in flexion and the needle is introduced (with a second syringe containing 10 ml of local anesthetic) opposite C5. An analogous maneuver is performed at the C5 level. The needle is then again withdrawn subcutaneously and now applied cephalad from this insertion site to the spinous process of C4, and the whole maneuver is repeated along this vertebra. This is facilitated by the skin gliding technique, allowing the operator to bring the dorsal cutaneous needle insertion site opposite the spinous process of the relevant vertebra to limit the number of cutaneous penetrations. Finally, the needle is withdrawn again subcutaneously and now directed caudad towards the spinous process of C6 and then C7. In this position it is not possible to slide the skin inferiorly and a diagonal approach is made to the (much larger) lamina and zygoapophyseal joints of the C6–7 and C7–T1 vertebrae. Contact is also made with the root of the first portion of the first rib from this particular maneuver. The remainder of the 10 ml of anesthetic is again applied to this whole area by droplet infiltration distributed to the two sides. The use of some local anesthesia with triamcinolone is discretionary, if the physician has made a diagnosis of a particularly inflamed area. The needle is now withdrawn. Suitable dressings are placed over the puncture site (there is no bleeding) and the patient is now placed in the supine position. The height of the couch is adjusted for the mobilization.

The initial mobilization is performed by Cyriax's technique with the assistant holding the lower limbs to avoid slippage and the patient positioned so that the shoulders are flush with the upper end of the couch. A straight pull is applied by Cyriax's technique. Firm continuous traction is applied to the cervical spine, the operator cradling the occipital portion of the head in the left hand and ensuring control with the right hand under the mandible. After traction is applied for about 10 seconds and the slack taken up, with slight maintenance of extension, the head is gently rotated to the unrestricted side and over-pressure is applied with very little movement. The maneuver is repeated to the other side and the patient then restored to the normal lying position (supine) on the couch. After this is completed, the height of the couch is readjusted and a lateral tilt chiropractic style mobilization applied in each direction to mobilize the atlanto-occipital joints. The patient is restored to the supine position, head-rolling exercises initiated on the low pillow. After recovery from the light conscious sedation the patient should be instructed in cervical exercises which facilitate complete movement of all the joints of the neck.

Prolotherapy is initiated the next day by a similar routine, also with light conscious sedation. The injection technique is the same as just described. It is not usual to exceed 20 ml of P2G for any one session.

The skill of performing this rather delicate routine can only be learnt by apprenticeship. It is recorded here for information only.

Mechanics and ligament proliferation

Prolotherapy has been shown to provoke hyperplasia of ligament tissue, with an increased amount of collagen. The mechanical effects of prolotherapy in human ligaments were studied through the treatment of the joint capsule and injured ligaments of the knees of athletes who had suffered injuries. During the enrolment period 30 patients with knee pain were seen, but in the cases of only 5 knees (in 4 patients) was it possible to obtain measurements after treatment, because the equipment was available only for 9 months and many of the athletes, after clinical improvement, failed to return for repeat measurements. All the selected subjects had substantial ligament instability. All measurements were taken by one researcher. The patients underwent multiple injections. The patients were followed routinely and within 9 months repeat measurements were obtained. Subjective symptoms were obtained at entry and exit from the study. Ligament stability was measured by a commercially available computerized instrument that measures ligament function objectively and reliably in three dimensions (Oliver and Coughlin 1985, Selsnick et al. 1986). It consists of a chair equipped with a six-component force platform and a electrogoniometer with six degrees of freedom. With computer-integrated force and motion measurements, a standardized series of clinical laxity tests can be performed and an objective report obtained. Earlier studies have compared clinical testing with objective tests (Daniel et al. 1985) and have established reproducibility (Highgenboten 1986). The proliferant solution used in these cases was P25G. The proliferant injections were 'peppered' into the lax ligament(s) usually at 2-weekly intervals, each offending ligament being treated an average of four times. A total of 30–40 ml of the proliferant solution is injected into the appropriate portion of the joint ligaments. Details of the injection technique can be found in the original publication (Ongley et al. 1988).

Prolotherapy in other parts

It will be evident to the reader, from the foregoing, that prolotherapy is a suitable injection treatment for treating any part of the fascio-ligamentous organ. A detailed style of needle placement, the selection of the needle, the volume to be injected at any one site, etc., vary and details of this have been given elsewhere (Dorman 1991).

References

Banks, A. (1991) A rationale for prolotherapy. *Journal of Orthopaedic Medicine*, 13, 54–9.

Cyriax, J. (1983) *Textbook of orthopaedic medicine*, 11th edn. W. B. Saunders, Baltimore. MD.

Daniel, D. M., Malcolm, L. L., Losse, G., Stone, M. L., Sachs, R., Burks, R. (1985) Instrument measurement of anterior laxity of the knee. *Journal of Bone and Joint Surgery*, 67A, 720–5.

DonTigny, R. L. (1993) Mechanics and treatment of the sacroiliac joint. *Journal of Manual and Manipulative Therapy*, 1, 1.3–12.

Dorman, T. (1991) *Diagnosis and injection techniques in orthopedic medicine*. Williams & Wilkins, Baltimore, MD.

Dorman, T. (1994) Failure of self bracing at the sacroiliac joint: the slipping clutch syndrome. *Journal of Orthopaedic Medicine*, 16, 49–51.

Gedney, E. H. (1937) Hypermobile joint. *Osteopathic Profession*, 4, 30–31.

Hackett, G. S. (1958) *Ligament and tendon relaxation treated by prolotherapy*, 3rd edn.: Charles Thomas, Springfield, IL.

Highgenboten, C. L. (1986) The reliability of the Genucom knee analysis system. 2nd European Congress of Knee Surgery and Arthroscopy, Basel, Switzerland.

Kayfetz, D. O., Blumental, L. S., Hackett, G. S. *et al.* (1963) Whiplash injury and other ligamentous headache – its management with prolotherapy. *Headache*, 3, 21–8.

King Liu, Y., Tipton, C., Matthews R. D. *et al.* (1983) An in situ study of the influence of a sclerosing solution in rabbit medial collat-eral ligaments and its junction strength. *Connective Tissue Research*, 11, 95–102.

Klein, R. G., Eek, B. J., DeLong, B., Mooney, V. (1993) A randomised double-blind trial of dextrose-glycerine-phenol injections for chronic low back pain. *Journal of Spinal Diseases*, 6, 22–3.

Oliver, J. H., Coughlin, L. P. (1985) An analysis of knee evaluation using clinical techniques and the Genucom knee analysis system. American Orthopedic Society for Sports Medicine interim meeting, Las Vegas, Nevada.

Ongley, M. J., Klein, R. G., Dorman, T. A. *et al.* (1987) A new approach to the treatment of chronic back pain. *Lancet*, 2, 143–6.

Ongley, M. J., Dorman, T. A., Eek B. C. *et al.* (1988) Ligament instability of knees: a new approach to treatment. *Manual Medicine*, 3, 151–4.

Selsnick, H., Oliver, J., Virgin, C. (1986) Analysis of knee ligament test-ing-Genucom and clinical exams. Presented at the American Orthopedic Society for Sports Medicine annual meeting, Sun Valley, Idaho.

Yeomans, F. C. (ed.) (1939) *Sclerosing therapy, the injection treatment of hernia, hydrocele, varicose veins and hemorrhoids*. Williams & Wilkins, Baltimore. MD.

4.3.7 The use of neurodynamics in pain management

David Butler

Introduction – a call for 'big picture' clinical decision-making

During the 1990s, management techniques using neural mobilization concepts became popular, even trendy. Now, with the rapid growth of neurobiological science, the hindsight of over a decade of practice, and the growth of evidence, a careful review of the role of neurodynamic tests in management is timely.

I propose that there is a number of ways in which tests such as the straight leg raise and slump test can be used in management. The first and most obvious is that they can be used as assessment and reassessment techniques, as is now common practice. Secondly, they have a role in active and passive neural tissue mobilization. Thirdly, and often forgotten, the tests can help explain some aspects of sensitivity; and finally, they have a role in postural and ergonomic adjustments. Under the heading 'active movements', consideration can be given to warmups, paced movements, integration into functional activities, and movement breakdowns. However, there is no recipe, prescription or protocol for use of the tests and I reject notions of 'neural stretches' or 'sciatic stretches' and the crudity of assessment which usually surrounds such techniques. To integrate neurodynamics, careful clinical judgement incorporating an evidence-based 'big picture' and a neurobiological viewpoint are necessary. This should engender an appropriate level of modesty in clinical use of the neurodynamic movements.

From Chapter 2.2.4, it should be clear that the physical abilities of the nervous system cannot be disregarded. It is impossible to engage in any activity without physically and thus physiologically affecting the nervous system. Also, it is impossible to ignore the many symptoms and signs which can be exhibited when the nervous system is injured or altered.

The evidence-based big picture

A very broad list can be made of management features that have been shown to help patients in acute and chronic pain states. This list is taken from diverse areas such as (in chronological order): Frank (1973), Gerteis *et al.* (1993), AHCPR (1994), Dworkin (1997), Kendall *et al.* (1997), Linton (1998), and Waddell (1998).

- Educate the patient and relevant associates about the nature of the whole problem including health status of the tissues, role of the nervous system, and results of investigative tests. Such information must make sense to the patient and be continually updated during management.

- Provide prognostication, and – with the patient – make realistic goals, which include clear recommendations about activities and progression.

- Closely related to the first two points is the promotion of self-care and patient control.

- Get patients active and moving as early as is possible and appropriate after injury, by any safe means possible. Utilize activities favoured by the patient.

- Decrease unnecessary fear related to movements, leisure, and work activities. This may mean challenging some beliefs and superstitions. It also requires that clinicians understand peripheral and central mechanisms of pain.

- Help the patient experience success and a sense of mastery of the problem. Guidance and supervision may be necessary.

- Perform a skilled physical evaluation which is likely to be more 'low tech' and functional in more chronic pain states and more specific in acute and tissue-based problems. Communicate the results to the patient. In some pain states specific exercises in specific population groups can help.

- Make any treatment strategy as closely linked to evidence of the biological nature of the patient's problem as possible, rather than syndrome, geography, or temporal nature.

- Use any measures possible to reduce pain, especially in the acute stage, and particularly patient-controlled analgesia.

- Minimize number of treatments and contacts with medical personnel.

Any manual therapy strategies that have a place in this 'big picture' could be said to be evidence based.

In this list, some suggestions are made that the use of tests and test responses may vary depending on the biological processes related to pain. The mechanisms behind sensitive human movement are varied. There could be a dominance of tissue involvement, including peripheral nerve damage, referred to as **primary hyperalgesia**. There could also be changes in neural activity, cooperation, and receptive fields in the central nervous system (CNS). This may lead to movement being reactive and not entirely due to damage to the underlying tissues. This is referred to as **secondary hyperalgesia** and forms a part of the central sensitization phenomenon. See Woolf and Doubell (1994), Cohen (1995), and Chapter 2.3.1 for further discussion.

When a movement such as the straight leg raise is sensitive and/or limited and a clinical decision is made that an improved straight leg raise would be beneficial to the patient's function, there are a number of ways in which the movement can be integrated into management. In the following discussion modes of examination, key points in a neurodynamic evaluation, and determination of the clinical relevance of a sensitive movement are considered.

Physical evaluation of the health of the nervous system

There are three ways, excluding electrodiagnostic testing and scanning, in which a physical evaluation of the nervous system can be carried out.

Palpation of the peripheral nervous system

Sites of abnormal impulse generation in peripheral nerves will usually be mechanosensitive (Devor and Seltzer 1999) and skilled palpation may assist clinical diagnosis by eliciting symptoms. Many nerves are easily palpable, even small ones such as the radial sensory nerve or the infrapatellar branch of the saphenous nerve. Where a nerve is not directly palpable, such as the median nerve in the carpal tunnel, pressure can be placed upon it to elicit symptoms that may be useful in diagnosis (Durkan 1991). Clinicians who are familiar with neurodynamic testing will often combine palpation with the neurodynamic tests (e.g. Novak *et al.* 1994). In this paper, palpation of the ulnar nerve at the cubital tunnel with the limb in a position that mechanically loads the ulnar nerve demonstrated good reliability in the diagnosis of cubital tunnel syndrome. For further details on the handling skills involved in nerve palpation see Butler (2000).

Physical examination of nerve conduction

A physical assessment of nerve conduction should involve an appropriately constructed sensory and motor evaluation of the CNS and peripheral nervous system. In the peripheral nervous system, root and trunk components can be tested. This will add data to an initial diagnosis, and provides part of a safety net. Unfortunately most clinicians don't do it, or limit the testing to the easily performed reflexes. A neurological examination requires manual handling skill. The testing is not only to assist diagnosis and for safety, but is also part of therapy in itself. Explaining findings, for example, 'that's strong', or 'these nerves are firing well' can be helpful therapy. There are many texts on this aspect of neurological examination including Mayo Clinic (1991), Nolan (1996), Butler (2000).

Neurodynamic tests

The third way, and a focus of this chapter, is to perform movements which place or presume to place a load on to the nervous system via neurodynamic tests such as the straight leg raise or the upper limb neurodynamic test.

The neurodynamic tests

The proposal is that certain movements preferentially challenge neural structures and create significant inputs into the CNS which, depending on CNS threshold control at the time of being tested, may be perceived as painful. Clinical and external data can be collected to support hypotheses that responses are neurogenic and these movements may be integrated into management with an eye to the 'big picture' proposed earlier. A base system has been proposed (Butler 1991) using a series of accepted tests such as straight leg raise, passive neck flexion and prone knee bend. Other, newer tests such as the upper limb neurodynamic test (Figure 4.3.71) and the slump test (Figure 4.3.72) are also proposed as base tests. These tests are places to start the evaluation and if there are clues in a subjective evaluation that the nervous system may be involved, further testing may be necessary. For further details on suggested protocols for these tests, see Butler (1991, 2000).

The base tests are not suggested for routine evaluation. In some patients the clinician may perform a number of tests including refined derivatives, in others, for various reasons, including pain severity, no tests are performed. Worthwhile clues to the amount of detail required in a physical evaluation may emerge from a subjective evaluation. For example, if a patient reported that their low back hurt while getting into a car, then I would be inclined to perform a slump test, a straight leg raise, even a passive neck flexion. In another patient where the history sounded like local lumbar spinal joint pathology, a straight leg raise alone may suffice.

A test is usually taken further by the addition of sensitizing manoeuvres. This is simply careful attention to the relation of nerve pathways to joint axes. For example, the most sensitive test for the peroneal nerve would be straight leg raise plus ankle plantar flexion/inversion plus hip adduction and medial rotation plus spinal lateral flexion and cervical flexion.

Key points in a neurodynamic assessment

A sensitive movement provides little information

The only information provided by a symptomatic straight leg raise is that your patient has a sensitive movement. Alone, it says nothing about anatomical sources of symptoms, nor does it impart any information about pathobiological mechanisms behind the symptoms, or where along the nervous system pathologies may lurk. The response may even be normal, and there may be other movements more sensitive. Perhaps a few evoked pins and needles or symptoms in a neural zone may point to a neural contribution, but further clinical data are necessary to make judgements on the clinical relevance.

At the time of physical evaluation, clinical data should already be at hand from a subjective evaluation and the use of external evidence such as scans. Indeed, if this is so, a reasoning clinician will have an expectation of certain findings on physical evaluation. Examples of support data include area of symptoms (e.g. neural zone symptoms), behaviour of symptoms (e.g. afterdischarge, symptoms on activities which pinch or elongate nerves) other physical findings (e.g. diminished reflex, stiffness in neighbouring joints) and tests such as a nerve conduction test. In-depth reasoning processes in orthopaedic evaluation are discussed elsewhere (Higgs and Jones 2000).

Determining the relevance of the test

The neurodynamic tests are not pathognomic, nor can they ever be called tests for syndromes such as the 'carpal tunnel test'. The tests will only provide information about one aspect of the big picture. Even the best researched of the tests, the straight leg raise, can only provide supporting evidence to a nerve root or discogenic problem (Supik and Broom 1994).

Everyone has varying sensitivity to the straight leg raise or the upper limb neurodynamic test. The following guidelines may help determine the relevance of a test.

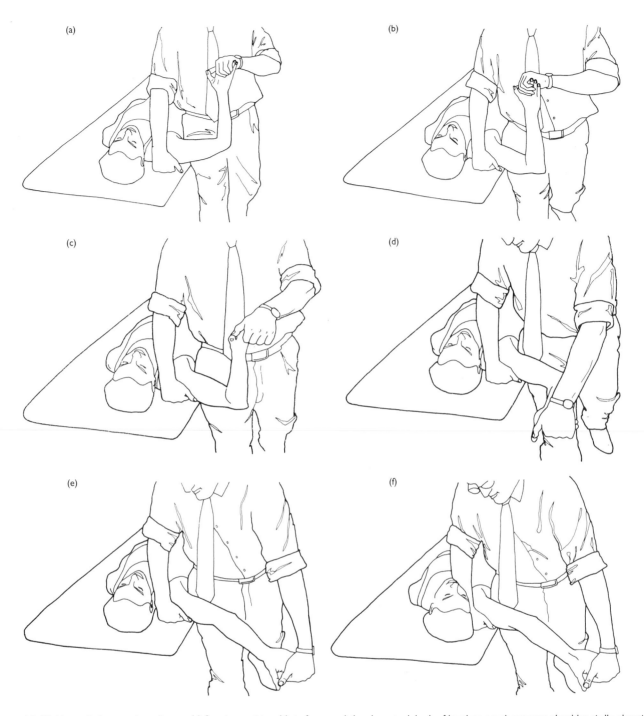

Figure 4.3.90 Upper limb neurodynamic test. (a) Starting position. Note finger and thumb control; back of hand on couch prevents shoulder girdle elevation during abduction; patient's arm rests on clinician's thigh. (b) Shoulder abduction. Take the arm to approximately 110 degrees or onset of symptoms. (c) Forearm supination and wrist extension. (d) Shoulder lateral rotation. (e) Elbow extension. (f) Neck lateral flexion. Lateral flexion away from test side usually increases symptoms; towards test side decreases symptoms.
Clinicians should be aware of symptoms evoked at each stage of the test. (From Butler, D. S. (2000) *The sensitive nervous system*. Noigroup, Adelaide. With permission.)

A test such as the straight leg raise can be considered positive if:

- it reproduces symptoms or associated symptoms, **plus**
- structural differentiation supports a neurogenic source, **plus**
- differences left to right and to known normal responses, **plus**
- support from other data such as history, area of symptoms and imaging tests.

However, this process of additive hypothesis support or rejection is just the first step to a clinical diagnosis.

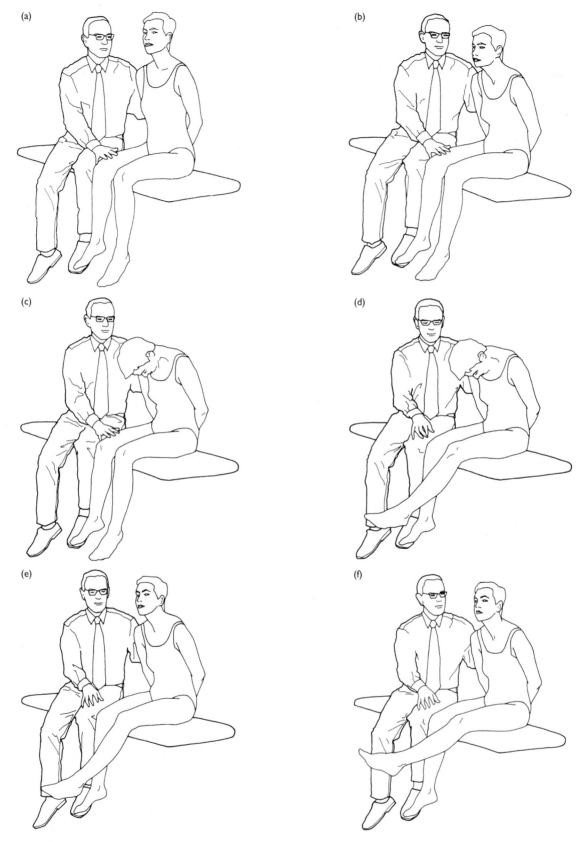

Figure 4.3.91 The Slump test. (a) Starting position. (b) Patient slumps. Clinician guides movement, keeping pelvis vertical. (c) Add cervical flexion. (d) Add knee extension. (e) Extend neck. Check if change of any evoked leg and spinal symptoms. (f) In this position, patients can often extend their knee further. Variations include adding ankle dorsiflexion, planterflexion/inversion, and adding hip flexion. Clinicians should be aware of symptoms evoked at each stage of the test. (From Butler, D. S. (2000) *The sensitive nervous system*. Noigroup, Adelaide. With permission.)

A test may appear positive but is it relevant, that is, is it a movement which would be worthwhile addressing to reduce sensitivity, improve quality and range of motion, and assist restoration of function? Also, if used as a reassessment tool, would a change in this movement be a worthwhile indicator of progression?

The following guidelines to the determination of test relevance are suggested:

- Base relevance on function. If this movement is improved, will it help the patient function better? To make this judgement, knowledge about current goals and activity levels is necessary. So is a skilled physical examination. So for example, minor limitations and hyperalgesia in a test which loads the radial nerve may well make the test relevant in a professional tennis player with lateral elbow pain. Similar minor findings in a patient with fibromyalgia may not be so relevant.

- A clinical judgement on pain processes in operation may help. For example, history and patterns of symptoms may allow a clinical judgement that a maladaptive central sensitization process is in operation and management may be better directed at threshold control of the CNS, rather than focusing on tissue health. More peripheral processes would suggest that more time be spent on tissue function and health. See Gifford and Butler (1997), Butler (1998, 2000), Gifford (1998) for further discussion on integrating pain mechanisms into practice.

- Finally, when considering which tissues are involved, consider all tissues. For too many years clinicians have had favourite hypotheses, usually focusing around one tissue. Any innervated tissue is a potential source of symptoms. Modern clinicians need clinical appreciation of all tissues and all processes related to pain.

The concept of structural differentiation

A response evoked by a straight leg raise, say in the buttocks, which is made worse by the addition of ankle dorsiflexion, is said to confirm the role of the nervous system in the disorder (Breig and Troup 1979). In the slump test, a hamstring area symptom response eased by neck extension is also said to be neurogenic (Maitland 1986, Butler 1991). This is an attractive and often exciting clinical finding for patients and clinicians. It does not mean much in terms of biological mechanisms. Such tests may well preferentially load one tissue and assist in a clinical diagnosis, but should not lead to an instant diagnosis of 'neural tension' or 'altered neurodynamics'. The finding is one more piece of data to add to others to infer that the nervous system is sensitive and/or physically compromised in a particular pain state. The problem occurs when there are multiple sensitive tissues, or in more chronic cases, additional inputs may well be normal inputs, even A beta inputs, which in the presence of a sensitized system have the ability to be upregulated and the patient then perceives pain. Thus a straight leg raise may evoke a back pain and the addition of dorsiflexion increases it by adding further normal input to an already sensitized system. Care in interpretation is therefore needed.

Structural differentiation can be used actively. A nice example is provided by Mackinnon and Dellon (1988). Some patients diagnosed with de Quervain's disease may have a local neuropathy of the musculocutaneous or superfical radial nerve rather than a tendon/tendon sheath disorder. Finkelstein's test of thumb flexion and wrist ulnar deviation is therefore a test of all lateral wrist tissues. However, if the 'Finkelstein position' is maintained and the elbow extended, shoulder girdle elevation should make neurogenic symptoms ease, and there should be little or no change if the local joints and muscles are involved.

Active and passive movements

Nearly all tests can be performed actively, although the straight leg raise may present some difficulties. As a routine I suggest that the tests, including structural differentiation, can be performed actively before passively. The observation of good range and movement quality in a particular movement that may preclude passive performance of a test. Where a passive evaluation follows, the patient will be better informed and allow better performance of the test. Protocols for active neurodynamic test evaluation are suggested in Butler (2000).

Pinch and stretch

The focus should not solely be on elongation of the nervous system. The system design is also such that it can adapt to compressive forces and the 'closing down' of tissues around the nerve. For example, spinal extension, lateral flexion, and rotation towards the test side closes down intervertebral foramina and may pinch contained neural tissues. This is especially so if there are degenerative changes in the structures of the spinal and intervertebral canals. These tests are known as quadrant tests (Maitland 1986) or Spurling's test in the case of the cervical spine. Whether they are reactive or not in the presence of neuropathy may depend on the dynamic roominess of the intervertebral foramen (Penning 1992). This should serve as a reminder that when considering the physical health of nerves, some thoughts must be given to the neighbouring structures around the nervous system in a static and a dynamic sense.

One base test may not be inclusive of other tests

It may seem that an all-inclusive test such as the slump test would preclude the necessity of testing straight leg raise and passive neck flexion. The slump test has been shown to be more sensitive than the straight leg raise in low back pain (Massey 1985) and it will often be noted in clinics that the responses will be different. It is possible to observe a patient who has a sensitive straight leg raise yet negative slump, and vice versa. Simply, the anatomy and neurobiomechanics involved in the tests and the performance environment of the tests are very different.

Precautions with neural mobilization

Patients with 'red flags' such as tumours and inflammatory diseases must be managed accordingly, but there are other clinical situations where some care and attention is warranted during exercise and management involving the nervous system. In hindsight and with modern neurobiological knowledge, it seems that care should be taken with repeated movements aggravating central sensitization, too early movements on acute nerve root disorders, and any examination processes that are not tolerated by the patient's CNS sensitivity threshold level. The possibility of aggravating disorders may be reduced if the patient's sensitivity levels can be reduced before any exercise or passive technique. There are many techniques or clinical processes which can do this, and most clinicians do it anyway. First, identify what it may be that is keeping the CNS sensitive and then try and address it if possible. Frequently, it will be beliefs and superstitions about the nature of the pain and disability; blame and anger directed at work, family, or clinical personnel; or simply the novelty of the manual therapy treatment experience.

Use of the tests in management

Once a reasoned judgement is made that a test is reflective of part of the patient's problem and worthy of incorporating into management, there are a number of ways in which they can be used.

Concepts of neurodynamics are useful to explain aspects of sensitivity and tissue health

In the slump test, neck extension frequently relieves evoked lumbar, pelvic, and hamstring area pain. Passively flexing the neck will evoke lumbar symptoms in approximately 25% of patients with low back pain (Troup 1986). If we were patients, we might find this odd and would want any physical examination finding to be explained. We might not even mention such symptoms, for fear of disbelief. These symptoms can be explained in terms of transmission of load through a continuous structure, and may well form part of a rationale for proposing that total spinal mobilizing exercises may be necessary for managing headache or lumbar pain. Findings such as foot movement evoking head and neck pain, which is not uncommon in acute whiplash trauma, or neck movements causing leg pain, may also provide a framework for explaining sensitivity related to the CNS.

Knowledge of neurodynamics is also linked to the art of listening and provision of appropriate empathy. The quality of interaction is enhanced when a clinician can listen to a patient's story because it makes sense rather than the patient feeling they have to prove something is wrong (Hadler 1996). Concepts of neurodynamics help, and so does a knowledge of modern pain neurobiology.

Neurodynamics tests and passive mobilization

In the current environment of emphasis on self-care, the role of passive movement therapies is being re-evaluated. Passive movement in its various forms may assist restoration of tissue health, and the handling may provide for a more acute patient memory of an active treatment prescription. Good handling, a supportive treatment environment and appropriate passive movement can be a collection of inputs into the CNS, signalling that it is possible to perform a certain movement and perhaps experience a little pain without evoking a stress response. Remember too, when education becomes a critical aspect of management the person who has skilfully touched and examined the sore areas may be the one whose advice is taken and adhered to.

Some suggestions related to passive techniques

- They should form part of a management strategy which is likely to include active movements, education, fitness, work adjustments, etc. They are unlikely to form treatments by themselves. Passive mobilization could be seen as part of the patient's education about their problem.

- Pick your patients. A passive movement prescription will depend on the healing state of tissues, the extent of damage, and likely operant pain mechanisms. See Gifford and Butler (1997), Butler (1998, 2000) for further details and discussion. Likely candidates will have a well-reasoned and supported clinical diagnosis of specific physical dysfunction of the nervous system.

- Start movements away from a presumed site of pathology. This was probably taken to extremes in the past (Butler 1989, 1991), but it is useful. It should enhance safety, and may allow less focusing on the painful area. For example, with a sprained ankle, as part of management, extending the knee in hip flexion may be useful. In more sensitive states, movements from the less painful side, which are likely to have more processing and reflexive effects than mechanical, could be useful.

- Where patients understand the rationale for mobilization, some movements can be coaxed into pain. Particularly, old and stable peripheral neurogenic pain states may be treated, challenging stiffness, although it is better to get the patients to progress actively and methodically into any vigorous movements. Many chronic pain patients will need to move with pain, at the same time equipped with knowledge that the pain does not signal a harmful experience.

- Where the nervous system is physically unhealthy, neighbouring structures are likely to be so also. For example, management of a patient with a carpal tunnel syndrome could involve (if assessed and deemed to be appropriate) active and passive mobilization of the carpal bones, massage of the skin across the tunnel, attention to a tight pectoralis minor and the postures which have lead to it, some scapular stabilization work, and attention to the cervical and thoracic spines.

The role of neurodynamic tests in active mobilization

Neurodynamic movements can be used in a number of ways in active movements. Passive techniques could be converted into specific, more functional and meaningful active exercises. The tests could be used as a warm-up/cool-down or as part of a paced movement programme. With integration of the movements, remember the big picture evidence list at the beginning of the chapter.

Active movements following on a passive programme

Consider active movements as a challenge both to the physical health of neural and other tissues and to the threshold controls of the CNS.

Activity is a better word than exercise. The term 'exercise' instantly evokes negativity in many people, particularly those in pain. The following are some examples of activities which challenge various nerve pathways and presumably their CNS receptive fields, based on anatomy and clinical observations. Throwing objects (graduating from small balls to large balls) and doing graded push-ups are median nerve challenges. It is possible to challenge the ulnar nerves, for example by drying the back with a towel, and adjusting collars. The radial and indeed all nerves are challenged during disco dancing, flamenco dancing, and movement activities such as tai chi. The 'baksheesh' position challenges the radial-based pathways. Walking and exaggerated walking is great for the straight leg raise. Many so-called muscle tests also challenge neural pathways, for example stretch tests for the iliopsoas group also elongate the femoral and genitofemoral nerves.

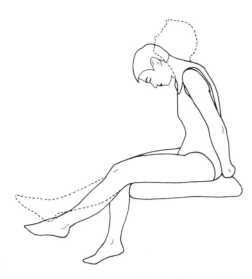

Figure 4.3.92 'Sliders and tensioners'. In the Slump position, if the neck is extended at the same time as the knee is extended this is conceptualized as a 'slider'. If the head is flexed at the same time as the knee is extended this is conceptualized as a 'tensioner'. The figure shows a 'slider'. (From Butler, D. S. (2000) The sensitive nervous system. Noigroup, Adelaide. With permission.)

Memorably, as Maitland (1986) said, 'technique is the brainchild of ingenuity'. From a close observation of the warm-up of many sporting teams, it appears that they have almost evolved to manoeuvres which load the nervous system, despite little knowledge of it.

For variety of movement, and to encourage large movements, the concept of 'sliders' and 'tensioners' can be useful. During the slump test, if the neck is flexed and the knee is extended at the same time, this is referred to as a 'tensioner', i.e. both ends are loaded. However, if the neck is extended at the same time the knee is extended, this is referred to as a 'slider' (Figure 4.3.73). Sliders allow a bigger range of motion, allow distraction, and should provide a multijoint, non-painful, hopefully fear-reducing input into the CNS. If a person extends an arm and then looks at the hand, this is more of a slider. If they were to do the same arm extension and look away, this would be a more aggressive tensioner.

Movement breakdowns and pacing

Neurodynamic tests are sensitive in many pain states, more so than in control groups. For examples, see Butler (2000). Perhaps this is due to the many tissues tested, likely dorsal root ganglion involvement, barrages of multiple input into the CNS, perhaps even their novelty. There are two aspects here. First, healing tissues need appropriate movement to assist healing and the nervous system, particularly its connective tissues, and receptive fields are probably no different. Gentle progressive movement with the body placed in varying degrees of nervous system load can be performed. For example, in a patient with a sensitive neck including neural structures, to exercise the neck, say in rotation, make sure their arms are folded and perhaps shoulder girdle elevated. Subsequent neck exercises can be performed with the arms by the side or even in a neurally loaded position. This is utilizing the concept of the continuum of the nervous system. Where patients cannot move their lumbar spine, movements of the head and feet will at least provide some neural movement in the lumbar area.

The patient with ongoing pain often loses movements and fitness and gets stiffer and often heavier, all of which leads to tissue ill health, probably altered CNS representations of tissues and movements, psychological distress at work and leisure, and sometimes curtailment of social pursuits. This can lead to a cycle of breakout overactivity attempts followed by underactivity which has been well described as a feature of the chronic pain sufferer (e.g. Sternbach 1987). An activity pacing programme may be relevant in these patients.

A pacing prescription involves determining a level of realistic pain-free activities followed by a gradual increase in activity, guided by agreements between patient and clinician. In those with more chronic pain, there is a need for a written exercise timetable and guidance over time and flare-up contingency plans. It is important that patients use time or number and not pain level as their guide to stopping and changing activity or posture (Harding and Williams 1995). Beneficial effects to tissue may initially be minimal, but the CNS has a chance to retrain. Movements that have always been painful, and perhaps learnt to be painful even by association to other inputs, will automatically cause stress responses. Many things can be paced, for example, taking a collar off, going for a walk, doing the ironing, a particular exercise, exposure to noise, even to psychosocial forces. Activity could be paced in regard to pain, sweating, nausea, or any other symptoms. Paced exposure to painful movements and stimuli happily accompanies continued provision of education (Vlaeyen et al. 1995).

Neurodynamic movements such as a slump test or part of a slump test could be paced either as a specific exercise or, even better, as part of a functional movement. In addition, altering the order of movement and 'trick' movements are useful here. Patients with sensitive slump tests often experience pain in getting out of a chair. Options here are to perform the movement a number of times short of pain and also to change the order of movement, almost a 'trick' movement. Most people initiate the movement from hip flexion. This may be a movement input which alerts the brain that a painful experience might be coming up. Do a foot movement first, or lead by the head. Removing gravity is another simple trick. To elevate the shoulder, get the patient to lean over and swing their arm as in a pendulum. Twisting the body while keeping the neck still is actually rotating the neck. The brain might get some novel, non-painful input from inputs which were once painful, and respond appreciatively with favourable output.

For further details and practical examples on pacing and associated education, see Caudill (1995), Harding (1998), Shorland (1998) among others. The description above forms just one part of numerous strategies for chronic pain management.

Use in postural/ergonomic advice

People adopt certain postures for a number of reasons. They may be forced into the posture by injury, there may be work or sporting postural demands, or they may have learnt to assume a particular posture or movement behaviour as a result of pain experiences. For example, a patient who has a lumbar problem and perhaps some root irritation may not want to flex forward and they may have developed a habit of lateral flexing while squatting to pick things up. Try to challenge these postures either by making the patient aware of them, using trick movements, or educating the patient that challenging postures assumed after injury will not be a harmful thing. A skilled examination may reveal some physical dysfunction in tissues, but in many cases the movement behaviours serve no beneficial purpose and are out of proportion to the local pathological changes.

Remember pinching as well as elongation. For example, a patient in a wheelchair who is resting their arms on the wheelchair table may have their cubital tunnels repeatedly compressed. Forward head postures in the presence of degenerative changes in the neck may pinch lower cervical nerve roots.

Some advice could be offered about sleeping positions. For example patients with non-resolving cubital tunnel syndrome may alter their nocturnal elbow flexion patterns by sleeping with a bean-bag cushion in the cubital fossa (Seror 1993). In acute states, for example, it may be as simple as keeping the knees flexed to enhance sleeping.

Conclusions

There is limited evidence-based work indicating that the inclusion of neurodynamics work will improve outcomes (although see Kornberg and Lew 1989, Rosmaryn 1997), and I consider it impossible to avoid neurodynamics in movement improvement strategies. Meanwhile, clinicians and researchers must continue to refine the specifics of individual tissue diagnosis and mobilization skills (e.g.Coppieters *et al.* 1999, Hall and Elvey 1999, Kleinrensink *et al.* 2000). However, there is plenty of 'big picture' evidence which suggests that patients can benefit if they can improve tissue and cardiovascular fitness and alter health-hindering beliefs, superstitions, and environmental forces. In this framework, concepts of altering neurodynamics have a place if they can be applied using uncorrupted clinical reasoning.

References

AHCPR (1994) *Clinical practice guideline number 14. Acute low back problems in adults.* Agency for Health Care Problems and Research. U.S. Department of Health and Human Services, Rockville, MD.

Breig, A., Troup, J. (1979) Biomechanical considerations in the straight leg raising test. *Spine*, **4**, 242–50.

Butler, D. S. (1989) Adverse mechanical tension in the nervous system: a model for assessment and treatment. *Australian Journal of Physiotherapy*, **35**, 227–38.

Butler, D. S. (1991) *Mobilisation of the nervous system.* Churchill Livingstone, Melbourne.

Butler, D. S. (1998) Integrating pain awareness into physiotherapy – wise action for the future. In: L. S. Gifford (ed.), *Topical issues in pain.* NOI Press, Falmouth.

Butler, D. S. (2000) *The sensitive nervous system.* Noigroup, Adelaide, Australia.

Caudill, M. A. (1995) *Managing pain before it manages you.* Guildford Press, New York.

Cohen, M. L. (1995) The clinical challenge of secondary hyperalgesia. In: M. O. Shacklock (ed.), *Moving in on pain.* Butterworth-Heinemann, Australia.

Coppieters, M. W., Stappaerts, K. H., Staes, F. F. (1999) A qualitative assessment of shoulder girdle elevation during the upper limb tension test 1. *Manual Therapy*, **4**, 33–8.

Devor, M., Seltzer, Z. (1999) Pathophysiology of damaged nerves in relation to chronic pain. In: P. D. Wall and R. Melzack (eds.), *Textbook of pain*, 4th edn. Churchill Livingstone, Edinburgh.

Durkan, J. A. (1991) A new diagnostic test for carpal tunnel syndrome. *Journal of Bone and Joint Surgery*, **73A**(4), 536–8.

Dworkin, R. H. (1997) Which individuals with acute pain are most likely to develop a chronic pain syndrome? *Pain Forum*, **6**, 127–36.

Frank, J. D. (1973) *Persuasion and healing.* John Hopkins University Press, Baltimore.

Gerteis, M., *et al.* (1993) *Through patient's eyes.* Jossey Bass, San Francisco.

Gifford, L., Butler, D. (1997) The integration of pain sciences into clinical practice. *Journal of Hand Therapy*, **10**, 86–95.

Gifford, L. S. (1998) *Topical Issues in pain.* NOI Press, Falmouth.

Hadler, N. (1996) If you have to prove you are well, you can't get well. The object lesson of fibromyalgia. *Spine*, **21**, 2397–400.

Hall, T. M., Elvey, R. L. (1999) Nerve trunk pain: physical diagnosis and treatment. *Manual Therapy*, **4**, 63–73.

Harding, V. (1998) Application of the cognitive-behavioural approach. In: J. Pitt-Brooke *et al.* (eds.), *Rehabilitation of movement.* Saunders, London.

Harding, V., Williams, A. de C. (1995) Extending physiotherapy skills using a psychological approach: cognitive behavioural management of chronic pain. *Physiotherapy*, **81**, 681–8.

Higgs, J., Jones, M. (2000) *Clinical reasoning in the health professions.* Butterworth-Heinemann, Oxford.

Kendall, N. A., S., Linton, S. J., Main, C. J. (1997) *Guide to assessing psychosocial yellow flags in acute low back pain: risk factors for long term disability and work loss.* Accident Rehabilitation & Compensation Insurance Corporation of New Zealand and the National Health Committee, Wellington.

Kleinrensink, G. J., Stoeckart, R., Mulder, P. G., H., Hoek, G. v. d. (2000) Upper limb tension tests as tools in the diagnosis of nerve and plexus lesions. *Clinical Biomechanics*, **15**, 9–14.

Kornberg, C., Lew, P. (1989) The effect of stretching neural structures on grade one hamstring injuries. *Journal of Orthopaedic and Sports Physical Therapy*, June, 481–7.

Linton, S. J. (1998) The socioeconomic impact of chronic back pain: is anyone benefiting? *Pain*, **75**, 163–8.

Mackinnon, S. E., Dellon, A. L. (1988) *Surgery of the peripheral nerve.* Thieme, New York.

Maitland, G. D. (1986) *Vertebral manipulation.* Butterworths, London.

Massey, A. (1985) Movement of pain sensitive structures in the neural canal. In: G. P. Greive (ed.), *Modern manual therapy of the vertebral column.* Churchill Livingstone, Edinburgh.

Mayo Clinic (1991) *Clinical examinations in neurology.* Mosby, St. Louis.

Nolan, F. M. (1996) *Introduction to the neurological examination.* F.A. Davis, Philadelphia.

Novak, C. B., Lee, G. W., Mackinnon, S. E., Lay, L. (1994) Provocative testing for cubital tunnel syndrome. *Journal of Hand Surgery*, **19A**, 817–20.

Penning, L. (1992) Functional pathology of lumbar spinal stenosis. *Clinical Biomechanics*, **7**, 3–17.

Rozmaryn, L., *et al.* (1998) Nerve and tendon gliding exercises and the conservative management of carpal tunnel syndrome *Journal of Hand Therapy*, **11**, 171–9.

Seror, P. (1993) Treatment of ulnar nerve palsy at the elbow with a night splint. *Journal of Bone and Joint Surgery*, **75B**, 322–7.

Shorland, S. (1998) Management of chronic pain following whiplash injuries. In: L. S. Gifford (ed.), *Topical issues in pain.* NOI Press, Falmouth.

Sternbach, R. A. (1987) *Mastering pain.* Ballantine Books, New York.

Supik, L. F., Broom, M. J. (1994) Sciatic tension signs and lumbar disc herniation. *Spine*, **19**, 1066–9.

Troup, J. D. G. (1986) Biomechanics of the lumbar spinal canal. *Clinical Biomechanics*, **1**, 31–43.

Vlaeyen, J. W., S., Kole-Snijders, A. M., J., Boeren, R. G., B., van Eek, H. (1995) Fear of movement/(re)injury in chronic low back pain and its relation to behavioural performance. *Pain*, **62**, 363–72.

Waddell, G. (1998) *The back pain revolution.* Churchill Livingstone, Edinburgh.

Woolf, C. J., Doubell, T. P. (1994) The pathophysiology of chronic pain – increased sensitivity to low threshold A beta fibre inputs. *Current Opinion in Neurobiology*, **4**, 525–34.

4.3.8 Trigger point injections

John Tanner

A trigger point is characterized by a focus of hyperirritability in a muscle that is locally tender when compressed, and if sufficiently hypersensitive gives rise to referred pain and tenderness (Travell and Simons 1983, 1998). A trigger point may produce autonomic phenomena. If the focus lies within a taut band of skeletal muscle and is active, it exhibits a local 'twitch' response when rolled under the palpating fingers. Each muscle tends to have characteristic locations of trigger points with typical patterns of referred pain (Figure 4.3.74).

Trigger points can be primary in the sense that they have become active as a result of direct influences on the muscle itself. This may follow a dynamic or a static postural strain. Indirectly these points may be triggered as part of a referral pattern, from other parts of the musculoskeletal system, or from visceral sources.

A final, and perhaps underestimated cause of trigger points with myofascial dysfunction is emotional distress, which may be mediated by increased sympathetic tone and circulating humoral factors.

Mechanical dysfunction of the spinal joints commonly cause referred pain with trigger point formation. When several trigger points can be found, the more peripheral ones tend to clear as range of motion improves with manipulative treatment (Fitzgerald 1991).

Microscopically the histology of these irritable foci of muscle reveal little abnormality. However, it has been observed that trigger points commonly seem to be quite closely related to the motor points (the point at which the motor nerve enters the underlying muscle) and in many instances they are close to traditional acupuncture points (Melzack *et al.* 1977). Thermography may show areas of increased skin temperature or, in more chronic situations, reduced skin temperature. Hubbard and Berkoff (1993) showed that fine-needle EMG produces insertional activity when the hyper irritable focus, which corresponds to an active muscle spindle, is directly penetrated.

The same authors have demonstrated the presence of direct sympathetic innervation of the muscle spindle. By using fine-needle EMG the trigger points are located and a small dose of phenoxybenzamine (an alpha-adrenergic blocker) is delivered through a stylet to block the sympathetic efferent stimulation: this effectively stops activity of the trigger-point. This procedure can give some significant soreness for up to 2 weeks. In therapeutic use, care must be taken not to inject too large a total dose in one session because of the risk of hypotension. For refractory trigger points this may prove to be a useful method.

Myofascial dysfunction can be treated in a variety of ways incorporating passive and active stretching techniques, improvement in posture, muscle balance, and attention to local joint or spinal dysfunction by appropriate mobilizing or manipulative techniques. If trigger points are persistent then one may apply direct ultrasound, digital pressure producing ischaemia and inhibition of the muscle, local anaesthetic injections with a small or large volume, and dry needling (intramuscular stimulation).

Different techniques of trigger point therapy for low back pain have been compared in two uncontrolled studies: Garvey *et al.* (1989) found stretching with a vapocoolant spray to be as effective as acupuncture or lidocaine (lignocaine) alone or with steroid, and Hong (1994) found that patients preferred lidocaine (lignocaine) trigger point therapy to dry-needling, as it was less painful (though equally effective). In a controlled study, Kovacs *et al.* (1997) used a skin device for stimulating the trigger points and found it effective.

The technique recommended by Travell and Simons (1983, 1998) is careful palpation of the active trigger point between two palpating fingers and inserting a fine (23- or 25-gauge) needle to a point where intense aching or soreness is noted by the patient, and then injecting 0.5–1 ml of a low-concentration local anaesthetic, such as 0.5% procaine or lidocaine (lignocaine) (Figure 4.3.93). The patient is recommended to perform stretching exercises actively and regularly over the next few days.

Fischer (1981) proposes a larger-volume local anaesthetic injection with multiple withdrawals and re-insertions in different directions to infiltrate larger bands of involved muscle (up to 10 ml 0.5% xylocaine).

References

Fischer, A. A. (1981) Thermography and pain. *Archives of Physical Medicine and Rehabilitation*, **62**, 542.

Fitzgerald, R. T. D. (1991) Observations on trigger points, fibromyalgia, recurrent headache and the cervical syndrome. *Journal of Manual Medicine*, **6**, 124–9.

Garvey, T. A., Marks, M. R., Wiesel, S. W. (1989) A prospective, randomised double-blind evaluation of trigger-point injection therapy for low-back pain. *Spine*, **14**, 962–4.

Hong, C. Z. (1994) Lidocaine versus dry-needling to myofascial trigger points. The importance of the local twitch response. *American Journal of Physical Medicine and Rehabilitation*, **73**, 256–63.

Hubbard, D. R., Berkoff, G. M. (1993) Myofascial trigger points show EMG activity. *Spine*, **18**, 1803–7.

Kovacs, F. M., Abraira, V., Pozo, F., *et al.* (1997) Local and remote sustained trigger point therapy for exacerbations of chronic low back pain. *Spine*, **22**, 786–97.

Melzack, R., Stillwell, D. M., Fox, E. J. (1977) Trigger points and acupuncture points for pain: correlations and implications. *Pain*, **3**, 3–23.

Travell, J. G., Simons, D. G. (1983) *Myofascial pain and dysfunction. The trigger point manual.* Williams & Wilkins.

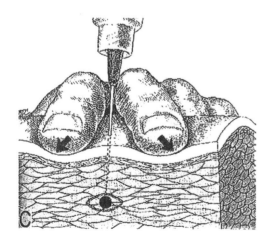

Figure 4.3.93 Muscle trigger points.

4.3.9 Soft tissue pain – treatment with stimulation-produced analgesia

C. Chan Gunn

It is critically important to understand and recognize the threefold nature of soft tissue pain, because it impacts on every musculoskeletal condition. This chapter reviews the three phases of pain, in order to establish that they are distinct physiological entities that call for individual diagnostic and therapeutic approaches. The chapter then examines myofascial pain syndromes, which are an assortment of chronic pain conditions affecting the musculoskeletal system. It explains how these seemingly unrelated conditions are merely symptoms of neuropathy and belong to the third phase of pain. Lastly, the chapter offers a rationale for the use of stimulation procedures, especially needling techniques.

The three phases of pain

Wall (1978) saw pain as a reaction pattern of three sequential behavioral phases: immediate, acute, and chronic. Each phase may exist independently, or in any combination and proportion with the others. In the immediate nociceptive phase, primary afferent nerves (with mechanosensitive or mechanothermal-sensitive and C-polymodal fibers) transduce specific forms of energy (mechanical, thermal or chemical) into electrochemical nerve impulses and transmit them to the central nervous system (CNS) via two main routes. One, the **spinoreticulothalamic tract**, has many synaptic relays and ends at the lower parts of the brain where it arouses the emotions and switches on the 'fight or flight' response. Its effects may, or may not, diffuse into the conscious brain; for example, nociceptive perception may not occur in the heat of battle (or the field of play) when there are other pressing distractions. The second tract, the **neospinothalamic**, evolved later and is more efficient, requiring only three relays to reach the sensory cortex that locates the pain. Thus, pain location occurs before its realization.

Nociception is usually transient, unless there is tissue injury and damaged cells result in the local release of algogenic substances (such as bradykinin, serotonin, histamine, hydrogen ions, potassium ions, prostaglandins, leukotrienes, nerve growth factors, and neuropeptides) to produce the inflammatory pain of Wall's acute phase. Anti-inflammatory drugs may have their application in this phase, but the abatement of inflammation with drugs can be counterproductive, because inflammation is the necessary prelude to healing.

After injury, most people heal rapidly and become pain free, but in some, pain persists beyond the usual time for the healing process and becomes intractable. Chronic pain, or Wall's third phase, is likely to occur if there is:

- **on-going nociception**, e.g. an unhealed fracture, or inflammation, e.g. rheumatoid arthritis

- **psychological factors** such as somatization disorders, depression, or adverse operant learning processes

- **abnormal function** in the nervous system.

The International Association for the Study of Pain defines injury in its definition of pain as 'an unpleasant sensory and emotional experience associated with actual or potential tissue damage, or described by the patient in terms of such damage'. But pain need not be linked causally to injury. Injury does not always generate pain, nor does pain always signal injury. Pain perception can also arise from within the body when there is a functional disorder in the nervous system. The most common functional disorder, by far, is peripheral neuropathy stemming from spondylosis. This large and mundane category of pain was first referred to as 'pain following neuropathy' (Gunn 1978), but the term **neuropathic pain** has now been extended to include any acute or chronic pain syndrome in which the mechanism that sustains the pain is inferred to involve aberrant somatosensory processing in the CNS or peripheral nervous system. Spondylosis and segmental dysfunction are no longer implicit in the present definition. Instead, the term **radiculopathic pain** is now used to refer to spondylotic pain (Gunn 1997).

Clinical features of neuropathic pain

The identification of chronic pain caused by ongoing nociception or inflammation is usually straightforward, but the clinical features of neuropathic pain are less well known.

Peripheral neuropathy may be defined as a disease that causes disordered function in the peripheral nerve. Although sometimes associated with structural changes in the nerve, a neuropathic nerve can – deceptively – appear normal. It still conducts nerve impulses, synthesizes and releases transmitted substances, and evokes action potentials and muscle contraction. All fibers can be damaged: sensory, motor, and autonomic. Some features of neuropathic pain are listed in the box overleaf; in radiculopathy, these features appear in the distributions of both anterior and posterior primary rami (Bradley 1974, Fields 1987).

Myofascial pain syndromes

Myofascial pain syndromes affect muscles and their connective tissue attachments in any part of the body and are customarily named according to the location of the painful part: e.g. 'tennis elbow', 'Achilles tendonitis', 'frozen shoulder', and even 'low back pain' (see Table 4.3.5). In neuropathy, muscles can shorten and mechanically stress their soft tissue attachments and joints. This can produce pain in many differ-

Neuropathic pain

Sensory

- Pain when there is no ongoing tissue-damaging process
- Delay in onset after precipitating injury. It takes about 5 days for supersensitivity to develop (Cannon and Rosenblueth 1949)
- Dysesthesia – unpleasant 'burning or searing' sensations
- Diffuse muscle tenderness and 'deep, aching' pain
- Pain felt in a region of sensory deficit
- Neuralgic pain – paroxysmal brief 'shooting or stabbing' pain
- Severe pain in response to a noxious stimulus (hyperalgesia)
- Severe pain in response to a stimulus that is not normally noxious (allodynia)
- Pronounced summation and after-reaction with repetitive stimuli

Motor

- Muscle shortening and pain caused by shortened muscle pulling on sensitive structures
- Loss of joint range

Autonomic

- Increased vasomotor, pilomotor and sudomotor activity (hyperhidrosis)
- Trophedema
- Causalgic pain, reflex sympathetic dystrophy or complex regional pain syndrome

Trophic

- Dermatomal hair loss
- Collagen degradation; weakness in tendons, offset by hypertrophy (enthesopathy)

When a unit is destroyed in a series of efferent neurons, an increased irritability to chemical agents develops in the isolated structure or structures, the effect being maximal in the part directly denervated.

lus, and sensitivity to catecholamines. These features are explained by a fundamental physiologic law: Cannon and Rosenblueth's (1949) law of denervation. This law points out that the normal physiology and integrity of all innervated structures are dependent upon the uninterrupted arrival of nerve impulses via the intact nerve to provide a regulatory or 'trophic' effect. When this flow – a combination of axoplasmic flow and electrical input – is obstructed, innervated structures are deprived of the vital factor that regulates cellular function. According to the law of denervation. atrophic structures become highly irritable and develop abnormal sensitivity. All denervated structures develop supersensitivity, including skeletal muscle, smooth muscle, spinal neurones, sympathetic ganglia, adrenal glands, sweat glands, and brain cells.

Cannon and Rosenblueth's original work was based on total denervation or decentralization for supersensitivity to develop: accordingly, they named the phenomenon **denervation supersensitivity**. It is now known that total physical interruption and denervation are not necessary. Any circumstance that impedes the flow of impulses for a duration of time can rob the effector organ of its excitatory input and disrupt normal physiology in that organ and in associated spinal reflexes (Sharpless 1975).

The importance of disuse supersensitivity cannot be overemphasized. Atrophic structures overreact to many forms of input, not only chemical, but physical as well, including stretch and pressure. Supersensitive muscle cells can generate spontaneous electrical impulses that trigger false pain signals or provoke involuntary muscle activity (Culp and Ochoa 1982). Supersensitive nerve fibers become receptive to chemical transmitters at every point along their length instead of only at their terminals; sprouting may occur, and denervated nerves are prone to accept contacts from other types of nerves including autonomic and sensory nerve fibers. Short circuits are possible between sensory and autonomic (vasomotor) nerves and may contribute to 'reflex sympathetic dystrophy' or the 'complex regional pain syndrome'.

Disuse supersensitivity is basic and universal, yet not at all well known. Many pain syndromes of apparently unknown causation can be attributed to the development of supersensitivity in receptors and pain pathways.

ent parts of the body. Although musculoskeletal pain syndromes appear to have an astounding diversity, the common denominator is muscle shortening. Myofascial pain syndromes can be puzzling, because they seem to arise and persist in the absence of detectable injury or inflammation. They are difficult to treat, because medications and physical therapies give only temporary relief. However, careful examination of myofascial pain conditions reveals them to be epiphenomena of neuropathy manifesting in the musculoskeletal system. Structural factors, such as muscle shortening and weakness of degraded collagen, also contribute to the pain.

The underlying problem is a functional disorder in the nervous system, and pain is a possible, but not inevitable, product of the neuropathy. The key to successful management of this important and widespread category of chronic pain is to understand neuropathy, how it can cause pain, and recognize it in its many disguises.

Electrophysiological features of neuropathy

Damaged primary afferent fibers demonstrate three electrophysiological features: spontaneous activity, exaggerated response to stimu-

Radiculopathy: its frequent relationship to spondylosis

It is not unusual for the flow of nerve impulses to be obstructed: peripheral neuropathy, often accompanied by partial denervation, is not exceptional. Of the numerous causes of nerve damage such as trauma, metabolic, and degenerative, spondylosis is easily the most prevalent.

Ordinarily, spondylosis follows a gradual, relapsing, and remitting course that is silent unless and until symptoms are precipitated by an incident often so minor that it usually passes unnoticed. The spinal

Table 4.3.5. Myofascial pain syndromes

Syndrome	Shortened muscles
Achilles tendonitis	Gastrocnemii, soleus
Bicipital tendonitis	Biceps brachii
Bursitis: pre-patellar	Quadriceps femoris
trochanteric	Gluteus maximus, medius, gemelli, quadratus femoris
Capsulitis (frozen shoulder)	All muscles acting on the shoulder, including trapezius, levator scapular, rhomboidei, pectoralis major/minor, supra- and infraspinati, teres major/minor, subscapularis, deltoid
Chrondromalacia patellae	Quadriceps femoris
De Quervain's tensynovitis	Abductor pollicis longus, extensor pollicis brevis
Facet syndrome	Muscles acting across the joint, e.g. rotatores, multifidi, semispinales
Fibromyalgia (diffuse myofascial syndrome)	Multisegmental, generally muscles supplied by cervical and lumbar nerve roots
Hallux vulgus	Extensores hallucis longus and brevis
Headaches: frontal	Upper trapezius, stenomastoid, occipitofrontalis
temporal	Temporalis, upper trapezius
vertex	Splenius capitis, cervicis
occipital	Suboccipital muscles
Intervertebral disc (early)	Muscles acting across the disc space, e.g. rotatores, multifidi semispinales
Low back sprain	Paraspinal muscles, e.g. iliocostalis lumborum and thoracis
Piriformis syndrome	piniformis muscle
Rotator cuff syndrome	Supra- and infra-spinatus, teres minor, subscapularis
Shin splints	Tibialis anterior
Temporomandibular joint	Masseter, temporalis, pterygoids
Tennis elbow	Brachioradialis, extensor muscles, anaconeus

nerve root is notably vulnerable to pressure, stretch, angulation, and friction, even from early prespondylosis (Gunn 1978). For pain to become a persistent symptom, affected fibers must have been previously irritated. After an acute injury to a healthy nerve, there is no prolonged discharge of pain signals, whereas injury to a neuropathic nerve can cause a sustained discharge (Howe *et al.* 1977). That is why some people develop severe pain after an apparently minor injury, and also why that pain can continue beyond a 'reasonable' period.

Physical irritation first entangles large-diameter nerve fibers – the axons of motoneurons and myelinated primary afferents from muscle proprioceptors. Muscle contracture with shortening is therefore an early feature of radiculopathy. Painless, tight knots can be felt in most individuals; not uncommonly, even in toddlers. Pain is not a feature until nociceptive pathways are involved. Many neuropathies are pain-free, such as hyperhidrosis and muscle weakness in ventral root disease.

Peripheral and central sensitization

Peripheral sensitization can follow tissue inflammation and peripheral neuropathy. There is increased transduction sensitivity of nociceptors caused by altered ionic conductances in the peripheral terminal. In inflammation, cells also produce growth factors and cytokines, which increase the sensitivity of nociceptors.

Central sensitization is a state of hyperexcitability in the dorsal horn. It can occur from damage to a peripheral nerve or from low-frequency repetitive C-fiber input, as in arthritis. The spinal cord is not simply a passive conveyer of peripheral sensation to the brain: it can modify or amplify incoming signals. There is increased spontaneous activity of dorsal horn neurons, increased response to afferent input, expansion of receptive field size, reduction in threshold and prolonged after discharges. Central sensitization leads to a cascade of molecular events, such as activation of the NMDA channel, increase in intracellular calcium, wind-up/wide dynamic range (WDR) neurone sensitization and other phenomena (Munglani *et al.* 1996).

In central sensitization, low-intensity stimulation can be perceived as painful, i.e. severe pain can occur in response to a stimulus that is not normally noxious (allodynia); and high intensity stimulation, which is normally painful, leads to hyperalgesia, i.e. there can be severe pain in response to a noxious stimulus. The receptive field size expands, and afterdischarges can occur. Pain often radiates several segments above and below the level of nociceptive input. This happens through propriospinal connections in adjacent layers of the dorsal horn where they make contact with WDR neurones. WDR neurones have immense fields compared to primary afferent neurones. Perceived pain can outlast the stimulus because a brief discharge from A delta or C fibers can generate prolonged activity in WDR neurones.

Fibromyalgia has recently become a popular diagnosis, and many doctors now apply the American College of Rheumatology (ACR)

1990 criteria. Is fibromyalgia a distinctive syndrome (Gunn 1995)? Or does it merely describe the most extreme and extensive of the aches, pains, and tender muscles that we all have, in various degrees, at one time or other? Mildly tender points are not unusual in most individuals, and moderate to extremely tender points are not unusual in those who have a vulnerable back. Other features of fibromyalgia such as articular pain, coldness of extremities, irritable bowel, and trophedema also point to a functional disorder in the peripheral nervous system with downstream changes in the spinal cord. For example, large-diameter afferent neurones that normally transmit non-noxious stimuli now start to express substance P (which is normally associated with small-diameter C-fibers that transmit pain and temperature). The exact significance of this phenotypic switch by large-diameter fibers is not known, but it may explain how light touch and proprioceptive information (carried by A-beta fibers) may be misinterpreted as pain by the spinal cord (Munglani *et al.* 1996). In the spinal cord, there are changes in neuropeptide levels, such as increase of substance P, glutamate, neurokinin A, and calcitonin gene-related peptide, and decrease of serotonin level.

Diagnosis

Pain from ongoing nociception or inflammation is usually promptly recognized and appropriately dealt with. But diagnosis of chronic neuropathic pain can be challenging, and depends almost entirely on the examiner's clinical experience and skill. The history gives little assistance. Pain frequently arises spontaneously with no history of trauma, and the degree of reported pain far exceeds that consistent with the injury.

Signs of neuropathy

The characteristic physical signs of neuropathy are different from the well-known ones of outright denervation, such as loss of sensation and reflexes (Gunn 1989). It is important to look for neuropathic signs because they indicate early neural irritation and dysfunction for which there is no satisfactory laboratory or imaging test. For example, thermography reveals decreased skin temperature, which is an indication of neuropathy, but does not by itself signify pain. Nerve conduction velocities usually remain within the wide range of normal values, and electromyography is not specific.

Diagnosis begins with a careful search for the signs of neuropathy: motor, sensory, and autonomic. Vasoconstriction differentiates neuropathic pain from inflammation pain: in neuropathic pain, the affected parts are perceptibly colder. There may be increased sudomotor activity, and the pilomotor reflex is often hyperactive and visible in affected dermatomes as 'goose bumps' (Figure 4.3.94). There can be interaction between pain and autonomic phenomena. A stimulus such as chilling, which excites the pilomotor response, can precipitate pain; vice versa, pressure on a tender motor point can trigger the pilomotor and sudomotor reflexes.

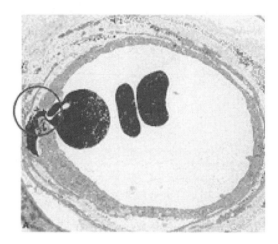

Figure 4.3.95 In neurogenic oedema, the permeability of small blood vessels is increased by transient gaps between endothelial cells, allowing fluid and plasma protein to escape into the extravascular space.

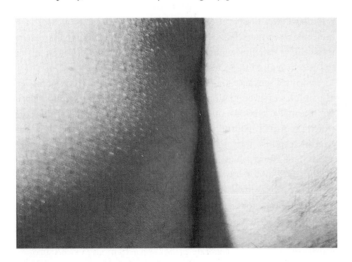

Figure 4.3.94 Goosebumps from a supersensitive pilomotor reflex on the left buttock, associated with muscle shortening in the gluteus maximus muscle.

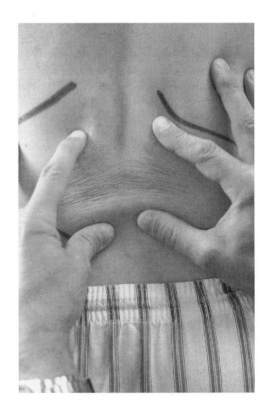

Figure 4.3.96 The peau d'orange sign indicating Neurogenic oedema or trophedema.

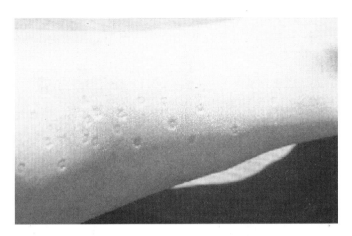

Figure 4.3.97 Gunn's Matchstick Test: Trophedema is non-pitting to digital pressure but the end of a matchstick produces a clear cut indentation that lasts for minutes.

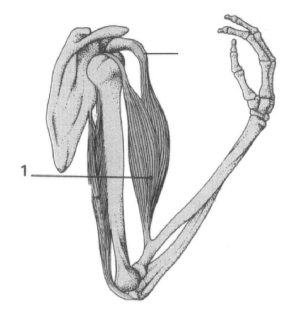

Figure 4.3.98 Muscle contracture can give rise to pain by its relentless pull on sensitive structures. Neuropathy degrades the quality of collagen, causing a tendon to thicken: enthesopathy. A shortened muscle pulling upon a tendon can produce 'tendonitis'. Increased tension in the synovial sheath causes tenosynovitis. Increased pressure of sesamoid bone on bone increases wear and tear, e.g. chondromalacia. Degraded collagen in a joint causes arthralgia and arthritis, eventually osteo-arthritis.

Increased capillary permeability can lead to local subcutaneous tissue edema – neurogenic edema or trophedema (Figure 4.3.95). This can be seen as *peau d'orange* skin (Figure 4.3.96) and can be confirmed by Gunn's 'matchstick' test. Trophedema is nonpitting to digital pressure, but when a blunt instrument such as the end of a matchstick is used, the indentation produced is clear-cut and persists for many minutes (Figure 4.3.97). This quick and simple test can demonstrate neuropathy earlier than electromyography. Trophic changes, including dermatomal hair loss, may also accompany neuropathy.

Muscle signs

Neuropathic changes are most apparent and consistently found in muscle. Even when symptoms appear in joints or tendons, changes can be found in muscle. There is increased muscle tone, tenderness at motor points, taut, tender, and palpable contracture bands (trigger points), and restricted joint range.

Each constituent muscle can and must be palpated, and its condition noted. Palpation requires a good knowledge of anatomy, and palpatory skill comes with practice. Paraspinal muscles are often compound; for example, the longissimus muscle extends throughout the length of the vertebral column. Even when symptoms appear to be localized to one level, the entire spine must be examined. A knowledge of the segmental nerve supply to muscles points to the level(s) of segmental dysfunction.

Muscle shortening from contracture

Muscle contracture – the evoked shortening of a muscle fiber in the absence of action potentials – is a fundamental part of musculoskeletal pain (Figure 4.3.98). Muscle shortening can give rise to pain by its relentless pull on sensitive structures (Gunn 1996) (Figure 4.3.98). Muscle contracture occurs from:

- **Increased susceptibility:** Lessened stimuli, which do not have to exceed a threshold, can produce responses of normal amplitude

- **Hyperexcitability:** The threshold of the stimulating agent is lower than normal

- **Super-reactivity:** The capacity of the muscle to respond is augmented

- **Superduration of response:** The amplitude of response is unchanged but its time-course is prolonged.

Supersensitive skeletal muscle fibers overreact to a wide variety of chemical and physical inputs, including stretch and pressure. In normal muscle, acetylcholine acts only at receptors that are situated in the narrow zone of innervation, but in neuropathy, it acts at newly formed extrajunctional receptors or 'hot spots' that appear throughout the muscle. Additionally, their threshold to acetylcholine is lowered because of reduced levels of acetylcholinesterase. Acetylcholine slowly depolarizes supersensitive muscle membrane. It induces an electro-mechanical coupling in which tension develops slowly, and without generating action potentials.

The role of the needle: the Deqi response

The fine, flexible acupuncture needle is a unique tool for finding and releasing muscle contractures. Contracture is invisible to radiography, CT, or MRI, and in deep muscles, it is beyond the finger's reach. The astonishing fact is that deep contracture can be discovered only by probing with a needle.

The needle transmits feedback information on the nature and consistency of the tissues it is penetrating. When penetrating normal muscle, it meets with little hindrance; when penetrating a contracture, there is firm resistance, and the needle is grasped by the muscle. This causes the patient to feel a peculiar, cramp-like, grabbing sensation which is referred to in acupuncture literature as the Deqi or Ch'i response (Gunn 1976). The intensity of the needle-grasp parallels the degree of muscle shortening, and it gradually eases off during treatment as muscle shortening is released. Release can occur in seconds or minutes.

The Deqi response is associated with proprioceptors that sense muscle shortening: it is an important finding because it confirms the presence of neuropathy. The traditional acupuncturist painstakingly elicits the Deqi response to differentiate between pain that has the Deqi response (neuropathic), and pain that does not (nociceptive). This distinction is vital because of the different nature and treatment of the two pains.

Treatment

Clinical trials have shown that the pharmacologic management of neuropathic pain is of limited effectiveness. Overall, there are no long-term studies of effectiveness to support the analgesic effectiveness of any drug beyond the short term (Kingery 1997).

Stimulation-induced analgesia

Physical therapy is widely used as a first line treatment for neuropathic pain. Early physical treatment is advocated because earlier treatment correlates with better outcome.

Neuropathic pain is a supersensitivity phenomenon and its treatment requires desensitization. Lomo (1976) has shown in animal experiments that supersensitivity and other features of denervated muscle are reduced or reversed by electric stimulation. Physical therapy also achieves its effect by stimulation. For example, massage stimulates tactile and pressure receptors. Heat and cold act on thermal receptors. Exercise, manipulation and dry needling stimulate muscle spindles and Golgi organs. These stimuli are sensed by their specific receptors, transduced into nerve impulses and relayed to the dorsal horn. Stimulation then spreads out reflexively to the entire segment. All forms of physical therapy, including dry needling, are effective only when the nerve to the painful part is still intact. When the nerve is not intact, neuropathic pain has been relieved by direct stimulation of the spinal cord (Howe *et al.* 1977).

All physical therapies have an inevitable limitation. They act as temporary substitutes for the body's own bioenergy, and their desensitization efforts do not persist. They last only as long as stimulation continues.

The current of injury

There is, serendipitously, an ideal source of energy: the body's own healing force, which can be tapped. Galvani, in a series of animal experiments that marked the beginning of electrophysiology, demonstrated in 1797 the existence of electricity in tissues. He was able to detect the electrical potential following tissue injury and called it the 'current of injury' (Galvani 1953). This intrinsic source of energy is the primary agent in promoting relief and healing. It is readily obtained, as in acupuncture and dry needling, by making minute injuries with a fine needle. Unlike extrinsic sources of energy, stimulation from the current of injury induced by the needle lasts for days until the miniature wounds heal. No injected medication is required.

The needle has another unique benefit offered by no other therapy: it promotes healing by releasing platelet-derived growth factor from blood. This substance induces cells to multiply and proliferate.

In chronic pain, fibrosis eventually becomes a major feature of the contracture: response to dry needle treatment is then much less dra-

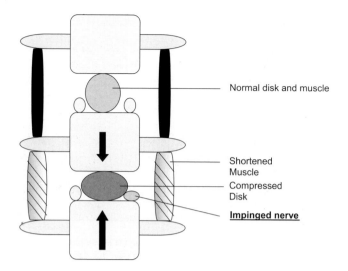

Figure 4.3.99 Muscle contracture across an intervertebral disk space can compress the disk which in turn can impinge on the spinal nerve.

matic. The extent of fibrosis does not correlate with chronologic age: scarring can occur after injury or surgery, and many older individuals have sustained less wear and tear than younger ones who have subjected their musculature to repeated physical stress. The treatment of extensive fibrotic contractures necessitates more frequent and extensive needling. To relieve pain in such a muscle, it is necessary to needle all tender bands. It is uncommon to encounter a muscle that is totally fibrotic and cannot be released by vigorous needling. Surgical release is usually unnecessary as the needle can reach deeply located shortened muscles.

Removing the cause of radiculopathy

For long-lasting pain relief and restoration of function, it is necessary to release muscle contracture in paraspinal muscle that is compressing a disc and entrapping the nerve root (Figure 4.3.99). Segmental dysfunction and pain are effectively resolved when pressure on the nerve root is relieved.

Treatment usually begins with simple measures such as heat and massage, escalating to more effective modalities such as TENS, manipulation, and ultimately needling. The outcome of treatment depends, not on the modality used, but on the skill and experience of the therapist.

The Multidisciplinary Pain Center has, since 1985, successfully used a dry needling technique called intramuscular stimulation (IMS). In IMS, diagnosis, treatment, as well as progress during therapy are determined according to physical signs of neuropathy. Effective IMS requires a sound background in anatomy and physiology (Gunn 1996). The efficacy of IMS for chronic low back pain has been demonstrated by a randomized clinical trial involving a large group of Worker's Compensation Board patients. At their 7-month follow-up, the treated group was clearly and significantly better than the control group (Gunn and Milbrandt 1978).

It is a convincing experience to diagnose neuropathic pain by finding its unmistakable physical signs, then to treat the patient with IMS and witness the signs disappear, often within minutes. Objective evidence, directly witnessed, is the best form of evidence-based medicine.

Conclusions

The traditional definition of pain as a consequence of injury is often invalid. Chronic pain is commonly a manifestation of neuropathy and unrelated to nociception or inflammation. Neuropathic pain is now widely accepted, but its near-constant connection to spondylosis is not widely known. Signs of neuropathy are subtle and differ from those of outright denervation. Neuropathic pain has a proprioceptive component – pain cannot exist without muscle shortening. Shortened muscles are often the unsuspected cause of many conditions, such as tension headache and low back pain (see Table 4.3.5). Neuropathy degrades the quality of collagen and contributes to degeneration in weightbearing and activity-stressed parts of the body.

The underlying problem is neuropathy, and therapy should be directed to its cause. Drug treatment is unavailing; physical therapy is the best approach. The needle is a unique and effective tool for diagnosing and treating neuropathic pain. It is not by happenstance that acupuncture is based on the relief of neuropathy.

References

Bradley, W. G. (1974) *Disorders of peripheral nerves.* Blackwell Scientific Publications, Oxford, pp. 129–201; 253–67.

Cannon, W. B., Rosenblueth, A. (1949) *The supersensitivity of denervated structures.* Macmillan, New York, pp. 1–22, 185.

Culp, W. J., Ochoa, H. (1982) *Abnormal nerves and muscles as impulse generators.* Oxford University Press, New York, pp. 3–24.

Fields, H. L. (1987) *Pain.* McGraw-Hill, New York, pp. 133–64.

Galvanni, A. (1953) *Commentary on electricity,* translated by Robert Montraville Green. Elizabeth Licht, Cambridge.

Gunn, C. C. (1976) Transcutaneous neural stimulation, needle acupuncture and 'Teh Ch'i' phenomenon. *American Journal of Acupuncture,* 4(4), 317–22.

Gunn, C. C. (1978) 'Prespondylosis' and some pain syndromes following denervation supersensitivity. *Spine,* 5(2),185–92.

Gunn, C. C. (1989) Neuropathic pain: a new theory for chronic pain of intrinsic-origin. *Annals of The Royal College of Physicians and Surgeons of Canada,* 22(5), 327–30.

Gunn, C. C. (1995) Fibromyalgia: letter to the editor. *Pain,* 60, 349–52.

Gunn, C. C. (1996) *The Gunn approach to the treatment of chronic pain – intramuscular stimulation for myofascial pain of radiculopathic origin.* Churchill Livingstone, London.

Gunn, C. C. (1997) Radiculopathic pain: diagnosis and treatment of segmental irritation or sensitization. *Journal of Musculoskeletal Pain,* 5(4), 119–34.

Gunn, C. C., Milbrandt, W. E. (1978) Early and subtle signs in low back sprain. *Spine,* 3(3), 268–81.

Howe, J. F., Loeser, J. D., Calvin, W. H. (1977) Mechanosensitivity of dorsal root ganglia and chronically injured axons: a physiological basis for the radicular pain of nerve root compression. *Pain,* 3, 25–41.

Kingery, W. S. (1997) A critical review of controlled clinical trials for peripheral neuropathic pain and complex regional pain syndromes. Pain, 73, 123–39.

Lomo, T. (1976) The role of activity in the control of membrane and contractile properties of skeletal muscle. In: Thesleff, S. (ed.) *Motor innervation of muscle.* Academic Press, New York, ,pp. 289–315.

Munglani, R., Hunt, S. P., Jones, J. G. (1996) The spinal cord and chronic pain. In: Kaufman, L. Ginsburg, R. (eds.) *Anaesthesia review* 12, pp. 53–75.

Sharpless, S. K. (1975) Supersensitivity-like phenomena in the central nervous system. *Federation Proceedings,* 34(10), 1990–1997.

Wall, P. D. (1978) The gate control theory of pain mechanisms – a re-examination and re-statement. *Brain,* 101, 1–18.

Wolfe, F., Smythe, H. A., Yunus, M. B., *et al.* (1990) American College of Rheumatology 1990 criteria for the classification of fibromyalgia: report of the Multicenter Criteria Committee. *Arth. Rheum.,* 33, 160–72.

4.3.10 Complementary therapies

Adam Ward

Complementary medicine, its use and clinical relevance

There is no simple definition of complementary medicine. It is a term that has evolved to describe therapies which were often previously considered 'fringe' or 'alternative', and because of this it may also be classified more generically as 'complementary and alternative medicine'. There have, of course, always been therapies that were considered to be outside the prevailing medical orthodoxy of the day. The British Medical Association Working Party in 1993 looking at complementary medicine defined it as 'treatments not widely used by orthodox health care professionals and which incorporated skills not routinely taught as part of orthodox medical training' (BMA 1993). However, medical schools are now increasingly providing exposure to complementary medicine within the undergraduate curriculum, and complementary therapies are frequently offered to patients in orthodox primary and secondary medical care.

Complementary medicine is of importance to orthopaedic and musculoskeletal medicine because it incorporates therapies that have particular relevance to the treatment of musculoskeletal problems. These include, among others, the manual therapies such as spinal manipulation, osteopathy, and chiropractic as well as acupuncture and dry needling. Studies in the UK and Europe (Fisher and Ward 1994) and in North America (Eisenberg *et al.* 1993) show that back problems and arthritis are one of the largest groups of clinical problems seen by practitioners of complementary medicine, and that manual therapies and acupuncture are some of the most frequently used treatments (Vincent and Furnham 1997). Complementary medicine also tends to take a holistic or whole-person approach, which is of particular value in chronic musculoskeletal problems.

A survey of 254 urban and inner-city general medical primary care practices in Birmingham (UK) revealed that, of the 175 practices which responded to the study, 94% offered at least one of acupuncture, osteopathy, chiropractic, hypnotherapy, or homoeopathy either in-house or by referral. These 5 therapies formed by far the largest group of complementary therapies out of a total of 17 which were defined as complementary by the practices themselves. Of these main 5 therapies, 64% of the practices offered acupuncture, 39% offered osteopathy, 33% offered chiropractic, 30% offered hypnotherapy, and 26% offered homoeopathy. The range of therapies offered by individual practices varied from 1 to 7, with a mean of 2.4 (Wearn and Greenfield 1998).

A separate study by Wharton and Lewith (1986) of 193 general practitioners in the Avon District of England showed that, of the 145 doctors who completed the questionnaire, spinal manipulation was considered to be useful or very useful by 89% and acupuncture useful or very useful by 57%.

Despite the fact that growth in the use of these therapies in Western countries is a relatively recent phenomenon, it is worth remembering that their origins often go back hundreds or even thousands of years. Manual therapies are as old as history. Spinal manipulation, for example, was practiced by bonesetters throughout medieval Europe. Similarly, acupuncture, in its various forms, goes back millennia and although its current popularity in developed countries is comparatively new, it was in fact probably in use in Europe 5000 years ago.

Holistic health care

The word 'holism' is generally associated with complementary medicine and thought of as a term that originated in antiquity. Although its underlying concepts go back at least as far as the earliest ancient Chinese literature, the use of the word itself is comparatively recent: it was first coined by General Jan Smuts (1870–1950), the South African soldier and statesman, in his book *Holism and Evolution*. In doing so he took a position outside scientific orthodoxy, stressing the tendency in nature to produce wholes, which were not explicable in terms of the sum of their parts. In its turn holistic medicine takes a 'whole person' approach to patient care that emphasizes the balance between the physical, psychological, social, and spiritual in the maintenance of health. This may be contrasted with the cartesian or reductionist scientific enquiry which is usually associated with modern Western medicine (named for René Descartes, 1596–1650, French philosopher).

Most complementary therapies encourage holistic, person-centred approaches to care which are of particular value, for example, when treating patients with medically unexplained symptoms presenting as symptoms of musculoskeletal pain and dysfunction.

Holism is now also used in a wider context in relation to the place of human society within the environment and global ecological systems. It is not, however, the sole property of complementary medicine and, indeed, has always formed an essential part of good medical care. This was enshrined in 1947 in the mission statement of the World Health Organization in which health is defined as 'a state of complete physical, mental and social well-being'.

A holistic approach can be of practical value in musculoskeletal medicine where an understanding of precipitating and perpetuating factors, whether related to lifestyle, occupation, or the environment, and the provision of continuing patient-centred support for more chronic conditions, can be crucial to the successful management of musculoskeletal dysfunction and pain.

There is no clear dichotomy

The classification of treatments as orthodox or complementary can sometimes be arbitrary and misleading. The complementary or alternative treatments of today influence the orthodox treatment of tomorrow. Clinical medicine is continuously evolving and incorporating different ideas and treatments while rejecting the ineffective or dangerous. This gives the key to the essential prerequisite of any therapy – whatever it may be called, whether orthodox or complementary – that it should be both **safe and effective**. In the rest of this chapter particular aspects of complementary therapies of special relevance to musculoskeletal disorders are described in greater detail.

Mind–body medicine

Overview

Mind–body medicine recognizes the importance of the relationship between physical and psychological health. It encourages an understanding of the functioning of the body as an integrated whole which is made up of interdependent systems that react in specific ways when exposed to stress. The body's response to stress depends not only on the event itself but on the way it is interpreted, and is a result of both physical and mental reactions to changes in the internal and external environments. Social and cultural support and previous experience can fundamentally affect specific responses to adverse events. Interactions between the individual and the environment lead to adaptive responses that, during the initial phase, can result in increased performance whether it is in terms of immunological function or productive activity (Selye 1956). The response to continuing stress may, however, lead to fatigue and failure of adaptive mechanisms with falling off of performance resulting in ill health (Figure 4.3.100).

Clinical relevance

There is now extensive evidence that continuing stress, particularly in those who have difficulty in coping, is a major risk factor for a range of both somatic and psychological illness. It is evident that the function of the brain has a key role in stress response and that it communicates through interdependent pathways linked with the mind and the body's reactive defences (Watkins 1997).

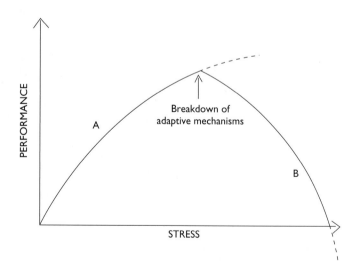

Figure 4.3.100 Performance stress graph. Performance can be enhanced in response to increased stress from a base of normal stress and good general health (A). Increasing stress, however, eventually reaches a point where adaptive mechanisms become fatigued and can no longer respond with further improvements in performance. Continuing stress beyond this point (B) can lead to decreased performance and ill health. Stress response curves will vary according to the individual and the environment.

Knowledge of mind–body pathways can lead to an improved understanding of functional somatic disorders that can be defined as somatic symptoms in the absence of detectable physical abnormalities. In the past such symptoms have often been described as psychosomatic, but this term has come to suggest that the cause is psychogenic. The term **medically unexplained symptoms** is better and less biased because it does not prejudge the nature of the symptoms and offers the open-minded possibility of better understanding in the future. No doubt, specific symptom patterns, previously labelled as medically unexplained symptoms, will come to be recognized and grouped in identifiable syndromes – as has happened, for example, with the musculoskeletal symptoms associated with fibromyalgia and chronic fatigue syndrome.

Such symptoms are of particular relevance to musculoskeletal medicine because of their frequent occurrence and the attendant risks of overinvestigation. The estimated lifetime prevalence in a population survey from the USA of somatic symptoms was: joint pains 37%, back pain 32%, and arm and leg pain 23%. One third of all the symptoms reported, however, were unexplained by organic disease (Kroenke and Price 1993).

Common medically unexplained symptoms include pain, tiredness, shortness of breath, insomnia, and dysthaesias. Similar symptoms accounted for almost half of all primary care consultations, of which only 10–15% were found to have an organic cause when followed up for 1 year (Katon and Walker 1998).

Medically unexplained symptoms are also common in secondary care, and present to most hospital specialties. A survey of hospitals in the south-east of England revealed that 21% of all consultation episodes were medically unexplained. Commonly these included abdominal pain, chest pain, headache, and back pain (Reid *et al.* 2001).

Patients with these symptoms are frequent users of musculoskeletal services, but they often feel that orthodox medical explanations fail to adequately recognize their distress. It is not surprising, therefore, that many seek help from practitioners of complementary medicine who may be able to make sense of symptoms in a way that better helps patients to understand and cope.

Extensive application

Mind–body medicine covers a wide field and incorporates current research in such specialist subjects as psychoneuroimmunology, in addition to traditional therapies such as the Chinese mind-body techniques of qigong and taijiquan as well as yoga, meditation, and a range of psychological techniques such as relaxation, hypnotherapy, biofeedback, guided imagery, and cognitive-behavioural therapy.

Of these, there is extensive evidence of the effectiveness of hypnotherapy in treating a range of psychological and physical disorders, and its use has now been approved by the American Medical Association as a clinical adjunct in the management of chronic pain.

Tinterow (1987) in an analysis of 178 chronic pain patients whose problems included amongst others, headaches, sciatica, and arthritis, reported that after hypnotherapy, 78% were pain free at 6 months, 44% at 2 years, and 36.5% at 3 years. Another study of chronic pain showed that after an 8-week course of meditation there was a 50% or greater reduction in pain in 61% of the participants (Kabat-Zinn 1990). Hypnotherapy was also shown to be beneficial in a controlled trial of patients with refractory fibromyalgia (Haanen *et al.* 1991). There is additional evidence of the beneficial use of biofeedback in migraine (Fahrion 1978), tension headache (Kondo and Canter 1977), and the pain and nausea associated with cancer treatment (Syrjala *et al.* 1992).

Qigong, a combination of meditation and movement, has been studied extensively in China (an estimated 5% of China's 1.3 billion people practice qigong) and is reported as being of value in patients with arthritis, pain, depression, and anxiety. It is not, however, without hazard: many reports of mental disorders associated with its use have been published in the Chinese psychiatric literature (Lee 2000). Yoga has also been shown to be of benefit in the management of pain (Nespor 1991).

Mind–body therapies are principally concerned with facilitating intrinsic healing mechanisms of the body through the restoration of psychoneuroimmunological balance. The importance of the endorphins in relation to pain is well known, but they are just one group of many neurotransmitters, which provide extensive links between mind and body. A wide range of therapies come under the general heading of mind–body medicine, some of which can be of value if used selectively as part of multidisciplinary rehabilitation schemes for patients with pain and associated anxiety and depression (Flor *et al.* 1992). Cognitive-behavioural therapy can help in improving daily functioning and quality of life for patients with chronic pain for whom conventional treatments have been unsuccessful.

A study of 212 patients with disabling chronic pain (mean duration 10.5 years) for whom no further medical or psychiatric treatment was appropriate were assessed after a 4-week programme which included education, behavioural and cognitive skills, stretch and exercise, and relaxation. All the patients had been referred to St Thomas' Hospital Pain Clinic in London from all over the UK and 68% had spinal pain. Assessment immediately after treatment showed significant improvements in all outcome measures, which were well maintained at 6 months (Williams *et al* 1993). Cognitive-behavioural therapy has also been found to be effective in reducing medically unexplained symptoms in a meta-analysis of six randomized controlled trials of chronic low back pain (van Tulder *et al.* 2000).

Future developments

Psychological stress is known to be associated with depressive disorders that are associated with neurochemical responses involving the triad of steroids, amines and peptides. Development in the treatment and understanding of depression is incorporating social, psychological and neurochemical information about stress and its effects on mental health (Herbert 1997). Levels of emotional well-being are also linked with physical disease. Medically unexplained symptoms are also associated with anxiety, depression, and distress. Epidemiological studies have shown that social and emotional support can protect against premature mortality, prevent illness, and aid recovery. The UK's green paper *Our healthier nation*, published by the Secretary of State for Health in 1998, defines health as 'being confident and positive and able to cope with the ups and downs of life'. The extent to which the emotional health of a nation can be regarded as the responsibility of its national health service is a debate that will tax health service providers and politicians for many years to come (Stewart-Brown 1998).

Acupuncture and dry needling

Chinese acupuncture and the West

Acupuncture is an English word used to mean puncture with a sharp object. It is commonly used to describe traditional Chinese medical needling, which is based upon ancient ideas that have evolved over several thousands of years about the flow of body energy and its rela-

tionship to health and disease. It is interesting to note, however, that similar needling techniques were probably being used in Europe 5300 years ago, as evidenced by tattoos found on the recently dated and well-preserved body of 'Oetzi', the iceman, who was discovered in a frozen gully high in the Oetzal Alps on the border between Austria and Italy in 1991.

The word acupuncture is also used to describe other needling techniques, which are based upon modern concepts of neurophysiology. In order to avoid confusion with traditional Chinese acupuncture, this Western form of acupuncture is now often referred to as **dry needling**, and over the last few decades it has evolved its own protocols and research base (Filshie and White 1998). The common link between the two is that they both use fine-gauge solid needles with atraumatic tips capable of providing graded and precisely positioned nociceptive stimulation. However, other approaches to nociceptive stimulation for the treatment of pain have been, and are still, used in many different cultures throughout the world over similarly long periods of time and include such techniques as cutting, scarification, cautery, and blistering.

Understanding needle effects

Traditional Chinese medicine is vitalistic and is concerned with the balance of energy (chi) within the body. Chinese acupuncture facilitates

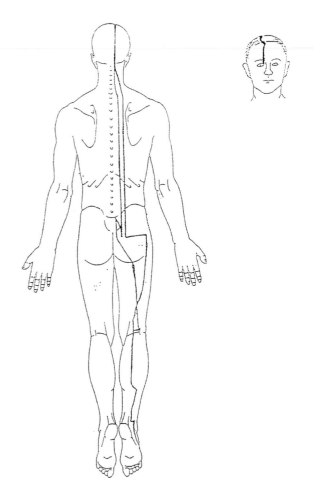

Figure 4.3.101 The urinary bladder meridian. This meridian contains many acupuncture points on the back and leg, which often correspond to the sites of trigger points. They are frequently used in the treatment of back and leg pain.

this balance by inserting needles through specific points in the skin (acupuncture points) to either enhance or subdue chi, which flows through channels or meridians. These meridians are not structural entities but functional pathways forming intercommunicating circuits of energy over which the majority of named acupuncture points lie (Figure 4.3.101).

Acupuncture skills in ancient China were usually passed on by apprenticeship from master to pupil. However, ancient books do exist, the earliest known being *The Yellow Emperor's Classic of Internal Medicine* (Huang Di Nei Jing Su Wen) which incorporates a wealth of knowledge gleaned over generations of practice. The oldest portions of this book date from the Han dynasty in the second century BCE, and describe the human body as a reflection of the universe with the physician's role being to maintain the body's harmonious balance with both its internal and external environments. This approach can be seen to be analogous with Western ideas of holism.

The details of the application of traditional Chinese acupuncture and its associated philosophy can appear excessively complicated and esoteric, and this may be one of the reasons why it has not, until recently, been widely accepted in the West. Although Western awareness of acupuncture dates back at least as far as the seventeenth century, and in the nineteenth century articles appeared in both the *British Medical Journal* (Ogier-Ward 1858) and the *Lancet* (Pridgin Teale 1871), it was not until President Nixon's visit to China in 1972 and the re-opening of China to foreign visitors after the Cultural Revolution that acupuncture made significant inroads into Western medical practice.

This was facilitated by the discovery in 1973 of the endogenous opioids, which were found to account for certain aspects of the analgesic effect of needling (Lewitt 1979). Current ideas about acupuncture's mechanism of action also include other neurotransmitters such as serotonin and noradrenaline (norepinephrine), which, by inhibitory control, can reduce the perception of pain. Part of this effect can be ascribed to the gate theory of Melzack and Wall (1965) and diffuse noxious inhibitory controls (DNIC) (Le Bars *et al.* 1991). These theories are expanding current understanding about how stimulation of A delta or group III small myelinated primary afferents and

associated small fibre afferents in skin and muscle by fine needles can lead to both segmental and more widespread (heterosegmental) analgesic effects.

DNIC and heterosegmental effects also help to explain why the insertion of a needle anywhere in the body causes a neurophysiological response, which can have a widespread therapeutic effect – one of the problems in designing adequate placebo controls for clinical trials. However, there is evidence to suggest that by concentrating the nociceptive needle stimulus in the affected pain segment (dermatome, myotome, or sclerotome), pain relief can be enhanced (Bekkering and van Bussel 1998). This needling technique, known as **segmental acupuncture**, is able to target the dorsal horns of the appropriate pain segment, the precise placing of the needle being based upon an analysis of each individual patient's pain pattern.

Other dry needling techniques include deep needling of muscles. This can include intramuscular stimulation (IMS), which is discussed in detail in Chapter 4.3.8, as well as specific needling of trigger points found in myofascial pain syndromes. There are interesting similarities between the locations of the Chinese acupuncture pain points (ah shi points) and myofascial trigger points. In one paper there was found to be 71% congruence between the sites of ah shi points and trigger points (Melzack *et al.* 1977). It has also been shown that the small, discrete areas of spontaneous electrical activity found in trigger points (Hubbard and Berkoff 1993) can also be found at sites common to both acupuncture points and trigger points, as shown in Figure 4.3.102 (Ward 1996). It seems probable that Chinese acupuncturists identified tender points associated with specific pain referral patterns, which in the West would be classified as trigger points, and incorporated them into their general philosophy and treatment protocols.

Western research into dry needling and trigger points, as well as contributing to knowledge about soft tissue pain and dysfunction, has helped to explain the possible ways in which needling techniques can lead to the resolution of musculoskeletal symptoms (Simons *et al.* 1999). It is seems likely that active trigger points, characterized by spontaneous electrical activity in small, circumscribed areas or points within muscles, are linked with abnormal motor endplate activity and associated with autonomic dysfunction. These hypersensitive points

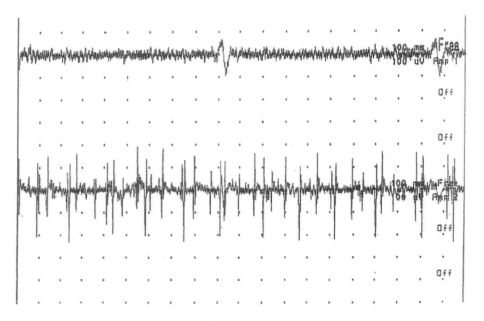

Figure 4.3.102 Spontaneous electrical activity (SEA) at the common site of a traditional acupuncture point on the small-intestine meridian and a myofascial trigger point in the infraspinatus. The lower tracing demonstrates SEA; the upper tracing is from an EMG needle placed within the same muscle to the same depth 1 inch (2.5 cm) away and demonstrates that the muscle as a whole is in a relaxed state.

in skeletal muscle are also associated with palpable taut bands, are painful on firm palpation, and can have widespread referral patterns. It is not unusual for trigger points around the shoulder or hip to refer into the arm or the leg; they may cause confusion with brachial neuralgia and sciatica. In addition, trigger points are associated with restricted muscle lengthening, which can cause stiffness and weakness as well as pain. Autonomic phenomena include changes in vasomotor, sudomotor, and pilomotor activity as well as changes in skin and subcutaneous tissues and can affect viscerosomatic reflexes. Autonomic effects include pain synthesis, and active trigger points have been found in reflex sympathetic dystrophy and other complex regional pain syndromes.

Relationship to wet needling

Wet needling (injection) is also used in the treatment of trigger points. This has included the use of local anaesthetics, saline, steroids, non-specific anti-inflammatories (NSAIDs), and *Botulinum* toxin. All have shown positive therapeutic results. There is evidence to indicate, however, that simple dry needling can be equally effective (Cummings and White 2001). It is intriguing to speculate how much of the therapeutic benefit of wet needling in the treatment of trigger points is due to the specific substance injected and how much is due to the needle effect and associated nociceptive stimulation.

The results of other wet needling techniques, not specifically related to the treatment of trigger points, are more dependent on the precise nature of the injection agent. Details of such procedures are covered elsewhere (see especially Chapters 4.3.3–6).

Clinical application

Pain is one of the commonest presenting symptoms in general medical practice, and individual studies have found significant relief of pain in patients of about 70% when acupuncture has been introduced into UK general practice clinics (Strauss 1989, Selly 1991, Wright 1991).

Randomized controlled trials have shown that acupuncture is of significant benefit for osteoarthritis of the knee (Christensen *et al.* 1992, Berman *et al.* 1995) and can be as effective as intra-articular steroid in osteoarthritis of the hip joint (McIndoe *et al.* 1995). The immediate analgesic effect of acupuncture in chronic tennis elbow pain (lateral epicondylalgia) was assessed after one treatment in a double-blind placebo-controlled trial where both pretreatment and post-treatment assessments were blinded. Overall reduction in the pain score was 55.8% in the verum group and 15% in the placebo group. The average duration of analgesia after one treatment was 20.2 hours in the verum group and 1.4 hours in the placebo group (Molsberger and Hille 1994). In another study of tennis elbow, 21 out of 34 patients who were treated with acupuncture became pain free, despite the fact that many had previously received steroid injections without improvement; 8 out of a control group of 26 patients who received only steroid injections reported a corresponding improvement (Brattberg 1983). A further study of tennis elbow compared different needling techniques consisting of superficial, no stimulation needling with 'classical' deep needling (usually 1.25–2.5 cm) with stimulation sufficient to cause obvious sensation and demonstrated a significant difference in favour of the more active treatment (Haker and Lundeberg 1990).

A systematic review of acupuncture for back pain (Ernst and White 1998) found 12 randomized controlled trials, of which 4 were placebo-controlled. Despite wide variability in their quality, it was possible to combine 9 of the studies in a meta-analysis of 377 participants. The overall odds ratio was 2.30 (95% confidence interval 1.28–4.13) in favour of active treatment, indicating that acupuncture was significantly better than the control interventions. However, the combined results of the four placebo controlled studies showed no significant difference between real and placebo acupuncture with an odds ratio of 1.37 (95% confidence interval 0.84–2.25).

It should be noted, though, that a later review of essentially the same studies using different assessment criteria concluded that the case mix and forms of acupuncture used were too heterogeneous to be included in a meta-analysis (van Tulder *et al.* 1999). This divergence of opinion highlights the need for further research, and the UK National Health Service is currently funding a pragmatic randomized controlled trial into the clinical and economic benefits of providing acupuncture to patients with low back pain in primary care (Thomas *et al.* 1999a).

A systematic review of acupuncture for neck pain found 14 randomized controlled trials with 7 positive and 7 negative outcomes. Of the positive studies, acupuncture was superior to waiting list in 1 study and in a further 3 was either equal to or better than physiotherapy (White and Ernst 1999). In another systematic review, which looked at acupuncture for osteoarthritis in any joint, 13 studies were found, 7 of which were positive and 6 negative. However, the majority of the positive studies failed to control for placebo effects. Of the 5 placebo-controlled studies within the group of 13, 4 showed no difference between real acupuncture and sham acupuncture (Ernst 1997). Systematic review of randomized controlled trials for migraine and tension headache found 22 studies of variable quality. Of the 14 studies comparing real acupuncture with sham, most showed a trend in favour of active treatment. Pooled results for the responder ratios were 1.55 (95% confidence interval 1.04–2.33) for migraine and 1.49 (95% confidence interval 0.96–2.30) for tension headache (Melchart *et al.* 1999).

Another systematic review of acupuncture for chronic pain looked at 50 trials with 2394 patients; 34 trials were of poor quality, scoring 2 or less on a 5-point scale. Controls included the use of waiting lists, sham acupuncture, and inert and active controls (usually transcutaneous electrical nerve stimulation). Of the 16 studies with a quality score of 3 or more, acupuncture was better than control in 3, there was no difference in 12, and acupuncture was worse than control in 1 study (Ezzo *et al.* 2000).

There is also an extensive research literature relating to myofascial trigger points which is discussed in Chapter 2.2.3 and is comprehensively surveyed by Simons *et al.* (1999, pp. 12–82, 150–55), who also discuss the efficacy of dry needling trigger points.

Current use

Although there is a need for further research to support the use of acupuncture, clinicians find that acupuncture/dry needling is a valuable tool in the successful treatment of many musculoskeletal problems. In 1996 the US Food and Drugs Administration graded acupuncture as a legitimate medical procedure, and the US National Institutes of Health concluded in a consensus statement (1997) that there was sufficient evidence of acupuncture's value to expand its use into conventional medicine and to encourage further studies.

A sample survey of chronic pain services in the UK found that acupuncture was available in 86% of clinics (Clinical Standards Advisory Group 1999). The most recent recommendations from the British Medical Association (BMA 2000), while calling for further research, felt that the currently available evidence was sufficiently supportive for healthcare purchasers to give consideration to including acupuncture in their patient services and singled out its use in the treatment of back pain.

Manual and physical therapies

Medical overview

Manual therapies have existed since the dawn of history. Many of the techniques have been passed down through successive generations and traditionally depended more on intuitive 'touch and feel', rather than any anatomical or analytical understanding of the underlying mechanisms involved.

From the general public's point of view the two best-known schools of manual therapy are osteopathy and chiropractic, but they are relative newcomers. Osteopathy, founded by Still in 1892, and chiropractic, founded by Palmer in 1895, both originated in North America. They used techniques that would not have been unfamiliar to the bonesetters who practised throughout medieval Europe and dealt not just with bony trauma but also a wide range of musculoskeletal and somatic pain and dysfunction. They even had their own specialist texts; there is a book by Robert Turner in the library of the Royal College of Surgeons in London dated 1656 entitled *The Compleat Bone Setter*, which is a revision of an earlier work by an Augustinian monk, Friar Moulton. The bonesetters were the orthopaedic surgeons of their day. Sir James Paget (1814–1899), a well-known British surgeon and President of the Royal College of Surgeons, writing in the *British Medical Journal* (1867) of cases that bonesetters cured, advised his colleagues to 'learn then to imitate what is good and avoid what is bad in the practice of bone setters'.

The first published book on manipulation written by a physician was printed in 1871 and entitled *On bone setting (so-called), and its relation to the treatment of joints crippled by injury, rheumatism, inflammation, etc.* (Hood 1871). The author, Dr Peter Wharton Hood (1833–1916), was a pupil of Hutton, a celebrated bonesetter who had treated Dr Hugh Owen Thomas (1834–1891) who himself came from a family of bonesetters dating back at least as far as 1740 when his great-grandfather was shipwrecked on the coast of Wales. Hugh Owen Thomas was the first of his family to gain a medical degree; he graduated from Edinburgh in 1858, going on to study in London and Paris. His nephew was Sir Robert Jones, regarded by many as the father of modern British orthopaedics, of whom it was said by John Ridlon, an American surgeon who knew both uncle and nephew, 'one of the greatest things Robert Jones ever did was to make the main principles of Hugh Owen Thomas acceptable to the medical profession'.

Hugh Owen Thomas had studied the writings of Thomas Sydenham, a seventeenth-century physician who advocated treating illness by working in concert with nature. In addition to his bone setting and manipulative skills, he believed in the benefits of fresh air and natural light. Tuberculosis was then the most common crippling disease of children and Sydenham treated his patients with rest, fresh air and splints; by so doing often enabling them to avoid amputation

or life as a cripple. Thomas made wide use of splints; one in particular which he developed for the stabilization of the femur and which came to be known as the Thomas splint, was estimated to have reduced mortality from femoral fracture during the First World War by 75% (Carter 1991).

The use of manipulation by the medical profession had a varied pattern of acceptance throughout the twentieth century. In the UK, even celebrated practitioners of international repute such as Dr James Mennell and Dr James Cyriax at St Thomas' Hospital (one of the oldest London teaching hospitals) were by some 'considered to be little better than outcasts' (Bourdillon *et al.* 1992).

In France, Dr Robert Maigne, convinced by the potential of manipulation, set out to present the indications and contraindications of reliable techniques in an objective way with clear rules of application. His theory and practice of manipulation achieved formal recognition from the Faculty of Medicine of the University of Paris in 1969 with the creation of a postgraduate specialist diploma for doctors in orthopaedic medicine and manual therapy (Maigne 1972). This has since been followed by teaching founded on the same model in other hospital centres throughout France.

The relationship between the medical profession and non-medically qualified practitioners has traditionally been difficult. Sir Herbert Barker, the celebrated lay bonesetter, when invited to demonstrate his manual skills in the physical exercise department at St Thomas' Hospital in the years before the Second World War, needed special dispensation to allow him to treat patients on hospital premises. In addition, because Sir Herbert was not a doctor, any anaesthetist assisting him was liable to disciplinary action by the General Medical Council: a special arrangement had to be made with

Table 4.3.6. Demonstration by Sir Herbert Barker of his methods of manipulative surgery Special Summer Meeting of the British Orthopaedic Association at St Thomas's Hospital, 22 July 1936

1	Recurrent dislocation of shoulder
2	Displaced semilunar cartilage
3	Adolescent hallux rigidus
4	Tennis elbow (2 patients)
6	Sacroiliac and lumbosacral pain
7	Hallux rigidus and stiff toes
8	Lumbosacral strain
9	Low backache
10	Stiff shoulder
11	Tennis elbow
12	Subluxating inferior radioulnar joint
13	Stiff hip following dislocation
14	Recurrent displacement of internal cartilage (2 patients)
16	Sprain of knee
17	Chronic arthritis of knee
18	Early flat foot
19	Indefinite painful foot
20	Arthritis of big toe joint

Dr Z. Menell, a senior anaesthetist at the hospital, to work with Sir Herbert for the purposes of the demonstrations. A list of the cases seen by him during the course of one of his demonstrations in 1936 is shown in Table 4.3.6. Mr. N. R. Barrett, honorary consultant surgeon at the hospital, subsequently wrote,

> Sir Herbert manipulated the affected joints forcibly and without hesitation. He knew what he was doing. A fortnight later the patients were examined in outpatients and almost all of them were clinically and symptomatically greatly improved. The Second World War intervened to stop these trials. As far as they went, Sir Herbert had established his abilities at St Thomas' Hospital and it was a pity that his untimely death prevented their resumption (Special Trustees for St Thomas' Hospital).

During those prewar years Sir Herbert was also working towards statutory recognition of osteopathy as a specialty in its own right, but this was another of his endeavours that was halted by the onset of war. It is salutary to note that such recognition by the British Parliament was finally achieved only in the last years of the twentieth century.

Osteopathic theory has always encompassed wider issues of health than simply manual therapy for musculoskeletal symptoms and has been concerned, for example, with broader issues such as somatic dysfunction (Ward 1997). These ideas have not, however, remained the sole preserve of the manual therapists; the interrelationship between viscera and soma (viscerosomatic and somatovisceral reflexes) have also long been recognized by orthodox medicine (Mackenzie 1909) and is illustrated by the somatic components of myocardial infarction (Ward 1985).

In addition to osteopathy and chiropractic, other types of manual therapies are legion and many fall into the general category of complementary medicine. Some do not require the use of mobilization or manipulation at all and rely on touch and massage. Some of these techniques are linked to other therapies or philosophies such as acupressure and shiatsu with acupuncture, reflexology with modified somatic homunculi on the feet, and aromatherapy, which makes use of plant-based extracts for body massage. Patients generally welcome hands-on therapies, but whether one particular school of massage is better than another is open to debate. A controlled trial of reflexology in asthma showed equal benefit for both real and simulated treatment. Despite the fact that, other than bronchial sensitivity, objective measures did not improve, patients in both groups felt better and it is likely that they were also more compliant with their drug treatment (*Respiratory Medicine* 2001).

Many manual therapies are based upon *vis medicatrix naturae* (nature's healing force) and the notion that benefits can be obtained by harnessing the body's inherent healing powers which is something that forms a common thread connecting the complementary therapies in general.

Manual therapies, as practised by medical doctors, continue to flourish, are used by physicians throughout the world, and have an extensive research base. Osteopathic training in the USA has become so thoroughly integrated within the medical health care system that degrees from osteopathic colleges carry equal status to those from orthodox medical schools.

Osteopaths in the UK, together with chiropractors, now have statutory recognition and protection of title and are increasingly recognized by the orthodox medical fraternity. Nevertheless, their training remains separate from the medical schools and there can still exist a degree of tension between the lay or non-medically qualified practitioners and the orthodox, medically trained physicians. There has been, and continues to be, a robust exchange of ideas between the orthodox and complementary which is healthy and to be encouraged.

More detailed discussion of the development, research and use of manual and physical therapeutic techniques are comprehensively covered in other chapters in this book.

Plant-based medicines

Historical development, taking NSAIDs as a practical example

The use of plant-based medicines by humans is as old as history. Many modern medicines were originally derived from phytochemicals, several of which have particular relevance to musculoskeletal treatments; the development of the non-steroidal anti-inflammatory drugs (NSAIDs) is a good example. The use of willow bark goes back nearly 2500 years to the Greeks, and Hippocrates used it to lower the fevers of

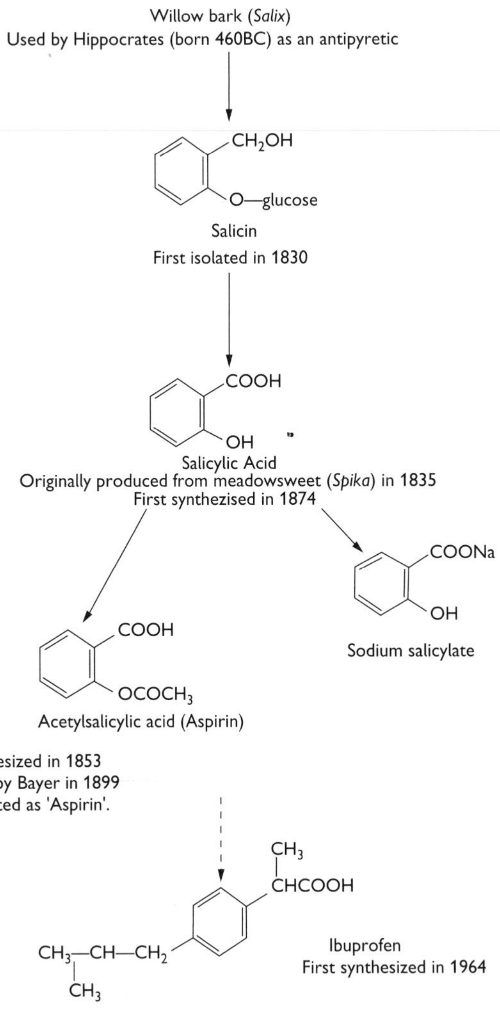

Figure 4.3.103 The historical development of NSAIDs from willow bark.

women in labour. The powdered bark of the willow tree, *Salix* species (Salicaceae), was described by the Rev. Edward Stone of Chipping Norton, England in 1763 as being used by the local people for the treatment of fevers. Its active principle, salicin, which is converted by the body into salicylic acid, was first isolated in 1830. Salicylic acid was originally produced in 1835 from an extract of meadowsweet (*Spiraea ulmaria*) but it only became generally available with the development of a synthetic process of manufacture in 1874. Acetylsalicylic acid was first synthesized in 1853 by Charles Gerhardt, and subsequently developed under the trade name of aspirin (*a* for acetyl; *spir* for *Spiraea*; and *in*, a common ending for drugs) by Bayer in Germany in 1899 as an alternative to sodium salicylate which, although effective, caused significant gastric irritation. The irritant action of the salicylates is, however, still made use of in topical plant-based rubs made from birch bark (sweet birch oil) or the leaves of wintergreen (*Gaultheria procumbens*) which act as counterirritants. Subsequent development by the pharmaceutical industry has led to a whole range of synthetic NSAIDs, including ibuprofen (Figure 4.3.103).

Although the modern synthetic NSAIDs are effective, they still cause significant upper gastrointestinal irritation, bleeding, and ulceration. Extrapolated figures indicate that side effects attributable to NSAIDs account for approximately 12 000 hospital admissions per annum in the UK with an estimated 2500 associated deaths (Bandolier 1998). Other unwanted side effects include the precipitation of heart failure, particularly in people with pre-existing heart disease, and renal dysfunction. The use of NSAIDs in the treatment of osteoarthritis should be carefully assessed especially as symptomatic osteoarthritis is more common in those aged over 65 years and it is in this group that unwanted effects are more common (Gotzsche, 2000). Osteoporosis is also more common in older patients who are more likely to be taking bisphosphonates. An endoscopic study found that alendronate when taken alone (10 mg once daily) was associated with an 8% incidence of stomach ulcers, naproxen (500 mg twice daily) taken alone gave a corresponding figure of 12%, and when the two were taken in combination the rate was 38% over the 14-day study period (Graham and Malaty 2001).

The anti-inflammatory, analgesic, and antipyretic effects of willow bark (salicin) and the NSAIDs depend on the inhibition of cyclooxygenase (COX) in the biosynthesis of prostaglandins (PGE 2). NSAIDs inhibit COX by simple blockade of the channel that leads to its active catalytic site. The difference between COX-1 and COX-2 is a single amino acid substitution, which produces a side pocket in the channel of COX-2. Selective COX-2 inhibitors are bulky molecules that fit into the COX-2 channel side pocket but are too large for the narrower COX-1 channel. It remains to be seen whether the newer, more selective COX-2 NSAIDs provide a significantly better safety profile in the long term.

Further examples of prostaglandin synthesis and herbs

In the mid-1960s, delta-9-tetrahydrocannabinol (THC) was isolated as the major active component of cannabis (marijuana). THC can now be synthesized and this has allowed pharmacological investigation of its effects. The use of cannabis is associated with anti-inflammatory and analgesic properties, and studies have indicated that THC and its non-psychoactive metabolite THC-11-oic acid may cause specific blockade of the COX-2 channel. Marijuana (*Cannabis sativa*) was con-

sidered by cultures of the ancient world to have anti-inflammatory and analgesic properties, and current research has indicated that, in addition to its other effects, it can act as a selective COX-2 inhibitor.

The prostaglandins PGE-1 and PGE-3, unlike PGE-2, provide anti-inflammatory benefits by moving the prostaglandin cascade away from series 2 products and by suppressing production by monocytes of inflammatory cytokines, suppressing synovial cell hyperplasia, decreasing platelet aggregation, and protecting the upper gastrointestinal tract from NSAID-induced injury. Synthesis of PGE-1 is supported by gamma-linolenic acid (GLA) and PGE-3 synthesis is supported by omega-3 fatty acids. Plant sources of GLA include the seed oils of the evening primrose (*Oenothera biennis*) with 7–9% GLA, borage (*Borago officinalis*) with 17–23% GLA, blackcurrant (*Ribes nigrum*) with 15–19% GLA, and hemp (*Cannabis sativa*) with 2–6% GLA.

Omega-3 fatty acids, in addition to being found in fish oils, are present in the seed oils of flax (*Linum usitatissimum*) with 58% alpha-linolenic acid (ALA), hemp with 15–25% ALA, and blackcurrant with 12–15% ALA. Only hemp and blackcurrant oil contain the precursors to PGE-1 and PGE-3, and the optimal anti-inflammatory ratio of 3 : 1 is found only in hemp oil (McPartland 2001).

Other plant-based analgesics

The corm of the autumn crocus (*Colchicum autumnale*) was first used more than 500 years ago. The active principle colchicine, which was first isolated in 1820, is still used in acute gout and, more recently, for the prevention of renal amyloid in familial Mediterranean fever. Its use is limited, however, because of unpleasant side effects and potential toxicity.

Morphine, the principal alkaloid of the opium poppy *Papaver somniferum*, derived from the latex exuded from the unripe plant capsule, still remains one of the most effective analgesics for the relief of severe pain, along with its more recent synthetic derivatives.

Treatment for depression

Patients suffering from chronic pain may become depressed, and over the last few years a plant-based antidepressant which is available over the counter has become particularly popular on the basis of its efficacy and relative freedom from side effects. Known as St John's wort (*Hypericum perforatum*), its use goes back thousands of years when it was used as a vulgary for the promotion of the healing of wounds.

The psychotropic activity of the plant was initially thought to be due to the presence of a reddish pigment called hypericin; however, more recent investigations suggest that the whole plant extract is responsible for its antidepressant action. It is thought to exert its therapeutic effects by a variety of mechanisms that include changes in the balance of neurotransmitters within the brain and spinal cord (Linde *et al.* 1996, Linde and Berner 1999, Philipp *et al.* 1999).

Unfortunately, it is not as free from side effects as was originally thought. Plant extracts can act as inducers of drug-metabolizing enzyme pathways, which may result in reduced blood levels and reduced therapeutic effects of medicines metabolized by these enzymes. Commonly used drugs that may be affected include warfarin, digoxin, oral contraceptives, theophylline, and some anticonvulsants. There may also be increased serotonergic effects with triptans and SSRIs. These interactions were considered sufficiently important for the chief medical officer to contact all health care professionals in the UK in 2000 and to provide a fact sheet for distribution to the general public (Breckenridge 2000).

Topical use of plants

A relatively novel approach to the topical use of plant-based chemicals has been the introduction of 0.025% capsaicin cream for the treatment of osteoarthritis. (It was already in use at 0.075% for the treatment of postherpetic neuralgia and diabetic neuropathy.) Studies indicate that it is effective for the joint pain of osteoarthritis, for which the American College of Rheumatology recommends its addition in the therapeutic ladder, after the use of paracetamol and before NSAIDs.

Capsaicin is a naturally occurring neuropeptide found in capsicum peppers and is the active ingredient that makes them taste hot. It appears to work by depleting substance P, a neurotransmitter for arthritic pain found in synovium and C fibre nociceptors. However, it takes a few weeks before full benefit is achieved. It also needs to be applied four times daily and benefit is maintained only as long as treatment is continued (*Prescriber* 1998).

Another plant that is used frequently in topical form is *Arnica montana* (Figure 4.3.104). It is used both by homoeopaths and herbalists and is approved by the Commission E under the German Drug Act of 1976 which has led the way in the authorization and processing of herbal drugs. Arnica is indicated for bruising, sprains, and rheumatic muscle and joint complaints.

Safety

In addition to interactions between herbal medicines and orthodox prescription medicines as illustrated by St John's wort, dangers associated with side effects as with *Colchicum* toxicity, and the risks of dependency with opium-based analgesics, there are also other potential safety hazards.

Traditional Chinese medicine makes extensive use of herbal preparations, often in complex combinations and some preparations have been associated with liver and kidney damage. The market is largely unregulated, and quality standards vary. For example, some products sold for the treatment of eczema have been found to contain synthetic steroids. There have also been reports not only of direct toxicity of known herbs but of poisoning due to the faulty identification or substitution of plants during harvesting and preparation. In Belgium in 1993, over 70 cases of renal failure were reported as a result of the substitution of *Aristolochia* for *Stephania* in a herbal slimming preparation (*Current Problems in Pharmacovigilance* 1999).

Plant-based medicines include some of the most potent therapeutic chemicals known. In the minds of the general public, herbal medicines are generally regarded as 'natural' and this is reinforced by the fact that they are classified as food supplements and can be sold without medical prescription (Ernst, 2000). Patients often do not consider them as 'drugs' and may fail to mention their use, or even forget it. Health professionals should, therefore, always specifically inquire about the use of herbal or complementary medicines when taking a drug history, and be constantly vigilant as to their appropriate and safe use.

Homoeopathy

Modern homoeopathy stems from the work of the German physician, Dr Samuel Hahnemann (1755–1843), who laid down the basic principles of classical homoeopathic prescribing that are still in use today.

The law of similars

A fundamental tenet of homoeopathic prescribing is that the medicines, or **remedies** as they are usually termed, are selected by their ability to cause similar symptoms in the healthy to those in the patient. This is known as the law of similars (*homoeo* – similar, *pathy* – disease). Although the notion of treating 'like with like' was not new, Hahnemann refined the process and conducted trials of a wide range of animal, mineral and plant-based substances, recording their effects on healthy volunteers. These trials or 'provings' were systematically recorded and combined with toxicological and empirical data to form detailed materia medica, many of which are still in use today. They record a wide range of psychological and physical symptoms and signs associated with each homoeopathic remedy, which can be matched to each individual patient. Nowadays specialized computer programs can facilitate this. Simple examples are the use of *Nux vomica* (the vomiting nut) for the treatment of nausea and *Allium cepa* (the onion) for the treatment of rhinitis and the common cold.

Use of dilutions

In addition, however, Hahnemann developed his prescribing techniques a stage further by using his remedies in highly dilute form. He produced them by a process of progressive serial dilutions (commonly 1 : 10 or 1 : 100) with each dilution being accompanied by vigorous shaking or 'succussion'. Hahnemann originally developed this technique in order to reduce the incidence of medical side effects, as many of the medicines

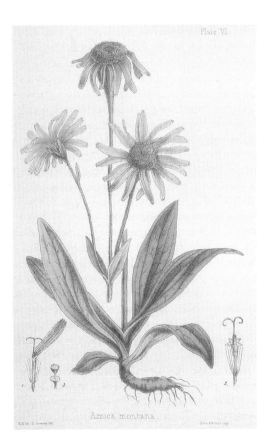

Figure 4.3.104 *Arnica montana*: a plant used extensively in both homoeopathic and herbal medicine to treat soft tissue trauma and arthritis.

of his day were derived from potentially toxic or poisonous substances. These included plant-based medicines such as aconite, belladonna, colchicum, and ipecacuanha as well as mercurials and arsenicals.

Interestingly, his clinical experience indicated that these progressively diluted and succussed medicines had powerful therapeutic effects even when dilutions went beyond Avogadro's number so that theoretically there was no longer any medicine left. It has been postulated that the liquid dilutions retain an 'imprint' or 'memory' of energy patterns which transmits the therapeutic effect of the original substance; although it should be noted that not all homoeopathic medicines are diluted beyond Avogadro's number and some are used undiluted, particularly in creams, ointments, and lotions. There has been much research into energy pattern transfer in liquids, and several hypotheses to explain such phenomena have been generated in the field of orthodox physics. Nevertheless, these mechanisms have yet to be unequivocally demonstrated and this remains one of the major blocks to the widespread acceptance of homoeopathic medicines by the orthodox community.

Evidence

There are a number of good-quality, randomized, double-blind clinical trials of homeopathy showing it to be more effective than placebo. A comprehensive summary of the evidence by Linde *et al.* (1997) was published in the *Lancet*. A total of 89 double-blind, randomized, placebo-controlled trials were analysed resulting in an odds ratio in favour of homeopathy of 2.45 (95% confidence interval 2.05–2.93). This indicated that the overall effects of homeopathy were approximately 2.5 times greater than placebo.

An earlier review, undertaken at the University of Limburg in the Netherlands by conventional epidemiologists, found that out of 105 trials with interpretable results, 81 were positive. A subgroup of 21 trials, selected on the basis of their methodological quality scores, found that homoeopathy was superior to placebo in 14 (Kleijnen *et al.* 1991).

A systematic review of homeopathy in the treatment of osteoarthritis (Long and Ernst 2001) yielded four randomized clinical trials, which although favouring homeopathic treatment, did not allow a firm conclusion to be made on effectiveness; although the authors go on to state that the evidence appears promising and that more research seems warranted.

Many patients with musculoskeletal symptoms request homoeopathic treatment and appear to benefit both in terms of pain and stiffness and overall well-being. However, more work is needed to examine the underlying mechanisms of action and to determine what conditions are likely to benefit from which specific interventions.

Diet and food supplements

The importance of a balanced diet

The importance of a well-balanced diet capable of providing all the essential nutrients is self-evident. Nevertheless, many patients can benefit from information about healthy eating.

It is salutary to note that the UK Ministry of Agriculture, Fisheries, and Food in a national food survey based on food diaries kept by 8043 households throughout Britain (MAFF 1993) showed that the average person was deficient in 7 out of 13 vitamins and minerals; 40% received less than the recommended daily allowance (RDA) of calcium. The average intake was deficient in vitamins B_1, B_2, C, and D,

as well as magnesium and iron, and more than 90% were receiving less that the recommended daily allowance for zinc (15 mg). Relatively simple changes in diet and lifestyle can have measurable benefits. Research suggests that diets rich in vitamin C may prevent the progression of osteoarthritis up to threefold. (*Ann Rheum Dis* 1977).

A well-balanced diet also includes consideration of energy intake, which is particularly relevant to weight control. Obesity is common and is a recognized risk factor for degenerative changes in weight-bearing joints, particularly the knees.

There are specific dietary intakes of special importance to musculoskeletal patients. For example, adequate intake of both vitamin D and calcium is recognized as one of the cornerstones in the prevention of osteoporosis, especially in postmenopausal women for whom dietary supplementation is almost mandatory. Population studies indicate that up to 40% of white women of European extraction over the age of 50 will sustain a fracture related to osteoporosis (Genant *et al.* 1999). It has been shown, however, that supplementation with 500 mg of elemental calcium and 700 IU of vitamin D reduces the risk of non-vertebral fractures in healthy people over 65 years old (Straus 2001). There is also evidence to suggest that the addition to the diet of omega-3 essential fatty acids (EFAs) present in fish oils is of benefit in rheumatoid arthritis (Fortin *et al.* 1995).

Essential fatty acids are also of general importance in inflammation. The two series of EFAs are the omega-6 series, derived from linoleic acid (LA), and the omega-3 series, derived from alpha-linoleic acid (ALA). Each of these precursors is converted by delta-6 desaturase (D6D). LA is converted to gamma-linoleic acid (GLA) and ALA is converted to eicosapentaenoic acid (EPA) and docosahexaenoic acid (DHA). The omega-3 EFAs are involved in the production of prostaglandin PGE 3, which is anti-inflammatory. The omega-6 series is important as it is involved in the production of both prostaglandin PGE 1 (anti-inflammatory) and prostaglandin PGE 2 (pro-inflammatory). PGE 2 is produced via arachidonic acid (AA), the dietary source of which includes offal and red meat.

The arachidonic acid cascade is also involved in the production of pro-inflammatory leukotrienes. Marine lipids which contain EPA and DHA have been shown to reduce inflammation by competitive inhibition of arachidonic acid. The enzyme D6D rate-limits the conversion of LA and ALA to their derived EFAs. A high intake of marine lipids can, however, inhibit this enzyme, resulting in less available GLA, and it is therefore better if EPA is taken together with GLA. The dietary sources of GLA include evening primrose, borage, and starflower oils (see section on plant-based medicines).

In addition, D6D can be blocked by a diet rich in saturated fats, cholesterol, *trans* fatty acids, and adrenal stress steroids. D6D also requires an adequate supply of cofactors, including zinc, pyridoxine, and magnesium. Putting all this together, current recommendations for dietary changes to reduce inflammatory activity in arthritis would reasonably include dietary supplements of GLA and marine lipids (EPA and DHA) combined with zinc, pyridoxine, and magnesium whilst avoiding offal, red meat, saturated fats, and *trans* fatty acids. And, of course, minimizing stress!

Many patients take multivitamin/mineral supplements or 'tonics' which contain iron. This may be relevant to patients with previously undiagnosed haemochromatosis, which affects approximately 1 in 200 of the UK population (Ryder and Beckingham 2001). Most patients usually present with cirrhosis or diabetes due to excessive iron deposits, but arthropathy can be a presenting condition in 45%. Patients can therefore be found in musculoskeletal clinics whose symptoms may have been unknowingly exacerbated by increased iron intake in their erroneous pursuit of better health.

Dietary changes and manipulations, including food sensitivities

Dietary changes and manipulations not specifically related to the intake of vitamins, minerals, or EFAs are common among patients with arthritis. A survey conducted by Arthritis Care (a large, nationwide UK charity) found that 32% of their members had tried some form of special diet (Freedman 1989). These included avoiding specific food combinations such as carbohydrates with proteins and acid fruits, known as the Hay diet, named after the American physician, Dr William Howard Hay (1866–1940). Hay also advised on the use of natural, unadulterated foods and the exclusion of white flour and sugar. Although there have been no rigorous trials of this regime, it is interesting to note that his contemporary, the Russian physiologist Ivan Petrovich Pavlov (1849–1936), showed in experiments that meat mixed with starch took twice as long to pass through a dog's stomach as either when given alone. At the very least, patients on this diet do usually pay more attention to the content of their meals which tend to contain less animal fat and refined sugars, more whole grains and fruit, and include 4-hour gaps between meals of a different character, thus tending to avoid 'grazing' and 'snacking' and consequent weight gain.

There are other diets, based on food sensitivities, which involve the exclusion of foods according to individual reactions (Lewith et al. 1992). The use of terminology is often confused and it is not unusual for patients to state that they are 'allergic' to certain foods when they are in fact describing symptoms of food sensitivities or intolerance. True food allergy is relatively uncommon and can usually be detected by assay of the immunoglobulins combined with a clear history. True food allergies can result in acute anaphylactic reactions, such as with peanuts, which can be life-threatening.

Many private clinics offer electrodiagnostic tests for food and environmental sensitivities/intolerance and allergies based upon electrodermal testing and there are now estimated to be more than 500 such electronic devices currently in use in the UK. The technique measures skin impedance over selected acupuncture points; the substance under test is inserted into an electrical circuit connected to the patient in series with a galvanometer. Despite its widespread use, the evidence base is limited and a recent well-designed study found that electrodermal testing was not able to distinguish between atopic and non-atopic individuals who had previously been assessed by skin prick testing for allergy to house dust mite or cat dander (Lewith et al. 2001). Electrodermal testing now needs to be evaluated to find if it has any role in the diagnosis of food sensitivities and intolerance. This is important, as there are many patients on restricted diets based on the results of such tests, which could prove to be invalid. Probably, the best clinical test currently available is based upon individual patient's reactions to dietary exclusion followed by blinded dietary challenge.

Further examples of other more general modifications of diet include:

- raw food diets, which avoid all cooked foods
- the 'stone age diet', which avoids grains, pulses, and other products of the agricultural revolution

- the macrobiotic diet, which mainly consists of grains and vegetables with foods chosen in accordance with traditional oriental principles
- veganism, which avoids all animal products.

They all have their followers and all have been claimed, at one time or another, to be of help in the treatment of arthritis.

One area where food sensitivities appear to be of some importance is in rheumatoid arthritis, and referring these patients a to a dietician with a special interest in the subject is often well worth while. It may be, however, that dietary changes in patients who are intolerant rather than allergic to certain foods work, at least in part, through changes in the microecologies of the gastrointestinal tract and the balance of micro-organisms (Hunter 1991). There is also evidence to support the beneficial effects of balanced communities of gut microflora in protecting against pathogenic bacteria and supporting immune function (Mcfarlane and Cummings 1999).

Glucosamine sulfate

An interesting food supplement for arthritis, which is widely available and relatively inexpensive, is glucosamine sulfate. This substance, which is made up of glucose with the addition of an amino and a sulfate group, is produced naturally within the body. It is of importance in the formation of hyaluronic acid, chondroitin, and keratin, all of which are found in cartilage. It is hypothesized that due to the accelerated breakdown and metabolic stress associated with degenerative joint change, normal anabolic processes cannot adequately maintain repair, and that dietary supplementation with glucosamine provides additional nutritional support. In addition, it has been hypothesized that inhibition of superoxide radical generation together with inhibition of inducible nitric oxide synthesis might explain some of its symptom-modifying effects. A literature search in 1997 (Bandolier 1997) found eight randomized trials involving oral or intramuscular glucosamine. Five trials compared glucosamine with placebo and all showed statistical superiority in favour of the active treatment in terms of reduced pain and tenderness with an overall number needed to treat of 5 (3.5 to 8.9). Three trials compared glucosamine with NSAIDs (phenylbutazone or ibuprofen). There was no difference between ibuprofen (1.2 g per day) and oral glucosamine (1.5 g per day).

Two further reviews, one for the Cochrane Library (Towheed et al. 2001) and the other a systematic quality assessment and meta-analysis (McAlindon et al. 2000), both reached positive conclusions. In addition, a long-term randomized placebo controlled study (Reginster et al. 2001) followed the long-term effects of glucosamine in the treatment of osteoarthritis of the knee over 3 years. The placebo group had a mean joint space loss of 0.31 mm, in contrast to no significant loss in the active group (−0.06 mm). The placebo group's symptoms worsened whilst the active group's symptoms improved and the glucosamine was generally well tolerated and free from side effects. This raises the intriguing possibility of using glucosamine as a specific preventive of joint degeneration.

Foods and enzyme systems

A diet that involves total exclusion of all food members of the Solanacae (a family which includes the deadly nightshade) has considerable anecdotal support in the relief of the symptoms of osteoarthritis. This food group includes potatoes, tomatoes, aubergines, red and green peppers, chillies, pimentos, paprikas, and tobacco. They all contain solanaceous glycoalkaloids, which are natural insecticides that remain in the body for several days after eating and are not altered by cooking. It is recognized by anaesthetists that dietary intake of even small amounts of these glycoalkaloids – most commonly derived from potatoes – can greatly slow the metabolism of muscle relaxant and anaesthetic agents such as suxamethonium, mivacurium, and cocaine. The solanaceous glycoalkaloids work by inhibiting butyryl cholinesterase, which breaks down many anaesthetic agents, as well as acetylcholinesterase, which breaks down acetylcholine, and is necessary for normal nerve and muscle function. Patients with a mutant form of butyryl cholinesterase may take 5–10 hours to recover from anaesthesia instead of the usual 40–90 minutes. It would be interesting to know whether those patients who respond to the solanacea exclusion diet possess the mutant form of butyryl cholinesterase.

Food-based binding proteins

It is also known that most plants, especially seeds and tubers, contain carbohydrate-binding proteins known as **lectins**. Many of these are toxic and/or pro-inflammatory as well as being resistant to cooking and digestive enzymes. Lectins have been implicated in a range of medical diseases. Wheat is one of the commonest trigger foods, and contains a lectin that is specific for N-acetyl glucosamine. The sugar N-acetyl glucosamine and its polymers can block wheat lectin, and this could be an intriguing additional explanation for the efficacy of glucosamine supplements. In addition, lectins have also been observed to strip away the mucus coat of the small intestine in rodents leading to imbalances in microbiological ecologies (Hunter 1991) which may also result in increased gut permeability, the consequences of which could exacerbate food intolerance and have effects on immune function. One way by which the 'stone age diet' might work, for example, is by its exclusion of starchy foods and therefore of most lectins (Freed 1999).

Future importance

There is still much to learn about the health consequences of what we eat and drink, not only in relation to adequate nutrition but also for the management of selected diseases. The mapping of the human genome of approximately 30 000–40 000 sequences paves the way for the genetic analysis of each individual's metabolic make-up and enzyme pathways, which will make it possible to determine the most appropriate diet both for the support of health and the prevention and treatment of illness for each person at different stages in their lives. In the UK the importance of diet and nutrition have been recognized both by the General Medical Council in their training document (GMC 1993) and by the formation of an Intercollegiate Group on Nutrition to promote both undergraduate and postgraduate education (Shenkin 2000).

Conclusion

The burden of musculoskeletal pain and dysfunction is enormous and has a worldwide impact. The first decade of the current millennium has been declared the 'bone and joint decade' and one of its aims is to improve the recognition and understanding of musculoskeletal con-

ditions. These conditions often cause long-term problems. In the USA, for example they are at the top of the list of chronic health impairments (Woolf and Akesson 2001).

Complementary and holistic approaches to health can offer significant clinical benefits. Musculoskeletal problems are often complex and multifactorial, and frequently require more than just biomechanical solutions. Psychosocial factors are of particular relevance, and studies of low back pain show that such factors can contribute both to consultation rates (Waxman et al. 1998) and the development of chronicity (Thomas et al. 1999b). Patients with somatic symptoms without specific physical cause (medically unexplained symptoms) are frequent users of musculoskeletal services. This group benefit from an open minded, patient-centred approach.

Straightforward division of therapies into either complementary or orthodox is often difficult. Patients with chronic pain particularly value holistic approaches to their care and these are now frequently incorporated into orthodox treatments. Mind–body medicine and 'whole person' care will continue to grow in importance, while the more specific and direct therapeutic interventions such as acupuncture/dry needling, manual therapy, therapeutic exercise, and others will continue to be incorporated into orthodox care as evidence of clinical effectiveness accumulates. An information pack on complementary and alternative therapies, produced collaboratively between the Department of Health, the Foundation for Integrated Medicine, NHS Alliance, and the National Association of Primary Care, has been distributed to doctors working in primary care and illustrates the importance now being placed on the management and provision of these services within the UK National Health Service (DoH 2000).

Musculoskeletal medicine, perhaps more than many other specialties, offers opportunities for combining orthodox and complementary approaches. The Royal London Homoeopathic Hospital is the largest public-sector provider of complementary therapies in Europe, and musculoskeletal patients form the largest single of diagnostic group seen at the hospital. Specialist orthopaedic and musculoskeletal physicians working with physiotherapists and nurse practitioners providing an integrated medical service for orthodox and complementary treatments staff the department of musculoskeletal medicine.

Change in clinical practice is a dynamic process and new ideas come from many different sources. Medicine in the twenty-first century will increasingly look to what is safe and effective, particularly with a view to minimizing both medical and social iatrogenesis. There will be increasing emphasis on prevention, encouraging individual responsibility and ways of working with the body's innate capacity for healing and self-regeneration.

Mr Andy Carr, Professor of Orthopaedic Surgery at Oxford writes that

> . . . most musculoskeletal complaints are influenced, if not caused, by circumstances of daily life . . . the commonest elbow complaint is tennis elbow. It is a considerable problem . . . symptoms are undoubtedly influenced by a range of factors . . . those affected should consider changing the pattern of their lives, reduce stress and seek advice from complementary and orthodox practitioners . . . (Carr 2001).

The way we approach our patients can also have significant effects. A comprehensive search of the research literature found that physicians who adopt a warm, friendly, and reassuring manner are more effective (Di Blasi et al. 2001). This was supported by a more recent study of 865 consecutive patients attending three general practices in the UK, which showed that patients attending doctors providing a positive, patient-centred approach are more enabled and may have less symptoms and lower rates or referral (Little *et al.* 2001).

The dichotomy between orthodox and complementary approaches to care will become increasingly blurred, and musculoskeletal medicine will continue to be one of the key specialties within this integrative, evolutionary process.

References

Bandolier (1997) Evidence-based health care. *Bandolier*, **46**, 1–2.

Bandolier (1998) Evidence-based health care. More on NSAIDs. *Bandolier*, **5**(7), no. 53, 5–6.

Bekkering, R., van Bussel, R. (1998) Segmental Acupuncture. In: *Medical acupuncture. A western scientific approach* (ed. Filshie, J., White, A.). Churchill Livingstone, London, pp. 105–35.

Berman, B. M., Lao, L., Greene, M., *et al.* (1995) Efficacy of traditional Chinese acupuncture in the treatment of symptomatic knee osteoarthritis: a pilot study. *Osteoarthritis and Cartilage*, **3**, 139–42.

BMA (1993) *Complementary Medicine. New approaches to good practice.* Oxford University Press, Oxford.

BMA (2000) *Acupuncture: efficacy, safety and practice.* Harwood Academic Publishers, Reading, UK.

Bourdillon, J. F., Day, E. A., Bookhout, M.R. (1992) *Spinal Manipulation.* Butterworth-Heinemann, Oxford, p. 5.

Brattberg, G. (1983) Acupuncture therapy for tennis elbow. *Pain*, **16**(3), 285–8.

Breckenridge, A. (2000) *Important interactions between St. John's wort* (Hypericum perforatum) *preparations and prescribed medicines.* Committee on Safety of Medicines CEM/CMO/2000/04, London.

Carr, A. (2001) Many orthopaedic surgeons do not think of patients just as malfunctioning elbows. *BMJ*, **322**, 1484.

Carter, A. J. (1991) Hugh Owen Thomas: the cripple's champion. *BMJ*, **303**, 1578–81.

Christensen, B. V., Luhl, I. U., Vilbek, H., *et al.* (1992) Acupuncture treatment of severe knee osteoarthrosis: a long-term study. *Acta Anaesthesiologica Scandinavia*, **36**, 519–25.

Clinical Standards Advisory Group (1999) *Services for patients with pain.* Department of Health, London.

Cummings, T. M., White, A. R. (2001) Needling therapies in the management of myofascial trigger point pain: a systematic review. *Archives of Physical Medicine and Rehabilitation*, **82**, 986–92.

Current Problems in Pharmacovigilance (1999) Renal failure associated with Chinese herbal medicines. *Current Problems in Pharmacovigilance*, **25**, 18.

Di Blasi, Z., Harkness, E., Erst, E., Georgio, A., Kleijnen, J. (2001) Influence of context effects on health outcomes: a systematic review. *Lancet*, **357**, 757–762.

DoH (2000) *Complementary medicine: information pack for primary care groups.* Department of Health, London (www.doh.gov.uk).

Eisenberg, D., Kessler, R. C., Foster, C. (1993) Unconventional medicine in the United States. *New England Journal of Medicine*, **328**, 246–52.

Ernst, E. (1997) Acupuncture as a symptomatic treatment of osteoarthritis – a systematic review. *Scandinavian Journal of Rheumatology*, **26**, 444–7.

Ernst, E. (2000) Herbal medicines: where is the evidence? *BMJ*, **321**, 395–6.

Ernst, E., White, A. (1998) Acupuncture for back pain: a meta-analysis of randomised controlled trials. *Archives of Internal Medicine*, **158**, 2235–41.

Ezzo, J. *et al.* (2000) Is acupuncture effective for the treatment of chronic pain? A systematic review. *Pain*, **86**, 217–25.

Fahrion, S. L. (1978) Autogenic biofeedback treatment for migraine. *Research and Clinical Studies in Headache*, **5**, 47–71.

Filshie, J. and White, A. (ed) (1998) *Medical acupuncture. a western scientific approach.* Churchill Livingstone, London.

Fisher P. and Ward A. (1994). Complementary Medicine in Europe. *British Medical Journal*, **309**, 107–11.

Flor, H., Fydrich, T., Turk, D. (1992) Efficacy of multidisciplinary pain treatment centres: a meta-analytic review. *Pain*, **49**, 221–30.

Fortin, P. R., Lew, R. A., Liang, M. H., *et al.* (1995). Validation of a meta-analysis: the effect of fish oil in rheumatoid arthritis. *Journal of Clinical Epidemiology*, **48**, 1379–90.

Freed, D. (1999) Do dietary lectins cause disease? *BMJ*, **318**(10), 23–4.

Freedman, D. (1989) *Arthritis – the painful challenge.* Arthritis Care, London.

Genant, H. K., Cooper, C., Poor, G. (1999) Interim report and recommendations of the World Health Organisation task-force for osteoporosis. *Osteoporosis International*, **10**, 259–64.

GMC (1993) *Tomorrow's doctors.* General Medical Council, London.

Gotzsche, P. C. (2000). Extracts from 'Clinical Evidence': Non-steroidal anti-inflammatory drugs. *BMJ*, **320**, 1058–61.

Graham, D., Malaty, H. (2001) Alendronate and naproxen are synergistic for development of gastric ulcers. *Archives of Internal Medicine*, **161**, 107–10.

Haanen, H. C. M., Hoenderos, H. T. W., van Romunde, L. K. J. *et al.* (1991). Controlled trial of hypnotherapy in the treatment of refractory fibromyalgia. *Journal of Rheumatology*, **18**(1), 72–5.

Haker, E., Lundeberg, T. (1990) Acupuncture treatment in epicondylalgia: a comparative study of two acupuncture techniques. *Clinical Journal of Pain*, **6**, 221–6.

Herbert, J. (1997). Stress, the brain, and mental illness. *BMJ*, **315**, 530–5.

Hood, W. P. (1871) *On bone setting (so-called). and its relation to the treatment of joints crippled by injury, rheumatism, inflammation, etc.* Macmillan, London.

Hubbard, D. R., Berkoff, G. M. (1993) Myofascial trigger points show spontaneous needle EMG activity. *Spine*, **18**, 1803–7.

Hunter, J. O. (1991) Food allergy or enterometabolic disorder. *Lancet*, **338**, 495–6.

Kabat-Zinn, J. (1990) *Full castrophe living: using the wisdom of your body and mind to face stress, pain and illness.* Delaware Press, New York.

Katon, W. J., Walker, E. A. (1998) Medically unexplained symptoms in primary care. *Journal of Clinical Psychiatry*, **59**(suppl 20), 15–21.

Kleijnen, J., Knipschild, P., Ter Riet, G. (1991) Clinical trials of homeopathy. *BMJ*, **302**(6772), 316–23.

Kondo, C., Canter, A. (1997) True and false electromyographic feedback effect on tension headache. *Journal of Abnormal Psychology*, **86**, 93–5.

Kroenke, K., Price, R.K. (1993) Symptoms in the community. Prevalence, classification and psychiatric comorbility. *Archives of Internal Medicine*, **153**, 2474–80.

Le Bars, D., Villanueva, L., Willer, J. C., Bouhassira, D. (1991) Diffuse noxious inhibitory controls (DNIC) in animals and man. *Acupuncture in Medicine*, **9**, 47–56.

Lee, S. (2000) Chinese hypnosis can cause qigong induced mental disorders. *BMJ*, **320**, 803.

Lewit, K. (1979) The needle effect in the relief of myofascial pain. *Pain*, **6**, 83–90.

Lewith, G. T., Kenyon, J., Dowson, D. (1992) *The complete guide to food allergy and food intolerance.* Green Print, London, pp. 65–75.

Lewith, G., Kenyon, J., Broomfield, J. *et al.* (2001) Is electrodermal testing as effective as skin prick tests for diagnosing allergies? A double blind, randomised block design study. *BMJ*, **322**, 131–7.

Linde, K., Berner, M. (1999) Commentary: has hypericum found its place in antidepressant treatment? *BMJ*, **319**, 1539.

Linde, K., Clausius, N., Ramirez, G., *et al.* (1997) Are the clinical effects of homoeopathy placebo effects? A meta-analysis of placebo controlled trials, *Lancet*, **350**, 834–43.

Linde, K., Ramirez, G., Mulrow, D., *et al.* (1996) St John's wort for depression – an overview and meta-analysis of randomised clinical trials. *BMJ*, **313**, 253–8.

Little, P. Everitt, H., Williamson, I. *et al.* (2001) Observational study of effect of patient centredness and positive approach on outcomes of general practice consultations. *BMJ*, **323**, 908–11.

Long, L., Ernst, E. (2001) Homeopathic remedies for the treatment of osteoarthritis: a systematic review. *British Homeopathic Journal*, **90**, 37–43.

Mackenzie, J. (1909) *Symptoms and their interpretation*. Shaw, London.

MAFF (1993) *The national food survey*. Ministry of Agriculture, Fisheries and Food. HMSO, London.

Maigne, R. (1972) *Orthopaedic medicine – a new approach to vertebral manipulations*. Charles C. Thomas, Springfield, IL.

McAlindon, T., Felson, D. T. (1997) Nutrition: risk factors for osteoarthritis. *Annals of the Rheumatic Diseases*, **56**, 397–402.

McAlindon, T. E. *et al.* (2000) Glucosamine and chondroitin for treatment of osteoarthritis. A systematic quality assessment and meta-analysis. *JAMA*, **283**, 1469–73.

Mcfarlane, G. T., Cummings J. H. (1999) Probiotics and prebiotics: can regulating the activities of intestinal bacteria benefit health? *BMJ*, **318**, 999–1003.

McIndoe, A. K., Young, K., Bone, M. E. (1995) A comparison of acupuncture with intra-articular steroid injection as analgesia for osteoarthritis of the hip. *Acupuncture in Medicine*, **13**, 67–70.

McPartland, J. M. (2001) Cannabis and eicosanoids: a review of molecular pharmacology. *Journal of Cannabis Therapeutics*, **1**, 71–83.

Melchart, D., Linde, K., Fischer, P., *et al.* (1999) Acupuncture for recurrent headaches: a systematic review of randomised controlled trials. *Cephalalgia*, **19**, 779–86.

Melzack, R., Stillwell, D., Fox, E. (1977). Trigger points and acupuncture points for pain: correlations and implications. *Pain*, **3**, 3–23.

Melzack, R., Wall, P.D. (1965). Pain mechanisms: a new theory. *Science*, **150**, 971–9.

Molsberger, A., Hille, E. (1994) The analgesic effect of acupuncture in chronic tennis elbow pain. *British Journal of Rheumatology*, **33**(12), 1162–5.

Nespor, K. (1991) Pain management and yoga. *International Journal of Psychosomatics*, **38**(1–4), 76–81.

Ogier-Ward, T. (1858) On acupuncture. *BMJ*, 8, August 2, 728–9.

Phillipp, M., Kohnen, R., Hiller, K.O. (1999) Hypericum extract versus imipramine or placebo in patients with moderate depression: randomised multicentre study of treatment for eight weeks. *BMJ*, **319**, 1534–8.

Prescriber (1998) *Topical capsaicin: a novel approach to osteoarthritis*. A&M Publishing, Guildford.

Pridgin Teale, T. (1871) On the relief of pain and muscular disability by acupuncture. *Lancet*, April 29, 567–8.

Reginster, J. Y., Deroisy, R., Rovati, L. C., *et al.* (2001) Long -term effects of glucosamine sulphate on osteoarthritis progression: a randomised placebo-controlled clinical trial. *Lancet*, **357**, 251–6.

Reid, S., Wessley, S., Crayford, T., Hotopf, M. (2001) Medically unexplained symptoms in frequent attenders of secondary healthcare: retrospective cohort study. *BMJ*, **322**, 767–9.

Respiratory Medicine (2001) *Respiratory Medicine*, **95**, 173–9.

Ryder, S., Beckingham, I. (2001) ABC of diseases of liver, pancreas, and biliary system. Other causes of parenchymal liver disease. *BMJ*, **322**, 290–2.

Selly, E. (1991) Use of acupuncture in a general practice: the first two years. *Acupuncture in Medicine*, **9**, 72–74.

Selye, H. (1956). *The stress of life*. McGraw-Hill, New York.

Shenkin, A. (2000) Unconventional approaches to nutritional medicine: Conventional doctors need more insight into nutritional medicine and can now get training in it. *BMJ*, **320**, 1538.

Simons, D. G., Travell, J. G., Simons, L.S. (1999) *Travell and Simon's myofascial pain and dysfunction. the trigger point manual, Vol. 1. Upper half of body*, 2nd edn. Williams and Wilkins, Baltimore, MD, pp. 11–178.

Stewart-Brown, S. (1998). Emotional wellbeing and its relation to health. *BMJ*, **317**, 1608–9.

Straus, S. (2001) Recent advances: geriatric medicine. *BMJ*, **322**, 86–9.

Strauss, S. L. (1989) Assessing the effectiveness of acupuncture: comparison and evaluation of four retrospective surveys of epicondylalgia patient's opinion. *American Journal of Acupuncture*, **17**, 229–39.

Syrjala, K.L. Cummings, C., Donaldson, G.W. (1992). Hypnosis or cognitive behaviour training for the reduction of pain and nausea during cancer treatment: a controlled trial. *Pain*, **48**, 137–46.

Thomas, K. J., Fitter, M., Brazier, J. *et al.* (1999a) Longer term clinical and economic benefits of offering acupuncture to patients with chronic low back pain assessed as suitable for primary care management. *Complementary Therapies in Medicine*, **7**, 91–100.

Thomas, E., Silman, A. J., Croft, P. R., Papageorgion, A. C., Jayson, M. I. V., Macfarlane, G.J. (1999b) Predicting who develops chronic low back pain in primary care: a prospective study. *BMJ*, **318**, 1662–7.

Tinterow, M. M. (1987). Hypnotherapy for chronic pain. *Kansas Medicine*, **6**, 190–2.

Towheed, T. E. *et al.* (2001) Glucosamine therapy for treating osteoarthritis (Cochrane Review). In: *Cochrane Library*, Issue 1. Update Software, Oxford.

van Tulder, M. W., Cherkin, D. C., Berman, B., Lao, L., Koes, B. W. (1999) The effectiveness of acupuncture in the management of acute and chronic low back pain. *Spine*, **24**, 1113–23.

van Tulder, M. W., Ostelo, R. W. J. G., Vlaeyen, J. W. S. *et al.* (2000) Behavioural treatment for chronic low back pain (Cochrane Review). *Cochrane Library*, Issue 4. Update Software, Oxford

Vincent, C., Furnham, A. (1997) *Complementary medicine: a research prospective*. Wiley, Chichester, pp. 45–70.

Ward, A. (1985) Somatic component to myocardial infarction. *BMJ*, **291**, 603.

Ward, A. (1996) Spontaneous electrical activity at combined acupuncture and myofascial trigger point sites. *Acupuncture in Medicine*, **14**, 75–9.

Ward, R. C. (ed.) (1997) *Foundations for osteopathic medicine*. Williams and Wilkins, Baltimore, MD. Sections I and X.

Watkins, A. (1997) Mind–body pathways. In: *Mind–body Medicine* (ed. A. Watkins). Churchill Livingstone, New York, pp. 1–18.

Waxman, R., Tennant, A., Helliwell P. (1998) Community survey of factors associated with consultation for low back pain. *BMJ*, **317**, 1564–7.

Wearn, A. M., Greenfield, S. M. (1998) Access to complementary medicine in general practice: survey in one UK health authority. *Journal of the Royal Society of Medicine*, **91**, 465–70.

Wharton, R., Lewith, G. (1986) Complementary medicine and the general practitioner. *BMJ*, **292**, 1498–500.

Williams, A. C. de C., Nicholas, M. K., Richardson, P. H. *et al.* (1993) Evaluation of a cognitive-behavioural programme for rehabilitating patients with chronic pain. *British Journal of General Practice*, **43**, 513–18.

Woolf, A. D., Akesson, K. (2001) Understanding the burden of musculoskeletal conditions. *BMJ*, **322**, 1079–80.

Wright, A. (1991) The first year of an acupuncture practice. *Acupuncture in Medicine*, **9**, 74.

4.3.11 Exercise therapy: limbs

Elva Pearson

Exercise prescriptions can and should be analogous to medicine prescriptions. The use of exercise as a therapeutic prescription is becoming much more commonplace and in fact the norm in many centres. A written prescription, rather than verbal advice to begin an exercise program, will provide better compliance in the short and the longer term (Swinburn 1997, 1998).

As 'exercise prescribers' then, physicians must become knowledgeable about the types of exercise, including their indications, contraindications, risks, and benefits. The combination of frequency, intensity, and duration of the desired exercise program effective for producing a training or restorative effect can then be prescribed. The recommendations should be given in the context of a patient's needs, goals, and initial abilities. The goals need to include consideration of the cardiorespiratory system, muscular strength, muscular endurance, and the flexibility components of the program. The goals must also include individual skill, and body mechanics.

Too frequently, an exercise prescription is equal to a physical therapy referral which states 'assess and treat'. In many centers physicians function to screen medical problems before having the patient referred to a physical therapist who makes a full evaluation of the musculoskeletal disorder, and provides the prescription for exercise. To provide the patient with the optimum benefit, physicians must consider the exercise prescription in the same light as the more familiar medical prescription. Just as 'assess and treat' is never written on the pharmacy prescription pad, so should it never be written on the exercise prescription pad.

Musculoskeletal physical therapists have become expert in their field of providing physical modalities, and exercise prescriptions to patients. When the musculoskeletal physician includes the patient as part of the team and works in concert with the physical therapist, the patient attains maximum benefit.

Goals of exercise therapy

In virtually every orthopedist's office, patients will have been heard to say, ' When I said the exercise was making my pain worse, I was told to just keep doing them'. The 'no pain, no gain' mentality of health care providers, patients, and insurance companies alike does not bode well for the success of exercise as a therapy for musculoskeletal injuries.

Treatment

The basic principles of rehabilitation after musculoskeletal injury include pain reduction by means of various modalities, prescribed medications, and rest: restoration of range of motion and flexibility of the injured limb is followed by therapeutic strengthening, and maximization of task-specific agility, coordination, and proprioception before return to sport or usual activity.

Rest of the injured limb is accompanied by relative rest of the overall person with the goal of maintaining aerobic conditioning and cardiovascular fitness by substituting usual exercise, which may not be possible with the current limb injury, by other aerobic activity that does not excessively use the injured limb.

In order to be therapeutic, which by definition means helpful or curative, exercise must be prescribed with appropriate timing and progression, and in combination with other therapeutic treatments. For example, subacromial bursitis will get worse, not better, if treated with 'rotator cuff' strengthening exercises alone. If the bursitis is not effectively treated, the rotator cuff exercises may cause further impingement and further pain, and the exercise prescription will have failed to help the patient.

In today's dollar-conscious, insurance-driven health care system in the USA, active therapeutic exercise prescriptions are at times the only prescriptions approved for payment. Therapeutic exercise for limb pain will not help the patient's pain go away, or prevent it from coming back. It is only after a specific diagnosis is made and the acute injury is treated that the exercise prescription comes into play as the appropriate therapeutic measure. This is not to say that therapeutic exercise is contraindicated early in the injury, but that a graduated exercise program for the injured limb, in concert with exercise for the non-injured body area, is more reasonable than 'active exercise' for the injured limb in isolation.

First and foremost, the goal of the exercise program must be clear. Exercises are used to increase muscular strength, muscular endurance, and musculotendinous and joint flexibility; and to improve cardiorespiratory conditioning and technique specific to a sport or occupation.

Exercises to increase muscular strength

The goal of all strengthening exercises is hypertrophy and the enhancement of recruitment and firing rates of the motor units. It is generally felt that a stronger athlete is overall a better athlete, and that a stronger muscle is less likely to be injured. It is for this reason that so much emphasis is put on strengthening the musculature in both injured and uninjured patients. Part of the exercise prescription must therefore include maintaining muscular strength in the uninjured limbs as well as the injured limb while an injury is healing, and then improving strength to hopefully prevent future injuries.

The general principle for improving muscular strength is for the muscle to adapt to the imposed demand. The imposed demand may be in the form of tasks specific to a sport or occupation, resistance against a set weight on a machine, resistance against free weights, or maximal contractions against an immovable weight.

Much has been written regarding muscle strengthening techniques. To better read and understand the literature, one must be familiar with some standard definitions.

Isometric contraction

Tension produced in a muscle without shortening of the muscle fibers. This implies that both ends of the muscle are fixed and therefore there is no motion in the muscle as a result of the contraction. A maximal isometric contraction can be held for only a few seconds. Isometric training is quite specific to the angle of the joint, and does not change muscle's ability to exert a force rapidly (Morrissey *et al.* 1995).

Studies which have evaluated the value of isometric techniques for improving muscle strength commonly are flawed in that the test used before and after the training regime is the one-repetition maximum test, which is of course not an isometric test. In studies where isometric tests are used following isometric training techniques, there is always improvement in the isometric strength after the training program. It is not always shown to be transferable to improved strength in other types of muscle contractions (Hickson *et al.* 1994). Isometric techniques may be most useful when there is a painful joint and thus provide the muscle with an imposed demand within the tolerance of the joint pain.

Isotonic contraction

Constant muscle contraction with constant tension. The muscle contraction that occurs against the constant tension may be produced as the muscle fibers shorten or lengthen. Because force produced during isotonic load is affected by the angle of pull, the muscle length at any given time during the range of motion, and the velocity of the muscle shortening, there is only one point during the motion where maximum capacity occurs during a one repetition maximum.

Concentric contraction

Shortening of the muscle fibers producing motion about a joint.

Eccentric contraction

Lengthening of the muscle fiber that is resisting a force producing motion about a joint. There is extensive literature comparing concentric vs. eccentric muscle contraction techniques in an effort to determine the optimum technique to produce muscle strength gains, and decrease post-exercise muscle soreness (Dillingham 1987, Wade *et al.* 1994, Mayhew *et al.* 1995, Brown *et al.* 1997a, 1997b, Asp *et al.* 1998, MacIntyre *et al.* 1998).

In the length–tension curve one can see that as the load becomes larger than the force able to be contracted against (concentric shortening) an isometric force is exerted and then eccentric lengthening of the muscle occurs. The ability for the eccentric contraction to produce the greatest force has stimulated interest, and the notion that eccentric contractions may be best at causing muscle strength gains has been considered, but has not consistently been borne out by study results.

Practically, it is difficult to prescribe and perform an eccentric contraction program exclusively if one wants to incorporate function into the program. It is difficult to find a functional activity that is performed exclusively eccentrically. However, in the rehabilitative phase, during supervised therapy exercise sessions, the therapist can incorporate eccentric exercises into the program. This allows the muscle as it is rebuilding to be stressed with larger force loads. Once the patient can control the given weight in an eccentric fashion, the same weight can then be added to the concentric program.

Isokinetic contraction

Dynamic contractions of the muscle fiber done at a constant velocity. The constant velocity may be produced as the muscle fibers shorten or lengthen. In contrast to isotonic contractions, during an isokinetic contraction the angular velocity is constant, loading the muscle equally at every point in the range of motion.

Kovaleski *et al.* (1995) compared strength gains after training with isotonic vs isokinetic contractions in the lower extremity. Post-exercise tests included both isokinetic and isotonic tests. They support the contention that isotonic contractions produced greater increases in muscle strength when tested both isotonically and isokinetically.

An explanation may be that isotonic contractions reflect more natural, functional motion of muscles and joints. In real life activities the velocity of the angular velocity about a joint is rarely held constant.

Overload

Taxing muscle beyond ordinary daily performance requirements. Overloading the muscle can be done by varying the intensity, volume, or frequency of the exercise. To increase intensity one can increase the weight lifted, or the time it takes to lift the weight. To increase volume one can increase the weight lifted, or the number of times the weight is to lifted, or the number of repetitions per set. To increase frequency, the number of training sessions per week should be increased.

The production of muscle tension is also influenced by the lever arm, angle of pull, insertion and origin of the muscles, fiber type, recruitment pattern, coordination, and speed of the cyclic pattern of agonist/antagonist. If training for strength, length determines speed of contraction and cross-section determines potential maximal force.

Numerous training systems are available to improve muscular strength. DeLateur (1994) has published extensively, and her technique of taking a relatively heavy weight which can be lifted by the individual approximately 4–10 times and increasing the repetitions to the point of muscle fatigue is simple, does not require extensive preliminary testing to determine one-repetition maximums, and is effective. Once 20 repetitions at this weight is mastered, the weight is increased. As she points out, the important factor is that the patient reaches muscle fatigue at the end of the session.

High volume vs low volume has been used in gymnasiums by individuals trying to improve muscle strength and girth. In the literature there is no support for the idea that high volume is necessary, and that one set of high-intensity resistance training is as effective as three sets for increasing isometric torque and muscle thickness in previously untrained adults. The limiting factor again is reaching muscular fatigue. Most studies look at adults who have previously not undergone a training program to improve muscular strength. It may be that to further improve muscular size and strength in trained individuals, higher volumes are necessary to produce the overload that is required to cause muscle adaptation (Starkey *et al.* 1996).

Open vs closed kinetic chain exercises – lower limb

Open chain refers to moving the distal limb with added weight and moves freely in space; closed chain refers to exercises where the distal limb is fixed. In the current literature there is little to support the use of open kinetic chain exercises vs closed kinetic chain exercises with relation to the effectiveness of objectively measured strength gains.

But there are significant differences biomechanically between closed and open kinetic chain exercises. In the lower extremity, the usual closed kinetic chain exercises are the squat and the leg press. Examples of open kinetic chain exercises include knee extension and thigh biceps curl. The squat generates approximately twice as much hamstring activity as the leg press and knee extensions. If co-contraction of hamstring and quadriceps is desired, then the squat is the exercise of choice in the lower extremity (Wilk *et al.* 1996, Escamilla *et al.* 1998).

The open kinetic chain exercises have been shown to cause greatest muscle activity in the rectus femoris, whereas the closed kinetic chain exercises produce more vastus muscle activity. In rehabilitative exercise prescriptions one needs to have a good understanding of which structures undergo the most stress with the different forms of exercise. The tibiofemoral compressive force is greatest in the closed kinetic chain exercise near full flexion and in the open chain kinetic exercise near full extension. Peak tension in the posterior cruciate ligament is twice as great in the closed kinetic chain exercise. Tension in the anterior cruciate ligament is present only in the open chain kinetic chain exercises and occurs near full extension. Patellofemoral compressive force is greatest in closed kinetic chain exercise near full flexion and in the mid-range of the knee extending phase in open kinetic chain exercises (Escamilla *et al.* 1998). In comparing two groups of patients with patellofemoral pain, both groups showed improved muscle strength with closed and open kinetic chain exercises, but only the closed kinetic chain group showed improvement in perceived functional status (Stein *et al.* 1996).

Generally, with closed kinetic chain exercises one gets co-contraction of agonists and antagonist muscles throughout the exercise which may be more physiologic and transferable to activities of daily living. It is well established that training a specific muscle or group of muscle for any one specific activity is very activity specific without a significant amount of cross-over. In the patient who is referred for general limb strengthening as a preventive measure, closed kinetic chain exercises would be recommended to gain the advantage of co-contraction, followed by functional exercise program to improve strength. The specifics of any individual strength training exercise program are too numerous to list due to the unlimited number of patient specific variables. There are, however, general principles which apply to both upper and lower limbs when considering therapeutic exercises to specifically strengthen the limb muscles:

- Maintain general conditioning while injury is healing. In the rehabilitation of an athlete or occupational worker, as the injury is healing maintaining strength in all muscles surrounding the injured limb is important in combination with maintaining cardio-respiratory fitness.

- Strengthen limb stabilizer muscles. Once the injury is healed and the specific limb is ready to be strengthened, beginning with the limb stabilizer muscles first should be followed then by either open or closed chain exercises and then by job/sport specific exercises.

The value of limb stabilizers cannot be overemphasized in the strengthening of both upper and lower limbs. By first ensuring the stabilizer muscles for the respective limb are working as a unit and are strong enough to support the specific exercises prescribed for the limb, a safe and more effective program will be developed. For example, if the hip girdle muscles are weak (gluteus medius is a prime example), it is difficult and indeed dangerous to prescribe leg squats to treat quadriceps/hamstring weakness.

Similarly in the shoulder, it is difficult to strengthen the deltoid muscles if the rotator cuff muscles are not working together to draw the head of the humerus into the glenoid fossa. If the rotator cuff has not been rehabilitated properly, strengthening the deltoid muscle with lateral, front, and rear arm raises will cause impingement and possibly bursitis, or tendonitis will result.

The following exercises are printed with copyright permission and give a basis of stabilizing exercises for both the shoulder and the hip girdle. From here individual muscle strengthening exercises can be added for the rest of the limb muscles.

Muscle strengthening summary

- Each exercise program is patient specific.
- Begin with joint stabilizer muscles first.
- Incorporate a home program early in the therapeutic exercise program.
- Ensure proper technique with each execution.
- Increase resistance in a planned, graduated progressive way to ensure safety.
- Incorporate occupation/sport-specific activity.

Exercises to improve endurance

In general, the stronger the individual the more endurance the muscle has. If the individual has a job or recreational activity that requires long periods of a particular motion, once the initial rehabilitation is complete, increasing the repetitions of the motion in a well-defined, graduated way will serve to successfully increase the endurance of the muscles involved.

Exercises to improve flexibility

Injuries occur more commonly if a joint is unable to move through its full range of motion. Flexibility is therefore an integral part of musculoskeletal fitness. Strength training does not by itself improve musculotendinous flexibility, but by the same token it does not, on its own, cause inflexibility. The flexibility of the musculotendinous unit is determined by the range of motion normally used by the individual. If the musculotendinous unit is tight, i.e. inflexible, injuries to the tendon, muscle, musculotendinous junction, or periosteal tendinous junction may occur. These are loosely termed 'pull' injuries and are more specifically tendinitis, muscle tears, or periostitis.

Intuitively then, one would think that each joint functions at its optimum, with the least chance of injury, if the musculotendinous segments around the joint are strong, and yet at the same time loose or flexible. This would produce a unit that is not under excessive stress during motion, and yet have good strength to produce work when required. This premise is really the basis for fostering rehabilitation programs where muscle imbalances around a joint are assessed and prescriptions to correct the imbalances are made. The muscle imbalances include part of the joints' musculotendinous structures that are tight, and usually the antagonist musculotendinous structures that are loose, i.e. stretched, or too flexible.

In the literature there are very few good studies that have looked at effective ways to improve the flexibility of the tight musculotendinous structures, which are part of the imbalanced joint unit. There is much more information on strengthening the lax or weakened structures by way of strength training.

In order to understand how to treat flexibility, one must have an understanding of those tissues that contribute to the soft tissue around a joint. These include the periarticular connective tissue, tendons, ligaments, and muscles. The mobile tissues of the body are separated by thin layers of loose areolar connective tissue. This allows the tendons, ligaments, muscles, and joint capsules to glide during normal motion. It is through immobilization studies that we have developed our understanding of the changes these tissues undergo, resulting in first inflexibility and finally contracture formation. When immobility occurs the loose connective tissue is reorganized, and is replaced by more dense material that contains a greater abundance of collagen cross-links. The collagen type is thought to remain the same (Akeson et al. 1987).

Ligaments and tendons are composed primarily of longitudinally arranged parallel, type 1 collagen fibers. This gives great strength in the direction of pull. In immobilization newly formed collagen is laid down in a haphazard array, decreasing the function of the structure. Stretching of the limb where the collagen is being formed is believed to promote linear alignment of the collagen which then has greater tensile strength (Gelberman et al. 1982).

Immobilization causes an increase in collagen turnover, a decrease in collagen mass, a decrease in glycosaminoglycan and water content, an increase in soft tissue stiffness, and an alteration in fibroblast function (Amiel et al. 1982). There is also loss of strength at the collagen–bone interface, with bone resorption directly below the insertion site (Newton et al. 1990).

Treatment to improve flexibility

Before the decision to treat a musculotendinous unit that is not flexible, one must be sure that the desired effect of improvements in the flexibility are, overall, what is most beneficial for the patient. Remember that the premise is that each joint is thought to function optimally when each musculoteninous unit around the joint is flexible and strong. Clearly in the case of some disease states in which muscle strength in compromised, limb support is obtained from the other periarticular structures. The prototype of this is in Duchenne muscular dystrophy; in this condition, the ability to stand and walk is achieved longer than muscle strength alone would allow, by soft tissue contractures balancing the limbs in the most energy-efficient way.

Even in people with healthy muscle, there is some evidence that certain musculotendinous inflexibility provides energy efficiency for movement. Craib et al. (1996) stated that sub-elite male runners who were less flexible in ankle dorsiflexion and standing hip rotation were more aerobically economical. Possibly inflexibility in these areas enhances running economy by increasing storage and return of elastic energy, minimizing the need for muscle stabilization activity.

Klinge et al. (1997) demonstrated that adding flexibility exercises had no significant effect on strength training responses. One wonders, then, if flexibility training is really important in the overall exercise prescription for limbs. As there is no scientifically based prescription for flexibility training, no conclusive statements can be made about the relationship of flexibility to athletic injury (Gleim et al. 1997). Despite the paucity of scientific evidence, however, I believe that a flexible musculotendinous unit is a more functional unit, and one that should undergo fewer injuries. In virtually all preventive exercise programs flexibility is listed as a component of the program, and it is felt to play a significant role in both sports medicine and occupational medicine (Laskowski, 1994). Janda et al. (1990) have shown that inflexible muscles can have an inhibitory effect on the antagonist muscle group.

Stretching technique

Frequency and duration

The result of frequency and duration of stretching techniques for the purpose of improving the flexibility of a specific musculotendinous unit has been assessed in very few scientific papers. Brandy et al. (1997) has shown that a 30-second stretch is just as effective at improving flexibility as a 60-second stretch. They also found that stretching once per day was equally as effective as stretching three times per day.

If stretching is done only once, it seems that stretching following some form of exercise is most beneficial. Lehmann and associates (1970) have shown in animal models that tendon length increase is greatest when the tendon is stretched at a temperature of 45°C compared with 25°C. After exercise, increased blood flow can increase tissue temperature far more than superficial heat. Jogging for even a short time can increase tissue temperature and aid in facilitating stretches (Martin et al. 1975). Deep heating modalities may also increase the tissue temperature and facilitate stretching.

Position of the limb

Many of the limb muscles cross not only one joint, but two. These are the muscles that are frequently found to be 'tight' and may contribute the most to limb girdle imbalance. Specifically, if the hamstring is tight, straightening the knee will stretch the insertion and transmit the stretch through the muscle belly to the origin at the ischial tuberosity. This can then put abnormal mechanical stress on the pelvis.

Many workers now find themselves in jobs where they are required to sit for most of the day. This puts the hamstring muscle in a flexed position at the knee and the quadriceps muscle in a flexed position at the hip for many hours. Conscientious stretching to avoid a chronically shortened musculotendinous unit is required.

Stretching methods

Static stretching occurs when the limb to be stretched is placed in a position such that the position itself provides a gradual stretch. Passive stretching is performed with a partner applying a stretch to a relaxed limb. This method has the inherent risk of injury as the partner may apply too sudden or too strong a force to the limb, resulting in musculotendinous injury. Provided there is excellent communication between the partners and a slow steady force is applied, it can result in an effective stretching technique.

Ballistic stretching employs a rapid, repetitive application of force. Most frequently the stretch is achieved by contracting the muscle group antagonistic to the muscle group desired to be stretched. As the antagonist muscle group relaxes, the momentum of the limb in combination with the force of gravity produces a strong force on the tight muscle group. This method of stretching, though effective at increasing range of motion, is generally not recommended. There is much less control over the amount of force applied and microtrauma to the muscle and connective tissue may occur. Athletic activities are predominantly ballistic in nature, and ballistic stretching techniques may be useful in a well-conditioned athlete, in order to maximize and condition the dynamic flexibility at the end of the athlete's available range of motion (Stone 1990).

Proprioceptive neuromuscular facilitation (PNF) technique is accomplished by a contract–relax sequence. A partner or therapist is required to position the limb in a stretched position. The antagonist muscle group then either isometrically or isotonically contracts against the therapist for approximately 10 seconds and then relaxes. During the relaxation phase the therapist moves the limb into a further stretched position (Sady et al. 1982).

Numerous studies have compared the difference stretching techniques (e.g. Sady et al. 1982, Etnyre and Lawrence 1986). Overall, if done consistently, all methods will increase the range of motion of the limb. The determination of which method to use depends on consideration of the safety of the technique, availability of a knowledgeable partner, age, experience, and motivation of the patient, and overall goal of the program.

Age-specific stretching

During adolescence when growth spurts occur, bone growth may occur at faster rates than musculotendinous lenthening. This results in a loss of flexibility and tension at the musculotendinous junction as well as the tendon–osseous junction. This can result in increased injuries in sports where extreme flexibility is required, such as gymnastics, and can also cause specific growth-related musculoskeletal problems such as Osgood–Schlatter disease. In older people, hip flexor inflexibility and hamstring tightness can limit mobility.

Kinetic chain exercises

Treating a specific injury in isolation, failing to give consideration to the entire kinetic chain, will prove to be frustrating, as the injury will tend to recur and the patient will not be successfully rehabilitated. At the shoulder, for instance, scapular stabilizers ensure that the humeral head maintains its center of rotation in the glenoid fossa. Injured tissue must be modified to deal more effectively with the loads and mechanics of the sport or activity and be reintegrated into the functional kinetic chain through a logical progression of sport-specific exercises. Gray (1991) uses the term 'integrated isolation' to describe the importance of understanding the site of injury, tightness, malalignment, or strength deficit and how integration of this region into the kinetic chain can contribute to excessive loading, overuse, or injury.

Various functional upper extremity and lower extremity exercises entail the use of multiple joints and muscle co-contraction. These exercises are sport- and life-specific and use muscle groups in a coordinated rather than an isolated fashion (Gray 1991).

Non-specific beneficial effects of limb exercises

It is generally thought that limb exercises are exercise-specific in that the improvements in performance are specific to the exercises done. It has been shown that besides the effect of improved strength in muscle groups trained, muscle strength training also has an effect on other components of motor performance. Healthy volunteers have been shown to improve performance of hand reaction time, speed of movement, tapping speed, and coordination after a strength training program (Kauranen et al. 1998).

Physical training not only improved muscle strength in elderly woman, but also beneficially influenced walking speed and endurance (Sipila et al. 1996). The frequency of falls in elderly people has also been reduced with strength training (Means et al. 1996). Exercise-based rehabilitation improves skeletal muscle capacity, exercise tolerance, and the health-related quality of life in men and women with moderate chronic heart failure (Tyni-Lenne'e et al. 1998).

Physiologic improvements in muscle strength without increasing tone in hemiparetic stroke patients also provided a psychological benefit associated with the physical activity. Gait velocity was also positively affected (Petrie et al. 1996).

Limb exercise and special populations

Elderly people

Good evidence exists that the sarcopenia, which is described as an age-related loss in skeletal muscle, is reversible with the use of the overload principle. In patients over 75 years of age the most common physically demanding activities, such as household work, walking, and gardening, may play an important role in maintaining the strength necessary for independent living. Adding a strength training program produced statistically significant improvements in muscle girth and size (Rantanen et al. 1997).

Young children

There is very little to support the concern that strength training by young children will cause early closure of the epiphyseal plates, or injury to developing tendons, bones, muscles, or ligaments. Strength training in preadolescents does not produce the hypertrophy seen after adolescence, but it does improve performance on motor tests. Injuries typically seen in the pediatric age groups are usually sports-specific and related to poor technique or overuse. Strength training using a spotter and good technique has resulted in very few injuries.

Women

With the explosion in the number of high-caliber female athletes, there has been a significant increase in strength training for women. There seems to be very little gender difference in the response to strength and flexibility training for the limbs. The overload principle applies to women as it does to men. There is some controversy as to whether estrogen has an ergogenic effect. Most data indicate that there is no evidence for an ergogenic effect of high estrogen status conferred by natural menstruation or hormonal replacement therapy (Bassey et al. 1996, Greeves et al. 1997).

Conclusion

Lack of exercise is a major contributing factor to many chronic diseases. Physicians are now prescribing exercises for patients just at they would drugs. Compliance with any exercise program depends on identifying the needs and goals of the individual. The fundamental principles of an exercise prescription apply to everyone, regardless of age, sex, or level of fitness. A systematic manipulation of the components of frequency, duration, intensity, and progression with periodic re-evaluation allows the program to be individualized. The guidelines for the program should include all the components of health-related physical fitness, cardiorespiratory endurance, body composition, muscular strength and endurance, and flexibiliity. The program for exercise should fit the lifestyle of the patient and be a life-long prescription (Petrie *et al.* 1996).

References

Akeson, W. H., *et al.* (1987) Effects of immobilization on joints. *Clinical Orthopedics*, **219**, 28–37.

Amiel, D., *et al.* (1982) the effect of immobilization on collagen turnover in connective tissue: A bio-chemical correlation. *Acta Orthopaedica Scandinavica*, **53**, 325–32.

Asp, S., *et al.* (1998) Exercise metabolism in human skeletal muscle exposed to prior eccentric exercise. *Journal of Physiology* (London), 26, 305–13.

Bassey, E. J., *et al.* (1996). Lack of variation in muscle strength with menstrual status in healthy women aged 45–54 years: data from a national survey. *European Journal of Applied Physiology*, **73**, 382–6.

Brandy, W. D., *et al.* (1997) The effect of time and frequency of static stretching on flexibility of the hamstring muscles. *Physical Therapy*, **77**, 1090–6.

Brown, S. J., *et al.* (1997a) Exercise-induced skeletal muscle damage and adaptation following repeated bouts of eccentric muscle contractions. *Journal of Sports Science*, **15**, 215–22.

Brown, S. J., *et al.* (1997b) Indices of skeletal muscle damage and connective tissue breakdown following eccentric muscle contractions. *European Journal of Applied Physiology*, **75**, 369–74.

Craib, M. W., *et al.* (1996). The association between flexibility and running economy in sub-elite male distance runners *Medicine and Science in Sports and Exercise*, **28**, 737–43.

DeLateur, B. J. (1994) Strength and local muscle endurance. *Physical Medicine and Rehabilitation Clinics of North America*, 269–293.

Dillingham, M. F. (1987) Strength training. *Physical Medicine and Rehabilitation: State of the Art Reviews*, 555–568.

Etnyre B. R., Lawrence, A. D. (1986) Gains in range of motion of ankle dorsiflexion using three popular stretching techniques. *American Journal of Physical Medicine*, **65**, 189–96.

Escamilla, R. F., *et al.* (1998) Biomechanics of the knee during closed kinetic chain and open kinetic chain exercises. *Medicine and Science in Sports and Exercise*, **30**, 556–69.

Gelberman, R. H., *et al.* (1982) Effects of early intermittent passive mobilization on healing canine flexor tendons. *Journal of Hand Surgery*, 7A, 170.

Gray, G. W. (1991) *Chain reaction*. Wynn Marketing, Adrian, MI, pp. 80–98.

Greeves, J. P., *et al.* (1997) Effects of acute changes in oestrogen on muscle function of the first dorsal interosseous muscle in humans. *J. Physiol.* (London), **500**, 265–70

Hickson, R. C. *et al.* (1994) Skeletal muscle fiber type, resistance training, and strength-related performance. *Medicine and Science in Sports and Exercise*, **26**, 593–8.

Janda, D. H. *et al.* (1990) A three-phase analysis of the prevention of recreational softball injuries. *American Journal of Sports Medicine*, **18**, 632.

Kauranen, K. J. *et al.* (1998) A 10-week strength training program: effect on the motor performance of an unimpaired upper extremity. *Archives of Physical Medicine and Rehabilitation*, **79**, 925–30.

Klinge, K. *et al.* (1997) The effect of strength and flexibility training on skeletal muscle electromyographic activity, stiffness, and viscoelastic stress relaxation response. *American Journal of Sports Medicine*, **25**, 710–16.

Kovaleski, J. E. *et al.* (1995) Isotonic preload versus isokinetic knee extension resistance training. *Medicine and Science in Sports and Exercise*, **27**, 895–9.

Laskowski, E. R. (1994) Concepts in sports medicine. In: *Rehabilitation* (ed. R. Braddom). Springer Verlag, New York, pp. 915–35.

Lehmann, J. F. *et al.* (1970) Effect of therapeutic temperatures on tendon extensibility. *Archives of Physical Medicine and Rehabilitation*, **51**, 481.

MacIntyre, D. L. *et al.* (1998) Fatigue of the knee extensor muscles following eccentric exercise. *Electromyography and Clinical Neurophysiology*, **38**, 3–9.

Martin, B. J. *et al.* (1975) Effect of warm-ups on metabolic responses to strenuous exercise. *Medicine and Science in Sports and Exercise*, **7**, 146.

Mayhew, T. P., *et al.* (1995) Muscular adaptation to concentric and eccentric exercise at equal power levels. *Medicine and Science in Sports and Exercise*, 27, 868–73.

Means, K. M. *et al.* (1996) Rehabilitation of elderly fallers: Pilot study of a low to moderate intensity exercise program. *Archives of Physical Medicine and Rehabilitation*, **77**, 1030–6.

Morrissey, M. C. *et al.* (1995) Resistance training modes: specificity and effectiveness. *Medicine and Science in Sports and Exercise*, **27**, 648–58.

Newton, P.O. *et al.* (1990) Ultrastructural changes in knee ligaments following immobilization. *Matrix*, **10**, 314–19.

Rantanen, T. *et al.* (1997) Physical activity and the changes in maximal isometric strength in men and women from the age of 75 to 80 years. *Journal of the American Geriatric Society*, **45**, 1439–45.

Sady, S. *et al.* (1982) Flexibility training: ballistic, static or proprioceptive neuro-muscular facilitation. *Archives of Physical Medicine and Rehabilitation*, **63**, 261–3.

Sipila, S. *et al.* (1996) Effects of strength and endurance training on isometric muscle strength and walking speed in elderly women. *Acta Physiologica Scandinavica*, **156**, 457–64.

Starkey, D. B., *et al.* (1996) Effect of resistance training volume on strength and muscle thickness. *Medicine and Science in Sports and Exercise*, **28**, 1311–20.

Stein, H. A. *et al.* (1996) A comparison of closed kinetic chain and isokinetic joint isolation exercise in patients with patellofemoral dysfunction. *Journal of Orthopedic and Sports Physical Therapy*, **24**, 136–41.

Stone, M. H. (1990). Muscle conditioning and muscle injuries. *Medicine and Science in Sports and Exercise*, **22**, 457–62.

Swinburn, B. A. *et al.* (1997) Green prescriptions: attitudes and perceptions of general practitioners towards prescribing exercise. *British Journal of General Practice*, **47**, 567–9.

Swinburn, B.A. *et al.* (1998) The green prescription study: a randomized controlled trial of written exercise advice provided by general practitioners. *American Journal of Public Health*, **88**, 288–91.

Tyni-Lenne'e, R. *et al.* (1998) Exercise-based rehabilitation improves skeletal muscle capacity, exercise tolerance, and quality of life in both women and men with chronic heart failure. *Journal of Cardiovascular Failure*, **4**, 9–17.

Wade, A. *et al.* (1994) Appropriate strength training. *Medical Clinics of North America*, (ed.) 457–75.

Wilk, K.E. *et al.* (1996) Comparison of tibiofemoral joint forces and electromyographic activity during open and closed kinetic chain exercises. *American Journal of Sports Medicine*, **24**, 518–27.

4.3.12 Exercise therapy: spine

Sarah Mottram and Mark Comerford

For many years clinicians have been convinced that movement dysfunction plays an important role in many painful conditions of the neuromusculoskeletal system (see Chapter 2.2.2 and Janda 1985, 1994, Richardson *et al.* 1999, Sahrmann 2000, Comerford and Mottram 2001a, 2002a). There is an improving understanding of the importance of dynamic joint stability and muscle balance in the management of neuromusculoskeletal disorders (Richardson and Jull 1995, Hides *et al.* 1996, Hodges and Richardson 1996, Lee 1996, Jull 1997, 1998, Mottram 1997, Mottram and Comerford 1999, Richardson *et al.* 1999, O'Sullivan 2000, Comerford and Mottram 2001a, 2002a, Sahrmann 2002). Research has demonstrated the need to consider dynamic joint stability and muscle balance in the treatment of low back pain (Hides *et al.* 1996, Hodges and Richardson 1996, O'Sullivan *et al.* 1997a, Richardson *et al.* 1999) cervical pain, and headaches (Beeton and Jull 1994, Jull *et al.* 1999).

The correction of movement dysfunction should be based on a sound clinical assessment and clinical reasoning. The approach in the clinic should include three points: the best skills from current therapies, the best information from science, and the best therapeutic relationship with a particular patient (Butler 1998). This chapter highlights an approach to managing symptoms, dysfunction, and disability through assessing movement dysfunction in the spine.

Concepts of muscle function and dynamic stability

It is useful to consider the classification of muscles in relation to function when considering dynamic stabilization. The concept of classifying muscles by function gained general acceptance with Rood's concept of stabilizer and mobilizer muscles (Goff 1972). Rood's concept of differentiating stabilizer and mobilizer muscles has been further developed by Janda (1985) and Sahrmann (1993, 2002). Stabilizer muscles are described as having the characteristics of being monoarticular or segmental, deep, working eccentrically to control movement, and having static holding capacities. Mobility muscles, on the other hand, are described as biarticular or multisegmental, superficial, working concentrically with the acceleration of movement and producing power. No other clinically accepted classification system was described

Table 4.3.7. Model of classification of muscle function

Local stabilizer	Global stabilizer	Global mobilizer
Local	Global	
Local stabilizer	Global stabilizer	Global mobilizer

Table 4.3.8. Classification of muscle function

Stabilizer		Mobilizer
Local	Global	
Local stabilizer	Global stabilizer	Global mobilizer

Table 4.3.9. Function and characteristics of the three classes of muscles

Local stabilizer	Global stabilizer	Global mobilizer
Increases muscle stiffness to control segmental motion Controls the neutral joint position	Generates force to control range of motion	Generates torque to produce range of movement
Contraction = little or minimal length change: does not produce range of motion	Contraction = eccentric length change \ control throughout range especially inner range ('muscle active = joint passive') and hypermobile outer range)	Contraction = concentric length change \ concentric production of movement (rather than eccentric control)
Activity is often anticipatory (or at the same instant) to functional load or movement to provide protective muscle stiffness prior to motion stress	Functional ability to: (i) shorten through the full inner range of joint motion (ii) isometrically hold position (iii) eccentrically control the return against gravity and control hypermobile outer range of joint motion if present	Concentric acceleration of movement (especially sagittal plane: flexion/extension)
Proprioceptive input re joint position, range, and rate of movement	Low load deceleration of momentum (especially axial plane: rotation)	Shock absorption of load
Continuous activity throughout movement	Activity is non-continuous	Activity is non-continuous (on–off phasic pattern)
Activity is independent of direction of movement	Activity is direction dependent	Activity is direction dependent

until Bergmark (1989) presented the concept of local and global muscle systems when describing mechanical modeling of the spinal system. In the local system all muscles have their origin or insertion at the vertebrae and this system is used to control the curvature of the spine and provide stiffness to maintain mechanical stability of the lumbar spine. In the global system the muscles are more superficial and link the thorax and pelvis. These muscles produce large torque or force.

Based on these concepts, a new model of functional classification into local stability muscles, global stability muscle, and mobility muscles has been proposed (Comerford 1997, Mottram and Comerford 1999, Comerford and Mottram 2001a, 2002a) (Tables 4.3.7, 4.3.8). The characteristics and function of these muscle categories are described in Table 4.3.9 and examples are listed in Table 4.3.10.

Physiology

All human muscles have both fast and slow motor units, and the function of the muscle is dependent on the recruitment of the motor units (Table 4.3.11). Dynamic postural control and normal low-load functional movement is primarily a function of low-threshold slow motor unit (tonic) recruitment (Rothwell 1994). Low-load exercise optimizes slow motor unit recruitment training (not high-load or overload). High-load activity or strength training (endurance or power overload training) is a function of both slow (tonic) and fast (phasic) motor unit recruitment.

Concept of articular translational and myofascial dysfunction

Movement dysfunction may present as a disorder of articular translational movements at a single motion segment, e.g. abnormal articular translational motion. Dysfunction may occur as a myofascial disorder in the functional movements across one or more motion segments, e.g. abnormal myofascial length and recruitment or as a response to neural mechanosensitivity. These two components of the movement system are interrelated, and consequently articular translational and myofascial dysfunctions often occur concurrently.

The inability to dynamically control movement at a joint segment or region may present as a combination of uncontrolled movement or **give**, which is defined as a lack of active, low-threshold control of the local or global muscle's ability to control motion (Comerford and

Table 4.3.10. Examples of muscle classification

Local stabilizer	Global stabilizer	Global mobilizer
Transversus abdominis	Oblique abdominals	Rectus abdominis
Deep lumbar multifidus	Superficial multifidus	Iliocostalis
Psoas (posterior fasiculii)	Spinalis	Hamstrings
Diaphragm	Gluteus medius	Latissimus dorsi
Pubococcygeus	Psoas (anterior fasiculii)	Levator scapulae
Longus colli (longitudinal)	Levator ani	Scalenae
	Longus colli (oblique fibres)	

Table 4.3.11. Key features of slow and fast motor unit recruitment

Function	Slow motor units (tonic)	Fast motor units (phasic)
Load threshold	Low (easily activated)	High (requires greater stimulus)
Recruitment	Primarily recruited at low % of MVC (<25%)	Increasingly recruited at higher % of MVC (40+%)
Speed of contraction	Slow	Fast
Contraction force	Low	High
Fatiguability	Fatigue resistant	Fast fatiguing
Role	Fine control of postural activity and low-load activity	Rapid or ballistic movement and high-load activity

Table 4.3.12. Articular translational and myofascial: give and restriction

	Give	Restriction
Articular translational	Uncontrolled intraarticular and interarticular joint hypermobility	Intraarticular and interarticular joint hypomobility
Myofascial	Myofascial inability to control range of motion	Lack of myofascial extensibility restricting range of motion

Mottram 2002a). The term can also be used to describe uncontrolled movement in myofascial, articular, neural, and connective tissue. This give can present as lack of control of normal functional motion or hypermobile range. It may be identified in the physiological or functional movements of joint range, or it may be identified in the accessory translational gliding movements of a joint. Give is usually associated with a loss of motion or **restriction** (Table 4.3.12; Comerford and Mottram 2002a).

The restriction may be associated with limitation of articular translation and a lack of extensibility of the connective tissue (intra-articular or periarticular) at a motion segment. This presents with a loss of translational motion at a joint and is confirmed with manual palpation (Maitland 1986). The restriction may be associated with a lack of extensibility of contractile myofascial tissue or neural tissue. The muscles may lose extensibility for three reasons (1) increased low-threshold recruitment (overactivity) (Janda 1985, Sahrmann 2002), (2) a lack of range due to length-associated changes (Gossman et al. 1982, Goldspink and Williams 1992) or (3) a lack of normal neural compliance and a protective response associated with abnormal neural mechanosensitivity (Edgar et al. 1994, Balster and Jull 1997, Hall et al. 1998, Hall and Elvey 1999). This restriction is confirmed by muscle extensibility tests. Myofascial dysfunction can result in abnormal movement about several motion segments. When a muscle contracts it generates tension across motion segments at both ends, and if there is inadequate stability or control at any segment, then inappropriate motion may develop at this site. There is frequently, but not always, a restriction of normal motion (loss of physiological or accessory movement) at one or more motion segments, which contributes to compensatory excessive movement at adjacent segments in order to maintain function.

Give often results from uncontrolled compensation for restriction. The give may be translational; that is, it is associated with laxity of articular connective tissue. Panjabi (1992) defined spinal instability in terms of laxity around the neutral position of a spinal segment called the **neutral zone**. Maitland (1986) has described joint hypermobility. The end result of this process is abnormal development of uncontrolled movement and a loss of functional or dynamic stability. Articular translational give can compensate for: (1) articular restriction in the same joint (give and restriction at an intra-articular level), (2) articular restriction in an adjacent joint (give and restriction at an inter-articular level), or (3) myofascial restriction (give and restriction at a regional level). The give may be myofascial; that is, it is associated with excessive length or poor control of contractile tissue. This is the usual compensation for: (1) myofascial restriction at an adjacent region (give and restriction at a regional level), (2) abnormal mechanosensitivity at an adjacent region (give and restriction at a regional level), or (3) segmental articular translational restriction at an adjacent joint (give and restriction at an interarticular level). Articular translational or myofascial give can present in isolation without restriction. Common examples of this type of presentation are: (1) a traumatic incident (capsular/ligamentous laxity or instability), (2) inhibition associated with pain and pathology, or (3) sustained postural strain positioning. The give may be due to muscle inhibition associated with abnormal neural mechanosensitivity.

In the functional movement system, the site of uncontrolled motion or give is the site of the **dynamic stability dysfunction** (Comerford and Mottram 2002a). The uncontrolled segment or region of give is the most likely source of pathology and symptoms of mechanical origin. The direction of give relates to the direction of tissue stress or strain and pain-producing movements (Sahrmann 2002). It is important in the assessment to identify the region and the direction of give (stability dysfunction) and relate it to the symptoms and pathology. The articular and myofascial give identify the segment and the direction of dynamic stability dysfunction and are related to the direction of symptom-producing movement. An articular or myofascial give into excessive uncontrolled flexion under flexion load may place abnormal stress or strain on various tissues and result in flexion-related symptoms. Likewise, excessive uncontrolled give into extension under extension load produces extension-related symptoms, whereas excessive uncontrolled give into rotation or sidebend/sideshift under unilateral load produces unilateral symptoms. Stiff or restricted segments are not usually the source of pain during normal functional

Table 4.3.13. Lumbar spine dynamic stability dysfunctions

Dynamic stability dysfunction	Direction of give (compensation)	Common symptom presentation
Lumbar flexion	Lumbar flexion under flexion load	Pain in lumbar spine (± referred) – aggravated or provoked by flexion load, movements or flexed postures
Lumbar flexion–rotation	Lumbar rotation and flexion under unilateral load	Unilateral pain in lumbar spine (± referred) – aggravated or provoked by unilateral load or flexion load, movements or flexed postures
Lumbar extension	Lumbar extension under extension load	Pain in lumbar spine (± referred) – aggravated or provoked by extension load, movements or extended postures
Lumbar extension–rotation	Lumbar rotation and extension under unilateral load	Unilateral pain in lumbar spine (± referred) – aggravated or provoked by unilateral load or extension load, movements or extended postures
Lumbar global (multidirectional)	Lumbar flexion and extension and rotation under related load tests	Pain in lumbar spine (central or unilateral) (± referred). Flexion symptoms provoked by flexion load or movements (especially prolonged sitting). Extension symptoms provoked by extension load or movements (especially prolonged standing). Unilateral symptoms provoked by unilateral load or movements (especially static asymmetrical postures)

Restriction ? Compensation ? Uncontrolled motion (give) ?
Pathology ? Pain

movement or loading, although pain may be elicited under abnormal movement or load. Generally, the stiff or restricted segment may be a cause of compensatory give at an adjacent joint.

Compensation that demonstrates good active control does not identify a stability dysfunction. Uncontrolled motion (give) identifies a dynamic stability dysfunction (Comerford and Mottram 2002a). It is important to relate the give to symptoms and pathology and to the mechanisms of provocation of symptoms. Management of the dysfunction that relates to the symptoms and pathology becomes the clinical priority. Give that may be evident, but does not relate to symptoms, is not a priority of pathology management, although it may indicate a potential risk for the future. The dynamic stability dysfunction can be labeled by the direction of give. Common patterns seen in the clinic are described in Tables 4.3.13 and 4.3.14.

Evidence of muscle dysfunction

Stability dysfunction can be identified in the local and global muscle systems (Table 4.3.15). It can occur as a dysfunction of the recruitment and motor control of the deep local muscle stability system, resulting in poor control of the neutral joint position (Hides *et al.* 1996, Hodges and Richardson 1996, O'Sullivan *et al.* 1997b, Richardson *et al.* 1999,

Table 4.3.14. Cervical spine dynamic stability dysfunctions

Dynamic stability dysfunction	Direction of give (compensation)	Common symptom presentation
Upper cervical extension ± rotation	Upper cervical extension under extension load Cervical extension or lateral flexion during rotation	Upper cervical pain (± headaches or referral) – aggravated or provoked by extension load, movements or postures Unilateral pain in upper cervical spine – aggravated or provoked by unilateral load or movements
Low cervical flexion ± rotation	Low cervical flexion under flexion load Cervical lateral flexion during rotation	Low cervical pain (± referred) – aggravated or provoked by flexion load, movements or postures Unilateral pain in upper cervical spine – aggravated or provoked by unilateral load or movements
Midcervical translation ± rotation	Mid cervical (usually translational shear C3–4 or C4–5) under extension load Cervical extension or lateral flexion during rotation	Mid cervical pain (± referred) – aggravated or provoked by extension load, movements or postures Unilateral pain in upper cervical spine – aggravated or provoked by unilateral load or movements
Upper cervical flexion ± rotation	Upper cervical flexion under flexion load Upper lateral flexion during rotation	Upper cervical pain (± headaches or referral) – aggravated or provoked by flexion load, movements or postures (often traumatic involving upper cervical ligamentous laxity, e.g. forced flexion injury) Unilateral pain in upper cervical spine – aggravated or provoked by unilateral load or movements

Table 4.3.15. Dysfunction in the three muscle classes

Local stabilizer	Global stabilizer	Global mobilizer
Motor control deficit associated with delayed timing or recruitment deficiency	Muscle lacks the ability to (i) shorten through the full inner range of joint motion	Myofascial shortening – limits physiological and/or accessory motion (which must be compensated for elsewhere)
Reacts to pain and pathology with inhibition	(ii) isometrically hold position (iii) eccentrically control the return	Overactive low threshold, low load recruitment
Decreased muscle stiffness and poor segmental control	Muscle active shortening ≠ joint passive (loss of inner range control)	Reacts to pain and pathology with spasm
Loss of control of joint neutral position	If hypermobile – poor control of excessive range	
	Poor low threshold tonic recruitment	
	Poor eccentric control	
	Poor rotation dissociation	

Result:

Local inhibition	Global imbalance	Global imbalance

Jull *et al.* 1999). The stedies have shown a motor control deficit associated with delayed timing or inefficient low-load recruitment in the local stability system. These changes may decrease muscle action around a motion segment and potentially result in poor segmental control and instability (Cholewicki and McGill 1996).

Inhibition of the local stability system has been demonstrated in subjects with headaches (Jull *et al.* 1999). Deep neck flexor muscle contraction was significantly inferior in the cervical headache group.

Hodges and Richardson (1996) investigated the contribution of transversus abdominis to spinal stabilization in subjects with and without low back pain. The delayed onset of contraction of transversus abdominis in subjects with low back pain indicates a deficit of motor control, so the authors hypothesize there would be inefficient muscular stabilization of the spine. From the evidence to date, it would appear that in all back pain subjects transversus abdominis is dysfunctional independent of the type or nature of pathology, while subjects who have never had significant back pain do not have this dysfunction (Hodges and Richardson 1996, Richardson *et al.* 1999). The dysfunction is related to motor control deficits, not strength.

There is evidence of lumbar multifidus muscle reduction in cross-sectional area ipsilateral to symptoms in patients with acute or subacute low back pain (Hides *et al.* 1994). This decrease in size of multifidus was seen on the side of the symptoms with the reduced cross-sectional area observed at a single vertebral level, suggesting segmental pain inhibition. This evidence suggests that pain and dysfunc-

tion are related. In acute-onset back pain this immediate inhibition of lumbar multifidus does not automatically return when symptoms settle. Recovery of symmetry was more rapid and more complete in patients who received specific, localized multifidus muscle retraining (Hides *et al.* 1996).

Dangaria *et al.* (1998) assessed the cross-sectional area of psoas major in unilateral sciatica caused by disc herniation. There was significant reduction in the cross-sectional area of psoas at the level and site of disc herniation on the ipsilateral side, perhaps caused by segmental inhibition due to pathology and pain.

A common model of stability in the lumbar spine relates it to a cylinder. Richardson *et al.* (1998) use a cylinder concept to describe the local stability system for the lumbopelvic region (Figure 4.3.105). They suggest the transversus abdominis and the spinal column make up the wall of the cylinder, with the diaphragm and pelvic floor muscles making up the top and bottom respectively. The model can be updated in the light of recent research: consider the spine as a flexible segmented structure embedded in the wall of the cylinder. The role of the cylinder is to support and stabilize this flexible structure while it moves. The cylinder can be portrayed as having an inner (local) core and an outer (global) shell (Comerford and Mottram 2003). The wall of the inner local core of the cylinder is made up of transversus abdominis, providing lateral control and resistance to segmental displacement laterally. The spine is stabilized posteriorly by segmental attachments of lumbar multifidus and stabilized anteriorly by segmental

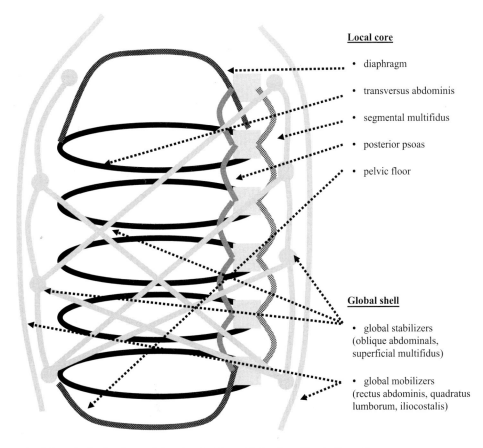

Local core

- diaphragm
- transversus abdominis
- segmental multifidus
- posterior psoas
- pelvic floor

Global shell

- global stabilizers (oblique abdominals, superficial multifidus)
- global mobilizers (rectus abdominis, quadratus lumborum, iliocostalis)

Figure 4.3.105 Functional stability cylinder for the trunk (reprinted with permission from Kinetic Control).

attachments of psoas. These two muscles provide sagittal and axial control and resistance to anteroposterior and rotatory segmental displacement. Their longitudinal fiber placement contributes to axial compression, to enhance stability throughout spinal range of motion. Tension generated by these three muscles also contributes to increasing fascial tension to improve the load-bearing ability of the spine.

The cylinder requires a top and bottom if it is to increase intra-abdominal pressure to enhance spinal stability. If intra-abdominal pressure is to perform a role in stability it must be able to generate pressure independently from respiratory and continence functions. It has been demonstrated that the costal part of the diaphragm has a stability role independent from respiration though it also contributes to respiratory function (Hodges *et al.* 1997, Hodges and Gandevia 2000). It is theorized that the puboviseral muscles (e.g. pubococcygeus) have the stability role within the pelvic floor (Sapsford *et al.* 1997, Jones and Gibbons 2001). Gibbons (2001) demonstrated a mechanical link between the crural portion of the diaphragm and pubococcygeus via the fascia of psoas major.

If the model of a local core of muscles is valid, then these muscles must have efficient recruitment and have sophisticated integration processes. It seems logical that if any one of these muscles is dysfunctional then the stability of the cylinder will be compromised unless the other muscles (or some other process) can adequately compensate.

The outer global shell of the cylinder consists of the global stabilizer muscles and the global mobilizer muscles acting around the trunk (Comerford and Mottram 2003). The global stabilizer muscles, such as the oblique abdominals, anterior fasciculus of psoas, superficial multifidus, and spinalis, act to eccentrically control range of motion and decelerate rotational forces across the trunk. The global mobilizer muscles, such as rectus abdominis, iliocostalis, longissimus, and quadratus lumborum, act to produce fast, large range and forceful movement. When the integrated local cylinder function can be achieved, then the local core and the global shell should be retrained to ensure coordinated normal function. The global stability of the trunk is essential for proximal control of the spine and girdles during limb motion and functional loading. If the local cylinder has re-established normal efficient function, then under low-load normal functional demands it should recruit automatically whenever the global system is required to work.

Dysfunction can occur globally as imbalance between the mono-articular stabilizers and the biarticular mobilizers or movement-producing muscles (Rood as reported by Goff 1972, Janda 1985, Sahrmann 1993, 2000, Kankaanpaa *et al.* 1998). This imbalance presents in terms of alteration in functional length tests and recruitment patterns of these muscles.

Clinically it can be seen that the global stability muscles lack the ability to shorten through the full range of joint motion. They also demonstrate poor low load or low threshold recruitment (Janda 1995,

Sahrmann 2002) and demonstrate poor low-load eccentric control of rotation (Sahrmann 2002, Comerford and Mottram 2002a–d). For example, gluteal dysfunction has been associated with lumbopelvic pain (Janda 1985, Kankaanpaa *et al.* 1998). With overactivity in the global mobility muscles, clinical examination demonstrates myofascial shortening which limits motion (Sahrmann 2002). For example, the overactivity of rectus abdominis, rectus femoris, tensor fascia lata, and the hamstrings can have a significant influence on the compensatory movement of the pelvis and lumbar spine. A similar influence can be observed in the cervical spine with overactivity or shortness of, for example, levator scapulae and scalanae.

Dysfunction in the global system may result in abnormal 'overtensioning' and 'undertensioning' by the muscles around a motion segment. The loss of ideal or normal local or global control may result in abnormal stress or strain being imposed on the joint, its supporting soft tissue structures, and related myofascial tissue and neural tissue. As a result of this dysfunction, pain may occur.

The assessment must identify recruitment changes in the local stability system and length changes in the global stability system.

Clinical examination

The clinical examination needs to identify any neuromusculoskeletal dysfunction and relate this dysfunction to the movement system. The movement system is made up of the articular, myofascial, neural, and connective tissue systems of the body. Good function requires the integrated and coordinated interaction of these systems. Each system needs to be examined and the influence of one system on the other needs to be considered. For example, pain, pathology, disuse, and abnormal proprioceptive input can inhibit muscle recruitment (Stokes and Young 1984, Hurley and Newham 1993, Brumagne *et al.* 1999, Taimela *et al.* 1999).

This inhibition can be noted in the local stability muscles and the global stability muscles. Noxious input, for example pain, may produce muscle 'spasm' (Schaible and Grubb 1993). Clinically this is frequently seen in the global mobility muscles. This dysfunction in motor recruitment is seen as a typical pattern in patients with low back pain, i.e. overactivity in the erector spinae and inhibition of multifidus. Proprioception can influence muscle function at peripheral joints (Hurley 1997) and may have an influence on spinal muscle function (Brumagne *et al.* 1999, Taimela *et al.* 1999). Pain, pathology, sensitized neural tissue, and altered proprioceptive input can all influence recruitment of stability muscles, thus affecting functional stability so it is important to assess function and dysfunction in all components of the movement system.

Sahrmann (1993, 2002) emphasizes the importance of considering the factor of cumulative microtrauma as a cause of musculoskeletal

Table 4.3.16. Differentiation between stability and strength dysfunction

Muscle dysfunction	Stability dysfunction	Strength dysfunction
Assessment	Identified by the failure of the movement system under low-load testing	Identified by the failure of the movement system under high-load testing
Result	Results in the development of pathology and pain	Results in weakness and loss of performance

pain and states, 'faulty movement can induce pathology, not just be a result of it'. This cumulative microtrauma can result from repetitive activities or from complex changes in patterns of multi-joint movements. For this reason movement patterns need to be examined in detail, and a history of activities and functional activities analyzed.

In view of the changes in muscle function in the local and global systems the physical examination must include an assessment of muscle function: local stability muscles, global stability muscles and global mobility muscles. Specific tests need to be considered (Table 4.3.16).

Local stability muscles: control of the neutral joint position

In the presence of regional pathology or pain, the local stability muscles demonstrate a recruitment dysfunction and specific tests have been designed to assess this dysfunction (Richardson and Jull 1995, Hides *et al.* 1996, Hodges and Richardson 1996, Jull 1998, Jull *et al.* 1999, Richardson *et al.* 1999). These tests must identify and exclude substitution strategies from the global muscles, e.g. during abdominal hollowing, excessive activity of the external obliques and rectus abdominis.

To test for the stability function of the deep neck flexors the subjects is positioned in supine with the spine, temporomandibular joint and scapula in a neutral position (head supported on towel). The subject is instructed to perform a very slight upper cervical flexion action, which causes a slight cervical flexion and flattening of the cervical curve. A pressure biofeedback unit can be used to measure function (Jull 1998, 2000, 2001) (Figure 4.3.106). There should be no substitu-

tion (for example from scalenae or sternocleidomastoid) or fatigue. A flattening pressure (6–8 mmHg in 2 mmHg increments) should be able to be sustained for 10 seconds by 10 repetitions (Jull 1998). There should be minimal range of movement.

Transversus abdominis will tension the low abdominal fascia and hollow the low abdominal wall. This 'drawing in' action should be specifically localized to the lower abdominal region and there should be minimal spinal or rib cage movement. It should not cause lateral flaring of the waist. A pressure biofeedback unit can be used to measure a function of transversus abdominis recruitment in prone lying (Hodges *et al.* 1996, Richardson *et al.* 1999, Cairns *et al.* 2000). For good motor control patterns the patient needs to be able to specifically activate, hold, and repeat the contraction; a 10-second hold with 10 repetitions has been suggested a useful guide (Richardson and Jull 1995) (Figure 4.3.107).

To test for lumbar multifidus function the multifidus is consciously activated against the facilitating pressure of a thumb/finger (Hides *et al.* 1996, Richardson *et al.* 1999) (Figure 4.3.108). This contraction should ideally be maintained for 10 seconds and consistently repeated 10 times. Substitution strategies, for example excessive activity of the erector spinae or lumbar extension should be avoided.

To test for psoas, the patient lies on one side with both legs bent. The top femur is supported horizontal with the spine, pelvis, and upper trunk all in neutral alignment. Psoas is facilitated by gently distracting the top leg longitudinally, and the patient is instructed to pull the hip back into the socket without moving the spine or pelvis. Facilitation may be localized segmentally. The therapist manually palpates the relative stiffness at that level by manually attempting to translate the spinous process side to side. The psoas activation is facilitated and resistance to manual translation (stiffness) is re-assessed

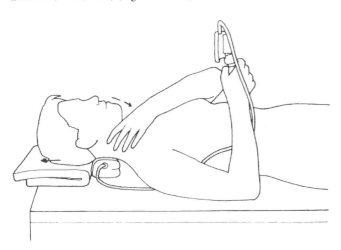

Figure 4.3.106 Deep neck flexor control of neutral (reprinted with permission from Physiotools).

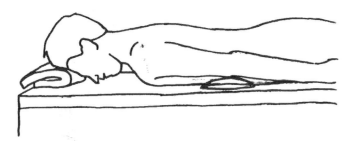

Figure 4.3.107 Transversus abdominus activation in neutral (reprinted with permission from Physiotools).

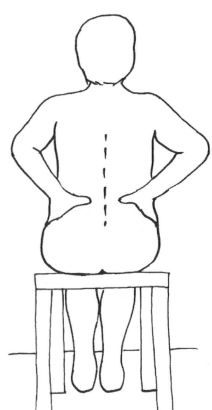

Figure 4.3.108 Lumbar bifidus activation in neutral (reprinted with permission from Physiotools).

(Comerford and Emerson, personal communication 1999). Ideally, a significant increase in resistance to manual displacement should be noted when psoas is activated. The contraction (and increased stiffness) should be able to be maintained for 10 seconds and consistently repeated 10 times. This response should be noted at all lumbar segmental levels. Segmental psoas dysfunction is identified by the level that does not increase resistance to manual translation when compared to adjacent levels (which do increase resistance to translation when psoas is activated). A lack of increased resistance to manual displacement during psoas activation indicates a probable loss of segmental control of the local stability role of psoas (Comerford and Mottram 2002b, 2002c).

Global stability muscles: direction control

The global muscles react to dysfunction with functional length and recruitment changes. The assessment of global muscle function consid-

ers the ability to dissociate direction and control of through range motion. The global stability muscles are required to control directional strain, i.e. control the excessive uncontrolled give into flexion/ extension or rotation. The assessment for the ability of the global stability muscles to dissociate direction involves actively maintaining the neutral position of the spine whilst moving the limbs independently into flexion, extension, rotation, and other directions. These movements are not normal functional movements but are movement patterns that everybody

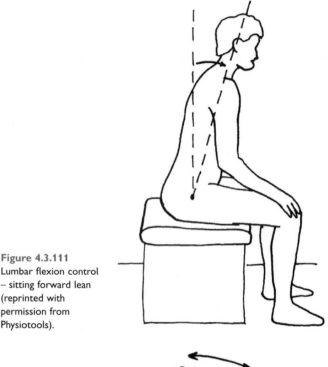

Figure 4.3.111
Lumbar flexion control – sitting forward lean (reprinted with permission from Physiotools).

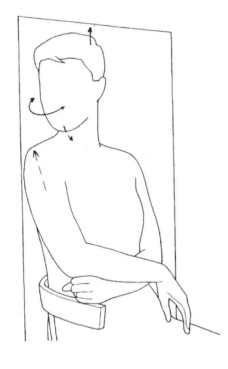

Figure 4.3.109
Cervical rotation control (reprinted with permission from Physiotools).

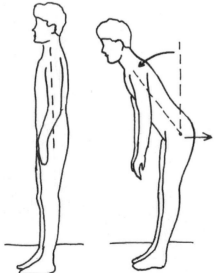

Figure 4.3.110
Lumbar flexion control – standing forward lean (reprinted with permission from Physiotools).

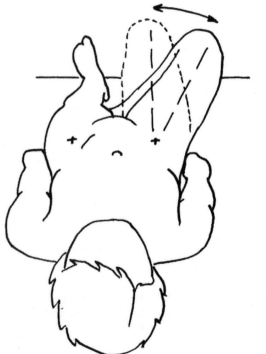

Figure 4.3.112 Lumbar rotation control – bent knee fall out (reprinted with permission from Physiotools).

should be able to perform (Sahrmann 2002, Hamilton 1998). Some examples of stability dysfunction are highlighted below.

In the cervical spine a symmetrical range of cervical rotation should be achieved. Symmetry is important but range is variable (80°; Kapandji 1982). The common directions of give are upper cervical extension (chin poke associated with poor stability of the deep neck flexors) and lateral flexion during rotation (associated with a coupling dysfunction in the articular system and/or poor stability of the deep neck flexors) (Figure 4.3.109). A significant asymmetry of rotation or an obvious decrease in range of motion is seen when the give is actively or passively controlled. Restriction may occur from articular translational dysfunction or myofascial dysfunction or related neural sensitivity.

Two useful tests for lumbar flexion stability dysfunction are the forward lean test standing (Sahrmann 2002; Figure 4.3.110) and the sitting forward lean test (Hamilton 1998; Figure 4.3.111). Bent knee fall out – supine (Figure 4.3.112) is a useful test to identify a lumbar rotation stability dysfunction.

Forward lean test – standing

The subject is instructed to stand tall and to bend or 'bow' forward from the hips, keeping the back straight (neutral spine). Ideally, the subject should be able to dissociate the lumbar spine from hip flexion, as evidenced by a 50° forward lean with maintenance of the lumbar spine neutral position. A positive test will demonstrate lumbar flexion, extension, or asymmetry.

Forward lean test – sitting

The subject is instructed to sit tall and to lean forward from the hips, keeping the back straight (neutral spine). Ideally, the subject should be able to dissociate the lumbar spine from hip flexion, as evidenced by 30° of forward lean with maintenance of lumbar spine neutral. A positive test will demonstrate lumbar flexion, extension, or asymmetry.

Bent knee fall out – supine

With the subject lying supine and with legs extended and the feet together, both anterior superior iliac spines (ASIS) are checked for symmetry in the anteroposterior plane. The subject is instructed to slide one heel up beside the other knee. Ideally the pelvis should not rotate and the ASIS should remain level. If the pelvis stays stable and does not rotate, the subject is instructed to allow the bent leg to slowly lower out to the side, keeping the foot supported beside the straight leg. There is usually some slight rotation of the pelvis at this stage. The subject is then instructed to repeat the 'bent leg fall out' but not to allow the pelvis to rotate at all. Ideally, the bent leg should be able to be lowered out through the available range of hip abduction and lateral rotation (at least 50°) and returned, without associated pelvic rotation. A stability dysfunction will demonstrate that the lumbar spine and pelvis have greater give into rotation relative to the hips

Global muscle imbalance: global stability muscle dysfunction

When dysfunctional, global stability muscles react less efficiently to low load stimuli and are unable to move the motion segment to full inner range. Through range control of the cervicothoracic stabilizing extensors is required to control segmental cervicothoracic extension and eccentric cervicothoracic flexion. Clinically, it is frequently observed that gluteus maximus loses the ability to control hip extension to inner range. The global stability muscles must have the ability to move the joint through the full available range in normal function. These examples are illustrated below.

Global muscle imbalance: global mobility muscle dysfunction

When the global mobility muscles lose extensibility, there may be changes in the contractile or connective tissue elements of the muscle.

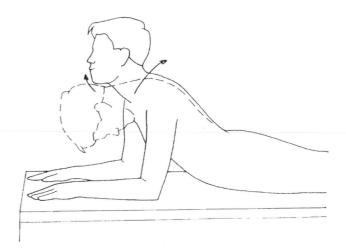

Figure 4.3.113 Cervicothoracic extensor stabilizers – through-range control (reprinted with permission from Physiotools).

Through range control of the cervicothoracic stabilizing extensors
(Figure 4.3.113)

The subject starts resting prone on elbows, with the scapulae and thoracic spine neutral and the head hanging in flexion. The subject is instructed to maintain the upper cervical spine in flexion or neutral and lift their head with independent extension of the low cervical spine through full range and lower the head to return to the starting position. Ideally, the subject should have the ability to independently extend the lower cervical spine through the full range of extension and hold in the shortened range position for 10 seconds without fatigue or substitution. Then return with eccentric control to the starting position in outer range without substitution. Activation of the mobility muscles under load is normal. When the movement is performed correctly (without substitution or fatigue) the range that can be controlled actively equals the available passive range of cervical flexion.

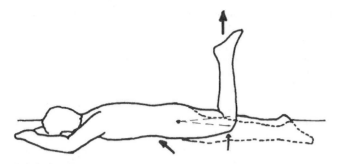

Figure 4.3.114 Gluteus maximus – inner-range control (reprinted with permission from Physiotools).

Hip extension with knee flexed – prone
(Figure 4.3.114)

With the subject lying prone and one knee flexed to past 90°, the lumbopelvic region is manually stabilized and the hip passively lifted into extension to check the available range of hip extension. The subject is instructed to lift the knee (hip extension) approximately 3–5 cm (1–2 inches). Note any lack of gluteal participation, cramping of the hamstrings or excessive lumbar extension or rotation under hip extension load. Ideally, the lumbopelvic region should maintain a neutral position as the hip actively extends (approximately 10–15°). Hip extension should be initiated and maintained by gluteus maximus. The muscle should have the ability to shorten sufficiently and hold limb load in the joint inner range position for 10 seconds and repeat the movement repeat the movement 10 times (without the inner range hold) and without substitution or fatigue. The hamstrings will participate in the movement but should not dominate. There will be paraspinal muscle activation (asymmetrically biased) but there should be no gross hyperextension, segmental shear (pivot) or rotation in the lumbar spine.

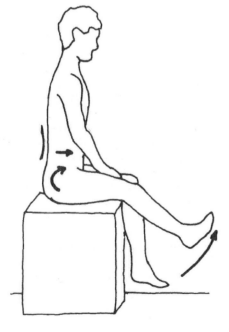

Figure 4.3.115
Hamstrings extensibility (reprinted with permission from Physiotools).

Assessment for levator scapula extensibility (Figure 4.3.116)

Position the subject with cervical spine and scapula in neutral (in lying). The cervical spine is flexed, the head rotated and laterally flex away from the side to be assessed. The head is moved until the extensibility limit of the levator scapula is reached or the scapula elevates to follow the muscle. Maintain this position and take tension off the muscle by passively elevating the shoulder. Then attempt to move the head into more range of lateral flexion. If there is no further available range, the cervical spine is at the limit of motion and the levator scapula muscle is not short. If there is more range available then the levator scapula is short and limiting function.

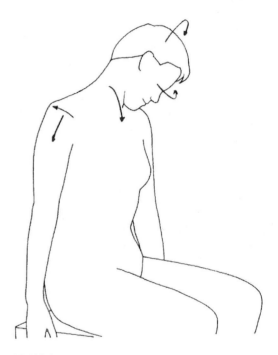

Figure 4.3.116 Levator scapulae extensibility (reprinted with permission from Physiotools).

Assessment for hamstring extensibility (Figure 4.3.115)

The subject sits with the spine and pelvis in neutral alignment, the acromion vertically positioned over the ischium, the hips flexed at 90°, and the feet unsupported. The operator monitors the lumbopelvic position and passively extends the knee until either resistance to extension is felt (stretch in the posterior thigh) or there is a loss of lumbopelvic neutral. Ideally, with maintenance of lumbopelvic neutral and the hip flexed to 90° the knee should be able to extend to within 10° of full extension. The lumbar spine should not flex and the pelvis should not posteriorly tilt or rotate. The shoulders should stay vertically aligned over the ischium and not lean back into hip extension.

Table **4.3.17.** Rehabilitation strategy for articular translational and myofascial give and restriction

	Articular translational	**Myofascial**
Give	Local stability muscle integration to control intersegmental motion – tonic recruitment	Global stability muscle training to control range of motion – tonic recruitment
Restriction	Mobilization of segmental articular restriction	Inhibition of overactivity and regaining extensibility of myofascial length

Recruitment issues or mechanical issues may influence these elements. The global mobility muscles need to be examined for length and recruitment changes.

Rehabilitation

The re-education of dysfunction will depend on the pattern of the dysfunction and the site and direction of the stability dysfunction. From the assessment, the articular translational and myofascial give and restriction will have been identified. Correcting motor control and recruitment patterns is the priority in the rehabilitation of the local stability system. Correcting length and recruitment dysfunction is the priority of the global system. Addressing the give and restriction is the key to rehabilitation (Table 4.3.17; Comerford and Mottram 2002a).

As well as dealing with mechanical components of movement dysfunction, the pathology must be addressed and non-mechanical issues identified and managed (Figure 4.3.117, Comerford and Kinetic Control 2000a). Fitness and exercise programs have been shown to be an effective treatment approach for chronic low back pain (Frost *et al.* 1998, Torstensen *et al.* 1998). Consideration of psychosocial factors is essential in the management of low back pain (Main and Watson 1999, Kendall and Watson 2000, Watson 2000, Watson and Kendall 2000). Cognitive behavioral approaches have a significant role in the man-

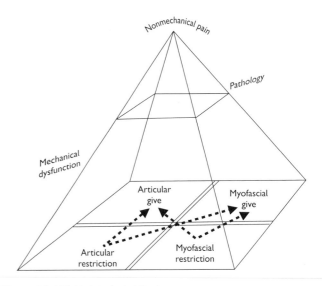

Figure 4.3.117 Model of rehabilitation.

agement of chronic low back pain (Waddell 1998, Klaber Moffet *et al.* 1999, Watson 2000).

A useful guide for rehabilitation has been described using the following four principles of low-load movement and stability rehabil-

Table **4.3.18.** Principles of stability rehabilitation

Principle I	Control of the neutral joint position	Retrain tonic, low threshold activation of the local stability system to increase muscle stiffness and train the functional low load integration of the local and global stabilizer muscles to control the neutral joint position
Principle II	Retrain control of the direction of stability dysfunction	Control the give and move the restriction. Retrain control of the stability dysfunction in the direction of symptom producing movements. Use the low load integration of local and global stabilizer recruitment to control and limit motion at the segment or region of give and then actively move the adjacent restriction. Only move through as much range as the restriction allows or as far as the give is dynamically controlled
Principle III	Rehabilitate global stabilizer control through range	Rehabilitate the global stability system to actively control the full available range of joint motion. These muscles are required to be able to actively shorten and control limb load through to the full passive inner range of joint motion. They must also be able to control any hyper mobile outer range. The ability to control rotational forces is an especially important role of global stabilizers. Eccentric control of range is more important for stability function than concentric work. This is optimized by low effort, sustained holds in the muscle's shortened position with controlled eccentric lowering
Principle IV	Regain extensibility and inhibit excessive dominance of the global mobilizers	When the two joint global mobility muscles demonstrate a lack of extensibility due to overuse or adaptive shortening, compensatory overstrain or give occurs elsewhere in the kinetic chain in an attempt to maintain function. It becomes necessary to lengthen or inhibit over-activity in the global mobilizers to eliminate the need for compensation to keep function

itation (low-threshold stability training) (Comerford and Mottram 2000a) (Table 4.3.18). The following section is confined to low-threshold stability training; the three principles of high threshold 'core' stability are not detailed here.

Principle I: control of neutral

To regain control of the local stability system requires specific activation of the stability system, without substitution strategies. There is evidence that transversus abdominis is controlled independently of other abdominal muscles (Hodges and Richardson 1999). The contraction needs to be sustained with the joint in neutral position and under low physiological load. This should be progressed and integrated into functional activities. The emphasis here is on motor control and recruitment and not strength and flexibility. The goal of Principle I is to regain the normal automatic functioning of the stabilizing system of the lumbar and cervical spines.

Teaching the specific activation of the local stability system is not easy and requires good clinical observation and teaching skills from the therapist and specific facilitation techniques as appropriate (Figure 4.3.118; Comerford and Mottram 2000a). Facilitation techniques will help to improve proprioceptive awareness and cognitive awareness, thus assisting in slow motor unit recruitment.

Re-education of the deep neck flexors requires the patient to learn a pure head nod, which the clinician must carefully teach (Jull 1998, 2000). The gentleness and precision of the action needs to be reinforced. The aim is to train 10-second holds by 10 repetitions with the appropriate pressure change (Jull 1998) (Figure 4.3.87). As control and stability improves, the ability to sustain the optimal pressure change without substitution 'feels easy'.

The specific activation of transversus abdominis is taught by asking the patient to gently draw in (hollow) the low abdominal wall (Richardson and Jull 1995, Hodges *et al.* 1996, Richardson and Hodges 1996, Richardson *et al.* 1999) (Figure 4.3.88). Facilitation and skill

learning techniques can be employed to assist the patient. These include visualization and instructional cues such as 'draw your lower abdomen up and in' to encourage conscious activation, tactile feedback, breathing control, and facilitation through a pelvic floor contraction or multifidus.

Recruiting a sustained and repeatable multifidus contraction needs specific instruction (Hides *et al.* 1996) (Figure 4.3.89). Again, visualization and cues are useful facilitators, as is achieving a joint neutral spinal position (Hamilton 1998, Richardson *et al.* 1999).

The re-education of the stability role of psoas involves the action of longitudinal compression, for example, 'shortening the leg' or attempting 'to pull the hip into the socket'. Psoas contraction should increase stiffness segmentally in the lumbar spine and should resist motion segmentally rather than produce it. Optimal facilitation and retraining requires providing an appropriate low-load facilitation and feedback. This training is best started in supine, side lying, or inclined sitting before progressing into function. Useful facilitation techniques are coactivation with the pelvic floor, breathing control, and low-effort lateral rotation of the femur. During active retraining of psoas it is also essential to identify and eliminate various substitution strategies and faults.

The patient must at all times be able to dissociate the specific recruitment of the stability system from their breathing pattern. Subjects with back pain have demonstrated difficulty in dissociating respiration from recruitment of the lumbar stability muscles (Cairns *et al.* 2000).

Once activation has been achieved in the clinic, the patient needs to practice so that the motor control pattern becomes integrated into all functional positions (see box). O'Sullivan *et al.* (1997a) have demonstrated the clinical effectiveness and importance of the integration of the deep stability muscle system into functional movements, activities of daily living, and even high loads and provocative positions.

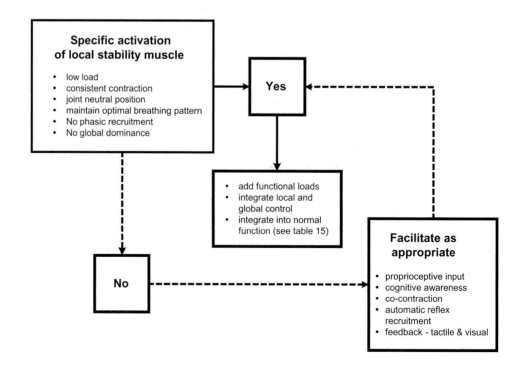

Figure 4.3.118 Specific recruitment of the local stability system.

Integration of local stability muscle recruitment into normal function

1 Activation in neutral alignment with a variety of different postures or positions (progression: supported → unsupported)
2 Activation in neutral alignment without co-contraction rigidity. (for the trunk: activation with normal relaxed breathing; for the limbs: activation without resistance to passive rotation)
3 Activation in neutral alignment on an unstable base (add a proprioceptive challenge)
4 Activation during directional control exercises (dissociation or recruitment reversals)
5 Activation during normal physiological movements (the trunk and girdles actively move away from neutral position)
6 Activation during functional activities (normal movements of the unloaded limbs and trunk – 'red dot' exercise)
7 Activation during stressful or provocative movements and positions (pathology and symptom specific)
8 Activation during occupational, recreational or sport specific skills

Key points for rehabilitation

Activation of local and global stability muscles to control the neutral joint position:

- Specific activation of the deep local stability muscles in the neutral joint position.
- The contraction is biased for the local stability muscles.
- The contraction is isometric.
- The contraction should be biased for slow motor unit recruitment (low force).
- It is a conscious activation requiring motor planning and proprioceptive feedback.
- The ability to sustain a consistent low force hold is paramount for rehabilitation of motor control deficits.
- Once cognitive control has been achieved, integrate the pattern into function (integrate local activity with the global function).
- Optimal facilitation is dependent on identification and elimination of substitution strategies and overload or fatigue.
- Maximum perceived effort is permissible initially, but as control and functional integration return low effort activation should dominate.
- There should be no fatigue or substitution.
- Recruitment of the stability muscles to control joint neutral must be non-provocative and pain free.
- Motor control, not strength, is the intention.

Principle II: direction control of global stability muscles

As soon as the patient has regained activation of the local stability system, the program can be progressed to regaining the control of the stability dysfunction (Tables 4.3.13 and 4.3.14), i.e. controlling the give. This requires activation of the global stability system along with integrated activation of the local stability muscles.

Specific recruitment and control exercise programs need to be practiced to restore normal muscle function (Sahrmann 2000, Comerford and Mottram 2002b–d). Failure of the dissociation test becomes the corrective exercise.

For example, for cervical rotation stability dysfunction the patient needs to regain control of cervical rotation (Figure 4.3.90). Position the cervical spine and scapula neutral, and rotate the head through the available range without substitution strategies (lateral flexion and chin poke). It may be useful to passively unload the ipsilateral scapula (taping, passive support). As range improves and symptoms decrease the patient should begin to actively control the scapula position. This exercise can be started in sitting with support but should be progressed into function.

The sitting bow and standing bow tests can be used to retrain lumbar spine flexion stability dysfunction (Figures 4.3.110 and 4.3.111). The bent knee fall out test can be used to retrain lumbar spine flexion stability dysfunction (Figure 4.3.112).

Key points for rehabilitation

Retrain control of the direction of stability dysfunction.

- Control the give and move the restriction.
- Use conscious activation of the stability muscles (both global and local stabilizers) to hold the dysfunctional region or segment in a neutral position (± assisted or supported) and move the adjacent joint or motion segment.
- Movement at the adjacent joint should be independent of the region of poor stability or control dysfunction.
- Movement must be controlled eccentrically as well as concentrically.
- Move at adjacent joint only as far as:
  – control of the dysfunctional region can be maintained
  – the restriction at the adjacent joint allows.
- Try to use low to moderate effort to facilitate tonic recruitment. Maximum effort (cocontraction rigidity) is to be discouraged
- The dynamic stability dysfunction is direction dependent and relates to the type and nature of pathology
- Direction control movements are not stretches or strengthening exercises: Low force! No stretch! No strain! No substitution! No fatigue! No pain!

Once spinal stability can be maintained during movements of the limbs into flexion, extension, rotation, or abduction, then the global stability muscles can be retrained to achieve through range control.

Through range control of the cervicothoracic stabilizing extensors is required to control the cervicothoracic spine (Figure 4.3.113). When movement is performed correctly (without substitution or fatigue) the range that can be controlled actively equals the available passive range of cervical extension. Train the holding time at the point that can be controlled without substitution (ideally 10-second holds by 10 repetitions, but if this is not possible for the time that can be controlled).

Through-range control of the hip stabilizing extensors is required to control hip extension and eccentric hip flexion.

Through-range control of the hip extensors

The patient supports their trunk on the edge of a bench, table, or bed with both feet supported on the floor and the knees slightly flexed. The lumbar spine is positioned in neutral alignment. The abdominal and gluteal muscles are coactivated to control the neutral spine and to prevent excessive lumbar extension. The patient is instructed to bend one knee to 90° and then lift that bent leg into hip extension. The hip extension must be independent of any lumbopelvic motion. The leg is extended only as far as the neutral lumbopelvic position can be maintained without cramping or over-activation of the hamstrings. At this point the leg is slowly lowered back towards the floor. Initially, the patient may only be able to dissociate the lumbar spine (neutral) from hip extension to within 40° flexion from horizontal. As the ability to control lumbopelvic extension gets easier and the pattern of dissociation feels less unnatural, the exercise can be progressed to hip extension level with the horizontal (0°) and eventually to 10–15° of extension above the horizontal. When the patient can lift the leg horizontal (to 0° hip extension), and control lumbopelvic neutral, the exercise can be progressed in prone (Figure 4.3.114). The patient is positioned prone with a pillow under the pelvis (hips flexed to approximately 10–15°) to allow the gluteals to work from an efficient length. The subject is instructed to bend one knee past 90° (to relax the hamstrings) and then lift that knee (hip extension) approximately 3–5 cm (1–2 inches). The leg may lift into extension only as far as the neutral lumbopelvic position can be maintained without cramping or overactivation of the hamstrings. At this point the leg is slowly lowered back towards the floor while also maintaining lumbopelvic neutral.

Principle III: through range control

Key points for rehabilitation

Low-threshold recruitment, through-range control of the global stability muscles.

- Low force to encourage slow motor unit recruitment.

- Increasing the holding time of muscles that have a stability function has priority over strengthening. This is to facilitate recruitment of tonic fibers and train specificity of antigravity holding function.

- Shortened muscle position: A basic requirement of stability function is that the global stabilizer muscles have the ability to move the limbs (functional load) through their available range; or at least move the limbs through the same range that the synergistic global mobilizers can.

- Eccentric control is important to control the joint through range.

- Because the global stabilizer muscles are the muscles that are anatomically and biomechanically best orientated to control rotation efficiently, it is important to have reasonable rotation dissociation ability before training the global stabilizer function. The rotatory component of global stabilizer muscle action must be controlled during the low force, sustained hold.

- Exercise in a closed kinetic chain environment (distal fixation or weightbearing) allows better tonic recruitment and also provides additional proprioceptive afferent information

- Coactivation of stability muscles may promote the recruitment of slow motor units.

- No phasic recruitment or dominance of global muscles should be allowed.

Principle IV: regain extensibility and inhibit the short or overactive global mobility muscles

The global mobility muscles need to regain their ideal physiological length and appropriate techniques can be employed to do this, e.g. muscle lengthening, soft tissue techniques, and myofascial release. Rehabilitation should ensure that they are not dominant synergists for postural stability. Their primary role is for high-load/high-speed activity.

Key points for rehabilitation

Regain extensibility and inhibit the short or overactive global mobility muscles

- The aim here is to target the tight contractile or connective tissue. Techniques for regaining length and inhibition of overactive muscles include myofascial release, proprioceptive neuromuscular facilitation, muscle energy techniques, and active inhibitory restabilizations.

- An inhibitory lengthening technique, active inhibitory restabilization, is a useful technique for regaining length. It involves the operator gently and slowly lengthening the muscle until the resistance causes a slight loss of proximal girdle or trunk stability (into the stability dysfunction). The operator then maintains the muscle or limb in this position. The subject is then instructed to actively restabilize the proximal segment that lost stability and sustain the correction for 20–30 seconds, repeated 3–5 times. This encourages reciprocal inhibition of the overactive muscle and a bonus proximal stability.

None of the corrective exercises to directly improve dynamic stability (Principles I, II, and III) should produce or provoke any symptoms at all. If any symptoms are aggravated or provoked by corrective exercises, first check that the exercise is being performed correctly with appropriate low load and control. Overload is the most common cause of provocation. If an appropriate exercise is performed correctly but is still provocative, then other issues must be considered – acute inflammatory pathology, gross segmental instability, neurogenic or neuropathic pain, visceral pain, or serious medical pathology.

Conclusion

There is a growing volume of evidence which suggests that improving muscle balance and function and assessing and correcting deficiencies is an integral part of the management of patients presenting with spinal pain of neuromusculoskeletal origin. Research evidence shows that patients with low back pain may demonstrate dysfunction in both the local and global stability systems. Local stability dysfunction presents as a change in the recruitment of the deep local stability muscles that have a role in maintaining dynamic stability at the spinal motion segments. Global dysfunction presents as a lack of global muscle control of direction especially rotation but also flexion, extension and

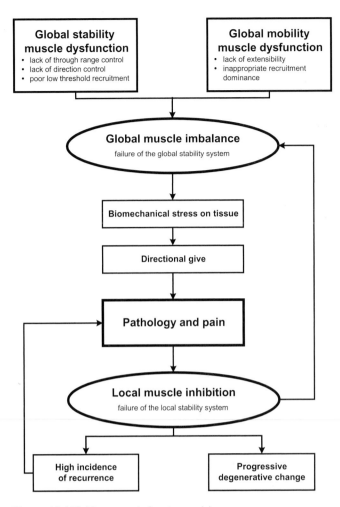

Figure 4.3.119 Movement dysfunction model.

other directions. Global stability dysfunction also presents as an imbalance between the global stability and mobility synergists. The stability synergists demonstrate a lack of through range control of a joint motion and poor low threshold postural recruitment. The global mobility synergists lack extensibility or demonstrate inappropriate dominance of low threshold postural function. These changes are associated with the presentation of spinal pain, disability, and dysfunction (Figure 4.3.119). Assessment procedures and rehabilitation protocols for stability dysfunction and muscle imbalance have been described (Richardson *et al.* 1999, Comerford and Mottram 2002a–e) and there is evidence of effectiveness for stability programs (O'Sullivan *et al.* 1997a, 1998, Hides 1998, Beeton and Jull 1994, Grant *et al.* 1997).

The ability to assess movement function and correct movement dysfunction is a key clinical skill required when managing neuromusculoskeletal dysfunction. Evidence suggests that clinicians would benefit from having the skills to assess and rehabilitate dynamic stability and muscle balance in patients attending the clinic with spinal pain, both acute and chronic.

References

Balster, S. M., Jull, G. A. (1977) Upper trapezius muscle activity during the brachial plexus tension test in asymptomatic subjects. *Manual Therapy*, 2(3), 144–9.

Beeton, K., Jull, G. A. (1994) The effectiveness of manipulative physiotherapy in the management of cervicogenic headache: a single case study. *Physiotherapy*, 80(7), 417–23.

Bergmark, A. (1989) Stability of the lumbar spine. A study in mechanical engineering. *Acta Orthopaedica Scandinavica*, 230(60), 20–4.

Brumagne, S., Lysens, R., Swinnen, S., Verschueren, S. (1999) Effect of paraspinal muscle vibration on position of lumbosacral spine. *Spine*, 24(13), 1328–31.

Butler, D. (1998) Integrating pain awareness into physiotherapy – wise action for the future. In: Gifford, L. (ed) *Topical issues in pain*. CNS Press, Falmouth, pp. 1–23.

Cairns, M. C., Harrison, K., Wright, C. (2000) Pressure biofeedback: a useful tool in quantification of abdominal muscular dysfunction? *Physiotherapy*, 86(3), 127–38.

Cholewicki, J., McGill, S. M. (1996) Mechanical stability of the in vivo lumbar spine: implications for injury and chronic low back pain. *Clinical Biomechanics*, 11(1), 1–15.

Comerford, M. (1997) Dynamic stabilisation – evidence of muscle dysfunction. Conference proceedings, British Institute of Musculoskeletal Medicine, London.

Comerford, M. J., Mottram S L (2001a) Functional stability retraining: Principles and strategies for managing mechanical dysfunction. *Manual Therapy*, 6(1), 3–14.

Comerford M. J., Mottram, S. L. (2002a) *Movement dysfunction focus on dynamic stability and muscle balance*. Course notes. Kinetic Control, Southampton.

Comerford M. J., Mottram, S. L. (2002b) *Dynamic stability and muscle balance of the lumbar spine and trunk*. Course notes. Kinetic Control, Southampton.

Comerford, M. J., Mottram, S. L. (2002c) *Dynamic stability and muscle balance of the cervical spine*. Course notes. Kinetic Control, Southampton.

Comerford, M. J., Mottram, S. L. (2002d) *Dynamic stability and muscle balance of the shoulder girdle*. Course notes. Kinetic Control, Southampton.

Comerford, M. J., Mottram, S. L. (2002e) *Dynamic stability and muscle balance for return to work and return to sport*. Course notes. Kinetic Control, Southampton.

Comerford M. J., Mottram, S. L. (2003) *Rehabilitation of movement and stability dysfunction within the human musculoskeletal system*. Course notes. Kinetic Control, Southampton.

Dangaria, T. R., Naesh, O. (1998) Changes in cross-sectional area of psoas major muscle in unilateral sciatica caused by disc herniation. *Spine*, 23(8), 928–31.

Edgar, D., Jull, G., Sutton, S. (1994) The relationship between upper trapezius muscle length and upper quadrant neural tissue extensibility. *Australian Journal of Physiotherapy*, 4, 99–103.

Frost, H., Lamb, S. E., Klaber Moffet, J. A., Fairbank, J. C., Moser, J. J. (1998) A fitness programme for patients with chronic low back pain: 2 year follow up after a randomized controlled trial. *Pain*, 75, 273–9.

Goff, B. (1972) The application of recent advances in neurophysiology to Miss Roods' concept of neuromuscular facilitation. *Physiotherapy*, 58(2), 409–15.

Goldspink, G., Williams, P. (1992) Muscle fibre and connective tissue changes associated with use and disuse. In: Ada, L., Canning, C. (eds) *Physiotherapy: foundations for practice. Key issues in neurological physiotherapy*, pp. 197–217.

Gossman, M. R., Sahrmann, S. A., Rose, S. J. (1982) Review of length-associated changes in muscle. *Physical Therapy*, 62(12), 1799–808.

Grant, R., Jull, G., Spencer, T. (1997) Active stabilisation training for screen based keyboard operators – a single case study. *Australian Journal of Physiotherapy*, 43(4), 235–42.

Hall, T., Zusman, M., Elvey R (1998) Adverse mechanical tension in the nervous system? Analysis of straight leg raise. *Manual Therapy*, 3(3), 140–6.

Hall, T. M., Elvey, R. L. (1999) Nerve trunk pain: physical diagnosis and treatment. *Manual Therapy*, 4(2), 63–73.

Hamilton, C. (1998) Active control of the neutral lumbopelvic posture, a comparison between back pain and non back pain subjects. *Proceedings of the 3rd Interdisciplinary World Congress on Low Back and Pelvic Pain, Vienna*.

Hides, J. A., Stokes, M. J., Saide, M., Jull, G. A., Cooper, D. H. (1994) Evidence of multifidus wasting ipsilateral to symptoms in patients with acute/subacute low back pain. *Spine*, 19(2), 165–77.

Hides, J. A., Richardson, C. A., Jull, G. A. (1996) Multifidus recovery is not automatic after resolution of acute, first-episode low back pain. *Spine*, 21(23), 2763–9.

Hides, J. A. (1998) The lumbar multifidus: evidence of a link to low back pain. *Proceedings of the 3rd Interdisciplinary World Congress on Low Back and Pelvic Pain, Vienna*.

Hodges, P. W., Richardson, C. A. (1996) Inefficient muscular stabilisation of the lumbar spine associated with low back pain: a motor control evaluation of transversus abdominis. *Spine*, 21(22), 2640–50.

Hodges, P. W., Richardson, C. A., Jull, G. A. (1996) Evaluation of the relationship between laboratory and clinical tests of transversus abdominis function. *Physiotherapy Research International*, 1, 30–40.

Hodges, P. W., Richardson, C. A. (1999) Transversus abdominis and the superficial abdominal muscles are controlled independently in a postural task. *Neuroscience Letters*, 265(2), 91–4.

Hurley, M. V., Newham, D. J. (1993) The influence of arthrogenous muscle inhibition on quadriceps rehabilitation of patients with early, unilateral osteoarthritic knees. *British Journal of Rheumatology*, 32, 127–31.

Hurley, M. V. (1997) The effects of joint damage on muscle function, proprioception and rehabilitation. *Manual Therapy*, 1(5), 11–17.

Janda, V. L. (1985) Pain in the locomotor system – a broad approach. In: Glasgow *et al.* (eds) *Aspects of manipulative therapy*. Churchill Livingstone, Edinburgh, pp. 148–51.

Janda, V. L. (1994) Muscles and motor control in cervicogenic disorders: assessment and management. In: Grant, R. (ed) *Physical therapy of the cervical and thoracic spine*. Churchill Livingstone, Edinburgh, pp. 195–216.

Jull, G. (1997) Management of cervical headache. *Manual Therapy*, 2(4), 182–90.

Jull, G. (1998) Physiotherapy management of neck pain of mechanical origin. In: Giles, L. G. F., Singer, K. P. (eds) *Clinical anatomy and management of cervical spine pain*. Butterworth-Heinemann, Oxford, pp. 168–91.

Jull, G., Barrett, C., Magee, R., Ho, P. (1999) Further clinical clarification of the muscle dysfunction in cervical headache. *Cephalalgia*, 19(3), 179–85.

Kankaanpaa, M., Taimela, S., Laaksonen, D., Hanninen, O., Airaksinen, O. (1998) Back and hip extensor fatigability in chronic low back pain patients. *Archives of Physical Medicine and Rehabilitation*, 79, 412–17.

Kendall, N., Watson, P. (2000) Identifying psychosocial yellow flags and modifying management. In: Gifford, L. (ed) *Topical Issues in Pain 2 – Biopsychosocial assessment and management* 4, pp. 131–9.

Klaber Moffet, J. A., Torgerson, D., Bell-Syer, S. (1999) Randomised controlled trail of exercise for low back pain: Clinical outcomes, costs, and preferences. *BMJ*, 319, 279–83.

Lee, D. G. (1996) Rotational instability of the mid-thoracic spine: assessment and treatment. *Manual Therapy*, 1(5), 234–41.

Main, C. J., Watson, P. J. (1999) Psychological aspects of pain. *Manual Therapy*, 4(4), 203–15.

Maitland, G. D. (1986) *Vertebral manipulation*, 5th edn, Butterworths, London.

Mottram, S. L. (1997) Dynamic stability of the scapula. *Manual Therapy*, 2(3), 123–31.

Mottram, S. L., Comerford, M. (1999) Stability dysfunction and low back pain. *Journal of Orthopaedic Medicine*, 20(2), 13–18.

O'Sullivan, P. B., Twomey, L., Allison, G., Sinclair, J., Miller, K., Knox, J. (1997a) Altered patterns of abdominal muscle activation in patients with chronic low back pain. *Australian Journal of Physiotherapy*, 43(2), 91–8.

O'Sullivan, P. B., Twomey, L., Allison, G. (1997b) Evaluation of specific stabilising exercises in the treatment of chronic low back pain with radiological diagnosis of spondylosis or spondylolisthesis. *Spine*, 22(24), 2959–67.

O'Sullivan, P. B. (2000) Lumbar segmental 'instability': clinical presentation and specific stabilizing exercise management. *Manual Therapy*, 5(1), 2–12.

Panjabi, M. M. (1992) The stabilising system of the spine. Part 1. Function, dysfunction, adaptation, and enhancement. *Journal of Spinal Disorders*, 5(4), 383–9.

Richardson, C., Jull, G., Hodges, P., Hides, J. (1999) *Therapeutic exercise for spinal segmental stabilization in low back pain: scientific basis and clinical approach*. Churchill Livingstone, Edinburgh.

Richardson, C. A., Jull, G. A. (1995) Muscle control – pain control. What exercises would you prescribe? *Manual Therapy*, 1, 1–9.

Rothwell, J. (1994) *Control of human voluntary movement*, 2nd edn, Chapman & Hall, London.

Sahrmann, S. A. (1993) Movement as a cause of musculoskeletal pain. *Proceedings of the 8th Biennial Conference of the Manipulative Physiotherapists Association of Australia, Perth*.

Sahrmann, S. A. (2000) *Diagnosis and treatment of management impairment syndromes*. Mosby, St. Louis.

Stokes, M., Young, A. (1984) The contribution of reflex inhibition to arthrogenous muscle weakness. *Clinical Science*, 67, 7–14.

Taimela, S., Kankaanpaa, M., Luoto, S, (1999) The effects of lumbar fatigue on the ability to sense a change in lumbar position. *Spine*, 24(13), 1322–7.

Torstensen, T. A., Ljunggren, A. E., Meen, H. D., *et al.* (1998) Efficiency and costs of medical exercise therapy, conventional physiotherapy, and self-exercise in patients with chronic low back pain. *Spine*, 23(23), 2616–24.

Waddell, G. (1998) *The back pain revolution*. Churchill Livingstone, Edinburgh.

Watson, P. (2000) Psychosocial predictors of outcomes from low back pain. In: Gifford, L. (ed.) *Topical issues in pain 2 – biopsychosocial assessment and management*, 5, 109.

Watson, P., Kendall, N. (2000) Assessing psychosocial yellow flags. In: Gifford, L. (ed.) *Topical issues in pain 2 – Biopsychosocial assessment and management*, 3, pp. 111–29.

4.3.13 Chronic pain management; cognitive–behavioural, pharmacological

Charles Pither

Chronic pain: systems, constructs, and paradigms

A physicist working in the late nineteenth century was practising in an enviably comfortable conceptual framework. Newton had set out the concepts upon which a secure scientific edifice had been constructed. Principles such as deterministic causation, the 'experimentum crucis', and the surety of the subjective/objective divide had no need to challenged. The observed phenomena fitted perfectly the described laws – the physics of the natural world was seemingly understood.

Then came the cataclysmic implications of the study of the nucleus. Bohr, Einstein, and Heisenberg made observations that were incompatible with Newtonian laws. Those laws that had seemed certain to fit for all time broke down in the special situations of the inside of particles. One rule would not suit all; new paradigms and theories were needed. Relativity theory and quantum physics emerged and even now, decades later, the parallel paradigms are not properly unified into a construct simple enough for the man in the street to fathom.

One could argue that twentieth-century physicians were in much the same position as their physicist counterparts of a century earlier. Virchow and the European protagonists of the scientific method were in no doubt that observation and scientific rigour would lead to the categorization and understanding of all disease processes and the development of curative treatments. Many physicians today would argue little differently – the elucidation of the biological and scientific basis of disease has led to the remarkable therapeutic advances that underpin modern high-tech medicine.

There are, however, other voices that would introduce a note of scepticism to such an analysis. Just as there were experimenters in the field of physics who could not reconcile their observation with the theories current at the time, so there are doctors trying to treat patients with chronic pain for whom a clinico-pathological analysis fails to help either explain or treat their difficulties. Many chronic pain syndromes just do not fit the conceptual paradigms of the biomedical model (Sullivan 1998). For every patient who clearly describes symptoms and signs of say, a rotator cuff lesion of the shoulder, there is another with vague complaints in and around the area, accompanied by inexplicable symptoms in the face or arm, that do not clearly fit within a precise diagnostic category. Such individuals occur within all medical specialities but are certainly common within the field of musculoskeletal medicine.

The ardent biologist believes that ultimately any experience or sensation will have a biochemical or electrical correlate within the individual's physiological system. Therefore a derangement of normal sensation – such as pain in a shoulder, for example – must be underpinned by an abnormality in the tissues as a primary event, and treatment should be delivered to the shoulder. The pain clinician's view is coloured by the frequent failure of imaging techniques to identify an abnormality, the temporal variability of symptoms, the interaction of mood and stress upon the symptomatology, the unpalatable frequency of treatment failure, and the positive experience of more holistic therapies. The reality of clinical experience is that even the vigorous pursuit of a biological endpoint will still leave some patients without resolution of their problems: another paradigm is needed.

Of course there are alternative paradigms, Chinese medicine, for example, or various psychoanalytic interpretations, but these often have little validity either pragmatically or scientifically. The problem is not the finding of an alternative paradigm, but finding one that can effectively integrate disparate views within an acceptable framework in a useful way. Numerous proposals have been put forward and variously been modified and updated. The most convincing propose the integration of psychological, environmental, and physical variables within an inclusive framework. This is usually termed the biopsychosocial model (Loeser 1989, Van Houdenhove *et al.* 1992), which although cumbrous as a term, has its attributes. The essence is that pain, which in many ways characterizes the complexity of the human experience, cannot simply be reduced to a biological phenomenon. Social and psychological aspects need also to be taken into account if the patient's difficulties are to be understood and resolved.

Unfortunately this dichotomy (biology versus a more holistic perspective) presents the pain specialist with very real dilemmas: does one yet again offer an alternative prescription for an analgesic when the first three drugs have not improved pain or function? Does one continue to order expensive investigations in spite of all previous examinations being negative? Does one perform an injection to try to eliminate local nociception even though previous attempts have not been helpful?

This dilemma has been categorized as being between what has been called the first person (I who have the pain) and the third person (the objective disease) perspectives (Sullivan 1999). Just as with nuclear physics, the reconciliation is difficult and incomplete. This chapter will not throw light into the dark corners of this uncertainty, but it will hopefully offer a more pragmatic approach to the treatment of pain from the perspective of the pain clinic. This can be summarized as attempting to help the person who has troublesome persistent pain without a detailed understanding of their mechanisms responsible for their symptoms.

A typical case is illustrated by the following vignette.

At the end of the treatment this man's radiographs or MRI would have looked no different from before the treatment started. The tissue damage (whatever it was) would not have miraculously been repaired after 7 years, and yet he is changed. He is changed because the pain has not been treated as a putative pathological source of nociception, but as an expression of a series of processes affecting a human being. Such an empirical approach, aimed at treating symptoms and addressing deficits of psychological and physical function, can be very helpful in reducing distress and disability.

A 43-year-old man is referred to the pain service for advice about his neck pain. He originally injured his neck some 7 years earlier in an accident at work when a shelf collapsed on him as he was reaching up to place a heavy item on it. Although he was bruised, radiographs were normal and he was sent home from the emergency department with analgesics and advice to rest.

This was the start of a problem of continuous pain in the neck and shoulder which has persisted in spite of multiple treatment approaches including physiotherapy, injections, medications, acupuncture, manipulation under anaesthetic, and a whole range of alternative treatments. All scans have been negative, and no clear cause for his pain has been identified. In spite of this he has been given lots of explanations and diagnoses including a soft tissue injury, disc degeneration, a frozen shoulder, tendonitis, and fibromyalgia. This array of possible causes has confused him considerably and left him frustrated and angry. This has fuelled his depression and left him desperate and at times suicidal. He cannot understand why no one can seemingly fix his problem.

He attends a 4-week interdisciplinary pain management programme which informs him that although he has pain this does not imply damage. The focus of the programme is learning new techniques to cope with the pain better in the future and to regain fitness and functionality. He is taught about the complex mechanisms of chronic pain, and how nervous system processes affect physical sensation. He commences a stretch and exercise programme and learns to pace up his tolerances in a range of activities. He learns a relaxation technique, starts to identify and challenge patterns of automatic negative thinking, and recognizes when he is catastrophizing.

Two months after the end of treatment he is taking no medications, is swimming once a week and stretching and exercising daily. He has less pain and reports his mood is better than it has been for years. He is getting on better with his spouse, and is looking at undertaking a retraining course. He is no longer frightened of his pain. All his family remark on the transformation and wonder why he had to wait 7 years for this type of treatment.

This review focuses on an approach to the treatment of chronic musculoskeletal pain using an interdisciplinary biopsychosocial approach, delivered by an interdisciplinary team.

Who gets chronic pain?

Chronic pain is extremely common in the community with telephone surveys revealing a prevalence of about 14% (Flor, Turk, and Rudy 1987, Maxwell, Gatchel, and Mayer 1998). Of this population there seems to be a greater than expected proportion of women and a loading for lower social class and poor education (Swimmer, Robinson, and Geisser 1992) However, the population attending pain clinics is further skewed: 70% female with high psychological distress and a significant number matching up to a psychiatric diagnosis (Kouyanou et al. 1998). The conclusion is that chronic pain is not a disease that strikes at random across all social demographic groups, but that it is a state that is influenced, at least in part, by psychosocial variables.

Various studies have attempted to examine the factors that predict the development of chronic pain following an initial injury or source of pain. Such studies are difficult to perform, and the setting and follow-up methodologies are crucial. From the data available it is clear that physical parameters or accessible measures of pathological process do not predict outcome or the development of chronic pain (Burton et al. 1995). Better predictors seem to relate to measures of distress, measured with psychological questionnaires, and fear avoidance models (Rose et al. 1992, Klenerman et al. 1995). Such findings are supported by the much-cited Boeing study (Bigos et al. 1992) which did not link back pain disability to physical tasks within the workplace, rather to the psychosocial environment.

It is also clear that there are complex and important links between chronic pain and various psychological difficulties and psychiatric syndromes (Chaturvedi 1987, Merskey et al. 1987). There is absolutely no doubt that pain that persists in spite of a wide range of treatments is a potent stressor. Any individual under stress may show signs of strain, and this commonly manifests itself in the form of an adverse psychological reaction. Traditional teaching would have it that while acute pain is more commonly associated with the emotional state of anxiety, chronic pain is more normally accompanied by depression. Many studies demonstrate that patients attending pain clinics have high levels of depression (Chaturvedi 1987, Merskey et al. 1987, Sullivan et al. 1991), and indeed psychiatric illness. In fact the percentage of patients referred to a pain clinic matching up to 'caseness' in psychiatric terms may be as high as 50%, certainly higher than comparable medical outpatients. However, it is overly simplistic to think that chronic pain sufferers are only depressed. First it must be realized that there is considerable overlap between the two poles of depression and anxiety (Kleinman 1988) and that many patients sit somewhere in between these traditional dichotomous classifications, with a condition best described by the term 'general dysphoria' (Goldberg and Huxley 1992). The question that begs to be asked is whether these levels of distress are simply a secondary reaction to the stress of pain or whether there was a tendency to the state prior to the onset of it.

The answer is that some individuals with symptoms of emotional distress do seem to be more likely to develop chronic pain problems given a potential source of pain. The problem with making a definitive link is the paucity of robust categorical diagnostic formulations from both the psychiatric and chronic pain perspectives. Because so many of the problems described by patients defy consistent classification it is very difficult to perform robust studies to disentangle cause and effect. However, clues do come from those patients who suffer from troublesome symptoms in more than one bodily area or system. These patients are often described as having symptoms that are medically unexplained or given the label 'somatizers', but it is clear that their difficulties are underpinned by excessive anxiety about bodily symptoms (Sharpe and Carson 2001). Given that frequently these patients' complaints include pain, it becomes clearer that excessive worry about any symptom can enhance attention to it and provoke a more vigorous psycho-physiological response, thus worsening the overall state. Neuroimaging techniques such as PET have enabled exploration of the different areas of the cortex responsible for pain sensation and pain unpleasantness (Price 2000). It is clear that the perceived threat associated with pain is expressed in the limbic system and must be seen as separate from the purely sensory detection of an unwelcome sensation. It is probable that activation of this area is influenced by experience and interpretation of the consequences of the situation, and is thus likely to be modified by upbringing and past experience. Such findings may provide the basis for an understanding of the interactions between general anxiety and pain distress and disability, especially in the chronic situation.

The conclusion is that among a group of patients with troublesome persistent pain, there will be a greater than expected number of individuals with a psychological vulnerability to stress expressed as high levels of depression and anxiety. This endorses the rationale for adopting interdisciplinary treatment approaches that incorporate psychological elements.

The process of chronic pain

Chronic pain is by definition of long duration. The precise time to a definition of chronicity can remain undefined, save to say that pain clinics seldom see individuals who have had pain for less than 6 months, and it is frequently much longer, with one programme reporting a mean pain duration of 10 years (Williams et al. 1996a). One aspect of such conditions that needs emphasis is the processes that occur during this time. Acute pain is certainly modified by the psychological situation of the individual; for example, postoperative morphine requirements have been shown to be related to preoperative anxiety (Feinmann et al. 1987). However, not only is such pain effectively treated with higher doses of opioid, but the healing process cures the underlying problem thus resolving the situation.

By definition, chronic pain has persisted even in the face of normal healing processes. The journey of the pain sufferer from the start of their problem to effective treatment in a pain centre is a long and arduous one, and this needs to be taken into account when attempting to provide treatment. The prolonged nature of the symptomatology influences the illness in a number of important ways, often overlooked by the general physician seeing a more acute spectrum of difficulties. The most crucial point is that after 5 years one is not just dealing with a specific pathology, but the consequences of the individual having that illness for that period of time. A person who has had pain for a long period of time will be different from a person with problems of more recent onset.

Such changes and processes can be summarized as follows:

- **Secondary musculoskeletal changes become more pronounced:** Chronic pain is very frequently accompanied by considerable degrees of disability. The individual may be resting for most of the day and walking with difficulty with sticks or crutches. Others become 'chair shaped' due to prolonged periods of chair or wheelchair use. It is inevitable that such prolonged rest leads to cardiovascular deconditioning, reduction in muscle bulk and general fitness, joint stiffness, and alterations to gait and posture. Although it is difficult to conclusively demonstrate that such changes contribute to the pain syndrome, with some studies finding it difficult to detect consistent changes between sufferers and non-sufferers (Waddell et al. 1992), it is inevitable that these changes make matters worse not better (Molin 1999). Furthermore the prospect for remediation are progressively decreased with the chronicity of symptoms.

- **Mood changes are more likely:** Although there is no linear relationship between the duration of pain and the level of psychological distress (as measured by depression inventories), in general the longer pain has persisted the more likely a negative impact on mental wellbeing. This may be partially mediated by loss of amenity, with for example a proven relationship between loss of work and depression (Dooley et al. 2000), or to treatment failure and a progressive fear that a cure or resolution of symptoms will not be found. Patterns of

negative thinking can without a doubt become stereotypic with the passage of time and thus habitual. Such thoughts often underpin chronic dysphoria and low mood.

- **Learnt and unhelpful patterns of behaviour become more relevant:** Behaviours are subject to learning influences, and these will be more pronounced and entrenched as time passes. Behaviours such as lying down and resting, bracing, rubbing the affected part, or verbalizing pain become established in the early phases in response to pain, but over a period of time but are progressively less clearly related to pathology. Similarly, solicitous interactions within families become habitual and 'set in stone' and so are extremely difficult to alter. Similar patterns of dysfunction can arise in areas such as sleep and medication consumption. Difficulty sleeping can be due to multiple causes, but once a pattern is established it can become self-perpetuating. A particularly troublesome development is the commencement of daytime napping with alteration in normal diurnal rhythm.

- **Treatment failures may influence mood and expectation:** If given the opportunity, chronic pain patients frequently voice dissatisfaction with medical services. This is partly because of the implicit failure of medical treatment to cure their pain, but is frequently related to a sense of not being believed or being dismissed as somehow imagining the symptoms (Walker et al. 1999). Furthermore, for a significant number of patients medical treatment has actually worsened their condition by overtreatment, overinvestigation, or overprescription (Kouyanou et al. 1997a). It would be surprising if such experiences were not to affect the overall outlook, behaviour, and presentation of the sufferer. It will also have an influence on the way the patient views further treatment, in some cases causing a withdrawal from medical systems with the refusal of further therapy, fuelling helplessness and depression.

The endpoint from the clinician's perspective – frequently that of a bizarre pattern of symptoms and behaviour, far removed from the pathoclinical entities of medical textbooks – represents a truly individual illness. Once again the distinction can be made between the impotence of the doctor to treat along logical scientific lines, and the palpable difficulties and needs of the patient. There comes a point when treatment aimed at addressing some of the above issues is more likely to benefit the patient than a persistent search for a categorical diagnosis or invasive treatment aimed at pathology that caused the initial symptoms many years before.

The role of the pain centre

Staff

A strand running through the approach set out in this chapter is that of interdisciplinary working (Gardea and Gatchel 2000). Such therapy is best delivered from within a service organized as a pain centre. The crucial feature is the recognition that single-modality treatment is less likely to be effective in chronic pain that multimodal therapy (Flor et al. 1992). The exact staffing complement of pain centres depends on local resources and varies substantially between units (see box).

The role of alternative therapies is less clear. There is all too little evidence for alternative therapies as being of benefit in chronic pain, but this implies neither that therapies are not commonly applied, nor that they cannot occasionally be helpful. However, there is often a distinction in terms of attitude. All too often the alternative practitioner

Possible disciplines involved in a pain centre

- Medicine
  - pain medicine
  - rheumatology
  - neurology
  - orthopaedic (musculoskeletal) medicine
- Surgery
  - orthopaedic surgery
  - neurosurgery
Psychology
Physiotherapy
Occupational therapy
Nursing
Acupuncture
Pharmacy
Social work

is still offering therapies as a means of curing the condition. This is accompanied by hypotheses of varying scientific credibility about the cause of the symptoms, and the rationale and benefits of the proposed treatment. The therapist is seen as the 'curer' and as such takes over ownership of the patient's problems. When the therapy fails the patient is left with regret, disbelief, and disappointment (Walker *et al.* 1999).

The aim of the pain centre, on the other hand, is to reduce pain and improve function while crucially restoring ownership of the illness to

Treatment modalities available in the pain centre

- Pharmacological management
  - analgesics
  - antidepressants
  - antiepileptics
  - others
  - implanted spinal infusion systems
- Stimulation techniques
  - TENS
  - acupuncture
  - dorsal column stimulation
- Physiotherapy and exercise
- Nerve blocks and injection
  - trigger point injections and infiltration
  - joint injections
  - nerve blocks
  - epidural and central neural blockade
  - sympathetic blocks
  - neurolytic and destructive procedures
- Psychological and rehabilitative approaches
  - cognitive–behavioural therapy
  - relaxation training
  - pain management programmes

the individual. Exaggerated claims are not made about potential cure, and theories are open ended and inclusive rather than specific and exclusive.

It is not the purpose of this chapter to detail all the therapeutic options and therapies available in a pain centre. Inevitably there is considerable overlap between those available to all physicians and therapists treating musculoskeletal problems, and many of these are covered in other sections of this volume. The interested reader is referred to the large range of textbooks devoted solely to chronic pain and its management (Abram and Haddox 1999, Loeser *et al.* 2000, Raj 2000).

Drug treatment

Reference has already been made to the many dilemmas facing those treating chronic pain, and one of the most problematic is to decide whether to increase or change medications or to reduce or stop them. It seems that the decisions made for a particular patient are predicated not by an informed evidence base but by the opinions and views of the prescriber. Seemingly such decisions are frequently random, inconsistent, and idiosyncratic (Turk and Okifuji 1997). The continued use of multiple medications can often produce unwanted adverse cognitive effects (McNairy *et al.* 1984).

In spite of the vast numbers of prescriptions issued yearly to sufferers from chronic pain and the huge costs associated with this and over-the-counter medications, the question has to be asked as to how effective any medication can be in chronic usage over a number of years. If medications were properly effective, individuals would not seek out the help of specialists nor pursue other more invasive therapies. The statistical notion of a drug providing 40% relief of pain is often of little benefit to the patient still left with 60%.

One of the major problems with assessing the long-term effects of medications is the difficulty of performing trials of sufficient duration, leading to contrary information about the merits of long-term prescribing (Halpern and Robinson 1985, McQuay 1999). The result is that there are very few studies demonstrating long-term beneficial effects of analgesics, with much of the data extrapolated from acute pain studies (Turk and Okifuji 1997).

With a greater understanding of the complex cortical interactions involved in pain processing comes a realization that for problems other than acute nociceptive pain the chances of developing a drug that will effectively abolish pain are slender. This is because chronic pain always has an evaluative and affective component. Even when a drug does reduce the intensity of the sensory experience, it does not alter the threat, implication, unpleasantness, and meaning of the pain.

Characteristics of the ideal drug for a chronic pain condition

- No side effects
- No problems with accumulation
- No toxic or active metabolites
- No problems with dependence, addiction or withdrawal
- Reduces or abolishes target pain only
- Once-daily dosage
- Allows functional restoration
- Cheap

It is interesting to note that patients presenting to pain centres are divided between those who try drugs and stop taking them because of an awareness that they are not ultimately helpful (Ralphs *et al.* 1994), and those who continue to take them swearing they couldn't live without the beneficial effect (Kouyanou *et al.* 1997b). The point is that both groups are still seeking help.

It is my view that medications are seldom the total answer to ongoing chronic pain of whatever cause. Patients should always be given the opportunity of exploring the benefits of a range of medications, but this should be done within the framework of rational prescribing as set out below.

- **Prescribe analgesics for pain, not distress:** Analysis of prescribing decisions reveals that prescription of stronger analgesics is driven by higher distress in patients. This is illogical, because analgesics do not treat distress. Increasing distress needs to be treated, but not with analgesics.

- **Let the patient be the arbiter of efficacy:** Given that pain is a subjective experience, there is no place for the physician enforcing continued use of a medication if the patient does not find it helpful.

- **Try to establish regular regimes:** Using medication on a 'prn' basis can provoke patterns of over- and underactivity, which are counterproductive in terms of rational pain management.

- **Remember compliance:** Even patients in pain often do not take their drugs. This is especially a problem with antidepressants. Many patients do not take the drugs once they realize they are antidepressants, no matter how much preparatory information is given in the clinic.

- **Monitor consumption and set a maximum:** Beware of the escalation of drug dosage beyond the recommended level. An individual who has taken excess doses of a weaker drug will be at risk of taking an excess of a stronger drug.

- **Try to avoid adding drugs of the same class:** There is little pharmacological sense in adding two or more drugs of the same type. The implication is that if one drug is not effective then it should be stopped before another is added. Combined therapy with different classes of drugs can be logical and provide added benefit.

- **Give clear indications of the expected effects:** In general, drugs should be seen as part of a portfolio of techniques rather than a single solution. With drugs such as antidepressants the effects may not primarily be in pain reduction and may take several weeks to develop fully. The patient must be fully aware of this.

- **Be prepared to treat side effects** if the positive effects of the regime are worthwhile.

- **Say no:** Doctors find it very difficult to say no to patients who ask for alternative or stronger drugs. If various drugs have been tried with little relief of symptoms and worsening distress and levels of function, it is extremely unlikely that an altered prescription will provide substantial benefit. Alternative treatment options should be pursued.

Stimulation analgesia

TENS

The gate theory of pain posits that input from both unmyelinated nociceptive C fibres and non-noxious myelinated cutaneous A sensory fibres impinge on the T cell in the spinal cord. The resultant rostral impulses are the balance of these two opposing systems. It has been shown that non-noxious cutaneous information travelling in the myelinated primary afferent A beta fibres activates inhibitory pathways in the superficial laminae of the dorsal horn which have an analgesic effect (Hansson and Lundeberg 1999). This was demonstrated experimentally, initially with vibration, and subsequently with electrical stimulation (Woolf 1979). The technique was given the name transcutaneous nerve stimulation (TENS).

Commercial devices followed rapidly, and a body of clinical experience demonstrated the effectiveness of the technique. Modern devices are smaller than a cigarette packet and produce a square wave pulse of 50–100 Hz. Output is varied by a simple amplitude control up to about 50 milliamps. The device is connected by cutaneous electrodes with conductive adhesive gel which are applied over the painful area or in an appropriate dermatome. When turned on, the device produces a sensation of tingling. Slower pulsed or burst modes can be used to stimulate muscles.

There is no doubt that TENS has a useful place in the therapeutic armamentarium of the pain clinic. It is possible to demonstrate significant analgesic effects with TENS in experimental and acute pain. A great many studies have been performed using TENS in a variety of different clinical conditions. These show that there is a beneficial effect in peripheral nerve disorders, spinal cord and root disorders, cancer pain, musculoskeletal pain, and numerous miscellaneous conditions. Initially more than 75% of patients will find the device helpful. For this reason a trial of TENS should be offered to those with persistent regional pain. It is usually necessary to explain and demonstrate the device to the patient in an educational visit. This is carried out by an experienced nurse. The patient is then given a device on loan to try at home for a 3-week period. They are instructed in electrode placement and given a suggested timetable to experiment with it. If they find the device helpful, they can then purchase one for themselves.

Although TENS frequently produces effective analgesia, there are some problems with the technique. First, it is difficult to predict who will benefit on the basis of disease categorization. It is clear from the large amount of research that has been carried out that TENS can be effective in a great many situations but not with a great deal of consistency. One patient with post-whiplash pain will find the device most helpful and use it as part of a multimodal treatment programme, while the next two will find that it aggravates their pain. A systematic review of TENS in low back pain could find no convincing evidence of efficacy (Milne *et al.* 2001).

The second problem is that the effectiveness of the technique tails of rapidly with time. By 3 months the number gaining benefit will have dropped from greater than 70% to less than 30%. However, there are still those who use the machines either occasionally or regularly, claiming significant ongoing benefit.

Acupuncture

Without a doubt acupuncture has a considerable effect in humans and indeed in animals. The effects of stimulation of certain anatomical points with manual pressure or needles has been part of the repertoire of Chinese medicine for thousands of years. Traditional Chinese acupuncture is only one therapeutic arm of a complex medical system based on an evaluation of the Qi (chi) or state of the fluxes within the individual (Turner *et al.* 1994). The formulation is made on the basis of a careful history, and analysis of the pulses and the tongue. The prescription of acupuncture may well be one component of a holistic therapy involving herbal remedies, exercise and a regime of activity to restore the balance of yin and yang. This holistic, multimodal therapy quite possibly has something to teach Western medicine about the treatment of musculoskeletal disorders that so often are not solved by primary care interventions (see Chapters 4.3.8 and 4.3.9).

Acupuncture has many effects and has been used widely for numerous conditions. The data supporting its effect in pain is better than for many other conditions (Vincent *et al.* 1989). It is less clear whether the needle insertion points need to be those traditionally described along the Chinese meridians. However, trigger points and areas of altered skin electrical impedance do show a close correlation with traditional Chinese acupuncture points.

The effectiveness of acupuncture in certain cases is without question (Lewith and Vincent 1996). It is still difficult to predict which patients will benefit. This, like so many aspects of chronic pain medicine, seems to depend on the patient more than the pathology.

Interdisciplinary pain management programmes

For many patients with chronic pain there comes a time when further conventional treatment is no longer logical. This may be because all possible treatment options have been tried without success, or that the elements of distress and disability are so pronounced that it is obvious they need treatment in their own right. It is in this situation that some form of pain management programme would be considered (Main and Spanswick 2000). The point must be made, however, that sufficient is now known about pain management programmes to make it clear that they should not be thought of solely as a last resort. Patients who will gain from a programme should not have to endure additional unhelpful and possibly harmful treatment in order to earn their place. Indeed, there is a case for treating needy patients as early as possible in their illness.

Aims of treatment

Interdisciplinary treatment programmes do not primarily aim to alter tissue pathology, rather they aim to diminish the impact of the pain on the individual. Frequently patients are told that the programme will help them cope better with the pain, but this denies the crucial conceptual link that acknowledges coping as intrinsic to the problem not external to it. The person who copes well with pain is not distressed by it and therefore the suffering caused by it is less. To say to a patient 'you will cope better' undervalues the potential benefit because it implies the pain remains unchanged, only the coping alters, and it suggests that this is only a psychological process. This is unhelpful for a number of reasons.

- First, pain does diminish (Williams *et al.* 1996b, Morley *et al.* 1999), albeit not hugely: 1 person in 6 will achieve a greater than 50% reduction in pain. Interestingly, but perhaps not surprisingly, pain distress diminishes more than pain intensity (Williams *et al.* 1996a).

- Secondly, interdisciplinary programmes for patients with rheumatoid and osteoarthritis can produce improvements in mobility and reductions in joint inflammation (Keefe and Caldwell 1997,

Scholten *et al.* 1999, Sharpe *et al.* 2001), a clear demonstration of the mind–body links that such treatment taps into. Furthermore, the diminution or elimination of secondary stiffness and weakness, accompanied by improvements in fitness, that usually occur during treatment, can be thought of neither as treatment of the primary pathology nor simply a psychological change, and yet they help to facilitate an overall improvement in function, self-esteem, and quality of life.

At its simplest the aim of treatment is to facilitate the sufferer to move towards a state of balance or equilibrium with their illness. Most pain sufferers who are referred to treatment centres are dysfunctional as a result of their pain, and are not in balance with their illness (as a competent diabetic might perhaps be, for example). Returning to a state of 'balance' sees this state alter to a level of acceptance and self-management, with a reduction in distress.

One helpful way to conceptualize this is to examine the person (not patient – because often they are not in contact with medical services) who has pain and yet who copes and lives a good quality life. Such individuals may at first glance seem to be distinguishable from patients by differences in tissue pathology, but this is not the case. Many studies have detected similar levels of MRI abnormalities in both symptomatic and symptom-free subjects (Jensen *et al.* 1994). Furthermore, such an analysis falls back to a dichotomous way of thinking that sees the pain as separate from the thoughts, emotions, and behaviours that accompany it.

Beliefs, strategies, and achievements of copers

- **Keeping mobile and flexible:** Copers keep physically active and mobile. They may not actively exercise, but they are not frightened of movement and they know that there are adverse consequences of rest and immobility. They frequently treat pain and stiffness with movement and stretch rather than rest and immobilization. The pain may well have limited their active participation in sports, but they often have kept up an interest or moved to less impacting and demanding hobbies such as golf or swimming. Underpinning this level of physical function is the overcoming of fear related to the pain. Clients of pain clinics are frequently found to be extremely fearful of the pain or its consequences (Vlaeyen *et al.* 1999). Avoidance of this is seemingly very important if normal function is to be maintained.

- **Managing a normal daily routine:** The copers' daily routine is normal in that they will be up for a full day with little use of resting or lying down. They may take a short rest or a nap after lunch, but they have a firm view that over-resting is harmful.

- **Living an active life:** Most individuals still have active interests that they pursue. These may not be physical but are often social such as voluntary work or being involved with a charity, local politics, or a society. They usually involve some intellectual activity. The adage 'people don't become disabled by chronic pain if they have something better to do' has a ring of truth to it. The importance of this psychologically is in the concept of distraction: these people recognize that keeping busy distracts them from their pain. They frequently court activity because they know they are 'better if they keep busy'. The implication is that, although perhaps an effort, physical and mental activity is necessary to stop them dwelling on their pain, and suffering the secondary problems associated with inactivity.

- **Using as few medications as possible:** The copers use minimal amounts of medications. Mostly they will have been prescribed tablets and may have purchased over-the-counter medicines, but they will have found that they produce minimal analgesia with unwelcome side effects. Such people often say 'I realized that tablets were not the answer'. If they are taking medications they will be taking single drugs in recommended dose. This is in marked contrast to many patients attending pain clinics, who frequently use medicines inappropriately (Kouyanou *et al.* 1997b).

- **Keeping a positive mental attitude:** These individuals are not depressed. They have a mental approach that favours coping and keeping a positive mood even in the face of pain. This does not mean that they have never known depression – some would admit that in the past they have been very low. They have recovered, however, and are aware that this has been due to taking an active approach to the pain. They pursue an active lifestyle and because of this they avoid becoming overwhelmed by the pain and are able to sustain their self-esteem. Some of this skill seems to entail avoiding catastrophic thinking. Catastrophizers, when given the option of two possible outcomes or eventualities, will tend to pick the most negative. Catastrophization can be characterized by three fundamental unhelpful ways of thinking: rumination, thinking the worst, and helplessness. Thus patients with intrusive pain (who have been shown to have a high likelihood of being expert catastrophizers – Sullivan *et al.* 2001a,b) tend to think about their pain for most of the day; tend to think that it will go on for ever, get worse, and render them an invalid; and think that there is nothing they or anyone else can do about it. There is now much in the literature on the links between catastrophizing and pain (Sullivan and D'Eon 1990; Sullivan *et al.* 2001a,b). It is clear that much of the low mood so frequently seen accompanying chronic pain is related to the generation of a series of awful and hopeless mental scenarios which can become automatic with the passage of time, prompted by routine everyday occurrences and events. Healthy copers tend to use more favourable psychological coping strategies involving active techniques such as distraction and challenging thoughts (which are the mainstays of cognitive therapy), as well as setting aside time for meditation and relaxation. Many patients report benefits from these techniques which underpin their continued use of the stratagems.

- **Accepting the pain:** Most of those who cope well with pain have truly accepted that it is a problem that has no medical solution. There are two implications of this. First, they realize that they have to take responsibility for their problem themselves and thus have a role in its management. Secondly, they are no longer actively seeking medical help for the pain. The importance of this aspect should not be underestimated. I believe that the major difference between the acceptance of many chronic illnesses such as diabetes and even spinal injury, and the distress of chronic spinal pain, is in the differing messages given by medical systems at the time of diagnosis. This is elegantly summed up by Ivan Illich (1976): 'Culture makes pain tolerable by interpreting its necessity; only pain perceived as curable is intolerable.'

Such successful ex-patients still have pain, and at times they may claim that it is severe. Furthermore, they never belittle the effort that they had to put in to take control of their pain. For the most part they continue to work hard at actively using various active techniques and strategies to maintain their performance. Thus the person who is not 'suffering' in the face of constant pain does not simply have less nociception, but has made a number of adaptations and employed active strategies to minimize the impact of the pain.

This group has been labelled 'adaptive copers' (Turk and Rudy 1990), as opposed to other response clusters characterized by greater levels of distress and disability. It is usually these latter groups who are referred to pain management treatment programmes. The aim of treatment is to help them move towards the optimal level of coping and function as set out above.

In sum, the aims of the interdisciplinary pain management approach is to help the sufferer to:

- keep mobile and fit
- live a rewarding active life
- avoid depression
- take as few tablets as possible
- understand and accept the pain
- use positive coping strategies including relaxation
- not seek further medical treatments with minimal chance of benefit.

Programme content

The commonality of the various different formats of focus and delivery of pain management programmes is the use of an interdisciplinary team providing an intensive fixed-length treatment package using a cognitive–behavioural framework.

Various other psychological approaches have been offered, but these are more often based on the individual therapist's own ideas rather than scientifically validated principles. As such, they should not be included within the rubric of pain management programmes, a term that has come to imply the use of cognitive–behavioural methodologies.

Cognitive–behavioural therapy

It is important to understand the principles of cognitive–behavioural theory and treatment, which are fundamental to this type of treatment.

Credit for the first practical demonstration that pain could be treated with behavioural approaches is rightly assigned to Wilbert Fordyce (Fordyce *et al.* 1968). It was he who applied quite rigid principles of reward and reinforcement to patients with chronic pain and demonstrated considerable reduction in what he described as 'pain behaviours' (Fordyce 1970).

Although these approaches were helpful in altering functional performance in the hospital setting, there were some doubts about the long-term maintenance of the changes. As could be expected from a purely behavioural methodology, old ways of behaving would recur on return to the previous environment once the reinforcement of the treatment was removed. Psychologists pursuing more cognitive approaches recognized this as a failure to address the underlying thoughts, fears, and beliefs, which need to be modified if lasting behaviour change is to occur. The cognitive–behavioural approach paid greater attention to the thoughts underlying the observed behaviour. For example, while Fordyce demonstrated that a patient's tendency to lie down for long periods could be reduced by the application of rewards for increasing their up time, the cognitive perspective would be interested in the thoughts that underpinned the need to lie down. These might be, for example, that rest was allowing the spine to heal and reduce the damage that the painful activities were causing. The cognitive therapist would seek to understand the pattern of thinking in the individual and modify such unhelpful thoughts with an alternative interpretation based on a more balanced and accurate perspective. The patient would then be taught to practice the technique in everyday situations. This self-correction would lead to a more permanent change in the thinking pattern and thus behaviour. Furthermore, because poor mood is linked to negative thinking, improvement is mood could be accomplished by correction of the harmful thought processes.

In fact the two constructs have become increasingly merged within the rubric of cognitive–behavioural therapy, which aims to harness the most effective principles of both. In essence, cognitive–behavioural theory states that all our behaviours and many of our emotions are predicated not directly by an event or experience, but by our perception of it. This was succinctly summarized by the Greek philosopher Epictetus when he said 'It is not things that trouble us but the views we take of them'. This observation is true for all human situations and contributes to making us the individuals we are. However, in the face of a situation that we have not come upon before, we need additional information to make sense of it, and to know what to do. We get this information from all sorts of sources including our own repertoire of experience, our family and friends, books and the Internet, and our medical advisors. To take an extreme example, consider the case of a patient with gradually worsening pain in the low back. When the patient was a child a relative had had tuberculosis of the spine and been put on bed rest and then in a cast for many months to 'prevent the spinal damage from progressing'. The patient's first thought is that perhaps their pain is due to the same cause. Although they may be relatively easily persuaded that this is not the case, the view that rest and immobilization will prevent the spine from degenerating and favour recovery may be deeply entrenched. So perhaps will be fears that there are potentially serious and harmful causes of back pain. Such an individual will respond completely differently from another back pain sufferer whose father used to swim twice a week because he found it the only way of keeping his back pain free and preventing it from 'seizing up'. In both these situations the patients' behaviour will reflect their beliefs, and these are unique to the individual.

It is not just visible behaviour that is predicated by such beliefs, but also the emotional response. Pain is surely unpleasant and many would say it is profoundly depressing. Modern imaging techniques have identified that pain can stimulate areas in the frontal lobe thought to modify mood and thus it may be that pain can, at least in some situations, lead directly to lowering of mood. Frequently, however, poor mood is contributed to by patterns of negative thinking. Thoughts, like many aspects of human behaviour, can become stereotypical and patterned in response to a particular situation. Persistent pain may be a constant reminder of the process going on at the site of the pain and the fears of permanent damage and the incurability of the problem. Past treatment failures, or the experience of others, may contribute to this. Further thoughts, such as the likelihood of never working again and the implications on mobility, will have a further negative effect on mood and lead to feelings of gloom and helplessness. This may amount to clinical depression. The alteration in psychophysiological processing that occurs in the depressed state alongside the lowering of energy levels and diminution of general motivation significantly worsen coping and pain experience.

The cognitive model posits that the patient's predicament is not simply dependent on the pathology in the tissues, the level of nociception, or afferent neural input, but the totality of the experience including the beliefs, fears, emotions, and helplessness that overwhelms them. The distress that follows is not caused solely by the tissue pathology but by the cessation of life-enhancing activities.

Cognitive therapy aims to alter the patient's view of their situation in a number of ways, but crucially by aiming to re-establish a more balanced perspective between the perceived and statistical likelihood of the worst option occurring. As has been suggested above the tendency to catastrophize has been identified as important in patients developing intrusive and limiting chronic pain (Sullivan *et al.* 2001b). Not only do many patients think the worst will happen, but they get into patterns of negative thinking that become habitual. Such processes have been given the label 'automatic negative thoughts' in the psychiatric setting. Cognitive therapy does not aim to direct the sufferer to simply replace their thoughts with more positive options, but to challenge the assumptions underlying their original thoughts and beliefs. 'Because I can't work I am useless and on the scrap heap' may be such a view. An appropriate cognitive therapeutic approach would be to help the individual consider whether this is always true, and to explore 'challenges' (alternative ways of looking at the problem) that make them feel less helpless and thus less miserable. The process is then completed by practice and rehearsal in different settings, and the generalization of these skills to other situations and scenarios.

Cognitive behavioural principles do not apply solely to the more psychological processes described above. Other aspects of the rehabilitative process crucially entail the use of techniques to overcome the physical limitations which the patients experience that have become entrenched over time.

Key principles are:

- **Graded exposure to feared tasks and activities:** Given that fear plays a major part in the avoidance of activities, the use of graded exposure can be effective at helping the individual to tackle feared activities and to gradually improve their performance. One currently favoured approach involves the establishment of a hierarchy of most feared activities, and assisting the patient to tackle the tasks starting with the easiest. Thus someone who rated lifting a saucepan as 3 out of 10, and lifting a shopping bag as 6 out of 10, would begin by lifting a small saucepan or equivalent on a regular basis (Vlaeyen *et al.* 2001). Once confidence for a certain level is attained, the load and perhaps frequency are increased. The crucial feature is the gradual progression, a factor that so often causes the failure of such programmes on an informal outpatient basis.

- **Active not passive learning:** It is an old adage that remembering a task or activity is more likely if it has been practised. The emphasis on behavioural learning is the repetition of tasks in the presence of the therapist or staff member: doing rather than talking. Cognitive–behavioural treatment sessions involve the repeated rehearsal of identified tasks or activities, within the therapeutic environment. Practically this distils down to the avoidance of procrastination and planning for the future, rather making a start while in the treatment programme, albeit at a lower level than might be desired in the longer term. Such practical aspects need to be closely integrated with other key areas such as setting goals and pacing. Thus sessions are not simply educational with a list of points identified on the flip chart or board, rather they are interactive with the group, or subgroups, generating the ideas and problem-solving within the framework set out by the therapist. A further crucial part of this type of interactive treatment is that of active listening. Unless the therapist takes the time to listen to where the patient is on their own learning curve, they will not be able to respond and fill the gaps or correct the erroneous assumption.

- **Group working:** Although it is not the case that group work is the only forum for cognitive–behavioural treatment (in fact probably most takes place in a one-to-one setting), the group environment provides important reinforcement for many of the principles outlined above. In the group setting patients share experiences and views which are often more meaningful than when described by a therapist. The common bond of shared difficulties is important in helping individuals to feel believed and not alone, but critically helps them move on. Often patients in the group can say things to each other that the therapist cannot. Perhaps the most crucial aspect of the group is the sense of shared endeavour. This phenomenon, perhaps exemplified by the 'Dunkirk spirit' of unity in a time of difficulty, often serves to bond a disparate group with a common aim, that of overcoming the pain. Changes made by one or two within the group are often the catalyst for the others to follow both in thought and in performance.

- **Reward and reinforcement:** Individuals whose pain increases when they attempt an activity are very unlikely to repeat the task. Behavioural principles recognize that a behaviour is much more likely to be maintained if there is some reward. While trying to generate behavioural change in patients with pain, the use of reinforcement and reward is crucial. Many chronic pain sufferers have had many years with little in their lives to make them feel good. Positive encouragement for trying new activities and working on their goals is crucial to aid patients contemplating changes. Initially the staff provides such reinforcement when the person attempts the activity. As they progress, so the reinforcement is directed to the increased level of attainment. Once the treatment is progressing and the individual is making gains, so they are instructed in ways to reward and reinforce themselves. This may involve a small treat or a 'pat on the back', or the coopting of a family member into the process. Alongside the recognition of reward is the concept of pacing. Pacing is crucial to the progressive attainment of desirable goals and is covered in more detail below. Pacing involves the breaking down of tasks into manageable fragments. Carried out effectively this avoids the pitfall of overdoing and so entering into a cycle of negative reinforcement (an activity being followed by an unpleasant 'reward' or punishment.)

Staffing

The essence of this type of therapy is the interdisciplinary nature of the treatment. The common disciplines involved are psychology, physiotherapy, occupational therapy, nursing, and medicine. The doctors, although crucial to the effective assessment and medical management of patients undergoing treatment, often find it difficult to adopt the same role as the other members of the team, and are for this reason less involved in the active delivery of treatment.

All disciplines bring their own skills and knowledge to the team, but this is not enough: the staff also need a core knowledge base and a range of core skills that relate to the area of cognitive–behavioural pain

Roles of staff members

- **Physiotherapists:** Assessment, supervising the exercise and stretch programme, problem-solving with individuals, follow-up and measurement of change of level of function.
- **Occupational therapists:** Goal setting, instruction in pacing techniques, postural retraining, ergonomics, and vocational evaluation. Also daily planning and activity scheduling.
- **Psychologists:** Cognitive behavioural therapy, instruction in the basics of behavioural change, individual therapy, and referral for ongoing work where necessary.
- **Nurses:** Medication adjustment and cut down, supervision of intercurrent medical problems, relaxation training.
- **Doctors:** Education about chronic pain mechanisms, management of intercurrent medical problems, dealing with individual patients' questions.
- **Pharmacists:** Assisting in medication cut-down regimes.

management. Many patients attending such a programme have had many years of failure in their voyage through the medical system. They are often quick to pick up on differences between doctors and therapists, and to explore inconsistencies in delivery of treatment. For this reason it is paramount that the therapy team are totally conversant with the concepts, principles, and content of the programme.

Treatment components

The exact content of programmes varies from centre to centre. Some will have additional components due to the enthusiasms of the

Relevant core knowledge and skills

Knowledge

- Biopsychosocial model
- Principles of cognitive behavioural theory and therapy
- Behavioural and contingency management
- Familiarity with common pain syndromes
- Understanding of spinal pain
- Understanding of chronic pain mechanisms
- Elements of exercise training
- Familiarity with common pain treatments such as TENS and nerve blocks
- Common drugs and their use in chronic pain
- Influence of benefits, compensation and legal system

Skills

- Communication and listening skills
- Cognitive restructuring
- Behavioural and contingency management
- Dealing with distressed patients
- Group working
- Team working

staff members or local availability, but the crucial elements are as follows:

- physical rehabilitation involving stretch and exercise
- cognitive–behavioural therapy, with an emphasis on identifying negative or unhelpful ways of thinking and learning to challenge thoughts
- identification of goals for future activities
- instruction in pacing techniques
- relaxation therapy
- education about the causes of pain, and the nature of chronic pain.

In addition, other components are often included with benefit, such as:

- reduction of excessive or unhelpful medication consumption
- vocational therapy.

This is not the place to go into detail of all aspects of the treatment programme, but three areas deserve further mention.

Stretch and exercise

Physical deconditioning is common among patients with musculoskeletal pain, many of whom are substantially disabled. They have usually had several attempts at treatment in the hands of physiotherapists, without success. This frequently leads to a view that physiotherapy cannot help their problem. Sometimes this is accompanied by even more unhelpful beliefs, with worsening symptoms being blamed on the therapist, with the perception that this was due to injury or damage. Furthermore, such patients have many years experience that activity provokes more pain. Suggesting that increasing activity is going to improve matters is met by at best scepticism and at worse frank hostility. As has been suggested above, one major reason for this is fear of pain, activity, or its consequences. A behavioural approach to any exercise programme is of paramount importance.

The aim of the exercise programme is to increase strength, range of movement, and fitness. At all stages during the programme the patient is in control of the number and range of exercises that they undertake. This is the essence of the cognitive–behavioural approach to exercise: the traditional 'stick' of encouragement and goading is replaced by the 'carrot' of reward and reinforcement. Giving the patient control of the rate and extent of activity transfers the responsibility for making change to the patient, and aligns better with the subjective nature of chronic pain. For the most part, therapy is not solely directed to the painful area. The aim is to improve general fitness and flexibility and overcome fear of movement rather than deal with specific deficits that individual therapists can often detect. Moving a therapist away from a target-specific manual therapy to the supervision of a more general approach is often a challenge for new physiotherapy recruits.

A useful protocol commences with simple stretching exercises with a small number of repetitions, to a series of simple isometric exercises followed by dynamic exercises when the time is right. This will vary from patient to patient.

A crucial part of the exercise programme is the overcoming of fear-avoidance mechanisms by graded exposure. Much pioneering work in this area has been carried out by Vlaeyen and colleagues in Maastricht (Vlaeyen et al. 2001). They make an initial hierarchical grading of the patient's most feared movements and then assist the patient to attempt these in a graded fashion. Results are encouraging.

Goal-setting and pacing up activity levels

All too often the chronic pain sufferer has had to stop pleasurable as well as necessary activities because of their pain. The world has closed in on them and the resultant impoverishment of repertoire of worthwhile activities causes reduction in self-esteem and lowering of mood. Crucial to rehabilitation is the identification of a range of activities that are meaningful for the patient and to which they wish to make a return. This process is formally termed **goal-setting** (Sternbach 1978), and although simple in concept it can require considerable skill to implement in practice in patients whose activity levels have been reduced to very low levels over a long period of time.

Goal-setting is typically the province of occupational therapists, although other disciplines also need to be involved. Traditionally goals should match up to the SMART acronym: specific, measured, achievable, relevant, and timetabled.

The use of pacing techniques is crucial to the successful implementation of a goal-setting programme is. The patient who says they will consider a return to work when they are fit enough, still is faced with the dilemma that work is impossible now and contingent upon events that may or may not happen in the future. Thus uncertainty prevails, with little to offer positive feedback or a sense of achievement in the meantime. Such an individual will need to be encouraged to think about what they can do at the present time to build up tolerances and skills to aid the return to work. They may thus start working on component building blocks such as sitting, standing, and walking as well as gradually increasing their time set aside for work-related activities. As they progress, consideration might be given to starting voluntary work, for example, or taking a part-time job in an undemanding field. In this way the individual can measure their performance over time and see a progressive move towards the desired end point.

Such principles can be applied to many areas of the rehabilitation, not only to the more practical tasks. Concentration and relaxation, for example, can be worked on in a very similar fashion.

Pacing up specific activities is best managed within the framework of a larger planning and quota-setting exercise, which is also important. Such an exercise would set a time scale for the integration of various components of function into more meaningful substantive activities.

Relaxation

Learning to relax can be a great help to pain sufferers (Carroll and Seers 1998). The initial hypothesis proposed that pain arose from increased muscle tension and that instruction in formal techniques to relax would help to ease symptoms. Many patients and not a few therapists refused to accept this, pointing out that they often still had pain when in an advanced state of relaxation. A better theory is that using the discipline of a variety of techniques of visualization and progressive relaxation many individuals can reduce the pain they experience (Buchser et al. 1994, Schofield and Davis 2000). Like similar techniques (yoga, meditation, etc.) practice is required in order to attain competence, and some give up trying long before this level is achieved. For those patients who have the right mind-set and can put in the time, the rewards can be an effective way of reducing pain that is cheap, always available, and has no side effects.

Relaxation is taught by an appropriate therapist using a flexible and adaptable range of techniques in a group setting (Grzesiak 1977). Once a patient has started to feel a benefit a tape can be made which they can continue to use at home.

Format

Pain management programmes as developed in the UK can be either outpatient or residential programmes.

Outpatient programmes

Typically therapy occupies a half-day, or slightly more, of therapy, once a week for 6–8 weeks (Rosen *et al.* 1990, Skinner *et al.* 1990). This approach is easy to organize and cheap to deliver. Staff can usually be found to participate from within the establishment. Such a programme can be easily put together and requires minimal space or administration. More importantly, because of the minimal resources required hospital management is usually supportive, thus a programme can be commenced without a great deal of political manoeuvring.

The disadvantages of this type of approach are that because of the part-time nature of the staff and the limited commitment, team members can remain only partly committed to the programme. This can have a detrimental effect not only in terms of staff turnaround, but also skill base and knowledge. Therapists may not feel that they need to enhance their knowledge and skill to the same extent as if they were working on the project full time. Unfortunately these aspects are important, because experience has shown that the patients accepted on to outpatient programmes are as severely distressed and disabled as those treated in residential programmes. Such patients are very demanding and require sophisticated management by all staff involved with their treatment.

A further drawback is that it is more difficult to develop a fruitful group dynamic with patients only being together for a few hours every week. They also have to make the decision whether to attend on 8–10 occasions. This may not simply be related to motivation. Many patients appropriate for this type of treatment have considerable disability and travel is difficult. Hospital transport is not generally efficient enough to guarantee patients' attendance on time, so they require family or friends to deliver them. This effectively debars some patients from attending.

Historically it is also the case that outpatient programmes have often suffered from unavoidable instability due to changes in personnel or environment. There are also differences in outcome (see below).

Residential programmes

Duration varies but the therapy is an intensive package delivered every day for 3–4 weeks. Patients stay either on the premises in hostel-style, self-caring accommodation, or nearby in an hotel. The core staff are employed full time on the programme. This usually ensures a high level of commitment and allows for the development of skills and experience. Aspects such as staff training and education can be properly addressed.

For the patients, daily therapy, both physical and psychological, is more effective in generating change. A positive group dynamic usually develops rapidly because the members are in close proximity. The removal of the patients from the home environment is not always helpful in the longer term, but does allow for a reduction in the negative influences of the home environment while treatment is taking place.

The main disadvantages of residential or inpatient pain management are the resources involved in setting up such a programme, not only in terms of staff salaries but also accommodation and space costs. The result has been a dearth of such programmes in the UK, although many would not argue with the practical and theoretical benefits.

Setting aside differences in efficacy, which are addressed below, I believe that the argument should move on from whether one type of treatment is better than another, to how needy patients should obtain high-quality treatment in the most convenient and expeditious manner. Undoubtedly there is a role for quality outpatient treatment programmes directed to the less distressed and disabled patients who will be able to attend on a daily basis over a number of weeks. There will still also be a need for residential treatment for those patients who are either too distressed or disabled to attend a local clinic, or for whom geography renders this impractical.

Outcome

The first question that needs to be resolved when discussing the outcome from pain management interventions is, what constitutes success? In an ideal world, nothing less than total relief of pain should be considered acceptable. Without a doubt, however, pursuit of this unrealistic end point would not only see virtually all chronic pain centres closing due to lack of efficacy, but would ultimately be damaging to pain sufferers because the relentless pursuit of relief at any cost frequently leads to therapies that are harmful.

Results are often reported for large diagnostic categories or for a particular mode of treatment. For example, it is possible to find reviews relating to the treatment of back pain by various therapies of the overall results of treatment within a multidisciplinary pain centre. Such evaluations, although important for both practitioner and consumer, are difficult to subject to the scrutiny of the randomized controlled study. As a result, although numerous retrospective evaluations of outcome have been performed over the years, these are often methodologically poor.

It must be said, however, that practitioners involved in pain management programmes and psychological therapies have been more ready to measure outcome than those involved in clinical procedures (Peat *et al.* 2001). This can be put down to an awareness of the need for decent outcome data if psychological therapies are to be accepted into the mainstream, and the statistical rigour of psychologists' training. It is now appreciated that if meaningful data are to be obtained consideration needs to be given to the choice of outcome measures, the time scale, the control condition, and the blindness of the observers.

Most of the results published relate to outpatient programmes, but these often have recruited patients of very variable functional level. The results indicate that worthwhile changes can be made in areas such as pain and activity level as well as mood (McCarberg and Wolf 1999, Becker *et al.* 2000, Moore *et al.* 2000, Peters *et al.* 2000).

Fewer results relate to inpatient intensive treatment. In general the results indicate larger changes for patients often more disabled by their symptoms (Peters *et al.* 2000). The St Thomas's unit demonstrated an approximate doubling of physical performance as measured by various tests, alongside a halving of psychological distress (Williams *et al.* 1993).

Only a few studies have directly compared inpatient treatment with outpatient therapy (Peters and Large 1990). Williams *et al.* (1996a) found that the inpatients made more substantial gains in a number of areas and that these changes were better maintained than for the outpatients. Further data analysis allowed a 'number needed to treat' (NNT) analysis to be performed, which demonstrated NNTs of between 2.8 and 5.6 for a range of outcomes for inpatient treatment being superior to outpatient treatment (Williams 2001). One is left with the impression that the clinical outcome is related to the time and intensity of treatment. Although it may be theoretically possible to achieve the same level of improvement with weekly treatment, the practical barriers are such as to render it largely inaccessible. A recent systematic review of multidisciplinary rehabilitation for chronic low back pain supports this observation by concluding that the treatment intensity was important, and could not recommend less intensive treatments (Guzman *et al.* 2001).

A number of meta-analyses and systematic reviews have also been performed examining the whole field of cognitive–behavioural treatment. Flor *et al.* (1992) concluded that such treatments were more likely to be of benefit than single-modality treatments. More recently Morley *et al.* (1999) in a systematic review found that cognitive– behavioural treatment was superior to no treatment or waiting list controls in most areas. When compared with active treatment, cognitive–behavioural therapy produced a significant reduction in pain and pain expression, and improvements in coping. Van Tulder *et al.* (2001) examined the efficacy of cognitive–behavioural therapy for low back pain. They concluded that there was strong evidence that it had a moderate positive effect on pain reduction and functional improvement.

Conclusion

Persistent musculoskeletal pain affects the whole person. Undoubtedly some individuals are more prone to the negative effects of pain, and this vulnerability is related to psychosocial factors. Those adversely affected find that the pain progressively limits function and has secondary effects on mood and quality of life. In order to understand and treat such individuals effectively multimodal treatment is required.

Various therapies have been shown to be effective in producing short-term pain relief, but longer-term improvements in function require a more holistic approach. This is best delivered by an interdisciplinary team. There are now numerous studies documenting the efficacy of cognitive behavioural approaches in the management of chronic musculoskeletal pain. The future will see an integration of the effective components of this treatment within the broader approaches being used by diverse therapists in the community at earlier stages in the development of chronicity.

References

Abram, S. E., Haddox, D. (1999) *Pain clinic manual.* Lippincott, Philadelphia.

Becker, N., Sjogren, P., Bech, P., Olsen, A. K., Eriksen, J. (2000) Treatment outcome of chronic non-malignant pain patients managed in a danish multidisciplinary pain centre compared to general practice: a randomised controlled trial. *Pain,* **84**(2–3), 203–11.

Bigos, S. J., Battie, M. C., Spengler, D. M. *et al.* (1992) A longitudinal, prospective study of industrial back injury reporting. *Clinical Orthopaedics,* **279**, 21–34.

Buchser, E., Burnand, B., Sprunger, A. L. *et al.*(1994) Hypnosis and self-hypnosis, administered and taught by nurses, for the reduction of chronic pain: a controlled clinical trial. *Schweizerische Medezinische Wochenschrift. Supplement,* **62**, 77–81.

Burton, A. K., Tillotson, K. M., Main, C. J., Hollis, S. (1995) Psychosocial predictors of outcome in acute and subchronic low back trouble. *Spine,* **20**(6), 722–8.

Carroll, D., Seers, K. (1998) Relaxation for the relief of chronic pain: a systematic review. *Journal of Advanced Nursing,* **27**(3), 476–87.

Chaturvedi, S. K. (1987) Prevalence of chronic pain in psychiatric patients. *Pain,* **29**(2), 231–7.

Dooley, D., Prause, J., Ham-Rowbottom, K. A. (2000) Underemployment and depression: longitudinal relationships. *Journal of Health and Social Behaviour,* **41**(4), 421–36.

Feinmann, C., Ong, M., Harvey, W., Harris, M. (1987) Psychological factors influencing post-operative pain and analgesic consumption. *British Journal of Oral and Maxillofacial Surgery,* **25**(4), 285–92.

Flor, H., Fydrich, T., Turk, D. C. (1992) Efficacy of multidisciplinary pain treatment centers: a meta-analytic review. *Pain,* **49**(2), 221–30.

Flor, H., Turk, D. C., Rudy, T. E. (1987) Pain and families. II. Assessment and treatment. *Pain,* **30**(1), 29–45.

Fordyce, W. E. (1970) Operant conditioning as a treatment method in management of selected chronic pain problems. *Northwestern Medicine,* **69**(8), 580–1.

Fordyce, W. E., Fowler, R. S., DeLateur, B. (1968) An application of behavior modification technique to a problem of chronic pain. *Behaviour Research and Therapy,* **6**(1), 105–7.

Gardea, M. A., Gatchel, R. J. (2000) Interdisciplinary treatment of chronic pain. *Current Review of Pain,* **4**(1), 18–23.

Goldberg, D., Huxley, P. (1992) *Common mental disorders.* Routledge, London.

Grzesiak, R. C. (1977) Relaxation techniques in treatment of chronic pain. *Archives of Physical Medicine and Rehabilitation,* **58**(6), 270–2.

Guzman, J., Esmail, R., Karjalainen, K., Malmivaara, A., Irvin, E., Bombardier, C. (2001) Multidisciplinary rehabilitation for chronic low back pain: systematic review. *BMJ,* **322**(7301), 1511–16.

Halpern, L. M., Robinson, J. (1985) Prescribing practices for pain in drug dependence: a lesson in ignorance. *Advances in Alcohol and Substance Abuse,* **5**(1–2), 135–62.

Hansson, P., Lundeberg, T. (1999) Transcutaneous electrical nerve stimulation, vibration and acupuncture as pain-relieving measures, in *Textbook of pain,* 4th edn, P. Wall and Melzack, R., eds., Churchill Livingstone, London, p. 1341.

Illich, I. (1976) *Medical nemisis.* Marion Boyars, London.

Jensen, M. C., Brant-Zawadzki, M. N., Obuchowski, N., Modic, M. T., Malkasian, D., Ross, J. S. (1994) Magnetic resonance imaging of the lumbar spine in people without back pain. *New England Journal of Medicine,* **331**(2), 69–73.

Keefe, F. J., Caldwell, D. S. (1997) Cognitive behavioral control of arthritis pain. *Medical Clinics of North America,* **81**(1), 277–90.

Kleinman, A. (1988) *Rethinking psychiatry.* Free Press, London.

Klenerman, L., Slade, P. D., Stanley, I. M. *et al.* (1995) The prediction of chronicity in patients with an acute attack of low back pain in a general practice setting. *Spine,* **20**(4), 478–84.

Kouyanou, K., Pither, C. E., Wessely, S. (1997a) Iatrogenic factors and chronic pain. *Psychosomatic Medicine,* **59**(6), 597–604.

Kouyanou, K., Pither, C. E., Wessely, S. (1997b) Medication misuse, abuse and dependence in chronic pain patients. *Journal of Psychosomatic Research,* **43**(5), 497–504.

Kouyanou, K., Pither, C. E., Rabe-Hesketh, S., Wessely, S. (1998) A comparative study of iatrogenesis, medication abuse, and psychiatric morbidity in chronic pain patients with and without medically explained symptoms. *Pain,* **76**(3), 417–26.

Lewith, G. T., Vincent, C. (1996) On the evaluation of the clinical effects of acupuncture: a problem reassessed and a framework for future research. *Journal of Alternative and Complementary Medicine,* **2**(1), 79–90.

Loeser, J. D. (1989) Disability, pain, and suffering. *Clinical Neurosurgery,* **35**, 398–408.

Loeser, J. D., Butler, S. H., Chapman, C. R., Turk, D. C. (2000) *Bonica's management of pain.* Lippincott, Philadelphia.

Main, C. J., Spanswick, C. C. (2000) *Pain management – an interdisciplinary approach.* Churchill Livingstone, Edinburgh.

Maxwell, T. D., Gatchel, R. J., Mayer, T. G. (1998) Cognitive predictors of depression in chronic low back pain: toward an inclusive model. *Journal of Behavioral Medicine*, 21(2), 131–43.

McCarberg, B. and Wolf, J. (1999) Chronic pain management in a health maintenance organization. *Clinical Journal of Pain*, 15(1), 50–7.

McNairy, S. L., Maruta, T., Ivnik, R. J., Swanson, D. W., Ilstrup, D. M. (1984) Prescription medication dependence and neuropsychologic function. *Pain*, 18(2), 169–77.

McQuay, H. (1999) Opioids in pain management. *Lancet*, 353(9171), 2229–32.

Merskey, H., Lau, C. L., Russell, E. S., *et al.* (1987) Screening for psychiatric morbidity. The pattern of psychological illness and premorbid characteristics in four chronic pain populations. *Pain*, 30(2), 141–57.

Milne, S., Welch, V., Brosseau, L., *et al.* (2001) Transcutaneous electrical nerve stimulation (TENS) for chronic low back pain (Cochrane Review). *Cochrane Database Systematic Review*, 2, CD.003008.

Molin, C. (1999) From bite to mind: TMD – a personal and literature review. *International Journal of Prosthodontics*, 12(3), 279–88.

Moore, J. E., Von Korff, M., Cherkin, D., Saunders, K., and Lorig, K. (2000) A randomized trial of a cognitive-behavioral program for enhancing back pain self care in a primary care setting. *Pain*, 88(2), 145–53.

Morley, S., Eccleston, C., and Williams, A. (1999) Systematic review and meta-analysis of randomized controlled trials of cognitive behaviour therapy and behaviour therapy for chronic pain in adults, excluding headache. *Pain*, 80(1–2), 1–13.

Peat, G. M., Moores, L., Goldingay, S., Hunter, M. (2001) Pain management program follow-ups. a national survey of current practice in the United Kingdom. *Journal of Pain and Symptom Management*, 21(3), 218–26.

Peters, J. L., Large, R. G. (1990) A randomised control trial evaluating in- and outpatient pain management programmes. *Pain*, 41(3), 283–93.

Peters, L., Simon, E. P., Folen, R. A., Umphress, V., Lagana, L. (2000) The COPE program: treatment efficacy and medical utilization outcome of a chronic pain management program at a major military hospital. *Military Medicine*, 165(12), 954–60.

Price, D. D. (2000) Psychological and neural mechanisms of the affective dimension of pain. *Science*, 288(5472), 1769–72.

Raj, P. P. (2000) *Practical management of pain*, 3rd edn. Mosby, Chicago.

Ralphs, J. A., Williams, A. C., Richardson, P. H., Pither, C. E., Nicholas, M. K. (1994) Opiate reduction in chronic pain patients: a comparison of patient-controlled reduction and staff controlled cocktail methods. *Pain*, 56(3), 279–88.

Rose, M. J., Klenerman, L., Atchison, L., Slade, P. D. (1992) An application of the fear avoidance model to three chronic pain problems. *Behaviour Research and Therapy*, 30(4), 359–65.

Rosen, G., Kvale, A., Husebo, S. (1990) [Group therapy of patients with chronic pain]. *Tidsskrift for den Norske Laegeforening*, 110(28), 3602–4.

Schofield, P., Davis, B. (2000) Sensory stimulation (snoezelen) versus relaxation: a potential strategy for the management of chronic pain. *Disability and Rehabilitation*, 22(15), 675–82.

Scholten, C., Brodowicz, T., Graninger, W., *et al.* (1999) Persistent functional and social benefit 5 years after a multidisciplinary arthritis training program. *Archives of Physical Medicine and Rehabilitation*, 80(10), 1282–7.

Sharpe, L., Sensky, T., Timberlake, N., Ryan, B., Brewin, C. R., Allard, S. (2001) A blind, randomized, controlled trial of cognitive-behavioural intervention for patients with recent onset rheumatoid arthritis: preventing psychological and physical morbidity. *Pain*, 89(2–3), 275–83.

Sharpe, M., Carson, A. (2001) Unexplained somatic symptoms, functional syndromes, and somatization: do we need a paradigm shift? *Annals of Internal Medicine*, 134(9:2), 926–30.

Skinner, J. B., Erskine, A., Pearce, S., Rubenstein, I., Taylor, M., Foster, C. (1990) The evaluation of a cognitive behavioural treatment programme in outpatients with chronic pain. *Journal of Psychosomatic Research*, 34(1), 13–19.

Sternbach, R. A. (1978) Treatment of the chronic pain patient. *Journal of Human Stress*, 4(3), 11–15.

Sullivan, M. (1998) The problem of pain in the clinicopathological method. *Clinical Journal of Pain*, 14(3), 197–201.

Sullivan, M. (1999) Between first-person and third-person accounts of pain in clinical medicine. In: *Pain (1999) an updated review. Refresher course syllabus*, IASP Press, Seattle.

Sullivan, M. D., Turner, J. A., Romano, J. (1991) Chronic pain in primary care. Identification and management of psychosocial factors. *Journal of Family Practice*, 32(2), 193–9.

Sullivan, M. J., D'Eon, J. L. (1990) Relation between catastrophizing and depression in chronic pain patients. *Journal of Abnormal Psychology*, 99(3), 260–3.

Sullivan, M. J., Rodgers, W. M., Kirsch, I. (2001a) Catastrophizing, depression and expectancies for pain and emotional distress. *Pain*, 91(1–2), 147–54.

Sullivan, M. J., Thorn, B., Haythornthwaite, J. A., Keefe, F., Martin, M., Bradley, L. A., Lefebvre, J. C. (2001b) Theoretical perspectives on the relation between catastrophizing and pain. *Clinical Journal of Pain*, 17(1), 52–64.

Swimmer, G. I., Robinson, M. E., Geisser, M. E. (1992) Relationship of MMPI cluster type, pain coping strategy, and treatment outcome. *Clinical Journal of Pain*, 8(2), 131–7.

Turk, D. C., Okifuji, A. (1997) What factors affect physicians' decisions to prescribe opioids for chronic noncancer pain patients? *Clinical Journal of Pain*, 13(4), 330–6.

Turk, D. C., Rudy, T. E. (1990) The robustness of an empirically derived taxonomy of chronic pain patients. *Pain*, 43(1), 27–35.

Turner, J. A., Deyo, R. A., Loeser, J. D., Von Korff, M., Fordyce, W. E. (1994) The importance of placebo effects in pain treatment and research. *JAMA*, 271(20), 1609–14.

Van Houdenhove, B., Vasquez, G., Onghena, P., *et al.* (1992) Etiopathogenesis of reflex sympathetic dystrophy: a review and biopsychosocial hypothesis. *Clinical Journal of Pain*, 8(4), 300–6.

van Tulder, M. W., Ostelo, R., Vlaeyen, J. W., Linton, S. J., Morley, S. J., Assendelft, W. J. (2001) Behavioral treatment for chronic low back pain: a systematic review within the framework of the Cochrane Back Review Group. *Spine*, 26(3), 270–81.

Vincent, C. A., Richardson, P. H., Black, J. J., Pither, C. E. (1989) The significance of needle placement site in acupuncture. *Journal of Psychosomatic Research*, 33(4), 489–96.

Vlaeyen, J. W., de Jong, J., Geilen, M., Heuts, P. H., van Breukelen, G. (2001) Graded exposure in vivo in the treatment of pain-related fear: a replicated single-case experimental design in four patients with chronic low back pain. *Behaviour Research and Therapy*, 39(2), 151–66.

Vlaeyen, J. W., Seelen, H. A., Peters, M., *et al.* (1999) Fear of movement/(re)injury and muscular reactivity in chronic low back pain patients: an experimental investigation, *Pain*, 82(3), 297–304.

Waddell, G., Somerville, D., Henderson, I., Newton, M. (1992) Objective clinical evaluation of physical impairment in chronic low back pain, *Spine*, 17(6), 617–28.

Walker, J., Holloway, I., Sofaer, B. (1999) In the system: the lived experience of chronic back pain from the perspectives of those seeking help from pain clinics, *Pain*, 80(3), 621–8.

Williams, A. (2001) NNTs used in decision making in chronic pain. *Bandolier*, 22, January 2001.

Williams, A. C., Richardson, P. H., Nicholas, M. K., *et al.* (1996a) Inpatient vs. outpatient pain management: results of a randomised controlled trial. *Pain*, 66(1), 13–22.

Williams, A. C., Pither, C. E., Richardson, P. H., *et al.* (1996b) The effects of cognitive-behavioural therapy in chronic pain. *Pain*, 65(2–3), 282–4.

Williams, A. C., Nicholas, M. K., Richardson, P. H., *et al.* (1993) Evaluation of a cognitive behavioural programme for rehabilitating patients with chronic pain. *British Jounral of General Practice*, 43(377), 513–18.

Woolf, C. J. (1979) Transcutaneous electrical nerve stimulation and the reaction to experimental pain in human subjects. *Pain*, 7(2), 115–27.

4.4 A pragmatic management strategy for low-back pain – an integrated multimodal programme based on antidysfunctional medicine

Stefan Blomberg

The STAYAC model of pain management

The **biopsychosocial model** (Waddell 1998) was an important move towards improved pain care. However, from the perspective of the extremely important somatically focused dysfunction theory (see below) it is unfortunate that the 'bio-' prefix is so closely associated with the structural/pathomorphological paradigm. Patients with dysfunctional conditions certainly constitute the largest group of pain sufferers to which this paradigm should be applied. Moreover, possibly aside from purely psycho-existentially based conditions in which pain is not a feature, dysfunctional pain causes more suffering in the population than any other medical state and, from a societal perspective, it is also the most costly pain condition. This is especially true in primary health care settings, although it is a significant problem in many other disciplines too.

Furthermore, the existential dimension of pain suffering – an issue associated with obvious clinical consequences for the management of pain patients – is severely underestimated. It is unfortunate that the term **'bio-dysfunctio-psycho-socio-existential paradigm'** is so cumbersome, as it accurately reflects the essence of the proposed model for pain management.

The aim of this chapter is to interest the reader in the successful treatment results at the Stockholm Clinic – Stay Active (STAYAC). The therapeutic model includes manual therapy, steroid injections, muscle stretching, medical exercise therapy, traction modalities, and prolo-therapy, closely incorporated in a cognitive behavioural and psychotherapeutic approach. The following constitute the key issues of the STAYAC method.

- **Profound pragmatism.** Since the real cause of (back) pain is rarely known, it is impossible to design high-precision target-based diagnostic measures as well as target-based treatment methods with an outcome that is satisfactorily predictable – all diagnostic measures have insufficient specificity, sensitivity, reliability, and validity. Consequently, it is impossible to satisfactorily identify in advance those patients who will respond to a specific single technique. This problem can only be resolved by pragmatic treatment approaches, together with the recognition that pragmatism in this context is ultimately a recognition of the fact that diagnostic measures are insufficiently precise.

- A truly **eclectic** approach.

- **Metacognitive processes,** i.e. the therapists' continuous review of their own thought processes, attitudes, and beliefs.

- **Dysfunction theory,** including the concept of markers of dysfunction ('green flags') and **antidysfunctional therapy/medicine.** With regard to the nature of dysfunction, and the beneficial effects achieved by manual therapy, the underlying theoretical models are adapted to modern rationales, supported by recent neurophysiological research; mechanically oriented theories are rejected, and terms such as 'locking', 'blockage', 'subluxation', 'hypermobility', 'instability', and 'micro-instability' are abandoned.

- **Manual therapy** is a fundamental part of the algorithm, regardless of the duration of the symptoms, even after years of severe suffering. Manual techniques range from forceful thrust techniques, in which the 'traditional' Scandinavian concept of locking is aimed at directing the therapeutic forces exclusively to the dysfunctional segment (in which muscle energy principles are integrated), to extremely gentle techniques in which 'pure' muscle energy principles are applied.

- Dysfunctional conditions are **treatable,** in spite of co-existent major pathomorphology such as clinically relevant herniated discs, spinal stenosis, spondylolisthesis, and neighbouring acute compression fractures. Numerous 'classical' contraindications for manual therapy are abolished.

- **Evidence-based steroid injections** are included as one of the major treatment modalities in dysfunction-free states. Of these, the **parasacrococcygeal injection** is unique, extremely potent, and one of the most important items in the treatment arsenal.

- The concept of **hyper-reactivity,** with essential clinical implications, is introduced.

- Specified indications for **prolotherapy** are outlined, increasing the efficacy of the method.

- It is proposed that manual therapy/medicine relies largely on systemized **palpatory illusions** – a manageable, not a major problem, but one with important clinical consequences.

- New pragmatic indications for the use of **antidepressants** are proposed. The benefits of high dosage are considered.

- **Antidysfunctional investigation** is undertaken over time.

- The '*ex juvantibus*' diagnostic principle (see explanation on page 516) is consistently and systematically applied in virtually all patients.

- A new, structured **classification process** is utilized.

- Therapies are **combined**, and a unique, **integrated approach** is shared by all members of staff: receptionists, nurses, physiotherapists, behaviourists, psychologists/licensed psychotherapists, psychiatrists, and physicians. The ambition is to combine all evidence-based and empirically supported specific treatment modalities, and therefore potentially valuable therapeutic contributions in a common concept, i.e. everything from psychoanalysis to fusion surgery (the ultimate '**black box**' concept).

- **The stay-active concept is paramount.** There is a powerful synergy in applying the stay-active approach and antidysfunctional treatments in parallel, in a systematic, consistent and integrated manner. The stay-active concept is not merely a matter of encouraging patients to increase activity simply by providing advice and prescribing physical exercise; another aspect, at least as important, is the effectiveness of the stay-active approach as a metacognitive method. Stay-active messages are conveyed while passive treatment, such as manipulation, is provided to the patients.

- The structured management protocol is aided by cost-effective routes of communication, with the aim of limiting the risk that patients remain at suboptimal levels for long periods of time, and reducing the likelihood that treatment possibilities are missed.

- The **evidence-based integrated algorithm** for pain management encompasses both specific and non-specific categories of pain with confounding/contributing psycho-existential and social factors, and the algorithm is utilized for all pain patients regardless of genesis, duration, localization, and character of the symptoms. Consequently, all patients are offered a true '**somatic chance**'.

- Potent synergistic effects are achieved from the integrated approach of antidysfunctional medicine, with manual therapy as its core, and cognitive–behavioural therapy. The 'bone setter'/**manual therapist and the (cognitive) behavioural therapist are the same person,** with the advantage that manual treatment may be replaced in appropriate patients by behavioural strategies.

- '**Patient education**' is a new methodology within STAYAC, with the aim of minimizing the consequences of persisting symptoms; modifying beliefs, attitudes, fears, and behaviour; and improving sense of coherence and coping skills. It takes the form of interactive cognitive group therapy. The authority of the 'lecturing' physician (and also the behavioural therapist) is strengthened during the antidysfunctional investigation. Circumstances are created in which the patients are much less hesitant to discuss sensitive topics such as 'long-term sick leave illness', the stay-active concept, primary benefits, secondary benefits, basic crisis psychology, insufficient coping abilities, fear-avoidance, catastrophizing, insufficient sense of coherence, pain behaviour, the pain-patient role, identity loss,

development of pain personality, and life-lies. One could say that the patient education is a qualified and powerful mode of '**mental manipulation**'.

- **New psychological perspectives** with respect to the interaction between psycho-existential/social factors and the patients' pain and suffering are identified, with important clinical implications; three different basic perspectives are defined. The psychological paradigm, in which denial of psycho-existential dimensions of pain suffering is considered the principal underlying psychological factor in pain syndromes, is promoted. In the analyses of the patients' psycho-existential status, psychodynamic dimensions of their suffering are considered ('cognitive therapy with psychodynamic overtones').

- **The pain is virtually always regarded as nociceptive,** and only rarely of pure psychological origin. A model (the 'third perspective') is promoted, in which the pain is frequently 'used' by the patients to control and to facilitate repression of denied psycho-existential crises, which are externalized outside their own responsibility and control, as are the responsibility and control of their condition and their recovery. In the 'third perspective', an unsatisfactory psycho-existential/social status of the patient at the onset of pain may induce inadequate consequences from the pain.

- The overriding objective of providing manual therapy initially in advanced chronic perception-disturbed pain patients is to create a **trusting doctor–patient relationship** and a satisfactory therapeutic basis for strategies based on psychodynamic theories, aiming at behavioural changes, improved coping strategies, and limited adverse consequences of the chronic pain. The manual therapy in these severe cases is more or less a **ritual** to achieve these psychological effects. Whether or not the patients benefit from the treatment, from a physical perspective, is really not important. This way of utilizing manual therapy, with these premeditated intentions, has not so far been described in the literature, as far as I know.

- Although patients with severe chronic pain frequently lack psychological awareness of important underlying factors such as their beliefs, attitudes, and behaviour, short-term psychotherapy is frequently very successful. **The fundamental reason is that, from the patients' perspective, the primary problem, namely their pain, is addressed throughout.**

- **Patience** is necessary. We 'give up' extremely rarely. Within the described concept, there is virtually always another move to be taken when one measure has failed; even when pain is therapy-resistant, the patients' life situations are habitually brought under control. In advanced cases, several **parallel processes** may be undertaken (for example by the physician, psychiatrist, psychotherapist, one physiotherapist providing manual therapy, another physical exercise, and a third acupuncture); intense communication between the therapists creates confidence and accelerates progress, and anxiety through separation is avoided compared with the patient being referred to therapists in other clinics.

- As a 'spin-off effect', knowledge of the STAYAC model and its benefits improves **professional confidence**, thereby affecting the treatment results positively. In an optimal situation, all therapists in the team attend individual psychotherapy and receive tuition in psychotherapy.

- In conclusion, a **new psychological paradigm** is introduced. The ultimate challenge is to manage unmotivated, psychologically unaware and perception-disturbed chronic pain patients.

These key issues form the basis for the algorithm on which this chapter focuses (Figure 4.4.1, p. 502).

Background, evidence-based medicine, clinical trials, and literature reviews

In developed countries the incidence of acute low back pain requiring sick leave of 1 week or more is extremely high (80%, according to Nachemson and Jonsson 2000). Although low back pain usually is self-limiting (most patients recover within weeks), it is a major diagnostic and therapeutic problem causing much suffering and large costs to the community (Nachemson and Jonsson 2000). Treatment has traditionally been conservative, consisting mainly of medication, prolonged bed rest, and the use of spinal supports. This passive regimen has been extensively criticized during the last decade (Nachemson and Jonsson 2000), but scientific support for the use of virtually all alternative treatment modalities has been considered to be insufficient (Nachemson, Jonsson et al. 1991). Nachemson, Jonsson et al. conclude that, apart from surgery in a minority of patients with herniated discs, the treatment of non-specific low back pain was not a concern of medical care. The authors stated that the consequences of low back pain were exclusively related to lifestyle conditions, social factors, circumstances at work, smoking habits, and so forth, not to the access to treatment.

For centuries, physicians have been expected to work according to the Galenic principle or Hippocratic oath, i.e. empirical observations (experience) and sound scientific principles. However, over time, scientific society has realized that experience cannot always be trusted; many firmly established therapeutic traditions have been shown not to fulfil expectations of efficacy, when evaluated according to rigorous rules. Consequently, since the late 1980s, the era of 'evidence-based medicine' has emerged. The therapeutic society, especially when financed by the state, is expected to prioritize medical methods that are demonstrated to be effective in randomized controlled trials (RCTs). In addition, the governmentally supported methods have to be cost-effective (Editor's note: see also Patijn, Chapter 1.2). A consequence of this is that the number of published RCTs increased exponentially during the 1990s and physicians have to rely on literature reviews performed by 'evidence-based medicine institutes' such as the Cochrane Collaboration, the RAND Institute, and the SBU (Swedish Council on Technology Assessment in Health Care). These institutes have an extremely important assignment – their reports have to be accurate, trustworthy, and unbiased.

Approximately 55 RCTs on manual therapy have been published since 1956. In the studies, as well as in the literature reviews, conclusions with respect to efficacy of treatment are contradictory. The complexity of this area is reflected by the fact that there are more literature reviews published within this field than RCTs. Two of the reasons for this extreme inconsistency in conclusions are the lack of a consensus concerning reviewing methodology, and inappropriateness of both study designs and reviewing methods. My thesis (Blomberg 1993) includes a 44-page systematic review, in which I concluded that manipulation was effective only in acute and subacute low back pain patients without radiating pain (Fisk 1979, Rasmussen 1979, Farrell and Twomey 1982, Nwuga 1982, Hadler, Curtis et al. 1987, Wreje, Nordgren et al. 1992). In my opinion, with respect to evidence, the additional studies published since then have strengthened the position of manual

therapy to a modest degree in acute neck pain and cervicogenic headache (Jull et al. 2002, Hoving 2002) and in chronic low-back pain (Aure, Nilsen 2003). Koes et al. (1992 a, b, c) claim positive results achieved by manipulation in chronic patients, but the results should be considered to be inconclusive in view of flaws in reviewing methods and bias (Blomberg 1993, pp. 28–9, 50–2). With respect to thoracic pain, low-back pain with radiating pain, and chronic neck pain there is still no evidence for the use of manual therapy. Bronfort, Evans et al. (2001) detected benefit from combined spinal manipulation and exercise for patients with chronic neck pain, but it was exercise that was evaluated by comparison with another group. This contradicts the recently published major literature reviews (see below), but in due course results will be published by the group I am working with, supporting the long-term efficacy of manual therapy in conjunction with steroid injections in acute, subacute, and chronic low back pain patients, plus corresponding data in a short-term study (10 weeks) of acute/subacute low back pain with radiating pain (Blomberg, Bogefeldt 2005). It is apparent that several high-quality studies on the use of manual therapy/manipulation are being conducted at the present time, hence the evidence for manual therapy/manipulation may become stronger in future years.

In recent literature reviews, produced by different evidence-based medical institutes, there is a clear trend for an increasing number of manual therapies to be identified as effective (van Tulder, Ostelo et al. 1996, Harms-Ringdahl, Holmström et al. 1999, Nachemson and Jonsson 2000, Bronfort and Haas 2004). By contrast, in a recent meta-analysis of manipulation and low-back pain, Assendelft and Morton (2003) concluded that 'there is no evidence that spinal manipulative therapy is superior to other standard treatments for patients with acute or chronic low-back pain'. (The meta-analytical approach has deep flaws when attempting to compare a variety of therapeutic approaches.) The stay-active concept is generally acknowledged as the basic treatment approach of choice for non-specific low-back pain. In addition, measures such as physical exercise, analgesics, non-steroidal anti-inflammatories (NSAIDs), manual therapy, behavioural therapy, and multidisciplinary treatment programmes are recommended, provided their respective indications and contraindications are considered. A further consideration is that not all of these identified treatment strategies are shown to be effective in patients suffering from acute, subacute, and chronic neck or back pain. Nevertheless, it is obvious that the existence of a large variety of evidence-based and non-evidence-based treatment methods for back pain has not solved this enormous societal problem. Virtually all modes of treatment are available in Stockholm, for example, but nevertheless the problem is expanding more rapidly than ever, not least from a cost perspective. Why is that? This chapter attempts to answer this question and offers an approach to management of spinal pain, and other localized or generalized pain, which is both evidence-based and pragmatic.

Gordon Waddell (1998) approached this problem in his thought-provoking and trailblazing book The Back Pain Revolution. He claims that (primarily) the physicians, but also their health care colleagues such as physiotherapists, chiropractors and osteopaths, actually created the Western back pain problem: 'Back pain, the medical disaster of the 20th century'. Of course he does not mean back pain per se; he is referring to the unreasonable consequences of back pain. He claims that epidemiological research demonstrates that the severity and prevalence of back pain is more or less the same in all countries in the world (Hoy, Toole et al. 2003, Wigley, Zhang et al. 1994, Anderson 1984). Waddell blames the biomedical paradigm for far-reaching negative consequences in developed countries. This

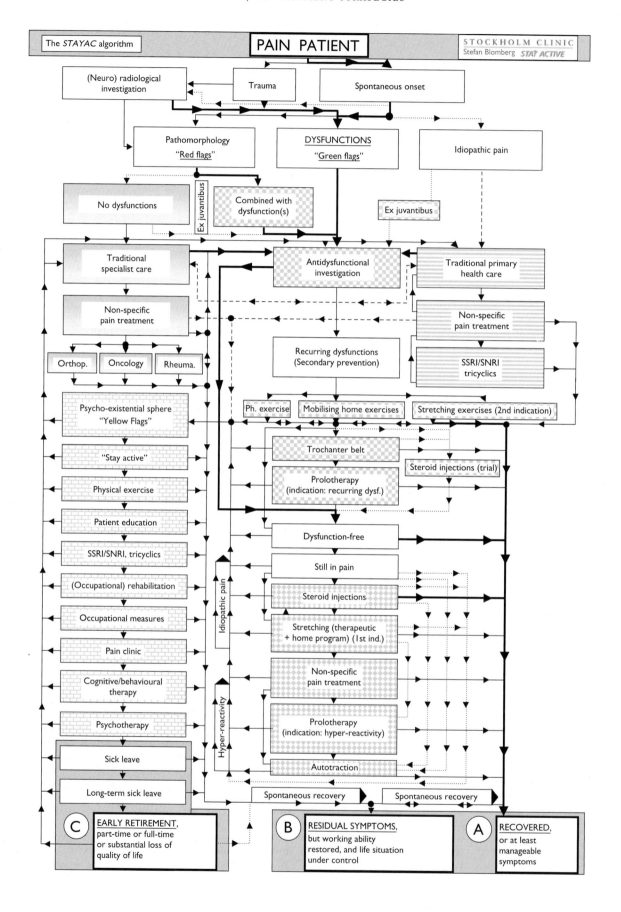

Figure 4.4.1 The STAYAC algorithm. A larger coloured version of the algorithm is found on STAYAC's website, **www.stockholmclinic.se**, and is available as printed copies (a plasticized version is also offered). It is indeed helpful to those who will utilize the algorithm in clinical practise. The patients 'start' at the top of the flowchart, and there are three possible outcomes at the bottom of the scheme; (A) No symptoms, or fully controllable minor symptoms; (B) Residual symptoms reducing some aspect(s) of quality of life and/or some daily activities to some degree; (C) Long-term sick leave or early retirement or a substantial loss of quality of life. In between the top and the bottom, there are four different domains:

- 'The specialist sphere' (upper left, grey-toned)
- 'The general health care' (upper right grey horixzontal stripes)
- 'The psycho-existential sphere' (to the left, grey bricked)
- 'The antidysfunctional domain': 'Yellow light A situation' ('secondary prevention', page 517) (upper middle, grey chequered)
- 'The antidysfunctional domain': 'Yellow light B situation' (pages 517 and 518) (lower middle, grey filled rhomboids)

The flows between the different spheres and boxes are described in the text. Apart from the standard arrows, there are three different special arrows:

- Dotted line: Unusual flows
- Dashed lines; Common, however unwelcome in a well developed algorithm
- main flows

---

paradigm has been extremely successful in numerous other medical fields, but it offers no solution to back pain patients except in a very few cases (*Editor's note:* see also Hutson, Chapter 1.1). A simplistic and pathomorphologically based paradigm was foisted not only on everyone with an interest in back pain management, but also on society in general. Waddell formulates the problem brilliantly; unfortunately, he does not offer a genuine solution to it.

In spite of being more complete than the biomedical paradigm, the biopsychosocial model does not, in my opinion, cover the entire problem complex either. I hope that this chapter will direct the reader, and in due course also health care in general, towards a solution of the problem.

All hitherto published systematic literature reviews apply a dichotomized system in which diverse treatments are listed exclusively as 'effective' or 'not effective'. However, apart from the classification of patients suffering from neck pain or low back pain, and division into acute/subacute versus chronic complaints, there have been no attempts to evaluate which therapies are effective in which patients, and during which periods of their 'sickness career'. Furthermore, virtually nothing is known about the effectiveness of different therapies with respect to specified efficacy variables, or about the next cost-effective move through the chain of therapy when a certain therapeutic modality has failed. Moreover, the efficacy of certain therapies is not analysed hierarchically, despite the obvious fact that, although two different therapies may indeed be effective in a defined patient group, one therapy may be substantially more powerful than the other. In addition, questions have to be asked regarding which combinations of treatment methods are useful.

Although no algorithms are to be found in the evidence-based medicine literature, they have been published in different consensus reports, in which some components are evidence-based, while others are supported by 'best available evidence' or by experience, treatment traditions, and common sense (AHCPR 1994, CSAG 1994, RCGP 1996, ACC 1997, Kendall *et al.* 1997, Waddell 1998). However, all these algorithms are incomplete with respect to important aspects of (back) pain management, not least regarding manual therapy and other factors emanating from the dysfunction theory. Consequently, there is a need for a new more comprehensive and inclusive algorithm.

Pragmatic treatment approach

Why pragmatic treatment approaches?

One reason for the lack of more specific data in current literature reviews is obvious – the information extracted from the pool of RCTs is insufficient. The required research has hardly begun, and the research field that emerges when these perspectives are considered is huge.

The real cause of back pain is rarely known (Nachemson and Jonsson 2000). Consequently, in 'non-specific' (back) pain, it is impossible today to design high-precision target-based diagnostic measures as well as target-based treatment methods with an outcome that is satisfactorily predictable. This is why all diagnostic measures have insufficient specificity, sensitivity, reliability, and validity, especially at an individual level, but also at group level. Different diagnostic instruments, including those with behavioural or psychological orientation, diagnostic imaging, laboratory tests, and clinical tests, are indeed valuable at a group level in RCTs, and in clinical epidemiological research, but their precision for the purpose of predicting treatment outcome of a specific therapy, particularly for the individual patient, is unsatisfactory. When a patient is examined manually, something tangible is being palpated. However, something other than what is believed is being palpated. In addition, it is likely that benefits accrue during manual treatment for more complex reasons than are usually believed. Consequently, manual therapy/medicine may to a large extent rely on **systemized palpatory illusions**. However, this is academic as long as the treatment proves to be beneficial to the patients and cost-effective in conclusive RCTs, while we are waiting for the true explanations for the underlying mechanisms, achieved by experimental research; evidence-based and cost-effective treatment models should be implemented in pain management even though they may be founded on incorrect theoretical models.

In conclusion, it is impossible to satisfactorily identify in advance those patients who will respond to a specific single technique. As long as we do not know the true cause of most low back pain, **this problem can only be addressed by pragmatic treatment approaches**. The essence of pragmatic treatment models is ultimately a recognition of the fact that diagnostic measures are insufficiently precise.

Why pragmatic trials?

In the context of RCTs, whatever measures are taken to select a patient group supposed to be susceptible to a specific treatment, the selected population will always contain a substantial subgroup of non-responders to the treatment in question. This may, in turn, seriously limit the power of the study, and may make it virtually impossible to detect the positive effects of a truly effective treatment modality. Consequently, when conducting RCTs in this field, there is a need for pragmatic studies, in which there is a flexibility to change treatment modality when the treatment response is poor, as a result of the insufficient precision in predicting treatment response to a certain treatment modality in the individual patient. The choice of therapies and the number of visits is determined by the provisional/working diagnosis and the response to treatment at each visit. Clinical trials using such approaches analyse the effect of a system of care, not the effect of single therapies or components of single therapies extracted from a complete treatment programme. In a pragmatic study, a multimodal therapeutic arsenal is utilized where the therapists are free to choose from the different treatment modalities according to need, after having assessed the patients at each consultation – the type, frequency, and duration of the treatment are at the discretion of the therapist, based on the patient's response. The treatment at each consultation is based on a functional diagnosis, which, in turn, generates a treatment hypothesis. This hypothesis is either confirmed or rejected at the subsequent consultation, depending on the treatment response – the treatment hypothesis may have to be reconsidered, and, consequently, the treatment strategy may be changed. **The unravelling of structural (i.e. pathomorphological), social, psycho-existential, or dysfunctional factors associated with the patients' suffering is a process over time, i.e. a mapping proced**ure (see subchapters 'The antidysfunctional investigation' and 'Idiopathic pain – *ex juvantibus* diagnosing', page 516). In conclusion, a true pragmatic system for investigation and treatment is a process of consistent and systematic *ex juvantibus* diagnosis. Consequently, recurrences are treated throughout the course of a pragmatic study, thereby allowing as many treatment sessions as are considered necessary. Thus, the termination of the therapy is based on the patients' needs rather than on a rigid schematic study protocol, and the design of the intervention is aiming at emulating clinical reality. Considering the difficulty of predicting the treatment outcome of single 'fastidious' therapies, it is reasonable to postulate that the different items of a pragmatic treatment arsenal do not merely have additive effects but rather that they have 'synergistic' effects. This statement is substantiated by the results of our group's studies (see below), and it is discussed more extensively in my thesis (Blomberg 1993, pp. 122–7), and by Blomberg, Svärdsudd *et al.* (1994).

Pragmatic trials are of the most immediate interest to the patients. However, this type of trial has a disadvantage: if one treatment is more successful than another it may be difficult to identify which item in the therapeutic arsenal is responsible for the positive effects.

Fastidious trials – shortcomings and advantages

In rigorous 'fastidious' trials, all conditions are the same in both groups, except for one variable: a patient-blinded active treatment versus placebo. Optimally, a fastidious trial answers only one question. There are three major blinding possibilities: the patient, the physician, and the evaluator. Thus, in pharmacology, the term 'triple-blind design' would be more accurate than 'double-blind'. However, within the field of manual therapy, only two of these blinding possibilities are achievable: the evaluator and the patient. (A standardized therapeutic manoeuvre may be compared with a similar placebo treatment – with this design, the patient should not be able to distinguish whether or not they received active treatment.) Consequently, fastidious double-blind evaluations of specific components extracted from a complete (pragmatic) treatment programme are possible. In pragmatic studies, only one blinding possibility is reasonable – the blinded evaluator. Consequently, these are open, observer-blinded studies. Fortunately, today, such designs are accepted, and are frequently found in the indexed journals. For many years, pragmatic studies were significantly more difficult to publish than fastidious trials; to a certain extent, this is still the case. In the literature, there are a couple of examples of trials (Bergquist-Ullman and Larsson 1977, Sloop, Smith *et al.* 1982) in which efforts have been undertaken to blind the patients. However, these study designs are very artificial. In fastidious trials the type, frequency, and duration of the treatment are strictly standardized in the study protocol, and equal in both groups – recurrences are not treated after the termination of the standardized treatment course. However, one of the important drawbacks is the obvious risk that fastidious trials of single therapies do not reveal detectable effects in controllable sample sizes. In addition, single treatments are of minor interest to the patients, which, in turn, creates substantial risks of high dropout rates, especially in long-term trials. Moreover, the results of single therapies may have only limited clinical applicability. Furthermore, using sham therapies as control intervention leads to methodological difficulties and ethical predicaments, and is far from clinical reality. Nevertheless, fastidious studies are necessary.

A pragmatic design is an advantageous first step in evaluating treatment programmes. If no differences in outcome between the groups in such a study are detected, the evaluation of the single items is of limited interest. Fastidious trials are needed to answer questions generated by pragmatic studies, such as the evaluation of separate treatment modalities extracted from a complete treatment programme. If a management algorithm is shown to be effective, further similar, but less pragmatic research will evaluate the importance of additions or elimination of certain treatment modalities, changing of paths through the chain of therapy, alterations of indications within the scheme, measures to optimize cost-effectiveness, and so forth. The subsequent studies may apply less pragmatic and more fastidious designs. However, in the subsequent research, it is important to consider the possible synergistic effects of a multimodal treatment programme – it may even be the case that long-term effects can only be detected in broad pragmatic treatment models (Blomberg 1993, pp. 122–7), or possibly in treatment programmes that change the patients' beliefs and attitudes in a fundamental manner (Blomberg 1993, p. 118). The longer the follow-up, the more valid is this statement. Moreover, it is reasonable to consider pragmatic studies more ethically acceptable for RCTs in the field of low back pain than fastidious studies. If a pragmatic multimodal algorithm provides long-term efficacy in a pragmatic RCT, short-term effects achieved by the isolated items of the management in question in fastidious trials are sufficient; their possible contributions to the long-term effects in the evaluation of the entire concept have to rely on assumptions.

Scientific basis of the STAYAC management strategy

There is evidence from two major studies of acute and subacute low back pain that a pragmatic approach incorporating a range of therapies is more effective than traditional care with respect to pain, disability, mobility, return to work, general (psychosomatic) symptoms, quality of life, and costs.

The original study and the partial cross-over study

In my thesis (Blomberg 1993, based on five papers: Blomberg, Svärdsudd et al. 1992, 1993a, 1993b, 1994, Blomberg, Hallin et al. 1994) it was demonstrated that a new pragmatic treatment of low back pain was superior to standardized and optimized conventional activity-based treatment by primary health care teams – the stay-active concept (Waddell 1998). The latter approach was the basic management in the experimental group also, but with the addition of a pragmatic multimodal treatment regime. The main items added were manipulation, specific mobilization, steroid injections, muscle stretching, and autotraction. After 1 month of follow-up, the proportion of patients on sick leave was six times larger in the conventionally treated group than in the experimental group. Furthermore, the 4-month follow-up showed considerable differences, again favouring the experimental group, in the two pain scores and the fifteen disability rating scores. Moreover, measurements of mobility and movements causing pain, as well as the results of quality-of-life measurements and the presence of general symptoms of a psychosomatic character, favoured the experimental intervention. Pain drawings also showed substantial differences favouring the experimental group (Grunnesjö, Blomberg et al. 2005).

The paper by Blomberg, Svärdsudd et al. (1992) provides the first indication in the literature of sick leave reduction (at 8 months) achieved by manual therapy. A 3-year follow-up showed that the reduction of sick leave in the experimental group remained (Bogefeldt, Blomberg et al. 2005a). In addition, the disability rating scores, followed for 2 years, indicated beneficial long-term effects as well. Such short- and long-term effects achieved by the pragmatic method in a population with chronic low back pain were also evident in a controlled partial crossover study of 'failures' from the control group of the original study (Bogefeldt, Blomberg et al. 2005b).

The reproducibility study

Because of the pragmatic design of the first trial, it was not possible to draw firm conclusions about which items in the therapeutic arsenal were responsible for the positive effects. Consequently, a reproducibility study with basically the same pragmatic design as the original study, but with randomization to four groups, was undertaken to evaluate separately some of the components of the complete treatment arsenal. The results were consistent and basically similar to the results of the original study, so it was concluded that the second study was a successful replication of the original study (Blomberg, Bogefeldt et al. 2005a, b, c, Grunnesjö, Blomberg et al. 2004, Grunnesjö, Blomberg et al. 2005, Bogefeldt, Blomberg et al. 2004). Consequently, the prag-

matic treatment programme can be communicated to other physicians and physiotherapists. In addition, the pragmatic concept, in combination with steroid injections, was shown to be superior to the corresponding treatment programme without steroid injections.

In our studies, not only do the differences favour the experimental treatment more substantially (even at 3 days) when compared with other RCT-evaluated treatment strategies, the experimental intervention was also substantially less costly than standardized traditional management based on the stay-active concept within primary health care (the original study) and orthopaedic care (our reproducibility study). In addition, since it was shown that the population studied in the second trial was representative of the most severely affected acute/subacute low back pain patients (Bogefeldt, Blomberg et al. 2004c), the results should be valid in other acute/subacute low back pain populations too. Long-term effects were indicated by the fact that many differences in outcomes between the two groups in both studies increased over time (Blomberg, Svärdsudd et al. 1993a,b), and by the persisting differences in favour of the experimental treatment in the long-term follow-up in the original study and in the partial cross-over study. The treatment programme is one of the few to be reproduced in two subsequent trials according to a state-of-the-art procedure.

In terms of cost-effectiveness and long-term effects in a group of patients with chronic low back pain, unrandomised, McGuirk et al. (2001) published their study of rural clinics. In this study, doctors who had postgraduate training in musculoskeletal medicine and who agreed to abide by evidence-based guidelines were compared with usual general health care with referral to physiotherapy or specialist if requested. There was less use of physiotherapy and opioid medication in the experimental group.

Behavioural aspects of manual therapy

When undertaken sensibly, manual therapy is a suitable starting point and a good basis for a trustful patient–doctor relationship. Unfortunately, excessive belief in manual therapy as a universal method, where the therapist believes (often subconsciously) that all pain problems can be solved by manual therapy, provided the therapist is skilful enough, is not uncommon. This attitude, often resulting in endless courses of passive treatment, may jeopardize the rehabilitation of the chronic 'perception-disturbed' patient by retaining or reinforcing their pain behaviour and the pain-patient role. It is crucial to prevent this, for example by broadening and improving the education in manual therapy, and by explaining to patients the basis, purpose, and scope of manual therapy.

Nevertheless, it is important to emphasize that **it is possible to incorporate modern behavioural therapeutic thinking into manual therapy**: the two approaches are definitely compatible. Once pathomorphological changes relevant to the symptoms have been ruled out (such as herniated disc, fractures, tumours, inflammatory disorders – altogether less than 5% of the patients; Nachemson and Jonsson 2000) it is essential that all patients presenting with symptoms that may be associated with the locomotor system are subjected to examination with the aim of identifying dysfunctions treatable with manual therapy. This should be done before measures based on socio-psychological/

psycho-existential considerations are undertaken. However, it is crucially important for the therapist to realize early when no further progress by manual therapy is possible. This is the point where psycho-existential factors must be taken into consideration.

I regularly meet chronic perception-disturbed pain patients whom I realize during the first consultation I will most probably not be able to help with manual therapy in a somatic sense. Despite this, I start by giving a short course (2–4 sessions) of manual treatment and/or steroid injections to give the patient a 'somatic chance'. In these patients, management from the beginning by physiotherapists trained in the stay-active concept parallels the investigation over time by the responsible physician, and a psychotherapist or psychiatrist may be included in the process early as well: the therapists communicate continuously and closely with each other. A small minority of these patients is treatable with antidysfunctional therapy alone, and since it is more or less impossible to predict these rare positive treatment responses, the only approach that avoids missing them is to perform the antidysfunctional investigation on all individuals in this patient category, regardless of severity and duration of pain. Since the antidysfunctional treatment, once learnt, is virtually free of additional costs, and since the associated risks are almost negligible (Nachemson and Jonsson 2000), this pragmatic approach is reasonable. However, the overriding objective of this process is to create a trusting doctor–patient relationship and a satisfactory therapeutic basis for strategies aiming at behavioural changes, improved coping strategies, and limiting the consequences of the chronic pain. This is achieved through subliminal communication and through transference/counter-transference mechanisms according to psychodynamic theories, sometimes in explicit verbal terms. Furthermore, often subconsciously, the patients are also made aware that it is pointless to rely on a chiropractor or other therapist providing manual therapy or other somatically focused therapies.

Whether or not the patients benefit physically from the manual treatment is really not important, even if it is extremely satisfying for the therapist in the few cases when they do. The manual therapy in these severe pain cases is almost a ritual to help achieve the psychological effects. I believe that using manual therapy this way, with these premeditated intentions, has not hitherto been described in the literature, even if some therapists may do this to some degree, at least subconsciously.

After this process, I consciously and abruptly change attitude; the 'bonesetter' identity is left behind and cognitive–behavioural therapeutic principles are applied instead. Frequently, I never touch the patient again, and the continuing management focuses exclusively on behavioural strategies.

Although these behavioural potentials in manual therapy were not applied in this premeditated manner in our group's RCTs, the positive effects of the experimental treatment, not least the conspicuous long-term outcome, may partly be attributed to the inherent behavioural therapy effect of the treatment strategy we used. This may be deduced, for example, from the fact that the experimental patients not only had less pain but also stated, to a significantly greater extent than the conventionally managed group, that the treatment made it easier to cope with their residual pain both at work and during their leisure hours (Blomberg, Svärdsudd et al. 1993b). This effect may have been achieved by the inherent behavioural therapeutic potential of the treatment.

Many differences in outcomes between the two groups in our RCTs increased between the follow-ups at 2 and 4 months (Blomberg, Svärdsudd et al. 1993a). The behavioural aspects of management may also be partly responsible for this (Blomberg 1993, p. 118). Differences between the groups persisted at the 2-year follow-up, and during the entire 3-year follow-up the experimental management gave better results in terms of work absenteeism (Bogefeldt, Blomberg et al. 2005a). In the long term, the experimental management may change the sick leave behaviour of the patients (Blomberg 1993, p. 118). The favourable long-term effects may also be explained by the perception of 'health', which was more positively influenced by the experimental management than the other 23 quality-of-life variables (Blomberg, Svärdsudd et al. 1993b). In another study (Eklund 1992), this measure was the most reliable predictor for an advantageous prognosis in occupational rehabilitation of low-back patients on extended sick leave. Even lifestyle changes may occur, leading to a persistently increased level of physical activity or even participation in new activities: 80% of the patients in the experimental group stated that they had increased their level of physical activities after 2 years, compared with 40% in the control group (Bogefeldt, Blomberg et al. 2005a). This indicates that we succeeded in reducing the 'passivizing' risks of providing passive treatments. In addition, during the 2 years' follow-up, the experimental group consumed less health care resources than the control group. In another study (Cherkin, Deyo et al. 1998), chiropractic care and management according to McKenzie (1981) increased the utilization of health care. This difference could be explained by the potential for favourable behavioural changes inherent in the STAYAC algorithm.

A sensible manual therapeutic approach should include stay-active messages at an early stage: for example, informing the patients of the generally benign character of their condition and the adverse effects of inactivity and sick leave; making them understand that bed rest usually makes the situation worse, and that it is generally not dangerous to work and take part in physical activities in spite of some pain.

Although manual therapy is a passive treatment modality, our therapeutic strategy seems to be an effective way to activate patients. This may seem paradoxical, but there are explanations:

- Pain creates anxiety and fear.

- Anxiety and fear create inactivity, leading to fear-avoidance behaviour and catastrophizing.

- This, in turn, generates increased sensitivity to loading of different soft tissues, decreased muscle strength, loss of fitness, postural control, and coordination.

- This process causes increased pain, and a vicious circle is established.

The evaluated treatment strategy might reduce and prevent the pain patient's anxiety, fear, and other phenomena such as personality changes. When patients notice that pain relief can be achieved by simple manual manoeuvres provided by a therapist, they may (subconsciously) realize that the symptoms cannot indicate dangerous tissue damage. Consequently, whether spontaneously or following encouragement from the physician and/or the physiotherapist, further moves towards more active behaviour are enhanced. To use behavioural therapeutic terminology, the physician and/or the physiotherapist become **reinforcers**.

Development of the STAYAC treatment algorithm

Continuous development has been in progress for many years at the STAYAC clinic, where the evaluated treatment programme originated. Since the two trials were completed, the applied method has broadened considerably. Although a behavioural approach has been an intrinsic part of the concept for a long time (Blomberg 1993, pp. 128–9), behavioural and psychological measures have subsequently been integrated into the programme in a more focused manner. Our occupational rehabilitation, managed over a period of 6 years by a physician, a behavioural therapist, and a specialized physiotherapist in a very special professional relationship, has had an important role in this process. One of the crucial characteristics of the STAYAC method is the close and integrated cooperation between all the staff members. A multidisciplinary team in itself is no guarantee of success. To achieve consistent results, a systematic algorithm, in which there is equal respect between the team members, has to apply.

Metacognition

The STAYAC model is largely a metacognitive approach. Metacognition (Flavell 1979, Jones and Rivett 2004) is a reflective process, and concerns the conscious (and, with time and experience, even pre- or subconscious) continuous scrutinizing and revising of the therapists' own thought processes, attitudes, and beliefs. Associated phenomena are **lateral thinking** (De Bono 1977) and **profound pragmatism**. In practice, this means that one has to be continually self-analytical, to reflect on whether one's actions and communication skills are optimal and of benefit for the patients. Although further discussion of this important aspect of management – in particular, the continuous scrutiny and revision of the therapist's own thought processes and beliefs – is outside the scope of this chapter, it should become apparent that the potential positive effects of metacognitive processes are identified in this chapter. In addition, there are numerous examples showing how inadequate metacognitive processes may affect the treatment results negatively. I believe that being aware of metacognition may optimize the treatment results more than any other factor. (An attempt to evaluate the impact on rehabilitation of physiotherapists' pain beliefs has been made by Daykin and Richardson (2004).) **One could even say that the STAYAC algorithm is a metacognitive method based on pragmatism.**

Pragmatic approach

Considerable efforts have been made at the STAYAC clinic to eliminate the potentially negative aspects (i.e. passivity) of manual therapy within the multidisciplinary team. An inherent problem in traditionally passive treatment methods, such as manipulation, is the risk of subliminal 'stay-passive' messages being transferred to the patients, usually non-verbally at a subconscious level but sometimes also by advice to limit activity. There are therapists whose 'treatment' strategies rely more or less exclusively on activity-limiting regimens, to avoiding pain at any price. One important reason for this is reliance on outdated, mechanistically oriented theoretical models. Perhaps the integration of manual therapy into the stay-active concept is one of the main reasons for the success of our programme, when compared with other similar, also pragmatic and fairly recent studies in which the results of different kinds of manual therapy were indifferent (Skargren, Öberg et al. 1997, Cherkin, Deyo et al. 1998, Seferlis, Németh et al. 1998, Rasmussen-Barr 2003). The dysfunction paradigm (see later) becomes an excellent pedagogical model, which is fundamental in achieving this synergy between activity and 'passive' manual therapy. For many patients, it is impossible to live pain-free lives. For these patients, the only way forward is to challenge the pain,

gradually increase their activity levels despite the pain, defeat it over time, and finally become able to live their lives normally as they once did. Preferably, during the entire process, a team of different therapists guides the patient, not infrequently over long periods of time – a tremendous pedagogical challenge. A distinctive trait of the STAYAC model is patience. There is almost always another move to be taken when one measure has failed. Our greatest success has been the successful management of unmotivated, psychologically unaware and perception-disturbed chronic pain patients who are no longer capable of managing the pressure of life or shouldering the responsibilities of their adult selves – the 'Peter Pan syndrome' (Kiley 1983).

One could say that our developmental project has led to the design of an 'ultrapragmatic' treatment programme, with the ambition of combining all evidence-based and empirically supported specific treatment modalities ('best available evidence' according to Waddell 1998), and therefore potentially valuable therapeutic contributions in a common concept, i.e. everything from psychoanalysis to fusion surgery. In fact, only a small minority of the treatment modalities is not evidence-based, and it is important to remember that the 'core package' (i.e. the 'antidysfunctional sphere') is evidence based. We also believe that the pragmatic principle, both with regard to the study design and the experimental intervention, has been another important key to the successful outcome of our group's trials. (Many types of manual therapy, although at first glance they may seem closely related to the mode of manual therapy developed in our clinic, suffer from an obvious lack of pragmatism.)

Our group's results indicate that it is reasonable not only to include the complete evaluated pragmatic treatment programme in a new algorithm; it should also play a major role from the beginning of the management of patients' back pain. Significant, clinically relevant differences in favour of our experimental intervention were demonstrated even after 3 days (Blomberg, Svärdsudd et al. 1994). This constitutes a major difference between the STAYAC algorithm and all other previously published algorithms – manual therapies play minor roles, if any, in these other algorithms, with the exception of the UK guidelines (RCGP 1996) in which manipulation is recommended as one of the options during the first 6 weeks. (However, this algorithm is unclear about why and when manipulation should be provided.) Moreover, current major literature reviews and algorithms recommend 'self-care' as the 'treatment' of choice during the first weeks, but STAYAC is opposed to this management philosophy. There are scientific and substantial observational data indicating that this strategy is not appropriate, so we suggest highly active management from the first day of pain. (Our studies indicate that this approach is cost-effective.) Manual therapy is a fundamental part of our algorithm, regardless of the duration of the symptoms.

In summary, the evidence-based integrated algorithm described in this chapter is used for all patients with locomotor system dysfunction, regardless of the genesis, duration, localization, and character of the complaints, regardless of whether or not the condition in question is complicated by psycho-existential or social factors, and regardless of whether the condition is specific or non-specific.

Evidence-based methods

What basically has been evaluated in our group's trials is the addition to the established stay-active concept of four treatment modes: manipulation/specific mobilization, steroid injections, muscle stretching, and autotraction. Individually, except for manipulation, these treatment modalities have a poor evidence base.

● According to the published systematic literature reviews, the overall results of manipulation are not very impressive, and its long-term effects remain to be demonstrated.

● There is only weak evidence for the benefit of epidural steroids for back pain (Nachemson and Jonsson 2000). (*Editor's note:* For their use in sciatica, see Bush, Chapter 4.3.4). The use of steroid injections is a non-evidence-based treatment method in patients with low back pain. Additionally, this type of intervention has a mixed reputation, both among the majority of patients in developed countries, and among many physicians.

● Muscle stretching, as a clinical method for low back pain, is non-evidence-based; on the contrary, available studies imply moderately negative clinical effects (Howell 1984, Bogefeldt, Blomberg *et al.* 2004c). In one of the four groups of our reproducibility study, muscle stretching was incorporated as a single addition to the basic stay-active concept, and recovery was postponed in comparison to the group in which neither muscle stretching, manual therapy, or steroid injections was added to the basic management. Nevertheless, in the manual therapy group and the manual therapy/steroid injections combination group, stretching was in fact even more frequently applied than in the stay-active/stretching group. (**However, the dysfunctions were treated before muscle stretching was applie**d.)

● Autotraction and other traction methods are not acknowledged as effective treatment modalities in any of the published systematic literature reviews (Harms-Ringdahl, Holmström *et al.* 1999, Nachemson and Jonsson 2000).

How is it possible that a combination of four treatment modalities, with more or less doubtful efficiency, brought together in a common treatment programme, can be strikingly helpful in patients with low back pain? This paradox must be explained before our group's scientific results can be regarded as trustworthy. Accordingly, we must define a treatment algorithm based on a pragmatic approach, which will allow its application to everyday clinical practice. This chapter aims to define such an algorithm on the basis of the available evidence.

The lack of evidence-based algorithms for the management of back pain is a substantial problem. Consequently, an 'ultrapragmatic' RCT is currently being planned at STAYAC. This study will not evaluate effects achieved by specific treatment methods. Its starting-point is the assumption that back pain is treatable, and, furthermore, that resources for effective care are available, at least in an urban setting like Stockholm. The hypothesis of the study is that the main problem of back pain care is the lack of 'infrastructure', i.e. an evidence-based multimodal algorithm for treatment/management of low back pain. All kinds of treatment modalities for back pain will be available in both groups (with no limitations in the control group), but care will be structured according to the STAYAC algorithm in the experimental group, whereas the control group will reflect the pathways according to poorly structured conventional care. Consequently, this infrastructure study will not evaluate the efficacy of any specific treatment modalities, but the possible effects of our treatment algorithm.

Dysfunction, markers of dysfunction, antidysfunctional treatment/medicine

The definitions used here are adapted to modern rationales, supported by recent neurophysiological research (Johansson 1981–1998, Johansson and Sojka 1991) on the nature of dysfunction, and the underlying mechanisms of the beneficial effects achieved by manual therapy.

Dysfunction – the dysfunction theory

The term dysfunction refers to disturbed function in musculoskeletal tissues (e.g. joints, muscles, ligaments, tendons), or in the neuromuscular reflex patterns within the 'operating system' of the postural muscles, probably also including higher levels of the central nervous system. **Dysfunctions occur in pathomorphologically damaged tissue, but also (and most frequently) in healthy tissues.** One of the many advantages of the dysfunction theory is that it is cause-neutral; the exact causes of pain are still unknown in most patients. Dysfunctions are diagnosed manually. Standard methods used within traditional health care for investigation of (back) pain including diagnostic imaging, scintigrams, sensory evoked potential, electromyography, electroneurography, and blood parameters (e.g. humoral markers of inflammation, hormones, etc.), aimed at identifying structural changes or abnormal biological processes, are of limited value. In the absence of a causal relationship between structural pathology and symptoms, the results of these investigations are frequently irrelevant: asymptomatic 'abnormalities' are common, particularly in diagnostic imaging. The dysfunction model makes it possible to understand momentarily restored mobility, resolved compensatory scoliosis, and immediate pain relief after antidysfunctional treatment.

Our pain patients usually have no disease, according to the biomedical definition: it is only a question of their backs or necks not functioning optimally. With this attitude, from a behavioural and psychological perspective, inherent positive effects are evident. It is logical to stay active, to move, and not to rest unnecessarily. Fear-avoidance and catastrophizing are counteracted, and the risk of subliminal stay-passive messages is reduced or even eliminated. The back is not 'worn out'; there is no real disease, and patients are reassured. There are even patients in whom there is no further need for treatment if the condition recurs, once the pain has disappeared after antidysfunctional therapy. The comforting subliminal message is: 'If the pain disappears (even if it is only a temporary effect) with a simple treatment manoeuvre, it cannot be anything serious or dangerous.'

The concept of dysfunction is also applied within other medical disciplines. For instance, it is now accepted today that 'gastritis' is an inappropriate diagnosis, since it is not an inflammatory condition: the mucosa of the stomach is dysfunctional, without pathomorphological/histological correlates, and the condition is now called 'dyspepsia'. Similarly, the dysfunctional 'irritable colon' was once thought to be an inflammatory disease. Dysfunctions are associated with many other relatively common symptoms, including numbness, paresthesiae, vertigo, tinnitus, ear problems, micturition disturbances, blurred vision, voice changes, and even cardiac arrhythmias (see Kuchera, Chapter 2.2.1).

Many dysfunctional musculoskeletal conditions frequently mimic symptoms from other organ systems. For example, bowel pain may be referred from iliopsoas muscle and pelvic dysfunctions, and chest pain is commonly referred from dysfunctions in the thoracic column or rib joints. In addition, women with pelvic pain frequently interpret their condition as gynaecological, and undergo unsuccessful gynaecological investigations or even laparoscopy without positive findings. Urologists frequently see analogous cases in male patients. At STAYAC, there is an ongoing RCT evaluating the addition of antidysfunctional treatment to gynaecological management in women with pelvic pain who attend gynaecologists, either spontaneously (interpreting their pain as gynaecological) or by referral from physicians (who suspect gynaecological origin), and in whom there is no gynaecological explanation for the pain or gynaecological care fails. Clearly, to prevent unnecessary, expensive and potentially stigmatizing investigations or even operations, education in antidysfunctional medicine should be made available not only to associated disciplines such as rheumatology, but also to other disciplines (for instance, cardiology, gynaecology, genitourinary medicine) in which patients may suffer from dysfunctional conditions that give rise to symptoms that mimic symptoms from other organ systems. Unfortunately, there appears to be little systematic high-quality research in this field.

There is a problem with the term 'functional'. Paradoxically, this once had a similar meaning to 'dysfunctional', as defined in this chapter. However, the meaning of the word has changed over time. In Sweden, as in other countries, the term has become a coded deprecatory diagnosis for conditions with a primary psychogenic/psychosomatic background but no real 'sickness' (see 'The first perspective', below), symptoms with an invented aspect, and even laziness. Consequently, I avoid the use of the term 'functional'. It should be appreciated that patients with dysfunctional conditions may present with symptoms that are as severe as, not infrequently worse than, those of patients suffering from pathomorphological conditions.

Dysfunction may sometimes be considered mechanical, insofar as it is caused by overuse, improper use, or strain, not least in dysfunctions of the extremities. However, it is my opinion that within manual therapy/medicine today, mechanical theories ('locking', 'blockage', 'subluxation', 'hypermobility', 'instability', etc.) are overemphasized and have to be balanced by more up-to-date rationales such as those suggested here. Many therapists get stuck in the 'biomechanical trap'. I believe that mechanical factors, as the primary cause of dysfunctions, are of minor importance especially in the spine and pelvis. This belief is substantiated by the fact that symptomatic clinical features and signs in the extremities frequently disappear with manual treatment to the spine or pelvis, or with injections applied in areas distant from these symptoms. This is exemplified by many cases of apparent tendalgias at the shoulder, epicondalgias (*Editor's note:* see also Hutson, Chapter 3.5), and plantar 'fasciitis'. Phenomena such as the momentary disappearance of paresthesiae, vertigo, blurred vision, and so forth can only be explained in a more general way, for instance as a reflex disturbance ('electrical chaos') localized in the postural operative system, rather than a mechanical dysfunction localized to a single vertebral segment (see below).

To avoid confusion of terminology, particularly in those countries in which the meaning of 'dysfunction' is equivalent to 'general dysfunction', indicating disturbance of activities of daily living (ADL) or impairment of functional capacity or disability, 'specific dysfunction' indicates the type of dysfunction defined in this chapter.

The nature of the dysfunction

The dysfunction perspective is specific to antidysfunctional medicine. According to the best available evidence from modern neurophysiological research, the dysfunction is most probably a relatively generalized disturbance (and not specifically localized, as suggested by the dominating mechanically oriented theories within manual therapy/medicine today). This generalized disturbance affects the intricate higher cerebral centres in addition to peripheral structures for postural control, with their complex, neuromuscular reflex patterns. The coordinating systems involved in postural control provide peripheral proprioceptive information to higher centres. The receptors situated in the vertebral

segments and the sacroiliac joints may be the most important proprioceptive information centres. The small movements in the sacroiliac joints (Egund, Olsson *et al.* 1978, Sturesson, Selvik *et al.* 1989, Tullberg, Blomberg *et al.* 1998) are necessary for optimized proprioceptive input to the postural system. However, from a biomechanical perspective, these minor movements are not necessary for everyday mobility and movement. According to Håkan Johansson's group's research in Umeå, Sweden, numerous proprioceptive receptors react to minor mechanical forces resulting in subtle, widespread, and complex modulation of muscle tension. Moreover, muscle spindles have virtually their own nervous system, the gamma system. The indications are that the ligaments function primarily as receptor organs, not as stabilizing structures; they are more or less an extension of the peripheral nervous system. Although the system Johansson's group suggests is not completely mapped out, there is scientific support for it (Johansson 1981–1998).

A dysfunction is a somatic cause of nociceptive pain in the locomotor system, most frequently not associated with simultaneous pathoneurophysiological or pathomorphological symptomatic manifestations in the back or its operative system. Of course, some type of abnormal electrical activity represents the dysfunction somewhere in the neuromuscular reflex systems. (This might be viewed as 'electrical chaos', meaning that a certain number of molecules are out of place, for instance on the 'wrong' side of cell membranes.) However, contrary to the situation in the wind-up-phenomenon and/or neuropathic pain, the symptoms are reversible and are not represented by any permanent pathoneurophysiological process, biochemical correlates, or, of course, by anatomical, morphological, or histological changes; otherwise, the immediate effects achieved by manipulation for instance could not be understood (an excellent example of pragmatism, according to the dictionary definition).

Alternative mechanisms of back pain and effects achieved by manual therapy are discussed in my thesis (Blomberg 1993, pp. 35–7 and 125–6).

Antidysfunctional treatment

Dysfunctions are reversible conditions and are, by definition, treatable by different modes of manipulation, specific or non-specific mobilization, muscle stretching, autotraction, and steroid injections. Within the antidysfunctional paradigm, such treatment aims to normalize the function of the affected neuromusculoskeletal structure as a consequence of (sometimes quite forceful) reflex patterns, and to maintain the improved or normalized function by means of home care programmes. Self-maintained disturbed pain-provoking reflex patterns in the postural system may be modified via gate-control mechanisms at the spinal level; additionally, as a consequence of (sometimes quite forceful) **proprioceptive** stimulation, 'reset' mechanisms may halt the electrical chaos triggered in the postural operative system. In the STAYAC model, the posturoproprioceptive dysfunction theory is more vital than the gate-control theory. Dysfunctions may also disappear spontaneously or with activation (including physical exercise and other home exercises), or indirectly by behavioural, cognitive or psychotherapeutically based approaches and other measures undertaken to modify the psycho-existential/social dimensions of the patients' suffering. Dysfunctions may also be positively and even causally influenced by drugs (for example, analgesics, NSAIDs, and antidepressants), and reflex therapy methods that inhibit vicious circles in neuromuscular reflex patterns (e.g. acupuncture, acupressure, massage). In fact, notwithstanding the relevance of the gate-control theory, it may be the case that all therapeutic modalities with positive effects act through 'reset buttons' interfering with the systems described above at different levels. This does not mean that they are equally effective; the efficacy of different modalities, or combinations of therapeutic modalities, has to be evaluated in RCTs. For back pain, particularly with radiating pain, it is my experience that the most effective 'reset button' is situated in the parasacrococcygeal structures, which are frequently injected with steroids at STAYAC.

Consequently, almost the entire treatment algorithm, even much of the specialist sphere, could be regarded as antidysfunctionally directed. There are many painful and dysfunctional conditions that are resistant to therapy before causal measures are undertaken for pathomorphological conditions, but treatable afterwards. An example is low back pain due to lumbar/pelvic dysfunction, obviously secondary to coxarthrosis. After surgery for the latter condition (and thereby cure of 'the disease component' of the patient's suffering), the dysfunctional component becomes treatable.

Antidysfunctional treatment may be passive (e.g. manipulation, steroid injection). However, it may also be active; most of the effects achieved by passive antidysfunctional treatments are also achievable by different kinds of home exercises. All physical exercises are antidysfunctional measures.

Markers of dysfunction

Dysfunctions are manifested by symptoms such as pain, stiffness, and disability. They are represented by 'markers of dysfunction' (i.e. non-pathomorphological physical signs) on manual examination, such as localized tenderness, disturbance of segmental mobility and joint play, and positive functional, positional, and provocative tests for e.g. spinal and pelvic dysfunctions (see Kuchera, Chapter 2.2.1). Positive manual diagnostic tests are sometimes referred to as 'pathological' tests. However, the validity of many of these tests, for instance those that are supposed to evaluate the mobility of the sacroiliac joint and the position of the pelvic bones in relation to each other, has been disproved (Tullberg, Blomberg *et al.* 1998). Consequently, the term '**markers of dysfunction**' is cause-neutral and more appropriate.

Pathomorphological conditions cannot be treated by means of antidysfunctional therapy. However, at STAYAC, patients with pathomorphological conditions frequently improve or become symptom-free; this is explained by successful treatment of dysfunctional components of the patient's symptoms. This means that in patients with clear pathomorphological features who progress to full recovery, the structural findings are asymptomatic. The most frequent examples of this are herniated discs, coxarthrosis, spinal stenosis, spondylosis, and spondylolisthesis.

Subjects with structural pathology whose symptoms are not controlled after a reasonable number of steps through the algorithm are referred to relevant specialists, provided the symptomatology is sufficiently profound. Cases in whom there is an unsatisfactory margin in terms of cost–benefit analysis (i.e. expected improvement achieved by surgery weighed against the risks taken) are preferably managed within primary health care.

Hyper-reactivity

In the STAYAC model, the concept of 'hyper-reactivity' supersedes concepts such as 'hypermobility', 'instability', and 'micro-instability', because it is more appropriate with regard to the pathogenesis of the 'classical hypermobility syndrome' than focusing on the mechanical properties of joints such as the degree of mobility and joint play. Experience of manual diagnosis suggests that the irritability of spinal segments is poorly related to mobility; the (hyper-reactivity) syndrome is more likely caused by seemingly 'permanent' distortion of proprioceptive afferents from the vertebral segment(s), which in turn, via misinformation, interfere with the operating system of the postural muscles. It is hypothesized that this operating system (including the cerebellum, the 'central computer') cannot interpret this misinformation and transform it into adequate instructions to the postural muscles, so that agonists counteract antagonists, causing overload of different structures, and a low-efficiency/energy 'crisis' of the entire system. Clinically, the hyper-reactivity syndrome has identical features to the 'hypermobility syndrome', including reliance on the history for diagnosis, and clinical signs such as delayed and prolonged stretch pain on provocation tests.

A hyper-reactive segment may in fact be hyper, normo-, or even hypomobile. It could even be that *hypomobility* is more common than hypermobility in the severe cases, and that these are the ones most frequently subjected to surgical fusion. On the other hand, many markedly hypermobile subjects have no symptoms of hypermobility syndrome. The term hyper-reactivity is applicable to all joints of the body, including the sacroiliac joint, the hip joint, and peripheral joints.

Hyper-reactivity is a pathoneurophysiological disturbance that gives the appearance of permanency. It may have a post-traumatic and/or a degenerative background. Unlike dysfunctional conditions, hyper-reactivity is not causally treatable. However, it is hypothesized and also empirically supported, that symptoms associated with hyper-reactivity in all joints of the body are frequently alleviated by muscle stretching (not least the iliocrural muscles in low back pain, an important indication for this treatment modality). Additionally, hyper-reactivity heals spontaneously over time, and the associated symptoms subside. (Unfortunately this may take years, even decades.) It is logical to believe that this healing process is attributable to the development of age-related spondylosis. This slowly decreases the mobility of the affected segment(s), resulting in less distortion of proprioceptive output, and finally, when there is little or no mobility, the postural control system is able to adapt to the abnormal situation, and the pain and other symptoms subside. This model could very well explain why virtually all back pain subsides with increasing age. I finish the 'Patient education' (see subsequent section) by presenting this model. Its behavioural potential (e.g. reassurance) is obvious:

> I can see on the X-ray that the so-called 'degenerative changes' in your back are more pronounced today than they were 4 years ago. This is very good – your irritated back is definitely healing! What I see on the X-ray is not 'wear and tear', it's a healing process: the body's own capacity for fusion, which is much better than surgical fusion. Just live your life as usual and be active, while this healing process continues. Eventually, you will become pain-free.

We can also understand from this model why, although surgical fusion may seem successful initially, months or years later patients may develop pain that is much worse than the condition that led to the operation: The fusion abolishes the distorted output (which is fine), but it also destroys other normal output that is needed for postural control. The mechanical rationales upon which fusion surgery is based are suspect, if one accepts the concept of hyper-reactivity. The same goes for the hypothesis that neighbouring segments become 'hypermobile' over time as a consequence of the stiff fused segment. In conclusion, rejecting mechanically oriented theories in favour of the 'posturoproprioceptive model' is a good example of fruitful metacognition.

This 'posturoproprioceptive model' may even have a more important role in the syndrome than the local pain factor; furthermore, it allows the dissemination of nociceptive pain and other symptoms from the original focus to other distant parts of the body to be better understood. (This mechanism is not equivalent to 'referred pain', which is a central mechanism in the CNS resulting from the inability of the pain-monitoring systems in the cortex to localize the pain to the proper part of the body – somatic 'pain' becomes 'pain' only at the point of time when nociceptive or neuropathic nervous input reaches the cortex. The posturoproprioceptive model, although including central nervous mechanisms in the form of the operative system of postural control, is a matter of peripheral nociceptive pain mechanisms.)

Psycho-existential dimensions of pain suffering

The usual term for psychological factors in the context of pain is 'psychosocial'. However, from the psychological and social perspectives, the overall health, prosperity, and social status of people in developed countries are comparatively good. I therefore prefer the term **psycho-existential**. I believe that the existential dimension of pain suffering is severely underestimated; as I perceive the world of back pain, it is the dominating factor with respect to the consequences of pain conditions (see 'The third perspective', below). This is not a matter of splitting hairs – the implementation of this paradigm in pain care, as an aspect of the metacognitive processes, is definitely associated with obvious clinical consequences. A good example of the denial of the psycho-existential dimensions of the suffering, and denial of the role of the life situation in general, as a confounding factor with regard to the consequences of pain, is loss of work. In a society such as Sweden, largely driven by Lutheran ideals and morals, loss of work activates the existential crisis of not being needed, not being seen, not being heard and, not infrequently, not feeling loved; and finally, the utmost existential crisis of all, having no right to exist. Unemployment is for many an unfathomable situation for which pain is 'convenient' in the short term but destructive and often disastrous for the individual patient in the long term. The mechanisms underlying 'long-term sick leave illness' (a condition/sickness caused by the long-term sick leave itself, a useful comprehensive term for all personality changes, behavioural changes, loss/distortion of identity, and loss of self-esteem and other psychological deviations that occur during long-term sick leave) are similar. Of course unemployment and long-term sick leave could be perceived as purely social problems. However, in Western society it is the profound existential dimensions of work loss and long-term sick leave, and their denial, that cause such destructive consequences.

Other relevant phenomena central to the STAYAC concept are poor quality of life, behavioural disturbances, insufficient coping strategies, and low sense of coherence (Antonovsky 1987).

Perception disturbances

The psychological phenomenon of perception disturbances develops in almost all patients with severe chronic pain, and frequently also in moderately affected subjects, during the destructive process of sick leave from the first day until the day of early retirement some years later. A stone becomes a mountain; it is as if numerous receptors in the perception system are turned to maximum volume, resulting in severe distortion. An illustrative situation arose during the early days of our occupational rehabilitation unit. When filling in questionnaires about their pain (after sitting quietly and apparently comfortably, listening

to a 2-hour lecture), patients repeatedly indicated high VAS scores for the item 'sitting for longer than a short period'. It was obvious that the instrument did not measure ability to sit; it was much more likely that existential anxiety was recorded, a cry for help. This dimension of pain suffering is frequently the main obstacle to successful rehabilitation. If we, as therapists, are not aware of this phenomenon, we will have huge difficulties in managing these patients.

A macro-perspective of the algorithm

The following description of the STAYAC algorithm takes the form of a macro-perspective; providing the details is not within the scope of this chapter. Our basic manual techniques are available in textbooks (Evjent and Hamberg 1985a, 1985b; Kaltenborn and Evjent 1993), but their modifications and many details have to be learnt in the STAYAC courses. Other authors have influenced the Scandinavian manual therapy model, and thereby also the STAYAC concept (Cyriax 1970, Janda 1976, Stoddard 1980, Lewit 1991). The reason for concentrating mainly on the wider perspective of the algorithm is that, to be able to improve pain care significantly, a better infrastructure in (back) pain care has to be developed; the details are less important.

The STAYAC algorithm is pragmatic and eclectic, and aided by cost-effective routes of communication. The intention is to limit the risk that patients remain at suboptimal levels (which might jeopardize their rehabilitation potential) for long periods of time, and to reduce the likelihood that treatment possibilities are missed. Central to the algorithm is a therapeutic philosophy emanating from dysfunction theory, which applies to most patients with neck and back pain, at least in the early stages of their pain. The therapeutic strategy directed by the dysfunction perspective is more scientifically based than other modes of treatment in an unselected patient group. In addition, the demonstrated effects appear more powerful in more important efficacy variables than other treatment approaches that have been evaluated in RCTs. The protocol allows unsatisfactory progress to be detected early, which is important from the psychological perspective.

The core of the algorithm – the antidysfunctional domain – is evidence-based, and so are most of its other components. However, some aspects, as reflected by a series of statements and assumptions in this chapter and as stated in other algorithms (AHCPR 1994, CSAG 1994, RCGP 1996, ACC 1997, Kendall *et al.* 1997, Waddell 1998), are not supported by hard evidence, but based on best available evidence, observational data and common sense. Patients' progress through the treatment protocol is based on the pooled experience of the clinic's staff members in mixing several management philosophies and methods over a 20-year period. Since the results of our algorithm are unique, it is important to publicize it to a broader circle of physicians, physiotherapists, and other people working with pain. To validate the results of our latest outcome study (to be published) an RCT evaluation of the entire algorithm is planned.

Possible outcomes

In terms of the diagram (Figure 4.4.1), all STAYAC patients enter the algorithm in the upper part of the figure and progress downwards to one of three possible outcomes (at the bottom of the figure):

- **No symptoms or fully controllable minor symptoms**, without negative consequences. Neither quality of life nor work capability is disturbed.

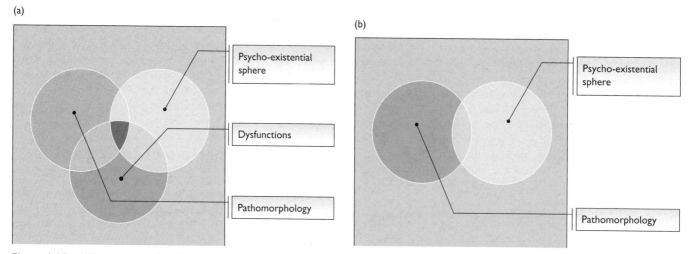

Figure 4.4.2 (a) The three basically different factors which can explain and/or influence pain, the perception of pain, and the consequences of pain. Any one factor may be the dominant (or single) factor, coexist in any combination, or all three may contribute simultaneously to the patient's condition (however, frequently with considerably different impact). Considering all three sectors is an essential requirement for optimal (back) pain care. (b) This figure signifies the basic structure of today's back (pain) care: managements based on the dysfunction theory are not systematically implemented in 'cultural' pain care; with their 'subcultural' character, antidysfunctionally related treatment models that exist are isolated from 'cultural' medicine.

- **Residual symptoms reducing some aspects of quality of life and/or some daily activities to some degree.** However, the ability to perform the patient's usual work is retained. Retention of work capacity is not only the most important target in rehabilitation from a societal perspective, it is also the most important issue regarding long-term well-being in a general sense, not least in Western societies, where a person's identity relies largely on the specific function they fulfil in society. Self-care will be appropriate as a short- and long-term strategy and the chances of spontaneous recovery with time are excellent. The provision of relevant information, reassurance, and reinforcement and, when needed, patient education help the long-term situation. In other words, the general life situation is not fully optimal, but under control; there are no major psychiatric disorders such as depression, and the patient's psychological state is satisfactory.

- **Long-term sick leave or early retirement (part- or fulltime) or a substantial loss of quality of life.** The patient may regard sick leave as a reasonable solution for a life situation that is no longer manageable by other means. However, although the prescription of sick leave may occasionally be appropriate, it should be avoided whenever possible. It has to be remembered that the sick leave instrument is one of the most dangerous treatments a physician can impose. This 'treatment' is associated with severe side effects and complications. In Western societies, largely driven by Protestant morals and ideals, long-term sick leave – or worse, early retirement – is almost always a virtual disaster for the suffering patient. **From a strictly somatic pain perspective, long-term sick leave is rarely indicated.**

The classification process

There are only three distinct factors that can explain and/or influence pain, the perception of pain, and the consequences of pain: the pathomorphological, the dysfunctional, and the psycho-existential spheres (Figure 4.4.2). In Figure 4.4.3 this is illustrated in another way and in more detail (see also Figure 4.4.4); the purpose is to illustrate the basis upon which the STAYAC concept relies.

The large square in Figure 4.4.3a represents a population and the large circle corresponds to the proportion of the population that, according to numerous epidemiological studies, has experienced low back pain during the last 3 months (30–40%). The smallest circle represents the small group (at the most, 5%) of patients with low back pain in whom the pain has a causal relationship with pathomorphological changes in the structures of the spine and/or pelvis (i.e. disease as defined according to the biomedical paradigm). The somewhat larger dashed circle indicates that this figure may, by scientific progress, increase in size to a modest degree in the future. In Figure 4.4.3b, the larger proportion of psycho-existential factors is shown. Figure 4.4.3c illustrates patho-neurophysiological conditions (in which, for simplicity, hyper-reactivity is included). Examples of patho-neurophysiological conditions are central sensitization and the wind-up phenomenon; it may be that segmental hyper-reactivity is a type of wind-up phenomenon. The large dysfunction sphere is illustrated in Figure 4.4.3d. Everyone working within manual therapy/ medicine knows that there are asymptomatic dysfunctions; opinions on whether or not they should be treated are usually represented by the extremes: 'never treat' or 'always treat'. In the STAYAC model, asymptomatic dysfunctions are treated in some situations, but not routinely. In terms of the posturoproprioceptive dysfunction theory, there is nothing strange in a patient promptly getting rid of headache after a lumbar/pelvic dysfunction has been treated (even when there is no low back pain), something that happens every now and then. There are many analogous examples, mostly associated with pelvic dysfunctions (such as groin pain interpreted as hip joint symptoms, knee problems, plantar fasciitis, and thoracic pain). Primary psychogenic pain is rare, and true simulators are even more infrequent (Figure 4.4.3c). From Figure 4.4.3f, in which all the basic conditions are brought together within a common outline, it is obvious that the adoption of the dysfunction paradigm decreases the proportion of pain patients whose pain cannot be understood or treated – idiopathic pain.

The first task of the physician (or the physiotherapist) is to consider the possibility of major red-flag conditions such as herniated discs,

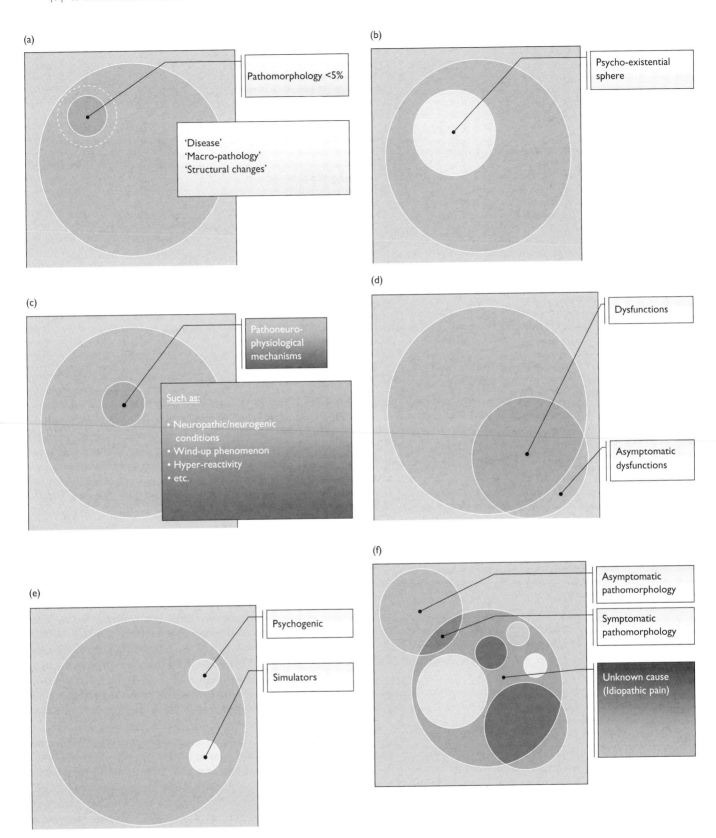

(a)

Pathomorphology <5%

'Disease'
'Macro-pathology'
'Structural changes'

(b)

Psycho-existential sphere

(c)

Pathoneuro-physiological mechanisms

Such as:

• Neuropathic/neurogenic conditions
• Wind-up phenomenon
• Hyper-reactivity
• etc.

(d)

Dysfunctions

Asymptomatic dysfunctions

(e)

Psychogenic

Simulators

(f)

Asymptomatic pathomorphology

Symptomatic pathomorphology

Unknown cause (Idiopathic pain)

Figures 4.4.3a–f The theoretical basis upon which the STAYAC concept relies. The squares represent a population and the circles different underlying factors with respect to pain (a larger sphere represents a larger proportion of the population). See text for details.

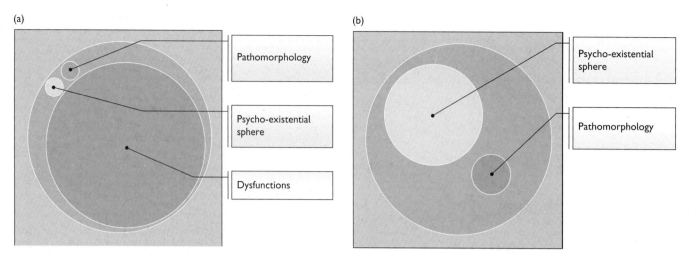

Figure 4.4.4 (a) In the acute phase, dysfunctions are the dominating cause of pain – pathomorphology and primary psychoexistentially based conditions are rare. Provided antidysfunctional treatment is carried out early, most patients in this category need only a few steps in the antidysfunctional sphere. (b) Psycho-existential dimensions of the pain suffering dominate in patients with severe chronic disease. Such patients with purely dysfunctional conditions (green flag conditions) and therefore treatable with antidysfunctional therapy are rare, and consequently are not represented here by a circle. With regard to chronic patients, the two figures represent the two extremes: there is an infinite variety of relationships between the three major spheres.

malignancy, fractures, and spondylolisthesis (see the corresponding box in the upper left corner of the algorithm). The history (anamnesis) given by the patient is the most important tool in identifying these conditions; the classical aspects of the history, alerting the therapist to potential red-flag conditions (Della-Giustina 1999), are described in several publications (Della-Giustina and Kilcline 2000, Deyo and Weinstein 2001). Laboratory or radiological investigations as a response to red flags may be initiated at the first visit or at any point throughout the algorithm. However, they are unnecessary in the majority of acute low-back pain patients after relevant screening questions for red flag conditions. (*Author's note*: Kuchera discusses features that suggest dysfunction(s) in Chapters 2.2.1 and 3.3.)

Another important issue is whether the condition in question is traumatic or spontaneous in onset. In this algorithm, as illustrated by the short but thick arrow from the 'trauma' box, a consequence of the first consultation is that the majority of the patients will be managed (in the 'dysfunctional' sphere) according to the same principles whether there is a history of trauma or not. This is because there are virtually always gentle manual techniques for which trauma is no contraindication, when they are adjusted to the specific situation. Only a small minority of the patients, particularly after major trauma, but also for instance when a herniated disc is suspected, needs to undergo radiological examination to confirm/reject red flags or exclude fractures before antidysfunctional treatment is begun. In most cases, after radiological examination, as illustrated by the thick arrow from the '(neuro)radiological investigation' box, the patients are allocated to the 'dysfunction' box, and will thereafter follow the same path through the algorithm as other patients with dysfunctional conditions.

In principle, with respect to radiography and neuroradiological imaging, we apply the criteria recommended in major evidence-based reports and consensus documents (Waddell 1998, Nachemson and Jonsson 2000). Neuroradiological imaging is regarded as a preoperative investigation. We use such investigations only if the clinical findings and history clearly indicate, for instance, a herniated disc. Furthermore, the expected benefit from an operation should be weighed against the risk taken (the 'cost/benefit' analysis). Not only does the demonstration of structural pathology such as disc prolapse by MRI *not* change the management strategy, pathomorphologically focused investigations also incur a specific risk of transferring fear and passivity to the patient. Routinely refraining from diagnostic imaging is in itself behavioural therapy, and the result of a well-developed metacognitive process. On rare occasions (neuro)radiological investigations are prescribed on psychological indications. However, such investigations should never be initiated just to satisfy the curiosity of the physician/physiotherapist or the patient.

At STAYAC, the antidysfunctional investigation over time is virtually always completed before any additional investigations are undertaken, and such measures are not needed when patients recover satisfactorily. This approach restricts the need for MR/CT, radiography, and laboratory tests to a minimum – neuroradiological investigations may of course be carried out at any point in the algorithm, not only at the first visit.

In the early phases only a few patients, whose complaints are not understandable or treatable from either a dysfunction or a pathomorphological perspective, i.e. their pain is unexplained, are allocated to the 'idiopathic pain' box. Since only a tiny minority of the trauma subjects are allocated to the 'pathomorphological' box, after the initial triage has been undertaken, almost all patients are allocated to the 'dysfunction' box. Note that the diagnosis 'non-specific' (benign) (back) pain – the dominating diagnosis within today's traditional (back) pain care paradigm, not least within primary health care and in other current algorithms – is not used at all in the STAYAC algorithm.

The 'pathomorphology' box

It is necessary to decide whether the pathomorphology is an isolated condition or if there are also markers of dysfunction. This step differentiates the STAYAC algorithm from other methods and is important because, even in the presence of pathomorphology (sometimes major, such as acute vertebral compression fractures), the dysfunctions are treated within this algorithm. In this context, suspected or confirmed herniated discs are the most frequent pathomorphology, but the same reasoning is also valid for spinal stenosis or spondylolisthesis. By contrast, in other manual treatment programmes, important dysfunctions and injection sites are not only left undiagnosed, they are also untreated. In these situations the possibility of referred pain from soft tissue irritations, mimicking true radicular pain, symptomatic spinal stenosis, or symptomatic spondylolisthesis is not considered. In traditional Swedish manual therapy, these patients are more or less exclusively treated by auto-traction (Lind 1974, Natchew 1984), and/ or by nerve mobilization techniques according to Elvey and Butler. (*Editor's note:* See Butler, Chapter 4.3.7.) At STAYAC, these techniques are rarely found to be effective if the dysfunctions and/or relevant sites of irritation are not treated first. Consequently, in the STAYAC algorithm, there is an important flow from the 'combined pathomorphology/ dysfunction(s)' box to the 'antidysfunctional (re-functional)' box, where the patients are managed in a similar fashion to those with dysfunctional symptoms only. This approach is controversial, since it goes against conventional manual treatment algorithms, where several pathomorphological conditions, especially herniated discs, are considered strong contraindications for manipulation and specific mobilization. Our manual techniques range from relatively forceful thrust techniques to extremely gentle techniques. The 'traditional' Scandinavian concept of locking techniques (Evjent and Hamberg 1985a, 1985b, Kaltenborn and Evjent 1993), aimed at optimizing the possibilities of directing the therapeutic forces exclusively to the dysfunctional segment, are applied and, in addition, muscle energy principles are integrated. As a consequence, these techniques may be applied to conditions such as herniated discs, spinal stenosis, spondylolisthesis, postoperative conditions, or even neighbouring acute compression fractures. Even patients with clinically relevant disc herniations, and in the presence of neurological signs from nerve root compression, and a classical positive Lasègue's sign of less than 30°, may be treated manually. When required, even rotational techniques in flexion and side-bending are applied in vertebral segments with MR-verified herniated discs. In these cases, gentle techniques are of course favoured, but, when indicated, thrust techniques may also be applied. It should be emphasized that this statement does *not* concern treatment manoeuvres outside the STAYAC algorithm – we use non-locking techniques infrequently, and we have no experience of treating patients with coexistent pathomorphological conditions by means of non-specific techniques or therapeutic manoeuvres in which locking techniques are *not* applied. These manual techniques act only by treating dysfunctions and are not believed to influence pathomorphological conditions *per se*. This approach to combined dysfunctional/ pathomorphological conditions may explain why our algorithm has been more successful than other related methods assessed in RCTs, not least those in which, as in our group's studies, unselected patient populations were recruited (Skargren, Öberg *et al.* 1997, Cherkin, Deyo *et al.* 1998, Seferlis, Németh *et al.* 1998, Rasmussen-Barr 2003).

The locking techniques referred to in this chapter are of Norwegian origin, and (to my knowledge) only published in Scandinavia (Evjent and Hamberg 1985a, 1985b, Kaltenborn and Evjent 1993) and only taught by Scandinavians (e.g. outside Scandinavia by Olav Evjent and the Ola Grimsby Institute). As these techniques may be important for our group's unique results, it is important to appreciate that the locking techniques used at STAYAC seem to be different from manipulation and mobilization techniques used elsewhere in the world.

Another important difference between the STAYAC algorithm and some other schools of manual therapy is that we almost always choose three-dimensional locking techniques in the most painful and movement-restricted direction (unlike some manual therapy philosophies, where treatment is preferably given in the pain-free direction). We state that treatment in the painful direction is more effective as well as timesaving. This is facilitated through the wide variety of different techniques including extremely gentle procedures with a combination of hold/relax, and muscle energy techniques, including coupled eye movements and synchronized breathing (Mitchel, Moran *et al.* 1979), in fact allowing patients to treat themselves with no application of external forces by the therapists whatsoever. Rarely, treatment in the painful direction is impossible; in those patients, according to the pragmatic principle, we simply try another direction first, and later the (previously) painful direction, by which stage the dysfunction has resolved. Since the dysfunction has not infrequently already resolved after treatment in the 'wrong' direction, this subsequent treatment in the 'painful' direction is not always necessary.

A common reason for therapeutic failures within manual therapy is over-emphasis on discogenic/true radicular symptoms. This is not only a problem in the lower back region, but also in patients with neck pain. In Sweden, this problem has paralleled the rapid dissemination of Butler's/Elvey's diagnostic and therapeutic principles among physiotherapists during the last decade. These principles have questionable validity with respect to reduced sliding of the nerves in their sheaths that they were at one time assumed to measure and treat. This statement is substantiated by the fact that, during the patient's progress through the STAYAC algorithm, positive 'nerve stretch tests' are frequently normalized even though no specific nerve 'mobilization' techniques have been applied. This normalization of the tests frequently is paralleled by disappearance of diffuse and complex peripheral, central, and general symptoms other than pain. Consequently, these observations suggest that positive 'nerve stretch tests' are not contraindications to manual treatment of symptomatic dysfunctions. Despite this (and the fact that there appears to be a limited evidence base for neural mobilisation), neural tension tests/treatment may indeed be useful (for instance in monitoring the progress of treatment, and sometimes as a therapeutic measure). However, therapists are often needlessly alarmed by positive 'nerve stretch tests', interpreting them as indicating true nerve impingement, as a consequence of which they refrain from treating symptomatic vertebral and pelvic dysfunctions. Undue reliance on these tests in deciding which type of treatment should or should not be applied may have a negative effect on the overall treatment results. Dysfunctional aspects of the patient's suffering may not even be considered. I do not claim that Butler and Elvey necessarily caused this problem; it may very well be the case that some physiotherapists have misinterpreted their therapeutic approach. Indeed, the Butler–Elvey methodology is included in the STAYAC algorithm, rarely as a primary method, but late in the algorithm. The reason for this is that our experience suggests that in the antidysfunctional sphere treatments such as manipulation, injections, and muscle stretching are considerably more effective. (*Editor's note:* For Butler's current thoughts on neurodynamics, see Chapters 2.2.4 and 4.3.7.)

In parallel with the popularity of neural mobilization in Sweden in recent years has been a heavy reliance on transversus abdominus exercises (Hodges 2004). However, they should be used within the stay-active concept, and not replace effective antidysfunctional therapy. In conclusion, within the STAYAC concept numerous 'contra-indications' to manual therapy have been abolished, of which only a few are mentioned here.

The 'antidysfunctional treatment' box – the antidysfunctional stack

The core, although not necessarily always the most important part, of the STAYAC algorithm is manual therapy. If there are markers of dysfunction, different kinds of manipulation and/or specific mobilization are applied as the first measure in virtually all patients. Of course there are exceptions. In some cases it is obvious that manual therapy is not the appropriate primary treatment measure – physical exercises may be the preferable basic treatment, and specific manual therapy may be undertaken later.

Virtually all subjects referred to a clinic like STAYAC are in need of exercise. Even though the basic principle has to be the elimination of markers of dysfunction before initiation of physical exercise, this means that physical exercise is frequently initiated from the beginning of the antidysfunctional investigation, in parallel with the measures in the antidysfunctional domain. In other patients, the main problem is depression or psycho-existentially based conditions, requiring anti-depressant medication and/or cognitive–behavioural measures res-pectively. Specific mobilizing exercises with the same intent as manipulation/specific mobilization, aiming at optimizing the treatment results and preserving increased mobility, are frequently taught to patients as an important part of the home care programme. All the other boxes under the 'antidysfunctional box' belong to the antidys-functional stack (situated centrally in the algorithm).

The term **green flags** (not found in PubMed, Cochrane Library, or Embase) is used here for markers of dysfunction and, consequently, implies dysfunctional conditions (see corresponding box in the algo-rithm). In addition, this term also covers features in the patients' history indicating dysfunctional conditions (Editor's note: see Kuchera, Chapters 2.2.1 and 3.3). Green flag conditions are therefore synonymous with dysfunctional conditions. One advantage of this term is avoidance of confusion in contexts where 'dysfunction' is equivalent to 'disability'.

The antidysfunctional investigation

A **trial treatment,** for instance a thrust manoeuvre, is provided accord-ing to identified markers of dysfunction (green flags); if an obvious positive treatment result is achieved, the provisional diagnosis is veri-fied – this is called a **green light**. The diagnostic procedure is carried out over time, during which a series of provisional working hypo-theses (i.e. functional diagnoses) are either verified (green light, yellow light A, yellow light B; see below) or disproved (red light), depending on the response to treatment. **Red light** means no improvement, or even deterioration. Provocation of symptoms after manual treatment is not uncommon; however, in most cases the post-treatment pain subsides rapidly, and in others the provoked pain disappears with steroid injections. The most frequent example in this context is (some-times radiating) pain after lumbar/pelvic manipulation, which is almost always a provocation of parasacrococcygeal structures and should not be misinterpreted as radicular pain, and which seems unavoidable. In these cases, steroid injections in the appropriate area are extremely effective. Rarely, the provoked pain persists for up to a few weeks, but in 20 years we have seen only a couple of long-term deteriorations, and none of them had demonstrable true radicular pain.

The **yellow light A** and **yellow light B** outcomes indicate that treat-ment is on the right track, i.e. a substantial or temporary improve-ment, but the symptoms are not yet entirely under control. In the yellow light A situation, the patient is improved or pain-free, but only for a limited period, for example a couple of days, and the markers of dysfunction (green flags) that disappeared immediately after the former treatment have recurred. The treatment may be repeated once or twice, but according to the STAYAC algorithm, not at subsequent visits without a reassessment of the functional diagnosis. In the yellow light B situation, the patient is persistently improved, the markers of dysfunction (green flags) at the previous visit are still absent, but there are residual symptoms still interfering with quality of life, everyday activities, or working capability. Again, the functional diagnosis and alternative strategies have to be reviewed.

Thus, the treatment hypotheses (i.e. the trial treatments) are continuously revised, and changed when needed. In patients with complex pain, the dysfunctional, pathomorphological, and psycho-existential dimensions of the condition are comprehensively mapped – this process is called the **antidysfunctional investigation**. The pro-cedure may take months. All available methods are tried in 'difficult' cases, as long as markers of dysfunction (green flags) persist. However, during this process, the passivizing risks have to be minimized by applying the stay-active concept from the first visit and, in addition, introducing physical exercises and the home care programme early. By contrast, a simple dysfunctional case is 'mapped' after a single treatment and a final consultation at which no further treatment is required (green light situation).

Our ultra-pragmatic approach recognizes that our tests can only determine in which order we try the different items of a complete treatment arsenal. In theory, all treatment modalities in the algorithm should be tried before concluding that there is nothing more to offer the patient in question, who thereby is entirely therapy-resistant; this process is in fact the only absolutely reliable manner to ensure that no treatment possibility is missed. In practice, this is not possible, but it is useful to keep in mind that the different items have to be tried systematically in a specified order according to the algorithm.

Idiopathic pain – *ex juvantibus* diagnosis

Another important, although relatively rare, pathway in the algorithm is from idiopathic pain to the antidysfunctional investigation box. The principle of *ex juvantibus* **diagnosis** is applied. The term '*ex juvan-tibus*' is applied when a diagnostic procedure/investigation does not lead to a clear diagnosis, but, despite this, a trial treatment is provided according to a hypothetical functional diagnosis; if an obvious positive treat-ment result is achieved, the provisional diagnosis is verified. In common with other antidysfunctional investigation, *ex juvantibus* dia-gnosis is a procedure that goes on over time during which a series of provisional/work hypotheses are either verified or disproved, depend-ing on the response to treatment. Otherwise, there are no differences between the regular antidysfunctional investigation and the ultra-pragmatic *ex juvantibus* principle.

In the pragmatically based STAYAC algorithm, the *ex juvantibus* diagnostic principle is applied consistently and systematically in vir-tually all patients. An example is pain with a distribution consistent with sacroiliac joint pain in a subject free from markers of dysfunction (green flags), and also no provocation pain from the sacroiliac joint. In this situation, a diagnostic injection (hopefully curative as well) of steroids and local anaesthetic may be given to the sacroiliac joint. A positive response, particularly if it persists, supports a diagnosis of sacroiliac joint 'irritation'. (A positive response to the injection does not indicate that a truly inflammatory condition has been treated.) An injection of 1 ml local anaesthetic and 1 ml steroid into the sacroiliac joint may eliminate pain not only momentarily, but even permanently. This is true for pain localized to the region of the sacroiliac joint as well as for radiating pain (sometimes as far as the foot) in the presence of a positive straight leg raising test. Consequently, where there has been a differential diagnosis of true radicular pain due to disc herniation, unnecessary (and therefore unsuccessful) surgery due to an asymptomatic disc herniation is avoided. In fact, this pragmatic measure may be the only reliable method to detect whether or not a herniated disc is symptomatic.

Another clinically important example of *ex juvantibus* diagnosis and treatment is the not unusual case of buttock pain, especially on sitting (particularly in a car), from the anatomical region of the ischial tuberosity. No remaining markers of dysfunction are present, there are no injection sites, range of movement in the hip joint is normal, there is no local tenderness and so forth. According to our stretching philosophy (Evjent and Hamberg 1985a, 1985b), there are four different stretching manoeuvres for the short extensors of the hip joint; these are tested, and the most painful and perhaps most restricted one is chosen. The corresponding home exercise is taught. Although we do not know which structures are affected in these cases – it could be the hip joint, capsule, muscle(s), or nerves – this may be the only effective treatment, and, in addition, an excellent example of pragmatically based therapy.

Another example is the situation in which the diagnostic signs do not confirm L5 dysfunction. In some obese patients and in patients with well-developed musculature, a reliable segmental manual functional diagnosis is impossible, but despite this, a manipulation in the four different possible three-dimensional physiological directions is undertaken. If this is effective, it verifies an L5 dysfunction. In other situations, a trochanter belt (Figure 4.4.5) is sometimes successfully tried in cases without recurring markers of pelvic dysfunction (see page 523). Autotraction may be tried in any patient with low back pain, sometimes most effectively in spite of the absence of clinical signs of a herniated disc including radiating pain. (According to conventional wisdom, autotraction is applied only in patients with radiating pain with a more or less clear nerve-root distribution and focal neurological signs.)

There are of course also patients with true idiopathic conditions in which the STAYAC concept cannot offer any specific treatment, because they do not respond positively to antidysfunctional investigation or to *ex juvantibus* treatment. They are represented by the vertical

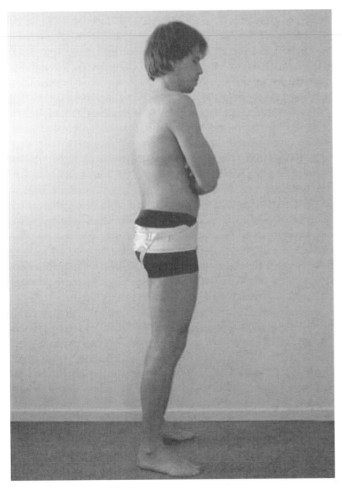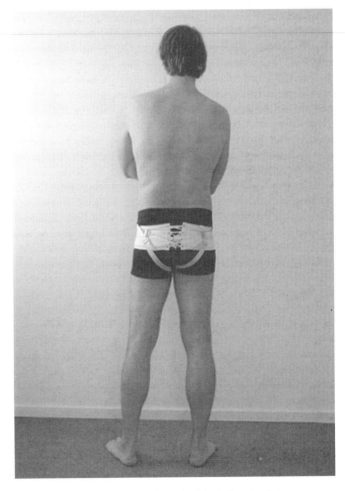

Figure 4.4.5 A trochanter belt is used following manipulation in both male and female patients with recurring markers of pelvic dysfunction. It is non-stretchable, strapped on with permanent fasteners, and with groin straps to prevent the belt from sliding upwards (Camp, 'Tro-Camp').

'idiopathic pain' box in the lower middle of the algorithm. In these patients only non-specific adjuvant treatment, the stay-active concept, behavioural strategies, physical exercise, and sometimes psychotherapeutic measures can be applied, with the intention of reducing the unwelcome consequences of the conditions. Applying the STAYAC algorithm in these patients consistently reduces to a minimum the risk of missing treatable conditions and thereby optimizes the number of patients whose symptoms cannot be brought under control.

In addition, there is a feedback flow from the 'psycho-existential sphere' to the 'antidysfunctional treatment' box: in Figure 4.4.1, all the arrows from the 'psycho-existential sphere' coalesce in a common long feedback loop far to the left, which continues all the way back to the 'antidysfunctional treatment' box; see the smaller descending arrow close to the left of the thick arrow from the 'dysfunction box' to the 'antidysfunctional domain'. This feedback loop takes account of patients in the 'psycho-existential sphere' in (renewed) need of antidysfunctional treatment, not least those who were subjected to physical exercise as the initial main management early in the antidysfunctional investigation.

Yellow light B situations

Steroid injections

Frequently, antidysfunctional treatment, such as manipulation, soon leads to a 'dysfunction-free state' followed by freedom from pain and other associated complaints. However, despite the apparent resolution of dysfunction, pain will persist in a group of patients. **This is when a steroid injection should be considered, not earlier.** Steroid injections undertaken in patients with ongoing dysfunctions are considerably less effective, and, in addition, long-term effects seem to be limited or non-existent. As indicated by the 'steroid injections (trial)' box (on the far right in the middle of the algorithm, Figure 4.4.1), there is one rare exception: steroid injections are sometimes tried as a 'secondary prevention' measure when other such moves have failed to achieving a dysfunction-free state; occasionally the phenomenon of recurring dysfunctions is brought to an end in this way.

Not all patients need steroid injections: approximately 40–50% of the most severely affected patients with acute/subacute low back pain are treated by steroid injections (Blomberg, Hallin *et al.* 1994, Grunnesjö, Blomberg *et al.* 2004c). Consequently, there is an important 'shortcut' from 'still in pain' to 'muscle stretching'. Moreover, as represented in the algorithm by the arrow in the reverse direction, some patients who have primarily been managed by physiotherapists are referred for steroid injections when treatment has not been sufficiently effective. The flow of patients between doctors and physiotherapists works best when both disciplines have been trained in the indications, limitations, and effectiveness of each other's treatment methods. This is achieved by training doctors and physiotherapists together in shared courses, covering the needs of both professional groups, an important approach within the STAYAC concept. Since, in spite of its complex structure, the STAYAC algorithm is still a simplification of the clinical reality in which therapists are educated in the pragmatic treatment programme, there are many more 'shortcuts' that are exceptions to the main flows, and which for simplicity are not included in the algorithm. Dotted arrows to the right of the antidysfunctional sphere indicate some of the less frequent shortcuts. The most important of these is the one on the far right: the small subgroup of patients suffering from significant idiopathic pain enters the antidysfunctional sphere, follows the thick arrow directly to the 'dys-

function free' and 'still in pain' boxes and, as indicated by the vertical 'idiopathic pain' box below in the middle of the algorithm, proceeds to the psycho-existential zone, via a connection to the ascending arrow collecting all the arrows from the different levels of the antidysfunctional sphere to the psycho-existential domain. A second fairly important shortcut is the one from 'still in pain' directly to 'autotraction'. This refers to the tiny minority of patients with verified herniated discs, but without any treatable dysfunctions; they are directed from the 'no dysfunctions' box (in the upper right corner of the algorithm) (see corresponding dotted arrow from this box connecting to the thick arrow from the box of 'combined with dysfunction(s)') to antidysfunctional treatment. Thereafter, the flow follows the main route to 'still in pain', and to autotraction. The patients are either non-surgical cases or candidates for operation, but, with the aim of avoiding surgery, autotraction and/or nerve mobilization are tried first. The *ex juvantibus* principle may be applied in cases with a suspected symptomatic herniated disc.

When steroid injections are applied in a dysfunction-free state, they are usually effective, and the effect is persistent. In the few cases that are refractory to steroid injections, or in whom the steroid effect is only temporary (some weeks), wet needling (i.e. with local anaesthetics, 5–6 times, 5–10 days in between, and with a steroid on the first occasion) to the structure(s) in question is provided. The most common sites for series of wet needling are the piriformis and the teres minor muscles, lateral epicondylalgia ('epicondylitis'), and the origin of the patellar tendon in the condition of apex patellae ('apicitis', 'patellalgia'). Although some authorities claim that this is incorrect, the periosteum should, in my opinion, be intensively needled, a procedure that definitely reinforces the treatment results. Dry needling without local anaesthetic (Lewit 1991) is infrequently applied at STAYAC, since it is less effective than wet needling. For optimized therapeutic effects of extra-articular injections (with the exception of parasacrococcygeal injections), wet needling should always combine local anaesthetic with steroid. In addition, the muscle in question is always stretched after injection with local anaesthesia. Combined treatments are a STAYAC trademark.

According to the literature (Zulian, Martini *et al.* 2003), triamcinolone hexacetonide is the drug of choice, often in combination with needling and local anaesthetics (prilocaine is normally used at STAYAC). The injections are given according to manual diagnostic findings, i.e. pain by palpation, isometric contraction, and/or stretching. However, according to the ultra-pragmatic approach, to avoid over-reliance on the predictive value of clinical findings, only one of these diagnostic requirements needs to be fulfilled, and sometimes not even that. Sometimes the *ex juvantibus* principle is applied, i.e. the treatment is given although none of these signs is present.

Several types of injection are undertaken at STAYAC. Some examples of important injection sites in the lower back region are listed in the box. (All these 'irritations' are rarely seen without a co-existent lumbar/pelvic dysfunction. According to the pragmatic STAYAC principle, in which dysfunctions are considered to represent disturbances of postural control organization, it is not possible to distinguish between lumbar and pelvic dysfunctions; they always come together).

The most important and most frequent injection, which is probably unique to the STAYAC concept is described in detail. This injection – to painful and sometimes spastic parasacrococcygeal structures – is responsible for a good deal of our treatment results. 'Parasacrococcygeal' is preferred to the more common term 'paracoccygeal' as the injection site is most frequently located more cranially in the area of the apex of the sacrum and near the cranial part of the coccyx, not

Some examples of injection sites in the lower back region

Dorsal aspect of the lower back and pelvis in order of frequency:

- Parasacrococcygeal structures
- Painful insertions on the greater trochanter of the piriformis muscle (also, less frequently, the origin/insertion of gluteus medius/minimus and the submedius bursa)
- Sacroiliac joint (provocation-positive but dysfunction-free)
- Muscle insertions and other structures on the ischial tuberosity
- 'Kissing spines' (i.e. interspinal tenderness, considered by some authors a bursitis)
- Origin of tensor fascia lata (lateral aspect)
- Transverse processes
- Iliolumbar ligaments*
- Posterior sacroiliac ligaments
- Epidural steroid injections**

Anterior aspect of the lower back and pelvis in order of frequency

- Hip joint
- Bursa iliopectinea
- All adductors (most frequently the adductor longus)
- Lateral femoral cutaneous nerve (in meralgia paresthetica)
- Ilioinguinal nerve.

* The iliolumbar ligaments attach to the anterior aspect of os ilia and are reachable with an 80-mm needle. Injections into tender soft tissues in this anatomical area are frequently to muscular structures. Nevertheless, they may sometimes prove beneficial. However, cases of significant hyper-reactivity in the lower lumbar spine usually manifest considerable tenderness here, resulting in only temporary effects from steroid injections. Despite this, injection may be tried, although not repetitively.

** Epidural steroid injections (through hiatus sacralis) are an important contribution to the STAYAC algorithm. However, this measure is introduced later than other steroid injections, after autotraction and never as a primary measure. Epidural injections are needed in only a tiny minority of the patients as a late move in the antidysfunctional investigation. The approach is pragmatic, i.e. it may, at an appropriate point of time, be applied in any patient with low back pain, not only when radicular pain or dural irritation is suspected.

only adjacent to the latter. Cyriax (1970) stated that the sacrotuberous and sacrospinal ligaments were common foci for pain, but it is obvious that contractile tissues also are involved. This anatomical region does indeed incorporate the origins of the sacrotuberous and sacrospinal ligaments, but also the musculus coccygeus and musculus levator ani pars iliaca and maybe also the origin of the piriformis muscle. To my knowledge, this area was first described as a site for (bimanual) injection by the late Sven-Otto Myrin (Myrin 1972), and the bimanual injection technique seems to have been developed by him in the 1960s (he taught me the technique in 1985). Originally the

patient lay on one side, but prone positioning seems more functional. The needle is usually introduced through the skin about 2 cm below crena ani and 1 cm lateral to the midline. To simplify the manoeuvre, the medial/upper part of the buttock is pushed away from the midline with the thumb of the hand palpating the rectum. In this way the distance from the surface of the skin to the bone is rarely more than 1 cm and a 0.7 mm × 50 mm needle is almost always sufficient. (On rare occasions, a 0.8 mm × 80 mm needle is needed.) After bone contact with the apex of the sacrum is made, the needle penetrates further laterally/caudally in the tissues. During this process, the tip of the needle is palpated by the gloved index finger of the other hand, which is inserted in the patient's rectum. The distance between the index finger and the tip of the needle is probably a few millimetres. A quick oscillation of the syringe and the needle with minimal amplitude makes it easier to palpate the tip of the needle *per rectum*. One millilitre of steroid and 5–10 ml of local anaesthetic is injected on the affected side. (Bilateral irritation is considerably more common than unilateral pain.) The injected fluid should be spread in the area while successively re-penetrating the needle in a fan-shaped pattern. Note that the skin is penetrated only once on each side. The most painful parts of the area are injected, which frequently means (a) the entire area as described above, but, not uncommonly, only (b) the tissue adjacent to the inferior lateral angle of the apex sacri or (c) the lateral and somewhat more distant parts. The bimanual injection technique seems necessary in order to enable the steroid to be injected deeply enough to affect the symptomatic tissue. In STAYAC, where nine different physicians altogether have provided at least 10 000 parasacrococcygeal injections since 1985, no complications have ever been observed. After the injection, the parasacrococcygeal structures are also stretched *per rectum* (Midttun, Bojsen-Traeden *et al.* 1983), a method that can be used as a primary alternative to the injection described above. However, parasacrococcygeal stretching seems to be less effective and frequently, in our experience, has to be repeated 4–5 times; in addition, applied as a primary measure, the stretching is considerably more painful than the injection. (Stretching the structures after local anaesthetic has been injected is not painful.) Tissue irritation in this region (the posterior part of the pelvic floor) is a common cause of pseudoradicular pain in the leg, frequently extending all the way down to the foot. Referred pain frequently emanates from irritable foci at the insertion of the piriformis muscle and from sacroiliac joints, in addition to the parasacrococcygeal structures. In some patients, particularly those who have not received appropriate treatment for a long time, all three irritable foci have to be injected. The clinical picture seems repeatedly to be misinterpreted as true radicular pain, and there is an obvious risk of operation for an asymptomatic herniated disc. **In fact this pragmatic measure may be the only reliable method of finding out whether a herniated disc is symptomatic.**

In patients in whom the steroids achieve merely temporary effects, the parasacrococcygeal structures may be re-injected once or twice, not more. If the tenderness persists, after a series of 5–6 parasacrococcygeal *per rectum* stretching sessions (habitually performed by our physiotherapists), the situation is usually resolved. Occasionally this procedure is extremely painful, and under these circumstances a physician takes care of the stretching series, each time after local anaesthesia (no steroid), administered in the same manner as the usual parasacrococcygeal injections. Botulinum toxin has recently been used instead of steroids but, despite seemingly good results (maybe even better than steroids), it is too early to be certain of its effectiveness.

Table 4.4.1. Needle sizes, volumes of steroid, and local anaesthetic for some of the most common injections

Structure	Triamcinolone (ml)	Prilocaine (ml)	Needle size (mm)
Lig. iliolumbale	1 (20 mg)	4–10 (unilateral injection)	0.8 × 80 (0.7 × 50)
Parasacrococcygeal inj.	1 per side	5–10 per side	0.7 × 50 (0.8 × 80)
Sacroiliac joint	1	1	0.8 × 80
Piriformis	1	4–6	0.7 × 50 (0.8 × 80)
Tensor fascia latae	1	4–6	0.7 × 50
Hip joint	2	3–4	0.8 × 80
Bursa iliopectinea	1	4–6	0.7 × 50
Adductor longus origin	1	2–6	0.7 × 50
Lev. scapulae, insertion	1	3–4	0.7 × 50
Teres minor, insertion	1	2–4	0.7 × 50
Supraspinatus, insertion	1	2–4	0.7 × 50
Subacromial bursa	1	3–4	0.7 × 50
Acromioclavicular joint	0.5–0.7	0[a]	Intracutanous needle
Lat. epicondalgia	1	2–4	0.7 × 30
Med. epicondalgia	1	2–3	0.7 × 30
Kissing spines	1	1–2	0.7 × 50

[a] There is no room for local anaesthetics in this small joint. Preferably, anesthetize the skin and deeper structures such as the periosteum with 2–3 ml of prilocaine before injecting the joint (particularly if you are not fully trained in injection techniques). Other small joints in which the same method may be applied are the finger joints, the toe joints, and the sacrococcygeal joint. In many joints, injection is facilitated by letting an assistant (physiotherapist or nurse) apply traction simultaneously with the injection procedure (not only in small joints, but also in the hip joint, shoulder joint and subacromial bursa, ankle joint, etc.)

From the general principles listed in Table 4.4.1, it should be possible to estimate reasonable procedures when injecting other locations. According to our latest outcome study (to be published) the average number of injections per patient, including the most severely troubled patient category, is 1.9 (0.29 injections per visit), a moderate number in comparison to what is provided in some pain clinics.

How do steroids exert their effects?

Only a tiny minority of extra-articular irritations are true inflammations, deserving an '-itis' suffix. Consequently, leading rheumatologists suggest the abolition of terms such as 'epicondylitis', and suggest 'epicondalgia' and 'tendalgia'. From a behavioural perspective, this is important. Using words stronger than necessary in communication with patients, implying that a patient is sicker than they actually are, may influence them negatively, i.e. in a stay-passive direction. Furthermore, if the physician/therapist thinks in terms of inflammation, the risk of subconscious transferring of stay-passive messages increases (insufficient metacognition and lateral thinking). Regrettably, limiting regimens due to this phenomenon are also frequently conveyed consciously. In communication with the patient, the word 'irritation' (of a muscle insertion, for instance) should be used. If a steroid injection is curative, it does not necessarily mean that a true inflammatory condition was eliminated; there are other, largely unknown, mechanisms suggesting that only a minor part of the entire inflammatory complex, e.g. antiprostaglandin effects, is involved. For the time being, as long as we have not identified a true inflammatory condition for sure, the soft tissue irritations are regarded as dysfunctions. Again, this illustrates the metacognitive aspects of the STAYAC approach.

Alternatives to steroid injections

There are numerous alternative treatment modalities that may be used instead of steroid injections at this stage although in general they are less effective: function massage, deep frictions, acupuncture, intramuscular stimulation (Gunn 1996), dry needling, wet needling (with local anaesthetics), transcutaneous nerve stimulation, transcutaneous electrical muscular stimulation, therapeutic ultrasound, etc. With the exception of needling they may be undertaken by physiotherapists with appropriate training. These methods are not infrequently used within the STAYAC concept, but never as primary methods; in the presence of ongoing dysfunctions, such management will certainly offer poor treatment results and is not cost-effective.

Which method is used is to a large extent a matter of personal preference. However, one has to be prepared to repeat the treatment, and in many patients a steroid injection will be necessary in the end anyway. Consequently, administering steroids from the beginning of this phase in the antidysfunctional investigation (in a dysfunction-free state) is obviously more cost-effective. Steroid injections may, however, be viewed as aggressive (not least by some patients). This is irrational; in reality, depot steroids have negligible side effects and complications (not least in comparison with the NSAIDs and opioids frequently used outside the STAYAC approach). Every physician has to develop an educational model to handle patients' scepticism. Preferably, this is done in the 'patient education' groups (see page 530).

Few physicians are adequately trained for these procedures: in order not to overload them, it is valuable for physiotherapists to have access to alternative treatments, which they may try before asking their cooperating physician to administer steroid injections.

Acupuncture

Acupuncture sometimes appears to be the only effective treatment, apart from graded physical exercise in moderate cases, especially in the cases of widespread regional muscle tenderness (dysfunction-free state), provided the acupuncturist is adequately trained and has satisfactory experience in this technique. Having scrutinized the results of different acupuncturists in the clinic for many years, I am now convinced that the original Chinese/Eastern mode of acupuncture is superior to acupuncture adapted to the Western biomedical paradigm, despite the lack of hard evidence indicating this.

The muscle tenderness referred to above is frequently described as 'myofascial' pain. Unfortunately, at least in Sweden, this term has become overused, and, according to our experience, too much focus on acupuncture (or intramuscular stimulation) as a single 'silver bullet' therapy yields poor and cost-ineffective treatment results. As usual within the STAYAC concept, other dysfunctions have to be treated first. In many patients all the trigger points in the back muscles, from the lower back up to the neck, disappear seconds after manual treatment of lower lumbar and pelvic dysfunctions. Consequently, within the STAYAC concept, trigger and tender points are considered a secondary manifestation of the more or less generalized electrical chaos in the postural system, not viewed as primary conditions.

Consistently disappointed by poor treatment results from dry needling of trigger points, I now inject trigger points with steroids (since triamcinolone hexacetonide is not to be administered intramuscularly, methylprednisolone is used), and local anaesthetics – but only when physiotherapists ask me to do so after having tried everything else without benefit.

In conclusion, in a fairly small subgroup of our patients, Chinese/Eastern acupuncture is an essential treatment method. Intramuscular stimulation is probably a useful alternative to acupuncture at this stage.

Muscle stretching: first indication

Muscle stretching, according to the 'first indication' (see corresponding box in the algorithm), is shown as an alternative or complementary treatment to the injections. The theoretical rationales for muscle stretching are that dysfunctionally shortened muscles may be an important source of pain (at their origin, belly, and/or insertion), and that they may secondarily cause joint, joint capsule, or ligament pain (or disseminated diffuse pain in a system of joints) by altering the biomechanics, even in the absence of diagnosable dysfunctions. Examples are pain from the thoracolumbar junction due to shortened iliopsoas muscle(s), and knee pain due to shortened muscles involved in knee function. The stretching approach applied within the STAYAC concept, which seems to be the most advanced one available, has been developed by Evjent and Hamberg (1985a, 1985b). Stretching is an important treatment in all regions of the body, including the hands and feet. An essential difference between this model and some other stretching philosophies is that even considerable pain in the muscle in question is allowed, as long as the patient can tolerate it, and in spite of the pain is able to relax the muscle during the stretching phase. This procedure is timesaving and more effective, particularly in patients with considerable shortening of muscles in whom it is impossible to make progress with pain-free stretching, whether therapeutic or as home exercises. Only dysfunctionally shortened muscles are stretchable. Contrary to what some authorities claim, it is virtually impossible to damage muscles or any other anatomical structures during muscle stretching. In contractures (i.e. pathomorphology with permanently changed plasticity), only

further shortening may be counteracted, and in spastic muscles e.g. due to disturbed (dysfunctional) complex neuromuscular reflex patterns in the postural control system, muscle stretching may provoke pain, and the treatment results are poor.

One important issue is whether or not we really stretch muscles. Analogous reasoning has to be applied as in the case of neurodynamics according to Elvey and Butler: a lot of structures may be stretched other than muscles: nerves, fasciae, veins, arteries, skin, fat, other subcutaneous tissues, and so forth. A further possible mechanism for the beneficial effects of muscle stretching is the posturoproprioceptive model (described in 'Antidysfunctional treatment, p. 509) in which it is logical to stretch muscles that may not even be shortened. If and when 'muscle stretching' becomes evidence-based, further fundamental research may be able to map out the underlying mechanisms.

Home exercises aiming at optimizing the treatment results and preserving the increased muscle lengths are almost always taught to the patients as an important part of the home care programme. This is true also with respect to muscle stretching according to the 'second indication'. The Evjent/Hamberg 'autostretching' book (Evjent and Hamberg 1990) covers advanced stretching techniques for iliocrural muscles and all muscles of the extremities, as well as specific mobilizing exercises for the entire spine including locking techniques. In addition, some other home exercises are included in our home programmes (Lewit 1991).

The 'non-specific pain treatment' box

The constituents of the 'non-specific pain treatment' box are primarily those associated with medical disciplines outside manual medicine/manual therapy. Since all these methods are considerably less effective than other items in the antidysfunctional sphere, especially if applied as primary measures, they have a comparably minor role in the STAYAC algorithm. Medication (for example, diazepam as a muscle relaxant, or opioids) is only occasionally used as a primary measure, usually to facilitate specific treatment in extremely acute cases of neck or back pain with significant regional muscle spasm. Other methods of handling such situations are strictly applied muscle energy principles (sometimes this works better than thrust techniques) and locking techniques, or using the autotraction couch as a primary measure, i.e. as a 'mobilization device'. This is a rather non-specific mobilization; however, despite significant muscle spasm, it is possible to move the dysfunctional segment(s) in the desired direction three-dimensionally during significant traction, simultaneously utilizing mechanical traction, gravitational traction, and traction applied by the patient himself/herself (the latter constituting the 'auto'-component of the autotraction method). Otherwise, non-specific pain treatment modalities are usually not applied until after manipulation, muscle stretching, and steroid injections have been tried.

Examples of non-specific pain treatments are analgesics, muscle relaxants, NSAIDs, transcutaneous nerve stimulation (TENS), transcutaneous electrical muscular stimulation (TEMS), therapeutic ultrasound, acupuncture, intramuscular stimulation (IMS) (*Editor's note: see Gunn, Chapter 4.3.8*), heat, cold, cryostretching (Travell 1983–1992) and so forth. With respect to NSAIDs (an evidence-based treatment modality), there is a tiny subgroup of pain patients, without confirmed inflammatory conditions, in whom NSAIDs are the only therapeutic measure that works, at least in combination with antidysfunctional treatment modalities. These patients are preferably identified during the selection process of the algorithm and NSAIDs should of course be prescribed for continuous use, over years if necessary, with relevant tests of blood parameters yearly. Over-enthusiasm for manual therapy may cause clinicians to overlook this small but important patient group.

Prolotherapy: first indication

In the few patients in whom the pain is not controlled at this stage, prolotherapy (see corresponding box in the algorithm) may be provided in relevant cases. The indication is **segmental hyper-reactivity.** The originator of prolotherapy (Hackett 1958) believed that it brought about proliferation of connective tissue in the spinal column, which, in turn, leads to 'stabilization' of 'hypermobile' vertebral segments or sacroiliac joints. Although I have experienced good treatment results from prolotherapy, when applied according to specific indications, my impression is that the spinal mobility of the patients increases, as supported by a dynamic radiography report (Tilscher 1995, 1996). I am convinced that the underlying mechanism is not mechanical: rather, I believe that this treatment, as is the case with other antidysfunctional treatment modalities, addresses the electrical chaos caused in central elements of the postural control system by disturbed proprioception from a damaged vertebral segment. In other words, prolotherapy is equivalent to a forceful and aggressive reset. It is important to avoid the 'hypermobility' model, in which rest is perceived as advantageous after prolotherapy. By contrast, most of our patients work as usual after treatment, except for some that have to stay at home for a day or two because of temporary post-treatment pain. They walk, exercise, ride on horseback, and so forth, and I am entirely convinced that the treatment results have improved considerably through this active approach. Being a fairly aggressive and expensive treatment method (lumbar/pelvic prolotherapy in STAYAC's protocol takes 10 treatment sessions), it is not appropriate for use as a primary approach, especially in patients with ongoing dysfunctions. (*Editor's note:* For a further discussion of prolotherapy, the reader is directed to Dorman, Chapter 4.3.5.)

Traction modalities, including autotraction)

Autotraction (Lind 1974, Ljunggren, Weber *et al.* 1984, Natchew 1984, Knutsson, Skoglund *et al.* 1988) and other traction methods are usually applied only in patients who are free from dysfunctions and after soft tissue foci of irritation have been injected with steroids. The elimination of 'pseudo-neurological' signs achieved by autotraction (which is an antidysfunctional treatment) is most probably not a question of reduction of nerve root pressure. Neuropathology caused by a herniated disc cannot be treated by autotraction or any other antidysfunctional therapy. In addition, the original theory that the herniation was 'sucked back into the disc' during autotraction, has been disproved (Gillström, Ericson *et al.* 1985). This retraction was attributed to a negative pressure during traction: on the contrary, it has been shown that the intradiscal pressure increases during autotraction (Andersson, Schultz *et al.* 1984).

The warning about the dangerous and passivizing regimen applied by some clinicians after prolotherapy goes for autotraction too. Unfortunately, the originator of this therapeutic modality (Lind 1974) and many autotraction therapists believed in mechanistically oriented models, and many therapists are still stuck in this 'biomechanical trap'. Patients were not allowed to leave their bed for weeks or even longer, and were transported by ambulance to and from the treatment sessions. The risk of the patients' perceiving this a dramatic procedure,

with potentially negative consequences, is evident. Adherence to these outmoded theories has contributed to the fact that this very useful treatment method, which flourished in the 1970s in Sweden and elsewhere, has today more or less disappeared outside manual therapy circles. Patients treated by autotraction should be encouraged to be active, and disabused of the previously applied passivizing regimens. Autotraction is perceived at STAYAC as an antidysfunctional treatment, with effects similar to manipulation (a reset manoeuvre), and combined with maintenance of activities of daily living.

Autotraction seems to be considerably less effective in patients with untreated dysfunctions, and with uninjected irritable soft tissue foci, not least in the presence of referred radiating pain mimicking true radicular pain (e.g. from parasacrococcygeal structures; from the sacroiliac joint; from musculus piriformis, gluteus medius/minimus). Since only a few patients need prolotherapy, there is of course an important shortcut from the 'non-specific pain treatment' box to the 'autotraction' box (see corresponding arrow).

Nerve mobilization

Nerve mobilization according to Elvey and Butler is included in the STAYAC concept. It is appropriate to introduce this treatment approach in the cases when autotraction is not applicable or successful, and of course in other parts of the body (e.g. extremities) when the patients have not responded to other antidysfunctional therapy, or in the few cases in which true dysfunctional nerve pain is suspected. (True neuropathic pain cannot be treated by means of nerve mobilization.) For simplicity, and since these techniques rarely provide additional positive treatment effects when the earlier measures in the antidysfunctional domain have been undertaken, this approach is not represented by a box of its own in the algorithm.

Yellow light A situations

Recurring dysfunctions

Patients whose dysfunctions recur despite 2–4 antidysfunctional treatments fall into the 'recurring dysfunctions' or 'yellow light A category'. The positive effect(s) of manipulations or specific mobilizations may be substantial, but short-lived, and more than 3–4 repetitions of similar specific treatment manoeuvres is inappropriate. The three, often parallel procedures that should be applied early in this instance are physical exercise, mobilizing home exercises, and muscle stretching. This last measure is applied according to its second indication in the algorithm, namely recurring dysfunctions (the first indication being primary muscle pain treatment). In the lower back/pelvic region, the most common muscles subjected to stretching are the hamstrings, rectus femoris, adductors, iliopsoas, tensores fasciae latae, and piriformis, but all muscles in the region are frequently stretched. A common name for this muscle group is the 'iliocrural muscles', even though a couple of them have an origin other than the os ilium.

The aim of the home exercise protocol is not only to maintain restored or improved function, achieved by the specific therapy; a proportion of the patients are even able to treat recurring dysfunctions themselves. Consequently, physical exercises, mobilizing home exercises, muscle stretching, the use of a trochanter belt, and prolotherapy for recurring dysfunctions are classified as secondary prevention measures for recurring dysfunctions. Two additional measures for secondary prevention are discussed in the section on antidepressants, and in the section on steroid injections respectively.

Trochanter belt

In patients with recurring lumbar pain with recurring markers of pelvic dysfunctions, in spite of regular physical exercises and normalized muscle lengths, a trochanter belt (Figure 4.4.5) is applied. The indication for this measure is simple and pragmatic. In recurring dysfunctions, the application of the belt is post-manipulative, and has nothing to do with 'sacroiliac joint instability', postpartum low back pain and so forth (i.e. the 'classical' indications for a trochanter belt in manual medicine). This means that the belt, originally developed for women with pelvic pain during or after pregnancy, is applied in male patients almost as frequently as in female patients. Thus, if the condition is not controlled at this stage, the belt should be applied following manipulation, and should be worn 24 hours a day for 6 weeks, and during the day only for another 6 weeks. Stretchable trochanter belts with self-adhesive straps are not firm enough to prevent recurrence of pelvic dysfunctions: the belt should be non-stretchable and strapped on with permanent fasteners. In most patients, groin straps are needed to prevent the belt from sliding upwards. The 'classical' mechanistic rationale for the use of this belt ('keeping the pelvic bones together in the correct position') is probably not valid – a proprioceptive effect (a slow continuous reset) is more likely. In most cases the dysfunctions resolve within 12 weeks, after which most patients remain free of dysfunctions for extended periods without the belt.

There are no corresponding measures for patients with neck or thoracic pain, although epicondalgia bandages and knee orthoses may have similar effects.

Prolotherapy: second indication

Prolotherapy is indicated in the few cases in which dysfunctions continue to recur despite the measures taken so far in the algorithm. This is the second indication for prolotherapy (the first indication being a primary treatment for hyper-reactivity, as previously described).

For treatment success with prolotherapy, strict indications are needed. At this stage, through the selection process within the algorithm, the patients frequently have been suffering for a long time, and psycho-existential/social dimensions/complications are common. This is also true for prolotherapy according to the first indication. An essential criterion that has to be fulfilled before prolotherapy is considered is that major psycho-existential dimensions to patients' symptoms are ruled out by means of a suitable psychological instrument – this could be done in many different ways. The patients should also have been undertaking continuous physical exercise for at least 6 months, and have pursued this in a well-motivated manner. Prolotherapy should never be carried through as an alternative to physical exercise – these two managements should always go hand in hand. Disappointing results for prolotherapy may be obtained if strict criteria are not used (Yelland 2004, Dechow 1999). Otherwise it is an excellent method. Although it is not yet considered sufficiently evidence based (Nachemson and Jonsson 2000), very few patients fail to benefit from it if provided at an appropriate stage. Substantive support for the use of prolotherapy is provided by Ongley, Dorman *et al.* (1987) who treated patients with chronic pain. Klein *et al.* (1989) demonstrated increased lumbar spinal mobility after prolotherapy, and Klein *et al.* (1993) also showed borderline differences in favour of prolotherapy in a double-blind RCT.

Note that in the algorithm (Figure 4.4.1) there are shortcuts to the 'dysfunction free' box from all the 'secondary prevention' boxes in the upper half of the antidysfunctional stack, indicating that only a minority of patients are in need of trochanter belt and prolotherapy respectively.

Dysfunction-free state

The dysfunction-free state is defined as follows: there are no remaining markers of dysfunction, no green flags conditions to be found, *ex juvantibus* treatment has not shed light on the situation, and/or there are no reasonable indications that *ex juvantibus* diagnosis would be meaningful. When the algorithm has been followed so far, a dysfunction-free state is almost always established. However, some patients are still in pain at this stage. These patients will follow the same pathways as those who became dysfunction-free during the early treatment steps of the algorithm without the described measures of secondary prevention.

Successful outcome: 'recovery' (alternative A) or a 'status of manageable symptoms' (alternative B)

From the 'stack' of antidysfunctional measures, there are pathways to the right at all levels, representing the recovered cases, or instances with minor symptoms, without the need for further treatment, and without significant consequences for the patients' quality of life and ability to work (outcome alternative A). In the acute phase, dysfunctions are the dominating cause of pain – see Figure 4.4.4a (pathomorphology and primary psycho-existentially-based conditions are rare). Consequently, according to our clinical trials (Blomberg 1993), in acute and subacute patients, after one or two treatments, the pathway leading to the dysfunction-free state is the most common scenario (an important shortcut in the algorithm), after which they progress to recovery (outcome alternative A) or to a status of 'manageable symptoms' (outcome alternative B). Another substantive group of patients make the same progress after steroid injections. A group of therapy-resistant chronic patients reaches this state over time, via the same route, through 'spontaneous recovery'/improvement. In addition, another group of chronic patients reaches outcome B (and finally also outcome A) according to a similar 'spontaneous recovery' pathway, after having been guided through the 'psycho-existential sphere'. As illustrated in Figure 4.4.4b, psycho-existential dimensions of pain suffering are dominant in severe chronic patients. Patients with purely dysfunctional conditions (green flag conditions), and therefore treatable with antidysfunctional therapy are rare; consequently, these patients are not represented by a circle in Figure 4.4.4b. There is an infinite variety of relationships between the three major circles: Figures 4.4.4a and 4b represent two extremes. Generally, chronic patients, in whom the dysfunctions and the relevant sites for injections have been untreated, sometimes for years, require on average more treatment steps than acute and subacute patients. Very few pain patients need to proceed through the entire antidysfunctional sphere or the entire algorithm. If antidysfunctional treatment is given early enough, most patients in this category need only a few treatment steps.

Outcome alternative B is somewhat less successful than alternative A, but still satisfactory. The ability to work is restored and circumstances are under control, although residual complaints still disturb everyday function and/or quality of life to some degree. In these patients the process of self recovery, facilitated by long-term and tailor-made self-care programmes, will finally lead to recovery over time.

The psycho-existential sphere (yellow flags)

The second important major 'stack' of therapeutic measures deals with the psycho-existential sphere (yellow flags). We know that the correlation between impairment (organ level) and perceived (dis)ability (individual level) is very weak (Waddell 1998). Consequently, we all meet patients who cope well with severe conditions and function well in most aspects including working ability, whereas others, whose impairment is minor (on objective assessment), perceive themselves as more or less completely disabled (see also the section on 'Perception disturbances'). **Nevertheless, patients with minor dysfunctional conditions, but who perceive themselves as disabled for instance with respect to working capability, should virtually always be treated in the first instance with antidysfunctional therapy before steps are taken to deal with the psycho-** existential dimensions of their suffering, although it is unlikely to be successful. (See the section on 'Behavioural aspects of manual therapy' for a discussion of antidysfunctional therapy for established chronic patents). Unfortunately, this rarely happens in today's health care; a premature psychological approach may even reduce a patient's chances of moving forward (see the section on 'The first perspective', below). The patient's pain must be addressed, but the risk of passivizing the patients with pointless courses of antidysfunctional treatment has to be continually kept in mind. Regrettably, as illustrated in Figure 4.4.6a, in manual therapy there is a widespread lack of awareness of psycho-existential factors, and endless series of passive treatments are too frequently provided. This leads to the reinforcement of pain behaviour and the development of pain identity, with adverse consequences.

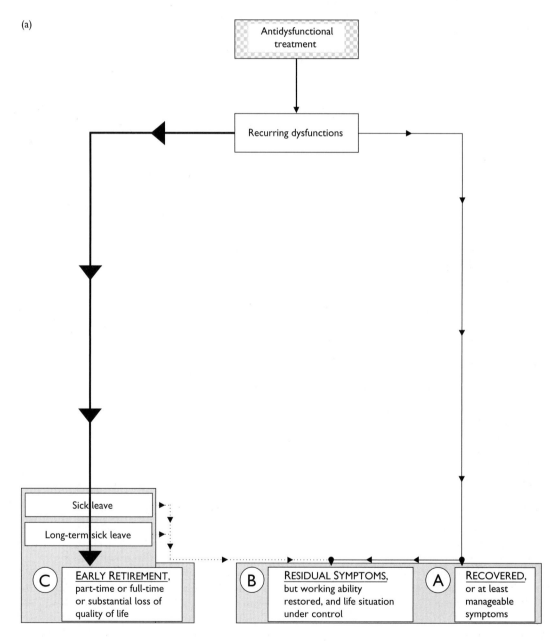

(a)

Figure 4.4.6 (a) Lack of awareness of psychoexistential factors and overreliance on antidysfunctional/manual therapy, too frequently resulting in an endless series of passive treatments.

Focusing on dysfunctional factors without attention to psycho-existential factors is not optimal, but the converse also applies (Figure 4.4.6b). As reflected by these two rudimentary algorithms, I believe that today's (back) pain care in general is simultaneously over-somatized and over-psychologized (see also 'The first and second perspectives').

Figure 4.4.7a–d constitutes a further series of rudimentary algorithms, also reflecting today's clinical reality. These are co-existing, but not connected or integrated, and in my opinion this total lack of infrastructure is the main reason for the complete failure of healthcare with respect to the management of pain. The schemes illustrated in Figures 4.4.7a–d are discussed in later sections.

Consequently, in all stages of the antidysfunctional exploration, it is important to be constantly aware of psycho-existential factors that may jeopardize the rehabilitation process. In the algorithm, this awareness is represented by a series of arrows on the left, each directed from the different steps of the antidysfunctional domain to the psycho-existential area (yellow flags). The lowest arrow from the autotraction box represents the point where the constituents of the psycho-existential sphere should be considered at the absolute latest. The need for such measures may be assessed by means of predictive questionnaires (Linton and Halldén 1998) and/or an algorithm specially designed for the identification of yellow flags (Kendall *et al.* 1997) but is not neces-

sary in the vast majority of cases. Failure to heed the psycho-existential factors early in the programme increases the risk of chronicity and progression to an unfavourable outcome such as early retirement. Theoretically, there is a possibility of spontaneous recovery, as represented by a flow from the C box to the A and B boxes in Figure 4.4.6a (see corresponding dotted arrow). However, probably as a result of the stigmatizing effect of long-term absence from work, this is rare. As illustrated in Figures 4.4.6a–b and 4.4.7a–d, the reason for this is the lack of coordination of the different therapeutic resources – slow and extended management at inappropriate levels of care, in incorrect periods of the patients' 'pain careers', and barriers hindering patients from entering appropriate levels. Their rehabilitation potential is eventually destroyed. In the more difficult cases, close cooperation between all the healthcare professionals involved, the family, workplace representatives, and social services, combined with well-defined behavioural attitudes, is necessary to avoid this slide into early retirement and its associated unhappiness.

The 'stay-active' box

The stay-active concept (see corresponding box in Figure 4.4.1) is not merely a matter of encouraging patients to increase their levels of activity just by providing advice and reassurance, and prescribing physical exercise. Another aspect, which is at least as important, is the

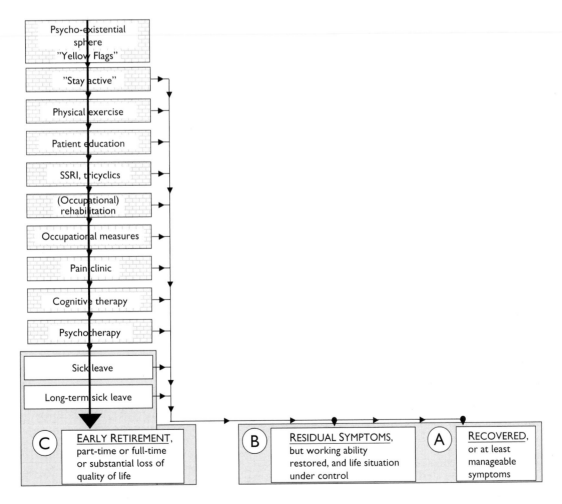

Figure 4.4.6 (b) The converse situation: a unidimensional focus on psychoexistential factors.

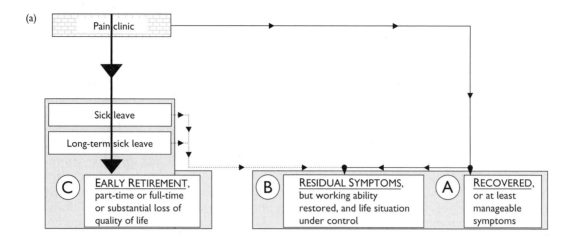

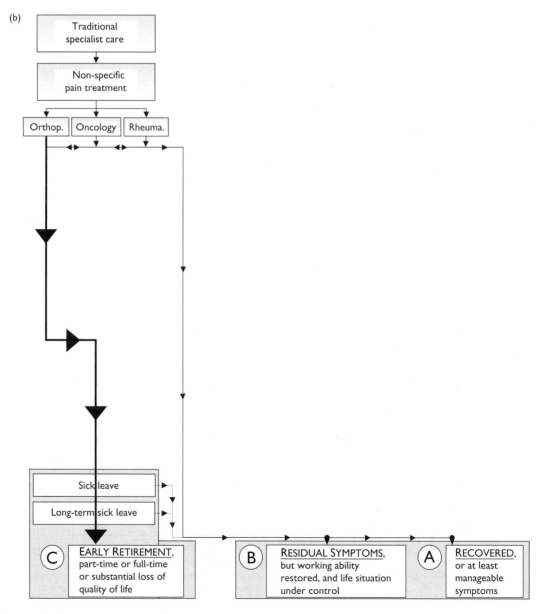

Figure 4.4.7 A series of rudimentary algorithms, reflecting today's clinical reality. See text for details.

(c)

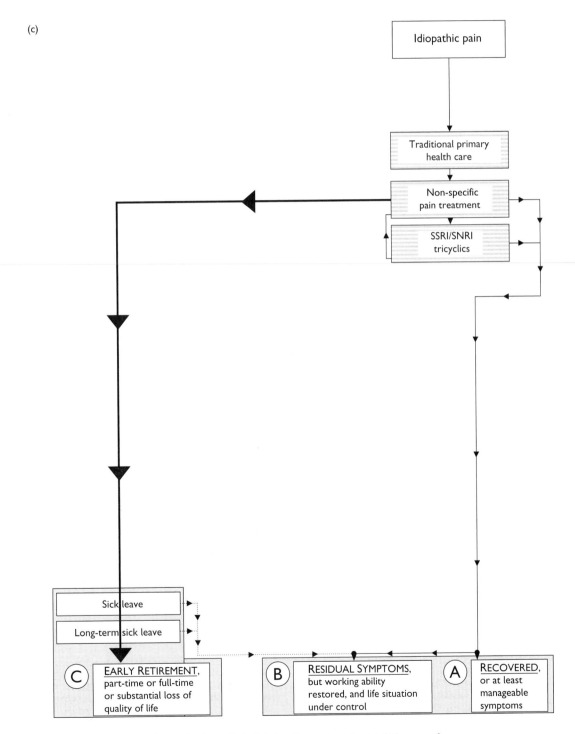

Figure 4.4.7 A series of rudimentary algorithms, reflecting today's clinical reality. See text for details (*continued*).

(d)

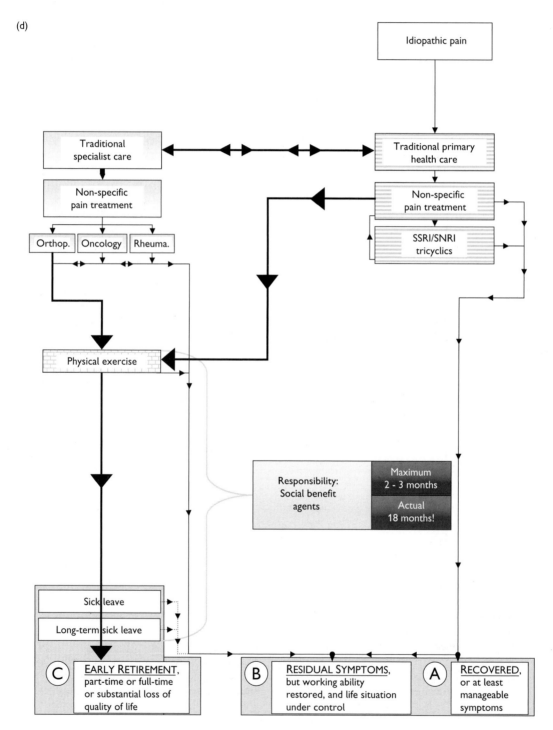

Figure 4.4.7 A series of rudimentary algorithms, reflecting today's clinical reality. See text for details (*continued*).

stay-active approach as a metacognitive method. Without metacognitive processes (see page 507), the activating strategies of the patients will never be optimal. In the STAYAC model, the metacognitive aspect means that every word communicated to the patient should contain (not infrequently subliminal) stay-active messages, not least while providing passive treatment such as manipulation.

Most pain management programmes focus on the stay-active approach, and it is now considered the most solidly evidence-based method of back pain care (Waddell 1998, Nachemson and Jonsson 2000, Koes, van Tulder *et al.* 2001). Nevertheless, the stay-active concept is insufficiently implemented in health care generally. All too often, management consists mainly of the passive prescription of medication and sick leave.

There is a synergy in a systematic and consistent parallel application of the stay-active approach, and antidysfunctional treatments: a therapeutic combination, which is all too infrequent today. The stay-active concept (evaluated by Indahl, Velund *et al.* 1995, Malmivaara, Hakkinen *et al.* 1995, and Torstensen, Ljunggren *et al.* 1998) includes encouraging patients to take part in physical and other activities. Providing information about the benign character of the condition, and the adverse effects of inactivity and sick leave, encourages the patient to be more active.

'Staying active' is not only a matter of increasing physical activity. Relatively 'passive' activities such as going to the movies (if the fear-avoidance thinking of the patient has hindered them from doing so), or going away on holiday for the first time in years, can be the key to rehabilitation success. Regrettably, these crucial but simple and frequently effective 'treatment' possibilities are often overlooked. The stay-active concept is a basic therapeutic principle, which is adopted from the first visit onwards. However, before it is applied, the possibility of dysfunctional factors must be considered. This is an important difference between the STAYAC approach and the widespread recommendation that only (unspecified) 'self-care' should be applied during the first weeks of acute low back pain. From our results (see earlier section) it is evident that active antidysfunctional treatment should be applied from the first visit, not least from a societal perspective; at this early stage, a decrease of only 2 days of sick leave on average per patient would be extremely cost-effective (Hadler 1987, Hadler, Curtis *et al.* 1987).

Physical exercise – another 'self-care' box

The STAYAC algorithm is basically an activity approach which includes physical exercises, enhanced by manipulation and steroid injections. The next box, 'Physical exercise' (see Figure 4.4.1), not only includes exercises under the supervision of physiotherapists, but also constitutes a 'self-care' box. It includes non-specific exercise, such as athletics or horse-riding, and stimulation to increase enjoyable, physically demanding leisure-time activities such as walking (Indahl, Velund *et al.* 1995) or any physical activity that the patient in question may have given up, frequently because of the pain. (Fear-avoidance is a frequent underlying factor.)

The most frequently applied exercise philosophy is medical exercise therapy (MET) (Holten, Torstensen 1991; Torstensen 1997, Torstensen, Ljunggren *et al.* 1998), but other models such as sequential exercises are also employed. Physical exercise is an evidence-based method (Waddell 1998, Harms-Ringdahl, Holmström *et al.* 1999, Nachemson and Jonsson 2000, van Tulder, Malmivaara *et al.* 2000). In a recent literature review, it was concluded that 'the reviewed trials

provided strong evidence that exercise significantly reduces sick days during the first follow-up year' (Kool, de Bie et al. 2004). Relaxation exercises, body awareness exercises, Alexander therapy, Rosen therapy, and Feldenkrais are other useful methods, which for simplicity have been allocated to this box but which are never used as primary measures and not applied in the (other) physical exercise box in the anti-dysfunctional sphere. The following are two important and different dimensions.

Physical exercise, indication moderate hyper-reactivity
When they have reached a dysfunction-free state and adequate steroid injections have been provided, patients suffering from slight to moderate hyper-reactivity normally do not need prolotherapy; their symptoms are usually controlled (outcome B) or eliminated (outcome A) by individualized exercises only. Although these patients do not express any obvious major psycho-existential dimensions to their suffering, they are managed within the psycho-existential sphere; hyper-reactivity is a matter of long-term suffering, which almost always has some psychological complication.

According to the dominant mechanically-oriented theories among physiotherapists, the apparent advantageous effects are achieved by, for example, 'stabilization' of 'unstable' vertebral segments. There is a huge variety of 'stabilization exercises' through which extreme positions of 'unstable' joints are supposed to be avoided in everyday life, and certain protective movement patterns are taught. There is an obvious risk of transferring subliminal and subconscious stay-passive messages to the patients. The net effect of the stay-passive messages weighed against the positive effects achieved by the exercises may even be negative. On the other hand, it is possible to convey stay-active messages while providing passive treatment, such as manipulation. An increased awareness of subliminal stay-passive messages is extremely important. This could be achieved, as in the STAYAC algorithm, by updating the rationales behind hyper-reactivity and improving the terminology. Mechanically oriented terms such as 'hypermobility', 'instability', and 'micro-instability' should be avoided. The exercises could instead be described as helping postural control and coordination, optimizing the control and operative system of the muscle spindles, improving peripheral proprioceptive functions, and compensating the impaired proprioceptive functions by improving the function of higher centres in the CNS. Within this paradigm of the 'operating system' of postural control organization, it becomes logical to stay active, move and so forth. Fear-avoidance and catastrophizing are counteracted, and the risk of subliminal stay-passive messages is reduced or even eliminated. In conclusion, the beneficial effects of physical exercises in hyper-reactivity may be achieved by optimizing the function of the 'software' in order to compensate for minor weaknesses in the 'hardware'. The contents of this section illustrate a metacognitive aspect of the STAYAC algorithm.

In addition, beneficial non-specific somatic effects may be achieved from increased strength, endurance, improved coordination, and fitness. (For alternative views on stabilization, see Mottram and Comerford, Chapter 4.3.12)

Of course there are patients with more severe hyper-reactivity syndromes that cannot be controlled or cured solely by individualized exercise (or prolotherapy). As indicated by the vertical 'hyper-reactivity' box (see Figure 4.4.1), by following the subsequent paths in the psycho-existential sphere (the stay-active concept, reassurance, behavioural measures, and so forth), the patients' coping strategies will become strengthened, while their conditions heal over time and the consequences of their suffering are reduced in various ways. At this point in the algorithm, these principles have to be applied in a more process-oriented manner. Fortunately, progression to chronic low-back pain is rare; only a tiny minority needs prolotherapy, and an even smaller number are referred to specialized orthopaedic surgeons for fusion surgery (see corresponding arrow to the left from the 'physical exercise' box). Except in clearly demonstrated pathomorphological cases (e.g. unstable and significant spondylolisthesis), fusion surgery is controversial. One study (Fritzell *et al.* 2001) provides only weak scientific support for surgery. In spite of this, I believe that surgery is appropriate for a tiny proportion of patients with chronic low-back pain. Unfortunately, moderate or even severe psycho-existential dimensions frequently seem to be overlooked by surgeons, leading to poor operation results. I believe that if patients for surgical treatment were preselected by careful and systematic application of the STAYAC algorithm, the results would improve considerably.

Physical exercise – the inherent potential for behavioural change

An underestimated aspect of physical exercise is its behaviour-modifying potential. Exercises carry positive subliminal messages. During the process of antidysfunctional analysis, the physician/therapist has built a platform of trust and mutual respect ('I respect and understand your pain, which has a physical component'; 'I have the competence to treat your pain'). By prescribing exercises, the therapist conveys to the patient their belief that the patient's condition is not dangerous. The patient's back is not 'worn out' – if it was, physical activities would aggravate the condition, and the therapist would not prescribe exercises. Tendencies to fear-avoidance and catastrophizing are thereby prevented. This inherent effect of physical exercise may be one of the reasons why no differences between the large numbers of different exercise modes have been demonstrated at group level in RCTs (Waddell 1998, Harms-Ringdahl, Holmström *et al.* 1999, Nachemson and Jonsson 2000, van Tulder, Malmivaara *et al.* 2000). Experienced physiotherapists may communicate this message to the patients more or less subconsciously, without the specific intention of altering the patients' behaviour. However, if a physiotherapist who is specially trained in both behavioural and manual therapy can invoke this dimension of physical exercise by a process-oriented (metacognitive) and premeditated application of exercises as a behavioural therapy, the ability of the method to stabilize the patient's life situations will probably be enhanced further. (A physiotherapist and a psychologist/licensed psychotherapist may also work together in group settings.) The patient's fear of pain associated with exercise, everyday life, and treatment is minimized or even eliminated. In many instances, the behavioural dimension of physical exercise is more important than improvement of strength, endurance, fitness, and even coordination and postural control.

The 'stay active' and the 'patient education' boxes

The education of patients – with the aim of modifying their beliefs, attitudes, fear, and behaviour – begins at the first visit. However, in the absence of sufficient therapeutic response at this stage of the algorithm, this approach has to be carried out using a new 'patient education' methodology that has been developed at STAYAC. A more focused and goal-oriented approach to influence various behavioural disturbances, long-term sick leave illness, coping skills, sense of coherence, learned helplessness (Miller, Seligman et al. 1975a, b), and poor

self-efficacy (Bandura 1977) are needed in a substantive subgroup of patients at this stage. The patients are usually in chronic pain and on extended sick leave; the diagnoses are idiopathic pain including somatoform pain syndromes, hyper-reactivity, fibromyalgia, whiplash-associated disorders (WAD), and so forth. The patient education takes the form of cognitive-behavioural group therapy, aiming to minimize the consequences of persisting symptoms (see the section on 'The third perspective'). This therapeutic method involves interactive sessions (of four hours on five occasions) by the responsible physician or physiotherapist, whom the patients have got to know during their antidysfunctional management. The basic idea is that the 'bone setter'/manual therapist, and the (cognitive) behavioural therapist are the same person. This approach increases the patients' confidence not only that the responsible clinician has the competence to take care of, or to initiate, all measures necessary to reduce the pain by means of somatically oriented treatment methods, but also that all such measures really have been carried through thoroughly or at least considered. In the analyses of the patients' psycho-existential status, psychodynamic dimensions of their suffering are considered, so this is **cognitive therapy with psychodynamic overtones**, but traditional psychotherapy is not provided at this level of the algorithm. Cognitive-behavioural therapy, as a stand-alone therapy, is considered solidly evidence-based (Nachemson and Jonsson 2000), and this cognitive-behavioural group therapy seems highly successful with regard to the enhancement of the patients' sense of coherence (Antonovsky 1991) and coping skills. Sometimes it is not even important for the preceding management to alleviate the somatic component of the patient's suffering. The patient's 'escape routes' are closed by the conveyance of the subliminal messages mentioned above, and circumstances are created in which patients are much less hesitant to discuss relevant matters. The 'teacher' can make a gradual shift from standard topics, such as pain mechanisms, anatomy, and the dysfunction perspective, to potentially controversial subjects such as long-term sick leave, the stay-active concept, primary and secondary benefits, the 'Peter Pan' syndrome (Kiley 1983), the 'Humpty Dumpty' syndrome ('Humpty Dumpty sat on a wall, Humpty Dumpty had a great fall, All the King's horses, And all the King's men, Couldn't put Humpty together again'; Carroll), and basic crisis psychology. Other sensitive topics include insufficient coping abilities, insufficient sense of coherence, pain behaviour, the pain patient role, identity loss, development of pain identity, and life-lies.

Much of the content of the lectures is too abstract for many patients. However, this does not matter, and it is not necessary for them to remember much from the lectures – basically, the patient education is a matter of repeating five or six basic stay-active messages, largely without the patients noticing. However, it is obvious to the clinician that, after these sessions, there are frequently dramatic changes in the patients' attitudes to work and sick leave, improved coping strategies and so forth, even in those who evidently disliked the lectures. Some of the most successful cases have been in patients who were clearly irritated and annoyed by the patient education. Irritating the patients is not a goal in itself, although the method may be experienced by some as partly provocative. In conclusion, one could even say that the core of the patient education is a qualified and powerful mode of 'mental manipulation'. (For another view on patient education, see Klaber Moffett, Chapter 4.2.)

Optimally, all therapists in the team should attend sessions of individual long-term psychotherapy, and/or individual guidance, by an experienced psychotherapist. This is at least as important as guidance for psychotherapists, where such supervision is considered a matter of course. At STAYAC, we have not yet reached this goal; however, we regularly have a Balint-type group conducted by our psychologist/licensed psychotherapist in which even secretaries, receptionists, and nurses take part.

Antidepressants

The next therapeutic principle, the use of antidepressants (see corresponding box in the algorithm), is well established. Low dosages of tricyclic antidepressants, such as clomipramine and amitriptyline are a well-documented treatment method for chronic pain. We have experience of the use of higher, antidepressive doses of tricyclic antidepressants for chronic pain since the mid 1980s. The dose–response curve seems linear: i.e. the higher the dose, the higher the therapeutic response. Supported by these observational data, I applied the same therapeutic principle, i.e. dosages towards the top end of the permitted range, when the selective serotonin/noradrenaline reuptake inhibitors (SSRIs/SNRIs) arrived in Sweden around 1990. After experience of this approach over many years, it seems obvious that the linear dose–response curve in the treatment of chronic pain is valid for SSRI/SNRIs as well. There is as yet no reliable evidence of efficacy for the use of SSRIs/SNRIs in chronic pain problems. However, only low dosages of SSRI/SNRIs (and tricyclic antidepressants) for pain have been evaluated in RCTs. Clearly, further RCTs using these drugs in higher dosages are required.

There are compliance problems with tricyclic antidepressants, because of relatively frequent adverse events. The SSRI/SNRIs have fewer side effects, and after a slow and gradual increase to maximum dosages, they may be as effective as tricyclics in chronic pain patients and even more useful. The apparent linear dose–response graph may be similar to the treatment strategies in patients with obsessive-compulsive disorders (OCD), social phobia, and panic anxiety syndromes, in which the linear dose–response relationship is well established. By contrast, the dose–side effect curve is apparently non-linear. Consequently, increasing the dosage of SSRI/SNRIs (after any initial side effects have subsided) rarely causes any further problems. In some patients the side-effects do not subside, and I have seen a handful of cases demonstrating moderate signs of too high levels of serotonin in the postsynaptic space, such as early wakening (early 'serotonergic syndrome'). However, these situations have been rapidly solved by reduction of the dosage or by a change to another SSRI/SNRI drug.

Generally, in the context of pain management, **the therapeutic potential of antidepressants is underestimated**, and, consequently, this type of treatment is underused. Aside from pain reduction/elimination, modulation of pain perception appears to be an important effect of SSRI/SNRI treatment in pain patients. Instead of focusing primarily on their pain, they may constructively plan their future return to a worthwhile life; the pain no longer rules their lives to the same extent. This frequently happens despite undiminished pain – a phenomenon which is exciting to observe. In our experience, this treatment approach is useful not only in advanced idiopathic somatoform pain syndromes, but also in other chronic conditions. In the STAYAC algorithm, when management at this stage has failed to provide sufficient pain control, antidepressants are tried in all pain patients whose quality of life, everyday functioning, and/or working capacity are reduced. Whether or not there is a co-existent depression

is not essential; the patient will report this after some weeks of medication (see also the section on 'ex juvantibus diagnosis'). Additionally, there are no reliable instruments with sufficient precision to predict accurately whether the pain will respond to this therapy. This is an excellent example of truly pragmatic management. Consequently, in the pragmatic approach, the method, when needed, is simply tried at a relevant stage, at full dosage, regardless of the patient's apparent psychiatric status. This seems to be a very fruitful approach, recently supported by one of the leading Swedish specialists in antidepressive medication, Lars von Knorring (personal communication): He considers SSRI/SNRIs not to be antidepressants, but rather a general restorative of the serotonergic/noradrenergic systems; these medications modulate numerous other aspects of perception, and depression is becoming merely one indication among many others. Certainly, antidepressants may be introduced at any level in the algorithm, and if the patient is obviously depressed, or has a chronic and severe pain condition, they may be recommended at the first visit.

In conclusion, according to the STAYAC algorithm, antidepressants are used frequently, and this type of therapy commonly resolves the patients' adverse life situation, not always by alleviating depressive symptoms, but often by relieving pain, and/or by modulating the perception of pain to a manageable level. However, patients' resistance to a trial of antidepressants is widespread. This seems to be especially valid for pain patients, but less of an issue in patients who spontaneously identify themselves as suffering from depression. To deal with the patients' concerns about antidepressant medication it is desirable to have a refined pedagogical model to provide an understandable explanation of potential benefits, rationales and side effects of antidepressants used for pain. This motivational process may be provided in individual consultations if necessary, but it is time-consuming and is preferably carried out in groups as part of the standard patient education procedure.

In some studies positive effects have been demonstrated with the use of SSRIs in non-depressive patients (Knutson, Cole *et al.* 1997, Knutson, Wolkowitz *et al.* 1998, Shores, Pascualy *et al.* 2001, Loubinoux, Pariente *et al.* 2002, Tse and Bond 2002, Harmer, Bhagwagar *et al.* 2003). For instance, there was improvement in coping with everyday situations, stress thresholds, and the ability to cooperate smoothly in groups, and a 'smoothing' of the less favourable aspects of their personalities. This suggests that our SSRI strategy may in fact bring about its positive effects by 'super-normal' levels of serotonin in the CNS, leading to biochemically induced, artificially strengthened coping strategies. Consequently, it seems that this strategy is not necessarily a matter of treating 'masked depressions' (see 'The first perspective'), even though that diagnosis is indeed relevant in some of the chronic pain patients. This hypothesis needs to be tested in experimental and clinical studies such as RCTs.

We have noticed another phenomenon that is not easily understood. In a subgroup of patients with recurring dysfunctions that are difficult to bring under control, after some weeks on antidepressants the situation is suddenly stabilized, and the markers of dysfunction do not recur. This phenomenon should be regarded as a measure of secondary prevention.

Occupational rehabilitation

The next step in the algorithm is occupational rehabilitation. The evidence that this approach is effective in the management of back pain is fairly recent (Bendix, Bendix *et al.* 1998a, 1998b, 2000). The fundamental difference between our approach and other multidisciplinary rehabilitation concepts is that all the previously discussed measures are undertaken before our patients are subjected to our occupational rehabilitation, and that the method itself is predicated upon the same fundamental principles as the rest of the algorithm, i.e. the inherent behavioural potential of the antidysfunctional approach, exploited (with respect to the content) in a process-oriented manner. A related approach, aside from the antidysfunctional management, is the pragmatic approach to low-back pain used at Volvo, Gothenburg (Lindström, Öhlund *et al.* 1992) in which a graded activity programme including a back school and graded individualized exercise programmes is the core, and the operant-conditioning behavioural concept is essential too. This concept was found to decrease sick leave and to increase mobility, strength, and fitness in comparison to unspecified uncontrolled 'traditional care'. It has been demonstrated that the elimination of dysfunctional factors from the patients' sufferings considerably enhances their ability to take part in physical activities (Blomberg, Svärdsudd *et al.* 1993c), and thereby of course rehabilitation programmes as well. This is substantiated by data from the reproducibility study: muscle stretching was the treatment most frequently considered painful by patients, which was expected (see pages 521–2). However, the second most painful treatment modality was the physical exercises in the two groups in which manual therapy (and steroid injections) were not provided. In these groups the physical exercises were experienced as painful more frequently than manipulation and injections in the experimental groups. The physical exercises were only rarely experienced as painful in the two groups in which manual therapy (and steroid injections) were allowed (Blomberg, Bogefeldt *et al.* 2005a). Accordingly, as much as possible of the antidysfunctional treatment/investigation is completed before occupational rehabilitation. These major differences from other rehabilitation programmes are probably the main reasons behind the extraordinarily successful results achieved by our 6-week/half-time rehabilitation programme with follow-ups after 1 and 3 months (and in some subjects continuous follow-up for longer periods of time) as evaluated in a hitherto unpublished outcome study. The population of this study suffered from advanced persistent pain syndromes refractory to earlier managements. The mean duration of pain in the first 76 patients was 4 years, and the pain debut averaged 10 years; 10% of the patients had suffered from pain for more than 20 years. The mean period of sick leave was 18 months, and only 10% of the patients had suffered periods of work absenteeism for less than 1 year. The quality-of-life score was extremely low, and the rating of symptoms, mainly of a psychosomatic character, was complex. The final assessment was performed between 6 months and 2 years after the rehabilitation period: From a societal perspective (with respect to reduction of sick leave), the rehabilitation was successful in 81% of cases. Consequently, the proportion of patients at definite risk of early retirement was only 19%, as compared with the realistic expected risk of early retirement of close to 100%. Most of the successfully rehabilitated subjects (81%) returned to their normal work, and the remainder returned to modified work tasks, or reduced their proportion of sick leave (in Sweden, 25%, 50%, 75%, or 100% sick leave can be prescribed), or were able to carry out different procedures with a realistic aim of returning to some type of work tasks that they could not do before the rehabilitation.

Occupational measures; blue and black flags

The next suggested step, occupational measures (see corresponding box in Figure 4.4.1) could be applied at any point in the algorithm. These measures include a graded return to work, light duties, retraining, re-education, further education, and referral to special establishments for people with permanently reduced working ability. It is not uncommon to discover during the first visit that this measure has been neglected. If the patient has been offered poor advice and lacks guidance and direction, this measure should be initiated promptly. At the other extreme, in Sweden occupational measures are unfortunately far too often initiated at early stages in individuals for whom a variety of treatment possibilities have not been taken into consideration. This is not a cost-effective strategy. For simplicity, there are no boxes in the algorithm representing blue flags and black flags. *Blue flags* include fear of being laid off, lack of job satisfaction, poor relationship with work colleagues, claim against employer, and organisational climate (Waddell 1998). *Black flags* comprise factors beyond individual influence such as governmental policies and work regulations, also workplace conditions associated with the onset of low back pain and the development of disability (Bartys, Burton 2002). These factors are often considered at this stage, not infrequently parallel to occupational measures.

Pain clinic

The fact that referral to a pain clinic (see corresponding box in Figure 4.4.1) is a late step in this protocol may antagonize some of the pain specialists. Depending on the medical management profile (which may vary considerably from unit to unit), pain clinics may or may not be included in the specialist sphere. In the current algorithm, for simplicity, pain clinics are included only in the psycho-existential sphere. Nevertheless, as a licensed pain specialist myself, I firmly believe that this, not earlier, is the appropriate point to refer a small minority of the pain patients, at least considering the structure of pain clinics in Sweden today.

There is no supporting evidence for the effectiveness of the (often extensive) series of blockades/injections that are provided more or less as a single-tool therapy at some clinics. In addition, such treatment strategies are expensive. The indications for injections within the STAYAC concept are very different from the indications within those pain management clinics in which a series of blockades are not supported by specific functional diagnoses. Consequently, within the STAYAC concept, with the exception of the few patients that are subjected to lumbar prolotherapy (10 treatments), costly series of injections are never provided. In addition, the injections in the STAYAC concept are evidence-based (Blomberg, Bogefeldt *et al.* 2005a). Cryostretching and IMS are two other methods that are frequently applied by Swedish pain specialists, but they have the same problems: the high cost, the lack of evidence, and their frequent appliance as single-tool 'silver bullet' therapy. In spite of this, these methods are used in the STAYAC concept, but never primarily and only at late stages in a tiny minority of the patients, because they are seldom needed. (*Editor's note:* For a contrasting view with respect to IMS, see Gunn, Chapter 4.3.9.)

However, **the essential problem in traditional pain medicine is the lack of the dysfunction perspective.** Although the underlying principles within this discipline are focused on (neuro-)physiological/biochemical peripheral and central pain mechanisms, rather than on structural factors, these are still in principle exclusively pathomorphologically oriented and an application of the biomedical paradigm. With respect to the diagnosis of '(pseudo)neuropathic pain', many patients with chronic pain have features of dysfunctional conditions (green flag conditions) that are treatable with antidysfunctional treatment. A number of clinical features that are regarded within traditional pain medicine as more or less pathognomonic for true neuropathic/neurogenic pain are frequently present in dysfunctional conditions, both axially (chest, lower back, and abdomen), and in the extremities. In addition, when of dysfunctional origin, symptoms such as hypoesthesia, hyperesthesia, dysesthesia, analgesia, paresthesia, and even reflex disturbances are reversible, resolving rapidly after antidysfunctional therapy, sometimes within seconds. In these situations that occur frequently during antidysfunctional management, it is obvious to the clinician that pathomorphological states or neuropathic diagnoses are of no relevance. Consequently, the lack of the dysfunction perspective within traditional pain medicine creates a risk of overdiagnosing of neuropathic/neurogenic pain and a corresponding overuse of medication such as antiepileptics. This is unfortunate, considering the frequent adverse effects, and the frequently unsatisfactory treatment results, especially in patients with symptoms of a dysfunctional origin. Furthermore, for the same reason, an over-reliance on psychological factors as the primary cause of pain is common ('psychogenic pain' – see 'The first perspective'). Another regrettable but frequent consequence is an insufficient application of the stay-active concept. Figure 4.4.7a illustrates the rudimentary algorithm of suboptimal pain clinics as described in this paragraph.

Thus, according to extensive observational data, in many cases **antidysfunctional investigation over time is the most reliable method of differentiating true neuropathic/neurogenic pain from 'pseudo-neurological' features of a dysfunctional origin**. Similarly, this reasoning is applied in the context of differentiation between true radicular pain and referred pain by antidysfunctional management, and in numerous other situations in which there is a differential diagnosis of pain syndromes, both with respect to the locomotor apparatus and within other medical disciplines. (Gynaecological issues for instance are discussed in the 'Nature of dysfunction' section). The mechanisms behind 'pseudo-neurological' signs may be related to the theories concerning the nature of the dysfunction that are postulated in this chapter: there may be dispersal effects between postural, proprioceptive, and sensory systems ('cross-talking', as in the case of referred pain). Patients with true neuropathic/neurogenic pain are sometimes, at least partly, treatable with SSRI/SNRIs and/or antiepileptics such as gabapentin or carbamazepine. Some pain specialists advocate double-blind injections of morphine, local anaesthetics, and placebo to differentiate neuropathic, peripheral nociceptive, central, and psychogenic pain, whereas others doubt the validity of this diagnostic method. There are indeed pain clinics that provide adequate occupational rehabilitation, and cognitive-behavioural therapies of different types.

A few patients need a referral to a pain specialist at this point in the algorithm, but premature and routine referral to pain clinics should be avoided. Other indications for referral to traditional pain clinics are the rare cases in which for instance stimulation of the dorsal horns, epidural infusions, rhizolysis, phenol, and alcohol blockades, and radiofrequency (heat) for destruction of the dorsal rami as indicated, for instance in some WAD patients. (*Editor's note:* See also Pither, Chapter 4.3.13.)

Figure 4.4.7 shows some further examples of malfunctioning, rudimentary, coexistent, but isolated, algorithms: over-reliance on pain medicine, specialist care, and primary health care respectively. Clinical reality today is no better than the one presented in Figure 4.4.7d.

Cognitive-behavioural therapy

The 'cognitive-behavioural therapy' box refers to extended therapy over a longer period of time, individually or in closed or open groups. At this stage, a few patients are in obvious need of such management, which indeed is available in some pain clinics, some psychiatric clinics, and within medical or occupational rehabilitation. The STAYAC concept underpins cognitive-behavioural therapeutic principles at all stages of the algorithm. Obviously, there are extremely potent synergistic effects in the integration of antidysfunctional medicine, with manual therapy as its core, and cognitive-behavioural therapy. Unfortunately, there is a widespread misconception that these two therapeutic principles are incompatible. Long-term behavioural therapy may be perfectly well executed by GPs or physiotherapists with appropriate insight and training: referral to a specialist is not always necessary.

Psychotherapy

The principal underlying psychological factor in pain syndromes is, I believe, denial of the psycho-existential dimensions of the suffering and denial of the role of the life-situation in general as a confounding factor with regard to the consequences of the pain. The pain is virtually always nociceptive (see the section on 'The third perspective'). However, the pain is 'used' by the patient to control and to facilitate repression of denied psycho-existential crises, which are externalized outside their own responsibility and control, as are the responsibility and control of their condition and their recovery; thus, this is the 'function' of the pain. However, the pain only rarely has a primary psychological origin.

The 'psychotherapy' box (lower left corner of the algorithm) is controversial. As a consequence of their lack of psychological awareness with respect to important underlying factors such as their beliefs, attitudes, and behaviour, most patients with severe pain are usually considered unsuitable for psychotherapy. Some degree of awareness of one's own situation is a requirement for successful psychotherapy of any kind. There is a definite risk that a patient whose pain is uncontrolled, and who primarily considers himself innocently stricken by pain outside his own control, may take offence and be further distressed by a therapeutic strategy that is too psychodynamically focused and/or introduced prematurely. This may also reinforce feelings of guilt and shame in some patients; being driven by these feelings is a common aspect of the pain-patient personality.

However, even powerful and profound psychotherapy, when indicated, is frequently very successful if undertaken at an appropriate stage of the algorithm. Even short-term therapies are commonly effective. At this point in the algorithm, most patients are 'mature' (i.e. well-motivated) for psychotherapeutic processes, and have no resistance to them. **The fundamental reason for this is that the primary problem as perceived by the patient, namely their pain, is addressed all the way through the algorithm.** This, in turn, facilitates the patients' understanding of psycho-existential, emotional, social psychodynamic, behavioural, and cognitive dimensions – the psychotherapeutic process is shortened and thereby cost-optimized. Another facilitating factor is that, at this stage, the patient's life-crises fre-quently have been controlled through cognitive-behavioural measures resulting in improved coping strategies, and some degree of reduction of pain is virtually always achieved by the antidysfunctional manage-ment. Moreover, an increased awareness of how ability to cope with everyday difficulties is connected to the patient's behaviour pattern is achieved. A feeling of hope is generated, and the patients develop confidence and self-respect. The importance of a complete picture when providing individuals with information has been stressed (Magnusson 2001). The multidimensional treatment of the patient, with touching and psychotherapy, creates parasympathetic reactions, thereby increasing motivation and trustfulness, facilitating the endur-ance of pain, and engendering a more positive attitude to life situa-tions (Arn 1999).

Several psychotherapeutic methods, both reality/cognitive and emotionally oriented, are used; these include traditional psycho-therapy, identity therapy, psychodrama, hypnotherapy, family therapy, and self-supporting therapy. The psychotherapy is both individual and group-based, sometimes combined with antidysfunctional physical therapy on the same occasion.

Pain-related syndromes – new psychological perspectives

According to a recent and so far unpublished outcome study (in preparation), we achieve excellent outcomes in a high percentage of patients with extremely complex problems, for whom numerous different approaches to pain management have failed.

Psychotherapy has an important role in the therapeutic process, in exploring the interaction between psycho-existential/social factors and the patients' pain and suffering. In the STAYAC concept, we have identified and defined three different basic perspectives with respect to the psychological approach:

- **The first perspective:** The first group comprises patients who present physical problems, with an underlying psychological trau-matic experience or a psychodynamic process resulting in pain instead of, for instance, open anxiety, which is thereby avoided (a primary benefit). This perspective could be exemplified by different kinds of **somatization syndromes**. Numerous models for pain are to be found in the psychosomatic/psychological/psychotherapeutic/ psychiatric literature, all apparently relating to the first perspective.

- **The second perspective:** The second group contains patients who have somatically based problems generating psychological disorders such as depression. This perspective is frequently adopted within different modes of manual therapy and musculoskeletal/manual medicine: 'If you have had pain long enough, you will of course be depressed and feel bad. Let me treat your (somatic) pain, and every-thing will become as it was before you were stricken by pain.' Manual therapists advocating this perspective as the fundamental approach frequently talk in terms of 'somatopsychic' conditions.

- **The third perspective:** The third group comprises patients in whom neither physical nor psychological problems are the dominating cause of the pain – both basic factors interact in a complex way: The pain is 'real', physical, nociceptive, and of somatic origin. Additionally, an unsatisfactory psycho-existential/social status of the patient at the debut of pain may induce inadequate conse-quences from the pain. Thus, 'consequences' is the key word in this paradigm; it is an essential concept for the success of treatment.

A conscious or subconscious over-reliance on, or incorrect appli-cation of, the first two perspectives is extremely common. For instance, mistrustful patient–therapist relationships are created by over-reliance on the first perspective (Figure 4.4.6b), and a destructive reinforcement of behavioural disturbances such as identity loss and development of a pain identity by over-reliance on the second per-spective (Figure 4.4.6a). Reinforcement in this context of the 'injury' or the 'lesion' and a reliance on continuing manual treatment can be extremely disadvantageous to the patient, leading to chronicity of symptoms (see also Main and Watson, Chapter 2.3.2).

In the STAYAC model, all three perspectives are relevant. How-ever, **the third perspective should be applied for most patients as** true 'psychogenic' pain (hysteria, conversion neuroses, pure somat-ization syndromes etc.) is rare, and the second perspective is over-emphasized, especially within manual medicine/therapy. The third perspective permeates the entire algorithm, as it does this entire chapter: attitudes, patient communication, metacognitive processes (the therapists' continuous review of their own thought processes) and so forth.

Unfortunately, in clinical reality, to the disadvantage of pain patients, the third perspective is rarely applied today – in general, pain care is extremely polarized between advocates of the first perspective and the second perspective.

Sick leave, long-term sick leave, and early retirement

The next phase is sick leave, long-term sick leave, and early retirement; see corresponding boxes, bottom left in the algorithm (Figure 4.4.1). Sick leave is in fact a treatment method, but its dangers are not uni-versally understood. It has a high risk of side effects and complications such as 'long-term sick leave illness' and alchoholism. Work absen-teeism is the most powerful risk factor for the development of alco-holism. A further predicament in this context is that it is largely the patients themselves and not the physicians who decide whether or not sick leave is necessary and/or adequate (Englund 2000).

Sick leave may of course be prescribed at any point of the algo-rithm, but should be used with the greatest caution and to the most limited extent possible. Not only may inappropriate sick leave be disastrous for individual patients, the danger of its widespread use is the legitimization of socio-cultural ills and problems. I am convinced that pain as a general societal predicament could be reduced to a minimum provided an appropriate infrastructure within pain care could be developed, departmentalization of the 'pain market' could be abolished, and the lack of knowledge with respect to possibilities as well as limitations within 'competing' and related disciplines could be taken care of.

Nevertheless, sick leave, including long-term sick leave and even early retirement, is sometimes therapeutic and is indicated for a tiny minority of pain patients.

Specialist domain: 'red flags without simultaneous dysfunction' box

On the upper left of the algorithm is the 'red flags without simul-taneous dysfunction' box (5% or less of patients with low back pain) (Nachemson and Jonsson 2000); see Figure 4.4.3a. This box is included in the 'specialist sphere'. In this context, the discussion within the 'Classification process' section has a clear relevance. In our concept the management of this patient group is consistent with other published guidelines for (back) pain. Consequently, there is no need here for an in-depth discussion of the management of symptoms of pathomorphological origin (i.e. 'red flags'). The algorithms and guidelines, currently available elsewhere, are mainly focused on management of such conditions, and therefore aiming at not overlooking them (AHCPR 1994, CSAG 1994, RCGP 1996, ACC 1997, Kendall *et al.* 1997, Waddell 1998). Consequently, they are indeed helpful in the management of the small subgroup of 'pure' red flag patients but of limited usefulness in the management of most patients who have benign, 'non-specific' (dysfunctional/green flags) pain. Nevertheless, it is essential not to miss treatable, potentially disabling, dangerous or life-threatening red flag conditions (e.g. herniated discs, tumours, spinal stenosis, true inflammatory conditions, infections), and there should be a continual awareness of these possibilities regardless of where the patient is in the algorithm at any moment in time, not least during the antidysfunctional investigation and in the psycho-existential sphere. In the figure, arrows from the different levels of the antidysfunctional and the psycho-existential spheres represent this awareness – all these arrows coalesce in a common feedback loop to the different modes of pathomorphologically-oriented management. The arrows from the antidysfunctional stack in the middle pass by the 'stay-active' box in the psycho-existential section.

The 'non-specific pain treatment' box

The other dominant therapeutic measures within this sphere are the different items in the 'non-specific pain treatment' box. This box is of course present in all three major domains of the algorithm (see also page 522). Basically, these are similar items to those applied in the antidysfunctional stack, but at a considerably earlier stage as basic core treatment modalities, and utilized to a far greater extent than in the STAYAC concept, where they are usually used only as adjuvant treatment, infrequently as a primary measure. However, the contents of this box are definitely more limited than the corresponding box in the STAYAC model, in which a larger variety of non-specific measures against pain is found. Traditional measures are NSAIDs, painkillers, and traditional physical therapy such as therapeutic ultrasound, heat, cold, TNS, and TEMS. With the exception of NSAIDs, none of them is evidence-based. (Although it is claimed in the latest back/neck pain SBU report (Nachemson and Jonsson 2000) that painkillers are evidence-based, unfortunately this conclusion is incorrect.)

The domain of 'traditional specialist care' includes referral to pathomorphologically focused specialists such as orthopaedic surgeons, rheumatologists, and oncologists. In addition, the sector covers neurologists and neurosurgeons, although they are not represented by boxes of their own in the scheme. Antidysfunctional filtering of the patients in this sector will substantively reduce unnecessary overloading of the specialists with patients to whom they cannot offer any relevant treatment. Their treatment results should then be improved by reducing excessive focus on pathomorphologically oriented rationales (which in turn frequently lead to nihilistic treatment attitudes and, paradoxically enough, also to overuse of sometimes aggressive therapeutic measures). If dysfunctional and psycho-existential factors have been taken care of before referral, the pathomorphological conditions will be more 'refined' at the start of the pathomorphologically oriented investigation, and the symptoms less 'diluted' by dysfunctional factors. This is true not only in the context of back surgery, neurology, and pain medicine. New green flag, easily treatable, conditions in patients with known inflammatory diseases are frequently, indeed automatically,

interpreted as manifestations of their basic inflammatory disease. These patients may be subjected unnecessarily to (sometimes aggressive) pharmacological treatments. A suboptimal specialist algorithm is presented in Figure 4.4.7b.

From the sphere of traditional specialist care there are two arrows pointing to the right, representing successful treatment outcomes.

Primary health care

The upper section on the right at the top of the scheme represents the GPs, conventional physiotherapists, occupational therapists, and sometimes psychologists within primary health care. Regrettably, pain management and corresponding referral strategies from within primary care are extremely variable, dependent to a large degree on a practitioner's postgraduate education in manual/musculoskeletal medicine and awareness of psycho-existential factors. The two thick arrows from the specialist sphere and the primary health care sphere respectively are important, and it is to be hoped that orthopaedic surgeons, rheumatologists, and GPs will make increased referrals for antidysfunctional treatment (see below). There are also patients who are referred back to primary health care after treatment in the antidysfunctional sector, for final management when control of pain and the patients' life situation is established, or when no further specialized management is required. (See the ascending long arrow on the far left of the algorithm, collecting all the feedback loops from the psycho-existential and antidysfunctional spheres to the specialist domain, which continues all the way back to the 'antidysfunctional treatment' box, and farther to the primary health care zone as well.)

Patients are usually referred directly to the specialist sphere (dashed arrow). Consequently, many patients are denied antidysfunctional management by (unnecessary) referral to the specialist sphere from the primary health care zone. In addition, a substantial subgroup of these patients, after referral from GPs, is referred back to their GPs and physiotherapists (according to the corresponding dashed arrow). Consequently, these patients too often remain somewhere in these two sectors until early retirement (often unnecessary). This is definitively not a cost-effective procedure, and is why the flows between these spheres are marked with dashed arrows: until education in antidysfunctional medicine within the specialist and primary health care sectors is sufficient, these flows should be avoided. In an optimized algorithm, the only reliable way in which to rule out dysfunctional and psycho-existential factors before referral to the specialist sphere (and vice versa) is by antidysfunctional investigation and, when indicated, psycho-existentially focused management in a unit like STAYAC.

In primary care, most patients are classified as idiopathic (very few patients, in STAYAC) or as having psychogenic conditions – see 'the first perspective', above. This is almost exclusively a group of patients with green-flag symptoms, and thus treatable conditions, provided they are referred for appropriate antidysfunctional management in time. Non-specific pain treatment, with limitations as discussed previously, constitutes the core treatment, but antidepressant medication is sometimes utilized – too rarely and most frequently in too low dosages. In spite of lack of supportive evidence, overall poor treatment results, and lack of cost-effectiveness, passive modalities such as therapeutic ultrasound, TNS and TEMS are frequently applied in pain patients as primary measures. Nevertheless, in a dysfunction-free state, these methods appear to be helpful in a small minority of patients. The suboptimal management of pain patients within primary health care is illustrated in Figure 4.4.7c. Figures 4.4.6a, 6b and 7a–d may of course be perceived as unfair, not least considering the thick arrows to the 'early retirement' boxes. This does not indicate that most patients are pensioned off early. However, it indicates that some may take early retirement unnecessarily, and that a large majority of those who do not – and are not subjected to causal-specific therapy in the different specialist spheres – heal spontaneously instead of having an accelerated recovery achieved by relevant antidysfunctional therapy or measures within the psycho-existential sphere. Nevertheless, clinical reality today is no better than the view presented in Figure 4.4.7d.

As demonstrated in the algorithm (Figure 4.4.1), there is also a flow of patients from the GP sphere to the psycho-existential sphere, together with a corresponding flow from the 'non-specific treatment' box in the pathomorphology sphere. Generally these routes do not function well today, and many patients 'get stuck' at inappropriate levels of the algorithm, managed passively with the prescription of medication and longer and longer periods of passive sick leave, without a plan for rehabilitation. Disappointingly, in many cases, a lot of adequate measures are never taken. Consequently, these flows are marked with dashed arrows, as are those between the primary health care sector and the specialist sphere (see above), the reason again being to assure the exclusion or confirmation of dysfunctional dimensions before premature referral to a psychologist, for instance. In a fully developed STAYAC model there will virtually be no patient flows along the dashed arrows in the algorithm.

In conclusion, there is a huge amount of developmental, education and scientific work to be done before health care will be able to offer an effective service for patients with pain from neuromusculoskeletal disorders – to reduce the suffering and to reduce costs to society of this patient group, costs that at the moment run riot.

Additional therapeutic measures

For simplicity, some constituents of the algorithm demonstrated in Figure 4.4.1 have been omitted. It should be noted, however, that in practice some of them are fairly frequently used, such as the following examples.

Cork wedges

The compensation of anatomical true leg-length differences (5–15 mm) by means of cork wedges (a secondary prevention measure), seemingly decreases the frequency of recurrence of pelvic/lumbar dysfunctions, or even eliminates recurrences. Differences larger than 15 mm have to be compensated by a combination of cork wedge inside the shoe, and building up the heel of the shoe, or preferably, the entire sole. It is important to appreciate that, since patients with ongoing dysfunction(s) in the pelvic/lumbar region always manifest false (dysfunctional) leg-length differences, measuring leg-length by means of a tape measure or by conventional radiography is meaningless. The final decision to compensate for leg-length differences should be undertaken in a stable and definite dysfunction-free state and, even better, when the patient is pain-free. The purpose of the cork wedge is to achieve a horizontal pelvis, and this can only be undertaken by means of relatively sophisticated manual techniques in the standing and the lying position. The difficulty of this procedure is severely underestimated, and, consequently, even more incorrectly prescribed cork wedges have to be discarded than new cork wedges prescribed.

Posture exercises and posture correction

However, to change posture permanently is rarely necessary, and it is also time-consuming, costly, and extremely difficult for the patient. Consequently, such measures have a minor role in the STAYAC concept. They are never undertaken as primary measures, but are occasionally appropriate for secondary prevention late in the antidysfunctional sphere. These cases may be referred to specialized physiotherapists who work with this exclusively.

Ergonomic advice

As secondary prevention this is also a late and fairly rare move in the algorithm, the reason simply being that it is rarely necessary when some steps in the antidysfunctional investigation have been undertaken. Adjusting the environment of the patient who has ongoing and treatable dysfunctions does not make sense. Indeed, when possible, enabling the patient to work in any workplace by means of optimizing their function is a preferable approach. However, sometimes a stable situation for the patient is achievable only in this way. Some of our physiotherapists visit workplaces for this purpose, but external specialists are sometimes engaged instead. The purpose of visiting workplaces, often in cooperation with the company's occupational care unit, is more often to analyse the workplace milieu from a social/psycho-existential perspective, involving colleagues, managers, and so forth.

Spinal supports, orthoses, special chairs, special, beds, etc.

Such measures are occasionally necessary, but only as one of the final measures that are undertaken within STAYAC, although in some other paradigms they constitute the core 'management'. We are especially disappointed with the use of spinal supports, which are virtually never used at STAYAC.

Oestrogen withdrawal

Although this is controversial, there is some support in the literature for the hypothesis that oestrogen therapy in women, for treatment of postmenopausal syndromes (Brynhildsen, Bjors *et al.* 1998) as well as for contraception (Wreje, Kristiansson *et al.* 1995, Wreje, Isacsson *et al.* 1997), increases the risk of lower back and pelvic troubles. Seemingly, in some therapy-resistant women with recurring lower lumbar/pelvic dysfunctions, withdrawal of such medications is the only correct move, at the right point of time and carefully weighed against the medication's significance for the quality of life. This measure is considered extremely late in the antidysfunctional investigation when it is absolutely necessary for the condition in question. Nevertheless, as it is frequently poss-ible to withdraw the oestrogen after some years of medication without recurrence of any postmenopausal symptoms, this may be the solution for this group of women. The indication for this move is recurring dysfunctions in the lower back and the pelvis. However, in both young and elderly women, it may take 6–12 months before the situation is stabilized after this measure.

Omissions from the algorithm

Dietary measures

With respect to pain management, very few therapeutic possibilities are not included in the STAYAC algorithm. As evident elsewhere in this chapter, some modalities have a minor role, and one or two are not included at all. In addition, we have not yet adopted dietary measures or antioxidants systematically, a strategy that is advocated by a growing number of physicians and physiotherapists, not least within manual therapy/ medicine. To gather experience from this field may be one of the future steps in the further development of the STAYAC algorithm, or we may wait for conclusive studies to support the inclusion of dietary measures in the management of pain patients.

Activity-limiting regimens

In the STAYAC concept, regardless of the condition (dysfunctional, WAD, herniated discs, coxarthrosis, and so forth), **no activity-limiting regimens at all are inflicted on the patients**. This essential part of the STAYAC algorithm will certainly be perceived as controversial within numerous medical fields including manual therapy/ medicine. Nevertheless, we have many years of experience of this approach. We probably practice the stay-active concept more extensively than in any other pain management paradigm. More or less all patients have already limited themselves unnecessarily, but extensively, when they first attend. Patients are encouraged to return gradually to their accustomed levels of activity. If an activity-limiting regimen is inflicted, the subliminal message will be that I, 'the expert', may believe that structures are 'injured', that doing this or that may be dangerous and so forth. This is a powerfully negative and unwanted message.

The expected benefit of inflicting activity-limiting advice is improvement of the short-term and long-term prognosis of the patient. Firstly, there is no evidence that this is possible. Secondly, the cost aspect of the measure is easily forgotten. All active medical measures are associated with calculated risks; if a physician prescribes penicillin for a sore throat, he takes a minimal risk that the patient dies from the medicine. Even seemingly innocent measures may be associated with considerable risk for the patients. Imagine that a patient has waited 20 years for his recent retirement enabling him to play golf full-time – in England during the summer, and in Spain in the winter. The quality of life of this patient is entirely dependent on his ability to play golf. If you advise him not to play golf (to avoid rotational movements in the back), you may more or less have destroyed his life, because you have overlooked the cost-benefit analysis. If a 35-year-old man who loves mogul skiing has a herniated disc, attempt to stimulate him to try! If he cannot do it, he will not do it. What could happen? In the worst case, surgery has to be undertaken, but there is no evidence that it is possible to heal a herniated disc by inactivity. In this patient, activities of daily living, such as lifting his child, are just as likely to precipitate surgery within a few weeks. In point of fact, I am still waiting for the first patient to come back to me, saying 'You told me that I could do anything in spite of my pain; see what happened!'

Conclusion

The STAYAC concept is definitely not finally developed once and for all; in clinical practice, we continually and systematically try to evaluate new treatment modalities, change the paths through the algorithm, and reconsider the indications within the scheme. A lot of research has to be performed to support such potential modifications. The first step will be the infrastructure study (page 509). In 10 years the algorithm will be different from the one presented in this chapter, but I am sure

that the core of the algorithm will continue to be the antidysfunctional sphere including manual therapy.

The STAYAC algorithm is usable in clinical management of all kinds of pain associated with the locomotor system. If a patient has not responded positively to any provided treatment, and you feel insecure about the next step, you can follow their path through the algorithm. This makes it easy to realize whether some box has been forgotten, or what should be the next reasonable step in the antidysfunctional investigation when the current measure has failed.

As some of the examples given in this chapter demonstrate, **numerous other medical disciplines would benefit from the application of the dysfunction/green flags paradigm and its consequences**. With appropriate and, in some instances, minor alterations, the algorithm could also be used in other medical fields outside pain management. The basic principle would be the same: with the exception of the few patients fulfilling indications for acute pathomorphologically focused specialist care, dysfunctional explanations for patients' symptoms should be considered before pathomorphologically or psychologically focused investigations are initiated.

References

ACC (1997) *New Zealand acute back pain guide*. Accident Rehabilitation & Compensation Insurance Corporation of New Zealand and the National Health Committee, Wellington, New Zealand.

AHCPR (1994) *Management guidelines for acute low back pain*. Agency for Health Care Policy and Research, U.S. Department of Health and Human Services, Rockville, MD.

Anderson, R. T. (1984) An orthopedic ethnography in rural Nepal. *Med Anthropol*, 8, 46–58.

Andersson, G. B. J., Schultz, A. B., *et al.* (1984) Intervertebral disc pressures during traction. *Scandinavian Journal of Rehabilitation*, 16, 88–91.

Antonovsky, A. (1987) *Unravelling the mystery of health: how people manage stress and stay well*. Jossey-Bass, San Francisco.

Antonovsky, A. (1991) *Hälsans mysterium*. Natur och Kultur, Stockholm.

Arn, I. (1999) A biopsychological analysis of functional gastrointestinal disorders and a clinical trial of its treatment with psychodrama. Dissertation, Division of Psychosocial Factors and Health, Department of Public Health Sciences, and the National Institute for Psychosocial Factors and Health, Karolinska Institute, Stockholm, Sweden.

Assendelft, W. J. J., Morton, S. C., Yu, E. I. *et al.* (2003) Spinal manipulative therapy for low back pain. A meta-analysis of effectiveness relative to other therapies. *Ann intern med*, 138, 871–81.

Aure, O. F., Nilsen, J. H. *et al.* (2003) Manual therapy and exercise therapy in patients with chronic low back pain. A randomized, controlled trial with 1-year follow-up. *Spine*, 28, 525–32.

Bandura, A. (1977) Self-efficacy: toward a unifying theory of behavioural change. *Psychol Rev*, 84, 191–215.

Bartys, S., Burton, K., Watson, P. J. *et al.* (2002) Organisational obstacles to recovery – the role of "black flags" in the implementation of an early psychosocial intervention for back pain. Paper presented at BritSpine, Birmingham.

Bendix, A. E., Bendix, T., *et al.* (1998a) A prospective, randomized 5-year follow-up study of functional restoration in chronic low back pain patients. *European Spine Journal*, 7(2), 111–19.

Bendix, A. F., Bendix, T., *et al.* (1998b) Functional restoration for chronic low back pain. Two-year follow-up of two randomized clinical trials. *Spine*, 23(6), 717–25.

Bendix, T., A. Bendix, *et al.* (2000) Functional restoration versus outpatient physical training in chronic low back pain: a randomized comparative study. *Spine*, 25(19), 2494–500.

Bergquist-Ullman, M., Larsson, U. (1977) Acute low back pain in industry. A controlled prospective study with special reference to therapy and confounding factors. *Acta Orthopaedica Scandinavica Supplement* 170, 1–117.

Blomberg, S. (1993) A pragmatic approach to low-back pain including manual therapy and steroid injections. A multicentre study in primary health care. Thesis, Uppsala University.

Blomberg, S., Hallin, G., *et al.* (1994) Manual therapy with steroid injections – a new approach to treatment of low back pain. A controlled multicenter trial with an evaluation by orthopedic surgeons. *Spine*, 19(5), 569–77.

Blomberg, S., Svärdsudd, K., *et al.* (1992) A controlled, multicentre trial of manual therapy in low-back pain, Initial status, sick-leave and pain score during follow-up. *Scandinavian Journal of Primary Health Care*, 10, 170–8.

Blomberg, S., Svärdsudd, K., *et al.* (1993a) A controlled, multicentre trial of manual therapy with steroid injections in low-back pain, functional variables, side-effects and complications during four months' follow-up. *Clinical Rehabilitation*, 7, 49–62.

Blomberg, S., Svärdsudd, K., *et al.* (1993b) Manual therapy with steroid injections in low-back pain. Improvement of quality of life in a controlled trial with four months' follow-up. *Scandinavian Journal of Primary Health Care*, 11(2), 83–90.

Blomberg, S., Svärdsudd, K., *et al.* (1994) A randomized study of manual therapy with steroid injections in low-back pain. Telephone interview follow-up of pain, disability, recovery and drug consumption. *European Spine Journal*, 3(5), 246–54.

Blomberg, S. E. I., Bogefeldt, J. P., Grunnesjö, M. I. *et al.* (2005a) A randomized clinical trial comparing four different treatment regimens: manual therapy including steroid injections, manual therapy, muscle stretching and orthopaedic care. Pain scores and functional variables. Submitted for publication.

Blomberg, S. E. I., Bogefeldt, J. P., Grunnesjö, M. I. *et al.* (2005b) A randomized controlled trial of stay-active care versus manual therapy combined with steroid injections in addition to stay-active care in low-back pain radiating to the leg(s), and below the knee(s) respectively. Functional variables and pain. In preparation.

Blomberg, S. E. I., Bogefeldt, J. P., Grunnesjö, M. I. *et al.* (2005c) A randomized controlled trial of stay-active care versus manual therapy combined with steroid injections in addition to stay-active care in low-back pain. Quality-of-life score and a general psychosomatic symptom profile. In preparation.

Bogefeldt, J. P., Grunnesjö, M. I., Wedel, H. *et al.* (2004) Sick-leave measures as outcome in a randomised controlled clinical trial of manual therapy combined with steroid injections for low-back pain. The Gotland low-back pain study. Submitted for publication.

Bogefeldt, J. P., Grunnesjö, M. I., Svärdsudd, K. F. *et al.* (2004c) Diagnostic differences between general practitioners and orthopaedic surgeons in a randomised controlled trial of manual therapy in low back pain. Submitted for publication.

Bogefeldt, J. P., Grunnesjö, M. I., Svärdsudd, K. F. *et al.* (2005b) A randomized clinical trial of manual therapy combined with steroid injections in chronic patients – a partial crossover study. In preparation.

Bogefeldt, J. P., Grunnesjö, M. I., Svärdsudd, K. F. *et al.* (2005a) A randomised clinical trial of manual therapy combined with steroid injections – The Säter low-back pain study. Results from the three-year follow-up. In preparation.

Bongers, P. M., de Winter, C. R., Kompier, M. A. J., Hildebrandt, V. H. (1993) Psychosocial factors at work and musculoskeletal disease. *Scandinavian Journal of Work and Environmental Health*, 19, 297–321.

Bronfort, G., Evans, R., Nelson, B. *et al.* (2001) A randomized clinical trial of exercise and spinal manipulation for patients with chronic neck pain. *Spine*, 26, 788–99.

Bronfort, G., Haas, M., Evans, D. C. *et al.* (2004) Efficacy of spinal manipulation and mobilization for low back pain and neck pain: a systematic review and best evidence synthesis. *Spine*, 4, 335–56.

Brynhildsen, J. O., Bjors, E., *et al.* (1998) Is hormone replacement therapy a risk factor for low back pain among postmenopausal women? *Spine*, 23, 809–13.

Carroll, L. (undated) *Alice In Wonderland and Through the Looking Glass.* Collins Clear Type Press, London.

Cherkin, D. C., Deyo, R. A., *et al.* (1998) A comparison of physical therapy, chiropractic manipulation, and provision of an educational booklet for the treatment of patients with low back pain. *New England Journal of Medicine*, 339(15), 1021–9.

CSAG (1994) *Report on back pain.* Clinical Standards Advisory Group. HMSO, London.

Cyriax, J. (1970) *Textbook of orthopaedic medicine.* Baillière Tindall, London.

Daykin, A. R., Richardson, B. (2004) Physiotherapists' pain beliefs and their influence on the management of patients with chronic low back pain. *Spine*, 29, 783–95.

De Bono, E. (1977) *Lateral thinking.* Penguin, London.

Dechow, E., Davies, R. K., Carr, A. J. *et al.* (1999) A randomized, double-blind, placebo-controlled trial of sclerosing injections in patients with chronic low back pain. *Rheumatology*, 38, 1255–9.

Della-Giustina, D., Kilcline, B. A. (2000) Acute low back pain: a comprehensive review. *Comprehensive Therapy*, 26(3), 153–9.

Della-Giustina, D. A. (1999) Emergency department evaluation and treatment of back pain. *Emergency Medicine Clinics of North America*, 17(4), 877–93, vi–vii.

Deyo, R. A., Weinstein J. N. (2001) Low back pain. *New England Journal of Medicine*, 344(5), 363–70.

Egund, N., Olsson, T. H., *et al.* (1978) Movements in the sacroiliac joints demonstrated with roentgen stereophotogrammetry. *Acta Radiologica Diagnosis*, 19, 833–45.

Eklund, M. (1992) Chronic pain and vocational rehabilitation: a multifactorial analysis of symptoms, signs, and psycho-socio-demographics. *Journal of Occupational Rehabilitation*, 2(2), 53–66.

Englund, L. (2000) Sick-listing – attitudes and doctors' practice with special emphasis on sick-listing practice in primary health care. Dissertation. *Acta Universitatis Upsaliens.* I.S comprehensive summaries of dissertations from the Faculty of Medicine, 956.

Evjent, O., Hamberg, J. (1985a) *Muscle stretching in manual therapy, a clinical manual, the extremities.* Alfta Rehab Förslag, Alfta.

Evjent, O., Hamberg, J. (1985b) *Muscle stretching in manual therapy, a clinical manual, the spinal column and the temporomandibular joint.* Alfta Rehab Förlag, Alfta.

Evjent, O., Hamberg J. (1990) *Autostretching. The complete manual of specific stretching.* Alfta Rehab Förlag, Alfta.

Farrell, J. P., Twomey L. T. (1982) Acute low back pain. Comparison of two conservative treatment approaches. *Medical Journal of Australia*, 1, 160–164.

Fisk, J. W. (1979) A controlled trial of manipulation in a selected group of patients with low back pain favouring one side. *New Zealand Medical Journal*, 10 (October), 288–291.

Flavell, J. H. (1979) Metacognition and cognitive monitoring: A new area of cognitive-developmental inquiry. *American Psychologist*, 34, 906–911.

Fritzell, P., Hägg, O., Wessberg, P. *et al.* (2001) Volvo award winner in clinical studies: lumbar fusion versus nonsurgical treatment for chronic low back pain: a multicenter randomized controlled trial from the Swedish Lumbar Spine Study Group. *Spine*, 26, 2521–32.

Gillström, P., Ericson, K., *et al.* (1985) Computed tomography examination of the influence of autotraction on herniation of the lumbar disc. *Archives of Orthopaedic and Trauma Surgery*, 104, 289–93.

Grunnesjö, M. I., Bogefeldt, J. P., Svärdsudd, K. F. *et al.* (2004a) A randomised controlled clinical trial of stay-active care versus manual therapy in addition to stay-active care; functional variables and pain. *J Manipulative Physiol Ther*, 27, 431–41.

Grunnesjö, M. I., Bogefeldt, J. P., Svärdsudd, K. F. *et al.* (2004b) The course of pain drawings relative to time and treatment in acute and subacute low back pain. Submitted for publication.

Grunnesjö, M. I., Bogefeldt, J. P., Svärdsudd, K. F. *et al.* (2005a) A randomised clinical trial of manual therapy combined with steroid injections – the Gotland low-back pain study. Pain drawings. In preparation.

Grunnesjö, M. I., Bogefeldt, J. P., Svärdsudd, K. F. *et al.* (2005b) A randomised clinical trial of manual therapy combined with steroid injections – the Säter low-back pain study. Pain drawings. In preparation.

Gunn, C. C. (1996) *The Gunn approach to the treatment of chronic pain– intramuscular stimulation for myofascial pain of radiculopathic origin.* Churchill Livingstone, London.

Hackett, G. S. (1958) *Ligament and tendon relaxation treated by prolotherapy,* 3rd edn. Charles C. Thomas Springfield, IL.

Hadler, N. M., Curtis, P. *et al.* (1987) A benefit of spinal manipulation as adjunctive therapy for acute low-back pain: a stratified controlled trial. *Spine,* 12(7), 703–6.

Harmer, C. J., Bhagwagar, Z. *et al.* (2003) Acute SSRI administration affects the processing of social cues in healthy volunteers. *Neuropsychopharmacology,* 28(1), 148–52.

Harms-Ringdahl, K., Holmström, E., *et al.* (1999) Evidensbaserad sjukgymnastisk behandling. Patienter med ländryggsbesvär. Rapport 102:99. SBU (Swedish Council on Technology Assessment in Health Care), Stockholm, Sweden.

Holten, O., Torstensen, T. A. (1991) Medical exercise therapy – the basic principles. WCPT congress, London 1991. Special issue of *Fysioterapeuten,* 58, 27–32.

Hoving, L. J. (2002) Neck pain in primary care – the effects of commonly applied interventions. Thesis. VU University Medical Centre, Amsterdam.

Howell, D. W. (1984) Musculoskeletal profile and incidence of musculoskeletal injuries in lightweight women rowers. *American Journal of Sports Medicine,* 12, 278–82.

Hoy, D., Toole, M. J., Morgan, D. *et al.* (2003). Low back pain in rural Tibet. *Lancet,* 361, 225–6.

Indahl, A., Velund, L., *et al.* (1995) Good prognosis for low back pain when left untampered: a randomized clinical trial. *Spine,* 20, 473–7.

Janda, V. (1976) *Muskelfunktionsdiagnostik.* Steinkopff, Dresden.

Johansson, H., Sojka P. (1991) Pathophysiological mechanisms involved in genesis and spread of muscular tension in occupational muscle pain and in chronic musculoskeletal pain syndromes: A hypothesis. *Medical Hypotheses,* 35, 196–203.

Johansson, H. and Sjölander, P. (1993) Neurophysiology of joints. In: V. Wright and E.L. Radin (Eds.), *Mechanics of human joints physiology, pathophysiology, and treatment,* pp. 243–90. Marcel Dekker Inc., New York.

Johansson, H., Pedersen, J., Bergenheim, M. *et al.* (2000) Pheripheral afferents of the knee: their effects on central mechanisms regulating muscle stiffness, joint stability, and proprioception and coordination. In: S.M. Lephart and F.H. Fu (Eds.), *Proprioception and neuromuscular control in joint stability,* pp. 5–22. Human Kinetics, USA.

Johansson, H., Arendt-Nilsson, L., Bergenheim, M. *et al.* (2003) Epilogue: an integrated model for chronic work-related myalgia "Brussels Model". In: H. Johansson, U. Windhorst, M. Djupsjöbacka et al. (Eds.), *Chronic work-related myalgia. Neuromuscular mechanisms behind work-related chronic muscle pain syndromes,* pp. 291–300. Gävle University Press.

Johansson, H., Windhorst, U., Djupsjöbacka, M. *et al.* (2003) *Chronic work-related myalgia. Neuromuscular mechanisms behind work-related chronic muscle pain syndromes.* Gävle University Press.

Jones, M. A. and Rivett, D. A. (2004) *Clinical reasoning for Manual Therapists.* Hodges P: Section 2; Clinical reasoning in action: Chapter 7; Chronic low back and coccygeal pain. Butterworth-Heinemann an imprint of Elsevier Science Limited, London.

Jull, G. *et al.* (2002) A randomized controlled trial of exercise and manipulative therapy for cervicogenic headache. *Spine,* 27(17), 1835–43.

Kaltenborn, F. M., Evjent O. (1993) *The spine, basic evaluation and mobilization techniques.* Olaf Norlis Bokhandel, Oslo.

Kendall, N. A. S., Linton, S. J., Main, C. J. (1997) *Guide to assessing psychosocial yellow flags in acute low back pain: risk factors for long term disability and work loss.* Accident Rehabilitation & Compensation Insurance Corporation of New Zealand and the National Health Committee, Wellington, New Zealand, pp. 1–22.

Kiley, D. (1983) *Peter Pan syndrome: men who have never grown up.* Dodd Mead, USA.

Klein, R. G. Dorman, T. A., Johnson, C. E. (1989) Proliferant injections for low back pain: histologic changes of injected ligaments and objective measurements of lumbar spine mobility before and after treatment. *J Neurol Orthop Med Surg,* 10, 123–6.

Klein, R. G., Eek, B. C., DeLong, W. B. *et al.* (1993) A randomized double-blind trial of dextrose-glycerine-phenol injections for chronic, low back pain. *J Spinal Disord,* 6, 23–33.

Knutson, B., Cole, S. *et al.* (1997) Serotonergic intervention increases affiliative behavior in humans. *Annals of the New York Academy of Sciences,* 807, 492–3.

Knutson, B., Wolkowitz, O. M. *et al.* (1998) Selective alteration of personality and social behavior by serotonergic intervention. *American Journal of Psychiatry,* 155(3), 373–9.

Knutsson, E., Skoglund, C. R., *et al.* (1988) Changes in voluntary muscle strength, somatosensory transmission and skin temperature concomitant with pain relief during autotraction in patients with lumbar and sacral root lesions. *Pain,* 33, 173–9.

Koes, B. W., Bouter, L. M., van Mameren, H. *et al.* (1992a) The effectiveness of manual therapy, physiotherapy, and treatment by general practitioner for chronic non-specific back and neck complaints: a randomized clinical trial. *Spine,* 17, 28–35.

Koes, B. W., Bouter, L. M., van Mameren, H. *et al.* (1992b) A blinded Randomized clinical trial of manual therapy and physiotherapy for chronic back and neck complaints: physical outcome measures. *Journal of Manipulative and Physiological Therapeutics,* 15, 16–23.

Koes, B. W., Bouter, L. M., van Mameren, H. *et al.* (1992c) Randomised clinical trial of manipulative therapy and physiotherapy for persistent back and neck complaints: results of one year follow-up. *British Medical Journal,* 304, 601–5.

Koes, B. W., van Tulder, M. W., *et al.* (2001) Clinical guidelines for the management of low back pain in primary care. An international comparison. *Spine,* 26(22), 2504–14.

Kool, J., de Bie, R., Oesch, P. *et al.* (2004) Exercise reduces sick leave in patients with non-acute non-specific low back pain: a meta-analysis. *J Rehab Med,* 36, 49–69.

Lewit, K. (1991) *Manipulative therapy in rehabilitation of the locomotor system.* Butterworth Heinemann, London.

Lind, G. A. M. (1974) *Auto-traction. Treatment of low back pain and sciatica. An electromyographic, radiographic and clinical study.* Linköping, Sweden.

Lindström, I., Öhlund, C., *et al.* (1992) Mobility, strength, and fitness after a graded activity program for patients with subacute low back pain. A randomized prospective clinical study with a behavioral therapy approach. *Spine,* 17(6), 641–52.

Linton, S. J., Halldén, K. (1998) Can we screen for problematic back pain? A screening questionnaire for predicting outcome in acute and subacute back pain. *Clinical Journal of Pain,* 14, 209–15.

Ljunggren, A. E., Weber, H., *et al.* (1984) Autotraction versus manual traction in patients with prolapsed lumbar intervertebral discs. *Scandinavian Journal of Rehabilitation Medicine,* 16, 117–24.

Loubinoux, I., Pariente, J., *et al.* (2002) A single dose of the serotonin neurotransmission agonist paroxetine enhances motor output: double-blind, placebo-controlled, fMRI study in healthy subjects. *Neuroimage,* 15(1), 26–36.

Magnusson, D., Mahoney, L. (2001) A holistic person approach for research on positive development. Report 76, Research Program on Individual Development and Adaption, Department of Psychology, Stockholm University.

Main, C. J. (2002) Concepts of treatment and prevention in musculoskeletal disorders. In: S. J. Linton (Ed.), *New avenues for the prevention of chronic musculoskeletal pain and disability.* Elsevier Science BV, Amsterdam.

Malmivaara, A., Hakkinen, U., *et al.* (1995) The treatment of acute low back pain – bed rest, exercises, or ordinary activity? *New England Journal of Medicine*, 332(6), 351–5.

McGuirk, B., King, W., Govind, J., *et al.* (2001) Safety, efficacy and cost-effectiveness of evidence-based guidelines for the management of acute low back pain in primary care. *Spine*, 26, 2615–22.

McKenzie, R. (1981) *The lumbar spine. Mechanical diagnosis and therapy.* Spinal Publications, Waikanae, New Zealand.

Midttun, A., Bojsen-Traeden, J., *et al.* (1983) Syndroma ligamenti sacrotuberalis – a case for manual therapy. Scandinavian Association for the Study of Pain, annual meeting 5.

Miller, W. R., Seligman, M. E. (1975) Depression and learned helplessness in man. *Journal of abnormal psychology*, 84, 228–38.

Miller, W. R., Seligman, M. E., *et al.* (1975) Learned helplessness, depression, and anxiety. *The Journal of nervous and mental disease*, 161, 347–57.

Mitchel, F., Moran, P., *et al.* (1979) *An evelution and treatment manual for osteopathic muscle energy procedures.* Mitchel, Moran and Prutzzo, Valley Park.

Myrin, S.-O. (1972) *Var rädd om ryggen.* Bokförlaget Robert Larsson, Täby, Sweden.

Nachemson, A., Jonsson, E., *et al.* (1991) *Ont i ryggen – orsaker, diagnostik och behandling.* SBU (Swedish Council on Technology Assessment in Health Care), Stockholm, Sweden.

Nachemson, A. L, Jonsson, E. (eds) (2000) *Neck and back pain: The scientific evidence of causes, diagnosis, and treatment.* Lippincott Williams & Wilkins, Philadelphia.

Natchew, E. (1984) *A manual on auto-traction treatment for low back pain.* Folksam Scientific Council, Stockholm.

Nwuga, V. C. B. (1982) Relative therapeutic efficacy of vertebral manipulation and conventional treatment in back pain management. *American Journal of Physical Medicine*, 61(6), 273–8.

Ongley, M. J., Dorman, T. A., *et al.* (1987) A new approach to the treatment of chronic low back pain. *Lancet* (18 July), 143–6.

Rasmussen, G. G. (1979) Manipulation in treatment of low back pain: a randomized clinical trial. *Manual Medicine, manuelle medizin*, 1, 8–10.

Rasmussen-Barr, E., Nilsson-Wikmar, L., *et al.* (2003) Stabilizing training compared with manual treatment in sub-acute and chronic low-back pain. *Manual Therapy*, 8, 233–41.

RCGP (1996) *Clinical guidelines for the management of acute low back pain.* Royal College of General Practitioners, London.

Seferlis, T., Németh, G., *et al.* (1998) Conservative treatment in patients sick-listed for acute low-back pain: a prospective randomised study with 12 months' follow-up. *European Spine Journal*, 7, 461–70.

Shores, M. M., Pascualy, M., *et al.* (2001) Short-term sertraline treatment suppresses sympathetic nervous system activity in healthy human subjects. *Psychoneuroendocrinology*, 26(4), 433–9.

Sjölander, P., Johansson, H. (1997) Sensory endings in ligaments: response properties and effects on proprioception and motor control. In: L. Yahia (Ed.), *Ligaments and ligamentoplasties*, pp. 39–83. Springer-Verlag, Berlin, Heidelberg.

Sjölander, P., Johansson, H., Djupsjöbacka, M. (2002) Spinal and supraspinal effects of activity in ligament afferents. *Journal of Electromyography and Kinesiology*, 12, 167–76.

Skargren, E. I., Öberg, B. E., *et al.* (1997) Cost-effectiveness of chiropractic and physiotherapy treatment for low back pain and neck pain. Six-month follow-up. *Spine*, 22(18), 2167–77.

Sloop, P. R., Smith, D. S. *et al.* (1982) Manipulation for chronic neck pain. A double-blind controlled study. *Spine*, 7(6), 532–5.

Stoddard, A. (1980) *Manual of osteopathic technique.* Hutchinson, London.

Sturesson, B., Selvik, G., *et al.* (1989) Movements of the sacroiliac joints. A roentgen stereophotogrammetric analysis. *Spine*, 14(2), 162–5.

Tilscher (1995 and 2004) A dynamic radiography report of spinal mobility before and after prolotherapy: the mobility of the lumbar spine is increased by prolotherapy. Personal communication (to be published).

Torstensen, T. A. (1997) The physical therapy approach. In: *The adult spine: Principles and practice*, ed. T. Whitecloud III. Lippincott-Raven, Philadelphia, pp. 1797–1805.

Torstensen, T. A., Ljunggren, A. E., *et al.* (1998) Efficiency and costs of medical exercise therapy, conventional physiotherapy, and self-exercise in patients with chronic low back pain. A pragmatic, randomized, single-blinded, controlled trial with 1-year follow-up. *Spine*, 23, 2616–24.

Travell, J. S. D. (1983–1992) *Myofascial pain and dysfunction – the trigger point manual.* Williams & Wilkins, Baltimore.

Tse, W. S., Bond, A. J. (2002) Serotonergic intervention affects both social dominance and affiliative behaviour. *Psychopharmacology (Berlin)*, 161(3), 324–30.

Tullberg, T., Blomberg, S., *et al.* (1998) Manipulation does not alter the position of the sacroiliac joint. A Roentgen stereophotogrammetric analysis. *Spine*, 23(10), 1124–9.

van Tulder, M. W., Ostelo, R., Vlaeyen, J. W. S. *et al.* (1996) Behavioral treatment for chronic low back pain. A systematic review within the framework of the Cochrane Back Review Group. *Spine*, 26, 270–81.

van Tulder, M. W., Assendelft, W. J. J., *et al.* (1997) Method guidelines for systematic reviews in the Cochrane Collaboration Back Review Group for Spinal Disorders. *Spine*, 22, 2323–30.

van Tulder, M., Malmivaara, A., *et al.* (2000) Exercise therapy for low back pain: A systematic review within the framework of the cochrane collaboration back review group. *Spine*, 25(21), 2784–96.

Waddell, G. (1998) *The back pain revolution.* Churchill Livingstone, Edinburgh.

Wigley, R. D., Zhang, N. C., Zeng, Q. Y. *et al.* (1994). ILAR-China study comparing the prevalence of rheumatic symptoms in northern and southern rural populations. *J Rheumatol*, 21, 1484–90.

Wreje, U., Isacsson, D., *et al.* (1997) Oral contraceptives and back pain in women in Swedish community. *International Journal of Epidemiology*, 26(1), 71–4.

Wreje, U., P. Kristiansson, *et al.* (1995) Serum levels of relaxin during the menstrual cycle and oral contraceptive use. *Gynecologic and Obstetric Investigation*, 39, 197–200.

Wreje, U., B. Nordgren, *et al.* (1992) Treatment of pelvic joint dysfunction in primary care – a controlled study. *Scandinavian Journal of Primary Health Care*, 10, 310–315.

Yelland, M. J., Glasziou, P. P., Bogduk, N. *et al.* (2004) Prolotherapy injections, saline injections, and exercises for chronic low-back pain: a randomized trial. *Spine*, 29, 9–16.

Zulian, F., Martini, G., Gobber, D. *et al.* (2003). Comparison of intra-articular triamcinolone hexacetonide and triamcinolone acetonide in oligoarticular juvenile idiopathic arthritis. *Rheumatology*, 42, 1254–9.

Index